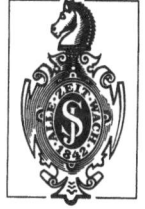

T. Takahashi (Ed.)

Recent Advances in Management of Digestive Cancers

Proceedings of UICC Kyoto International Symposium
on Recent Advances in Management of Digestive Cancers,
March 31–April 2, 1993

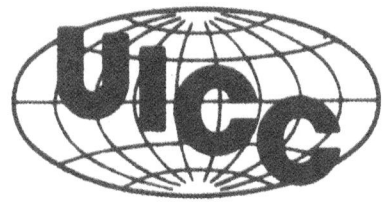

With 530 Illustrations, Including 3 in Color

Springer-Verlag
Tokyo Berlin Heidelberg New York London
Paris Hong Kong Barcelona Budapest

Toshio Takahashi, M.D.
Professor and Chairman
The First Department of Surgery
Kyoto Prefectural University of Medicine
Kyoto, 602 Japan

ISBN-13:978-4-431-68254-7   e-ISBN-13:978-4-431-68252-3
DOI: 10.1007/978-4-431-68252-3

Printed on acid-free paper

Preface

Cancer is the leading cause of death in many countries, and digestive cancer is one of the most common types of neoplasms. Advances in research on the management of digestive cancer therefore represent an important contribution to the welfare of humankind throughout the world.

The UICC Kyoto International Symposium on Recent Advances in the Management of Digestive Cancer was held in Kyoto from March 31 to April 2, 1993 under the presidency of Dr. T. Takahashi of the Kyoto Prefectural University of Medicine. At this event, leading researchers and clinicians presented new findings and the latest results of clinical trials concerning digestive cancers. The UICC President and other members of the Executive Committee of the UICC also gave speeches on their own fields, and more than 1000 participants from 28 countries were very well received. This book presents the proceedings of this symposium.

In addition to 30 selected papers presented at special lectures and symposia by invited speakers, this book contains 230 free papers presented at poster sessions during this conference.

The book provides an overview of the global aspects of digestive cancers, which are closely related to dietary habits, socioeconomic conditions, and environmental hygiene. It also reports on the early detection of digestive cancer, which has been increasing through the use of newly developed diagnostic tools such as video-endoscopy, ultrasonography, CT scanning, and MRI. The results of treatment have improved correspondingly, although pancreatic cancer is still associated with a poor prognosis. In recent advances in the management of digestive cancers, endoscopic treatment, rather than open surgery, has provided favorable outcomes in early superficial esophagus, stomach, and colon cancer. Further reports on newer strategies in treating cancer patients, such as organ transplantation, immuno-guided surgery, computer-assisted surgery, missile therapy, and inhibition of neovascularization in cancer should likewise elicit great interest in this book.

In the publication of these proceedings of the UICC Kyoto International Symposium, I wish to thank the President of UICC, the Executive Committee of the UICC, Dr. Aoki, the Aichi Cancer Center, Dr. Inokuchi, Kyushu University, Dr. Sugano, the Cancer Institute, and the Organizing Committee of the UICC Kyoto International Symposium for their various contributions.

May this book become a milestone toward the great goal of conquering digestive cancers.

July, 1993

TOSHIO TAKAHASHI, M.D.
President of the Kyoto UICC Symposium

Organizing Committee

UICC Council

S. ECKHARDT (Hungary)
G.P. MURPHY (USA)
C.G. SCHMIDT (Germany)
CH. R. EBERSOL (USA)
M.M. BURGER (Switzerland)

UICC National Committee

K. AOKI (Nagoya)
K. INOKUCHI (Fukuoka)
H. SUGANO (Tokyo)

Japanese Organizing Committee

President of the Meeting:
T. TAKAHASHI (Kyoto)

Vice-President of the Meeting:
K. KAWAI (Kyoto)

Honorable Advisors

O. ABE (Tokyo)
S. FUJITA (Kyoto)
H. ICHIKAWA (Tokyo)
G. KOSAKI (Tokyo)
S. MAJIMA (Kyoto)
T. MAKI (Sendai)
T. NAGAYO (Nagoya)
M. NISHI (Tokyo)
H. SATO (Sendai)
T. SATO (Sendai)
T. SHIRATORI (Akita)
K. SUEMASU (Tokyo)
T. SUGIMURA (Tokyo)
T. TAGUCHI (Tokyo)
T. TOBE (Kyoto)

Committee Members

S. ABO (Akita)
T. AOKI (Tokyo)
S. BABA (Hamamatsu)

M. ENDO (Tokyo)
M. FUJIMAKI (Toyama)
K. HAMANO (Tokyo)
F. HANYU (Tokyo)
Y. HIKI (Kanagawa)
K. HIOKI (Osaka)
T. HIRAYAMA (Tokyo)
Y. IDEZUKI (Tokyo)
K. ISONO (Chiba)
T. IWANAGA (Osaka)
K. KASHIMA (Kyoto)
N. KAIBARA (Tottori)
T. KAKEGAWA (Kurume)
K. KIMURA (Tokyo)
S. KIMURA (Ehime)
H. KINOSHITA (Osaka)
M. KITAJIMA (Tokyo)
M. KODAMA (Shiga)
M. KONN (Hirosaki)
M. KONDO (Kyoto)
K. KOYAMA (Akita)
M. KURIHARA (Tokyo)
M. MAI (Kanazawa)
M. MAKUUCHI (Matsumoto)
K. MARUYAMA (Tokyo)
S. MATSUNO (Sendai)
Y. MISHIMA (Tokyo)
M. MITO (Asahikawa)
T. MITOMI (Kanagawa)
I. MIYAZAKI (Kanazawa)
R. MIZUMOTO (Mie)
S. MORI (Sendai)
T. MORI (Osaka)
R. MOTOKI (Fukushima)
T. MUTO (Niigata)
T. MUTO (Tokyo)
K. NABEYA (Tokyo)
Y. NAGAMACHI (Maebashi)
G. NAKAGAWARA (Fukui)
T. NAKAJIMA (Tokyo)
H. NAKANO (Nara)
H. NAKAZATO (Nagoya)

Table of Contents

Part 3

Recent Advances in Early Detection and Treatment of Digestive Cancers

Part 4

Recent Strategies in the Treatment of Cancer Patients

— Endoscopic and Laparoscopic Surgery

— New Technology for Cancer Surgery

— New Strategies for Cancer Therapy

Stomach

— Carcinogenesis

— Clinical Analysis

— Lymphnodes and Surgery

— Chemotherapy

— Immunotherapy

XVIII

Peritoneum

Endoscope

— Diagnosis

— Treatment

Colon and Rectum

— Carcinogenesis

— Histopathology

Liver

Primary

— Carcinogenesis

— Diagnosis

— Surgery

— Others

Pancreas

— Surgery and/or Radiation

Biliary

Immunotherapy

Others

Special Lectures

The Role of UICC in the Management of Cancer Patients

SÁNDOR ECKHARDT

National Institute of Oncology, Budapest, Hungary

The International Union Against Cancer (Union Internationale contre le Cancer, UICC) is a voluntary, non-governmental organization active in the fight against cancer. It was created in 1934 after a successful International Cancer Congress held in Madrid (1933). It had several aims : a) to study the basis of an anatomo-clinical classification of tumours, b) to set up a permanent international documentation centre on all matters relating to cancer, c) to publish an international bulletin, d) to prepare future international cancer congresses, e) to publish an illustrated tumour nomenclature, f) to prepare a survey of cancer control societies and institutes. In order to reach these goals a structure of this organization was established. Basically, during the past, this structure did not change much and nowadays both the aims and means of the UICC are very similar to the original ideas. Therefore we are featuring the present UICC structure for a better understanding. For the time being UICC has the General Assembly consisting of more than 250 members from over 80 countries, the Council Members elected by the Member States and the Executive Committee. Besides, UICC set up a permanent Office for continuous functioning in Geneva, headed by the Executive Director. The General Assembly meets at the Business Meetings jointly held with the International Cancer Congresses every four years, while Business Meetings of the Council occur every two years. Both events take place in order to determine the policy of UICC in the coming period. Moreover, Council Members play a leading role in deciding action in cancer research and patient care. Executive Committee members meet twice yearly and their responsibility is to run activities decided by the Council. They do it through Program Chairmen elected by the Council and they supervise their aims and funding. Program Chairmen are initiating projects for shorter or longer duration and appointing Project Chairmen as well as members to carry out action. The Project Chairmen stands as a head of a Project and might run or close any activity according to his scientific and professional expertise. At the same time he has to report to the Program Chairman on the outcome of his action. The Program Chairman is obliged to survey his Program (composed of various Projects) to the Executive Committee and the Council. Thus, a feedback of successes and failures is possible in the existing structure and the quality control is constantly assured.

Actually, UICC runs nine Programs. Moreover, it possesses the wellknown scientific journal entitled "International Journal of Cancer" and three Special Projects, those of oral, cervical cancer and melanoma. The Programme of Epidemiology and Prevention (Chairman: K.Aoki) lists the following objectives: a) to review and evaluate the causative factors of cancer and to search for the most practical and effective ways of prevention, b) to encourage collaboration in accumulating data and information exchange between member organizations, c) and to provide and to spread useful knowledge and technology. The Program is composed of the following Projects: familial cancer and its prevention, information exchange in developing countries, nutrition, diet and cancer, evaluation and effectiveness of primary prevention, publication of cancer mortality statistics in the world and various other publications, follow-up of Chernobil atomic accident. The Tumour Biology Programme (Chairman: R.Brentani) focuses on the following objective: en bloc transfer of practical research know-how from experienced practitioners to group of young scientists from various regions of the world, especially the less developed regions. For this reason, it organizes courses with special emphasis to techniques which can be used in research of UICC Special Projects (Oral, cervical cancer, melanoma). The Detection and Diagnosis Programme (Chairman: F.Badellino) enumerates the following objectives: a) to provide an internationally agreed and uniform TNM program including pathological aspects and prognostic factors, b) to assist in the evolution and evaluation of international trials, screening programmes and computer-assisted techniques. In order to reach these goals Projects were initiated and activated as follows: TNM classification of malignant tumours, computer aid for patient management, evaluation of screening programmes. The Program of Treatment on Cancer (Chairman: D.Hossfeld) summarizes its objective as such: a) to publish guidance on the current treatment of cancer and b) to advise clinicians on the future prospects of cancer treatment. In order to fulfil these tasks the following projects are in progress: current treatment of cancer and prospects of treatment. The former activity is a survey of a constantly updated knowledge of the cancer patient care and the latter project deals with experimental and clini-

cal approaches which are ongoing or under evaluation. For this reason expert committee meet-

ings are invited and several publications appear. In the Program of Professional Education

(Chairman: C.Sherman) the goal has been set to raise the capability and effectiveness of pro-

fessionals involved in the treatment, management and care of cancer patients. The following

projects are directed towards this task: cancer education for medical students, clinical onco-

logy courses, manual of clinical oncology, cancer nursing, professional education project

chairmen coordination meetings, regional coordinating meetings. Among these widespread acti-

vities the sixth edition of the Manual of Clinical Oncology has to be stressed, which will be

finished and published next year on the occasion of the XVI.International Cancer Congress. So

far, five editions have been published and translated into eleven languages. In the Program of

Cancer Organization and Public Education Services (COPES, Chairman: K.Horsch) the main object-

ive has been chosen to establish a worldwide network of collaborating voluntary cancer control

agencies. A further task is to assure that these agencies are efficiently organized in order

to carry out their mandate in cancer control. Furthermore, this Program is aimed at providing

a service directly to the cancer patients. The Program is composed of the following projects:

behavioural science, cancer education in schools and communities, health professional involve-

ment in public education on cancer, patient support and rehabilitation, COPES progress reports,

COPES regional coordination, cancer education at the workplace, COPES project chairmen meeting

and the William Rudder grants projects. From this impressive list of projects it is easy to

conclude that this Program is playing a key role of UICC in the community. In order to support

the UICC activities an adequate manpower is needed which is expert in both research and care

of cancer patients. Therefore the Program of Fellowships (Chairman: G.McVie) instituted se-

veral types of fellowships to fulfil this task. The objective is the administration of four

international cancer fellowships for investigators, clinicians and success to support original

cancer research, to facilitate technology transfer, augment and disseminate research, clinical

and nursing skills throughout the world. Accordingly, the Program has four projects: American

Cancer Society International Cancer Research Fellowship for more advanced research workers,

Yamagiwa-Yoshida Memorial International Cancer Research Grants generously supported by the

Japanese Cancer Society for the same purpose, International Cancer Research Technology Transfer (ICRETT) for both investigators and clinicians on a more basic scale, International Oncology Nursing Fellowships which is a new project jointly organized with the Professional Education Program. The objective of the last fellowship segment can be elucidated as such: to enable English-speaking nurses caring for cancer patients in their home institutes and who come from countries where specialist cancer nursing training is not yet available, to observe specific oncology nursing skills at North American or UK-based comprehensive cancer centres so that these skills may be practised and disseminated to other patient care staff upon return. "Reserve" awards of qualified oncology nurses to teach their skills, where it is needed, is also possible. Special attention of UICC was always directed towards playing a leading role of the antismoking campaign. Consequently, the Program of Tobacco and Cancer (Chairman: M.Wood) was established with the clearcut objective to change attitudes to tobacco use in the society and to promote regional strategies to eradicate production, sales, promotion and use throughout the region. In favour of reaching this goal numerous projects were launched. Tobacco Control Africa, Tobacco Control Asia (Pacific North), Tobacco Control Asia (Pacific South), Tobacco Control Europe, Tobacco Control Indian Subcontinent, Tobacco Control Latin America, Tobacco Control North America, Smoking Cessation, Resources and Support. In addition, recently Globalink, an uptodate information system to coordinate these efforts was transferred to UICC and there is good hope that with the aid of the EC further successes can be reached. The Program of the Committee of International Collaborative Activities (CICA, Chairman: P.Desai) has one objective of major importance: to facilitate international collaboration in cancer research, care and management. The following projects serve this purpose: various publications including an International Directory of cancer establishments, the International Cancer Patient Data Exchange System (ICPDES) compiling uniform minimum requirement data sets of cancer patients for basic comparison among different regions (i.e. Europe, North America, China, Latin America), establishment of National Cancer Plans in order to assign priorities in the fight against cancer.

The UICC was always taking efforts for being in the centre of dissemination of information related to cancer. For this reason, it edited a Bulletin and in the last two decades the "International Journal of Cancer", a very wellknown and distinguished scientific journal, was established for reaching this goal. For the time being it is a monthly scientific review read and appreciated as one of the best cancer research information sources by the cancer community all over the world. In recent years specific tumour localisations were chosen for topics of Special Projects. Those cancers are priorities for UICC which are worldwide killers in which causative factors are known and prevention is possible. They are oral cancer (Chairman: P.Desai), cervical cancer (Chairman: J.Pontén) and melanoma (Chairman: R.Marks). Various meetings and publications are sponsored by UICC related to the knowledge of these malignancies, and progress is expected in the near future.

Mechanisms for Organ Specific Metastasis, in Particular from the Gastro-Intestinal Tract to the Liver

MAX M. BURGER

Friedrich-Miescher-Institute and Biocenter of the University of Basel, 4002 Basel, Switzerland

ABSTRACT

Highly metastasizing cells display some general characteristics compared to poorly metastasizing cells. They adhere less to each other, they produce and release enzymes which degrade their surroundings and they have a tendency to deform easier. Any of these properties or several of them together could be shown to promote metastasis in animal model systems. Organ-specific metastasis, as e.g. to the liver, was thought to be due to increased adhesion to the endothelial cells, the vascular basal membrane or the parenchymal cells of the target organ liver. Here an additional mechanism could be identified, namely liver-specific growth promotion by a liver cell membrane-specific growth factor. In the final section the recent literature on liver-specific metastasis mechanisms was reviewed including some comments on a possible cross-talk between metastasizing cells and their surrounding host organ cells.

INTRODUCTION

Paget's concept from 1889 that tumor cells metastasize into a particular organ since they have a preference to survive and grow there as compared to other organs [1] has been challenged by Ewing in 1928 [2] who was convinced that the vascular connections between primary tumor and host organ of metastasis are the key factor determining the dissemination pattern. Today, there is no question that both mechanisms have their significance.

A similarly dogmatic concept prevailed for the last 20 years as to the molecular and cell biological mechanism leading to organ specific metastasis: primary tumor cells adhere to the target organ specifically, be that organ specific endothelial cells, basal membranes or organ parenchymal cells [3]. We have challenged this concept and provided evidence that primary tumor cells may not adhere preferentially to the target organ but disseminate fairly randomly and then receive specific growth signals only in one or a few target organs [4]. Most likely both specific adhesive as well as specific growth promoting mechanisms determine the outcome of the metastatic dissemination pattern. In some cases it may be adhesive forces [5], in some cases growth promoting forces [4,6,7], and in some cases both [8]. In order to understand organ specific metastasis better, a survey of mechanisms leading to increased metastasis in general will be discussed first.

TUMOR ALTERATIONS LEADING TO INCREASED METASTASIS IN GENERAL

Loss of Cohesion

Loss of cohesion in the primary tumor is certainly a factor contributing to the loss in containment of the tumor cell mass leading to extravasation into lymph and blood vessels as well as into body cavities. Earlier on this loss of containment was thought to be due to the 'pressure' developped by the expansion in tumor cell numbers. Now there is evidence that many tumor cells adhere less to each other or to the surrounding extracellular matrix. Such alterations have been shown to be due to glycoprotein changes, in particular also carbohydrate changes. Thus very subtle decreases in sialic acid terminals [9] due to decreases and increases in sugar transfering enzymes [10] can alter the adhesive properties among tumor cells [11]. Exactly the same changes in sialic acid [12] do alter also the interactions of integrin-like cellular receptors [12] for extracellular matrix molecules like laminin [13] and thereby seem to alter the degree of metastasis. Recently a human oncogene-dependent (c-Ha-ras) increase of the sialyl transfer enzyme was detected [14] and correlated with metastasis [15] which lends further support to the concept that these fine alterations in sialic acid terminals on tumor cell surface glycoproteins have a role in metastasis.

Degradation of the Extracellular Matrix

Degradation of the extracellular matrix can be achieved by metastatic tumor cells through various means, each of which has been observed in highly metastatic tumor cells. Thus proteolytic enzymes (urokinase-type plasminogen activator, collagenase type IV, tissue-type plasminogen activator, cathepsins, etc.) are increased in many human and animal metastatic tumor cells, though not in all. Tissue inhibitor of metalloproteases (TIMP) is decreased in a variety of metastatic tumors. A manipulated decrease in TIMP (antisense RNA in TIMP) has been shown to render none-tumorigenic cells invasive, tumorigenic and metastatic [16]. For some metastatic cells an increase in extracellular carbohydrate degrading enzymes could be demonstrated as well [17].

Deformability

Deformability has been shown to increase the potential of a tumor cell to metastasize. Thus if a strain of poorly metastasizing tumor cells is exposed to a filter (2µ) the few cells which have acquired the capability to deform easier and penetrate the filter turn out to metastasize better [18,19]. Their cytoskeleton shows similar changes (loss of microfilament bundles) as in highly metastatic human tumor cells which may be the reason for the increase in deformability. To what degree increased tissue motility of metastatic cells is due to cytoskeleton or/and membrane and adhesion changes is not yet clear.

SPECIFIC MECHANISMS LEADING TO INCREASED LIVER METASTASIS IN GASTROINTESTINAL NEOPLASMS

Plenty of speculations filled the literature about possibilities why tumor cells metastasize into a given organ. We felt therefore that a comparison of tumor cell strains of identical origin which would have the stable characteristics of metastasizing into two different organs may provide clues as to the mechanisms of organ specific metastasis in man.

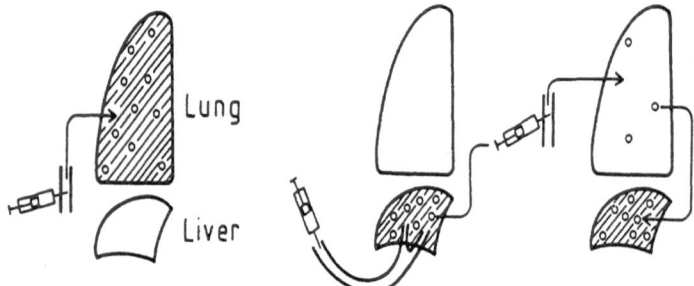

Fig. 1 Selection of Melanoma Cells with a Preference to Metastasize into the Liver. The parent B16 melanoma cells produce almost exclusively lung tumors if injected into the tail vein (see left part of figure). If injected into the portal vein system primarily liver tumors will be found. If these cells are grown in tissue culture for one passage (not shown) and then injected into the tail vein, a few liver tumors can be found beside the lung tumors. Repetition of such liver cycles leads to cells with a clearly detectable tendency to colonize the liver if administered intravenously. (Reprinted with permission from Burger MM (1983) Experimental Models for Metastasis. In: Fortner JG, Rhoads JE (eds) Accomplishments in Cancer Research, 1983 Prize Year General Motors Cancer Research Foundation. Lippincott, Philadelphia, p 179) [20]

The Liver Can Promote The Growth Of Liver Specific Metastasizing Cells.

A mouse melanoma line which was injected into the tail vein and resulting lung colonies were reinjected i.v. several times until it had the characteristics to metastasize preferentially into the lung (F-10). The same or similar lines were then selected for liver specificity by injecting them into the portal vein [20]. Colonies growing in the liver were then reinjected into the portal vein again another eight times (Fig.1) and finally tested for organ specificity by injecting them again into the tail vein. Regardless whether a typical melanoma line with low lung specificity (F-1) or a non-typical melanoma line with high lung specificity (F-10) was chosen, lines could be isolated which now always metastasized into the liver (Tab. 1) [21]. Similar selections were successful for melanoma cells going preferentially into the brain by injecting them into the a. carotis [22] and there the dogma that organ specificity is based on preferential adhesion to the target organ could be confirmed.

Cells	Passage through the liver	No. of animals with hepatic tumors following IV injection.[1] Total No. of animals
F1	—	2/50
L1-F1	1st	4/12
L2-F1	2nd	6/12
L4-F1	4th	8/12
L5-F1	5th	12/13
L6-F1	6th	16/16
L8-F1	8th	18/18
F10	—	0/20
L5-F10	5th	4/8
L8-F10	8th	12/12

[1] 4×10^4 cells were injected intravenously. Animals were examined for macroscopically visible nodules 2-3 weeks later.

Tab. 1 Selection of Melanoma Cells Showing Increasing Capacity to Form Tumors in the Liver (Reprinted with permission from Burger MM [20])

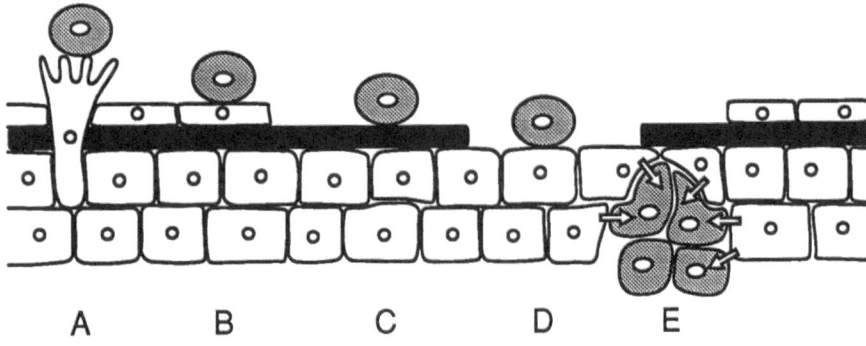

Fig. 2 Possible Mechanisms Leading to Liver-Specific Metastasis. Some tumor cells arriving in the liver (hatched cells) are not deposited in the liver due to specific adhesion to Kupffer cells (A) or to liver endothelial cells (B) or to the liver vascular basal membrane (C) or to liver parenchymal cells (D), but they receive directly or induced growth promoting signals preferentially in the liver (E).

Adhesion tests of these melanoma cells metastasizing into liver were therefore carried out in vitro. They did, however, not adhere preferentially to Kupffer cells or to liver parenchymal cells neither in rosetting tests nor in monolayer adhesion tests [4, 20]. Injection of these liver-specific cells intravenoulsy and following their organ distribution with isotopic label showed no preference of settling in the liver for these liver-specific cells as compared to the lung specific cells [4, 20]. Preferential binding to liver endothelial cells as much as to any other cells in the liver could therefore be ruled out (Fig.2). We had to consider thus other mechanisms than adhesion or lodging which could lead to organ specific metastasis of these cells. We found good support for the concept that these cells had a growth advantage in liver confirming Paget's concept of a preferential soil [1]. Co-culture of these melanoma cells with liver cells stimulated the growth of the liver-specific melanoma cells (Fig.3). Later on, a more detailed analysis showed that liver cells had a better survival effect on liver specific melanoma cells than on lung specific melanoma cells [23]. The stimulatory effect necessitated pores of larger than 0.2μ if liver cells were plated on one side of a Nuclepore filter and liver-specific melanoma cells on the other side, thus indicating that physical contact was necessary for the two cells to allow the growth signal to proceed [7]. A liver membrane-bound growth factor could now be isolated which is different from the well known scatter or hepatic growth factor [23], and which promote the growth of liver specific melanoma cells better than lung-specific melanoma cells.

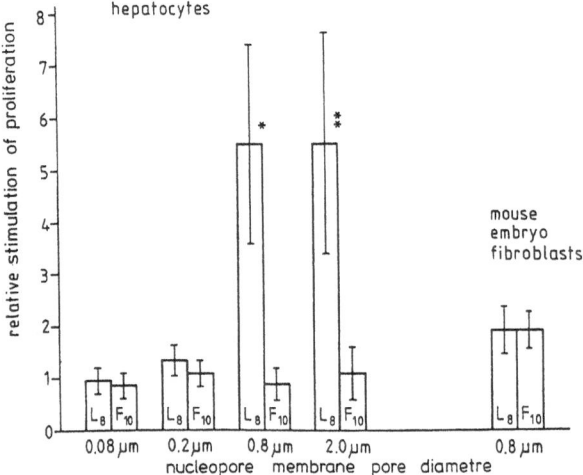

Fig. 3 Growth Promotion of Liver-Specific Melanoma Cells by Liver Cells on the Other Side of a Nuclepore Filter. L8: Melanoma cell metastasizing into liver, F10: Melanoma cell metastasizing into lung. In the first four experiments on the left hepatocytes were plated on the other side of the filter. In the last experiment mouse embryo fibroblasts were plated on the other side of the filter. After 4 days of coculture, hepatocytes or fibroblasts were wiped from the filters with paper tissues, and melanoma cells were counted in a Coulter Counter after detachment with EDTA. *, P<0.001; **, P<0.002.(Reprinted with permission of Burger MM [7].)

Adhesive and Other Mechanisms Can also Participate in Liver-Specific Metastasis

The contribution of adhesion to organ specific metastasis in general has been reviewed [24, 25, 26, 27]. Here we want to summarize gastrointestinal liver-specific aspects only.

Adhesion to Endothelial Cells

If stimulated with Tumor Necrosis Factor (TNF) human colon carcinoma cells begin to attach to human endothelial cell surfaces via a defined endothelial glycoprotein, endothelial leukocyte adhesion molecule-1 (ELAM-1) [28]. Such receptors have first been found to guide homing of lymphocytes but seem to be used by tumor cells as well.

Adhesion to the Basal Membrane

Since endothelial cells are easily sheared off by hemodynamic forces or actively scooped off by tumor cells or leukocytes, the basal membrane beneath may often be exposed to tumor cells. Extracellular matrix molecules of this membrane may then be attachment hooks for tumor cells provided they have the appropriate receptors. Integrins which are such receptors have recently been shown by the Kobata group [12] to display exactly the same partial loss in terminal sialic acid as we described above and earlier in poorly metastatic cells [9]. These same poorly metastasizing cells turned out to adhere less to the basal membrane component laminin [13]. A correlation between increased laminin receptor concentrates on human colon carcinoma cells, and an increased metastatic potential shows that such observations on animal models may have significance for human tumors as well [29]. Such differences explain general changes in metastatic properties but quantitative and particularly qualitative changes in both extracellular matrix and tumor cell receptors may turn out to explain organ-specific metastatic patterns as well.

Adhesion to Liver Parenchymal Cells

The vascular system of the liver differs from many organs insofar as there are many windows in the vascular wall, devoid not only of endothelial cells but also of basal membrane. Tumor cells passing through the liver can thus contact liver parenchymal cells directly through the Dissé space. Liver cells have unique galactose-sensing receptors which have the duty to fish glycoproteins from the blood stream which are defect in sialic acid and have the galactose which lies below the sialic acid in glycoproteins or N-acetylgalactosamine residues exposed. These same receptors may therefore bind tumor cells with exposed galactose/N-acetylgalactosamine residues. Schirrmacher's group has provided support to this concept when they found highly liver-metastasizing murine lymphoma cells to bind to liver cells while low liver-metastatic lymphoma sublines do not bind [30]. It is, however, unlikely that in all cases where more galactose is exposed on surface glycoproteins liver-specific metastasis begins to increase as well. Thus the lectin (WGA) resistant melanoma cells described at the beginning of this article [9] have specific glycoprotein galactose residues exposed but seem not to metastasize specifically to the liver. Furthermore, the liver-specific mouse melanoma cells described above seem not to show drastic changes in exposed galactoses on their cell surfaces [31].

Not Yet Defined Adhesion Molecule Changes

Recently, cell membrane changes in gastrointestinal tumors could be detected where the pathogenic mechanism involved is not yet clear. A tumor suppressor gene which seems to be absent in some human colon cancers (Deficient in Colon Cancer, DCC) codes for a cell adhesion molecule (N-CAM) which has the characteristics of the immunoglobulin superfamily [32]. It seems to be missing rather late in the ontogenesis of a tumor and one assumes therefore that it prevents some step(s) in metastasis. Rat pancreas and mammary carcinoma cells display an additional aminoacid loop in the CD44 general adhesion molecule [33]. Introduction of this loop into non-metastasizing rat cells renders them metastatic. Since the parent molecule is under normal circumstances involved in mediating adhesion to some vascular endothelial cells one can speculate that the additional loop alters simple functions like general adhesion and cell migration or more sophisticated functions like organ distribution, but here again the molecular alteration has no exact functional correlate as of yet.

Cross Talk Between Tumor and Host Organ

Tumor cells may not only depend on growth signals and growth factors already available in the host tissue [4,20], but there may be a close reciprocal interaction between the tumor cell and its host tissue where the tumor induces growth stimulatory phenomena in its surrounding tissue [26, 27]. Thus invasive human breast carcinoma cells do not express extracellular matrix degrading proteases like stromelysin-3 while the surrounding stromal cells do [34]. Since proteolytic enzymes do not only loosen up the tumor cell aggregate but were earlier found to promote cell growth [35], the induction of proteolytic enzymes in tumor surrounding tissues by tumor cell factors like Fibroblast Growth Factor may lead to a powerful cascade of paracrine growth stimulation [26, 27]. If such cross talk via growth promoting proteases [35] is restricted between tumor cells and only certain host tissues, then organ-specific metastasis pattern can ensue from selected tumor/host organ interactions. A good example for this line of thought is the fact that human colon carcinoma only produce increased collagenase and metastasize to the liver when implanted in the colon wall of nude mice, but not when implanted ectopically under the skin [36].

Both Growth and Adhesion Determine Organ Specificity

In most cases the outcome of organ specific dissemination is dependent on more than one factor. A good example are the F-9 murine teratocarcinoma cells which efficiently colonize the liver, but can hardly be found in the lungs after tail-vein inoculation [37]. These cells both adhere better to liver extracellular matrix and are stimulated to grow better by liver extracts as compared to lung extracellular matrix and lung extracts [38]. When they are treated with retinoic acid the lungs become the main target for the same cells. In this case they are also better growth stimulated by lung extracts, and - although they do not adhere now better to lung extracellular matrix - they are still better trapped by the lung capillary bed since the retinoic acid treated cells are larger [39]. This then illustrates well the multifactorial causes for organ-specific metastasis. Correlations between metastatic phenotype and alterations in various molecular and cellular characteristics will always be incomplete as long as not all factors influencing organ-specific dissemination are defined. For the time being, we will have to consider seriously besides target organ adhesion target organ-specific growth promotion.

REFERENCES

1. Paget S (1889) Lancet 1: 571-573
2. Ewing J (1928) A Treatise on Tumors. W.B. Saunders, Philadelphia
3. Hart IR (1982) Cancer Metast Rev 1: 5-16
4. Burger MM, Madnick HM (1983) Liver in Metabolic Diseases. MTP Press Ltd., Boston, pp 351-365
5. Auerbach R, Lu WC, Pardon E, Gumkowski F, Kaminska G, Kaminski M (1987) Cancer Res 47: 1492-1496
6. Nicolson GL, Dulski KM (1986) Int J Cancer 38: 289-294
7. Sargent NSE, Oestreicher M, Haidvogl H, Madnick HM, Burger MM (1988) Proc Natl Acad Sci USA 85: 7251-7255
8. Rusciano D, Lorenzoni P, Burger MM (1991) Int J Cancer 48: 450-456
9. Finne J, Tao TW, Burger MM (1980) Cancer Res 40: 2580-2587
10. Finne J, Burger MM, Prieels JP (1982) J Cell Biol 92: 277-282
11. Tao TW, Jenkins M, Vosbeck K, Matter A, Miller M, Jockusch BM, Shenz Z, Burger MM (1983) Int J Cancer 31: 239-247
12. Kawano T, Takasaki S, Tao TW, Kobata A (1993) Int J Cancer 53: 91-96
13. Oz OK, Campbell A, Tao TW (1989) Int J Cancer 44: 343-347
14. Le Marer N, Laudet V, Svensson EC, Cazlaris H, Va Hille B, Lagrou C, Stehelin D, Montreuil J, Verbert A, Delannoy P (1992) Glycobiology 2: 49-56
15. Le Marer N, personal communication
16. Khoka RP, Waterhouse P, Yagel S, Lala PK, Overall CM, Norton G, Denhardt DT (1989) Science 243: 947-950
17. Niedbala MJ, Madiyalakan R, Matta K, Crickard K, Sharma M, Bernacki RJ (1987) Cancer Res 47: 4634-4641
18. Tullberg KF, Burger MM (1985) Invasion Metastasis 5: 1-15
19. Ochalek T, Nordt FJ, Tullberg K, Burger MM (1988) Cancer Res 48: 5124-5128
20. Tao TW, Matter A, Vogel K, Burger MM (1979) Int J Cancer 23: 854-857
21. Burger MM (1983) In: Fortner JG, Rhoads JE (eds) Accomplishments in Cancer Research, 1983 Prize Year General Motors Cancer Research Foundation. Lippincott, Philadelphia, pp 174-182
22. Brunson KW, Beattie G, Nicolson GL (1978) Nature 272: 543-544
23. Rusciano D, Lorenzoni P, Burger MM, unpublished observation
24. Hart IR (1982) Cancer Metastasis Rev 1: 5-17
25. Nicolson GL (1988) Biochim Biophys Acta 948: 175-224
26. Rusciano D, Burger MM (1993) In: Molecular Genetics of Nervous System Tumors. Wiley-Lyss, New York, pp 356-369
27. Rusciano D, Burger MM (1992) Bioessays 14: 185-194
28. Rice GE, Bevilaqua MP (1989) Science 246: 1303-1306
29. Cioce V, Castronovo V, Shmookler BM, Garbisa S, Grigioni WF, Liotta LA, Sobel ME (1991) J Natl Cancer Inst 83: 29-36
30. Cheingsong-Popov R, Robinson P, Altevogt P, Schirrmacher V (1983) Int J Cancer 32: 359-366
31. Burger MM, unpublished observation
32. Fearon ER, Cho KR, Nigro JM, Kern SE, Simons JW, Ruppert JM, Hamilton SR, Preisinger AC, Thomas G, Kinzler KW, Vogelstein B (1990) Science 247: 49-56
33. Günthert U, Hofmann M, Rudy W, Reber S, Zöller M, Haussmann I, Matzku S, Wenzel A, Ponta H, Herrlich P (1991) Cell 65: 13-64
34. Basset P, Bellocq JP, Wolf C, Stoll I, Hutin P, Limacher JM, Podhajcer OL, Chenard MP, Rio MC, Chambon P (1990) Nature 348: 699-704
35. Burger MM (1969) Proc Natl Acad Sci USA 62: 994-1001
36. Nakajima M, Morikawa K, Fabra A, Bucana CD, Fidler IJ (1990) J Natl Cancer Inst 82: 1890-1898
37. Terrana B, Rusciano D, Pacenti L (1987) Cancer Res 47: 3791-3797
38. Rusciano D, Lorenzoni P, Burger MM (1991) Int J Cancer 48: 450-456
39. Rusciano D, Lorenzoni P, Burger (1992) Int J Cancer 52: 471-477

Part 1

Present and Prospective Trends of Digestive Cancers in the World

Present and Prospective Trends of Digestive Cancer in Germany

CARL G. SCHMIDT

West German Tumor Center, University of Essen, 4300 Essen 1, Germany

The present situation of digestive cancer patterns in Germany follows more or less the distribution pattern within the Western European countries. Age distribution, incidence rates, biological behaviour, and the therapeutic results are similar within the Western European countries.

New trends in epidemiology in certain European areas point to a possible decrease in incidence rates of cancer of the oesophagus in spite of the fact that the risk factors smoking and drinking are still present. By analysing the environmental facts there is the possibility that the increased consumption of green and yellow vegetables could play a role in explaining this interesting tendency. We acknowledge, of course, the pioneer work which Japanese epidemiologist have been able to perform in the important field of diet and cancer and I should like to add that there is a controversial discussion because some people think that recent data indicate an increase.

When it comes to a therapeutic approach surgical removal has remained the traditional and accepted treatment for cancer of the oesophagus but it is well known that the cumulative 5 years-survival rate after the huge operation in major series is rather disappointing. The majority of patients will be incurable by current means. I am not dealing with improved surgical techniques, importance of tumour stage, grading and biological risk factors in relation to the prognostic outcome but I would like to address the design of modern chemotherapeutic regimes for oesophageal cancer and how they can be integrated into combined modality treatment plans. Adjuvant chemotherapy (following surgery) has a demonstrated role in breast cancer, colon cancer, certain sarcomas and several cancers of childhood. Neo-adjuvant therapy (prior to surgery) has theoretical advantage over adjuvant therapy. One of them is the possible downstaging of the primary tumour, facilitating the operation in marginal cases.

So far results with local treatment alone are disappointing, an improvement of the prognosis of patients with locally advanced disease can at best be expected by the integration of chemotherapy with combined modality programmes.

Several single-agent and combined chemotherapy trials preceding surgery have been performed. In this context I would like to present some recent results on trials of the West German Tumor Centre Essen. Chemotherapy programmes for oesophageal cancer are usually Cis-platinum-Bleomycin or Cis-platinum-5-Flurouracil based. In loco-regional disease they induce approximately 50 to 60 % of objective remissions (major response) but usually less than 40% in extensive disease. In a new phase II-trial a new combination consisting of folinic acid, 5-Flurouracil, Etoposide and Cis-platinum (FLEP) was performed, the rationale being the effectiveness of the 3 single agents, the synergistic interaction between the 3 drugs, the well-known enhanced cytotoxicity of 5-Flurouracil by the biochemical modulator folinic acid, and the results of a pilot study with FLEP.

Fig. 1 FLEP-regime

TREATMENT PLAN - STUDY WTZ/ECN/1

Part 1:
Folinic acid	300 mg/m^2	10 min. iv,	d 1,2,3
Etoposide	100 mg/m^2	50 min. iv,	d 1,2,3
5-FU	500 mg/m^2	10 min. iv,	d 1,2,3
Cisplatin	30 mg/m^2	60 min. iv,	d 1,2,3

Repeat d 22 for 3 cycles

Part 2:
Irradiation	42 Gy, d 1-29 (2 Gy/fraction)		
Cisplatin	50 mg/m^2	60 min. iv,	d 2,9
Etoposide	100 mg/m^2	60 min. iv,	d 4,5,6

Part 3. Transthoracic esophagektomy, 4 weeks after end of irradiation.

14

Fig. 2   Results after chemotherapy

RESULTS AFTER CHEMOTHERAPY (N=35)

Complete remission	2	(6%)
Partial remission	16	(46%)
CR + PR	18	(51%)
Minor regression/No change	11	(31%)
Progression	5	(14%)
Toxic death	1	(3%)

So far 38 patients with advanced oesophageal carcinoma were treated with the FLEP-protocol, the majority with locally advanced disease (LAD). Oesophagectomy was planned for patients with LAD in case of tumour regression after chemotherapy, while patients with M1 disease received chemotherapy only. The overall remission rate was 45% including 4 clinical and 2 pathological confirmed complete remissions. Sixteen patients underwent oesophagectomy. The medium survival time of LAD patients was 13 months and actuarial survival time was 31%. Patients with tumour resection had a medium survival time of 17 months and a two years-survival rate of 44%. I should like to point out that in patients with locally defined tumours the CR/PR rate was 47%, the medium survival time reached 12 months. After RO/R1-resection 40% remained continuously disease-free after 25 to 43 months' follow-up. At the first hint, these results do not seem to be superior to those being reported in other phase II-studies but I would like to emphasize that we entered only patients with locally defined tumours judged to be irresectable by an experienced surgeon and that despite these unfavourable preconditions 62 % of our LAD patients underwent successful tumour resection after chemotherapy alone or for 4 patients after subsequent chemo-radiotherapy. The 2 years-survival rates of 31% of all LAD patients and of 44% for patients with tumour resection are promising and suggest in accordance with other phase II-trials that an effective pre-operative chemotherapy contributes to higher resection rates and improve survival. However, this apparently positive impact of pre-operative chemotherapy in the treatment of oesophageal cancer remains to be proven by randomized trials.

In conclusion, FLEP is a feasible and active combination for oesophageal cancer, especially for locally advanced disease. Due to these results a new combined protocol was designed in March 1991 including 3 cycles of FLEP, followed by one cycle of simultaneous chemo-radiotherapy followed by surgery in a similar patients' population. The first experiences with this approach confirm the efficacy of FLEP because in this ongoing study the preliminary results demonstrate that about 50% of these patients had CR/PR after treatment whereas more than three quarters of these patients were rendered disease-free.

Fig. 3   Results of Surgery & Final Results

RESULTS AFTER SURGERY (N = 27)

Thoracotomy; not resected due to complications; biopsies tumor negative	1	
Tumor resection	26/35	(74%)
Pathologic CR ($T_x N_x M_0$)	11/26	(42%)
RO-resection/NED	13/26	(50%)
pCR/RO= rate	24/26	(92%)
R2-resection	2/26	(8%)

2 postoperative deaths (7%)

FINAL RESULTS OF ALL PATIENTS (N = 35)

Clinical CR	3	(9%)
Pathologic CR	11	(31%)
RO-Resection	13	(37%)
cCR/pCR/RO	27	(77%)

Fig. 4 Summary

SUMMARY - WTZ/ECN/1

This intensive preoperative combined-modality program induces an unusually high local tumor control rate (cCR/pCR/NED = 77%)

Of special note is the 31% pCR-rate of all off-treatment patients and that an additionally 18% only had microscopic disease in the resected material.

The impact of this high local tumor control rate on median and long term survival can not be estimated yet.

Turning to the problem of gastric cancer the Japanese pioneer work regarding early gastric cancer is well known and admired. In the Western European countries most cases are diagnosed beyond that early stage. In this context the question of radical surgery including lymphadenectomy arises. I should like to refer to a recent clinical study including 319 patients with gastric cancer (mostly intestinal type) performed at the Medical School at Hanover. 75,9% of these patients underwent surgical resection (mostly gastrectomy) whereby a medium number of 36,8 lymph nodes were removed. Without going into details the prognostic outcome was remarkably influenced by the tumor stage, of course, and furthermore by the number of lymph nodes involved. In patients with a maximum number of 3 positive lymph nodes there was no significant prognostic difference compared with lymph node-negative cases. The number of lymph nodes involved is crucial because there was a definite decline in the outcome for cases with more than 3 nodes involved.

In locally advanced cases chemotherapy has shown effectiveness in recent years. The widely used FAM protocol includes 5-Flurouracil (F), Adriamycin (A) and Mitomycin-C (M). In 1982 Klein from the University of Cologne reported of 63% response rate in patients with advanced gastric cancer treated with sequential high dose Methotrexate (MTX) and 5-Flurouracil (F) combined with Adriamycin (A) = (FAMTX). In order to confirm these data a prospected randomized comparison with the standard FAM regime was performed. The EORTC (European Organization for Research and Treatment of Cancer) GI tract operative group including the Medical Department of the University of Cologne, The EORTC Data Center in Brussels/Belgium and the Laurentius Hospital, Roermond/The Netherlands has produced multicenter phase III trials to compare the new FAMTX with FAM. Both protocols are reviewed in the following figures.

Fig. 5 FAM and FAMTX protocol for advanced gastric cancer

FAMTX

MTX 1500 mg/m^2 i.v.
followed after 1 h by
5-FU 1.500 mg/m^2 i.v. day 1
Leucovorin rescue 15 mg/m^2, orally
after 24 h, every 6 h for 48 h
Adriamycin 30 mg/m^2 i.v. day 15
repeated every 4 weeks

FAM

5-FU, 600 mg/m^2 i.v.
days 1,8,29,36
Adriamycin 30 mg/m^2 i.v.
days 1 and 29
Mitomycin C 10 mg/m^2 i.v.
day 1
repeated every 8 weeks

Fig. 6 response rate of FAM and FAMTX

response

	FAMTX	FAM
	(n=81)	(n=79)
CR	5	0
PR	28	7
NC	25	25
PD	16	34
early deaths	7	13
Response rate	41%	9%

Although all drugs combined in FAMTX show an activity in gastric cancer, the new rationale for this regime is based on the enhanced cytotoxicity of 5-FU obtained by means of pretreatment with MTX, which is presumed to act as a modulating agent. The synergistic concept of schedule-dependent anti-tumor effect of MTX and 5-FU has a sound biochemical basis, however, the clinical applicability remains to be investigated. Doses of MTX in several protocols were mostly in intermediate range, and time intervals ranged from 0 to 24 hours. 213 patients with advanced gastric cancer were randomized (108 FAMTX; 105 FAM). The results show a significantly superior response rate, 41 versus 9% (p < 0,0001) and survival for FAMTX. This EORTC study demonstrates that FAMTX regime offers a superior response and survival rate as opposed to FAM while the hematological toxicity is less. The 1 year survival in FAMTX was 43 vs. 22% in FAM.

The 2 years survival figure were 10 vs. 4%, respectively. I would like to point out that response to FAM in this study was lower than generally reported, which is probably due to differences in the methods used to assess the response. In conclusion, FAMTX has demonstrated a priority over FAM and is a step ahead in the treatment of advanced gastric cancer but it is obvious that these results are still modest. It would be interesting to see the results of further treatment after the downstaging, especially of those cases which respond with complete remission (8 out of 81 cases in the FAMTX regime).

The major problem within the tumours of the digestive tract concerns the tumours of the large bowel. Within the European Community the annual incidence rate includes 130000 cases, the death rate being about 90000. Within the Federal Republic of Germany (before unification) the annual incidence rate amounted to about 78000. It is not surprising to see a remarkable age-related distribution pattern and within Europe a typical north-south gradient, which is regarded as a reflection of industrialization. The age-related incidence rate is still increasing in the industrialized countries. I am not referring to the interesting investigations regarding the high fat consumption and the related incidence rate of colorectal cancer, but I'd like to stress that during the last 15 years the 5-year survival rate of colorectal cancer - being the second most common tumour type -has gradually increased in the FRG. It is still a matter of discussion whether this beneficial result is due to the results of screening methods using the test for fecal blood. So far the present results are preliminary and it will take some years for further follow-up to come to a definite answer. The test cannot be regarded as very sensitive but it seems that screening will allow an earlier diagnosis which means operation at a curable stage compared with operation of symptomatic patients and furthermore detection of great polyps before undergoing malignant transformation. The tendency of a 10-percent mortality reduction seems to be realistic.

More than 50 percent of patients with large bowel cancer develop disseminated disease and will finally succumb. Since no chemotherapy with a curative potential is available for these patients, the question arises whether adjuvant chemotherapy for high-risk patients may be useful, because the only realistic hope for cure may be in the setting of minimal tumour burden. I am not referring to the well-known multiple randomized international trials involving several thousands of patients but I should like to refer to a recent trial within the Federal Republic of Germany. Some trials involving fluorinated pyrimidines alone have induced no statistically significant survival advantage compared to untreated controls. A meta-analysis of 17 trials using combined chemotherapy produced moderate evidence for small advantage in overall survival. The German GI group is especially interested to compare 5-FU plus folinic acid versus 5-FU plus Levamisole in the adjuvant setting. It is well-known that Verhaegen and co-workers reported of a striking and statistically significant survival advantage for the Levamisole-treated group in 1982. Since Levamisole has been widely used as an anti-helminthic drug for more than 20 years some immune stimulating effects are under discussion. Patients within the large American trial with Dukes' B- and C-large bowel cancer received either treatment for one year with 5-FU plus Levamisole or Levamisole alone or no treatment. The very significant reduced risk of recurrence and a remarkable death reduction in the combined treatment group with stage C was the background information to compare 5-FU plus folinic acid against 5-FU plus Levamisole in the Federal Republic. The combination of 5-FU plus folinic acid as a biochemical modulator is justified because of higher remission rates induced by the combined regime in advanced cases. The

German GI group has recently been able to confirm the prolongation of survival in disseminated disease under these circumstances. The ongoing prospected randomized German trial includes patients with colon cancer stage TNM III which includes cases with involvement of all areas of the bowel wall and loco-regional involved lymph nodes. Using the log rank test it has been calculated that about 650 patients will be needed to prove a significant difference between the 2 arms. It is too early to present even preliminary results but the question whether Levamisole instead of folinic acid in combination with 5-FU might produce an improvement is expected with great interest.

Chemotherapy plays a major role in the advanced stage. So far chemotherapy produces remission and palliation but no cure is available. I am not discussing the well-known effect of 5-FU or new treatment strategies including combination with other drugs or biochemical modulators but like to refer to some recent German studies dealing with regional chemotherapy for hepatic metastases of colorectal cancer by investigating continuous intra-arterial versus continuous intra-arterial/intravenous therapy. Hepatic artery infusion with 5-Fluorodeoxyuridine (FUdR) by implanted pumps did not improve the results compared with the other group reaching about 50% complete and partial remissions in both arms. The advantage of this type of therapy has remained controversial mainly because extra-hepatic metastases are less influenced.

With regard to systemic chemotherapy the poor results with single agent 5-FU are disappointing. Even the biochemical modulation with 5-FU + FA is producing a relatively small improvement only. We therefore need to continue to evaluate novel therapeutic approaches for metastatic colorectal cancer. One of them might be the chance of improving the effect of 5-FU by using the   pharmocokinetic pattern of the drug. The plasma half-life of 5-FU is very short. Further- more Thymidine   labeling studies with human colon carcinoma demonstrate an uptake in only about 3% of cells. Thus for each bolus injection of 5-FU, only a small fraction of the tumor cells would be susceptible which represents a fundamental limitation to the efficacy of the bolus application. For that reason continuous infusion schedules of 5-FU have been explored as a possible means for increasing the percentage of tumor cells exposed to the drug, especially during S-phase and thereby improving the effectiveness of the therapy. First results have been published in the USA. Our protocol includes continuous infusion of 5-FU by using a pump system where 300 - 350 mg/m^2/d as a maximum tolerated dose-rate has been used which could lead to a total dose of about 3g/m^2/7d. At this dose about 30 patients with advanced colorectal disease have been treated, the overall response-rate being 80%. We have not seen CR but PR ratie being about 30% including advanced liver metastases. So far the prolongation of survival reaches 11.3 months as compared to conventional application. Altogether this regime is remarkably well tolerated, using the WHO-gradient the toxicity is rather minimal. The advantage being prolongation of survival, good palliation, low risk of side-effects and a remarkable reduction in hospitalization days because most patients are able to continue their daily work without being in hospital during the infusion.

Present and Prospective Trends of Digestive Cancers in Korea

JUNG-HYUN YANG[1] and JIN-POK KIM[2]

[1]National Medical Center, Seoul, Korea
[2]Seoul National University, Seoul 100-196, Korea

(Abstract)

In Korea, cancer has been the leading cause of death since 1988. Digestive cancers comprise nearly half of all sites with stomach cancer and liver cancer ranked first and second respectively in frequency. Korean dietary habits are probably related to their high incidence. Traditionally Koreans like spicy and salty vegetables and baked meats. Also the high prevalence of hepatitis seems to result in frequent hepatoma.

Because Korean lifestyles are very rapidly becoming westernized in diet, it is predicted that the incidence of stomach cancer and liver cancer will decrease. Instead, colon cancer might increase in the coming decade.

(Key words: Trend, Digestive Cancer, Korea)

Since 1988, cancer is the first ranking cause of death in Korea following CVA and accidents.(1) The annual incidence rate of cancer is 134.8/100,000 persons according to one population-based cancer registry, at Kangwha Island. Crude mortality rate of cancer in 1991 was 105.3/100,000 persons by nationwide mortality statistics. Table 1 shows that current statistics on cancer including incidence and mortality rates of various populations in Korea. Now cancer is becoming a major health problem in Korea, along with social and economic growth. Based on this data, estimated new cancer cases in Korea total about 60,000 per year, and deaths number about 45,300 per year. (Total population of Korea is about 43,000,000) In 1991, the mortality rate of stomach cancer was 29.5/100,000 persons ranking first among all sites and followed by liver cancer in second place. The mortality rate of all digestive cancers was 64.1/100,000 persons in 1991. Cancer of digestive organs is proving to be a heavy burden in Korea rather than genitourinary and respiratory organs.

A nationwide cancer registry (Central Cancer Registry, Republic of Korea) was started in 1980, with the support of WHO to collect information on all hospitalized cases of cancer in Korea. The government instructed every teaching hospital to establish a medical record room and to send a completed report form for each tumor case to the Central Cancer Registry located in the National Medical Center in Seoul(2). Table 2 shows the relative frequencies of cancers among registered cases (total number = 50,078) in 1991. Even though the Korean government has expended much effort on the cancer registry program for more than 10 years, the registration is not at present complete, nor does it extend throughout the country. However the registry presumed to cover more than 85% of new cancer cases in the country. In males, stomach, liver, lung and colorectum are the most common sites of cancer. In females, uterine cervix followed by stomach, breast and colorectum are the top four sites since the registry started. Overall, digestive cancers comprise nearly half of all cancer sites for the ten years from 1981 to 1990. During this period, registered cancer cases totaled 277,492(male:150,755, female:126,737), including 131,598(47.4%) digestive cancers. Male cases number 88,815(58.9% of total male cases), and female cases total 42,783(33.8% of total female cases). The proportion of digestive cancers in females is relatively small because uterine cervical cancer and breast cancer are still frequent. Considering individual digestive cancers, esophagus and liver cancers have relatively higher frequency in males, and colorectal and gallbladder cancer occur more frequently in females than males.(Table 3) These patterns are not changed in 1991.(3) Age distribution of digestive cancers shows that the 6th decade is the most vulnerable period followed by the 7th and 5th decade, for all cancer sites. Table 4 snows annual incidence rates of each digestive cancer among inhabitants of Kangwha Island from 1983 to 1987. However generalization of this result to the national population is not plausible, because of many constraints in case detection and its coverage.

Stomach cancer ranked first in incidence and mortality in Korea as in Japan. The epidemiologic studies on stomach cancer suggest that environmental factors such as diet and lifestyle play a dominant role. Traditionally, Koreans like spicy and salty vagetables (for example Kimchi which is a very important side dish on Korean dining tables), and smoked meats and pickled fishes. The average Korean uses 25gm of salt per day, whereas ideal daily intake is 10gm. Studies of risk factors for digestive cancers are very scarce in Korea; most of them are simple case reviews in relation to some hypothesized factors. Seel(4) thought that Korean diet contributes to the high incidence of gastric cancer. He reported that in the late 1970's cereals and tubers together comprised about 60% of Korean diet by weight, whereas fresh vagetables provided only 18%, meats and seafood 2%, and friuts 2%, Two case-control studies on stomach cancer show that spicy or hot foods and salted or baked fishes have some impact on the high incidence and mortality rates of stomach cancer among Koreans. Refrigerators are now indispensable for the Korean's daily life but 20years ago they were luxuries in Korea. In one study, a man who has used the refrigerator for more than 20years has a lower relative risk of stomach cancer with 1/10 fold.(5)

Before 1980, gastric cancer was diagnosed in its early stages in less than 10 percent of cases. By 1989, detection rates of early gastric cancer were approaching 20% in large hospitals in metropolitan areas. But the range of frequency for the past ten years was reported from 6.6% to 15% in rural areas. Mass screening for gastric carcinoma is not well organized in Korea because economic development is still the main concern of Korean government. However, we have a medical insurance system which covers all citizens since late 1980 and it will help early detection of cancers.

The radical lymphadenectomy is standard surgical treatment for operable stomach cancer in Korea. Postoperative chemoimmunosurgery(ImmmunoChemoSurgery) for advanced stomach cancer is widely accepted. This multimodality treatment contributed to improve survival rates. Kim(6) reported 5 year-survival rate of 45.5% in the treated group (ImunoChemoSurgery), while it was 24.4% in the contol group(Surgery only) among stage III stomach cancer patients.

Liver cancer is the second-ranking cancer in Korea. The population attributable risk of hepatitis B virus for hepatoma is reported to be as high as 70%. Hepatitis B forms more than 60% of acute hepatitis and slightly more than 85% of chronic liver diseases such as chronic hepatitis and liver cirrhosis. Ahn(7) reported positive rate as 8.0% in general Korean male population and chronic carrier rate as 3.3% in females. Recent reports have shown decreases, but improvement in medical services (for example, disposable syringes and needles, strict screening tests for donated blood, etc.) and introduction of cheap domestic vaccines for HBV after 1982 could be partly responsible. Liver resection for hepatoma is sometimes difficult because cirrhosis is frequently present in more than 75% of hepatoma cases.

Incidence of colorectal cancer, panreas cancer and esophagus cancer show increasing numbers in the Central Cancer Registry annually but they haven't played a major role in prior years.

Changes in dietary patterns are now taking place in Korea because of the improvement in Korean economy, and Korean dietary patterns are changing to increase intake of meats and popular usage of refrigerators. Therefore, we might anticipate a substantial decrease in gastric cancer occurrence in due time based on comparisons of the patterns of cancer incidence rates between kangwha Island inhabitants(8) and Koreans who were living in Los Angeles of the U.S.A.(9).(table 5) The incidence rate of all cancer was somewhat higher in Los Angeles than on Kangwha Island; however stomach,liver, and cervical cancer incidence rates, were higher on Kangwha Island than in LA. The lower incidence of stomach and liver cancer rates in Los Angeles may originate from changes in environmental factors such as dietary changes. According to a study of beneficiaries by Korean Medical Insurance Corporation(10), lung and breast cancer are expected to increase. A national nutritional survey in Korea has shown that carbohydrate intake per capita is decreasing year after year and intake of protein and fat is increasing with animal foods instead of vegetables, thus increasing the tendency toward colon cancer(11). Observing the trends in distribution of digestive cancer cases which were registered in Central Cancer Registry of Korea, it could be said that there were continued increasing tendencies for most of gastrointestinal cancers except stomach and rectum(table 6). So the proportion of digestive cancers might be unchanged or decrease because breast and lung cancer incidence is expected to increase in the future in Korea the same as in other developed countries.

Table 1. Current statistics on cancer in Korea

unit: /100,000 persons per year

Rate	Crude		Standardized **	
	M	F	M	F
Incidence				
nationwide*	140	115	225	140
Kangwha	185.4	183.0	115.4	99.5
Mortality				
nationwide	131	77	211	92
Kyungnam	129	65	212	69

* KMIC beneficiaries-based
** standardized to world population

Table 2. Relative frequencies of cancers(Korea, 1991)

unit: %

Organ	Total	Male	Female
Stomach	23.5	28.2	17.5
Liver	11.1	15.8	5.1
Lung	10.9	15.4	5.2
Cervix	9.8	-	22.3
Colorectum	6.9	6.6	7.2
Breast	4.6	-	10.5
Hematopoietic	3.2	3.3	3.1
GB & EBD	2.9	2.7	3.1
Thyroid	2.6	0.6	5.1
Esophagus	2.2	3.5	0.4
Digestive organs	49.4	59.8	36.0

Central Cancer Registry
MOSHA

Table 3. Distribution of digestive cancers by site(Korea, 1981-1990)

Total registered No.   : 277,492
No. of digestive cancers : 131,598

ICD-O	Sites	Total	Male	Female
150	Esophagus	3.9	5.2	1.2
151	Stomach	51.0	50.0	53.1
152	Small intestine	0.7	0.7	0.9
153	Colon	5.7	4.6	8.0
154	Rectum-anus	7.5	5.7	11.1
155	Liver & IBD	21.5	25.4	13.4
156	GB & EBD	4.6	3.8	6.2
157	Pancreas	4.0	3.7	4.5
158	Retro & peri	0.8	0.7	1.2
159	Others & ill-def	0.3	0.2	0.3

Male : Female = 2.7 : 1, unit :%
Central Cancer Registry, MOSHA

Table 4. Incidence rates of digestive cancers (Kangwha 1983-1987)

unit : / 100,000 per year

Site	Male	Female
Esophagus	8.7	0.9
Stomach	69.1	29.5
Small intestine	-	-
Colon	7.8	4.5
Rectum	6.9	3.6
Liver & IBD	20.6	11.2
GB & EBD	2.3	2.3
Pancreas	2.7	3.6
Retro & peri	-	-
Other & ill-def	-	-
Total	117.7	55.6

Table 5. Cancer incidence rates among Koreans in Kangwha and LA, U.S.A.

unit : 100,000 per year

Primary site	Male		Female	
	Kangwha	LA	Kangwha	LA
All sites	183.0	196.5	99.5	129.9
Stomach	67.7	44.8	22.8	18.6
Liver	19.7	15.8	9.1	5.7
Lung	26.8	34.7	4.3	10.5
Cervix	-	-	22.5	17.5
Breast	-	-	5.8	14.1
Colon	7.8	4.5	4.5	3.6
Rectum	6.9	4.3	3.6	10.3

Table 6. Trends in distribution of digestive cancers in Korea

Year Organ	unit : % of total cancer cases		
	1983	1987	1991
Esophagus	1.6	2.0	2.2
Stomach	23.5	24.2	23.5
Small intestine	0.3	0.4	0.4
Colon	2.3	2.8	3.1
Rectum-anus	3.6	3.6	3.1
Liver & IBD	9.6	10.4	11.1
GB & EBD	1.6	2.3	2.9
Pancreas	1.7	2.0	2.0
Retro & peri	0.5	0.4	0.4
Other, ill-def.	0.1	0.2	0.1
Digestive cancers	44.6	48.3	49.4

Central Cancer Registry, MOSHA

References

1. National Statistical Office, Republic of Korea(1991) Annual report on the cause of death statistics. National Statistical Office. Seoul

2. BH Lee, JH Yang, MH Park,(1986) Central Cancer Registry of Republic of Korea(1982-1983), In: DM Parkin(editor) Cancer occurence in developing countries IARC Lyon pp 281-285.

3. Ministry of Health and Social Affairs, Republic of Korea(1991) Cancer registry programme in Republic of Korea. Ministry of Health and Social Affairs. Seoul

4. DJ Seel(1980) Observed cancer incidence in Southwest Korea. Cancer 46:852-858

5. YO Ahn (1992) Case and prevention of stomach cancer. Journal of Korean Medical Association. 35:820-825

6. JP Kim(1992) Surgical treatment and Immunochemosurgery of stomach cancer. Journal of Korean Medical Association. 35:843-850

7. YO Ahn, YS Kim, MS Lee, MH Shin(1992) Hepatitis B virus infection rate among Koreans. Seoul Journal of Medicine. 33:105-114

8. IS Kim, I Suh, HC Oh, BS Kim, Y Lee(1989) Incidence and survival of cancer in Kangwha county. Yonsei Medical Journal 30:256-268

9. International Agency for Research on Cancer (1987) Cancer incidence in five continents Vol.5,Lyon

10. KY Yoo, YO Ahn, BJ Park(1988) Changing patterns of cancer in Korea: Six-year experience of cancer admission in the beneficiaries of Korean Medical Insurance Corporation. Seoul Journal of Medicine. 29:45-53

11. Seoul National University Publishing Co. (1992) Oncology 2nd ed. Seoul

Rise and Fall in Environmental Cancer Mortality and Suggestion to Prevention Programs

KUNIO AOKI

Aichi Cancer Center, Nagoya, 464 Japan

INTRODUCTION

It is well known that secular trends in cancer mortality by site in various countries reflect chronological changes in socio–environmental backgrounds and in lifestyle habits. Age adjusted death rates of stomach cancer have been decreasing for the last four decades in most countries and marked differences in the mortality between countries seem to largely depend on the year starting decline in the death rates. The earlier the year started to decline, the lower the mortality at present. The peak rate of stomach cancer mortality was different from country to country, which seemed to closely be related to lifestyle habits in the young and changes in socio–medical conditions including economical growth, migration, war and disasters, etc.

Secular trend in cancer mortality, especially for stomach cancer in Japan, showed an interesting changing pattern for the last 80 years. Comparing secular trends in cancer mortality of the US–White and other countries, epidemiological characteristics of the trends like cyclic variation were discussed in this paper.

MATERIALS AND METHODS

Cancer mortality statistics in the world complied firstly by Segi[1-3] and succeeded by the authors[4-7] were used for this analyses. Basic data in the countries of the world were also obtained from WHO[8] data base of cancer mortality statistics since 1950 and complied by the authors. Segi–Doll's world population[1-3] was used for standardization of death rates. Vital statistics in Japan[9] was used for calculating death rates of cancer by site and prefecture in 1968 to 1990, and crude death rate of stomach cancer in 1910–1954[10] were standardized by Segi's world population. Vital statistics in the United States and England–Wales, and other statistics monographs[11-16] were referred in the analyses.

RESULTS

1. Trends in stomach cancer mortality

Figure 1 shows trends in age adjusted death rates of stomach cancer in six countries between 1950–51 to 1983–87[7]. Gradual declining trends in the rates were observed since 1950 in the US–White and England–Wales which rates were already low in 1950. Japan, Poland and Portugal showed monomodal trend curves with high peak after 1950, and then the downward curves were similar to those of other countries. These rise and fall trends in the death rates suggest that stomach cancer mortality may have cyclic change and also the US–White with lower rate at present should have a certain high peak in the past. It is suggested that the time lag of the peak year for stomach cancer

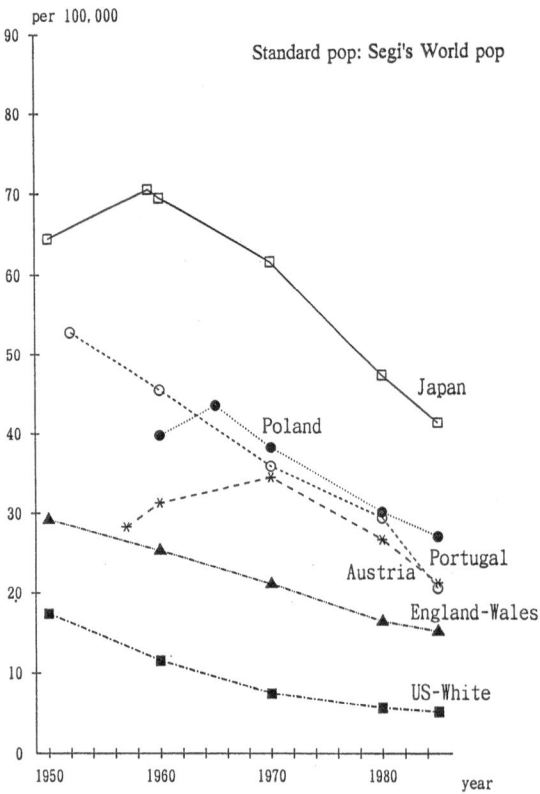

Figure 1. Trends in age adjusted death rates of stomach cancer in several countries

24

between countries might mainly be due to socio-medical conditions in the past. Comparing disease patterns in the past, the delay in reduction of deaths from tuberculosis and other infections in the younger closely be associated with higher mortality from stomach cancers in the above three countries[17], although this association might be incidental. Reduction in death rates for younger age group were closely related to socio-economical status in a community, and the increased aged population has elevated cancer incidence.

2. Trend in stomach cancer mortality in Japan since 1910

Figure 2 shows trend in stomach cancer mortality in Japan, US-White and England-Wales for the decades. Solid line was the curve related to observed age adjusted rates, and dotted curves were estimated rates calculated from crude rate of stomach cancer or exterpolated from the observed death rates.

Crude death rate of stomach cancer between 1910 and 1932[10] in Japan were estimated from the combined rate of cancers of the stomach and liver, which were not separately classified in the published data, under the assumption that proportion of stomach cancer to liver cancer in this period was the same as that of the average proportion in 1933-39, where two sites of cancer

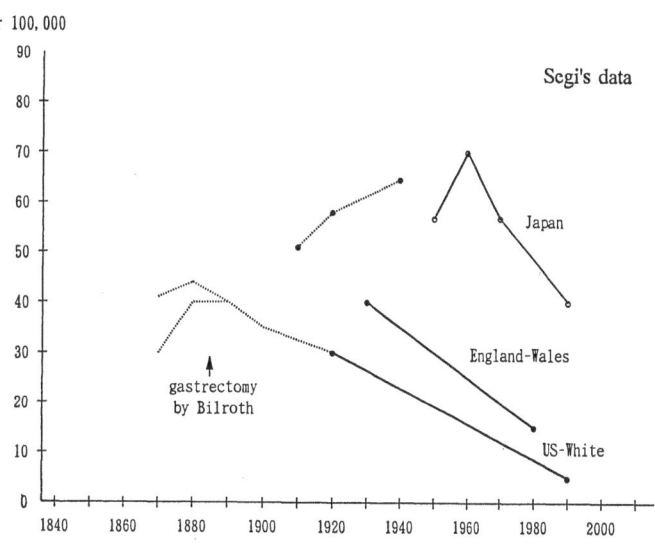

Figure 2. Observed trends in stomach cancer mortality in three countries and roughly predicted secular trends in the US-White

were separately recorded in the statistics. Cancers of the stomach and duodenum were, however, in one category of the ICD from 1933 to 1943[10]. The death rates of duodenal cancer were very low, so that the combined rates of stomach and duodenum were regarded as stomach cancer in 1933 to 1943, although the rate was slightly higher than that of stomach alone. These crude death rates of stomach cancer in 1910 to 1943 were standardized using Segi-Doll's world population.

In Japan, the death rate of stomach cancer in 1910 was estimated as 44 per 100,000, and the death rate had gradually been increased and recorded around 60 per 100,000 in 1943. Mortality statistics in 1944-1946 were destroyed by war hazards. Very high mortality from tuberculosis, diseases in digestive and respiratory organs mainly due to infections were estimated in 1944-46[9,17]. In 1947, the death rate of stomach cancer was 57 per 100,000 and increased to 70 per 100,000 until around 1960. In spite of better diagnosis and increased aged population, the rate turned to go downward after 1960, and in 1980 the rate decreased to 50 per 100,000. It takes about 50 years from 40 per 100,000 in 1910 to reach the peak rate of 70 in 1960. If the World War II did not occur, the peak year, however, might be recorded between 1945 and 1950. It is estimated about 70 years from 50 per 100,000 in 1980 to reach 10 per 100,000 in the future, when the reduction rate be 40% per 20 years. These estimation indicate that the duration of a cyclic change from the increased period to the lower level of 10 per 100,000 via the peak, may exceed 150 years.

3. Stomach cancer in Japanese American in Hawaii

Hirohata[18] reported time trends in stomach cancer mortality from 1920 to 1970 among major ethnic groups in Hawaii. Japanese American and indigenous Hawaiian showed high peak of stomach cancer around 1930 and then turned to steep declining way in males. Caucasian in Hawaii recorded more than 50 per 100,000 in 1920 and decreased to around 15 in 1970, which was higher than that of US-White in whole country. It indicates that US-White could reach to the higher rate of 50 per 100,000, if they were living like in Hawaii. Japanese migration to Hawaii started in 1868 and majority of them migrated until 1920[19], because of the restriction of migration from Japan by legislation. Hard labour and poor living conditions might increase stomach cancer mortality in earlier days for the migrants. It seemed to take more than 70 years for Japanese American in Hawaii to reach to level of 10 per 100,000 from the peak rate of around 90 in 1930.

4. Trends in stomach cancer mortality in the US–White

Reviewing age specific death rates for stomach cancer by birth cohort in the US per 100,000[8,14], the age groups more than 80 years in the birth cohort born in 1878–1883 marked around 220 per 100,000, and that of 75–79 years was 177[8], where were very low compared with those of England–Wales at that time. And the successive younger birth cohorts showed lower and lower rates for stomach cancer. It is suggested that a declining trend in stomach cancer mortality for the US–White started at least in the birth cohort born in 1860–65[14], reviewing down trends in stomach cancer mortality in female population.

Predicted stomach cancer mortality in US–White males in Figure 2 were calculated under the following assumption.
1) Peak rate of stomach cancer mortality was between 40 and 50 per 100,000 before 1920.
2) A declining trend in stomach cancer mortality be similar to that of 1920–1940, as large population traces a gradual declining slope in general.
3) Higher death rates from tuberculosis or other diseases in the young had given little effect on the trend in stomach cancer mortality before 1920.

Dotted lines were curves related to calculated trends in mortality, if the peak rate be 40 per 100,000, the year starting to decline in Whole US–White is around 1890, and if the peak rate be 45, the year starting declining be around 1880. External stimuli related to carcinogenesis seem to be very effective to the younger ages less than 20. Millions of young people had migrated to the USA between 1820 to 1920[20]. Some year marked about 8 millions migrants. These group had higher birth rate after immigration, and population growth since 1820 was very high in the US. These rapidly increased younger generation may accelerate declining trend in stomach cancer, in addition to reduction effect by economical growth and dietary changes since 1820. If a secular trend for the US–White in Figure 2 is acceptable, the duration from the peak year to that of 10 per 100,000 becomes 70 to 80 years, and the duration from rise to fall in the mortality may not exceed 150 years.

Possible factors contributing to very low rate of stomach cancer mortality in the US–White are summarized as:
1) Improved food production and increased imported foods, and good supply and hygienic supervision.
2) Changes of labour conditions from physical labours to sedentary/mental works, and increase in income under economical growth since 1800 as a result of developing modern industries.
3) Improved public health and medical care.
4) Promoted education for children in 19 century.
5) Inflow of young migrants since 1820 and growing population with relatively lower rate of aged people.

These results will be of great use for understanding current trends in cancer mortality and also for planning stomach cancer control programs.

Reduction speed in stomach cancer seems to be lower in the countries with few young migrants, in general. It may be one of the causes for occurring about 30 years gap in epidemiological phases in stomach cancer mortality between US–White and England–Wales. The rapidly increased aged population in England–Wales[21] seems to prevent a declining trend, as the aged group have had higher rate from stomach cancer. (Figure 3)
Japan have ever had little migrants and birth rate has been low for the last decades. The rapidly increased aged population may slow down a declining speed in stomach cancer mortality in Japan.

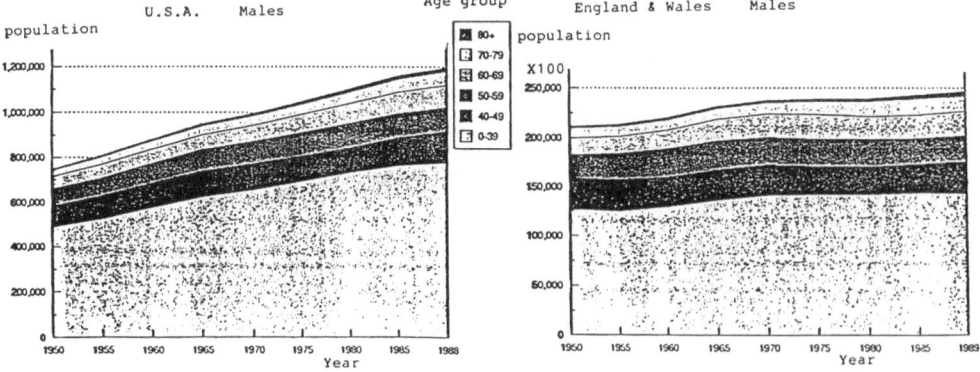

Figure 3. Trends in number of resident population by age group

5. Other Cancer

Increased mortality from colon cancer has been observed in many countries for the last decades, but US–White tends to level down recently[7,8]. England–Wales showed a similar trend to the US–White[7,8]. In spite of clear findings of genetic factors on colon cancer, majority of colon cancer seems to be occurred due to environmental factors, reviewing familial cancer studies by Ogawa et al[22,23]. Lung cancer has continuously been increasing in most countries. However, England–Wales, a country with one of the highest death rates, seems to reach the peak rate in males and tends to decline after 1985[8]. Anti–smoking movement and regaining clearer outdoor air may contribute to reduction in lung cancer in man. These epidemiological findings suggest that environmental cancers like lung and other cancers have possibility to decrease in mortality, and they might show cyclic variation like epidemic diseases, even though the duration of a cycle may be more than one century.

6. Decrease trend in cancer mortality in the aged more than 80

It is well known that age–specific cancer mortality has in general been levelling off around at the age of 80 in many countries including Japan[6,8]. We suspected it may be due to error of diagnosis or other information biases due to the old. The author observed lower metastasis rate among lung cancer patients autopsied in Japan. Recently Sato[24] revealed that the autopsied cancer cases aged more than 80 have had lower rate of remote metastases, although proportion of cancer among the aged in the autopsy series was small. and this may partly explain a fact of levelling off in mortality rate from stomach cancer in the age groups of more than 80 years. It also suggests that aged society may, at first, increase cancer deaths, but cancer mortality in matured aged society with high proportion of the aged group more than 80 will be levelling off and down.

EPILOGUE

It needs more concrete evidences to confirm the hypothesis that common cancer mortality may have a secular change –rise and fall based on mortality statistics. Similar living conditions results in similar cancer pattern, and time lag of declining trend in cancer mortality may largely be due to time lag of changing lifestyles between countries. But, it requires longer observation on incidence and mortality from cancer by site and then the conclusion should be drawn. Secular changes in cancer mortality, however, may suggest policy and way of effective cancer control programs in each country.

This study in partly supported by Ministry of Education and Ministry of Health and Welfare, Grant–in–Aids Cancer Study, 1990–1992.

REFERENCES

1. Segi M (1960) Cancer Mortality for Selected Sites in 24 Countries (1950–1957). Dept of Public Health, Tohoku Univ, School of Med, Sendai, Japan
2. Segi M, Kurihara M Cancer Mortality for Selected Sites in 24 Countries. No.2 (1958–1959), 1962, No.3 (1960–1961), 1964,   No.4 (1962–1963), 1966, No.5 (1964–1965), 1969, No.6 (1966–1967), 1972, Dept of Public Health, Tohoku Univ, School of Med, Sendai, Japan
3. Segi M, Kurihara M, Matsuyama T (1966) Mortality for Selected Causes in 30 Countries (1950–1961) – Age–adjusted death rates and age–specific death rates –. Dept of Public Health, Tohoku Univ, School of Med, Sendai, Japan
4. Segi M, Tominaga S, Aoki K, Fujimoto I (1981) Cancer Mortality and Morbidity Statistics. Japan and the World, Japan Scientific Societies Press, Tokyo
5. Kurihara M, Aoki K, Tominaga S (1984) Cancer Mortality Statistics in the World. University of Nagoya Press, Nagoya, Japan
6. Kurihara M, Aoki K, Tominaga S (1989) Cancer Mortality Statistics in the World, 1950–1985. University of Nagoya Press, Nagoya, Japan
7. Aoki K, Kurihara M, Hayakaya N, Suzuki S (1992) Death Rates for Malignant Neoplasms for Selected Sites by Sex and Five–year Age Group in 33 Countries, 1953–57 to 1983–87. UICC, Lyon/Univ Nagoya COOP Press, Nagoya
8. WHO data base obtained by courtesy of Dr. Lopez AD, Global Epidemiological Surveillance and Health Situation Assessment and Projections, WHO
9. Health and Welfare Statistics and Information Department, Ministry's Secretariat, Ministry of Health and Welfare. Vital Statistics, Japan, 1947–1990. Kosei–Tokei Kyokai, Tokyo 1942–1992, annually (in Japanese)
10. Segi M (1955) Cancer Mortality Statistics in Japan, 1900–1954. Dept of Public Health, Tohoku Univ, School

of Med, Sendai, Japan

11. Segi M (1970) Mortality by Causes of Death and Prefectures in Japan (1953–1967) – Death Rates by Age-groups and Age-adjusted Death Rates. Dept of Public Health, Tohoku Univ, School of Med, Sendai, Japan

12. US Dept H,E,W, Pub Hlth Serv. (1968) Vital Statistics Rates in the United States, 1940–1960, by Robert D Grove, Alice M Hetzel

13. Office of Population Censuses and Surveys (1978) Trends in Mortality, 1951–1975. England & Wales, Series DHI No.3, Her Majesty's Stationary Office, London

14. US Dept of Health, Education and Welfare, Public Health Service (1961) End Results and Mortality Trends in Cancer. NCI Monograph, No.6 Part 1: End Results in Cancer, eds Sidney J Cutler, Fred Ederer, Part 11: Cancer Mortality Trends in the United States, 1930–1955, eds Tavia Gordon, Margaret Crittenden, william Haenszel

15. Pickle LW, Mason TJ, Howard N, Hoover R, Fraumeni JFJr Atlas of US Cancer Mortality among Whites: 1950–1980, US Dept of Health and Human Health Service, NIH, Bethesda, DHHS Publications No(NIH), 87–2900

16. Segi M, Kurihara M, Matsuyama T (1965) Cancer Mortality in Japan (1899–1962), Dept of Public Health, Tohoku Univ, School of Med, Sendai, Japan

17. Okada H (1967) Global Epidemiology of Tuberculosis. Dept of Preventime Med, Nagoya University School of Med, Nagoya

18. Hirohata T (1980) Shifts in cancer mortality from 1920 to 1970 among various ethnic groups in Hawaii. In Genetic and Environmental Factors in Experimental and Human Cancer, eds, Gelboin et al, pp341–350, Japan Sci Soc, Press, Tokyo, 1980

19. The Publication Committee (Okahata JH, Chairman) (1971) A History of Japanese in Hawaii. United Japanese Society of Hawaii, Honolulu

20. Madden TA. Turner IR, Eckenfels EJ (1982) The Health Almanac, Raven Press, New York

21. Kuroishi T: Personal Communication

22. Ogawa H, Kato I, Tominaga S (1985) Family history of cancer among cancer patients. Jpn J Cancer Res (Gann), 76:113–118

23. Aoki K, Ogawa H (1992) Familial cancer among cancer patients registered at the Aichi Cancer Registry – heterogeneity of aggregation of familial cancer. In Familial Cancer Control, ed, Weber W, pp119–122, Springer–Verlag, Berlin

24. Sato T: Personal Communication

Present and Prospective Trends of Digestive Cancers in the World (USA)

GERALD P. MURPHY[1] and BERNARD LEVIN[2]

[1]American Cancer Society, Atlanta, GA, USA
[2]The University of Texas, MD Anderson Cancer Center, Houston, TX, USA

ABSTRACT

The American Cancer Society and the Commission on Cancer of the College of Surgeons have conducted national surveys of cancer sites since 1976. Several surveys of colorectal cancer have been conducted. For the past two years, the American Cancer Society has also produced an annual patient review. This was possible since over 85% of the 1300 participants have computerized registries. It was possible to evaluate the treatment results of the cancer and the diagnostic and treatment results and tumor stage of the various cancers. Most recent data indicate an increase in cancers of the colorectal diagnosed in the cecal and ascending colon area as contrasted to the rectosigmoid and descending colon.

KEY WORDS

Colon cancer; colon, treatment; colon, epidemiology; colon, diagnosis; colon, research

Digestive cancers, for the sake of this report from the United States, will focus on colorectal cancers because these are the major digestive cancers by site and number, although cancers of the esophagus, stomach, and pancreas continue to present significant problems both in early diagnosis and treatment[1].

Over 156,000 new cases and 58,200 deaths from colorectal cancer are projected in 1992[1]. A recent report suggests that mortality rates for cancer of the rectum decreased among white and black people of each gender, in most age categories, and all regions of the United States[2]. This may not be a feature limited to the United States but rather generally, as a similar improvement in rectal cancer in France was recently described[3].

Colorectal cancer occurs mainly in the middle and later years of life (Fig.1)

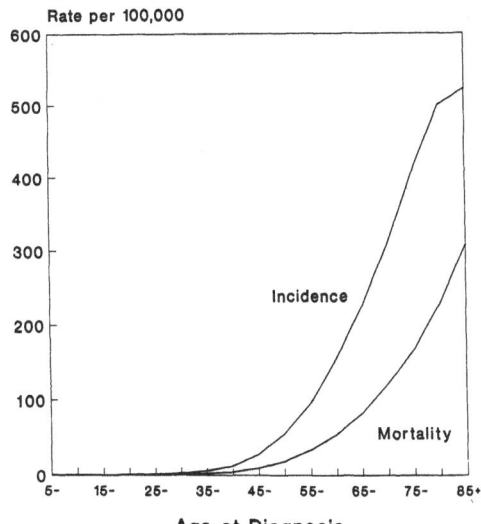

Figure 1. Age-specific incidence and mortality rates for colorectal cancer. Source: SEER Program, National Cancer Institute and NCHS Vital Statistics, 1984–88.

However, an earlier age of onset is more common in those at high risk by virtue of inherited susceptibility or in those with a long history of inflammatory bowel disease[4].

Other data suggest that a slow decline in the U.S.A. in the mortality rate has been occurring since 1985 (Fig. 2).

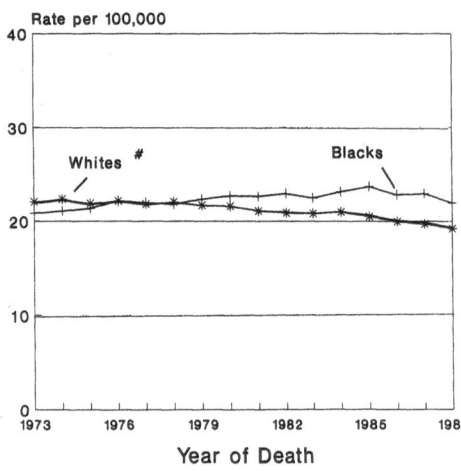

Mortality rates (age-adjusted to 1970 standard) for colorectal cancer according to race and year. Rates for total indistinguishable from rates for whites. Source: NCHS Vital Statistics, 1973–88. —: Total; —*—: whites; —+—: blacks.

There has been a shift towards earlier diagnosis as well. The relative survival rate has been reported to increase from 49% among those whose cancers were diagnosed during the mid 1970's, to 56% in those diagnosed during the early 1980's[5].

There are also significant age differences in the incidence of colorectal cancer. In a recent study, younger patients (less than 40 years) waited significantly longer to seek medical attention than did their older counterparts[6]. The report cited had a higher incidence of right-sided tumors, in contrast to a predominance of well-differentiated, less advanced, rectosigmoid lesions in older patients (more than 40 years)[6].

UNITED STATES NATIONAL CANCER DATA BASE (NCDB)

The American Cancer Society and the Commission on Cancer of the American College of Surgeons have jointly developed computer-based registries in over 1300 hospitals and annually report on patient care[7]. The 1992 report included colon cancer, as defined by all cases being 15 centimeters proximal to the anal orifice. Other previously published patient care evaluations were used to compare the results[8].As shown in Table I of this report, previous data from 1971 suggested the colon cancers exhibited a cephalad migration. The NCDB 1985 and 1988 data (Table I) show a continuing increase in cancers of the ascending colon and cecum with a corresponding decrease in the transverse colon, descending colon, and sigmoid. The majority of these cases were Grade I and II adenocarcinomas.

Table 1
Percent of Cases of Colon Cancer by Subsite

Subsite	1971 (PCE)*		1985 (NCDB)**		1988 (NCDB)**	
	N	%	N	%	N	%
Ascending/Cecum	11047	28.6	3599	37.6	8777	39.7
Transverse	6240	16.2	889	9.3	1923	8.7
Descending/ Sigmoid	20477	53.0	4309	44.9	9405	42.5
Other	857	2.2	89	0.9	288	1.3
NOS***	–	0.0	703	7.3	1737	7.8
Total	38621	100.0	9589	99.9	22130	100.0

* Patient Care Evaluation Studies
** National Cancer Data Base
*** Not otherwise specified

Among patients with distant metastases at the time of presentation, the most common site of distant spread was the liver (Table 2). Contrary to previous reports[8], the peritoneum was the next most common site of spread, and the lung was the third most common site (Table 2).

Table 2

Percent of Cases by Subsite and 1st Distant Metastasis Site, Stage IV, (pAJCC), 1988

Distant Metastasis	Ascending/ Cecum	Transverse	Descending/ Sigmoid	Other/NOS*	Total
Liver	55.1	56.9	57.5	57.8	56.5
Peritoneum	11.7	9.7	8.3	8.4	9.8
Lung	5.3	4.8	4.9	1.9	4.9
Lymph Nodes	3.5	2.2	2.2	4.5	2.8
Other, NOS*	24.4	26.4	27.1	27.4	26.0
Total	100.0	100.0	100.0	100.0	100.0
Number of cases	1001	274	1102	154	2534

* Not otherwise specified

From the NCDB, survival differences by anatomic subsite were reported (Fig. 3) with a three-year survival of 63% for descending sigmoid tumors, compared to 52% and 54% for the ascending cecum and transverse tumors respectively.

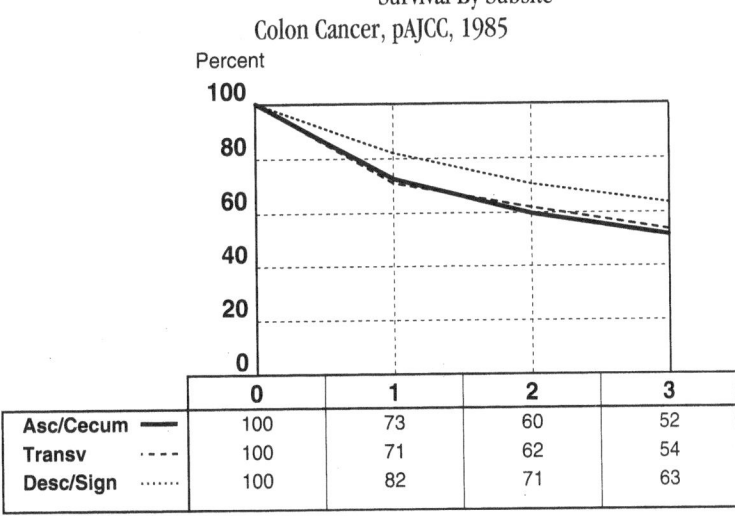

Survival By Subsite
Colon Cancer, pAJCC, 1985

	0	1	2	3
Asc/Cecum	100	73	60	52
Transv	100	71	62	54
Desc/Sign	100	82	71	63

Years

These data support the hypothesis that, within the colon, cancers are moving to the right side. Females tend to have more right than left-sided disease and males have more left-sided disease. Distal left-sided tumors may be more accessible to local management techniques such as local excision coupled with radiation therapy[7,8].

GUIDELINES FOR COLORECTAL CANCER SCREENING

A recent study combined fecal occult blood testing with rigid sigmoidoscopy. In this study, a 43% reduction in mortality was observed after 10 years of followup in the screened group who had not been examined previously[9].

Although a randomised prospectively controlled study on sigmoidoscopy has not been performed, two recent case control studies have provided evidence that rigid sigmoidoscopy reduced mortality from colorectal cancer[10,11].

A major criticism of the current fecal occult blood tests are that they lack sensitivity. The test itself may be flawed because many cancers or adenomas bleed intermittently[12]. Genetic alterations may precede or accompany neoplastic progression in the colon. These events primarily involve the mutation of oncogenes and the inactivation of suppressor genes. The detection in the stool of Ras oncogene mutations has been facilitated by the application of the polymerase chain reaction technique[13]. If this finding can be extended to large scale screening efforts, it may be more useful than occult blood testing.

Based on more recent information, the Colorectal Cancer Task Force of the American Cancer Society recently revised its guidelines for the detection of colorectal cancer in asymptomatic individuals. These guidelines also extend to issues such as the follow-up of those with pre-neoplastic lesions (adenomas). Such guidelines need to be reasonably flexible and the American Cancer Society will assuredly be willing to make modifications if new data is presented in the future which substantially alters the value of the current recommendations.

The National Board of Directors of the American Cancer Society, at its June 1992 meeting, approved the following revisions in the Society's guidelines for the early detection of colorectal cancer in asymptomatic individuals, as recommended by the Colorectal Cancer Task Force:

1. Flexible Sigmoidoscopy

That the American Cancer Society Guidelines for the early detection of cancer in asymptomatic people be revised to recommend sigmoidoscopy, preferably flexible, for males and females, age 50 and over, every three to five years, based on advice of physician. The addition of the words "preferably flexible" to the recommendation for the sigmoidoscopy places emphasis on the greater comfort with the flexible scope compared with the rigid scope and the likelihood of greater patient compliance with the recommended guidelines.

The American Cancer Society encourages the wide-scale availability of flexible sigmoidoscopy performed by primary care physicians and/or highly trained paramedical personnel at affordable costs. Recent data suggest that it may be possible to increase the recommended interval between flexible sigmoidoscopic examinations to every five years or longer. However, before making a change in its current recommendations the American Cancer Society requires additional evidence.

The feasibility of screening double-contrast barium enema or colonoscopic examinations at five- or 10-year intervals, so as to visualize the entire colon of average-risk persons over age 50 years, warrants careful study as to efficacy, availability, patient acceptance, safety, and cost. These examinations are not currently recommended for screening purposes.

2. Occult Blood Tests

That the term "fecal occult blood test" be substituted for the term "stool guaiac slide test" so that the American Cancer Society recommends a fecal occult blood test for males and females age 50 and over every year. While the guaiac-based stool blood test is currently under evaluation in large-scale screening programs and is widely used in clinical practice, newer tests such as the immunochemical method are also under study for possible use. In the future, molecular genetic technology, which provides the ability to detect aberrant genes in the stool or blood, will require prospective clinical validation.

3. High Risk Groups

Certain asymptomatic persons have higher risks for developing colorectal cancer. These include those with a family history of colorectal cancer (defined as colorectal cancer in one or more first-degree relatives); those with chronic inflammatory bowel disease (ulcerative colitis or Crohn's disease); those with familial polyposis syndromes; those with a history of prior colorectal, breast, endometrial, or ovarian cancers; and those with a history of adenomas of the large bowel. Surveillance of such persons should be determined on an individual basis after discussions between the patient and physician. Surveillance may be required at an earlier age than for average-risk persons, and additional examinations may be required.

The American Cancer Society places great emphasis on the importance of the family history in assessing risk if the age of onset of colorectal cancer in the affected relative is 55 years or below. First-degree relatives include blood-related parents, siblings, and children[14].

An examination of the entire colon and rectum is advised; colonoscopy or double-contrast barium enema should be performed every five years in men and women, beginning at age 35 to 40 years for those with one or more first-degree relatives with colorectal cancer with an age of onset of 55 years or younger[15]. The finding of a radiological abnormality on barium enema will usually necessitate colonoscopy.

Members of families with a history of familial adenomatous polyposis require earlier screening utilizing flexible sigmoidoscopy. Members of families with a history of hereditary nonpolyposis colorectal cancer require earlier and more intense surveillance utilizing colonoscopy.

Persons with inflammatory bowel disease syndromes are at exceptionally high risk for colorectal cancer and require individualized management.

4. Previous Colorectal Adenomas.

Persons with a history of colorectal adenomas may be at higher risk for cancer of the colon and rectum. Interim recommendations for postpolypectomy surveillance include the following:

- When a polyp has been identified in the colon and rectum, it should be removed for histological examination.
- Individuals with an adenomatous polyp detected by sigmoidoscopy, colonoscopy, or barium enema need to have the entire colon cleared of all polyps considering the high rate of additional (synchronous) adenomas. Individuals found to have only a single or several small tubular adenomas (less than 1 cm) at the initial flexible sigmoidoscopic examination may not need to have the entire colon examined[16]. More confirmatory evidence of this point is being sought by the the American Cancer Society Colorectal Cancer Task Force.
- Individuals need a follow-up program of surveillance to identify subsequent (metachronous) adenomas if the initial endoscopic

findings include a single or several adenoma(s) over 1 cm and/or adenoma(s) with villous changes. Most patients can have subsequent follow-up by colonoscopy at intervals of every three to five years, provided the entire colon has been satisfactorily examined and cleared. Individuals who have had a single or several small tubular adenoma(s) (less than 1 cm) removed by colonoscopic polypectomy may not require repeated follow-up surveillance examinations[17]. More confirmatory evidence on this point is being sought by the Colorectal Task Force.

Surveillance needs to be individualized for those with a malignant adenoma, numerous adenomas, or large sessile adenomas. In the aged, individual considerations such as general health and comorbid conditions will help to determine when follow-up surveillance should be discontinued.

5. Previous History of Colorectal and Other Cancers.

Persons with a personal history of colorectal cancer are at high risk for developing another colorectal cancer and require periodic evaluation of the large bowel as well as examination for evidence of metastases.

Persons with a history of breast, ovarian, or endometrial cancers are at some increased risk but their risk is probably lower than that of the high-risk groups mentioned above. These people should follow the standard American Cancer Society recommendations for the detection of colorectal cancer in average-risk asymptomatic persons.

The development of new techniques and the availability of more information concerning the cost-effectiveness of screening tests will undoubtedly require modifications of these guidelines in the future.

In summary, this is a current report on the current cancer control aspects in the United States for colorectal cancers, from the perspective of the American Cancer Society. A good deal of change and progress has been noted.

In addition, a secondary prevention trial is underway in our Virginia Division of the American Cancer Society. Patients who have had polyps removed are randomized to a high fiber diet vs a non high-fiber diet. This demonstration project has been underway for 3 years but it is too soon, at this time, to describe any results.

REFERENCES

1. Boring CC, Squires TS, Tong T (1993) Cancer Statistics, Ca 43(1):7-26.
2. Funkhouser E, Cole P. (1992) Declining rates for cancer of the rectum in the United States: 1940-1985. Cancer 70:2599-2601.
3. Laundy G, Gignoux M, Pottier D, Lefort F, Soumrany A, Maurel J, Beck A (1993) Prognosis of rectal cancer in France: Eur J Cancer Clin Oncol 29A(2):263-266.
4. Lynch HT, Smyrk T, Watson P (1991) Hereditary colorectal cancer: Semin Oncol 19:337-366.
5. Levin B. (1993) Colorectal cancer screening. Cancer (in press).
6. Marble K, Banerjee S, Greenwald L (1992) Colorectal cancer in young patients: J Surg Oncol 51:179-182.
7. Steele GD, Winchester DP, Menck HR, Murphy GP (1992) National Cancer Data Base Annual Review of Patient Care 1992. Amer.Cancer Society/Amer.Coll.Surg. Comm. on Canc. Joint Publication, 1992: chap.5, Colon Cancer. Beart, W.R., pgs.41-46.
8. Evans JT, Vana J, Aronoff BL, Baker HW, Murphy GP (1978) Management and survival of carcinoma of the colon: Results of a National Survey by Amer Coll of Surg: Ann Surg 188:716-720.
9. Winawer SJ, Schottenfeld D, Flehinger BJ (1991) Colorectal Cancer Screening. J Natl Cancer Inst 83:243-253.
10. Selby JV, Friedman GD, Queensberry CP, Weiss NS (1992) A Case-control study of screening sigmoidoscopy and mortality from colorectal cancer: N Engl J Med 326: 653-657.
11. Newcomb PA, Norfleet RG, Storer BE (1992) Screening sigmoidoscopy and colorectal cancer mortality: J Natl Cancer Inst 84(20): 1572-1575.
12. Ahlquist DA (1992) Occult blood testing. Cancer 70: 1259-1265.
13. Sidransky D, Tokino T, Hamilton SR s(1992) Identification of Ras oncogene mutations in the stool of patients with curable colorectal tumors. Science 256:102-105.
14. Cannon-Albright LA, Skolnick MH (1988) Common inheritance of susceptibility to colonic adenomatous polyps and colorectal cancers. N Engl J Med 319:533-537.
15. Bishop DT, St. John DJB (1992) Genetic susceptibility to common colorectal cancer: How common is it? Gastroenterology 102(4) Part 2:A346.
16. Atkin WS, Morson BC, Cuzick J (1992) Long-term risk of colorectal cancer after excision of rectosigmoid adenomas. N Engl J Med 326:658-662.
17. Ransohoff DF, Lang CA, Kuo HS (1991) Colonoscopic surveillance after polypectomy: Considerations of cost effectiveness. Ann Intern Med 114:177-182.

Part 2

Avoidability of Digestive Cancer

Prevention of Digestive Cancers
— The UICC Project on Evaluation of Primary Prevention

MATTI HAKAMA, VAL BERAL, and MAX PARKIN

Finnish Cancer Registry and University of Tampere, Finland; University of Oxford, UK;
International Agency of Research on Cancer, France

In the following prevention will be considered from the point of view of primary prevention. Screening, sometimes called secondary prevention, will not be covered. This paper is based on the work by the UICC project on Evaluation of Primary Prevention which has focussed on the effect of specific interventions on cancer risk. The project belongs to the UICC Epidemiology and Prevention Programme chaired by K. Aoki.

Evaluation of preventive efforts is done mainly in terms of follow-up and monitoring for changes in the exposures (risk factors) believed responsible for cancer. Much less is known about the relationship between the preventive intervention and the final outcome, cancer occurrence. Efforts to evaluate the effectiveness of primary prevention measures are limited particularly because of the lack of relevant data.

It has been well established that diet and nutrition affects the risk of digestive cancer and cancers at several other anatomical sites (1). The Japanese study by Hiraymama is classical in this respect (2). In early 1980's Doll and Peto estimated that about one third of all cancers are attributable to diet (3). Optimal in many ways to show the role of dietary factors in the etiology of cancer is through linkage of a serum sample bank and a cancer regisry. one of the largest studies was run in Finland, a bank of 40,000 serum samples established in late 1960's was linked with the Finnish Cancer Registry early 1980's. More than 700 cancers with 1400 controls were analysed for several vitamins and trace elements (4). Table 1 shows the risk of cancers among those with low levels (lowest quintile except three lowest quintiles for alpha-tocopherol for males) of retinol, beta-carotene, alpha-tocopherol and selenium. The relative risks for stomach cancer were high but also for breast and lung cancer there were associations with most of the biochemical substances studied. The risk of total cancer increased with the number of the subtances with low level. The estimates for population etiologic fractions were close to the estimate of one third by Doll and Peto (Table 2).

The UICC-Project brought together results of the relatively few studies that were performed where specific, documented preventive interventions could be evaluated with respect to their effect on cancer risk(5). Most of the studies involved preventive programmes against cardiovascular disease. The interventions mainly aimed at reduction in cigarette smoking and changes in diet, the major risk factors for cardiovascular disease, and also the most important known causes of cancers. Twelve studies were described; essentially new analyses were done for seven of them, for five studies results relating to cancer were previously published in some detail. All but two were randomized experiments. Also all but two were aimed at change in diet or nutrition as the only intervention or the dietary interventions were combined with the efforts to quit smoking. The interventions itself were health education sometimes supported by community services.

The randomized preventive trials varied in size form about 200 to 30000 subjects. The community trials were considerable larger in size. The period of follow-up varied form 6 to 14 years. Among the populatons subjected to any type of intervention, more than 2000 cancers occurred. The effects of the diet-related interventions on cancer risk were expected to affect mainly gastrointestinal cancers. Gastric cancers were the most frequent cancers of digestive organs. The total number in the six studies with detailed information enough was 162 stomach cancers in the intervention groups and 160 cancers among the controls. Table

Table 1. Smoking-adjusted relative risks of cancers at selected primary sites for low levels of biochemical substances (lowest quintile except three lowest quintiles for alpha-tocopherol among men): The cancer Registry follow-up of the Mobile Clinic Health Survey in Finland in 1968-1977 (4).

Substance	Stomach men	women	Lung men	Breast women
Retinol	0.6	1.1	1.8	1.2
Beta-carotene	1.0	1.0	1.0	0.4
Alpha-Tocopherol	2.5	2.2	1.1	1.1
Selenium	6.7	2.0	1.8	3.1

Table 2. Relative risks (RR) and population etiologic fractions (PEF) of all cancers by the number of low levels of alpha-tocopherol, beta-carotene and selenium (lowest decile except three lowest deciles for alpha-tocopherol for males). The Finnish Cancer Registry follow-up of the Mobile Clinic Health Survey in Finland (4).

number of substances with low level	Males RR	PEF	Females RR	PEF
None	1.0	0	1.0	0
One	1.5	6	1.3	6
Two	2.0	13	1.7	7
All Three	3.0	14	1.1	0

3 gives a summary of the results. A similar analysis reselted in 164 colorectal cancers in the intervention groups and 168 cancers among the controls (Table 4). There was little evidence of a reduced risk of total cancer in the intervention groups either. The risk ratios varied between 0.5 and 1.3, with these extreme estimates derived from the smallest trials. The median of relative risk estimates was one.

All the studies demonstrated a substantial to moderate change in intensity and prevalence of the risk factors (smoking and diet) in the target populatons, indicating the success of such intervention programmes in achieving behaviour change. It might therefore be expected that changes in risk of cancer would follow an intervention which was successful in these terms. However, the efficacy of the preventive trials in reducing the risk of cancer seems to be low. Several possibilities for the negative results should be taken into consideration, however, before such a conclusion is drawn.

None of the studies was designed to examine the prevention of cancer. However, it seems probable that some of the diet-related interventions (for example, a low-fat diet) are cancer-preventing and is not clear that the interventions would by and large have been very different if cancer had been a predesigned endpoint.

Table 3. Summary of cases of stomach cancer among intervention and control groups in the preventive trials (5).

Country, study	sex	Inter-vention	Control	Relative risk
Finland				
North Karelia	M	72	66b	1.1
	F	53	50b	1.1
Italy				
collaborative WHO	M	8	11	0.7
Poland				
collaborative WHO	M	25	22	1.0
Spain				
collaborative WHO	M	2	7	0.3
UK				
collaborative WHO	M	31	25	1.1
USA				
MRFITa	M	24	29	0.8

a Including digestive cancers other than colorectum
b Expected number

Table 4. Summary of cases of colorectal cancer among intervention and control groups in the preventive trials(5).

Country, Study	sex	Inter-vention	Control	Relative risk
Finland				
North Karelia	M	57	55b	1.0
	F	63	66b	1.0
Italy				
collaborative WHOa	M	9	10	0.8
Poland				
collaborative WHOa	M	10	10	1.0
Spain				
collaborative WHOa	M	2	4	0.5
UK				
collaborative WHOa	M	13	10	1.0
USA				
MRFIT	M	10	13	0.8

a Including also pancreatic cancer
b Expected number

Because the main focus of the studies was on the prevention of cardiovascular disease, the accuracy of the follow-up and of recording the incident cases of cancer or cancer deaths was not necessarily of the same quality as that for cardiovascular events. Even if less accurate, the comparability of the cancer death certificates was probably valid between the intervention and control groups.

Cancer is a group of diseases which usually have a long latent period between first exposure and diagnosis. Where the risk factor in question acts late in the carcinogenic process, reduction in exposure might be expected to have a relatively rapid effect. Migrant studies suggest that colorectal cancer risk changes relatively rapidly after change in the environment. However, because evaluation was based on all cases of deaths within the follow-up period, the results were greatly dominated by cases with short latent periods during the first years of follow-up. Furthermore, if a study was based on mortality, there was the further delay between diagnosis and death.

It should also be noted that health education in some of those studies was of relatively short duration and of low intensity. Compliance with life-style changes is inevitably far from perfect and deteriorates with time-this will be more marked with low-intensity interventions. Furthermore, most efforts were undertaken in countries where health consciousness tends to spread rapidly; it is likely that , over a longer period of time, the control populations would be exposed to similar information to that offered in the intervention group, and sometimes also to similar services. Dilution of the information in the control group does not imply that such information is ineffective or unnecessary.

In many countries primary prevention is multifactorial and based not only on health education. Tobacco-related legislation, price policy and food additives are examples on interventions in terms of regulative actions. The effect of one relatively limited intervention is likely to be indistinguishable when combined with other preventive measures. Because the broad basis of the preventive activities, it is feasible to consider the trends and differentials of cancer risk at population level as indicators of the success of cancer control. Sir Richard Doll recently made such a proposal and focussed on young adults in his analysis (6). He emphasized that cancers among young adults have been produced in the near past by environmental factors (such as personal behaviour) whereas cancers occurring later in life are likely caused by a combination of agents that existed many years before and of more recent exposures. Furthermore, prediction of future assumes examination of recent changes in the relatively young. Doll found that for many primary sites of cancer the mortality trends were the more favourable the younger was the age. Mortality reflects the infuence of both the success in clinical activities and the success of prevention.

It is well known that for several primary sites of cancer the long term incidence rates have been increasing at old ages and decreasing at young ages also in many of the Nordic Countries (7) i.e. the finding of Doll on mortality can be fund on incidence of several cancers. Whereas the mortality trends are an indicator of the success of the total cancer control, both prevention, diagnosis, treatment and after care, the incidence trends relate more directly to the changes in etiology i.e. in the environmental (such as behavioural) exposures.

Finland has long term and accurate cancer registration and we report here the very recent trends of both incidence and mortality for cancers of digestive organs. We elected to use three most recent 5 year time periods: 1977-81, 1982-86 and 1987-91; it was assumed that focussing on the recent trends in incidence also recent trends in causes could be established.

The trend in incidence of and mortality from total digestive cancer were decreasing in all age groups form 30 to 69 years. The changes were small but according to the expectation: They

Figure 1   Cancer of the digestive organs in Finland in 1977–1991. Males

(Finnish Cancer Registry, 1993)

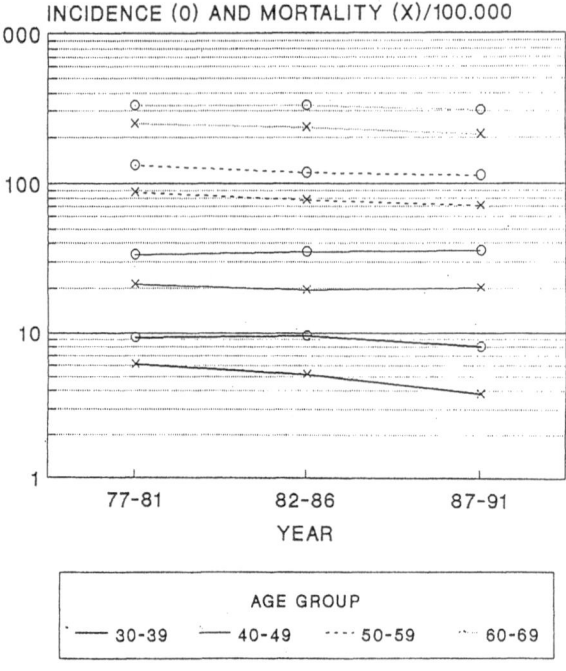

Figure 2   Cancer of the digestive organs in Finland in 1977–1991, Females

(Finnish Cancer Registry, 1993)

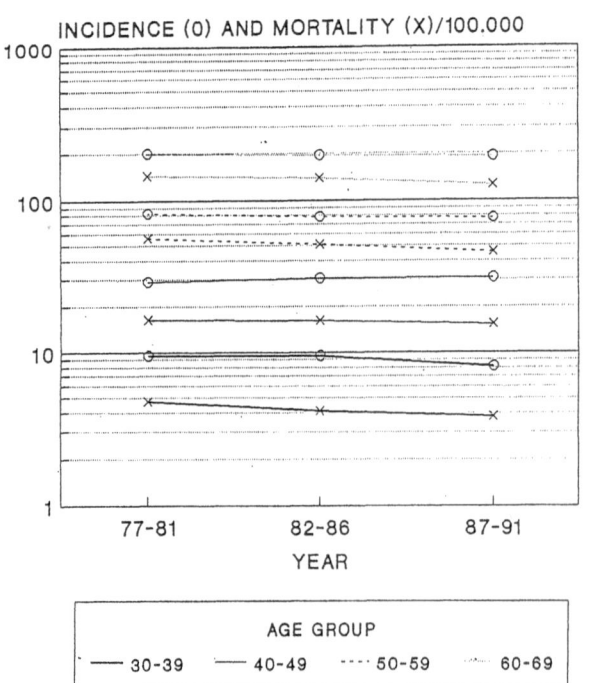

Figure 3   Cancer of the colon in Finland in 1977–1991. Males

(Finnish Cancer Registry, 1993)

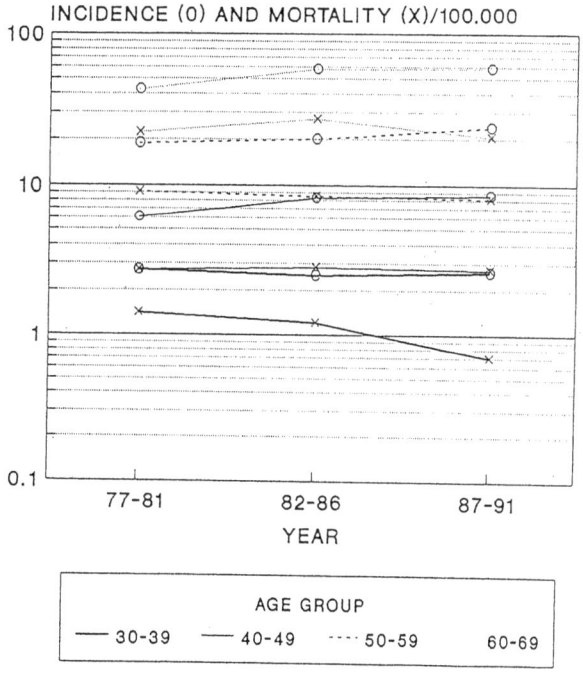

Figure 4   Cancer of the stomach in Finland in 1977–1991. Males

(Finnish Cancer Registry, 1993)

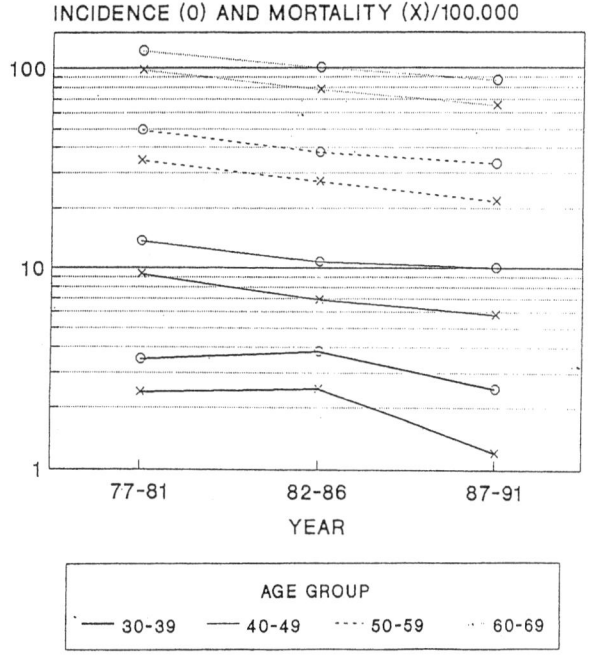

Figure 5   Cancer of the rectum in Finland in 1977–1991. Females

(Finnish Cancer Registry, 1993)

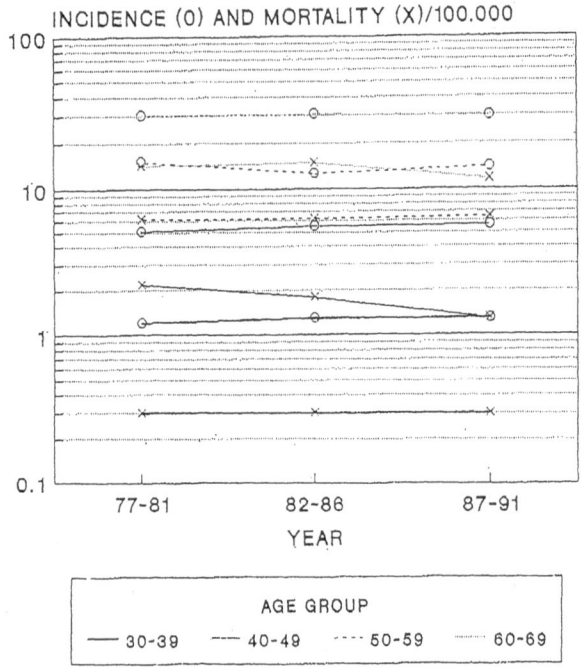

were more substantial among the young and more substantial during the last period. The changes in incidence were smaller than for mortality. (Figures 1 and 2)

 For individual primary sites two examples consistent with the hypothesis of a progress in cancer control are given (stomach cancer rand colon cancer in males) and one example, rectal cancer in females, is given that do not show any consistent trend. (Figures 3, 4 and 5) Especially for the male stomach cancer there was a downward trend for ages 30 to 39 which got more steep during the more recent period and which was consistent for incidence and for mortality but bigger for mortality than for incidence. Such trends support the hypothesis that the cancer control became more effective by time and there were relatively recent progress in control of the causes of stomach cancer as well as progress in clinical care or diagnosis.

 Gastrointestinal cancers are strongly dependent on diet nd nutrition. There is some evidence on basis of the time trends in risk in western countries, including Finland, that progress has occurred in the control of these cancers. The changes were small, however, and smaller than the changes for many of the other primary sites than digestive organs. It is not clear, furthermore, whether the progress was due to health services and to specific preventive actions. Globally, most people eat to survive. Some people eat for pleasure, they enjoy the meal socially and culinarilly. In western countries many eat to keep slim, to look beautiful according to the social standards. It may be that relatively few eat to prevent cancer and it may be a pure coincidence, that the dietary changes as a result of food fashions are also preventive for cancer. In such circumstances it is important design well controlled studies and it is likely that three areas in research on prevention of digestive cancers deserve special emphasis: long term effects of regulative actions, effect of combination of different interventions based both on health education and regulative actions, and chemopreventive trials.

References

1 Mettlin C, Aoki K (eds) (1990) Recent proress in Research on Nutrition and Cancer. Progress in Clinical and Biological Research Volume 346. Wiley–Liss, Inc., New York

2 Hirayama T (1990) Life–style and mortality: a large–scale census–based cohort study in Japan. Contributions to epidemiology and biostatistics, vol.6. Karger AG, Basel

3 Doll R, Peto R (1981) The causes of cancer. Oxford University Press, Oxford, New York

4 Hakama M, Aaran RK, Alfthan G, Aromaa A, Hakulinen T, Knekt P, Maatela J, Nikkari T, Peto R, Teppo L (1990) Linkage of serum sample bank and cancer registry in depidemiological studies. In: Mettlin C, Aoki K (eds) Recent Progress in Research on Nutrition and Cancer, Wiley–Liss, Inc., New York, pp. 169–178

5 Hakama M, Beral V, Cullen JW, Parkin DM (eds) (1990) Evaluationg Effeciveness of Primary Preventin of cancer. IARC Scientific Publications No 103, Lyon

6 Doll R (1990) Are We Winning the Fight Against Cancer? An Epidemiological Assessment, EACR–Muchlbock Memorial Lecture, Eur J Cancer 26: 500–508

7 Hakulinen T, Andersen AA, Malker B, Pukkala E, Schou G, Tulinius H (1986) Trends in Cancer Incidence in the Nordic Countries. A Collaborative Study of the Five Nordic Cancer Registries. Acta Pathologica Microbiologica et Immunologica Scandinavica, Supplement No 288, Helsinki

The Role of Nutrition in the Cause and Prevention of Digestive Cancers

CURTIS METTLIN

Department of Cancer Control and Epidemiology, Roswell Park Cancer Institute, Buffalo, NY 14263, USA

ABSTRACT

The nutritional factors associated with digestive cancers are numerous and vary widely by geographic region and cancer type. The factors related to risk include micronutrients such as beta-carotene, vitamin C, riboflavin, calcium, and zinc. Macronutrients such as dietary fat and fiber have been studied mainly in association with colorectal cancers but because different aspects of the human diet are complexly interrelated, the role of these factors in other digestive cancers can not be excluded. Non-nutritive exposures in the diet such as alcohol or carcinogens and mutagens resulting from poor food preservation also show association to digestive cancer risk, particularly cancers of the upper gastrointestinal tract. The evidence linking diet to cancer risk is strong and world-wide trends in stomach cancer suggest to many that large scale prevention by dietary change may be feasible.

Chemoprevention, diet, fat, fiber, prevention, vitamins.

INTRODUCTION

Cancers of the digestive tract account for a large proportion of cancer mortality world-wide and it is likely that dietary factors are involved in etiologies of the most of these cancers. The laboratory, epidemiologic and clinical study of diet and digestive cancers are major fields of inquiry which have been very productive in recent years. In this chapter some of the most prominent associations between nutrition and cancer at different digestive sites and the prospects for effective cancer prevention are reviewed.

ORAL CANCER

Oral cancers share the etiology of lung cancer in that tobacco use enhances risk significantly. Oral cancers, however, involve potentially a wider range of etiologic factors. They are much more common in persons with histories of alcohol abuse and poor nutrition. In India, oral cancer is the most common type of cancer and its high frequency there is related to the practice of betel nut chewing. Nutritional deficiencies, however, also have been related to increased risk. Low levels of fruit and vegetable intake have repeatedly been linked to greater risk of head and neck cancers and these findings have been taken to suggest that vitamin A and/or vitamin C play a protective role [1,2].

The Syrian golden hamster has served as an animal model to human oral carcinogenesis [3]. Its cheek pouch is sensitive to a number of carcinogens and cancers develop at this site in a way analogous to human tumors. This model also serves as a model for chemoprevention in that tumors can be prevented or inhibited by administration of a different agents including beta carotene, vitamin E or, the synthetic vitamin A 13-*cis*-retinoic acid.

Another relevant laboratory tool is the study of micronuclei in exfoliated cells [4]. These microscopic anomalies are believed to reflect chromosomal aberrations occurring in proliferating tissue and elevated micronuclei frequency has been found in smokeless tobacco users, betel nut chewers and other similar high risk populations. Stich and colleagues [5,6] have demonstrated that micronuclei frequency can be reduced by administration of chemopreventive agents such as beta-carotene and retinyl palmitate.

46

ESOPHAGEAL CANCER

Esophageal carcinogenesis has been linked to excesses and deficits of dietary exposure that may act through several different mechanisms. As with other upper digestive cancers, vitamins A and C have been studied in association with cancer of the esophagus. Several of the regions with high rates happen to be undeveloped and have primitive and often unsanitary food storage facilities. Mutagens or carcinogens from molds, from pickling or, from smoked preservation of foods are suspect. Finally, because of the relatively direct exposure of the esophagus to undigested dietary components, the role of direct physical trauma in the form of thermal or mechanical irritation has been hypothesized and investigated.

Esophageal cancer patients report less frequent historical intake of fruits and vegetables that usually are sources of vitamin A in the diet [7,8]. A study in the Washington D.C. area examined plasma vitamin A levels of esophageal cancer patients relative to those of a control group [9]. The cancer patients were observed to have significantly lower levels of plasma vitamin A compared to either group. A major problem is assessing the effects of vitamins A or C is that they do not occur in isolation in the diet. The foods that are sources of vitamin C often are also sources of vitamin A as well as other nutrients. Many of the epidemiologic findings linking vitamin A to esophageal cancer risk could equally relate vitamin C to the observed risks.

Deficiencies in riboflavin and zinc intake have been linked epidemiologically to increased risk along with low vitamin A. To study the possibility of preventing esophageal cancer in a high risk region Munoz and colleagues [10] conducted a double blind randomized trial of riboflavin, retinol and zinc supplementation on the prevalence of precancerous lesions of the esophagus. After over a year of intervention in 305 subjects in Henan Province, PRC, the overall prevalence of esophagitis in the population was unaffected. The feasibility of chemoprevention of esophageal cancer is, to date, unproven.

GASTRIC CANCER

The international variations in risk for stomach cancer and the trends during migration suggest a major role for some aspect of culture in determining risk for this disease. Stomach cancer generally is more common in poor populations. It has been assumed that poor persons consume a simple diet high in content of "starchy" foods, e.g., potatoes and rice, and low in protein. There is some support for this hypothesis from retrospective studies [11,12]. It also has been noted that gastric cancer rates have been decreasing parallel to decreasing reliance on such staples as bread and potatoes .

The possible role of salt intake in stomach cancer etiology has been examined. The biologic rationale for salt as a source of risk is that salt solutions can damage the gastric mucosa leading to atrophic gastritis. This, in turn, results in altered gastric pH permitting the production of carcinogenic nitrosamides. Salt intake has been shown to be correlated with stomach cancer risk across regions and across time [13].

Before the advent of modern refrigeration, the preservation of meat by smoking was common. Smoking and singeing meats may impart polycyclic aromatic hydrocarbons to food. Smoked fish consumption is high in Japan and in Iceland, both regions of high stomach cancer incidence. Smoked foods in Iceland have been demonstrated to contain significant levels of benzopyrene, a known carcinogen [14]. Smoked meats also have demonstrated the capability of inducing cancers in laboratory animals. A study in Canada revealed a twofold increase in stomach cancer risk associated with more frequent reported consumption of smoked meats and a similar level of risk elevation for consumption of smoked fish [15]. In a prospective study in Japan, consumption of broiled fish was found associated with a 70 percent increased relative risk for gastric cancer [16].

The inverse association of vitamin A intake with gastrointestinal cancer risk has not been as great as has been observed for other epithelial sites, and the significance of the role of vitamin A in the etiology of stomach cancer must be regarded as doubtful. The relatively weak associations that have been demonstrated must also be considered in light of the fact that vitamin A occurs predominantly in foods that may confer protection due to other nutritional properties. Low vitamin A intake may reflect other nutritional deficiencies that may be of greater significance.

One model of stomach carcinogenesis is that involving the *in vivo* formation of nitrosamides from nitrate and nitrite ingestion [17]. Preformed N-nitroso compounds may occur in the diet but, nitrosamides are believed to be formed mainly in the stomach, promoted by a low pH environment, from the presence of nitrite and amines. Internationally, there is a substantial correlation between per capita nitrate intake and risk of gastric cancer [18]. This process is subject to inhibition by ascorbate (vitamin C) and other nutrients [19]. Fresh fruit and vegetable consumption repeatedly has been linked to gastric cancer risk reduction. In the Roswell Park and other series, stomach cancer patients reported less frequent consumption of raw vegetables than did controls [20,21]

In addition to differentiating case and control patients in analytic studies, the vitamin C risk reduction hypothesis is consistent with the secular trend for stomach cancer. Modernization of the food distribution and storage system and the household use of mechanical refrigeration have changed fruit and vegetable availability from a highly seasonal phenomenon to one of routine availability. Refrigerator ownership has been observed in case-control comparisons to be a protective factor for gastric cancer although this association may be confounded by the role of socioeconomic status [15]. The long-term decline of stomach cancer in the United States is correlated with a similar long-term increase in per capita fruit and vegetable consumption. Similar changes in the postwar diet of Japan may account for the more recent downturn in stomach cancer mortality there.

Given the large number of investigations of diet and stomach cancer, it is inevitable that many different food items will show some association with risk in one region or another. Many of these findings may be relatively isolated and of unclear etiologic significance. For example, consumption of chocolate was found in a retrospective study to be reported more often by stomach cancer patients than controls [15]. Hirayama [22], in a large cohort study, found that more frequent consumption of a popular soybean paste soup (miso) was associated with reduced stomach cancer risk.

LARGE BOWEL CANCER

Epidemiologic data reveal that where diets include little fiber, the incidence of colorectal cancer is higher. Migration from a low risk region to high risk region has the effect of increasing risk. Other types of observational research have supported the associations of high dietary fat and low fiber to increased risk to varying degrees. Willett has observed significant correlation between red meat consumption and colon cancer rates internationally and in large prospective study, both red meat and animal fat intake were significantly associated with risk [23]. Others have found the international correlation data .mainly to support the hypothesis that cereal intake is protective [24]. Trock and colleagues carried out a meta-analysis of a large number of studies of diet and colon cancer and reported that a fiber rich diet was associated with an average 43% reduction in risk [25].

Prevention of nonmalignant large bowel polyps may be used as an indicator of the potential usefulness of intervention, since polyps often ultimately progress to cancer. Polyps removed from the large bowel frequently reappear within three years, and these high risk patients may be good candidates in which to study dietary as well as chemopreventive interventions. DeCosse and his colleagues [26] conducted a randomized, placebo controlled trial of wheat fiber, vitamin E and vitamin C supplementation and recurrence of polyps in a group of familial polyposis patients. They found evidence of significant reduction of polyp formation.

The American Cancer Society is conducting a trial using wheat bran to determine whether the effects observed DeCosse in familial polyposis patients can be replicated in the general population of patients experiencing adenomatous polyps. The National Cancer Institute is conducting a study the effects of a diet high in fruit and vegetable fiber on polyp recurrence [27]. This study, the Polyp Prevention Trial, is a multi-institutional intervention trial which is testing the ability of a low-fat high-fiber vegetable and fruit enriched eating plan to reduce the recurrence rate of adenomatous polyps.

Other possible large bowel chemopreventive agents include calcium, beta-carotene, vitamin C and vitamin E. Although supported by some epidemiologic observations there are few other data are to indicate the preventive effectiveness of any of these substances. Supplements of vitamin C and vitamin E were studied in a randomized trial of prevention of colorectal polyp recurrence but significant protective effects were not observed [28].

CONCLUSION

Dietary factors are among the most important factors in the etiology of digestive cancers. Many uncertainties about the associations remain but, there are numerous findings that suggest causal associations. The relationships between diet and digestive cancers, however, vary markedly across geographic regions and sites of cancer and few generalizations about the totality of the relationship are valid. On the other hand, there are data for several digestive cancers that fruit and vegetable consumption has beneficial effect. These effects may occur as a result of the properties of the food such as their fiber or micronutrient content. Alternatively, plant food intake may have benefit by displacing food types that may enhance risk such as animal fat sources.

The future opportunities for prevention are two-fold. First it is possible that changes in diet can lead directly to reduced risk. The world-wide decline of stomach cancer would seem to indicate that changes in dietary may lead to large reductions in risk. It also is possible that study of the association of diet and digestive cancers will lead to identification of effective chemopreventives. Large controlled trials are being conducted to determine the effectiveness of this approach.

REFERENCES

1. Marshall J, Graham S, Mettlin C, Shedd D, Swanson M (1981) Nutr Cancer 3:145-149

2. Notani PN, Sanghvi LD (1976) Indian J Cancer 13:156-160

3. Gimenez-Conti IB, Slaga TJ (1992) Adv Exp Med Biol 320:63-67

4. Rosin MP (1992) Adv Exp Med Biol 320:95-104

5. Stich HF, Stich W, Rosin MP, Vallejera MO (1984) Int J Cancer 34:745-750

6. Stich HF, Rosin MP, Hornby AP, Mathew B, Sankaranarayanan R, Nair MK (1988) Int J Cancer 42:195-199

7. Mettlin C, Graham S Priore R, Marshall J, Swanson M (1981) Nutr Cancer 2:143-147

8. Ziegler RG, Morris LE, Blot WJ, Pottern LM, Hoover R, Fraumeni JF (1981) J Natl Cancer Inst 67:1199-1206

9. Mellow MH, Layne EA, Lipman TO, Kauslik M, Hostetler C, Smith JC (1983) Cancer 51:1615-1620

10. Munoz N, Wahrendorf J, Bang LJ, Crespi M, Thurnham DI, Day N, E, Ji ZH, Grassi A, Yan LW, Lin LG, Quan LY, Yun ZC, Fang ZS, Yao LJ, Correa P, O'Connor GT, Bosch X (1985) Lancet, 2 (Pt. 1):111-114

11. Graham S, Schotz WW, Martino P (1972) Cancer 30:927-938

12. Modan B, Lubin F, Barell V, Greenberg RA, Modan M, Graham S (1974) Cancer 34:2087-2092

13. Joosens JV, Geboers (1981) Nutr Cancer 2:250-257

14. Thorsteinsson T (1969) Cancer 23:455-457

15. Risch HA, Jain M, Choi NW, Fodor JG, Pfeiffer CJ, Howe GR, Harrison LW, Craib KJP, Miller AB (1985) Am J Epidemiol 122:947-959

16. Ikeda M, Yoshimoto K, Yoshimura T, Kono S, Kato Hiroo, Kuratsune M (1983) Gann 74:640-648

17. Mirvish S (1983) J Natl Cancer Inst 71:629-634

18. Armijo R, Gonzalez A, Orellana M, Coulson AH, Sayre JW, Detels R (1981) Int J Epidemiol 10:57-62

19. Graham S, Lilienfeld AM, Tidings J (1967) Cancer 20:2224-2234

20. Bjelke E (1974) Scand J Gastroenterol 9:1-235

21. Weisburger JH, Marquardt H, Mower HF, Hirota N, Mori H, Williams G (1980) Prev Med 9:352-361

22. Hirayama T (1982) Nutr Cancer 3:223-233

23. Willet W (1989) Nature 338:389-394

24. McKeown-Eyssen GE, Bright-See E (1984) Nutr Cancer 6:160-170

25. Trock B, Lanza E, Greenwald P (1990) J Natl Cancer Inst 82:650-661

26. DeCosse JJ, Miller HH, Lesser ML (1989) J Natl Cancer Inst 81:1290-1297

27. Greenwald P (1992) Cancer 70:1206-1215

28. McKeown-Eyssen G, Holloway C, Jazmaji V, Bright-See E, Dion P, Bruce WR (1988) Cancer Res 48: 4701-4705

Epidemiology of Stomach Cancer in Japan with Special Reference to the Relationship Between Atrophic Gastritis and Stomach Cancer

S. Tominaga[1], I. Kato[2], Y. Ito[3], S. Kobayashi[3], and A. Matsuura[3]

[1]Aichi Cancer Center Research Institute, Nagoya, 464 Japan; [2]Director's Office, International Agency for Research on Cancer, 150, Lyon Cedex 08, France; [3]Department of Gastroenterology, Aichi Cancer Center Hospital, Nagoya, 464 Japan

ABSTRACT

A clinico-epidemiological study on the etiology and natural history of atrophic gastritis and stomach cancer was conducted in Nagoya, Japan. The study subjects were 5,399 patients who received gastroscopic examination and questionnaire survey between April,1985 and March,1989 at the Aichi Cancer Center Hospital. From a cross-sectional study involving 427 patients with stomach cancer, 1,414 patients with moderate to severe atrophic gastritis and 3,014 patients with normal stomach mucosa or mild atrophic gastritis, several risk factors of stomach cancer were identified, but no special risk factors were identified for moderate/severe atrophic gastritis. Patients with atrophic gastritis had an increased risk of stomach cancer, especially of intestinal type.

KEY WORDS: stomach cancer, atrophic gastritis, epidemiology, etiology, natural history

INTRODUCTION

Stomach cancer is one of the most common cancers worldwide[1] and in Japan it is still the leading cancer despite a declining trend[2]. Previous pathological and epidemiological evidence has suggested intestinal type of stomach cancer is predominant in high risk areas and closely associated with atrophic gastritis and intestinal metaplasia[3-5]. Correa et al.[6-7]proposed a hypothesis linking stomach cancer to chronic atrophic gastritis and intestinal metaplasia and to the conversion of nitrate to N-nitroso compounds. In their hypothesis, the development of atrophic gastritis is the first important stage caused by environmental agents that injure the gastric mucosa. According to their hypothesis, it is considered that identification of risk factors for atrophic gastritis may lead to a more effective primary prevention of stomach cancer in high risk populations. Furthermore, identification of specific and common risk factors for both atrophic gastritis and stomach cancer may provide useful information to interrupt each part of the sequence to stomach cancer. In order to identify risk factors of atrophic gastritis and stomach cancer and to study the natural history of atrophic gastritis and stomach cancer, we have conducted a clinico-epidemiological study on atrophic gastritis and stomach cancer risk among subjects who received gastroscopic examination. This report summarizes the major results of this study reported elsewhere[8-10].

MATERIALS AND METHODS

Details of this study were described elsewhere[8-10]. From April, 1985 to March, 1989, a questionnaire survey was conducted for the patients who received gastroscopic examination at Aichi Cancer Center Hospital. A total of 7,019 questionnaires were distributed and 6,226 were collected (88.7%). After excluding prevalent cases of cancer and the subjects with resected stomach, a total of 5,859 subjects comprised the original cohort of this study. The gastroscopic findings were evaluated by the six gastroenterologists of the Aichi Cancer Center Hospital with respect to presence of atrophic gastritis, degree and extension of atrophy, and presence of gastric ulcer, polyps and other lesions. The degree of atrophy was classified into three groups; mild, moderate and severe, according to the size of transparent blood vessels and discoloration of the gastric mucosa.
The questionnaire was self-recorded and included items on medical history, family history, diet, smoking and drinking habits. Frequency of intake of the 10 food items including salty food (pickled vegetable, salted or dried fish, salted fish gut or cod roe, food boiled down in soy and pickled Japanese apricot) and other foods (soy bean paste soup, raw vegetable, green-yellow vegetable, fruit and meat) was divided into the three categories; 'almost daily',' 2-3 times per week' and 'once or twice per month or less'. Frequency of alcohol and cigarette consumption was divided into the four categories; 'almost daily', 'occasionally', 'formerly' and 'never'. Consumption of rice and cigarettes was reported as amounts consumed per day. Family history of cancer was restricted to parents and siblings.

After the baseline survey, incidence of cancer and deaths among the study subjects have been identified through linkage to gastroscopic records at the Aichi Cancer Center Hospital, the data from the Aichi Cancer Registry and death certificates. Additional mail surveys have been conducted to identify cancer incidence and death among all subjects including those living outside of Aichi Prefecture. Nine cases of stomach cancer that developed within 3 months of the initial survey and 1,472 subjects who had never responded to mail surveys and never received gastroscopic examination after the initial examination but whose death and cancer incidence had not been identified were excluded from the analyses. As a result, 3,914 subjects were used in the analyses of follow-up data. Walker–Duncan logistic regression model[11] was used in the cross–sectional case–control analysis and Cox's proportional hazards regression model[12] was used to estimate the relative risks(RR) and their 95% confidence intervals(CI) associated with various baseline characteristics, adjusted for age and residence. A test for trend in the log of the relative hazard was also performed by Cox models.

RESULTS

Risk Factors of Atrophic Gastritis and Stomach Cancer Risk: Cross–sectional Case–control Analysis.

Various baseline characteristics of 427 patients with newly diagnosed stomach cancer and 1,414 patients with moderate to severe atrophic gastritis were compared to those of 3,014 control patients with normal gastric mucosa or mild atrophic gastritis. No special risk factors of atrophic gastritis were identified, however, several risk factors of stomach cancer were identified. The factors which were significantly associated with stomach cancer risk in males were: a frequent intake of salted fish guts or cod roe(RR=1.52, CI=1.08–2.15), smoking 20 or more cigarettes per day(RR=2.84, CI=1.79–4.51), Western–style breakfast(RR=0.68, CI=0.48–0.96). Several environmental factors, such as daily intakes of green–yellow vegetables(RR=0.53, CI=0.28–0.99), fruit(RR=0.28, CI=0.09–0.84) and meat(RR=0.28, CI=0.08–0.93), and a family history of stomach cancer(RR=2.33, CI=1.17–4.67) were only associated with intestinal types of stomach cancer in females, whereas a clear difference between diffuse and intestinal types was not observed in males.

Atrophic Gastritis and Stomach Cancer Risk: a Case–control Analysis.

The relationship between atrophic gastritis and stomach cancer risk was investigated in case–control analyses involving 387 cases with newly diagnosed stomach cancer and 5,422 control subjects. The prevalence of atrophic gastritis increased with age and was higher in males than in females(Table 1). The prevalence of any type of atrophic gastritis was 82.9%(86.8% in males and 79.1% in females) and the prevalence of moderate to severe atrophic gastritis was 33.0%(38.1% in males and 28.1% in females).

Table 1. Sex- and age-specific prevalence (%) of atrophic gastritis in total study subjects

Age	Male All types	Male Moderate /severe	Female All types	Female Moderate /severe	Total All types	Total Moderate /severe
-29	59.7	9.0	54.7	5.7	57.5	7.5
30-39	81.8	21.9	68.2	17.8	74.1	19.6
40-49	83.6	36.1	75.9	22.2	79.6	28.9
50-59	89.4	41.8	84.2	32.6	86.6	36.8
60-69	92.8	46.9	87.7	38.9	90.3	43.1
70+	95.8	51.0	86.5	42.9	92.3	47.9
Total	86.8	38.1	79.1	28.1	82.9	33.0

Data source: Kato I et al.[9]

Table 2 shows the sex- and age-adjusted relative RRs associated with various types of atrophic gastritis in the total subjects. There was a five-fold increased risk of stomach cancer among subjects with any type of atrophic gastritis(RR=5.13, CI=2.79-9.42). The risk further increased with advancing degree of atrophy and increasing extension on the greater and lesser curvatures. The presence of granularity and erosion did not much affect the risk associated with atrophic gastritis. Females had slightly higher RRs than males. The RR associated with any type of atrophic gastritis was 6.34(CI=2.33-17.23) among females and 4.44(CI=2.07-9.53) among males. The increasing trend in risk with degree of atrophy was also clearer among females than among males. The increasing risks associated with various types of atrophic gastritis were also observed among both younger(=<59) and older(=>60) age groups and they were a little higher in the younger age group.

Table 3 shows RRs associated with any type of atrophic gastritis according to the histologic type of stomach cancer. The risk of intestinal type of stomach cancer was specifically increased in relation to the presence of atrophic gastritis. The RR associated with any type of atrophic gastritis was 24.71(CI=3.46–176.68) and that associated with severe atrophic gastritis was 42.74(CI=5.75–317.99). There was a moderately, but statistically significantly, increased risk of diffuse type of stomach cancer in relation to the presence of atrophic gastritis. The RR associated with any type of atrophic gastritis was 3.49(CI=1.77–6.87) and that associated with severe atrophic gastritis was 4.62(CI=2.05–10.40).

Table 2. Sex- and age-adjusted relative risks (RR) and 95% confidence intervals (CI) of gastric cancer according to the presence of various types of atrophic gastritis

Type of atrophic gastritis	No. of cases /controls	RR	95% CI
Presence/absence			
No	11/ 985	1.00	
Any type	376/4437	5.13	2.79- 9.42
Degree of atrophy[a]			
Mild	170/2671	4.22	2.27- 7.84
Moderate	134/1372	5.34	2.85-10.01
Severe	56/ 330	7.73	3.95-15.12
Extension on the greater curvature[a]			
Lower third	33/ 737	3.18	1.58- 6.36
Middle third	152/2047	4.69	2.51- 8.74
Upper third	167/1450	6.08	3.26-11.36
Extension on the lesser curvature[a]			
Lower third	155/2636	3.95	2.13- 7.35
Middle third	124/1223	5.50	2.93-10.32
Upper third	36/ 189	8.90	4.39-18.04

[a] Reference category is subjects with no atrophic gastritis

Data source: Kato I et al.[9]

Table 3. Sex- and age-adjusted relative risks (RR) and 95% confidence intervals (CI) of gastric cancer by histological type according to the presence of various types of atrophic gastritis

Type of atrophic gastritis	Intestinal type		Diffuse type	
	RR	95% CI	RR	95% CI
Presence/absence				
No	1.00		1.00	
Any type	24.71	3.46-176.68	3.49	1.77- 6.87
Degree of atrophy[a]				
Mild	20.64	2.84-149.93	2.78	1.39- 5.57
Moderate	25.78	3.53-188.11	3.68	1.81- 7.52
Severe	42.74	5.75-317.99	4.62	2.05-10.40
Extension on the greater curvature[a]				
Lower third	15.40	2.01-117.80	2.24	0.99- 5.04
Middle third	23.19	3.19-168.83	3.12	1.55- 6.30
Upper third	31.40	4.31-228.63	3.79	1.86- 7.71
Extension on the lesser curvature[a]				
Lower third	18.73	2.58-135.94	2.71	1.35- 5.43
Middle third	27.34	3.75-199.38	3.67	1.79- 7.55
Upper third	47.28	6.23-358.84	5.26	2.18-12.67

[a] Reference category is subjects with no atrophic gastritis.

Data source: Kato I et al.[9]

Multivariate analyses in the total subjects revealed that the extension on both curvatures and the degree of atrophy had independent effects on the stomach cancer risk.

Atrophic Gastritis and Stomach Cancer Risk: Results of a Prospective Study.

The relation of atrophic gastritis, other gastric lesions and lifestyle factors to stomach cancer risk was prospectively studied among 3,914 subjects. During the follow-up period representing 17,289 person-years at risk, a total of 45 incident cases of stomach cancer (35 males and 10 females) were identified.
The incidence markedly increased with advancing age, especially after age 65 in both sexes combined(Table 4).

Table 4. Age- and sex-specific incidence rates of stomach cancer per 100,000 person-years

	Male	Female	Total
Age	Rate (No)	Rate (No)	Rate (No)
-44	49.6 (1)	77.5 (2)	65.3 (3)
45-49	261.9 (3)	238.6 (3)	249.7 (6)
50-54	380.6 (5)	67.3 (1)	214.4 (6)
55-59	671.6 (8)	0.0 (0)	286.9 (8)
60-64	666.9 (7)	0.0 (0)	312.3 (7)
65-69	733.4 (5)	326.9 (2)	541.2 (7)
70-74	1013.1 (5)	0.0 (0)	619.3 (5)
75+	381.3 (1)	2023.6 (2)	830.8 (3)
Total	429.3 (35)	109.5 (10)	260.3 (45)

Data source: Kato I et al.[10]

Table 5 shows the sex- and age-adjusted relative RRs of stomach cancer associated with various types of atrophic gastritis in the total subjects. If the baseline endoscopic findings indicated the presence of atrophic gastritis, the risk of developing stomach cancer increased 5.73 fold, compared with no indication at the baseline. The risk further increased with advancing the degree of atrophy and increasing the extension of atrophy on lesser curvature. These trends in the relative risks were statistically significant (P=0.027 and P=0.041, respectively). The increasing trend in the relative risks associated with extension on the greater curvature was neither clear nor statistically significant. The risk of developing stomach cancer was statistically significantly increased among subjects with gastric polyps (RR=2.43, CI: 1.12-5.27), but not among those with gastric ulcer.
There was an increased risk of stomach cancer among current smokers who smoked 20 or more cigarettes per day, daily alcohol drinkers, subjects who consumed three or more cups of rice per day, daily pickles consumers, subjects who ate salted fish gut or cod roe at least twice a week and subjects with a family history of stomach cancer. But, none of these relative risks and their trends was statistically significant. Conversely, there was a decreased risk of stomach cancer associated with frequent intake of fruit and raw and green-yellow vegetables, although these relative risks and their trends were not statistically significant.

DISCUSSION

Atrophic gastritis has long been suspected to be a precursor lesion of stomach cancer. A close geographical correlation between prevalence of atrophic gastritis or intestinal metaplasia and stomach cancer has been reported in addition to the histological observation that carcinoma developed frequently in areas of intestinal metaplasia. Although many epidemiological studies on stomach cancer have been conducted in various countries and suggested associations with some dietary habits, little is known about the etiology of atrophic gastritis. If the sequence from atrophic gastritis to stomach cancer is common, some of the risk factors identified in the previous studies of stomach cancer may also be related to the risk of atrophic gastritis. In the present study, however, no specific environmental risk factors were identified. There are several possible interpretations of these results[8]. The present clinico-epidemiological study has demonstrated a close statistical relationship between gastroscopically diagnosed atrophic gastritis and stomach cancer risk, especially of intestinal type. The follow-up on the study subjects is still continuing and updated results of this study will be reported in the future.

ACKNOWLEDGEMENTS

This study was supported by Grant-in-Aid for a Comprehensive 10-year Strategy for Cancer Control, Japan, from the Ministry of Health and Welfare.

Table 5. Sex-, age- and residence-adjusted relative risks (RR) and 95% confidence intervals (CI) of stomach cancer by baseline endoscopic findings

Gastroscopic findings	No. of cases /person-years	Rate[a]	RR	95% CI
Atrophic Gastritis				
Absence	1/ 2931.0	34.1	1.00	
Presence	44/14321.2	307.2	5.73	0.78-41.90
Degree of atrophy				
No	1/ 2931.0	34.1	1.00	
Mild	19/ 8566.0	221.8	4.50	0.60-33.78
Moderate/severe	23/ 5558.7	413.8	6.69	0.89-50.11
			P=0.027[b]	
Extension on the greater curvature				
No	1/ 2931.0	34.1	1.00	
Lower third	6/ 2310.0	259.7	5.47	0.66-45.62
Upper two thirds	33/11303.3	291.9	5.28	0.72-38.96
			P=0.130	
Extension on the lesser curvature				
No	1/ 2931.0	34.1	1.00	
Lower third	21/ 8413.6	249.6	5.09	0.68-37.96
Upper two thirds	19/ 4496.3	422.6	6.87	0.90-51.94
			P=0.041	
Gastric ulcer				
Absence	41/16046.5	255.5	1.00	
Presence	4/ 1242.6	321.9	0.97	0.35- 2.72
Gastric polyp				
Absence	37/15957.9	231.9	1.00	
Presence	8/ 1331.2	601.0	2.43	1.12- 5.27

[a] per 100,000 person-years
[b] P-value for trend   Data source: Kato I et al.[10]

REFERENCES

1. Muir C, Waterhouse J, Mack T, Powell J and Whelan S(1987) Cancer incidence in five continents V, IARC Scientific Publication No.88. IARC, Lyon
2. Kurihara M, Aoki K and Hisamichi,S(1989) Cancer mortality statistics in the World 1950–1985. The University of Nagoya Press, Nagoya
3. Munoz N, Correa P, Cuello C and Duque E(1968) Int J Cancer 3:809–818
4. Correa P, Cuello C and Duque E(1970) J Natl Cancer Inst 44:297–306
5. Correa P, Sasano N, Stemmermann GN and Haenszel W(1973) J Natl Cancer Inst 51:1499–1459
6. Correa P, Haenszel W, Cuello C, Tannenbaum S and Archer M(1975) Lancet ii:58–60
7. Correa P, Haenszel W and Tannenbaum S(1982) Natl Cancer Inst Monogr 62:129–134
8. Kato I, Tominaga S, Ito Y, Kobayashi S, Yoshii Y, Matsuura A, Kameya A and Kano T(1990) Cancer Res 50:6559–6564
9. Kato I, Tominaga S, Ito Y, Kobayashi S, Yoshii Y, Matsuura A, Kameya A and Kano T(1992) Jpn J Cancer Res 83:1041–1046
10. Kato I, Tominaga S, Ito Y, Kobayashi S, Yoshii Y, Matsuura A, Kameya A,Kano T and Ikari A(1992) Jpn J Cancer Res 83:1137–1142
11. Walker SH and Duncan DB(1967) Biometrika 54:167–179
12. Cox DR(1972) J R Stat Sect B 34:187–220

Pathogen Oriented Prevention
of Hepatocellular Carcinoma in Japan

Kusuya Nishioka[1], Shigeru Kobayashi[2], and Noburu Sakakibara[2]

[1]The Japanese Red Cross Central Blood Center, Tokyo, Japan
[2]First Department of Surgery, Juntendo University School of Medicine, Tokyo, Japan

ABSTRACT

Annual mortality of HCC in Japan was $21.1/10^5$ in 1990. Less than 25% of them were due to persistent HBV infection and 77% to HCV infection including 10% double infection. Main route of persistent HBV infection was perinatal and that of HCV was blood transfusion. Immunization with HBIG and HB vaccine of newborn babies made 98% protection and HCV blood screening 99% protection. Improvement of general hygienic and nutritional states significantly prevented both virus infections. Together with interferon therapy and early stage diagnosis, more than 92% of HCC in Japan can be prevented.

KEY WORDS: Persistent hepatitis B virus infection, persistent hepatitis C virus infection, hepatocellular carcinoma.

INTRODUCTION

Hepatocellular carcinoma (HCC) has long been recognized as one of the most prevalent and most lethal cancers in Asia, Africa, the Pacific, southern Europe and Latin Ameria. The epidemiological and clinical studies based on serology and molecular biology in a defined population provided important answers to etiology of this type of cancer. Not only persistent hepatitis B virus (HBV) infection but also chronic hepatitis C virus (HCV) infection play important etiological roles in a great majority of HCC in the HCC prevalent area of the world. For prevention of HCC, prevention of persistent HBV and HCV infection is the most rational approach and strategies in Japan will be reviewed.

PERSISTENT HBV AND HCV INFECTION IN HEPATOCELLULAR CARCINOMA

When sensitive tests for the detection of the surface antigen (HBsAg) of hepatitis B virus (HBV) were developed [1], a series of studies in Africa and Asia consistently showed a much higher frequency of persistent HBV infection in patients with HCC than in appropriate controls [2]. Encouraged by these findings, studies in Africa, Asia, Europe and America were proceeded to test the hypothesis that HBV infection was required for the development of HCC and the hypothesis was supported by seroepidemiological surveys, clinical follow up study, immunohistochemical analysis and molecular biological studies [3]. It is now substantially established that persistent HBV infection is required for the development of a large percentage of HCC cases through disease progression from asymptomatic carrier, chronic hepatitis and liver cirrhosis [4].
It is well known that HCC occurs commonly in regions where chronic HBV carriers are prevalent and much less frequently in areas where they are not. However, in our early collaborative studies on 439 cases of HCC patients' sera from Ghana, Kenya, Burma, India, Thailand, Indonesia, Philippines, Hong Kong, China, Japan and Papua New Guinea, 212 (48.3%) were HBsAg positive and the other half (51.7%) were negative. Since then, these HCC cases whose sera were HBsAg negative, became important problems to be solved.
In Japan, 37.3 to 40.7% of the HCC cases have been shown to be positive for HBsAg between 1968 and 1977, even when employing sensitive detection system. On the other hand, the vital statistics of Japan indicate that the numbers of fatal cases of liver cancer reported to the Ministry of Health and Welfare have been dramatically increasing from 1978 to 1987, as compared with those from 1968 to 1977. The number of deaths with liver cancer per year per 10^5 populations were 9.5 in 1968 to 1977 and increased yearly since then. However, the ratio of HBsAg - positive individuals among HCC patients examined by the liver cancer study group of Japan, have decreased from 1968 to 1987, 40.7% (1968-77), 34.1 (1978-79), 31.4% (1980-81), 27.5% (1982-83), 24.6% (1984-85), down to 22.4% (1986-87). Based on these figures, it is estimated that the mortality rate in association with liver cancer, and exhibiting HBsAg positivity is 3.9 (1968 to 77), 4.0 (1948 to 79), 4.0, (1980 to 81), 4.0

56

(1982 to 83), 4.0 (1984 to 85) and 4.0 (1986 to 87) per year per 10^5 populations, respectively [5].

In striking contrast, the mortality rate with respect to HBsAg negative liver cancer per year per 105 populations has increased significantly by 2.5 times from 5.6 (1968 to 77), to 7.7 (1978 to 79), 8.8 (1980 to 81), 10.5 (1982 to 83) 12.1 (1984-85) and up to 14.0 (1986 to 87)[5]. Therefore, elucidation of the causative agent(s) of HBsAg negative HCC cases, which are 78% of the HCC cases reported in recent years becomes prime importance.

Recently a candidate agent of PT-NANBH has been reported and carries a single-stranded RNA viral genome of at least 10,000 nucleotides. This agent, termed the hepatitis C virus (HCV), encodes an antigen that is associated specifically with PT-NANBH infections both in man and experimentally infected chimpanzees. Using a viral antigen synthesized in recombinant yeast, a capture assay for circulating antibodies was developed [6].

Accordingly, the antibody to HCV antigen (HCVAb) assays have been performed on some 180 serum samples from clinically and pathologically confirmed cases of HCC in Japan to investigate further the role of HCV in HCC [5].

Of the 180 cases, 105 samples were found to be HBsAg negative and of these, 80 cases (76.2%) were HCVAb positive. Of the remaining 75 cases who were HBsAg positive, 11 cases were HCVAb positive (14.7%). Twenty-five cases (13.9%) of HCC were negative for both HBsAg and HCVAb. The observed prevalence of HCVAb present in patients with HCC is extremely high in comparison with that found in random blood donors (1.18%).

In a 6-month follow-up study of acute hepatitis in Japan, 31 out of 41 (75.6%) cases of PT-NANBH and 14 out of 40 (35.0%) cases of sporadic non-A non-B hepatitis were found to be positive for anti-HCV. After 12 months of follow-up, 30 cases (81.1%) became chronic among 37 HCVAb positive acute NANB hepatitis cases. This figure shows a significantly higher rate of chronicity as compared with HCVAb negative acute non-A non-B hepatitis [7]. The prevalences of HCVAb in HBsAg negative cases of chronic hepatitis and liver cirrhosis were 76.3% (200/262) and 66.7% (106/159), respectively, which were significantly different from the values of 5.1% (13/255) and 10.6% (13/123) observed in HBsAg positive cases [7].

HCVAb positive rates in patients with HCC in Japan using second generation test [8], Spain [9], Italy [10] and Mongol [11] are extremely high (77.4%, 75.0%, 65.2% and 62.1% respectively) and HBsAg positive rates in these countries are 25.0%, 9.4%, 31.1%, and 48.2%. Both HBsAg and HCV positive cases were observed in 10.0%, 5.2%, 16.6% and 24.1%.

In China [11], Indonesia [11], Taiwan [11], Korea [11] and South Africa [12], the positive rates of HBsAg in HCC patients are as high as 64.6%, 35.5 - 58.6%, 83.5%, 57.3% and 48.8%. It should be noticed that in patients in these areas, HCVAb positive rates are around 30 - 40% and both HCVAb and HBsAg positive rates were observed in 26.0%, 12.9% - 17.1%, 22.3%, 9.3% and 12.3%. Thus, the magnitude of HCV infection in these districts where HBV infection was known to predominate in HCC patients is unexpectedly high as compared with lower rate in U.S.A [13]. Also double infection of HCV and HBV showed much higher risk of disease progression from asymptomatic HCV carrier to cirrhosis and HCC as observed in Japan, China, Mongolia and Taiwan.

TIME AND ROUTES OF PRIMARY EXPOSURE TO CAUSE PERSISTENT HBV INFECTION

To move towards a prevention against a persistent HBV infection, it is essential to acquire an understanding of the times of primary exposure and the routes by which the virus is transmitted. A persistent HBV infection occurs following the primary exposure of an immunologically immature host to the HBsAg. With respect to transmission of the virus, both vertical transmission, i.e. HBV carrier mother to child, and horizontal transmission, i.e. from HBV carriers to infants, have been considered.

In 1972, Ohbayashi et al [14] described the clustering of the HBsAg in three families through the maternal line. In their study, HBsAg was present in sera from 20 out of 24 children (83%) of female siblings, whereas only 1 out of 7 children of male siblings was HBsAb positive. In these families, some members developed hepatic disease and the spectrum ranged from chronic hepatitis to liver cirrhosis and to HCC. The subtype of HBsAg within a family was always the same. These results suggested that the familial distribution of HBV infection and the cases of chronic hepatitis, liver cirrhosis, and HCC, could be explained by transmission of HBV from mother to child.

Following this, 7 cases of maternal perinatal transmission of HBV infection to newborn infants were reported [15, 16]. One of the maternal factors that determines whether infection will occur, or not, is the presence of the HBeAg, in the mother's blood which is a marker of high infectivity. In some cases, HBsAg has appeared within 2 weeks after birth, which is too short an incubation period for the HBV infection to have been perinatal. In these cases and in cases where a moderate amount of HBsAg is detectable in cord serum, viral transmission is recognized as being antenatal, suggesting an intrauterine infection with HBV. Such cases are less than 5% of the total cases of vertical transmission and so most of the cases result from perinatal infection.

Family members or community members who are carriers for HBV, may infect infants after birth (postnatal transmission). This may also be true for infection of infants of 4 years of younger. This is more common in an HBV endemic area, where the levels of social and personal hygiene are poorly maintained.

PREVENTION OF PERSISTENT HBV INFECTION

As for the causes of persistent HBV infection, in the nineteen seventies in Japan, two thirds of all HBV carrier infants resulted from a horizontal HBV transmission of the virus. The remaining one third was as a consequence of maternal transmission (vertical transmission). Later in the nineteen eighties, there was a switch over and more than 90% were due to maternal transmission. The horizontal mode for virus transmission had decreased significantly most probably due to an improvement in general hygiene. A nation-wide policy to adhere to a single use of sterile needles in the health care environment, especially for mass vaccination of infants, in an HBV endemic area (such as Japan), contributed most effectively towards this general trend in improvement. In 1972, HBsAg positive rate in general population in Japan was 2.7% [2]. In 1991, it was reduced to 0.92% especially in age group 6-15 was 0.40%.

Many factors, such as improvements in sanitation and the decreasing number of members in each household, may have contributed to such dramatic reduction in HBV carrier state. However, one of the most important factors is an increased immunological competence in Japanese young generation due to improvement of nutritional state. It is worth drawing attention to the fact that from 1946 to 1970 the intake of protein, which is the most important factor in immunological competence, had increased from 40 g/capita/day to 80 g rapidly.

Epidemiological surveys carried out over the past two decades have shown that the greatest source of persistent HBV infection is perinatal infection from HBeAg positive mothers to their neonates. Other mechanisms for transmission of HBV are now greatly reduced. The most effective procedure to prevent perinatal infection of the selected high risk group babies has been adopted. At present, this is a combined passive and active immunization of neonates, born to HBeAg positive mothers, at the earliest possible stage, this being at the latest 24 hours after birth.

First success of combined passive and active immunization, to prevent perinatal transmission of the HBV carrier state, was reported by Tada et al [17]. A one year follow-up study of 146 infants born to HBeAg positive mothers, and treated as above showed that only 3 infants (2.1%) became HBV carriers. In an incident where 200 babies born to HBeAg positive mothers remained untreated, 170 (80%) were found to become carriers for HBV.

Based on these facts, the Ministry of Health and Welfare in Japan initiated a nation-wide prevention programme in June 1985. The programme was set into action in January 1986 and the protocol stipulates that all the pregnant women are to be tested for HBsAg and all babies born to HBeAg positive carrier mothers, are to be treated with HBIG and HB vaccine. According to this programme, the infants born to HBeAg positive carrier mothers were injected with 1 ml (200 IU) of HBIG intra-muscularly at birth. At the age of 2 months, a second injection of HBIG was given, and at the same time, or at least before 3 months of age, the first dose of HB vaccine was injected subcutaneously. The second and the third doses of HB vaccine were given at 4 and 12 weeks after the first injection of HB vaccine, respectively. The costs for the prevention programme are covered by the government.

To date, almost all pregnant women in Japan were tested for HBsAg. 23.4% of HBsAg positive mothers are found to be HBeAg positive and neonates born to HBeAg positive mothers will receive immunoprophylaxis as described above. The protective efficacy rate of persistent HBV infection by this program is given as 98%. In 1991, HBsAg positive rate among infants younger than 6 years, those born after initiation of nation wide prevention program, was 0.04%. This was 98.5% reduction as compared with that in two decades before.

Now the problems to be solved are how to minimize the number of cases that become carriers, in spite of the preventive measures currently undertaken. It may need to determine the optimum time for the booster vaccination. It is also important to develop a new vaccine to prevent perinatal infection of S gene mutants of HBV which transmit from mother to child immunized with HBIG and conventional vaccine [18].

For infants born to HBeAg negative carrier mothers, it has been advised that some preventive measures should be taken. This is because, in rare cases, the babies born to HBeAg negative HBV carrier mothers have developed infantile fulminant hepatitis due to prescore mutant HBV [19].

ROUTES OF HCV INFECTION

Following the report that HCC had developed in individuals 23.8±10.8 years after PT-NANBH [20] and that in 40% (43 out of 108) of cases with liver cirrhosis and HCC without HBs antigenemia [21] there was a prior history of blood transfusion, attention has been drawn to the fact that a relationship may exist between PT-NANBH and HCC and history of blood transfusion was examined.

Whereas 36 (39.6%) of the 91 HCC patients were positive for HCVAb and had a prior history of blood transfusion, only three (4.7%) of 64 HCC patients, who were negative for anti-HCV and positive for HBsAg, were found to have been transfused previously. This represents a significant statistical difference (P<0.001). The time interval between the diagnosis of HCC and the blood transfusion, in the patients who were positive was 26.9±10.0 years [5]. Moreover, in chronic liver diseases positive for HBsAg and negative for HCVAb, only 3.7% (13/352) had a history of blood transfusion, whereas, in HCVAb positive chronic liver diseases cases with or without HBsAg, 45.8% (152/322) (48.8% in chronic hepatitis and in 40.3% in liver cirrhosis) had a history of blood transfusion before development of the chronic liver disease [7].

Kiyosawa et al [22] analyzed 231 patients with chronic Non-A Non-B hepatitis cases (96 with chronic hepatitis, 81 with cirrhosis and 54 with HCC). A history of blood transfusion was documented in 52%, 33% and 42% of HCVAb positive cases of chronic hepatitis, cirrhosis and HCC. The mean intervals between the date of transfusion and date of diagnosis of HCVAb positive chronic hepatitis, cirrhosis and HCC were 10, 21.2 and 29 years respectively. In 21 patients with transfusion associated HCC, HCVAb was present in each serial sample available for testing. A history of blood transfusion was observed in 61 out of 280 (21.8%) HCVAb positive blood donors surveyed (Iino S, et al. personal communication). These data demonstrate the slow, sequential progression from acute posttransfusion hepatitis C through chronic hepatitis and cirrhosis to HCC and this chronological sequence supports a causal association of HCV and HCC.

It is obvious that transfusion of blood or blood products are major route of HCV infection. However, for prevention of HCV infection especially cases with sporadic non-A non-B hepatitis, routes of transmission other than blood transfusion should be clarified and studies are now going by collaborative the Non-A Non-B Hepatitis research group of the Ministry of Health and the Welfare Japan [23]. Striking differences were observed with regard to the age distribution among the first time donors in 10 blood centers. Among 1,224 presumably healthy 5-15 year old school children tested, none were HCVAb positive [24]. On the other hand, 63.6% (7/11) of PTNANBH infants were anti-HCV positive. Therefore, it is more likely that the presumably healthy school children have not had any exposure to HCV infection, rather than that they cannot develop an antibody response to HCV because of some immaturity of their immune system. Thus, vertical transmission, known as the most predominant mode of HBV transmission to induce an HBV carrier state, does not play major role in HCV transmission. Horizontal transmission of HCV must predominate.

The anti-HCV positive rate in family members of patients with NANB hepatitis was examined by Drs. Suzuki and Furuta. For HCVAb negative patients, only one family member among 40 cases was HCVAb positive. Among HCVAb positive patients, 4 spouses of 48 (8.3%) patients were HCVAb positive: only one case each of a child of 58 patient fathers and 33 patients mothers was positive, indicating little vertical transmission. On the other hand, 7 siblings out of 40 HCVAb positive patients (17.5%) were HCVAb positive also, strongly suggesting the possibility of horizontal transmission along with the positive percent (8.3%) of data on spouses of HCVAb positive patients.

Therefore, family clustering data in siblings and spouses plus the age distribution pattern noted of anti-HCV positivity suggest that horizontal transmission of HCV among persons under similar environmental conditions is the predominant mode of transmission.

HCVAb positive rates in various groups tested in Japan are as follows. Male homosexuals: 2.0% (8/409 Mizogami): Female prostitutes: 7.9% (23/290, Minamidani); Tattooed patients with liver diseases: 70.6% (12/17, Iwamura); Drug addicts: 42.9% (18/42, Isomura): Long term hemodialysis patients: 21.7% (88/406, Furuta and Yoshizawa): Hemophilia patients treated with domestic anti hemophiliacs: 71.4% (5/7) and those treated with imported anti hemophiliacs: 74.4% (64/86, Yamada). After introducing a liquid heating of antihemophiliacs, new infections have not been observed. These data all suggest transmission of HCV is mainly due to blood borne infection and partially to sexual contact.

PREVENTION OF HCV INFECTION

Since blood transfusion has been documented as a major transmission route of HCV, elimination of donated HCVAb positive blood from blood transfusions becomes most important not only for prevention of PTNANBH but also for prevention of its chronic sequela, chronic hepatitis, cirrhosis and HCC.

Despite screening donated blood for HBsAg and serum ALT levels higher than 35 Karmen units, over the 11-year period from 1976 to 1987, 621 (18.1%) of 3,437 transfused patients studied developed posttransfusion PTNANBH. In order to reduce the PTNANBH common throughout Japan at that time, the screening of donated blood for HCVAb started in November 1989 in all Japanese Red Cross Blood Centers nationwide.

Since November 1989, the Japanese Red Cross blood Centers all over Japan began screening donors for antibody to C100-3 recombinant protein of HCV using HCVAb ELISA (Ortho Diagnostics, Japan). At the same time, the Blood Center also began screening for high titer ($\geq 2^6$) antibody to HBcAg with negative HBsAb.

Prospective follow-up studies have been carried out by the Japanese Red Cross non-A non-B Hepatitis Research Group, after screening of HCVAb and high titer HBcAb with negative HBsAb.

Incidence of PTNANBH in the patients who received 1 to 10 unit blood transfusions was 4.9% (58/1, 189) before the 1989 screening program began, but only 1.9% (15/784) after screening. The incidence of those who received 11 to 20 blood transfusions was 16.3% (64/392) before screening but only 3.3% (4/124) after screening [25].

This reduction of PTNANBH demonstrates the usefulness of the screening programme that we began in November 1989. The programme is also important for the prevention of hepatocellular carcinoma, liver cirrhosis, and chronic hepatitis, which are closely linked to PTNANBH, and particularly linked to posttransfusion HCV infection in HCV endemic areas such as Japan.

As previously noted, even after the introduction of this HCV screening programme using C100-3 antigen of HCV, the incidence of PTNANBH in Japan is still 1.9% to 3.3%. In hopes of providing more complete protection from posttransfusion hepatitis C, we are now investigating more sensitive screening methods using other HCV related antigens.

In our analysis of such tests, we compared the results of serological tests on 16,500 blood donors in 11 blood centers using HCV core antigen-related reagents (GOR and N14), the second generation ELISA kits (Ortho 2, and Abbott 2) and agglutination tests using the 2nd generation antigens (PA and PHA) with the results of HCV RNA detection using the PCR technique [26] standardized across 3 separate laboratories.

The effectiveness of each serological screening test to predict reduction of PTHC can be shown as the serologically positive ratio in HCV PCR positive donors. The first generation C100-3 test was positive in 62% of HCV RNA positive sera, which corroborates our previously reported data that 61% of PTNANBH was prevented by C100-3Ab screening in patients who received 1-10 unit transfusions [25]. The HCV core-related reagents (GOR and N14) were positive in 75 to 86% of these sera, indicating superior effectiveness compared to C100-3. The 2nd generation ELISA and agglutination tests pick up 99% of PCR positives.

Based on these results, since February 1992, we began using routine PHA tests to screen donated blood for HCV viremia and clinical follow up study is now under way.

Route of HCV infection other than blood transfusion still remained to be solved. However, as mentioned above, HCV infection rate decreased naturally and nearly unrecognizable in generation younger than 16 years old. Improvement of nutritional state and general hygienic condition, especially a nation wide policy to adhere to a single use of sterile needles in the health care environment may have contributed significantly as in the case of HBV injection.

DISCUSSION

The strategies for pathogen oriented prevention of HCC are now summarized into four steps :
(1) Primordial Prevention (0次予防): To avoid exposure of the viruses to general population by improvement of hygienic environmental condition and proper medical care system including blood screening for transfusion.
(2) Primary Prevention (1次予防): To enhance immunological competence against primary exposure to the viruses by both non-specific measures such as improvement of nutrition or immunodulators and specific measures such as HBIG and HBV vaccine.
(3) Preclinical Prevention (1.5次予防): To intervene disease progression from persistent viral infection to chronic sequelae such as liver cirrhosis and HCC by antivirals.
(4) Secondary Prevention (2次予防): Early stage diagnosis by ultrasonography, computed tomography or tumor markers such as AFP or PIVKA II followed by non invasive or surgical treatment.

All these strategies are now translated into action and we can predict more than 92% of HCC in Japan can be prevented in several decades.

REFERENCES

1. Nishioka K, Hirayama T, sekine T, Okochi K, Mayumi M, Sung JL, Hui LC, Lin TN (1973) Gann Monograph Cancer Res. 14:167-175
2. Nishioka K, Levin A, Simons MJ (1975) Bull W.H.O 52:293-300
3. Blumberg BS, London WT (1981) N Engl J Med. 304:782-784
4. Nishioka K (1985) Advances in Viral Oncology 5:173-199
5. Nishioka K, Watanabe J, Furuta S, Tanaka E, Iino S, Suzuki H, Tsuji T, Yaho M, Kuo G, Choo QL, Houghton M, Oda T. Cancer 67:429-433
6. Kuo G, Choo QL, Alter HJ, Gitnick GL, Redeker AG, Purcell RH, Miyamura T, Dienstag JL,

Alter MJ, Stevens CE, Tegtmeier GE, Bonino F, Colombo M, Lee WS, Kuo C, Berger K, Shuster JR. Overby LR, Bradley DW, Houghton M (1989) Science 244:362-364

7. Nishioka K, Watanabe J, Furuta S, Tanaka E, Suzuki H, Iino S, Tsuji T, Yano M, Kuo G, Choo QL, Houghton M (1991) Liver 11:65-70

8. Suzuki H, Akahane Y, Matsushima T, Iino S, Hino K, Furuta S, Kuroki T, Yano M, Watanagbe J, Nishioka K (1991) Igaku to Yakugaku 26:303-312

9. Bruix J, Barrera JM, Calvet X, Ercilla G, Costa J, Sanchez-Japais JM, Ventura M, Vall M, Bruguera M, Bru C, Custiro R, Rodes J (1989) Lancet 2:1004-1006

10. Colombo M, Kuo g, Choo QL, Donato MF, Ninno ED, Tommasin MA, Dioguard N, Honghton M (1989) Lancet 2:1006-1008

11. The Japanese Society of Gastroenterology: Seroepidemiology of hepatitis C virus (1991) Gastroenterologia Japonica. 26:Suppl. 3 152-223

12. Kew MC, Houghton M, Choo QL, Kuo G (1990) Lancet 335:873-874

13. Di Bisceglie AM (1991) In Etiology, pathology and treatment of hepatocellular carcinoma in North Amnerica eds by Tabor E, Di Biscegli AM, Purcell RH (1991) Gulf Publ Co. Houston USA.

14. Ohbayashi A, Okochi K, Mayumi M (1972) Gastroenterology 62:618-625

15. Nishioka K, Mayumi M, Okochi K, Okada K, Hirayama T (1973) Analytical and experimental epidemiology of cancer ed by W. Nakahara 137-146. Univ. Park Press Baltimore

16. Okada K, Yamada T, Miyakawa Y, Mayumi M (1975) 87:360-363

17. Tada H, Yanagida M, Mishina J, Fuji T, Baba K, Ishikawa S, Aihara S, Tsuda F, Miyakawa Y, Mayumi M (1982) Pediatrics 70:613-619

18. Okamoto H, Yano K, Nozaki Y, Matsui A, Miyazaki H, Yamamoto K, Tsuda F, Machida A, Mishiro S (1992) Pediatric Res 32:264-268

19. Terazawa S, Kojima M, Yamanaka T, Yotsumoto S, Okamoto H, Tsuda F, Miyakawa Y, Mayumi M (1991) Pediatric Res 29:5-9

20. Kiyosawa K, Akahane Y, Nagata A, Furuta S (1984) Am. J. Gastroenterol. 79:777-781

21. Ohbayashi A, Tanaka S, Ohtake H (1983) Acta Hepat. Jap. 24:521-525

22. Kiyosawa K, Sodeyama T, Tanaka E, Gibo Y, Yoshizawa K, Nakano Y, Furuta S, Akaahane Y, Nishioka K, Purcell RH, Alter HJ (1990) Hepatology 12:671-675

23. Nishioka K (1991) Gastroenterologia Japonica. 26 Suppl 3:152-155

24. Tanaka E, Kiyosawa K, Sodeyama T, Hayata T, Ohike Y, Nakano Y, Yoshizawa Y, Furuta S, Watanabe Y, Watanabe J, Nishioka K (1991) Am. J. Trop. Med. & Hyg 46:460-464

25. The Japanese Red Cross NANB Hepatitis Research Group (1991) Lancet 338:1040-1041

26. The Japanese Red Cross NANB Hepatitis Research Group (1993) Vox Sang. in press

Part 3

Recent Advances
in Early Detection and Treatment
of Digestive Cancers

Recent Advances in the Diagnosis and Treatment of Superficial Esophageal Cancer

Mitsuo Endo, Kunihide Yoshino, and Tatsuyuki Kawano

The First Department of Surgery, Tokyo Medical and Dental University, Bunkyo-ku, Tokyo, 113 Japan

ABSTRACT

I have described the present state of diagnosis and surgical treatment of superficial esophageal cancer (Tis and T1 cancer). Better long-term survival rate was obtained in mucosal cancer cases, negative nodal involvement cases and negative vascular invasion cases. Regarding lymph node metastasis and vascular invasion, mucosal cancer was superior to submucosal cancer in terms of ability to perform curative treatment among T1 cancer cases. Thus I would like to stress that detection and treatment of mucosal cancer is most important to improve the long-term survival of esophageal cancer.

KEY WORD: superficial esophageal cancer, lymph node metastasis, endoscopic resection, mucosal cancer of the esophagus

MATERIALS

Lymph node metastasis and prognosis in superficial esophageal cancer

A total of 235 cases of superficial esophageal cancer, that is Tis and T1 cancer, were resected between 1965 and 1992 in our hospital. With respect to lymph node metastasis 170 cases (72%) were negative for metastasis, that is stage 0 and stage 1 cancer, whereas 65 cases (28%) were positive for metastasis. Stage 0 and Stage 1 cancers are referred to as early esophageal cancer in the Japanese Guidelines for Studies on Esophageal Cancer[1]

The long term survival rate of superficial esophageal cancer was studied in relation to lymph node metastasis, including all deaths apart from operative deaths. The 5-year and the 10-year survival rate of negative nodal involvement cases were 74% and 53% respectively. However, those of positive node cases were 36% and 28% respectively. There was a significant difference between the two groups.

Depth of invasion and prognosis in superficial esophageal cancer

With respect to the depth of invasion, 22 cases were epithelial cancer (ep cancer), 57 cases intramucosal cancer invading as far as the muscularis mucosa (mm cancer) and 156 cases were submucosal cancer (sm cancer). Mucosal cancer (ep + mm cancer) consisted of 79 cases (34%) in total.

The 5-year and the 10-year survival rate of mucosal cancer were 86% and 54%, otherwise those of submucosal cancer were 56% and 40% respectively. A significant difference was observed in the long-term survival rate of m cancer and sm cancer.

Vascular invasion and prognosis in superficial esophageal cancer

As for the vascular invasion of superficial esophageal cancer, the 5-year and the 10-year survival rate of negative vascular invasion cases were 83% and 62% respectively. However those of positive vascular invasion cases were 41% and 27% respectively, showing the significant negative effect of vascular invasion.

Relation between depth of invasion and lymph node metastasis and vascular invasion

Considering the relation between the depth of cancer invasion with regard to lymph node metastasis or vascular invasion, lymph node metastasis was observed in 4% of mucosal cancers, but in 40% of submucoal cancers. Vascular invasion was observed in only 10% of mucosal cancers, but in 70% of submucosal cancers.

From these points of view, a better long-term survival rate of superficial esophageal cancer was obtained in mucosal cancer cases, negative nodal involvement cases and negative vascular invasion cases. In practice, recurrence was seen most frequently in submucosal cancer cases with vascular invasion, even in cases without lymph node metastasis. Mucosal cancer was superior to submucosal cancer in terms of the ability to perform curable treatment.

Symptoms of superficial esophageal cancer

A catching feeling or feeling of a narrowed esophagus were the most common symptoms, followed by retrosternal pain and food causing tingling in the esophagus. However, 45% of cases showed no symptoms. The diagnosis of esophageal cancer was occasionally made in periodic mass surveys or in the course of investigation of some unrelated abdominal complaints.

Endoscopic diagnosis

Endoscopic examination played a large role in the diagnosis of mucosal cancer of the esophagus. The macroscopic classification of esophageal cancer is as shown in Table 1[2]. Superficial type (0-type) is defined as are esophageal lesions which are considered to be mucosal or submucosal cancer at the time of examination. 0-type is further classified into five subtypes; 0-I type, 0-IIa type, 0-IIb type, 0-IIc type and 0-III type. When more than two basic types are found in one lesion, the category of combined type is recommended. The 0-IIb type and 0-IIc type lesions were detected more easily by endoscopic staining with Lugol's solution than by the gross appearance. Normal epithelium is stained dark brown, and pathologic mucosa can be recognized as an unstained area. Thin non-cancerous epithelium covering cancerous tissue is also not stained by Lugol's solution.Thus malignancy in thebasal layer of the epithelium or dysplasia is also demonstrated as an unstained area.

Table 1. Endoscopic Classification of Esophageal Cancer

0.	superficial type
0-I	superficial and protruding type
0-II	superficial and flat type
0-IIa	slightly elevated type
0-IIb	flat type
0-IIc	slightly depressed type
0-III	superficial and distinctly depressed type
1.	protruding type
2.	ulcerative and localized type
3.	ulcerative and infiltrative type
4.	diffusely infiltrative type
5.	unclassifiable type

To detect early stage cancer, especially mucosal carcinoma of the esophagus, examination is performed as follows; when patients present with slight esophageal complaints, esophagoscopy should be performed. A periodic examination may be appropriate for high risk populations, such as males more than 50 years of age. Long-term follow-up in cases of achalasia and Barrett's esophagus is necessary. Our experience demonstrated that double esophageal and gastric, colonic or head and neck cancer is by no means uncommon in Japan. Some 0-IIb type lesions could only be recognized after staining with Lugol's solution. Therefore the endoscopic staining technique with Lugol's solution should be actively applied for periodic examinations or mass surveys in high risk subject. Biopsy is necessary to confirm pathological diagnosis. The most common mucosal cancer lesions detected were 0-IIb type and 0-IIc type. Small sessile lesions (0-IIa type) were less commonly observed. Lymph node metastasis was infrequent in the 0-II type. The 0-I type and 0-III type of lesions were mostly submucosal cancer even when the lesions were small.
Considering changes in invasion of superficial esophageal cancer according to chronological period, the detection of ep and mm cancers increased in the last 8 years. This is due to endoscopic examination has being applied widely in upper GI screening.

DISCUSSION

A less extensive operation can be indicated when mucosal cancer is suspected and extensive examinations reveal no lymph node metastasis. Usually transhiatal or endoscopic resection is performed in such cases, even when combined thoracotomy is performed, lymph node dissection is only performed in the most important nodes.

For submucosal cancer of the esophagus, however, transthoracic esophagectomy and lymph node dissection are performed, because lymph node metastasis in superficial esophageal cancer is frequently found in the upper and lower mediastinum and through the upper abdomen.

When a lesion suspectd to be mucosal cancer is less than 2 cm in size and the absence of lymph node metastasis is shown pre-operatively, endoscopic resection is indicated.

Endoscopic resection was performed in 12 cases. Histologically, all cases were mucosal cancer. The resected mucosa consisted of 1/5 to 4/5 of the circumference of the esophagus. The endoscopic type of most lesions was 0-IIb or 0-IIc. In all cases complete response (CR) was obtained locally. The longest period of follow up is 3 yrs and 2 months, and no recurrence has been observed in any case. No postoperative complication has been experienced with endoscopic resection.

REFERENCES
1. Japanese Society for Esophageal Disease: Guide Lines for the Clinical and Pathologic Studies on Carcinoma of the Esophagus (8th edition) Kanehara Co. Tokyo 1992
2. Endo M., Takeshita K., Yoshino K.: Oesophagoscopy for the diagnosis of superficial oesophageal cancer. Surg. Endosc. 1988 2: 205-208

Recent Advances in Early Detection and Treatment of Gastric Cancer

MITSUMASA NISHI

Department of Surgery, Cancer Institute Hospital, Tokyo, Japan

ABSTRACT

The detected number of early gastric cancer has been markedly increasing due to the progress in various diagnostic method, including double contrast radiography, conventional and electronic endoscopy with biopsy. Dye- spraying method has enabled the exact definition of lateral extension of cancer, and the advent of endoscopic ultrasound has made it possible to accurately estimate its invasive depth. In addition, the establishment of the mass screening system has contributed to the detection of gastric cancer with favorable prognosis. To determine whether the recent advances in early detection and treatment of gastric cancer are effective, and contribute to change the cumulative 5-year-survival rate we retrospectively studied a consecutive number of patients with gastric cancer who underwent surgery at the Cancer Institute Hospital. We correlated the endoscopic resection and surgery. In recent years early cancer has accounted for approximately 45% - 50% of the total of 350 to 400 patients with gastric cancer who were treated annually at our institution. Endoscopic resection can be applied to about 28% of early cancer limited to the mucosal membrane. Similarly, the preoperative staging of cancer has been made possible by the progress in the integrated diagnostic imaging , and appropriate operation method can be selected according to its stage estimated.. The operation method has also been improved in the terms of reductive, standard, and extended surgery. However, the chronological changes of cancer staging and treatment method have been brought about in most part by the progress in the methodology of the diagnosis The limit of surgical treatment was noted in terms of extended radical surgery and adjuvant chemotherapy. Efforts should be directed to the detection of early cancer which can be radically treated by reductive and function preserving surgery or by endoscopic resection.

KEY WORDS: Early gastric cancer, Reductive and function preserving surgery

History of cancer detection

There are three major factors which contributed to founding the basis for the detection of early gastric cancer in early 1950s. They are the advent of gastrocamera, the commencement of mass survey, and the development of double contrast radiography.

The definition and classification of early gastric cancer was first proposed at the annual meeting of Japan Gastroenterological Endoscopy Society in 1962. The number of operated early gastric cancer started to gradually increase soon after the definition and classification of early gastric cancer was approved in 1963. Fiberscope was introduced into clinical use in early 1960s, and biopsy under direct vision through fiberscope has become a reliable tool for making a definitive diagnosis of early cancer since 1964.

In early 1970s microcancer measuring less than 1cm became a target for challenging the limit of the diagnosis. Histogenesis of gastric cancer was discussed and elucidated at the same time.

Endscopic surgery for early cancer has been getting popular since end of 1970s and segmental resection in surgery for early cancer has frequently been tried since early 1980s. It is needles to mention that these new trials aimed at reductive and function preserving surgery in considering the quality of life of patients treated.

In Japan we have recently been confronted with the situation in which early cancer surpasses advanced cancer in their annually detected number. Such a phenomenon appeared around 1987 in many institutions of Japan which specialized in the management of gastrointestinal cancer. In our institution the annual rate of operated early gastric cancer has been nearly 60% of the total number of operated gastric cancer since 1988.

The change of cancer staging
There has been a remarkable increase in stage I cancer since 1960s, and early cancer has accounted for more than 50% since 1980. As a consequence, stage II, III, and IV cancer has reduced in number. Especially, stage IV cancer has reduced markedly.
Extended combined resection has been tried for the purpose of obtaining the better prognosis of advanced cancer. Especially, for advanced cancers located in the upper to middle third of the stomach left upper abdominal evisceration has been enforced.

Cumulative survival rate of gastric cancer with combined resection of neighboring organs Splenectomy cases showed a favorable prognosis with the 5-year-survival rate of 55%. However, extended combined resection resulted in poor prognosis, revealing 13% in left upper abdominal evisceration and 8% in pancreatoduodenectomy. This result may indicate the limit of surgical treatment for advanced gastric cancer.

The change of lymph node dissection
The extension of lymph node dissection has been changing recently. R_0 and R_1 dissection has decreased in number while R_3 dissection has gradually increased. Recently nodal dissection has been extended as far as to the forth group of paraaortic lymph nodes. This is R_4 dissection.
The retropyloric, celiac, and subpyloric node is considered to be a sentinel node in cancer located in the lower portion of the stomach whereas the para-aortic nodes just above the renal vein plays a role of a sentinel node in cancer located in the upper portion and gastric cardia. These lymph nodes should be dissected very carefully.

The change of operation method
The rate of distal resection reduced from 83.8% to 57.5% in a period of about 40 years. Total gastrectomy showed little change in its rate. The number of proximal and segmental resection has increased in recent years, and wedge resection has been tried very recently for a small number of early gastric cancer cases. The various reconstruction methods in surgery for early cancer which has been employed in our institution. Each method has its design to minimize the occurrence of stenosis, leakage, reflux, and dumping symptoms. It has been a recent trend to consider the reduction in the extent of resection as well as that of lymph node dissection in a surgery of early gastric cancer. We have tried to preserve the hepatic and celiac branch of the vagal nerve in segmental resection for small early cancer. The dietary life is reported to be satisfactory in patients who underwent the function preserving surgery.
Adjuvant chemotherpy was started in 1960, and revealed 10% improvement in the survival rate of stage III cancers, and it was statistically significant.

Five-year-survival rate of surgical cases

The 5-year-survival rate of the curative resection cases in the first period of 14 years from 1946 to 1959 was 45.2%, and it improved as high as to 76% in the third period of 6 years from 1980 to 1985. At the present time, the 5-year-survival rate of all surgical cases is estimated to be 61.6% (Fig. 1).

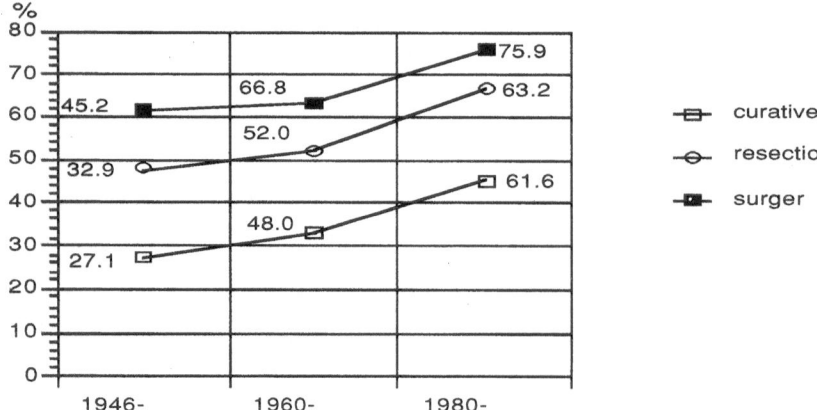

Fig. 1. The change of five-year-survival
in surgical cases

Endoscopic resection

Endoscopic resection or endoscopic mucosectomy has established its methodology as a radical treatment method for a very small early cancer. In recent years cases of early cancer which is indicated for endoscopic resection has gradually been increasing in accordance with the increasing number of early cancer as shown in this slide. Now, it is the time to make the more precise assessment of the indication for endoscopic surgery in order to avoid unnecessary surgery.

Summary

The chronological change of cancer staging and treatment method was described, and it has been brought about in most part by the progress in the methodology of the diagnosis. There was the limit of surgical treatment in terms of extended radical operation and adjuvant chemotherapy. Finally it was emphasized that our efforts should be directed not only to the detection of early cancer which can be radically treated by reductive and function preserving surgery but also by endoscopic resection.
BIBLIOGRAPHY.

1. Ohta K, Nakajima T, Yamada H, Ishihara S, Nishi, M (1993) KARKINOS 6: 25-32
2. Takekoshi T, Fujii A, BabaY, Takemoto N, Kaku S, Shimizu H, Koizumi K, Tomimatsu H, Murakamami Y, Takano K, Nagatani K, Ohta H, Ueno M, Ishihara, S, Nishi M, Kato Y, Yanagisawa A, Takagi K (1992) Shokakinaishikyo 6: 847-856, 1992.

Early Detection of Colorectal Cancer and Advancement in Its Treatment in Japan

MASAYUKI YASUTOMI

The First Department of Surgery, Kinki University School of Medicine, Osaka-Sayama, Osaka, 589 Japan

ABSTRRACT

Japanese research society for colorectal cancer defined early cancer as mucosal and submucosal cancer. of 22,652 cancers registrared with the society up to 1983, 1,585cases or 7% were early cancers Flat and depressed type early cancer (FDEC) accounted for only 0.5%, though 98% were protruded and elevated types.Due to recent advances in endoscopy, early cancer has incerased 20-30% of overall cancer, and FDEC accounted for 10-15% of rarly cancer. 90% of FDEC is 10mm or smaller in size, and higher rate of invasion. If FEDC is found 10mm or larger, surgical treatment should be considered. Screening started in 1992 using the immunological fecal occult blood test in Japan. According to joint study of 864,652 asymptomatic subjects, positive rate was 8.0%. Cancer was found in 0.17%, and 53.2% of cancer detected was early cancer. Efficasy of this screening, however, remains uncertain.

KEY WORD: colorectal early cancer, flat and depressed type, rapid invasion, screening by fecal occult test, immunological reaction.

INTRODUCTION

With increased consumption of westernized foods, the incidence of colorectal cancer has been increasing rapidly in Japan. The number of deaths from colorectal cancer has increased more than 5-fold over the last 30 years. Furthermore, the disease is expected to rank third highest after lung and gastric cancer in the year 2000. With such a background, there has been great concern about the early detection and treatment of colorectal cancer, and some advances have been achieved during the past two decades.

Definition of the early cancer and its classification

In 1974, the Japanese Research Society of Colorectal Cancer was established, and it worked out "General rules for clinical and pathological studies" [1]. These general rules are very detailed and are characterized by their having been much influenced by the concept of gastric cancer. At present, 80% of colorectal cancer cases in Japan are being recorded according to the general rules. The general rules define early colorectal cancer as mucosal (m) cancer and submucosal (sm) cancer, as in gastric cancer. As for macroscopic classification of the early cancer, the general rules give the following classifications: Type I: protruded type, Type II: superficial type, and Type III: excavated type. Protruded type is further subclassified into Ip: pedunculated type and Is: sessile type. Superficial type is further subclassified into IIa: superficial elevated type, IIb: flat type, and IIc: depressed type. This subclassification is the same as in gastric cancer.
In 1974, major surgical institutions across the country started registration of

colorectal cancer according to the Japanese general rules, and a total of 24,652 cases were registered during a period of 10 years up to 1983. There were 1,585 cases (7%) of early cancer, of which 631 were m cancer, and 954 sm cancer. The 5-year survival rate of these early cancer patients was 88% in m cancer (Table 1), and 86% in sm cancer, with 87% in early cancers as a whole. In cases of stage I cancer (Dukes A), the survival rate was 85%. In our institution, the 5-year survival rate in patients with colorectal cancer was 90% in stage I, and 80% in stage II. Thus, from the viewpoint of survival, stage I may be taken as early cancer.

Table 1. Early Cancer Registration
         Jpn. Research Sciety(1974~'83)

m	631
sm	954
m+sm	1,585

(7% of 22,625 cancer cases)

The advantages of this definition of early cancer of the mucosal and the submucosal type in Japan are: (1) it is defined under the same concept as gastric cancer which has the highest incidence, (2) it is curable by endoscopic or minimized treatment, (3) it has a lower incidence of metastasis, (4) it provides important information on carcinogenesis. However, the problem is the histological diagnosis of mucosal cancer. Difficulty is often experienced in distinguishing the mucosal cancer from the atypical epithelium [2.3]. The second problem is that there is less cost-benefit with regard to reduction of mortality. It can be said that, in Japan, early cancer is defined focusing on research into carcinogenesis rather than the clinical results.

Advances in endoscopic detection and treatment

The main role in the detection and treatment of early cancer shifted from surgeons to endoscopists as colonoscopy began to be widely used at the end of the 1970. Nowadays, colonoscopy is the standard technique commonly used at ordinary hospitals, and patients with symptoms are examined by total colonofiberscopy. Then, lesions suspected to be cancerous are totally removed, followed by histological examination. Of 1,585 registered cases of macroscopic type early cancer; pedunculated type (Ip): 47.0%, sessile type (Is): 27.8%, flat elevated type (IIa): 18.7%, IIa+IIc: 6.0%, while flat or depressed types (IIb or IIc) account for only 0.5% (Table 2). As almost all the early cancers were protruded type or superficial elevated type, it was necessary to look for a polypoid lesion, and to determine whether it was cancerous or not, based on the histological examination of the polypectomized tissue.

Table 2. Macroscopic Classification of 1,585 Early Cancer

Ip	47.0%
Is	27.8%
IIa	18.7%
IIa+IIc	6.0%
IIc	0.5%

Flat type (IIb) and depressed type (IIc) of early cancer (FDEC)

In the past, it was considered that incidence of early cancer was 7-10% of overall colorectal cancer, and that 98% or more of early cancer cases were protruded type and elevated type. However, as a result of recent advances in endoscopic diagnosis, early cancer accounts for 20-30% of all colorectal cancer. Furthermore 10-15% of detected early cancers are reported as flat or depressed type (IIb or IIc) [7.8.9]. In the detection of protruded type of early cancer in polyps, the possibility of cancer is determined by tumor size and the character of its mucosal surface. In FDEC, however, the cancer possibility of cancer is judged by the redness or faded color of the mucosa and any irregularity in the mucosal surface. Through a dye-spraying technique, mucosa is stained with methylene blue or crystal violet, then slight depressed or elevated areas, or irregular pit-patterns are revealed more clearly. A strip biopsy is performed after saline is injected into the submucosal layer (8). The removed specimen is examined histologically. Electronic fiberscope, mucosal staining by dye-spraying, and the analysis of pit-patterns on the mucosa by magnifying fiberscope are important techniques in the detection of FDEC.
Kudo (1993) reports that of 673 cases of early cancer, 553 (82.0%) were protruded or elevated type, and 81 (12.0%) FDEC. Of these 81 cases of FDEC, 76 (92.7%) were 10mm or smaller in size, and few were larger than 10mm. As to the rate of sm-invasion, 8 cases (14.3%) out of 56 of 5mm or less showed invasion, and 9 cases (45%) out of 20 of 10mm or less showed invasion. In protrued type cancer, however, the number of cases showing invasion from cancers of 5mm or less was 0 (0%) out of 40 cases, and of those of 10mm or less, 16 (8.0%) out of 174 cases [9] showed invasion (Table 3). Toyonaga (1992) reported the same results of the early cancer (Table 4).

Table 3. Submucosal Invasion from Early Cancer

macroscopic type	size(mm) -5	6-10	11-15	16-20	21-	Total
porotruded	40(0)	174(16)	84(16)	67(17)	30(8)	395(55)
%	0	8.0	19.0	25.4	26.7	13.9
flat elevated	82(3)	53(9)	11(7)	9(8)	3(3)	158(30)
%	3.6	17.0	63.6	8.9	100	19.0
flat depressed	56(8)	20(9)	2(1)	1(0)	2(1)	81(19)
%	14.3	45.0				23.5

(   )   No. of sm cancer
Total invasion rate : 673(111) 16.5%   Kudo(1993)

Table 4. Submucosal Invasion from Early Cancer

macroscopic type	size(mm) -5	6-10	11-15	16-20	Total
porotruded	18(0)	85(7)	59(8)	28(9)	210(29)
%	0	8.2	13.6	32.1	13.8
flat elevated	11(1)	33(4)	19(1)	8(3)	78(9)
%	9.1	12.1	5.2	37.5	11.5
flat depressed	32(3)	8(5)	1(0)	2(2)	44(11)
%	9.4	62.5	0	100	25.0

(   )   sm incasion   Toyyonaga(1992)
Total invasion rate : 332(49) 14.8%

Thus, invasion from FDEC showed a higher incidence than that in protruded type.Moreover, in FDEC, the invasion takes place at an earlier stage. In addition, when the cancer exceeds 10mm, it is handled as advanced cancer and is not considered as an early cancer. Surgical treatment must therefore be considered, because sm-invasion is likely when FDEC is found to be 5mm or larger in diameter. FDEC occurs regardless of adenoma, and develops into sm-invasion at an early stage, leading to advanced cancer in a short time. An unexpectedly large number of such FDEC are found in Japan, and this is a problem in the early detection and treatment of colorectal cancer.

Submucosal invasion and nodal involvement

In endoscopic treatment, it is important to make a distinction between m cancer and sm cancer. According to the nationwide registration, the incidences of sm invasion in early cancer cases were: Ip: 12%, Ips: 18%, Is: 25%, IIa: 36%, and IIa+IIc: 80%. Thus, Is, IIa and IIa+IIc are most likely to be sm cancer.
It is stipulated in the general rules that if any of the following is found in the polypectomized tissue, it should be removed by subsequent surgery: (1) positive surgical margin, (2) strong vascular invasion, (3) massive invasion into sm-layer, (4) poorly differentiated cancer.
According to Muto's collection of 858 of sm cancer cases in 1991 [10], 223 cases out of the 858 underwent subsequent surgery because of positive surgical margin or possible nodal involvement after polypectomy. Out of these 223 cases, the rate of residual cancer was as follows: Ip: 4.8%, Ips: 7.9%, Is: 8.3%, IIa: 16.0%, and IIa+IIc: 12.5%. Of these, cases of IIa and IIa+IIc were diagnosed as m cancer before the treatment, and polypectomy was performed (Table 5).
However, these were actually sm cancer, and they had positive cut-margin.
Next problem is nodal involvement in early cancer. According to the nationwide registration, the rate of nodal involvement was 3.0% in m cancer, 9.9% in sm cancer, and 24.4% in pm cancer. It is generally known that m cancer shows no metastases. The reason why 3% metastasis was noted in m cancer is probably because, in those days, resected specimens might not have been properly prepared at some institutions, with the result that invasive cancer might have been taken as m cancer. According to Muto's statistics (1991), of 776 cases of sm cancer, nodal involvement was seen in 8.8%, and liver metastasis in 1.0%. In addition, in 223 cases operated on by excision of the intestine after polypectomy, the rate of nodal involvement was as follows: Ip: 8.1%, Ips: 9.2%, Is: 16.7%, and IIa-IIa+IIc: 25%. Thus, sessile and flat-elevated type shows a high metastatic rate. The metastasis of early cancer was limited to the lymph nodes adjoining the tumor according to nationwide registration (Table 6).
Of the 776 collected cases of sm cancer, although over a short period of observation, death occurred in 36 cases (4.6%).

Table 5. Residual cancer of 223 sm-cancer requiring subsequent surgery after polypectomy

macroscoic type	residual cancer
Ip	4.8%
Ips	7.9%
Is	8.3%
IIa	16.0%
IIa+IIc	12.5%

collected by Muto(1991)

Table 6. Node involvement of 223 sm-cancer requiring surgery subsequent to polypectomy

macroscopic type	node cancer
Ip	8.1%
Ips	9.2%
Is	16.7%
IIa	12.0%
IIa+IIc	25.0%
IIc	25.0%

collected by Muto(1991)

Screening for early detection of cancer:

In Japan, screenings have been conducted for early detection of stomach, uterine cervix, lung and breast cancer. Screenings for stomach and uterine cervix cancer are considered to have contributed to a reduction in the mortality rate. As to lung and breast cancer, however, sufficient evaluation has not been made as yet. In the U.S. and European countries, screenings for colorectal cancer are being conducted by means of fecal occult blood test as a randomized controlled trial, using a biochemical method. However, it seems that the screenings have not been so successful as to reduce the mortality in these groups.

Table 7. Efficacy of Fecal Occult Blood Testing for Screening

Subject	Reaction	
	biochemical (%)	immunologiccal (%)
sensitivity		
m.ca	12.9-13.8	44.1-50.0
sm.ca	7.7-21.0	50.0-55.6
advanved ca	60.8-68.0	73.9-84.3
specificity		
nomal	84.3-89.2	99.1

Hisamichi '89

Table 8. Screening for gastrointestinal Cancer (1989)

	Coloectal ca	Gastric ca
subjects	n=864,652	n=5,393,941
positive screening	8.0%	12.2%
further exam.	53.0%	71.8%
cancer detected	0.17%	0.10%
early cancer	53.2%	53.5%

In Japan, nationwide screening for colorectal cancer was started in 1992 using immunological fecal occult blood tests. As to the differences between the biochemical and immunological methods, there is a report by Hisamichi (1989). Sensitivity in the biochemical method was lower with 12-13% in m cancer, 8-21% in sm cancer, and 60-68% in advanced cancer, while the immunological method was higher with 44-50%, 50-55%, and 74-84% respectively (Table 7). Specificity by the immunological method is also higher than the biochemical method. Sensitivity was further increased by making tests over two consecutive days, the results being 74% in m cancer, 61% in sm cancer, and 85% in advanced cancer. The immunological fecal occult blood test was performed on 864,652 asymptomatic subjects in 1989, and the overall positive rate was 8.0%. As a result of further examination by colonoscopy, colorectal cancer was found in 0.17% of subjects and 53.2% of cancer detected was early cancer (Table 8). The results of this screening were fairly good. However, as mentioned earlier in this paper, a number of problems still exist with regard to histological over-diagnosis for mucosal cancer, length bias of early cancer, low positive reaction in FDEC and cost-benefit. Thus, no conclusion has yet been reached as to whether the screening program will lower the mortality rate of colorectal cancer patients.

REFERENCES

1. Japanese Research Society for Cancer of the Colon and Rectum (1983) General Rules for Jpn. J. Surg.
2. Morson B.C. and Jass J.R. (1985) Precancerous lesions of the gastrointestinal tract. Bailliere Tindall, London. 104-159
3. Muto T.,Bussey H.J.R., Morson B.C. (1975) The evolution of cancer of the colon and rectum.Cancer 36:2251-2270
4. Crauford B.E., and Stromeyer F.W. (1983) Small nonpolypoid carcinomas of the large intestine. Cancer 51:1760-1763.
5. Kuramoto S., Oohara T. (1983) Minute cancers arising novo in human large intestine. Cancer 61:829-834.
6. Adachi M., Muto T. and Morioka Y. (1984) Flat adenoma and flat mucosal carcinoma (IIb type); A new precursor of colorectal carcinoma? Report of two cases. Dis. Colon Rectum, 31:236-243.
7. Ikegami M. (1987) A pathological study on colorectal cancer. Acta Pathol. Jpn. 37:21-37.
8. Toyonaga A., Arima N., Tsuruta O. etal (1992) Diagnosis of depressed type early colorectal cancers from the endoscopic and pathological point of view. (in Japanese) Stomach and Intestine 27:911-923.
9. Kudo S. (1990) Detection of colo-rectal minute cancer.(in Japanese) Stomach and Intestine 25:801-812.
10.Kudo S. (1993) Personal comunication.
11.Muto T., Nishisawa M.,Kodaira S. A report of the collected sm cancer of the large intestine. (in Japanese) Stomach and Intestine 26:911-913.

Long-Term Results of a German Prospective Multicenter Study on Colo-Rectal Cancer*

PAUL HERMANEK

Department of Surgery, University of Erlangen, 8520 Erlangen, Germany**

ABSTRACT

Between 1984 and 1986 2347 patients with invasive colorectal carcinoma were registered in a prospective multicenter observation study in which seven German institutions participated. The 5-year survival following tumor resection primarily is influenced by the residual tumor (R) classification. Within the R0 patients prognosis can be well estimated by pTNM and pTNM based stage grouping. Stage III is inhomogeneous and should be subdivided into pN1 and pN2,3. The 5-year survival rates for the individual institutions showed significant differences for the total, but also for the individual stages. This reflects the importance of the surgeon as "prognostic factor".

KEY WORDS: Colorectal carcinoma / Interdepartment variation / Long-term prognosis / pTNM / Residual tumor (R)

INTRODUCTION

In 1984 started a multicenter observation study on patients with invasive colorectal carcinoma. The aims were
-to evaluate prospectively the 4th edition of the UICC TNM classification(1),
-to obtain an overview on clinical practice in diagnosis and treatment,
-to analyze treatment results.

PATIENTS AND METHODS

Data of 2347 unselected patients with invasive colorectal carcinoma were

 * Supported by grant no. 071910-9/9A from the German Federal Ministry for Research and Technology.
 ** For the Study Group Colo-Rectal Carcinoma (SGCRC) collected by the

Study Group Colo-Rectal Carcinoma (SGCRC) during 1st August 1984 an 30th November 1986. Seven departments of surgery (5 universitary, 2 municipal) participated in the study which was conceived as prospective clinico-pathological observation study where different treatment forms could be freely chosen. Initial presentation, diagnosis, pathology, classification, treatment and follow-up were documented using uniform criteria. Residual tumor (R) and pTNM classification as well as stage grouping were performed according to UICC 1987/1992 (1). The resection rate was 1185/1126 (96.7 %) for colon and 1056/1121 (94.3 %) for rectum carcinoma.

All patients were followed-up until death or at least 5 years. Observed survival rates were calculated according to Kaplan-Meier, surgical mortality not excluded. Also relative survival rates were calculated as ratios of the observed to the expected rates considering sex, age and period of observation. The twofold standard error (corresponding to the 95 % confidence interval) is added to the survival rates.

PROGNOSIS IN RELATION TO R AND pTNM CLASSIFICATION

The 5-year survival rates following tumor resection primarily are influenced by the R classification (Table 1).

Table 1: Prognosis in relation to R classification

Patient group		n	5-year survival rates (%)	
			Observed	Relative
Rectum carcinoma	R0	887	55.2 ± 3.5	68.4 ± 4.3
	R1,2	169	9.6 ± 4.9	12.0 ± 6.1
Colon carcinoma	R0	947	58.4 ± 2.5	76.9 ± 4.4
	R1,2	238	3.1 ± 2.5	4.1 ± 3.3

Within the R1,2 patients only absence or presence of distant metastases significantly influences prognosis (Table 2).

Table 2. Prognosis of patients with R1,2 tumor resection. Relation to M classification. Observed survival rates (%).

	Rectum carcinoma		Colon carcinoma	
	M0 (n= 48)	M1 (n= 118)	M0 (n= 33)	M1 (n=205)
2-year survival	43.9 ± 14.3	16.3 ± 6.8	48.5 ± 17.4	11.3 ± 4.4
5-year survival	23.0 ± 13.4	2.6 ± 2.9	19.9 ± 15.9	0.5 ± 1.0
Median survival time (months)	21.4	11.4	19.4	8.6

The prognosis of R0 patients shows a wide range and can be well estimated by pTNM and stage grouping (Table 3)

Table 3. Prognosis following R0 resection.

Patient group	n	Rectum carcinoma 5-year survival rates (%)		n	Colon carcinoma 5-year survival rates (%)	
		observed	relative		observed	relative
pT1	80	74.3 ± 10.0	93.4 ± 12.9	84	79.7 ± 9.1	98.4 ± 11.3
pT2	231	70.9 ± 6.2	87.1 ± 7.6	118	74.2 ± 8.4	96.6 ± 11.0
pT3	518	48.7 ± 4.5	60.6 ± 5.7	602	58.0 ± 4.1	77.0 ± 5.5
pT4	58	24.2 ± 11.2	29.7 ± 13.8	143	34.7 ± 8.2	46.4 ± 10.9
pN0	464	68.1 ± 4.5	84.8 ± 5.6	552	70.0 ± 4.0	92.4 ± 5.3
pN1	160	46.6 ± 8.0	58.0 ± 10.0	195	48.3 ± 7.4	65.0 ± 10.6
pN2	74	31.1 ± 10.8	38.4 ± 13.3	95	34.9 ± 10.0	45.7 ± 13.0
pN3	132	32.7 ± 8.5	38.2 ± 9.5	88	30.0 ± 9.9	37.9 ± 12.4
Stage I	256	73.6 ± 5.8	91.5 ± 7.2	166	79.9 ± 6.5	100 - 5.9
Stage II	258	61.7 ± 6.4	77.8 ± 8.1	389	66.8 ± 4.9	88.3 ± 6.6
Stage III	351	39.8 ± 5.3	48.8 ± 6.4	354	42.8 ± 5.4	56.6 ± 7.2
Stage IV	22	9.1 ± 12.3	10.9 ± 14.7	38	23.7 ± 13.8	29.8 ± 17.4

Stage III is inhomogenous with regard to prognosis and should be subdivided into any pT pN1 M0 and any pT pN2,3 M0 (Table 4).

Table 4. Prognostic subdivision of stage III.

Subgroups	n	Rectum carcinoma 5-year survival (%)		n	Colon carcinoma 5-year survival (%)	
		Observed	Relative		Observed	Relative
Any pT pN1 M0	159	46.9 ± 8.1	58.5 ± 10.0	187	50.1 ± 7.6	67.8 ± 10.3
Any pT pN2,3 M0	192	33.8 ± 7.0	41.0 ± 8.5	165	34.3 ± 7.5	44.3 ± 9.7
Difference (p)		0.05			0.01	

The reported results were achieved predominantly by surgery alone, only 13.5 % of R0 rectum and 8.4 % of R0 colon carcinoma patients received adjuvant or neoadjuvant therapy. Any significant survival differences in relation to additional non-surgical treatment could not be observed.

INTERDEPARTMENT VARIATIONS IN SURVIVAL

The 5-year survival rates for the individual institutions showed significant differences. This applies to the total and to stages II and III, while the difference in stage I and IV are statistically not significant (Table 5).

Table 5. Interdepartment variation in 5-year survival rates after tumor resection (any R).

Tumor site	Stage	5-year survival rates (%)				
		Observed		Relative		
		Total	Variation[1]	Total	Variation[1]	
Rectum	any	47.9 ± 3.2	31 – 52 % *	59.5 ± 4.0	40 – 63 % *	
	I	73.0 ± 5.7	67 – 87 %	91.6 ± 7.1	81 –100 %	
	II	59.4 ± 6.3	41 – 70 % *	75.2 ± 7.9	52 – 85 % *	
	III	38.1 ± 5.1	13 – 53 % *	46.8 ± 6.3	16 – 66 % *	
	IV	3.7 ± 3.2	0 – 7 %	4.4 ± 3.9	0 – 8 %	
Colon	any	47.3 ± 3.0	27 – 54 % *	62.2 ± 3.9	37 – 69 % *	
	I	79.9 ± 6.5	56 – 87 %	100 – 7.3	70 –100 %	
	II	66.0 ± 4.9	39 – 87 % *	88.3 ± 6.6	49 –100 % *	
	III	41.1 ± 5.3	21 – 52 % *	54.7 ± 7.0	27 – 65 % *	
	IV	4.1 ± 2.6	0 – 12 %	5.3 ± 3.3	0 – 16 %	

[1] Statistically significant variations marked by an asterisk

The considerable interdepartment variations of 5 -year survival rates reflect the importance of the "prognostic factor surgeon". While the ratio R0 / R1,2 did not significantly differ between the departments, in other surgeon-related variables significant variation could be detected.

For rectum carcinoma there were significant differences in the frequency of inadvertant perforation of or incision into tumor during surgery (6 - 30 %, mean 12.2 %). Also the incidence of locoregional recurrences shows a highly significant interdepartment variation: any stage: 12 - 35 %; mean 21.7 %, stage II: 13 - 40 %, mean 20.2 %; stage III: 14 - 52 %; mean 31.4 %. The completeness of the removal of the mesorectum (2) and avoidance of intraoperative locoregional spillage of tumor cells (3) are the decisive challenges in rectum cancer surgery.

With regard to colon carcinoma significant differences in the frequency of multivisceral resections (0-23 %, mean 12.0 %) could be noticed. Also, the extent of regional lymph node dissection in carcinomas of the transverse colon and the colonic flexures was significantly different in the various institutions: in elective surgery for solitary sporadic carcinomas of these sites the frequency of extended surgery (right and transverse colectomy, left and transverse colectomy) varied between 15 and 68 %.

DISCUSSION

The presented interdepartment variation of long-term results emphasizes the necessity of consideration of the details of surgical procedures and of identification of the surgeon as variable as proposed in 1991 by the International Documentation System (IDS) for Colorectal Cancer (4). The data also recommend the following requirements for clinical trials on adjuvant treatment of colorectal carcinoma (5):data collection according to IDS (4); pTNM classification 1987/1992 (6); stratification according to pN (pN1 vs pN2, 3) and extent of surgery (limited vs radical, conventional vs extended); consideration of the surgeon.

REFERENCES:

1. Hermanek P, Sobin LH (eds) (1992) UICC TNM classification of malignant tumours. 4th ed, 2nd revision 1992. Springer, Heidelberg Berlin New York Tokyo, pp 52-55
2. Heald RJ (1988) Holy place of rectal surgery. J Roy Soc Med 81: 503-508
3. Zirngibl H, Husemann B, Hermanek P (1990) Intra-operative spillage of tumor cells in surgery for rectal cancer. Dis Colon Rectum 33: 610-614
4. Fielding LP, Arsenault PA, Chapuis PH, Dent O, Gatright B, Hardcastle JD, Hermanek, P, Jass JR, Newland RC (1991) Clinicopathological staging for colorectal cancer: An International Documentation System (IDS) and an International Comprehensive Anatomical Terminology (ICAT). J Gastroenterol Hepatol 6: 325-344
5. Hermanek P (1991) Data collection aspects for the design of adjuvant treatment protocols in colorectal carcinoma. Onkologie 14: 491-497
6. NIH (1990) Consensus conference adjuvant therapy for patients with colon and rectal carcinoma. JAMA 264: 1444-1450

Evaluation of Early Detection and Treatment of Hepatocellular Carcinoma

ZHAO-YOU TANG, YE-QIN YU, BING-HUI YANG, XIN-DA ZHOU, ZHI-YING LIN, JI-ZHEN LU, and ZHEN-CHEN MA

Liver Cancer Institute, Shanghai Medical University, Shanghai 200032, China

ABSTRACT

During 1972-1991, 1443 patients with hepatocellular carcinoma (HCC) were studied. Comparison between screening (n=522) and nonscreening (n=921) groups revealed higher small HCC percentage (49.4% vs. 12.4%), higher resection rate (75.10% vs 45.9%) higher 5-year survival (42.1% vs. 24.8%) and bigger number of 5-year survivors (71 vs. 53). The increase of series 5-year survival (11.5% in 1970s to 43.4% in 1980s) coincided to the increase of screening in the series (25.3% to 41.2%). The increase of 5-year survival in screening group (29.0% in 1970s to 47.4% in 1980s) was a result of increasing resectability. The 5-year survival of 391 patients with subclinical HCC after resection was as high as 60.5%. It is concluded that screening using AFP and/or ultrasonography in high risk population and treated with resection is of proved merit to improve survival of patients with HCC.

KEY WORDS

hepatocellular carcinoma, screening, alphafetoprotein, subclinical hepatocellular carcinoma, small hepatocellular carcinoma

INTRODUCTION

Hepatocellular carcinoma (HCC), the third killer of malignancies in China, has long been regarded as a hopeless disease. The discovery of subclinical HCC in early 1970s, however, has opened a new field in clinical research of HCC. The advances in the study of alphafetoprotein (AFP) has provided possibility for early detection of HCC[1]. Unfortunately, the early trial by Masseyeff in Senegal was disappointed[2]. In 1975, Okuda et al reported five cases of small HCC detected during routine clinical follow-up[3]. In China , the value of early detection using AFP screening with low sensitive assays during 1971-1973 was not satisfactory. However, unquestionable results were shown in AFP screening of 343999 people and reported in the 2nd International Symposium of Cancer Detection and Prevention[4]. Substantial progress in early detection was achieved by using more sensitive assay - passive reverse hemagglutinaton assay and radiorocket electrophoresis autography [5]. The earliest report concerning small HCC resection in a high risk area - Qidong County of Jiangsu Province was made in 1975[6]. Two years latter, 48 patients of subclinical HCC (SCHCC) were reported in the same area, and resection was done in 33 (68.7%) of them, the 2-year survival was 77.0%[7]. In Shanghai, during 1971-1976, 1967511 persons were screened,

134 (44.7%) of the 300 cases of HCC detected were SCHCC, the 3-year survival was 57.1% after resection [8]. Data of 30 cases of small HCC were reported, the 3-year survival after resection was as high as 70.5% [9]. In authors's institute, during the 1970s and 1980s, efforts have been made to define high risk population, to combine ultrasonography in the screening, to make early diagnosis at relatively low AFP level, to increase resectability by using limited resection in cirrhotic liver, to prolong survival using re-resection for subclinical recurrence, to determine cell origin of recurrent lesions, to investigate natural history of HCC, etc [10-21]. In Alaska, an encouraging result of HCC screening was also reported [22]. This paper will try to make an evaluation of early detection and treatment of HCC based on 20 years' follow-up study.

PATIENTS AND METHODS

A twenty years' (January 1972- December 1991) materials comprising 1443 patients with pathologically proven HCC treated in Liver Cancer Institute of Shanghai Medical University were analyzed. The median age was 49 years (ranging from 13 to 82). Male and female ratio was 8:1. The positivity of serum HBsAg was 70.4% (424/1170) and antiHBc 72.1%, whereas antiHCV was only 11.1% (46/416). Co-existed cirrhosis was present in 86.7% of patients, macronodular cirrhosis amounted to 71.4% (775/1085) of patients with cirrhosis. Of the entire series, 36.2% of patients were discovered by screening, in the screening group, 72.0% (376/522) being discovered by screening in natural population or health checkup, whereas the rest (28.0%, 146/522) was pick up by high risk population screening. Clinical patients amounted to 63.8% of the whole series. Abnormal serum AFP (>20ug/L) was found in 70.5% of patients. Of the entire series, asymptomatic subclinical HCC amounted to 27.1% (391/1443). Survival rate were calculated by life table method. Comparison was made between screening and nonscreening groups, between patients in 1970s and 1980s in the entire series and in screening groups as well.

RESULTS

1. Comparison between Screening (n=522) and Nonscreening (n=921)Groups

As shown in Table 1, Screening group when compared with nonscreening group, the median tumor size was smaller (5cm vs. 10cm), percentage of small HCC higher (49.4% vs 12.4%), resulted in higher resectability (75.1% vs. 45.9%), higher 5-year survival in the entire series (42.1% vs. 24.8%), and bigger number of 5-year survivors (71 vs. 53 patients).

2. Comparison between 1970s and 1980s in the Entire Series

The 20 years' materials were divided into two groups, the 1970s group (1972- 1981) and the 1980s group (1982-1991), When these two groups were compared , it is clearly shown in Table 2, that with the increasing patients from screening in the series (from 12.5% to 31.5%), and resulted in marked increase of resectability (from 28.1% to 69.55), decrease of operative mortality (from 4.7% to 2.5%), and led to encouraging improve of prognosis (5-year survival from 11.5% to 43.4%).

Table 1. Comparison between screening and nonscreening groups

	Screening (n=522)	Nonscreening (n=921)
Median tumor size (cm)	5	10
Small HCC (<=5 cm)(%)	49.4	12.4
Resection (%)	75.1	45.9
Palliative surgery other than resection (%)	19.5	30.7
Conservative treatment (%)	4.4	19.5
No treatment (%)	1.0	3.9
Limited resection and left segmentectomy (%)	67.6 (269/392)	56.7 (240/423)
Operative mortality (%)	2.3 (9/392)	3.3 (14/423)
Re-resection (n)	57	37
5-year survival (%)		
Entire series	42.1	24.8
Resection	54.0	43.9
5-year survivor (n)	71	53

Table 2. Comparison between 1970s and 1980s in the entire series

	1972-1981 (n=455)	1982-1991 (n=988)
Screening (%)	25.3	41.2
Small HCC (%)	12.5	31.9
Resection (%)	28.1	69.5
Operative mortality (%)	4.7	2.5
Re-resection	19	75
5-year survival (%)	11.5	43.4

3. Comparison between 1970s and 1980s in Screening Group

The screening group was subdivided into 1970s(1972-1981) and 1980s (1982-1991) groups. Comparative study of these two groups was shown in Table 3. The median tumor size was same (5 cm) in both groups, however, the series 5-year survival was 47.4% in 1980s, whereas it was only 29.0% in 1970s. The possible correlated factors might include: the increase of resectability (from 53.9% to 81.1%), the increase proportion of limited resection (from 33.0% to 55.8%) and increase number of patients received re-resection for subclinical recurrence (from 11 patients to 46 patients).

Table 3. Comparison between 1970s and 1980s in screening group

	1972-1981 (n=115)	1982-1991 (n=407)
Screened in high risk Population (%)	15.7	27.8
Median tumor size (cm)	5	5
Resection (%)	53.9	81.1
Limited resection and left segmentectomy (%)	33.0	55.8
Re-resection (n)	11	46
5-year survival (%)	29.0	47.4

4. Subclinical HCC and Subclinical Recurrence

Of the entire series, 391 (27.1%) patients were asymptomatic subclinical HCC, which amounted to 74.9% (391/522) of the screening group. In patients with subclinical HCC, 77.6% of them had their AFP>20ug/L, the rest was detected by ultrasonography. In the whole series of subclinical HCC, 61.1% of them were small HCC. Resection was done in 81.4% of patients. Operative mortality was only 1.9%. The 5-year survival of subclinical HCC was 50.7% in the entire series and 60.5% in resection group. The 10-year survival was 35.6% in the entire series and 44.2% in subclinical patients with resection. Of the 1443 patients in this series, 815 patients received resection, re-resection was done in 94 patients with subclinical recurrence. The 5-year survival was as high as 53.3% calculated from first resection and 39.8% from time of re-resection.

DISCUSSION

1. Evaluation of Early Detection and Treatment of HCC

In early 1980s, evaluation of screening for HCC had been made by the authors[10,12,15]. In this series, data continued to reconfirm the conclusion made decade's ago . As shown in Table 1, the differences of clinical, therapeutic and prognostic patterns between screening and nonscreening groups were clear. In screening group, median tumor size was smaller (5 vs 10 cm), proportion of small HCC in the series was higher (49.4% vs 12.4%), this resulted in higher resectability (75.1% vs. 45.9%) and higher series 5-year survival (42.1% vs. 24.8%). It is particularly interest that the absolute number of 5-year survivor was bigger (71 vs. 53) even they have smaller number of patients in the series (522 vs. 921). Table 2 also clearly showed that screening has played important role to the improvement of series 5-year survival from 11.5% in 1970s to 43.4% in 1980s. The marked increase of resectability from 28.1% in 1970s to 69.5% in 1980s was mainly a result of increasing proportion of small HCC in the series (from 12.5 to 31.9%). which was a result of increasing patients from screening (from 25.3% to 41.25). Re-resection of subclinical recurrence was of proved merit to prolong survival further after curative resection [14]. The marked increase of number of re-resection (from 19 to 75 patients) also added weight to the improvement of series 5-year survival, which was actually a special form of screening using AFP and ultrasonography monitoring at 3 months interval to a very high risk group, because the 5-year recurrent rate after curative resection of small HCC was as high as 61.5% [14].

2. Approach to Improve Ultimate Outcome of Patients from Screening

Table 3 showed an increase of 5-year survival of screening patients from 29.0% in 1970s to 47.4% in 1980s. However, the median size of tumor was similar in these two periods, there should be some other factors involved. In Chinese patients with HCC, 86.7% of patients associated with cirrhosis, therefore, the increase of limited resection (from 33.0% to 55.8%) instead of lobectomy has resulted in marked increased of resectability (from 53.9% to 81.1%). The second approach was re-resection for subclinical recurrence, which was done in only 11 patients in 1970s, but went up to 46 patients in 1980s. It has been proved that 10-20% further prolong of 5-year survival could be achieved by re-resection in subclinical stage of recurrence after a curative resection [14]. It was also the opinion in the literature that re-resection was superior to that treated by transarterial embolization for recurrence, the 2-year survival being 34.3-92.3% versus 30.0-64.9% [23].

3. Limitation and Problems Pertaining to HCC Screening

Despite advances made in early detection and treatment of HCC, the limitation, however, includes problem of "cost-effectiveness", the high recurrent rate after resection, as well as the multicentric origin. Instead of natural population screening in 1970s, high risk population(people who has history of hepatitis or serum HBsAg and in the age of 40-65) screening has been conducted in 1980s ; instead of active screening with high cost, regular health checkup including AFP and ultrasonography has been advocated. The accurate evaluation of HCC screening is currently undertaken by a better design after a workshop on screening for HCC [24]. In accordance to the literature, using analysis of integrated HBV-DNA structure, the authors also demonstrated that both unicentric and multicentric origin of recurrence of lesions occurred [26]. The recent findings in authors' institute that immunohistochemistry revealed HBxAg in 59.4% of HCC and surrounding hepatocyte [27], and that the high p53 mutation in HCC was correlated to the site of HBxAg expression, indicating strong background of high recurrent rate even after curative resection.

CONCLUSION

Screening using AFP and/or ultrasonography in high risk population of HCC remained important approach to get early stage HCC. Resection of subclinical HCC has resulted in marked increase of 5-year survival and improve series prognosis. The problems of cost-effectiveness and multicentric origin remained to be investigated.

ACKNOWLEDGEMENT: The authors would express appreciation to Dr. Hong-Wei Wang and Dr. Xue-Sheng Feng for their help in preparing data and manuscript.

REFERENCES

1. Abelev GI (1971). Adv Cancer Res 14: 295-358
2. Masseyeff RF (1973). Gann Monogr Cancer Res 14: 3-18
3. Okuda K, Kotoda K, Obata H, Hayashi N, Hisamitsu T, Tamiya M, Kubo Y, Yakushiji F, Shimokawa Y (1975). Gastroenterology 69: 226-234
4. Coordinating Group for Research on Liver Cancer , China (1974) In Maltoni C (ed) Proc 2nd Internatl Symp Cancer Detection and Prevention. Excerpta Med, Amsterdam pp655-658
5. Sun TT, Wan LC, Chang YL (1979) Clin Med J 92: 17-22
6   Yu YQ, Sang LA (1975) Tumor Prevent Treat Study 3:1-5 (Chin)
7. Tang ZY, Qian SQ (1977) Jiangsu Med 3:501-505 (Chin)
8. Shanghai Coordinating Group for research on Liver Cancer (Tang ZY, Yu EX, Wu CE, Gu XY) (1978) In Canonico A, Estevez O, Chacon R (eds) Adv Med Oncol Res Educ. Pergamon, Oxford. 4: 285-289
9. Tang ZY, Yu YQ, Lin ZY, Zhou XD, Yang BH, Cao YZ, Lu JZ, Tang CL (1979) Chin Med J 59: 35-40
10. Tang ZY, Yang BH, Tang CL, Yu YQ, Lin ZY, Weng HZ (1980) Chin Med J 93: 795-799
11. Tang ZY (1981) Chin Med J 94: 585-588
12. Tang ZY, Ying YY, Gu TJ (1982) In Popper H, Schaffner F (eds) Progress in liver diseases. Vol 7. Grune & Stratton, New York pp637-647
13. Tang ZY, Yu YQ, Zhou XD, Zhou NQ (1983) J Exp Clin Cancer Res 93: 261-268
14. Tang ZY, Yu YQ, Zhou XD (1984) J Exp Clin Cancer Res 3: 359-366
15. Tang ZY (ed) (1985) Subclinical hepatocellular carcinoma. Springer, Berlin pp1-188
16. Tang ZY, Yu YQ (1986) Gann Monogr Cancer Res 31: 185-190
17. Tang ZY, Yu YQ, Yang BH (1987) In Wagner G, Zhang YH (eds) Cancer of the liver, esophagus, and nasopharynx. Springer, Berlin. pp 64-72
18. Tang ZY (1987) In Okuda K, Ishak KG (eds) Neoplasms of the liver. Springer, Tokyo. pp 367-373
19. Tang ZY (1989) In Tang ZY, Wu MC, Xia SS (eds) Primary liver cancer. Springer. Berlin. pp 191-203
20. Tang ZY, Yu YQ, Zhou XD, Ma ZC, Yang R, Lu JZ, Lin ZY, Yang BH (1989) Cancer 64: 536-541
21. Tang ZY (1992) In Tobe T et al(eds) primary liver cancer in Japan. Springer, Tokyo. pp 437-443
22. Heyward WL, Lanier AP, McMahon BJ, Fitzgerald MA, Kilkenny S, Paprocki TR (1985) JAMA 254: 3052-3054
23. Uchino J, Une Y, Nakajima Y, Sato N, Matsuoka S, Kamiyama T, Misawa K, Ishizu H, Ogasawara K (1992) In Tobe T et al (eds) Primary liver cancer in Japan. Springer, Tokyo. pp 353-361
24. McMahon BJ, London T (1991) J Natl Cancer Inst 83: 916-919
25. Sakamoto M, Hirohashi S, Tsuda H, Shimosato Y, Makuuchi M, Hosoda Y (1989) Am J Surg Path 13: 1064-1067
26. Liang XH, Loncarevic IF, Tang ZY, Yu YQ, Zentgraf H, Schroder CH (1991) J Gastroenterol Hepatol 6: 77-80
27. Liang XH, Tang ZY, Shi DR, Ho GP, Hu SQ (1992) Chin J Microbiol Immunol 12: 302-304 (Chin)

Recent Advances in Diagnosis and Surgical Treatment of Pancreatic Cancer

SEIKI MATSUNO[1], MASAO KOBARI[1], YOICHI SAITOH[2], and OSAMU OHASHI[2]

[1]First Department of Surgery, Tohoku University School of Medicine, Sendai, 980 Japan
[2]First Department of Surgery, Kobe University School of Medicine, Kobe, 650 Japan

ABSTRACT

In the present study, we reviewed the recent advances in diagnosis and surgical treatment of pancreatic cancer in Japan. During the period from 1981 to 1990, 11317 patients were collected and analysed at registration commitee of pancreatic cancer in Japan Pancreas Society(JPA). 3743patients(33%) were resected. There were 435 patients(3.8%) with T1 tumors less than 2cm in size and the diagnosis of StageI tumors was made in 274(2.4%)patients. Thirty eight percent of T1 tumors and 38% of StageI tumors were detected by US. Three year survival and 5-year survival according to JPS staging were 64% and 46% in StageI, 35% and 28% in StageII, 24% and 20% in StageIII, and 12% and 8% in StageIV respectively.

KEY WORDS: pancreatic cancer, Stage, Survival rate

INTRODUCTION

In spite of advances in tumor imaging technique and the increase in the resection rate, the prognosis of pancreatic cancer has not been improved as much as expected. The purpose of this study is to review the recent advances in the diagnostic methods and surgical techniques for pancreatic cancer in Japan.

PATIENTS AND METHODS

From 1981 to 1990, 11,317 patients were accumulated for the analysis at the registration commitee of pancreatic cancer of Japan Pancreas Society(JPS). In 4811 patients with head cancer, resection rate was 50%. Resection rate in 1212 patients with body or tail cancer was 42%. Consequently, total resection rate was 33%. Usefulness of each diagnostic methods and survival ratse were compared between each stage of pancreatic cancer.

RESULTS

Table 1 shows the stage classification pancreatic cancer proposed by JPS. Distant metastasis including hepatic metastasis and peritoneal dissemination is classified into stageIV. T indicates size of tumor. No means no lymph node metastasis. N1 is involvement of primary group of lymph nodes situated close to the tumor. N2 is involvement of secondary group of lymph nodes between N1 and N3. N3 is involvement of tertiary group of lymph nodes regarded as juxta-regional lymph nodes. S means anterior serosal invasion. Rp means retroperitoneal invasion. PV indicates invasion to portal vein. Zero is absence of invasion. One is suspected of invasion. Two means definite invasion and threemeans severe invasion. Figure 1 shows the methods of diagnosis according to stage. The most reliable method to make a diagnosis of pancreatic cancer was ultrasonography. In all stages, about 40% of tumor were first detected by US. ERCP was also useful to detect StageI tumor. CT had no advantage in screening the small cancer. In the StageI patients, more than 40% of patients were accompanied with high CA19-9 level of high serum amylase level. As stage progresses, the positive rate of CEA and CA19-9 increased to 80% and 50% respectively.

Table 1. Stage Classification of Japan Pancreas Society

Stage I	T1(<2cm)	No	So	Rp0	PV0
Stage II	T2(2-4cm)	N1	S1	Rp1	PV1
Stage III	T3(4-6cm)	N2	S2	Rp2	PV2
Stage IV	T4(>6cm)	N3	S3	Rp3	PV3

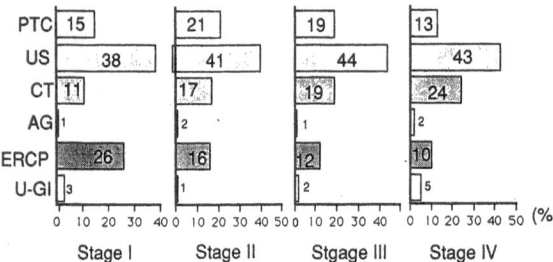

Fig. 1 Method of diagnosis according to stage

The change of resection rate from 1981 until 1991 is shown in Table 2. Resection rate was significantly increased to 41.9% from 25.7% during the last 10 years.

Table 2. Chronological Change of Resection Rate

Type of Operations	1981	1991
	Number of Patients	Number of Patients
Resection	292(25.7)	398(41.9*)
Palliative Operation	545(47.9)	270(28.4)
Exploratory Laparotomy	104(9.2)	73(7.7)
Non-Operation	196(17.2)	209(22.0)
Total	1137(100)	950(100)

( ): %   *: p<0.01

Chronological change of stage in resected cancer is shown in Table 3. The incidence of StageI tumor increased to 8.3% from 4.5% during the last 10 years, furthermore, the number of StageI patients increased to 33 from 10. Total number of patients who underwent cancer resection also increased to 398 from 292.

Three year survival rate was increased from 12.5% in 1983 to 22.9% in 1991 and 5-year survival rate rate was also improved to 16.9% in 1991 from 12.5% in 1985. It is speculated that the increasing number of StageI patients brought about this improvement(Table 4).

In Fig.2 survival rate on the basis of the type of operation. Three year survival rate and 5-year survival rate after resection were 22.4% and 16.6% respectively. Those of palliative surgery or exploratory operation were low as compared with resection. Without resection, most patients were lost within one year. Cancer resection seems to be a only way to get the long survival.

Table 3. Chronological Change of Stage in Resected Pancreatic Cancer

Stage	1981 Number of Patients	1991 Number of Patients
I	13(4.5)	33(8.3**)
II	76(26.0)	94(23.6)
III	86(29.5)	110(27.6)
IV	114(39.0)	152(38.2)
Unknown	3	9
Total	292(100)	398(100)

( ): %   **: p<0.05

Table 4. Chronological Change of Survival Rate in Resected Pancreatic Cancer

3-Year Survival Rate		5-Year Survival Rate	
1983	1991	1985	1991
12.5%	22.9%	12.5%	16.9%
(602)	(3279)	(1148)	(3279)

( ): Number of Resected Patients

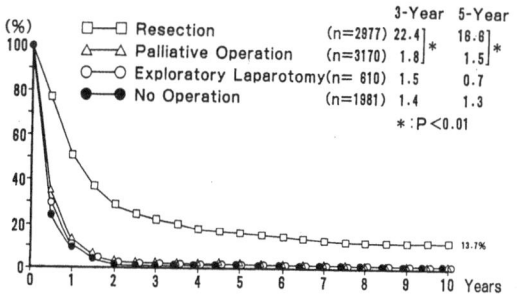

Fig. 2 Survival rate according to type of operation

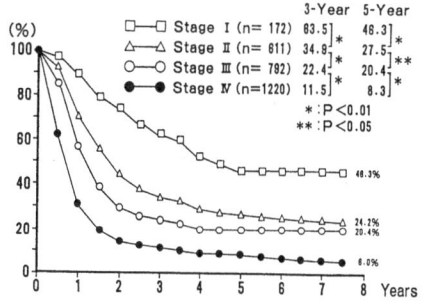

Fig. 3 Survival rate according to stage

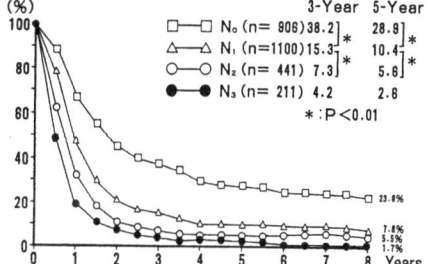

Fig. 4 Survival rate according to lymph node metastasis

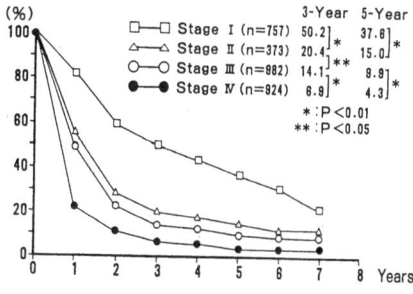

Fig. 5 Survival rate according toUICC stage

Figure 3 shows the survival rate on tne basis of JPS staging. Three year survival rate were 63.5% in StageI, 34.9% in StageII, 22.4% in StageIII, and 11.5% in StageIV. Five year survival rate were 46.3% in StageI, 27.5% in StageII, 20.4% in StageIII, and 8.3% in StageIV. Prognosis was significantly better in the early stage of pancreatic cancer and these differences were statistically significant. Therefore, it is demonstrated that JPS staging is practical to forecast the prognosis of the patients with pancreatic cancer. Total number who survived for more than 5 years reached to 540. In Fig. 4, survival rate according to lymph node metastasis is shown. Five year survival rate were 28.9% in N0, 10.4% in N1, 5.6% in N2, and 2.6% in N3. Survival time of the patients without lymph node metastasis and patients with involvement of only primary group of lymph nodes were significantly longer than that of the patients with involvement of secondary or tertiary group of lymph nodes. These results suggested that the extent of lymph node metastasis was consistent with the prognosis.

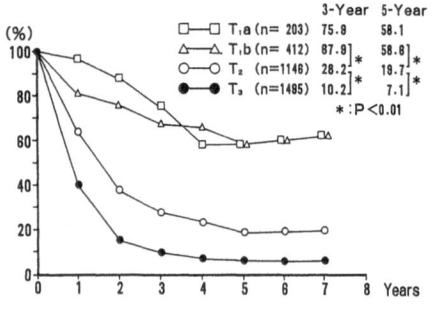

Fig. 6 Survival rate according to UICC T factor

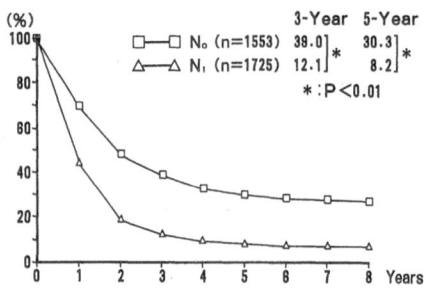

Fig. 7 Survival rate according to UICC N factor

In UICC staging, 3-year survival rate were 50.2% in StageI, 20.4% in StageII, 14.1% in StageIII, and 6.9% in StageIV. As compared with the survival rate analyzed by JPS staging, UICC staging did not bring about distinct differences among 4 groups(Fig. 5).
In Fig. 6, survival rate according to UICC T factor. Three year survival rate in T1a tumor of 75.9% was not significantly higher than that in T1b tumor of 67.9%. However, the rate were 28.2% in T2 tumor and 10.2% in T3 tumor. Survival rate became lower as the T number increased from T1b to T3. There was the same tendency in the 5-year survival rate. UICC T factor also did not coincide with the survival rate. In survival rate according to UICC N factor, 5-year survival rate in N0 patients of 30.3% was significantly higher than 8.2% in N1 patients. If the extent of lymph node metastasis was analyzed more in detail, UICC staging would be more useful to foretell the prognosis(Fig. 7).

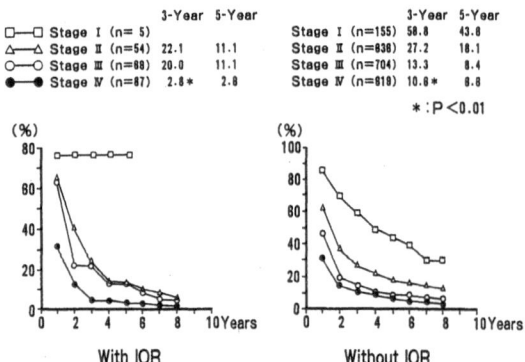

Fig. 8 Survival rate according to intraoperative radiation(IOR)

Effect of intraoperative radiation(IOR) therapy after resection of tumor was shown in Fig.8.In patients with IOR just after tumor resection, 5-year survival rate were 11.1% in StageII, 11.1% in StageIII, and 2.8% in StageIV. On the other hand, without IOR, 5-year survival rate were 43.8% in StageI, 18.1% in StageII, 8.4% in StageIII, and 6.8% in StageIV. So that, IOR is not effective to improve the prognosis in the patients with cancer resection.

DISCUSSION

In this study, it was suggested that as the result of advances in tumor imaging technique, especially ultrasonography, the increasing number of StageI early cancer can be detected, consequently, resection rate has been increasing remarkably to more than 40% which improve the survival rate markedly. It was also indicated that cancer resection is the only modality which result in longer survival, but other treatment modalities such as IOR does not improve survival so far.
Therefore, it is important to make effort to find patients with StageI early pancreatic cancer who can undergo cancer resection.

REFERENCES

1. Japanese Pancreatic Society.(1982) General Rules for Surgical and Pathological Studies on Cancer of the Pancreas. 2nd ed. Tokyo: Kanehara Publishing.
2. Registration Commitee of Pancreatic cancer in Japan Pancreas Society.(1990) Report of registeration during last 10 years. Kobe: Registration Commitee of Pancreatic Cancer.

Part 4

Recent Strategies in the Treatment of Cancer Patients

Endoscopic Mucosal Resection for Early Carcinomas of the Esophagus

HIROYASU MAKUUCHI, TAKAO MACHIMURA, KYOICHI MIZUTANI, KOHJI KANNO, TAKASHI SUGIHARA, YUTAKA TOKUDA, TOMOO TAJIMA, and TOSHIO MITOMI

Department of Surgery, Tokai University School of Medicine, Isehara, Kanagawa, Japan

ABSTRACT

Recently, the rate of detection of early and superficial esophageal cancer has increased particularly with the development of panendoscopy and endoscopic staining techniques in Japan. The intra-epithelial and intra-mucosal carcinomas not extending to the muscularis mucosae did not have vascular invasion or lymph node metastases. Thus we have employed endoscopic mucosal resection for these patients. In this paper, we explained the technique of endoscopic mucosal resection in detail, focusing on the endoscopic mucosal resection tube(EEMR-tube) method which we devised originally. This method was employed in more than 85 cases and 107 lesions of early esophageal cancers.

KEY WORDS: early esophageal cancer, endoscopic treatment, endoscopic mucosal resection

INTRODUCTION

The recent development of endoscopic technique has greatly improved the diagnosis of esophageal carcinoma. Therefore, the number of patients with early and superficial carcinomas of the esophagus have markedly increased in Japan. The factors contributing to the diagnosis of these early stages of esophageal carcinomas include: (1) widespread use of direct esophageal visualization by the slender-diameter fiberscope, and (2) widespread use of chromoendoscopy, especially iodine staining as well. Formerly we had employed surgical resection for all esophageal cancer patients without major operative risk. But the surgical operation for esophageal cancer is highly invasive and the post operative quality of life is often poor. In this paper, we examined the indication of endoscopic mucosal resection, established the technique for early esophageal cancer using the endoscopic mucosal resection tube(EEMR-tube), and analyzed the results.

MATERIALS AND METHODS

The Relationship Between the Depth of Invasion and Lymph Node Metastasis and Vascular Invasion

The relationship between the depth of invasion and lymph node metastases and also vascular invasion was examined in 99 cases who underwent radical surgical operation. Each of the proper mucosal layer and the submucosal layer was divided into three as mm1, mm2, and mm3 of the proper mucosal layer, and sm1, sm2, and sm3 of the submucosal layer. The prognosis was also analyzed.

Invention of Endoscopic Mucosal Resection Tube (EEMR-tube)

We devised the silicon rubber tube for esophageal mucosal resection. The tube is 60 cm in length, 14 mm in internal diameter and 18 mm in external diameter. The tube is equipped with a side channel to pass a snare and with a balloon at the proximal end of the tube to keep the air tight inside the tube.

94

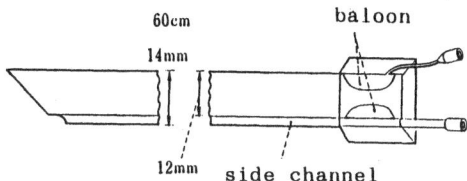

Fig.1 EEMR-tube

Procedure of the EEMR-tube Method

1: A fiberscope is first passed through the EEMR-tube and the fiberscope alone is inserted into the esophagus. The EEMR-tube is then passed along the fiberscope into the esophageal lumen. Staining with iodine is performed to confirm the site of the lesion and then, saline is injected to swell the submucosa. (Fig 3-a)

2: A snare is passed through a side channel of the tube and is opened to enclose the lesion. (Fig 3-b)

3: Using suction through the fiberscope, the lesion is drawn into the guide tube by negative pressure. (Fig 3-c)

4: Then the snare strangulates the mucosa surrounding the lesion and current is passed to resect it. (Fig 3-d)

5: The resected specimen is retrieved by grasping forceps or basket forceps. (Fig 3-e)

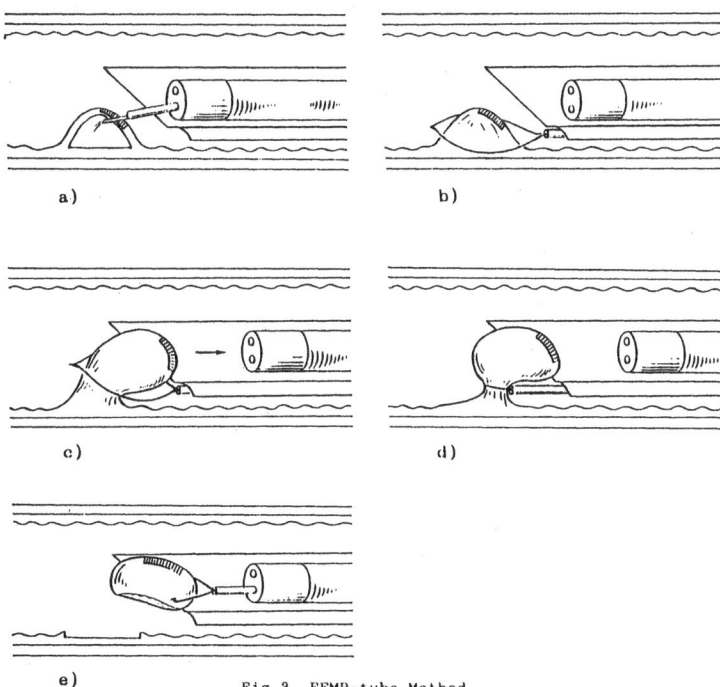

a) b) c) d) e)

Fig.3 EEMR-tube Method

Application of Endoscopic Mucosal Resection

The endoscopic mucosal resection was employed in more than 85 cases and 107 lesions. Among them, 92 lesions were superficial esophageal cancer, 6 lesions were dysplasia, 3 lesions of erosion at the esophagogastric mucosal junction were suspicious of esophageal carcinoma, one was a case of a protrusion in Barrett's esophagus, and remaining 5 lesions were benign tumors.

RESULTS

The Relationship Between The Depth of Invasion and Lymph Node Metastasis and Vascular Invasion

The majority of intra-epithelial and intra-mucosal carcinomas did not have vascular invasion or lymph node metastases, with only four exceptions of which three had vascular invasion and one had lymph node metastasis. These lesions invaded very near to the muscularis mucosae. However, in carcinomas which invaded the submucosal layer, 31.7% had lymph node metastases and 73.3% had vascular or lymphatic invasion, thus increasing the likelihood of metastasis. Actually, the prognosis of the lesion which was limited within the mucosal layer, the 5-year survival rate was 100%. But in contrast for the submucosal carcinoma the survival rate fell down to 55.1%.

depth of invasion	no. of cases	vessels invasion		lymph node metastases	
		(−)	(+)	(−)	(+)
ep	14	14	0 (0%)	14	0 (0%)
mm	25	22	3 (12.0%)	24	1 (4.0%)
sm	60	16	44 (73.3%)	41	19 (31.7%)

Table 1. Depth of Invasion vs Vessels Invasion and Lymph node Metastases in Superficial Esophageal Cancer

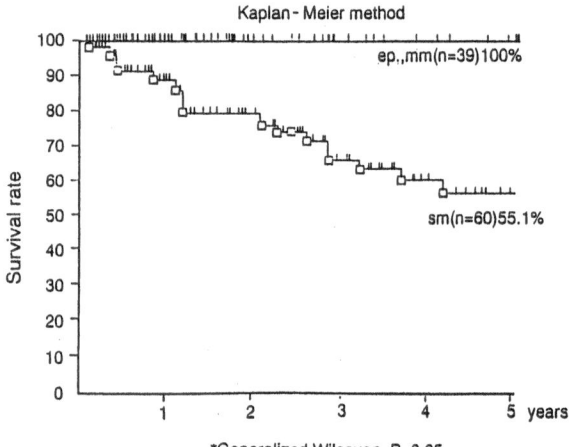

Fig.2 Survival rate of the patients with superficial esophageal cancer

The Results of Endoscopic Mucosal Resection

Eighty-eight lesions were resected completely, and incomplete resections were in 10 lesions, which were added irradiation or heater probe therapy. As for complications, esophageal perforation was occurred in 2 cases and subcutaneous emphysema was caused in 1 case. However, they were successfully treated conservatively. There were 4 cases with arterial bleeding controlled easily by endoscopy and in addition, one case, in which bleeding from an esophageal varix could be controlled by endoscopic sclerotherapy. There was no case with complications requiring surgery. No recurrence was recognized within 5-year observation.

DISCUSSION

From the year 1986, the number of cases of superficial esophageal carcinoma have started to increase and the incidence accelerated even more in the last three years. Furthermore, this increase not only refers to the number of cases of superficial esophageal carcinoma, but also reflects recently an increase in the number of intra-epithelial carcinomas and intra-mucosal carcinomas. Out of 703 cases of thoracic esophageal carcinomas that were treated at the Department of Surgery, Tokai University School of Medicine,

180 cases (25.6%) were superficial carcinomas. Among these 180 patients, 52 cases were intra-epithelial cancers, 51 were limited within the proper mucosal layer, and 70 were submucosal cancers. Thus, the treatment strategy of superficial esophageal carcinoma in our institution is as follows. If we preoperatively diagnose that a lesion is limited to the mucosal layer, namely, if a lesion exists in the epithelial layer or the proper mucosal layer not extending to the muscularis mucosae, we employ an endoscopic mucosal resection. And if a lesion is invading to the muscularis mucosae or the submucosal layer, we would perform a radical surgical operation with wide lymph node dissection in the neck, thorax and abdomen. The indications for endoscopic mucosal resection of esophageal cancer are as follows:(1) intra-epitherial or mucosal cancer not extending to the muscularis mucosae, (2) 2cm or less lesion invading part in the proper mucosal layer, and (3) not more than 5 lesions in the esophagus. And as relative indication, in operative submucosal cancer cases with high operative risks can be applied, if swollen lymph nodes are not recognized on endoscopic ultrasonogram and / or CT.

There are 3 methods of trans-endoscopic mucosal resection of the esophagus. The first is double channel method. Using a 2-channel fiberscope, the lesion is grasped by grasping forceps and the snare is strangulated, then current is passed through the snare to resect. This method is popular to be employed for early gastric carcinoma in Japan. The second is cutting polypectomy method. The area surrounding the lesion is cut with a high frequency cutter, the lesion is lifted up by the forceps, and a snare is used to electrosurgically resect it. This method is very difficult and also dangerous. The third is our original guide tube method. Using a silicon rubber guide tube for esophageal mucosal resection, the lesion is drawn into the tube by aspiration and the area including the lesion is resected using a snare. This method is the best because this method is : (1) extremely simple and time saving, requiring about 10-15 minutes to resect one lesion, (2) a 4-5 cm mucosal specimen can be obtained in one piece, (3) the lesion is not damaged compared to the double channel method, (4) if necessary, resections can be repeated, and (5) there is little danger of complications. Surgical procedures for cancer of the esophagus are highly invasive, requiring thoracotomy, laparotomy, and lymph node dissection of the three fields such as cervical, intrathoracic, and abdominal, and as a result, the postoperative quality of life can be seriously impaired. It would be likely to increase the detectability of early stage lesions which could be endoscopically treated.

REFERENCES

1. Makuuchi H.,Machimura T.,Mizutani K.,Shimada H.,Kanno K.,Tokuda Y.,Sugihara T.,Tajima T.,Mitomi T. (1992) Diagnostic accuracy of endoscopy in estimating the depth of invasion of superficial esophageal carcinoma. Stomach and Intestine 27: 175-184
2. Makuuchi H., Machimura T.,Soh Y.,Mizutani K.,Shimamura H.,Tokuda Y.,Sugihara T.,Sasaki T.,Tajima T.,Mitomi T. (1991) Endoscopic mucosectomy for mucosal carcinomas in the esophagus. Jpn J Gastroenterol Surg. 24: 2599-2603
3.   Makuuchi H.,Machimura T.,Mizutani K.,Shimada H.,Kanno K.,Sugihara T.,Sasaki T., Mitomi T. (1992) Endoscopic surgery for superficial esophageal cancer. Operation 46: 603-609

Endoscopic Surgery for Gastric Cancer

Yoshiki Hiki, Hitoshi Shimao, and Hiroyoshi Mieno

Department of Surgery, Kitasato University School of Medicine, Sagamihara, Kanagawa, 228 Japan

ABSTRACT

Application of endoscopic treatment for early gastric cancer seem to have been widely accepted in the recent years. To establish the indication of endoscopic therapy for early gastric cancer, results of 2072 surgery were reviewed:survival rate, complication, and lymph node metastasis. Local treatment by surgical endoscopy can eradicate early gastric cancer without lymph node metastasis. 631 cases of operated single early gastric cancer were studied to confirm which type of early gastric cancer has no lymph node metastasis.
In using the mucosal resection method, a physiological saline solution is injected by means of a needle into the periphery of the lesion, thus inflating the lesion. Forceps are applied to the building portion to further raise the lesion and snare is set around for resection by high frequency coagulation. The Nd-Yag Laser with a power output of 50-70 Watt and irradiation time of 0.5 to 1.0 second was employed in the endoscopic laser therapy. We concluded that our endoscopic treatment is the ideal method for currative treatment of special type of early gastric cancer. Especially small tumor less than 1cm in size, ca.in situ and with no associated ulcer, those cases are most suitable, and absolute indication for the endoscopic treatment, and I think it is very excellent procedure as a minimally invasive surgery for gastric surgery.

KEYWORDS: early gastric cancer, endoscopic surgery, endoscopic resection,
          laser irradiation, minimally invasive surgery

INTRODUCTION

Why is endoscopic tretment necessary in the treatment of early gastric cancer? What motivated us to develop this procedure? We developed this technique with the expectation that it will circumvent the various problems that are encountered after conventional gastrectomy for early gastric cancer[1]. The various problems encountered during the post-operative period in 331 patients who underwent conventional gastrectomy for early gatric cancer within the past 5 years. The 3 factors evaluated were as follows:1) complications, 2) operative deaths, and 3) post-operative complaints. Which kinds of operations constitute the so-called "minimally invasive" surgeries? First, there is modified gastric resection which is a conventional surgical technique (open abdominal surgery). The original technique included total omentectomy[2], but the modified version leaves a portion of the omentum intact. Second, there is local resection. Local resection can be performed either by open abdominal surgery or by the recently developed laparoscopic surgical technique[3]. Both approached involve full-thickness resection of the focus of cancer and its surrounding tissues. Third, there is endoscopic treatment. This method approaches the cancer endoscopically. The lesion is removed or eradicated from inside the stomach by resection of cancerous tissues including the mucosa[4] or by destroying the cancer using lasers or microwaves[1,5].

MATERIALS AND METHOD
From July, 1971, over the following 19 years, the operations performed at the Department of Surgery at Kitasato University Hospital on gastric

cancer have totalled 2072 cases, of which 788 were in their early stage. In all of these 788 cases, especially a total of 631 cases of the single early gastric cancer, we performed a pathological examination with the aim of studying the metastasis in the lymph nodes. Further, from 1981 and over the subsequent 10 years, our Department of Endoscopy has performed endoscopic resection on 53 early stage gastric cancer cases; and in 100 cases, we carried out a laser therapy. The steps to be followed in endoscopic resection are outlined below:

1) Methylene blue is sprayed on the gastric mucosa endoscopically using the dye scattering method[Figure.1,2].
2) Tumor size is measured by a 6mm rubber disk.
3) The tissues surrounding the lesion is marked by the tattoo method.
4) To facilitate resection of the lesion, saline solution is injected into the submucosa layer.
5) A snare is applied to the tissues surrounding the lesion, and the lesion is elevated using grasping forceps. The snare is then tightened at the root of the lesion.
6) The lesion is resected using an electrotome[Fig.3].

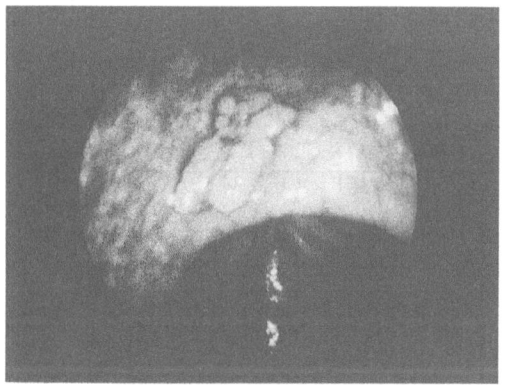 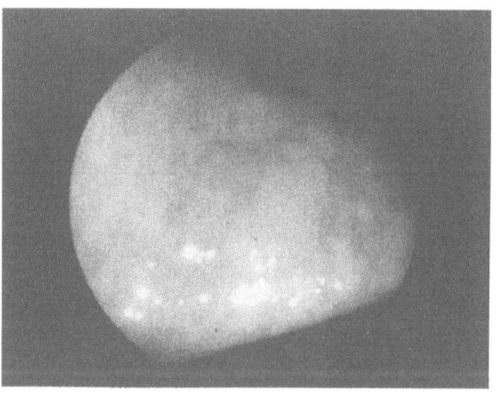

Fig.1 Dye scattering method for gatroscopy. The elevated lesion clearly in this picture.

Fig.2 Normal endoscopic view of the same lesion. It is not so easy to exactly identify the lesion.

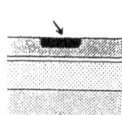 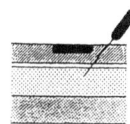 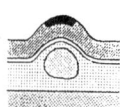 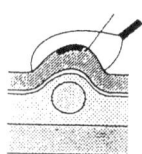 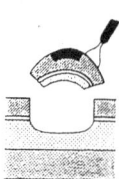

Fig.3 The method of endoscopic resection for early gastric cancer.

Next, I will describe laser endoscopy.
The first 3 steps are identical to those of the resection method as described in the previous section. The last step, laser irradiation is initiated from the margins of the lesion and continued circumferentially and toward the center of the lesion. Finally, the whole lesion is irradiated. Laser treatment is conducted by using a Nd.Yag Laser. The optical-fiber is passed through the Biopsy Channel of the Endoscope, inserted into the abdomen, and the laser beam is then irradiated on the cancer lesion. The laser can be placed directly on the surface of the mucos membrane (the contact method), or it can be irradiated from 2cm away (the non-contact method). It is essential that the laser beam be irradiated at 70w to 100w/1 sec., and that the therapy be performed by repeated irradiation.

RESULTS

A metastasis in the lymph node of an early gastric cancer

Table 1 shows, relationship between lymph node metastasis and endoscopic type. Among the protruted type of early gastric cancer, if tumor size is less than 2.5cm in diameter, there was no lymph node metastasis. In contrast to that, among the depressed type cases, with lesion size less than 2.0cm associated with no ulcer or no ulcer scar, ulcer minus there was no metastasis. In mixed type cases with lesion size less than 1.5cm in diameter, there was no metastasis. This is the retrospective study at our university hospital. A total of 631 cases of the simple E.G.Ca., not multiple cancer, which was operated has been examined[Table 2].

Table 1. Lymphnode metastasis in early gastric cancer resected early gastric cancer 631 cases -size and macroscopic type-

(mm)	1-5	6-10	11-15	16-20	21-25	26-30	31-	Total(%)
Type ⌐‾⌐	0/ 1	0/ 2	0/ 6	0/ 7	0/ 5	1/12	5/ 35	6/ 68 (8.8)
Type - ‾⌐_	0/13	0/33	0/44	0/23	1/17	1/11	5/ 41	7/182 (3.8)
+	0/ 2	1/17	1/27	2/24	1/37	3/33	31/160	39/300(13.0)
Mixed Type	-	0/ 3	0/ 4	2/10	3/10	0/12	10/ 42	15/ 81(18.5)
Total	0/16	1/55	1/81	4/64	5/69	5/68	51/278	67/631
(%)	(0.0)	(1.8)	(1.2)	(6.3)	(7.2)	(7.4)	(18.3)	(10.6)

-:without associated ulcer   1971-1990.12, Kitasato Univ.
+:with associated ulcer

Table 2. Lymphnode metastasis in early gastric cancer resected early gastric cancer 631 cases -size and depth of invasion-

(mm)	1-5	6-10	11-15	16-20	21-25	26-30	31-	Total (%)
m	0/16	0/39	0/49	0/38	1/32	0/37	5/118	6/329(1.8)
sm	-	1/16	1/32	4/26	4/37	5/31	46/160	61/302(20.2)
Total	0/16	1/55	1/81	4/64	5/69	5/68	51/278	67/631
(%)	(0.0)	(1.8)	(1.2)	(6.3)	(7.2)	(7.4)	(18.3)	(10.6)

1971-1990.12, Kitasato Univ.

Problems of surgical treatment

We examined the problem of surgical treatment of the stomach cancer that we operated 322 cases ourselves during this 5 years period.

1. Operation death
The operation death, that is death within a month after the operation, there is one case of 322 patients, that was 0.3% in insidence.

2. Post-operative complication
The second problems post-operative complication. The post-operative ileus on early gastric carcinoma. Number of post-operative ileus was 49 cases among those operative early gastric carcinoma, 322 cases during this 5 years period. The rate of occurrence for post-operative ileus was 15.2%.

3. Post-operative complaint
We examined, change of food intake, change of body weight, and performance status after the conventional operation for early gastric cancer.

Especially, we must draw attention to change of body weight. The decrease of post-operated body weight was remarkable to an advanced age of over eighty.

The results of endoscopic resections(over all)

All patients had been followed up for more than 1 year. Endoscopic
resection was performed in 79 patients (81 lesions) as initial treatment.
Of those, tumor removal was complete in 51 lesions (62.3%) resected.
Pathological examination revealed that tumor removal was incomplete in
31 resected lesions. Although many of the patients in this group
subsequently underwent open abdominal surgery (gastrectomy), surgery could
not be performed in 13 patients. These 13 patients underwent laser
irradiation, and complete tumor removal was successful in 12 of them.

The results from laser treatment(over all)

56 lesions were initially treated by laser irradiation. Of these lesions,
complete tumor eradication was successful in 42 lesions(75%). 14 patients
from this group are either still undergoing treatment or have died from
other diseases.

The results of tumor size and procedure

The relationship between size of the early gastric tumors and treatment
results was evaluated. Results were from patients who had been followed
up for more than a year. When the tumor size was within 10mm, the tumor-
free rate after the procedure was 81.4% with endoscopic resection. With
laser treatment the tumor-free rate after the prodedure was 100%. The
tumor-free rate after the prodedure for tumor 11mm to 15mm in size was
59.1% for endoscopic resection, and 76.9% for laser treatment[Table 7].

Table 3. Results(Tumor size and procedure)

	<10 mm	11-15 mm
ER	35/43 (81.4%)	13/22 (59.1%)
Laser	14/14 (100.0%)	10/13 (76.9%)

DISCUSSION

What are some of the advantages of endoscopic treatment?
First, endoscopic treatment is much less invasive than conventional surgery.
Furthermore, the required period of stay in the hospital after the procedure
is much shorter compared to conventional surgery.
Moreover, endoscopic treatment is more advantageous from a cost-benefit
standpoint because it is less costly. Are there any drawbacks to this
prodedure? The technique, unfortunately, cannot be used in all stages
of gastric cancer. The technique is only indicated for treatment of early
gastric cancer, particularly that of microcancer. Second, unlike in open
abdominal surgery, lymph node cannot be removed. Third, the operator must
have highly sophisticated endoscopic skills; he must be experienced not
only in a single technique but in many techniques. Several new diagnostic
techniques are being used in selecting patients who can be treated by
endoscopic surgery.
First, there is the dye scattering method[6]. This diagnostic method
accurately evaluates the horizontal spread of the cancer. Second, there
is endoscopic ultrasonography (EUS)[7].
This diagnostic method is used to assess the depth of tumor invasive; it
is also useful in detecting the presence of ulcerations or scars in the
cancerous lesion[8].
Indecations for treatment by endoscopic surgery should be evaluated from
the perspective of spread of the cancer to the lymph nodes. Two factors
have to be considered when determining indications for endoscopic surgery.
The 2 factors are: 1) tumor size, and 2) type of endoscopic classification
of the tumor. The relarionship among these 2 factors and extent of spread
to the lymph nodes will also have to be clinically explored. Now, I would
like to describe the principles on which we base our clinical decisions

regarding endoscopic treatment. Our technique of first choice for curative treatment is endoscopic resection. This way a specimen for histopathological examination can be obtained at the same time[Fig.4].

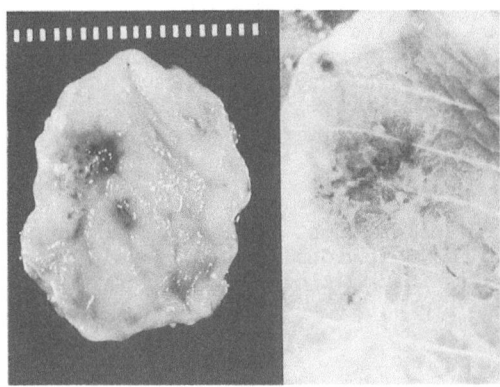

Fig.4 A speciment after endoscopic resection. After observation using binocular scope,the speciment is cutten each 2mm to examine a histo-pathological findings.

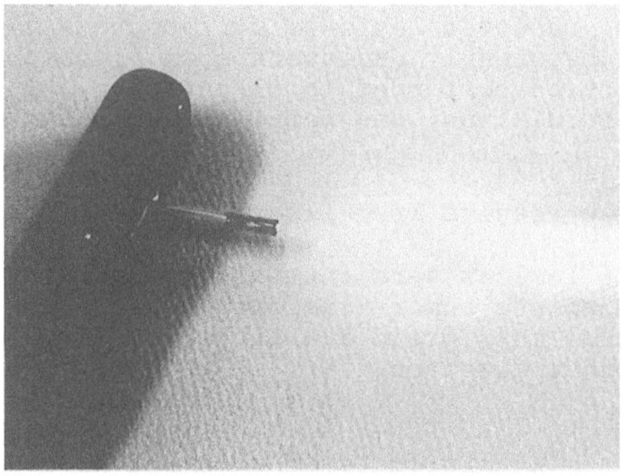

Fig.5 We developed a new laser optical fiber to use for side view endoscope.

If tumor cells stil remain after the initial treatment, conventional open abdominal surgery will have to be performed for resection of the remaining tumor. However, when the clinical status of the patient does not allow for such an option, the remaining tumor cells will have to be laser-irradiated endoscopically. If both endoscopic resection and open abdominal surgery are impossible in a patient due to reasons of tumor location[Fig.5] or size, the first choice intial treatment is laser irradiation. If initial treatment was by lasr irradiation, endoscopic biopsy is repeated at regular intervals. Additional laser treatment is performed when required. Laparoscopic operations for early gastric cancer stand somewhere between modified gastrectomy and endoscopic resection in terms of invasiveness. More precise but less invaseve surgical techniques will surely be developed in the future.

CONCLUSION

1. Endoscopic treatment is a useful mode of therapy for early gastric cancer because from our experience, complications and patient complaints are less frequently encountered after it than after conventional gastric resection.
2. while the results of modified gastric resection are still being evaluated, treatment techniques with less invasiveness are being developed.
3. Endoscopic resection for early gastric cancer is the least invasive technique so far developed for that purpose. We here report the results from our study in which we evaluated endoscopic treatment for early gastric cancer.
4. Naturally, there are limitations regarding treatment indicatinos as well as the effectiveness of this technique.
5. We have begun our research in laparoscopc gastric resection. We believe that laparoscopic gastric resection can overcome many of the limitations encountered with endoscopic resection. Larger tumor sections can be resected by this method than by the intraluminal approach (endoscopic resection).
6. The laparoscopic procedure will widen the indications of endoscopic therapy for treatment of early gastric cancer.

Soon, removal of regional lymph nodes will be possible by this method.

REFERENCES

1.Hiki Y (1991) Endoscopic Treatment for Gastric Cancer from the Surgical perspective. Gastroenterological Endoscopy 33:2285-2299
2.Kajitani T (1992) Kajitani's Surgical Atlas of the Gastrointestinal Tract Cancer. Kanehara Co.Ltd. Tokyo
3.Ohgami M, Kumai K, Kitajima M (1993) Laparoscopic Wedge Resection of the Stomach for Early Gastric Cancer(Lesion Lifting Method). Progress of Digestive Endoscopy 42:in press
4.Tada M, Takemoto T (1989) Endoscopic treatment for early gastric cancer by "strip biopsy method". Gastroenterological Endoscopy 1:155-159
5.Nagai Y, Katsumi M, Tabuse K (1986) Endoscopic treatment for early gastric cancer using microwave coagulation. Gastroenterological Endoscopy 28:1511-1517
6.Hiki Y, Shimao H, Mieno H, Sakakibara Y (1991) Endoscopic treatment of gastric cancer. Surgical Endoscopy 5:11-13
7.Hiki Y, Shimao H, Mieno H, Sakakibara Y (1992) Laser Therapy for Early Upper Gastrointestinal Carcinoma. Surgical Clinics of North America 72:571-580
8.Kida M, Saigenji K, Hiki Y (1988) A study on the hearing process of gastric ulcer using endoscopic ultrasonography(EUS). Stomach and Intestine 23:502-510

Radio-Immunoguided Surgery for Large Bowel Cancer

Ian C. Lavery

Cleveland Clinic Foundation, Cleveland, OH 44195, USA

ABSTRACT

The intra-operative detection of metastatic disease in colorectal cancer depends on tumor-associated antigen and antibodies a- well as detection technology. A hand-held gamma detecting probe is capable of detecting as few as 6×10^5 labelled cells in vitro.

In a multicentre phase 1-11 study using B72.3 with 1^{125} 105 patients (26 primary, 72 recurrent, 6 no tumor) were enrolled. There was 78% localization - 24/32 primary tumors 126/199 recurrent sites. Occult tumor was detected in 30 sites in 26 patients. There was an impact on management in approximately 1/3 of recurrent cases.

Of 17 patients for complete excision of recurrent tumor, 10 had complete excision and 7 recurred in 1 year. Four with elevated CEA had no tumor found, 2 had widespread metastases (no resection), 1 had bilateral radio uptake and biopsy -negative tumor-free at 3 years.

A current Phase II study is being conducted using MoAle CC49 labelled with 1-2 Mci with primary tumor localization 86% and 97% in second look metastases.

DISCUSSION

The use of monoclonal antibodies in surgery is founded on the work of Kohler and Milstein who described a technique to produce monoclonal antibodies in 1975.[1] It is hoped the development of monoclonal antibodies to the epitopes of tumor cells will enable investigation of the cellular elements of tumors, improved detection and therapy of cancer. Antibodies to various tumors have been produced. These are, however, not tumor specific. Antigens from tumor cells may be from the cytoplasm or the cell surfaces, and may be found in normal cells of a number of different tissues. The antigens do occur in higher concentration in neoplastic cells than normal cells. This allows quantification and differentiation of cells. The hybridoma technique allows the production of isolated antibodies to specific antigens.

Gold and Freedman[2] isolated carcinoembryonic antigen in 1965. CEA is found in large bowel cancer and since it was isolated, numerous studies using antibodies to CEA have been reported. Hundreds of monoclonal antibodies to neoplasms have been identified and the number of potential antibodies is probably unlimited. As tumor-associated antigens occur on normal cells, the successful application of antibody techniques will depend on the selection of antigens that occur in much larger quantities on tumor cells than normal cells. Neoplastic cells are heterogeneous. This creates problems in selecting antibodies within the same tumor and results in problems in detection and therapy of metastatic lesions. Poste, et al.[3] have shown in a mouse model using an uncloned melanoma line that some of the metastases had different metastatic properties from the original neoplasm.

When an antibody is labelled, the immunoreactivity must not be destroyed. Advantages and disadvantages exist for different isotopes. Iodine is distributed evenly, but deiodination of the antibody may take place as it is sequestered in the thyroid or attaches to other circulating proteins. Indium is more stable, but is selectively concentrated in the liver, making it unsuitable

for the detection of hepatic metastases. There are also questions relating
to the use of whole tumor-associated antigens or fragments of IgG. One might
anticipate that molecules of a larger molecular weight might be less permeable
to the vascular wall and have more difficulty reaching the receptor sites.
Fragments of immunoglobulin are smaller than whole igG and there is indirect
evidence that antibody fragments localize in tumor in greater numbers than the
whole immunoglobulin.[4] This may be due to the finding of O'Connor and Bale[5]
that the neovascularity of tumor is more permeable than normal vessel walls.

Murine monoclonal antibodies used in colorectal cancer are anti-CEA, B72.3
19.9, 17.1A, SP-25, 79 IT/36, 250 - 30.6. All have varying capabilities of
identifying colon cancers dependent on their individual characteristics.

17-1A antibodies are specific for membrane-bound antibodies while anti-CEA
antigen and B72.3 detect colon cancer and shed antigen in the blood stream.
The clinical use of radio-immunoguided surgery is a new field which was first
described in an experimental model in a nude mouse.[6] Following this, in early
clinical studies[7], colon cancer not identified by conventional means of detection was found in 18% of patients. Using immunohistochemical assays and radio-
immunoassays, monoclonal antibody B72.3 identified 80% of colon cancers.[8] The
monoclonal antibody is not specific, reacting with ovarian, breast and other
gastrointestinal cancers to varying degrees. The in vitro studies were consistent with clinical data generated in intra-operative studies by Martin, et
al.[9]

The ability to detect radiolabelled isotopes intraoperatively is provided by
hand-held devices which have auditory and visual signals. Aitken, et al.[6]
described its successful experimental use and a case report in 1984. The
probe is hand-held and easily directed to tumors or suspicious areas and placed
in close proximity to the tumor. The ability to be as close as possible is
important when one considers the inverse square law which is important in measuring the intensity of radiation detected from a small source of radiation.
The design of the detector and the inverse square law allow detection of these
small sources against the presence of circulating isotope in the background.
The ability to bring the probe within a few millimeters of the source allows
high ratios of source to background to be achieved.

Important in the consideration of intra-operative scanning with a hand-held
gamma probe is the isotope used. The isotope chosen is different from that
used for external imaging. The radiation emitted from the high energy isotopes ^{111}In and ^{131}I used in external imaging is very penetrating, and the
hand-held gamma detecting probe cannot accommodate detector crystals sufficiently thick to be efficient. The hand-held probe has a small detector and
will register a low energy isotope more efficiently. ^{125}I is a low energy
isotope that has several advantages. It has a comparatively long half-life
(60 days) and has a tissue half-length of approximately 2.5 cm. Emissions
from the background are absorbed in layers of tissue which helps to improve
tumor to background ratio. The longer half-life allows the clinician to wait
longer until the background levels are excreted to improve tumor-to-background
ratios. This makes the assumption that the antibody-isotope conjugate remains
attached to the tumor or is lost at a slower rate than circulating conjugate.
Clinically this is apparent. The optimum time between injection and probing
is influenced by the type of monoclonal antibody and fragments. Circulating
immune complexes and antigen shedding from the tumor cell surface may be variables that alter the time.

The monoclonal antibody B72.3 with ^{125}I as the radionuclide is now being
investigated. B72.3 has been studied in tissue sections, nude mouse xenografts and patients.[10,11] The antibody is an IgG_1 sublcass and recognizes
mucin glycoprotein TAG-72. ^{125}I is a weak gamma emitting isotope, with a 60-
day half-life suitable for use with the Neoprobe^R unit with its sophisticated
micorprocessor that eliminates background counts. The system has been evaluated in phase I/II and Phase III studies. I mgm of B72.3 combined with 2 mCi
of ^{125}I has been shown to be relatively non-toxic. The mechanism used in
clinical studies has been to obtain baseline evaluations, including history and
physical examination as for any large bowel cancer. CBC, CEA and coagulation
studies and T_3 uptakes and TSH are documented. Because of the use of ^{125}I,
SSKI is administered to block the thyroid gland. It is given 10 drops bid for
2 days prior to the injection of ^{125}I B72.3 monoclonal antibody.

Vital signs are taken before the injection and at intervals for 1 hour after injection. After the injection, external probe counts are taken, using the hand-held gamma detecting probe. The thyroid, breast, liver, spleen and abdomen are counted using two-second counts. Counting is done one week, two weeks and three weeks after injection. This counting measures the activity of the blood pool background. When the average of three two-second counts is $\leq$ 20 counts/2 seconds, it is considered that conditions are favorable for obtaining the appropriate 2:1 ratios at laparotomy.

At operation, conventional laparotomy is performed to assess the extent of the disease and stage the tumor clinically. Obvious tumor sites are assessed using the probe. The tumor site and adjacent tissue are counted for two seconds. This establishes the tumor to normal tissue ratio. A complete exploration of the abdomen is undertaken scanning with the probe. All node bearing areas are examined. This includes regional lymph nodes, para aortic nodes, and periportal lymph nodes. The liver is also examined. Any areas showing increased radioactivity uptake ($\geq$ 20 counts per 2 seconds) compared with normal adjacent tissue are regarded as being suspicious for containing tumor. Biopsies are taken.

Judgments on the most appropriate treatment are made based on clinical and probe findings. If technically possible, and there are no other contraindications, the planned resection may be extended to allow removal of all detectable tissue. If the probe detects tumor in an area that is not able to be removed, indicating the disease is incurable, the planned procedure is again reassessed. There may be lesser procedures performed and adjunctive therapy instituted.

Following a preliminary study by Martin at Ohio State University,[12] a multi-center study was performed. One hundred and five patients with colorectal cancer were entered into the study, 104 were able to be evaluated. One patient had an acute hypersensitivity reaction to the skin test and was not injected with the antibody. There were 26 patients with primary cancer and 78 recurrent or suspected recurrent cancers. In the recurrent group, no tumor was found in 6 patients. Insufficient time has elapsed to allow further meaningful follow-up evaluation of these six patients. HAMA developed in 40% of patients within 5 weeks.

Using the gamma detecting probe, tumor localization occurred in 78% of patients. This was in 24/32 (75%) of sites in primary tumors and 126/199 (63%) with recurrent colorectal cancers. Of all tumor sites, 9.2% were clinically occult. These sites were identified with the probe and confirmed histologically. In the 26 patients with primary tumors, additional occult tumors were detected and resected in eight instances. Thirty-seven patients with recurrent cancers were unresectable. In 27% of these patients, the decision not to perform a resection was based on data derived with the probe during the operative procedure. Thirty-five patients with recurrent tumor underwent resection. Twenty-three percent had the procedure extended based on information obtained with the probe.

The more conventional and readily available means of testing for disease remote from the primary tumor are effective in identifying gross disease. There are a large group of patients who develop a rising CEA with no disease detected on C.T. scans and M.R.I. scans. Laparotomy is frequently unrewarding in these cases also. Intraoperative use of the gamma detecting probe enhances our ability to detect tumor in these cases but has not been 100% effective.

A more recent study using CC_{49} MoAb has been undertaken. Seven of 8 primary tumors localized with histological confirmation. In the 8 patients, 10 sites which were away from the regional drainage were detected. These were liver, pancreas, supra pancreatic LN and gastrohepatic lymph nodes, positive to the probe. Eight of the sites were not confirmed histologically, though further sections are being taken.

Future uses of monoclonal antibodies in colon surgery include: Immunolymphoscintigraphy which shows some promise of imaging. The technique is similar to colloid lymphoscintigraphy. A radiolabelled antibody is administered in the lymphatic drainage field and sequesters in the metastatic tumor in the draining lymph nodes.[13,14] This technique has been used in breast cancer and raises a number of questions of clinical significance. Early studies injecting MoAb cc49 labelled with 1^{131} adjacent to rectal cancer has not been rewarding. The conjugate did not disperse to the lymph nodes, but remained at the site of ingestion.

The results of using antibodies to tumor-associated antigens for therapy have so far been disappointing. The development of antibodies raised many hopes and possibilities for cancer therapy, but more investigation is needed to realize what appears to be theoretically possible. Antitumor antibodies labelled with ^{131}I have been used most frequently. The basis for this has been that the emission from the ^{131}I may cause lysis of cells. Specific localization of the isotope to neoplastic cells is necessary to prevent damage to normal tissue. With several different isotopes for a variety of tumor types, there are reports of remission, but no cures.

Significant progress has been made in the preparation and development of antibodies. Methods of antibody-nuclide conjugation have improved, but no tumor specific antibody has been found. Further success may be found in the concurrent use of biologic response modifiers or in genetically-engineered monoclonal antibodies.

REFERENCES

1. Kohler G, Milstein C (1975) Continuous cultures of fused cells secreting antibody of predefined specificity. Nature 256: 495-497

2. Gold P, Freedman SI (1965) Demonstration of t-mor specific antigens in human colonic carcinomata by immunologican tolerance and absorption techniques. J Exp Med 121: 439-462

3. Poste G, Doll J. Brown AE, et al. (1982) Comparison of the metastatic properties of B16 melanoma clones isolated from cultured cell lines subcutaneous tumors and individual lung metastases. Cancer Res 42: 2770-2778

4. Herlyn D, Powe J, Alavi A, et al. (1983) Radioimmunodetection of human tumor xenografts by monoclonal antibodies. Cancer Res 43: 2731-2735

5. O'Connor SW, Blae WF (1984) Accessibility of circulating immunoglobin G to the extravascular compartment of solid rat tumors. Cancer Res 44: 3719-3723

6. Aitken DR, Hinkle GH, Thurston MO et al. (1984) A gamma detecting probe for radioimmune detection of CEA producing tumors: Successful experimental use and clinical case report. Dis Colon Rectum 27: 279-282

7. Martin DT, Hinkle GH, Tuttle S, et al. (1985) Intraoperative radioimmunodetection of colorectal tumor with a hand-held radiation detector. Am J Surg 150: 672-675

8. Thor A, Ohuchi N, Szpak CA, Johnston WW, Schlom J (1986) The distribution of oncofetal antigen TAG-72 defined by monoclonal antibody B72.3. Cancer Res 46: 3118-3124

9. Martin EW Jr., Mojzisik CM, Hinkle GH, et al. (1988) Radioimmunoguided surgery using monoclonal antibody. Am J Surg 156: 386-392

10. Colcher D, Esteban JM, Carrosquillo JA et al· (1987) Quantitative analyses of selective radiolabelled monoclonal antibody localization in metastatic lesion of colorectal cancer patients. Cancer Research 47: 1185-1189

11. Schlom J, Colcher D, Roselli M, et al. (1988) Tumor targeting with monoclonal antibody B72.3. Nul Med Biol 16: 137-142

12. Sickle-Santanello BJ, O'Dwyer PJ, Mojzisik CM, et al. (1987) Radioimmunoguided surgery using the monoclonal antibody B72.3 in colorectal tumors. Dis Colon and Rectum 30: 761-764

13. DeLand FH, Kim EE, Corgan RL, et al: Axillary lymphoscintigraphy by radioimmunodetection of carcinoembryonic antigen in breast cancer. J Nuc Med (1979) 20: 1243-1250

14. Thompson CH, Lichtenstein M, Stacker SA et al. (1984) Immunoscintigraphy for detection of lymph nodes metastases from breast cancer. Lancet 2: 1245-1247

Computer Assisted Surgery for Gastric Cancer

KEIICHI MARUYAMA, MITSURU SASAKO, TAIRA KINOSHITA, TAKESHI SANO, and
KUNIO OKAJIMA

Gastric Surgery Division, National Cancer Center Hospital, Chuo-ku, Tokyo, 104 Japan

ABSTRACTS

Lymph node (LN) dissection is an effective procedure in surgical treatment of gastric cancer. For the rational LN dissection, it is essential to know the incidence of metastasis at each LN station and effectiveness of the dissection. In 1984 we created the computer program using our data of 3,785 primary gastric cancer patients. Pre-operatively seven data of an individual patient are input; sex, age, location, macroscopic type, size, depth of invasion, and histological type. The computer informs us the expected 5 year survival rate, incidence of metastasis at all regional LN stations, type of recurrence. Accuracy of the system was very high; false positive was only 14 cases (1.8%) in the prospective study of 774 patients. This system was also evaluated in Germany, and the sensitivity was 100%, specificity was 78%, and accuracy was 89% for N2 compartment.

KEY WORDS: Gastric cancer, Lymph node metastasis, Computer assessment

INTRODUCTION

In the last 30 years period since 1962, 6,652 primary gastric cancer patients were treated surgically in National Cancer Center, and its five year survival rate (5YSR) was 55.1% in all cases, 57.8% in resected cases, 69.2% in curatively resected cases. 5YSR was 42.5% in the first 5 year period (1962-66) and it was improved to 74.9 in the last 5 year period (1987-91). Between the two periods the 5YSR was improved from 84.6% to 94.3% in Stage I, from 57.7% to 77.9% in Stage II, from 33.6% to 58.1% in Stage III, and from 1.7% to 11.8% in Stage IV. This improvement was mainly produced by the progress of surgical treatment, particularly by systematic lymph node dissection.

It is well known that it is quite hard to diagnose whether a LN is metastatic or not. However it is essential to know the incidence of metastasis at each LN station for reasonable node dissection. Moreover the effectiveness of dissection should also be considered. The effectiveness was demonstrated by 5 year survival rate of the patients with metastasis at the lymph node (5YSR+meta). These data can only be obtained by a computer analysis using high quality database. A computer program was created by us in 1984 using data of 3,785 primary gastric cancer patients treated at our Center. Background of the computer assisted surgery and its accuracy were stated in this paper.

REGIONAL LYMPH NODES OF THE STOMACH

The lymphatic flows from the stomach and the Lns along the streams were clarified by anatomical (1) and lymphographic studies (2) (Fig. 1). These studies showed clearly that the location of LN metastases depend significantly on the location of the main tumor. Based on these studies, regional LNs were anatomically classified in sixteen stations by the Japanese Research Society for Gastric Cancer in 1963 (3). They were grouped as N1, N2, N3, and N4 according to the location of the tumor (Fig. 2).

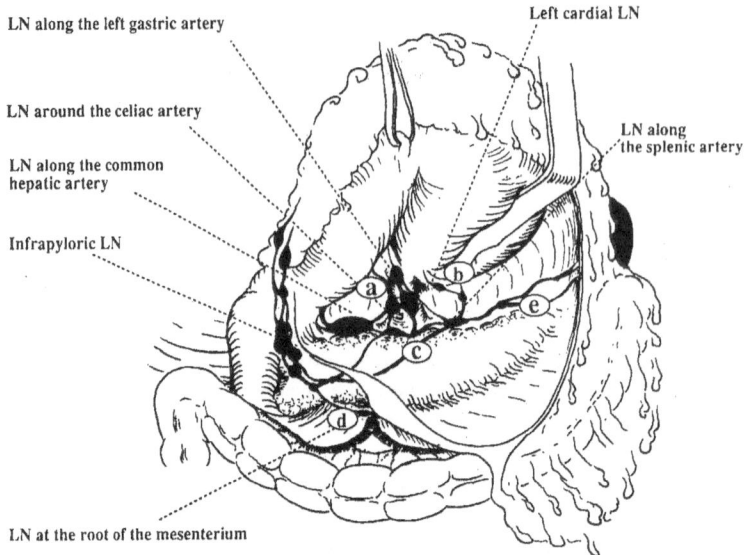

Fig. 1 Schema of five major lymphatic flows (a-e) from the stomach

From the lesser curvature, a stream flowed along the left gastric artery to the upper border of the pancreas (a), and the other flowed along the left subphrenic artery to the upper part of para-aortic LN (b). From the greater curvature, the first channel runs passing through the subpyloric LN and the pancreas surface to the upper border of the pancreas (c), the second runs along the superior mesenteric artery to the para-aortic LN (d), and the third runs through the splenic hilus to the upper border of the pancreas (e).

Location of tumor Lymph node station	A AM	M MA MC	C CM	AMC MAC MCA CMA
Nr. 1 right cardial LN	N2			
Nr. 2 left cardial LN	N3	N2		
Nr. 3 LN along the lesser curvature			N1	
Nr. 4 LN along the greater curvature				
Nr. 5 suprapyloric LN				
Nr. 6 infrapyloric LN				
Nr. 7 LN along the left gastric artery				
Nr. 8 LN along the common hepatic artery			N2	
Nr. 9 LN around the celiac artery				
Nr.10 LN at the splenic hilus				
Nr.11 LN along the splenic artery				
Nr.12 LN in the hepatoduodenal ligament				
Nr.13 LN behind the pancreas head			N3	
Nr.14 LN at the root of the mesenterium				
Nr.15 LN along the middle colic artery				
Nr.16 para-aortic LN			N4	

A: Distal third   M: Middle third   C: Proximal third   LN: lymph node

Fig. 2 Regional LN of the stomach and the N Classification

Regional LNs were anatomically classified and numbered in sixteen stations by the Japanese Research Society for Gastric Cancer in 1963. They were grouped as N1, N2, N3, and N4 according to the location of the tumor.

REQUIRED FACTORS FOR REASONABLE LYMPH NODE DISSECTION

Three factors should be considered when making a plan for LN dissection for an individual patient (4). The first is the incidence of metastasis at each LN station (5), the second is the effectiveness of LN dissection (5YSR+meta), and the third is the improvement of surgical technique for the dissection. The incidence of metastasis is shown by gray bar at Fig. 3, and the 5YSR+meta by black bar at the same figure. The results were obtained from a statistical analysis using data from 2,212 patients treated by gastric resection in the 23 year period from 1969 to 1991 excluding patients with early cancer and distant metastasis.

Surgical techniques of LN dissection had remarkably been improved in the last 10 years in Japan (6). Techniques for complete removal of N1 and N2 were established and popularized in 1962. This procedure is called "R2 dissection, and it is considered as the standard operation for gastric cancer. One of the latest progresses in LN dissection was extended systematic LN dissection for advanced cancer. The retroperitoneal LNs were widely and completely removed under the extensive mobilization of the head of pancreas (Fig. 4) and the spleen and distal pancreas (Fig. 5). LN in the hepatoduodenal ligament (No. 12), behind the pancreas head (No. 13), at the splenic hilus (No. 10), along the splenic artery (No. 11), and at the para-aortic area (No. 16) can easily be dissected by these exposures. These figures demonstrate also the incidence of metastasis and the 5YSR+meta at each LN station.

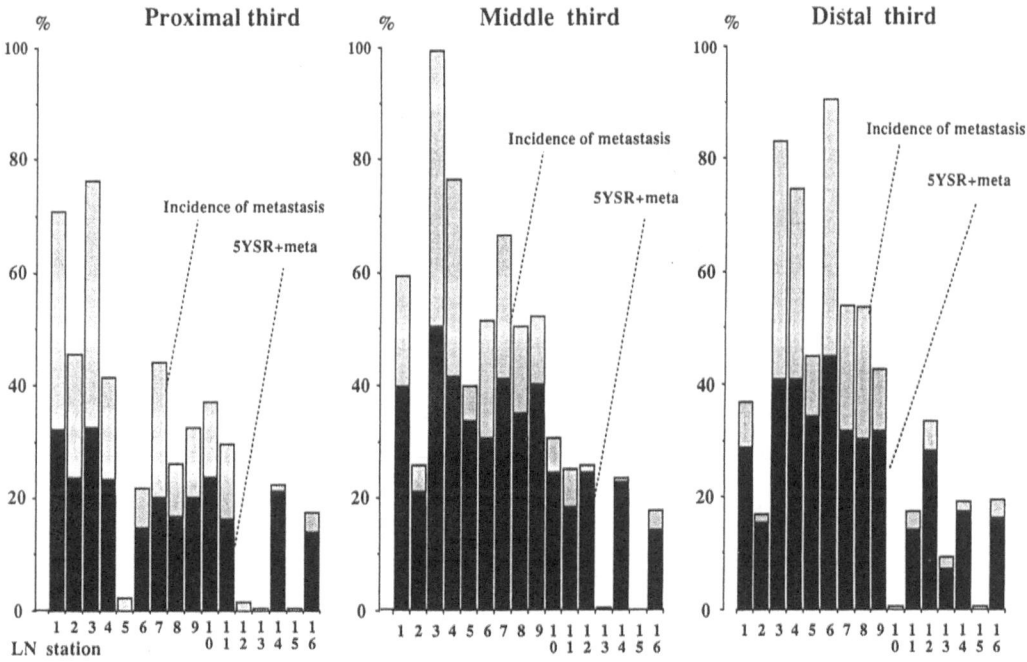

Fig. 3 Incidence of metastasis at each LN station and 5YSR of the node positive patients treated by node dissection (5YSR+meta)

Gray bar shows the incidence of metastasis and black bar shows 5YSR+meta. For example, the incidence was 12% and the 5YSR+meta was 41% at LN along the celiac artery (No. 9) in middle third cancer. Dissection of these nodes was indicated because of the high incidence of LN metastasis and apparent effectiveness of LN dissection. The figure shows also the effectiveness of LN dissection in the para-aortic area (No.16); the 5YSR+meta was 14%, 14%, and 16% for proximal, middle, and distal cancer respectively.

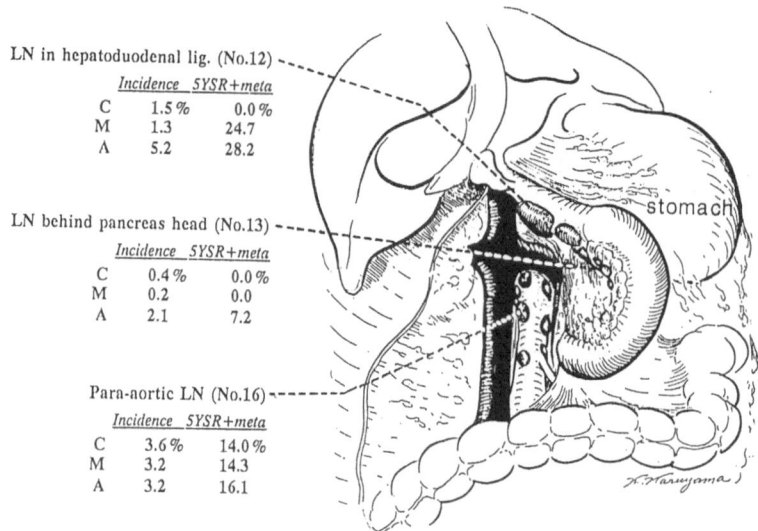

LN in hepatoduodenal lig. (No.12)

	Incidence	5YSR+meta
C	1.5%	0.0%
M	1.3	24.7
A	5.2	28.2

LN behind pancreas head (No.13)

	Incidence	5YSR+meta
C	0.4%	0.0%
M	0.2	0.0
A	2.1	7.2

Para-aortic LN (No.16)

	Incidence	5YSR+meta
C	3.6%	14.0%
M	3.2	14.3
A	3.2	16.1

Fig. 4 Extensive mobilization of the pancreas head (Kocher's maneuver) and LN dissection

This procedure is used to remove the right retroperitoneal LNs. The 5YSR+meta of LN No. 12 was 22.0% and 29.7% in the middle and distal cancer respectively, and the dissection was therefore considered effective. However the effectiveness of LN No. 12 in the proximal third and LN No.13 dissection was doubtful due to low 5YSR+meta. Incidence of the lower part of the para-aortic LN (No. 16b) was low but the effectiveness was not. The incidence was 2.5%, 1.3% and 1.4% in the proximal, middle and distal third cancer respectively, and the 5YSR+meta was 13.8%, 12.0% and 20.0%. It is noteworthy that these incidence and effectiveness figures are not altered by the location of the tumor.

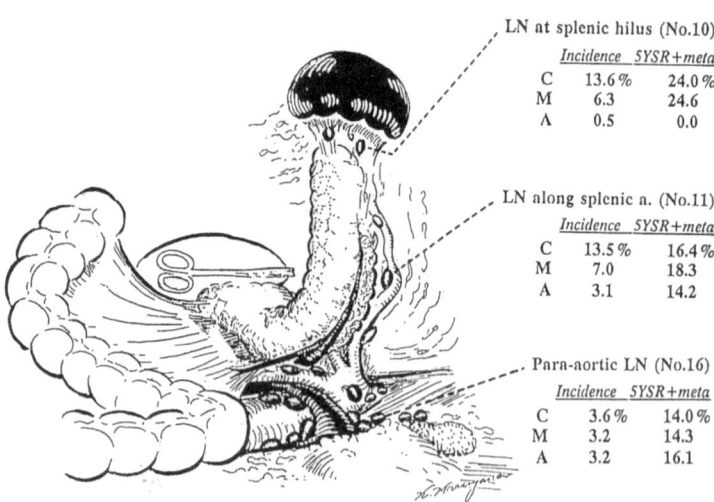

LN at splenic hilus (No.10)

	Incidence	5YSR+meta
C	13.6%	24.0%
M	6.3	24.6
A	0.5	0.0

LN along splenic a. (No.11)

	Incidence	5YSR+meta
C	13.5%	16.4%
M	7.0	18.3
A	3.1	14.2

Para-aortic LN (No.16)

	Incidence	5YSR+meta
C	3.6%	14.0%
M	3.2	14.3
A	3.2	16.1

Fig. 5 Extensive mobilization of the distal pancreas and LN dissection

This procedure is used to remove the left retroperitoneal LNs. The incidence of metastasis and 5YSR+meta were shown in the figures.

COMPUTER PROGRAM FOR A PREOPERATIVE ASSESSMENT OF SURVIVALS AND LYMPH NODE METASTASES

In the above figures, the incidence and effectiveness of node dissection at each LN station were shown according to the location of tumor. However they are also significantly influenced by macroscopic type, depth of invasion, size of tumor, histological type, sex, and age. To resolve this complicated problem, a personal computer program was provided by the Gastric Surgery Division of National Cancer Center Hospital in 1984 (7). The seven above mentioned variables of individual patient were input preoperatively into the computer, then it estimated statistically the 5YSR, incidence of metastasis at the 16 LN stations, causes of death, and probable curability by surgery (Fig. 6). The most rational operation plan could be made for individual patient by reference to this report.

```
PROGNOSIS AND LN-METASTASES OF THE PATIENTS WITH SAME BACKGROUND
treated by resection in National Cancer Center Tokyo, 1969-1983


         PATIENT            92-352122    K. YAMAMOTO
-----------------------------------------------------------------
         SEX and AGE        M    63 (+5/-5)
         TYPE and DEPTH     B3   S1
         LOCATION           A    L
         MAX DIAMETER       6.0 cm  (+2.5/-2.5)
         HISTOLOG TYPE      POR

[ DEPTH OF INVASION ] PM              S1                  S2
-----------------------------------------------------------------
TYPE OF CANCER       B3               B3                  B3
5 YEAR SURV RATE     78.1%            50.1%               42.8%
GREENWOOD 5% ERR     22.6%            23.6%               18.0%
NUMBER OF CASES      20               19                  34

[ LYMPH NODE METASTASIS ]  meta/dissect (meta% in group)
-----------------------------------------------------------------
    LN- 1      1/20 (  5.0%)    3/18 ( 16.0%)    7/31 ( 21.0%)
    LN- 2      0/ 0 (  0.0%)    0/ 4 (  0.0%)    0/ 7 (  0.0%)
    LN- 3      6/20 ( 30.0%)   10/19 ( 53.0%)   28/33 ( 82.0%)
    LN- 4      1/20 (  5.0%)    8/19 ( 42.0%)   17/33 ( 50.0%)
    LN- 5      3/20 ( 15.0%)    2/18 ( 11.0%)    4/31 ( 12.0%)
    LN- 6      8/20 ( 40.0%)   10/18 ( 53.0%)   20/32 ( 59.0%)
    LN- 7      3/20 ( 15.0%)    7/19 ( 37.0%)   15/31 ( 44.0%)
    LN- 8      3/20 ( 15.0%)    7/19 ( 37.0%)   14/29 ( 41.0%)
    LN- 9      3/20 ( 15.0%)    3/18 ( 16.0%)    7/29 ( 21.0%)
    LN-10      0/ 0 (  0.0%)    0/ 3 (  0.0%)    0/ 0 (  0.0%)
    LN-11      0/ 8 (  0.0%)    2/ 7 ( 11.0%)    2/13 (  6.0%)
    LN-12      0/10 (  0.0%)    1/ 7 (  5.0%)    2/20 (  6.0%)
    LN-13      0/ 3 (  0.0%)    0/ 3 (  0.0%)    0/ 6 (  0.0%)
    LN-14      0/ 1 (  0.0%)    1/ 3 (  5.0%)    2/ 4 (  6.0%)
    LN-15      0/ 1 (  0.0%)    1/ 1 (  5.0%)    0/ 0 (  0.0%)
    LN-16      0/ 5 (  0.0%)    2/ 4 ( 11.0%)    1/ 7 (  3.0%)
-----------------------------------------------------------------
[ CAUSE OF DEATH ]
LIVING NOW        15 ( 75.0%)      7 ( 37.0%)     10 ( 29.0%)
UNKNOWN            1 (  5.0%)      1 (  5.0%)      2 (  6.0%)
PERIT DISSEMI      4 ( 20.0%)      4 ( 21.0%)      7 ( 21.0%)
HEPATIC META       0 (  0.0%)      2 ( 11.0%)      2 (  6.0%)
LOCAL RECURR       0 (  0.0%)      3 ( 16.0%)     10 ( 29.0%)
DISTANT META       0 (  0.0%)      1 (  5.0%)      0 (  0.0%)
RECURRENCE         0 (  0.0%)      0 (  0.0%)      0 (  0.0%)
DIRECT DEATH       0 (  0.0%)      0 (  0.0%)      0 (  0.0%)
OTHER CANCER       0 (  0.0%)      0 (  0.0%)      1 (  3.0%)
OTHER DISEASE      0 (  0.0%)      1 (  5.0%)      2 (  6.0%)
-----------------------------------------------------------------
[ CURABILITY AT SURGERY ]
ABS CURATIVE      13 ( 65.0%)      8 ( 42.0%)     10 ( 29.0%)
REL CURATIVE       7 ( 35.0%)      6 ( 32.0%)     16 ( 47.0%)
REL NON-CURA       0 (  0.0%)      3 ( 16.0%)      2 (  6.0%)
ABS NON-CURA       0 (  0.0%)      2 ( 11.0%)      6 ( 18.0%)
-----------------------------------------------------------------
```

Fig. 6 An example of report from the computer system for a preoperative assessment of survival and LN metastases of individual patient

In case of 63 year old male with Borrmann type 3 cancer 6.0 cm in diameter invading the serosal surface locating at the distal third at the lesser curvature, poorly differentiated carcinoma, the estimated 5YSR was 50.1% and LN No. 1, 3, 4, 5, 6, 7, 8, 9, 11, 12, 14, 15, and 16 should be dissected due to the possibility of metastasis.

The accuracy of the program was very high in a prospective study at our department. The initial database was data of 3,785 patients treated in 1969-1983. False negative results were found only in 14 cases (1.8%) in our prospective study of 774 patients treated in 1984-1987. This program has been in use at many hospitals abroad. A study evaluated the computer program using data of 222 German patients in Munich (8). It revealed also high sensitivity and accuracy of the program (Table 1).

Table 1   Sensitivity, specificity, and accuracy of the computer program studied using data of 222 German patients

Lymph node station	No.1-6	No.7-12	No.13-16
Sensitivity (%)	97	100	100
Specificity (%)	43	78	95
Positive predictive value (%)	80	83	86
Negative predictive value (%)	94	100	100
Accuracy (%)	82	89	96

Bollschweiler E. et al. Br. J. Surg. 1992

In conclusion, our experience of the computer assisted surgery for gastric cancer showed that detailed data are essential to make a rational surgical treatment for individual patient. Such data can be obtained only from huge and high-quality database not from limited personal experience. This computer system is one of the new strategies for cancer treatment.

This work was supported in part by the Grant-in-Aid for Cancer Research (91-03) from the Japanese Ministry of Health and Welfare, and by the Princess Takamatsu Cancer Research Fund (1992).

REFERENCES

1.   Inoue Y (1936) Jpn. J. Anatomy. 9: 35-117
2.   Sawai K, Takahashi S, Kato G, Takenaka A, Tokuda H (1985) Jpn. J Gastroenter. Surg. 18: 912-917 (in Japanese)
3.   Japanese Research Society for Gastric Cancer (1981) Jpn J Surg. 11: 127-145
4.   Maruyama K, Sasako M, Kinoshita T (1992) Arch für Chirurg Suppl (Kongressbericht). 130-135
5.   Maruyama K, Gunven P, Okabayashi K, Sasako M, Kinoshita T (1989) Ann Surg. 210: 596-602
6.   Maruyama K (1986) National Cancer Center Press, Tokyo
7.   Kampschöer G H M, Maruyama K, van de Velde C J H, Sasako M, Kinoshita T, Okabayashi K (1989) Br. J. Surg. 76: 905-908
8.   Bollschweiler E, Boettcher K, Hoelscher A H, Sasako M, Kinoshita T, Maruyama K, Siewert J R (1992) Br. J. Surg. 79: 156-160

Targeting Chemotherapy for Digestive Cancer Using Monoclonal Antibody Drug Conjugate

Toshio Takahashi, Toshiharu Yamaguchi, Kazuya Kitamura, Akinori Noguchi, Eigo Otsuji, Takuya Miyagaki, and Akira Noguchi

Department of Surgery, Kyoto Prefectural University of Medicine, Kyoto, 602 Japan

ABSTRACT

Murine monoclonal antibody A7 against human colon cancer was conjugated with the anticancer agent Neocarzinostatin (NCS) to form the conjugate A7–NCS. Using this conjugate, immunotargeted chemotherapy, (missile therapy), was administered to 80 patients with digestive cancers. This missile therapy produced tumor reductions on CT scans in some patients with liver metastasis. In a non–randomized clinical trial, the survival rate for patients with liver metastasis treated with A7–NCS was higher than for patients treated with conventional chemotherapy and was approximately the same for patients receiving chemoembolization. Patients who received A7–NCS experienced no serious adverse effects. Human anti–mouse antibody (HAMA) was detected in all A7–NCS–treated patients. To overcome HAMA, early repeated injections, preparation of human–mouse chimeric antibody, and chemical modification of monoclonal antibody were carried out.

Key words: monoclonal antibody–drug conjugate, A7–NCS, colon cancer, chemotherapy, missile therapy.

INTRODUCTION

Although chemotherapy has been effective in the treatment of many malignancies, results with gastrointestinal cancers have been disappointing. A major problem with chemotherapy for gastrointestinal cancers is the toxic effect of the anticancer agents on normal cells of the digestive tract."Missile " or "Targeted" therapy is specifically directed at cancer cells and is designed to overcome adverse effects in normal cells. There have been several reports on experimental[1,2] and clinical [3,4] missile therapy, but the general utility of this therapy is as yet unknown.

Since 1980, we have been engaged in the studies of missile therapy using monoclonal antibody drug conjugates[5,6] directed at digestive cancers[7]. This paper describes the outline of our studies and the results of clinical trials for patients with digestive cancers.

Monoclonal Antibody (A7)

The monoclonal antibody, A7, was produced by a hybridoma obtained after fusion of splenocyte from a mouse immunized against a human colon cancer with murine myeloma cells. Monoclonal antibody A7 is an IgG directed to a glycoprotein antigen with a molecular weight of 40,000.[8] A7 reacted with 70 to 80 percent of colon, pancreas and stomach cancer in surgically resected specimens, but it did not react with malignant melanoma or brain tumor.

Specific Localization of Monoclonal Antibody A7 to Human Colon Cancer

Patients with colon cancer were injected with ^{131}I–A7 intravenously three days before surgery. Autoradiography of resected specimens demonstrated that A7 localized specifically in colon cancer cells which invaded into a whole layer of the colon, while there was little localization in normal tissues of the colon(Fig.1). Therefore, A7 was selected as a suitable drug carrier to colon cancer in human.

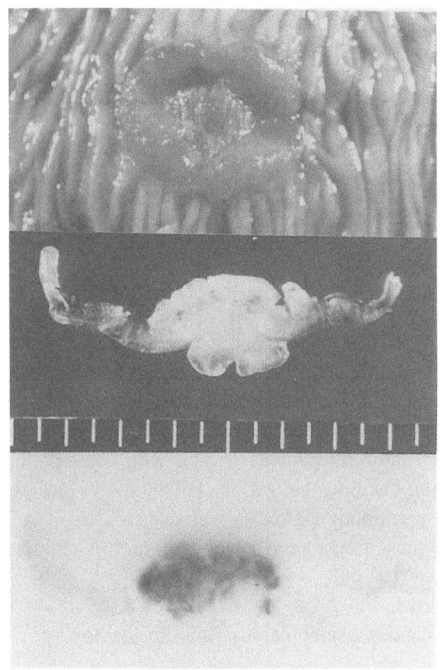

Fig. 1

Resected specimen of colon cancer forming cancerous crater with marginal elevation (Type II). This patient was injected with $_{131}$I–A7 intravenously 3 days before operation.

Cut section of the above specimen.

Autoradiography of the specimen. A7 was localized specifically in tumor cells which invaded into whole coat of the colon. There was little localization of A7 in the normal mucosa.

Monoclonal Antibody Drug Conjugate

Mitomycin C (MMC Kyowa Hakko, Tokyo), Adriamycin (ADM Pharmacia, Italy) and Neocarzinostatin (NCS Pola, Tokyo) were used to prepare conjugates with monoclonal antibody A7. These drugs were covalently bound to A7 to form A7–MMCD, A7–ADM and A7–NCS by previously described methods[9,10] (Table 1).

After in vitro and in vivo studies of these conjugates, we administered A7–NCS to patients with colon and pancreatic cancer because of one mole of A7 to one mole of NCS resulted in a potent anticancer protein containing 15 mg of A7 per 1,000 units of NCS.

Table 1. Monoclonal Antibody–Drug Conjugates

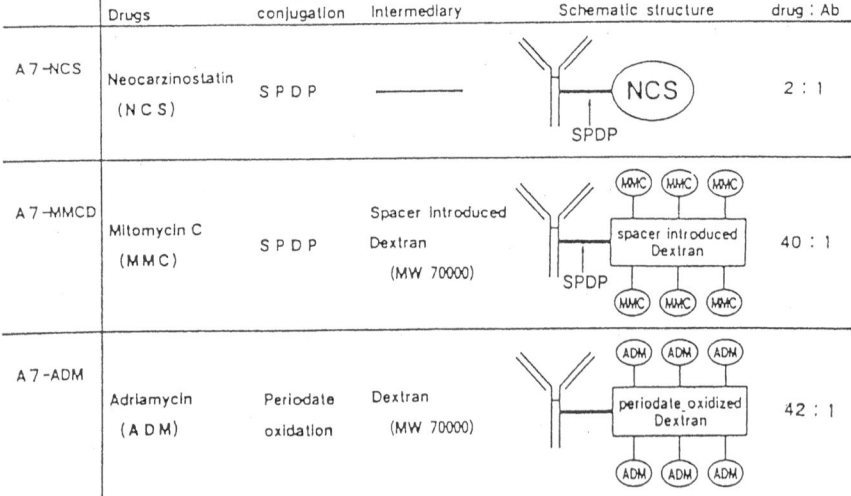

Clinical Trial of Missile Therapy
Patients receiving A7-NCS:
A total of 80 patients with advanced colorectal and pancreatic cancer admitted to the Department of Surgery, Kyoto Prefectural University of Medicine from 1985 to 1990 were treated with A7-NCS. Fifty-five patients had advanced colorectal cancer and they underwent surgery for tumor removal. Nineteen patients had multiple liver metastases after surgery, two had multiple lung metastases after surgery and one had peritoneal metastasis after surgery for colorectal cancer(Table 2).

Table 2. Patients given A7-NCS Conjugate

Target lesion	No. of Patients	Route of Admistration	Dose {A7(mg)/NCS(units)}		
			<30/2,000	45/4,000	45/4,000<
Colorectal Ca.					
Primary & Local Recurrence	57	i.a. (53)	21	3	29
		i.v. (3)			3
		local (1)		1	
Liver metastasis	19	i.a. (19)	5		14
Lung metastasis	2	i.v. (2)			2
Peritoneal meta.	1	i.p. (1)		1	
Pancreatic Ca.	1	i.a. (1)			1

Clinical effects of A7-NCS on inoperable cancer patients:
Of 19 patients with postoperative liver metastasis, four responded clearly to A7-NCS on CT scan. Two cases were shown in Fig. 2 and 3. Patient with pancreatic cancer and patients with lung or peritoneal metastasis did not have any clinical response to the conjugate.

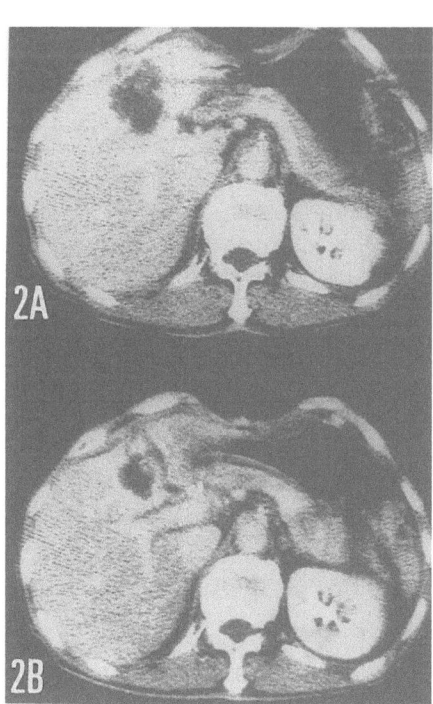 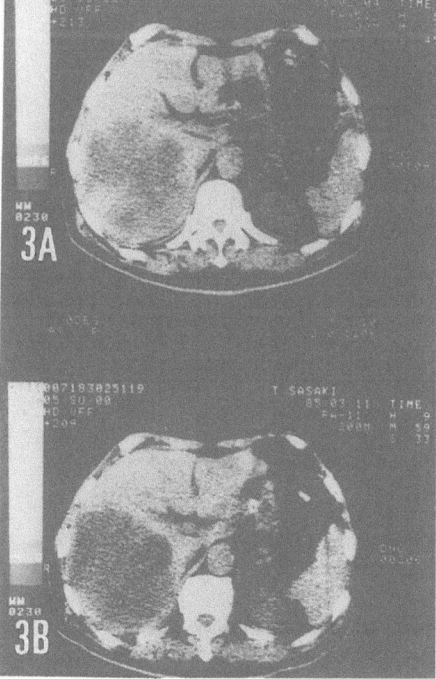

Fig. 2A: CT scan of a patient with liver metastasis 5 years after surgery for colon cancer. This patient was given a single dose of A7-NCS (A7:90 mg, NCS:6,000 units) through hepatic artery. Fig. 2B: CT scan taken 3 weeks later showed a 67 % tumor reduction. Fig. 3A: CT scan of a patient with liver metastasis 3 years after surgery for rectal cancer. This patient was given a single dose of A7-NCS (A7; 60mg, NCS; 4,000 units). Fig. 3B: CT scan taken 3 weeks after the treatment revealed a reduced density which meant that the tumor became necrosis.

Adverse effects:

Patients who received the conjugate experienced no serious adverse effects. A fever greater than 38.0 C was the most common adverse effect and was evident in 36 patients immediately after the injection. Other side effects were leucocytosis greater than 10,000/um in 30 patients and slight hypotension with a systolic pressure from 80 to 100 cm Hg in three patients.

End-Result of the Patients Given the Conjugate

(1) Survival of patients with liver metastases:

Twenty-five patients with liver metastasis from colorectal cancer were given the conjugate. The survival curve for patients receiving the conjugate was compared with that for patients with liver metastasis treated with intra-arterial infusion chemotherapy using 5-FU and mitomycin C (MMC) aqueous solution and with that for patients with liver metastasis treated with intra-arterial chemoembolization using multiple anticancer agents suspended in a lipid contrast medium containing 5-FU, MMC and adriamycin (ADM).

Fig. 4 shows the survival curves for patients with liver metastasis, treated with these three modalities. The group of patients given A7-NCS had the highest survival rate. The median survival times were as follows: 328 days for the A7-NCS group, 128 days for the chemoembolization group, and 205 days for the conventional intra-arterial chemotherapy group. The survival rate of the A7-NCS group was statistically higher than that of the group given conventional chemotherapy from 490 to 850 days (p<0.05). However, there was no statistically significant difference between the group receiving A7-NCS and the chemoembolization group.

Although comparisons with patients who received NCS alone were not performed in this study, the literature indicates that patients receiving NCS alone do not experience significant prolongation of survival. Therefore, treatment with the monoclonal antibody drug conjugate A7-NCS appears to be superior to conventional chemotherapy and allowed longer survival for patients with liver metastasis from colorectal cancer. Survival of patients receiving A7-NCS, however, did not exceed that of patients receiving chemoembolization, which is the most powerful targeting chemotherapy for liver metastasis currently available[11].

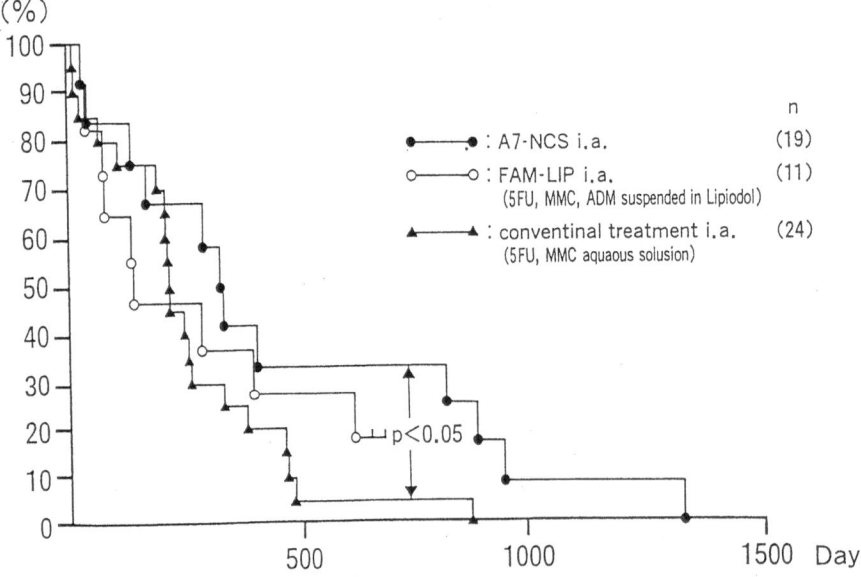

Fig. 4 Survival curves of the patients with inoperable liver metastasis treated with A7-NCS, FAM-LIP and conventional chemotherapy.

(2) Survival of patients undergoing tumor resection:

In the patients who underwent tumor resection, the five year survival rate was 44.4% for the patients given A7-NCS and 46.4% for those not given A7-NCS. There was no difference between these two groups.

Human Anti-Mouse Antibody (HAMA)

Human anti-mouse antibodies (HAMA) and antibodies against NCS in sera were investigated in 14 patients given A7-NCS (A7: 45mg, NCS: 4,000 units). As shown in Table 3, IgG HAMA was detected in all 14 patients.

IgM antibodies were detected in nine patients, and IgE antibodies were not found in any of the patients. Anti–NCS antibodies were not found in any of the patients. HAMA could be detected from one week after the administration of A7–NCS, peaked at three to five weeks, and lasted for more than 35 weeks.

Table 3. Human Anti–Mouse Antibody (HAMA) in Patients
Given A7–NCS

	No. of Patients Examined	No. of Patients with HAMA
		%
IgG	14	14 (100.0)
IgM	14	9 (64.3)
Ig E	14	0 (0)

Trials Overcoming HAMA

(1) Early multiple injections of A7–NCS:
Six patients with liver and/or lung metastasis were injected with A7–NCS (A7: 45mg, NCS: 4,000 units, i.e. a total dose of 225 mg of A7 and 20.000 units of NCS) for five successive days before the HAMA appeared. There were no adverse effects from these repeated injections, but responses of the metastases were not valuable.

(2) Preparation of chimeric antibody:
We successfully prepared a human–mouse chimeric Fab of A7. This chimeric Fab A7 reacted with stomach, colon and breast cancer, but did not react with esophagus, lung and kidney cancers, showing identical reactivity to that of parent monoclonal antibody A7(Table 4).

Table 4. Reactivity of Fab of human–mouse chimeric A7 and mouse A7 against human cell lines by ELISA

Human Cancer Cell Lines		Chimeric A7 Fab (Human/Mouse)	Mouse A7 Fab
Esophageal Ca.	TE-1	−	−
	TE-2	−	−
Lung Ca.	PC-1	−	−
	PC-3	−	−
Stomach Ca.	MKN-28	+	+
	MKN-45	+	+
	KATO-Ⅲ	+	+
Colon Ca.	COLO-201	+.	+
Breast Ca.	ZR-751	+	+
Kidney Ca.	NRC-15	−	−

(3) Chemical modification of the monoclonal antibody:
The murine monoclonal antibody A7 was chemically modified with polyethylene glycol (PEG)[12]. PEG–substituted A7 showed less organ uptake in liver and spleen, compared with the parent A7. Tumor localization was enhanced by REG modification for the $F(ab')_2$. Multiple i.v. injection of this PEG–modified antibody to rabbit did not appear to elicit a measurable immune response.

DISCUSSION

Although there have been several promising reports on experimental missile therapy, there is little information on clinical effects or adverse effect in a large sample of cancer patients. Our study was conducted in 80 patients with digestive cancer during 5 years period.

Missile therapy with A7-NCS produced tumor reductions on CT scans in some patients with liver metastasis. To evaluate this treatment, it will be necessary to undertake a randomized control study. However, we were not able to generate an accurate randomized control for this clinical trial because the treatment is not established as a common drug therapy. Accordingly, A7-NCS was given to a limited number of patients with considerably advanced cancers, and comparisons were made between patients who received A7-NCS and those who underwent conventional treatments during the same five year period. The survival rate for patients with liver metastasis treated with A7-NCS was higher than for patients treated with conventional chemotherapy and was approximately the same as that for patients receiving chemoembolization.

There were no serious adverse side effects in patients receiving the conjugate. However, HAMA was detected in all patients examined for the IgG class. IgG HAMA appeared from one week after the administration of A7-NCS, and reached a peak level at 3 to 5 weeks after injection, lasting for more than 35 weeks. These results suggest that missile therapy using murine monoclonal antibodies is limited by the presence of HAMA in the patient's blood when injected more than one week after the initial injection.

In order to overcome the adverse effects of HAMA, we attempted to inject a sufficient dose of the conjugate for five successive days before the HAMA reached its peak level. Despite the initial administration of a large dose of the conjugate, there were no adverse side effects from the antibody. Therefore, early multiple injections of a large dose of conjugate may be one of the ways to overcome HAMA.

We prepared a human-mouse chimeric antibody which exhibited identical reactivities as the parent antibody. We have also made chimeric antibody-drug conjugate which showed promising effects in human colon cancer transplanted in nude mice.

The chemical modification of murine monoclonal antibody by polyethylene glycol apparently reduces the host immune response against monoclonal antibodies. This modified form of the antibody may have clinical applications in missile therapy.

In conclusion, missile therapy with monoclonal antibody drug conjugates will become a novel modality for patients with digestive cancer.

This work was supported by Grant-in-Aid for Cancer Research and for the Comprehensive 10-Year Strategy for Cancer Control from Ministry of Health and Welfare.

REFERENCES

1.Mathe, G., BaLoc, T., Berunaed, F.(1958)JCR Acad Sci 246:1626-1627
2.Hurwitz E, Maron R, Bernstein A, Wilchek M, Sela M, Arnon R.(1978) Int J Cancer 1978; 21: 747-755
3.Tjandra JJ,Pietersz GA, Cuthberton AM et al.(1989) Surgery 106:533-545
4.Elias SJ,Klinel KW,Killman RO. et al.(1990) Antibody Immunoconjugates and Radiopharmaceutical 3:60.
5.Takahashi T, Yamaguchi T, Kohno K(1980) In: Hellmann K, Hilgard P, Eccles S (eds) Metastasis. Martinus Nijhoff, London, pp 441-445.
6.Kotanagi H, Takahashi T, Masuko T(1986) Tohoku J exp Med 148: 353-360
7.Takahashi T,Yamaguchi T, Kitamura K, et al.(1988) Cancer 61: 881-8889.
8.Kitamura K, Takahashi, T, Yamaguchi T, et al.(1988) Tohoku J exp Med 157:83-97
9.Fukuda K(1985) Akita J Med 12:415-468.
10.Noguchi A,Takahashi,Yamaguchi T et al.(1992) Bioconjugate Chemistry 3:132-137
11.Taniguchi H, Takahashi T, Yamaguchi T. et al.(1989) Cancer 64:2001-2006.
12.Kitamura K, Takahashi T, Yamaguchi T et al.(1991) Cancer Res 51:4310-4315

Hepatocellular Carcinoma: Hepatic Resection Versus Transplantation

Juan R. Madariaga, Rick Selby, Shunzaburo Iwatsuki, Brian Carr, and Thomas E. Starzl

University of Pittsburgh Medical Center, Pittsburgh Transplant Institute, Pittsburgh, PA 15213, USA

ABSTRACT

From 1980 to 1989, 76 patients with hepatocellular carcinoma were treated by subtotal hepatic resection (HX) and 105 by orthotopic liver transplantation (TX). The overall 1 to 5 year survival rates of the HX group were 71.1%, 55.0%, 47.2%, 37.2% and 32.9% respectively, and those of the TX group were 65.7%, 49.0%, 39.2%, 35.6% and 35.6%, respectively. The survival was similar stage by stage in both groups and correlated well with the pTNM classification. Tumor recurrence was high in both groups after HX (50%) and TX (43%) particularly in stages IV-A ($\geq$ 60%). Twelve patients after HX and 13 patients after TX lived more than 5 years.

KEYWORDS: TNM classification and hepatocellular carcinoma

INTRODUCTION

It has been recognized that subtotal hepatic resection and liver transplantation can be effective in the treatment of hepatocellular carcinoma (HCC), especially in the early stages of the disease (1-5). In this report we analyze the results of 181 patients who were treated either by liver transplantation (TX) and or by subtotal hepatic resection (HX) during a 10 year period (6), using pTNM staging for HCC.

MATERIAL AND METHODS

From 1980 to 1989, 76 patients with HCC were treated by subtotal hepatic resection (HX) and 105 patients by liver transplantation (TX) at the University of Colorado Health Science Center (1980) and at the University of Pittsburgh (1981 to 1989).

Whenever possible hepatic resection was carried out and liver transplantation was reserved for the cases of poor functional reserve, liver cirrhosis or whenever the anatomic location of the tumor precluded a safe resection.

All cases were staged according to the pTNM classification (7).

I Subtotal Hepatic Resection Group (HX Group):
Among the 76 patients, 53 were male and 23 were females with an age range from 9 to 86 years with a mean $\pm$ SD of 51.4 $\pm$ 17.4 years. In 22% of the cases there were associated cirrhosis, 10% were chronic hepatitis B carriers and 4% had hepatitis B surface and/or core antibody. Twelve of 76 patients with HCC were of fibrolamellar variant (FL-HCC).

II Liver Transplantation Group (TX Group):
There were 105 patients, 76 were male and 35 female with an age range from 3 to 69 years with a mean $\pm$ SD of 43.5 $\pm$ 18.2 years. Liver cirrhosis was present in 67% of the patients. Hepatitis B surface antigen (HBsAg) was positive in 21% of the patients and in 11 HBsAb and/or HBcAb was positive. Ten of the 105 patients had fibrolamellar HCC's.

FOLLOW-UP:
In both groups the follow-up periods ranged from 16 to 131 months with a median follow-up of 53 months in the resection group and of 37 months in the transplant group.

STATISTICAL ANALYSIS:
Actuarial survival rates were calculated by the life-table method. Univariate and multivariate analysis across different groups were made by the method of Mantel-Cox and the Cox proportional hazard regression model. A p value of less than 0.05 was considered significant.

RESULTS

There was no difference in the overall survival rates between the subtotal hepatic resection group (HX group) and the liver transplant group (TX group). Patients with FL-HCC had better 5 year survival than those with HCC in the HX group (64.8% versus 26.3%) but was similar in the TX group (37.5% versus 36.5%).

Survival rates were similar between the HX group and the TX group in each stage of the pTNM. It is worth noting that there was no patient with stage I disease in our HX group. (Table 1).

Table 1. Survival Rates After Resection and Liver Transplantation According to the pTNM Staging System

	1 year	2 years	3 years	4 years	5 years
RESECTION					
Stage I (n=0)					
Stage II (n=19)	100% (18)	84.2% (15)	78.6% (13)	58.2% (8)	43.7% (4)
Stage III (n=25)	76.0% (19)	68.0% (14)	53.4% (9)	46.8% (6)	46.8% (5)
Stage IV-A (n=32)	53.1% (17)	26.9% (7)	22.4% (4)	16.8% (3)	16.8% (3)
TRANSPLANTATION					
Stage I (n=4)	75.0% (3)	75.0% (3)	75.0% (2)	75.0% (2)	75.0% (2)
Stage II (n=19)	79.0% (15)	68.4% (12)	68.4% (12)	68.4% (8)	68.4% (5)
Stage III (n=23)	78.3% (18)	59.8% (11)	59.8% (8)	52.3% (4)	52.3% (4)
Stage IV-A (n=59)	55.9% (33)	36.6% (15)	16.3% (4)	10.9% (2)	10.9% (2)

When cirrhosis was present the survivals of the HX group were lower than those of the TX group (Table 2).

Table 2 Survival Rates After Resection and Liver Transplantation for Hepatocellular Carcinoma

	1 year	2 years	3 years	4 years	5 years
Hepatic Resection (n=17) (Cirrhosis)	35.3% (6)	23.5% (4)	5.9% (1)	0% (0)	--
Hepatic Resection (n=59) (Noncirrhosis)	81.4% (48)	64.3% (32)	60.2% (25)	49.5% (17)	43.7% (12)
Liver Transplantation (Cirrhosis) (n=71)	63.4% (45)	48.6% (28)	42.9% (21)	40.7% (12)	40.7% (10)
Liver Transplantation (Noncirrhosis) (n=34)	70.6% (24)	50.0% (16)	32.5% (6)	26.0% (4)	26.0% (3)

Stage by stage the survival rates of the TX group were significantly better (p< 0.05) than those of the HX group (Table 3).

Table 3. Survivals after Resection and after Transplantation in Patients with Hepatocellular Carcinoma in the Cirrhotic Liver.

	1 year	2 years	3 years	4 years	5 years
RESECTION GROUP					
Stage 1 (n=0)					
Stage 2 (n=2)	100% (2)	50.0% (1)	50.0% (1)	0% (0)	
Stage 3 (n=5)	40.0% (2)	40.0% (2)	0% (0)		
Stage IV-A (n=10)	20.0% (2)	0% (0)			
TRANSPLANT GROUP					
Stage 1 (n=4)	75.0% (3)	75.0% (3)	75.0% (2)	75.0% (2)	75.0% (2)
Stage 2 (n=16)	81.3% (13)	75.0% (11)	75.0% (11)	75.0% (7)	75.0% (5)
Stage 3 (n=19)	79.0% (15)	56.1% (8)	56.1% (7)	48.1% (3)	48.1% (3)
Stage IV-A (n=32)	43.8% (14)	26.2% (6)	0.(0)		

Prognostic factors that adversely affected the survival in both groups and achieved statistical significance (p< 0.05) were: (1) associated cirrhosis (2) infiltrative shape (3) bilobar involvement (4) microscopic positive tumor margin (5) metastasis to regional lymph nodes (6) vascular invasion.

The overall tumor recurrence rate was similar in both groups but in the early stages (II and III) tumor recurred more often in the HX group (42.1% and 28.0% in the HX group versus 5.3% and 13.0% in the TX group). Both groups had a very high incidence of recurrence in stage IV-A (53.1% in the HX group and 64.4% in the TX group). Two thirds of the deaths were related to tumor recurrence.

DISCUSSION

In the past the comparison of results among various reports of different therapies for HCC was not possible because there was not a unified staging classification. For the past 10 years we have used the pTNM staging classification in the patients treated by subtotal hepatic resection and transplantation for HCC. We have found that the pTNM classification predicts quite well the survival after subtotal hepatic resection and liver transplantation.

Our survival rates after hepatic resection in the noncirrhotic liver were similar to those of other reports, even though we did not have patients with Stage I disease (67.1% at one year, 47.2% at 3 years, and 32.9% at 5 years). When cirrhosis was present, however, our results of hepatic resections were inferior to those from Asia probably because our patient population fell into advanced stages. The survival after liver transplantation in the cirrhotic liver (63.4% at 1 year, 42.9% at 3 years, and 40.7% at 5 years) were superior to those reported in Asia (3). We had only a few patients in early stages who underwent hepatic resection in the cirrhotic liver, therefore we could not have a meaningful comparison between liver resection and transplantation in the early stages. Tumor recurrence of stage II and III were higher after hepatic resection than after liver transplantation. On the other hand, two thirds of the recurrence occurred in stage IV-A in both groups. Late death was usually the result of tumor recurrence in those patients.

For the last two years intrahepatic arterial (I/A) chemotherapy has been utilized in our service as a means to improve survival in these patients.

REFERENCES

1. Iwatsuki S, Starzl TE. Personal experience with 411 hepatic resections. Ann Surg 1988; 208:421-434.

2. Bismuth H, Houssin D, Ornowski J, Meriggi F. Liver resection in cirrhotic patients: a Western experience. World J Surg 1986;10:311-317.

3. Lin TY, Chen KM, Chen CC. Role of surgery in the treatment of primary carcinoma of the liver: a 21-year experience. Br J Surg 1987; 74:839-842.

4. Nagasue N, Yukaya K, Ogawa Y, Sasaki Y, Chang Y and Niimi K. Clinical experience with 118 hepatic resections for hepatocellular carcinoma. Surgery 1986; 99:694.

5. Yamanaka N, Okamato E, Toyosaka A, Mitunobu M, Fujihara S, Kato T, Fujimoto J, Oriyama T, Furukawa K and Kawamura E. Prognostic factors after hepatectomy for hepatocellular carcinoma. Cancer 1990; 65:1104.

6. Iwatsuki, S, Starzl TE, Sheahan MB, Yokoyama H, Demetris AJ, Todo S, Tzakis AG, Van Thiel DH, Carr B, Selby R and Madariaga J. Hepatic resection versus transplantation for hepatocellular carcinoma. Ann Surg, 1991; 221-223.

7. American Joint Committee on Cancer. Manual for Staging of Cancer, 3rd Edition. Philadelphia: JB Lippincott, 1987, pp 87-92.

Inhibition of Vascularization in Cancer

KATSUICHI SUDO

Pharmaceutical Research Laboratories III, Takeda Chemical Industries, Ltd., Osaka, 532 Japan

ABSTRACT

Recent advances in the study of angiogenesis and angiogenesis inhibitors resulted in the establishment of a new field of cancer treatment with great potential, anti-angiogenic therapy. Angiogenesis is involved in tumor progression from the beginning of tumorigenesis to its final stage, metastasis. Thus, angiogenesis seems to be a good indicator of diagnosis, prognosis and therapeutic response. Furthermore, tumor vasculature appears to be a good target for antitumor agents. Some angiogenesis inhibitors are now under evaluation in clinical trials. This paper reviews recent findings on tumor angiogenesis and angiogenesis inhibitors, and discusses the possibility of anti-angiogenic therapy.

KEY WORDS: anti-angiogenic therapy, angiogenic factor, angiogenesis inhibitor

ANGIOGENESIS AS A DIAGNOSTIC, PROGNOSTIC AND THERAPEUTIC INDICATOR

In the early stage of solid tumor progression, there is a prevascular phase during which no angiogenic activity is shown by tumor cells. Such tumor cells cannot expand the tumor population beyond a few cubic millimeters [1,2]. These small tumors in the prevascular phase may remain dormant without any clinically detectable signs. Some of them may disappear after being exposed to immunosurveillance by the host. Therefore, a switch to the vascular phase must occur in small, dormant tumors in the early stage. This switch to the angiogenic phase may occur either by mutation of tumor cells causing them to secrete angiogenic factors, phenotypic changes in response to the microenvironment or by accumulation of angiogenic activity [3].

Table 1. Angiogenesis in cancer

1) Indicator of Clinical Significance
    a) Elevation of Angiogenic Factors in urine/Diagnosis
    b) High microvessel density in tumors correlated
        with early recurrence/Prognosis
    c) Reduction of urine Angiogenic Factors by effective
        therapy/Therapeutic Response

2) Target for Antitumor Agents
    a) High dependence of tumor growth and metastasis
        on neovasculature
    b) Rapid proliferation of endothelial cells only in
        tumors

Elevated levels of a representative angiogenic factor, bFGF, have been demonstrated in the urine of bladder cancer patients (Table 1)[4]. Patients with metastatic active disease had the highest levels of urinary bFGF, followed by medium levels in the urine of patients with local active (restricted to the bladder) disease, in comparison with levels indicating no evidence of disease following complete surgical resection of previously local tumors. Increase in levels of urinary bFGF is not restricted to patients with urogenital cancers, but also those with a wide variety of other tumors, suggesting that urinary bFGF may be a good diagnostic indicator [5]. Angiogenic factors are released either by tumor cells directly or by tumor-associated host cells, indicating that markers of angiogenesis could also be used as an indicator of therapeutic response after surgical and medical treatment.

Microvessel density in breast and non-small-cell lung tumors seems to be a good prognostic indicator of metastasis and survival of patients (Table 1)[6,7]. Microvessel density in invasive breast carcinoma, a measure of tumor angiogenesis, is associated with metastasis, and thus with overall and relapse-free survival. The likelihood of metastasis increases as the vessel count increases. Metastasis frequency also differs significantly between the prevascular and vascular phases. The prevascular phase is characterized by local invasion, associated with limited tumor growth, and seldom results in metastasis. All these observations suggest the importance of angiogenesis in metastasis, and the possibility that determination of microvessel density in surgically removed tumors is of prognostic value for appropriate patient follow-up.

Tumor cell malignancy is associated with a high content of cellular angiogenic factors in some of the human cell lines established from highly malignant tumors [8,9,10]. The presence of a large quantity of angiogenic factors is highly likely to contribute to malignant properties of tumors such as invasiveness and metastatic capability. It must also be noted that angiogenic factors are generally multi-functional, stimulating the proliferation of tumor cells, and enhancing tumor cell motility and basement membrane degradation. Taken together, it can be said that angiogenic factors stimulate tumor growth, invasion and metastasis either directly by stimulation of cell growth and motility, or indirectly by increased vessel formation and basement membrane degradation. Thus, markers of angiogenesis or levels of angiogenic factors would be a good diagnostic indicator of tumors in the early stage, for prediction of survival, which is markedly affected by metastasis, and for therapeutic response. The indicators seem to have a causal relationship with malignancy, rather than being merely parallel markers.

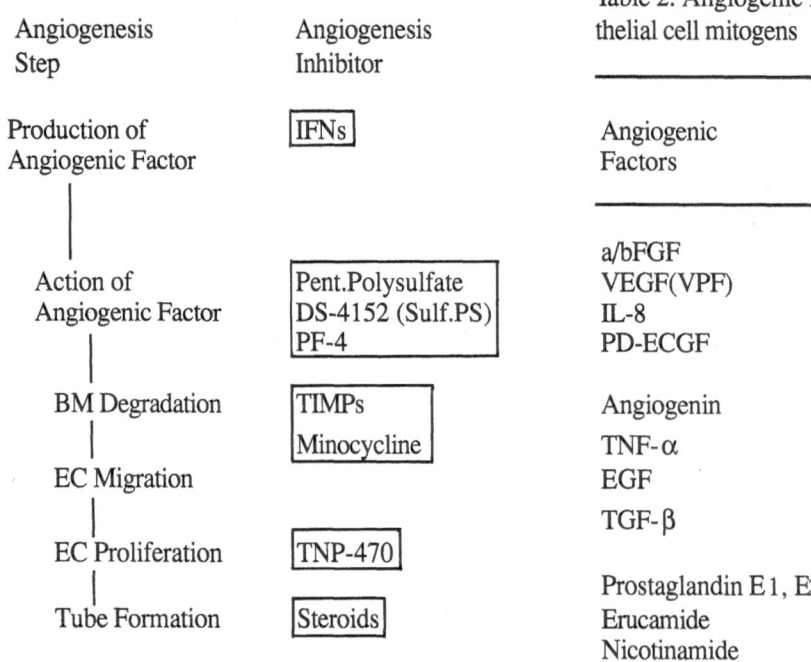

Angiogenesis Step	Angiogenesis Inhibitor
Production of Angiogenic Factor	IFNs
Action of Angiogenic Factor	Pent.Polysulfate DS-4152 (Sulf.PS) PF-4
BM Degradation	TIMPs Minocycline
EC Migration	
EC Proliferation	TNP-470
Tube Formation	Steroids

Fig. 1 Angiogenesis process and possible action sites of representative angiogenesis inhibitors

Table 2. Angiogenic factors and endothelial cell mitogens

Angiogenic Factors	Endothelial Cell Mitogen
a/bFGF	IL-4
VEGF(VPF)	Endothelin
IL-8	G/GM-CSF
PD-ECGF	HGF
Angiogenin	
TNF-α	
EGF	
TGF-β	
Prostaglandin E 1, E2	
Erucamide	
Nicotinamide	

ANGIOGENIC PROCESS AND ANGIOGENIC FACTORS

New capillary formation begins with local dissolution of the basement membrane of an existing microvessel by proteases released from the tumor or from host cells under the influence of angiogenic factors (Fig. 1)[1,2]. This is followed by endothelial cell migration and proliferation. Finally, tubular structures are formed; two microvascular structures anastamose, blood flow commences, and a new capillary is thus completed. Table 2 lists the reported angiogenic factors and endothelial growth factors [2]. The most intensively studied factor is FGF, now known to be a member of a family of eight, all of which are potentially angiogenic. FGF stimulates multiple steps of the angiogenic process [11]. bFGF is contained in most tumor cells and many host cells, such as macrophages and endothelial cells which play important roles in the response to tumors.

Vascular endothelial cell growth factor (VEGF, VPF) is of particular interest in that it appears to be a specific growth factor for endothelium, in contrast to the FGF family which are mitogens for a wide range of cells [10]. Receptors for VEGF are expressed specifically in endothelial cells. This angiogenic factor is secreted by many types of tumor cell, and its expression is enhanced by hypoxia. These factors along with IL-8 [12] and PD-ECGF are also mitogens of endothelial cells [1,2]. Many other polypeptides and small molecules have been reported to be angiogenic although their direct action on endothelial cells and physiological significance are not clarified. They may indirectly induce angiogenesis under influence of major angiogenic factors. In addition to these factors, IL-4, G/GM-CSF, endothelin, and hepatocyte growth factor variant are also reported to be mitogenic for vascular endothelial cells [1,2]. These factors may work as additional ones in concert with major angiogenic factors in some types of tumor. The release or leakage of these many angiogenic factors and endothelial cell mitogens may indicate a difficulty in blocking tumor angiogenesis by competing with any one of the factors. More reasonable approach to blocking angiogenesis would be to interfere with endothelial cell growth at the site common to pathways of various factors, rather than inhibition of receptor binding.

ANGIOGENESIS INHIBITORS

Tumor vasculature is characterized by its unregulated structure, which is quite different from the highly organized networks of vessels in normal tissues. In chemotherapy, chemotherapeutic drugs must reach a much higher concentration in the blood than that needed to be effective, in order to penetrate sufficiently into the target tumor cells distant from the vessel (Table 3). Thus, a poor vascular network in tumors is believed to confer upon them a resistance to both chemotherapy and radiotherapy. Further, tumor cells, the target of chemotherapy, are heterogeneous, responding to drugs in different sensitivity, acquires drug-resistance.

Table 3. Comparison of chemotherapy and anti-angiogenic therapy

	Chemotherapy	Anti-angiogenic Therapy
Target	Growing Tumor Cells	Growing Endothel. Cells (Quiescent in Normal)
	Heterogeneity	Homogeneity
	Multi-Drug Resistance	No MDR Expression
Access of Drug	Diffusion from Vessel	Direct Contact
Side Effects	Severe	Mild

In anti-angiogenic therapy, the main target is growing endothelial cells. It is calculated that one endothelial cell supports more than one hundred of tumor cells [13]. Growth of tumors can be inhibited by growth inhibition of endothelial cells which are in direct contact with drugs in the bloodstream. Furthermore, endothelial cells in normal tissues are largely quiescent except for those in reproductive organs [13]. P-glycoprotein for multi-drug resistance is not expressed in endothelial cells except for a few organs. These observations assure long-term effectiveness with mild toxicity for angiogenic inhibitors if they are specific for endothelial cell growth. The concept that inhibition of angiogenesis leads to inhibition of tumor growth has been supported by animal studies using antibody against bFGF, a representative angiogenic factor. Monoclonal anti-bFGF antibody inhibited both angiogenesis and tumor growth of bFGF gene-transfected tumor cells, even though they are resistant to the antibody *in vitro* [14].

Recently, many angiogenesis inhibitors have been reported in animal studies both *in vivo* and *in vitro*. Despite the many reports on angiogenesis inhibitors, only a few of them have been demonstrated to act at a certain step in the angiogenic process. If we take into consideration that many of the currently used anti-angiogenic assays are not sufficiently specific to detect true angiogenic inhibitors, it may be safe to choose angiogenic inhibitors whose action sites have been clarified. Figure 1 lists angiogenesis inhibitors currently under evaluation in clinical trials, or about to be evaluated in the near future, each corresponding to respective step of angiogenesis. Interferon-α, an inhibitor of growth and migration of vascular endothelial cells causes regression of hemangioma and inhibits subretinal neovascularization [15,16]. Inhibition of angiogenesis by interferons seems to be exerted by modulation of signal transduction independent of the antiproliferation activity of the cytokine [17]. Pentosan polysulfate [18] and DS-4152 (D-gluco-D-galactan sulfate, a fermentation product)[19] are heparin-like compounds. They along with Platelet Factor-4 (30 kDa recombinant protein) [20] inhibit angiogenesis induced by heparin-binding growth factors such as FGF. TIMPs (Tissue inhibitors of metalloproteinase) and minocycline inhibit degradation of collagen, a major component of the basement membrane [2]. TNP-470 (AGM-1470, a semisynthetic analog of a fermentation product, fumagillin)[21,22] inhibits growth of endothelial cells with relative specificity. At least, a part of action sites of angiostatic steroids seems to be at the tube formation. As an example of angiogenesis inhibitors, some results of TNP-470 along with new assays are shown below.

TNP-470 specifically inhibits the formation of capillary-like structure with minimal effect on growth of non-endothelial cells at a wide range of concentration in fibrin gel culture of blood vessel fragments (Fig. 2)[22]. This specific inhibition of *in vitro* angiogenesis is now thought to be due to

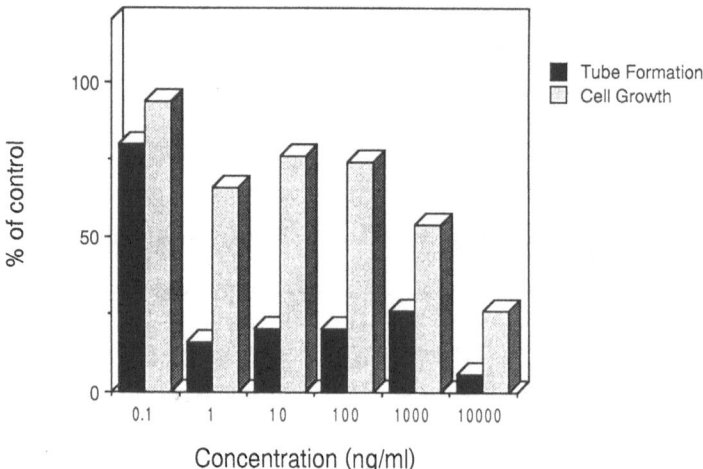

Fig. 2 Specific inhibition of capillary-like tube formation *in vitro*
Rat vessel fragments were cultured in a fibrin gel for 12 days in the absence or presence of TNP-470. Growth of capillary-like tube formation in the gel and growth of cells in monolayer was evaluated on the next day.

the highest sensitivity of endothelial cells to this angiogenesis inhibitor when compared with other types of cells *in vitro*. Chemotherapeutic agents such as adriamycin did not exhibit such specific inhibition of angiogenesis in this assay.

The specific inhibition of endothelial cell growth was confirmed *in vivo*. TNP-470 was given to tumor (mouse M5076 reticulum cell sarcoma)-bearing mice, and growing tumor and endothelial cells were labelled with BrdU. From comparison of the BrdU-labelling index, TNP-470 was found to inhibit the growth of endothelial cells in tumor vessels much earlier and more extensively than that of tumor cells, in contrast to chemotherapeutic agents such as adriamycin and cisplatin (in preparation). TNP-470, as being characteristic to the angiogenesis inhibitor, exhibits antitumor actions against a wide variety of tumor models. These include tumor growth inhibition, antimetastasis and survival prolongation of tumor-bearing animals in various models. Angiogenesis-rich human tumors such as choriocarcinoma [23], hormone-refractory breast [24] and nerve-sheath [25] tumors well responded to TNP-470 in nude mouse systems. Angiogenesis inhibitors may be favorably used for chemoembolization in a controlled-release formulation against cancers such as those of the liver which induce prominent neovessels upon recurrence [26]. These tumors known to be resistant to conventional chemotherapy may be good targets for anti-angiogenic therapy.

CONCLUSIONS

Anti-angiogenic therapy seems to have great potential. Angiogenesis inhibitors highly specific to endothelial cell growth would be promising antitumor drugs with long efficacy and low toxicity. Angiogenesis and metastasis share mechanisms in common: requirement of basement membrane degradation: involvement of cell motility and invasion, dependence on some growth factors in common etc.[27]. Thus, some angiogenesis inhibitors are also likely to act directly on metastatic tumor cells in addition to their inhibitory action on angiogenesis. Synergistic action is expected in combination with chemotherapy [28]. All these findings suggest that anti-angiogenic therapy is especially promising in areas where chemotherapy and radiotherapy cannot exert satisfactory effects, such as hormone refractory cancers, metastasis and recurrence after surgery.

REFERENCES

1. Folkman J, Shing Y (1992) Angiogenesis. J Biol Chem 267: 10931-10934
2. Bicknell R, Harris AL (1991) Novel growth regulatory factors and tumor angiogenesis. Eur J Cancer 27: 781-785
3. Kandel J, Bossy-Wetzel E, Radvanyi F, Klagsbrun M, Folkman J, Hanahan D (1991) Neovascularization is associated with a switch to the export of bFGF in the multistep development of fibrosarcoma. Cell 65: 1095-1104
4. Nguyen M, Watanabe H, Budson AE, Richie JP, Folkman J (1993) Elevated levels of the angiogenic peptde basic fibroblast growth factor in urine of bladder cancer patients. J Natl Cancer Inst 85: 241-242
5. Nguyen M, Watanabe H, Budson AE, Folkman J (1992) Basic fibroblast growth factor (bFGF) is elevated in the urine of patients with a wide variety of neoplasms. Mol Biol Cell 3 (suppl): 234a
6. Weidner N, Folkman J, Pozza F, Bevilacqua P, Allred EN, Moore DH, Meli S, Gasparini G (1992) Tumor angiogenesis: A new significant and independent prognostic indicator in early-stage breast carcinoma. J Natl Cancer Inst 84: 1875-18875.
7. Macchiarini P, Fontanini G, Hardin MJ, Squartini F, Angeletti CA (1992) Relation of neovascularization to metastasis of non-small-cell lung cancer. The Lancet 340: 145-146
8. Wellstein A, Fang W, Khatri A, Lu Y, Swain SS, Dickson RB, Sasse J, Riegel AT, Lippman ME (1992) A heparin-binding growth factor secreted from breast cancer cells homologous to a developmentally regulated cytokine. J Biol Chem 267: 2582-2587
9. Nakamoto T, Chang C, Li A, Chodak GW (1992) Basic fibroblast growth factor in human prostate cancer cells. Cancer Res 52: 571-577

10. Ferrara N, Houck K, Jakeman L, Leung DW (1992) Molecular and biological properties of the vascular endothelial growth factor family of proteins. Endocr Rev 13: 18-32

11. Gospodarowitz D, Ferrara N, Schweigerer L, Neufeld G (1987) Structural characterization and biological functions of fibroblast growth factor. Endocr Rev 8: 95-114

12. Koch AE, Polverini PJ, Kunkel SL, Harlow LA, DiPietro LA, Elner VM, Elner SG, Strieter RM (1992) Interleukin-8 as a macrophage-derived mediator of angiogenesis. Science 258: 1798-1801

13. Denekamp J (1984) Vasculature as a target for tumour therapy. Prog Appl Microcirc 4: 28-38

14. Hori A, Sasada R, Matsutani E, Naito K, Sakura Y, Fujita T, Kozai Y (1991) Suppression of solid tumor growht by immunoneutralizing monoclonal antibody against human basic fibroblast growth factor. Cancer Res 51: 6180-6184

15. Fung WE (1991) Interferon alpha 2a for treatment of age-related macular degeneration. Amer J of Ophthalmol 112: 349-350

16. Ezekowitz RAB, Mulliken JB, Folkman J (1992) Interferon alfa-2a therapy for life-threatnening hemangiomas of infancy. New Engl J Med 326: 1456-1463

17. Sidky YA, Borden EC (1987) Inhibition of angiogenesis by interferons: Effects on tumor- and lymphocyte-induced vascular responses. Cancer Res 47: 5155-5161

18. Zugmaier G, Lippman ME, Wellstein A (1992) Inhibition by pentosan polysulfate (PPS) of heparin-inding growth factors released from tumor cells and blockage by PPS of tumor growth in animals. J Natl Cancer Inst 84: 1716-1723

19. Nakayama Y, Iwahana M, Sakamoto N, Tanaka NG, Osada Y (1993) Inhibitory effect of a bacteria-derived sulfated polysaccharide against basic fibroblast growth factor-induced endothelial cell growth and chemotaxis. J Cell Physiol 154: 1-6

20. Sharpe RJ, Byers HR, Scott CF, Bauer SI, Maione TE (1990) Growth inhibition of murine melanoma and human colon carcinoma by recombinant human Platelet Factor 4. J Natl Cancer Inst 82: 848-853

21. Ingber D, Fujita T, Kishimoto S, Sudo K, Kanamaru T, Brem H, Folkman J (1990) Synthetic analogues of fumagillin that inhibit angiogenesis and suppress tumour growth. Nature 348: 555-557

22. Kusaka M, Sudo K, Fujita T, Marui S, Itoh S, Ingber D, Folkman J (1991) Potent anti-angiogenic action of AGM-1470: Comparison to the fumagillin parent. Biochem Biophys Res Commun 174: 1070-1076

23. Yanase T, Fujita K, Igarashi H, Tanaka K (1992) The inhibition of metastasis of human chorio-carcinoma cell line by angiogenesis inhibitor, AGM-1470. Proceedings of 83rd Annual Meeting of American Association for Cancer Research 33: 69p

24. Sugita T, Gottardis M, Lippman ME, Itoh C, Ueda N, Fukunishi R (1992) Proceedings of the Japanese Cancer Association 51st, 36p (in Japanese)

25. Takamiya Y, Friedlander RM, Brem H, Malick A, Martuza RL (1993) Inhibition of angiogenesis and growth of human nerve-sheath tumors by AGM-1470. J Neurosurg 78: 470-476

26. Kamei S, Okada H, Inoue Y, Yoshioka T, Ogawa Y, Toguchi H (1993) Antitumor effects of angiogenesis inhibitor TNP-470 in rabbits bearing VX-2 carcinoma by arterial administration of microspheres and oil solution. J Pharmacol Experiment Therap 264: 469-474

27. Liotta LA, Steeg PS, Stetler-Stevenson WG (1991) Cancer metastasis and angiogenesis: an imbalance of positive and negative regulation. Cell 64: 327-336

28. Teicher BA, Sotomayor EA, Huang ZD (1992) Antiangiogenic agents potentiate cytotoxic cancer therapies against primary and metastatic disease. Cancer Res 52: 6702-6704

Part 5

Evaluation of Multidisciplinary Treatment of Patients with Digestive Cancers

Evaluation of Efficacy of Chemotherapy/Radiation Therapy in the Treatment of Inoperative Gastric Cancer with Primary Foci

M. Kurihara and M. Matsukawa

Department of Gastroenterology, Toyosu Hospital, Showa University, Koto-ku, Tokyo, 135 Japan

ABSTRACT

In the "Criteria for Evaluating Efficacy of Chemotherapy/Radiation Therapy in the Treatment of Gastric Cancer with Primary Foci" described in the 11th Revised Edition of the General Rules for Gastric Cancer Study, the primary foci of inoperative gastric cancer are classified into three subtypes by X-ray or endoscopic findings, i.e., measurable lesion (a-lesion), not measurable but evaluable lesion (b-lesion), and diffusely infiltrated lesion (c-lesion). PR (partial response) defined for c-lesion required a minimum of 100% enlargement of the affected area in X-ray films for a minimum for 4 weeks. With respect to this requirement for a minimum of 100% of enlargement of the affected area, we have analyzed the results of inoperative cancer study by the Gastric Cancer Study Subgroup under a Grand-in-Aid for Cancer Research from the Ministry of Health and Welfare, and reached the conclusion that it is appropriate to redefine the said cPR requirement as a minimum of 50% enlargement of the affected area for a minimum of 4 weeks.

KEY WORDS: response criteria, gastric cancer, chemothrapy, c-lesion

INTRODUCTION

For the purpose of adequate evaluation of efficacy of chemotherapy/radiation therapy of gastric cancer, the Criteria for Evaluating Efficacy of Chemotherapy/Radiation Therapy on the Treatment of Gastric Cancer [1] (Table 1) were established by the Japanese Research Society for Gastric Cancer, which are described in the 11th Revised Edition of the General Rules for the Gastric Cancer Study. It was already translated into English and explained the details with case reports [2].

Table 1. Criteria for Evaluating efficacy

Type of Primary Lesion	Measurable lesion(a)		Not measurable, but evaluable lesion(b)		Diffusely infiltrated lesion(c)	
Evaluating Scale	Tumor shrinkage rate		Macroscopic change Margin:flattening Ulcer:decrease		extention rate of affected area	
CR	not detected(aCR)		not detected(bCR)		not detected(cCR)	
PR	≥ 50% (aPR)	≥	≥ 50% evaluated(bPR)	≥	≥ 100% (cPR)	≥
NC	< 50% (aNC)	4wks	< 50% evaluated(bNC)	4wks	< 100% (cNC)	4wks
MR	≥ 25% < 50% (aMR)		≥ 25% < 50% (bMR)		≥ 50% < 100% (cMR)	
	≥ 50% (< 4wks)(aMR)		≥ 50% (< 4wks)(bMR)		≥ 100% (< 4wks)(cMR)	
PD	≥ 25% increase (aPD)		progression(bPD)		progression(cPD)	

One of the features of these criteria is that the primary foci of inoperative gastric cancer are classified into three subtypes according to their X-ray or endoscopic findings, i,e.,measurable lesion (a-lesion), not measurable but evaluable lesion (b-lesion), and diffusely infiltrated lesion (c-lesion). CR (complete response) of all three types of lesions a, b and c is common in that it is defined as nondetectability of cancer. Efficacy evaluation of chemotherapy/radiation therapy by PR response of the three types of lesions is made as follows. For a-lesion, the efficacy is evaluated by the rate of reduction in the lesion, and its PR requires a minimum of 50% reduction in the sum of the products of the greater perpendicular diameters of measurable lesions. For b-lesion, the efficacy is evaluated by the macroscopic change in the focal form, and its PR requires more than 50% regression and flattening of elevated or ulcerated lesions on X-ray or endoscopy for a minimum of 4 weeks. For c-lesion, the efficacy is evaluated by the extension rate of the affected area, and its PR requires a minimum of 100% enlargement of the affected area in X-ray films for a minimum of 4 weeks. NC (no change) and PD (progressive disease) are defined as shown in the said table. NC of c-lesion is defined as less than 100% enlargement of the affected area in X-ray films for a minimum of 4 weeks. This evaluation method is widely accepted in Japan because it offers the possibility of grasping the efficacy of chemothrapy/radiation therapy as a real image. However, PR of c-lesion (cPR), which requires a minimum of 100% enlargement of the affected area at present, is relatively easy to obtain from pyloric stenosis type lesions, but is rarely obtained from linitis plastica type lesions. Accordingly, the minimum extension rate of the affected area of cPR has been an outstanding question since the aforementioned Criteria for Efficacy Evaluation were established.

In view of the situation mentioned above, we have analyzed the results of two inoperative cancer studies performed by the Gastric Cancer Study Subgroup under a Grand-in-Aid for Cancer Research from the Ministry of Health and Welfare, i.e, a randomized comparative study based on two treatment regimens of Tegafur + MMC and UFT + MMC [3] , and a pilot study using one regimen of 5'-DFUR + CDDP. The results of analysis are described below.

DISCUSSION

Distribution of Patients and Efficacy by Type of Primary Lesion

Table 2 show the distribution of patients and efficacy ratings by type of primary lesion in the said two studies. In both studies, the eligibility determination of patients for the study and therapeutic efficacy evaluation were performed by an outside organization under a strict control system. As a result, it was found that c-lesions accounted for about 30% of all primary lesions in both studies, or about 1/3 of primary lesions of all inoperative cancer patients. Therapeutic efficacy as judged according to the present cPR criterion was 3.2%, 8.3% and 5.0%, respectively, which were all lower than the values for a- and b-lesion.

Table 2. Ratio and efficacy rate in advanced gastric cancer by type of primary lesion

(1)Comparative study of Tegafur + MMC and UFT + MMC in randomization

Tegafur + MMC (90 cases)

Type of lesion	No. of cases (ratio)	Response				Efficacy rate
		CR	PR	NC	PD	
a (measurable)	26 (28.9%)	0	3	16	7	11.5% (3/26)
b (not measurable but evaluable)	33 (36.7%)	0	3	14	16	9.1% (3/33)
c (diffusely infiltrated)	31 (34.4%)	0	1	23	7	3.2% (1/31)

UFT + MMC (79 cases)

Type of lesion	No. of cases (ratio)	Response				Efficacy rate
		CR	PR	NC	PD	
a (measurable)	27 (34.2%)	0	10	11	5	40.7% (11/27)
b (not measurable but evaluable)	28 (35.4%)	0	7	15	6	25.0% (7/28)
c (diffusely infiltrated)	24 (30.4%)	0	2	15	7	8.3% (2/24)

(2)Pilot study of 5'-DFUR + CDDP (64 cases)

Type of lesion	No. of cases (ratio)	Response				Efficacy rate
		CR	PR	NC	PD	
a (measurable)	17 (26.6%)	0	8	8	1	47.1% (8/17)
b (not measurable but evaluable)	27 (42.2%)	2	8	16	1	37.0% (10/27)
c (diffusely infiltrated)	20 (31.1%)	0	1	16	3	5.0% (1/20)

Survival Curves by Type of Primary Lesion

Figures 1 shows the survival curves by type of primary lesion. These curves indicate that the prognostic progress was specifically serious for patients with c-lesions alone. It was therefore considered likely that efficacy rating were low for c-lesions because the criteria for efficacy evaluation were too strict. The survival curves were also examined by the efficacy evaluation of a-, b- and c-lesions covered by the comparative study of two treatment regions (tegafur + MMC and UFT + MMC)in which a large number of patients were registered.

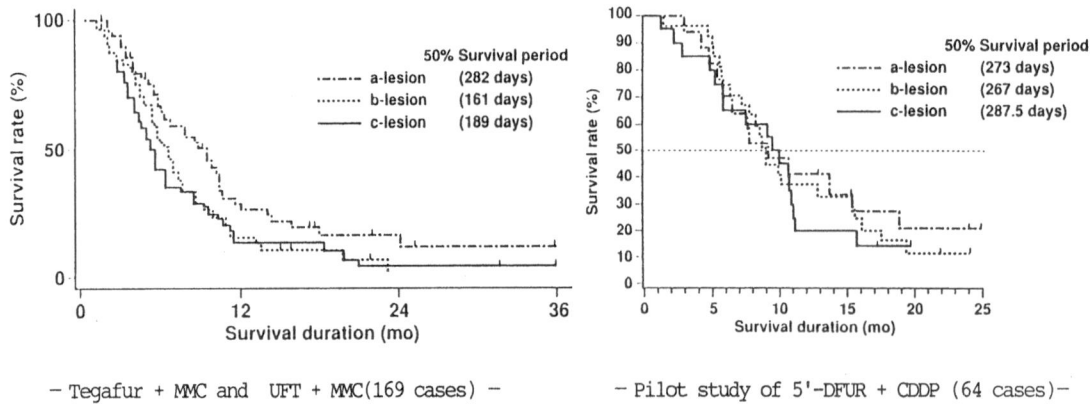

– Tegafur + MMC and UFT + MMC(169 cases) –   – Pilot study of 5'-DFUR + CDDP (64 cases)–

Fig.1 Suvival curves by type of primary leison in gastric cancer

As shown in Figure 2, this examination disclosed that 50% survival time after initiating the treatment was 411 days and 233 days, respectively, for PR and NC of a-lesions, and 295.5 days and 165 days, respectively, for PR and NC of b-lesions, thus showing a significant difference between PR and NC, but it was 213 days and 193 days, respectively, for PR and NC of c-lesions, thus showing no significant difference.

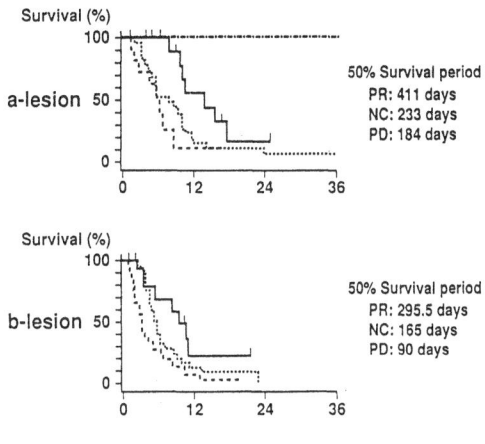

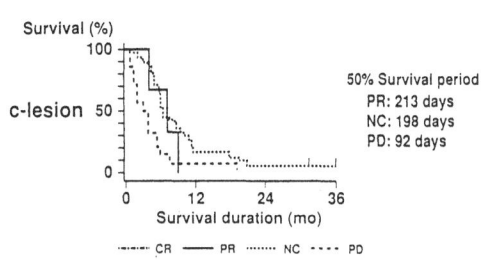

Fig.2 Suvival curves by response
(Tegafur + MMC and UFT + MMC)

Proposed Revision of cPR Criterion

We made the following study by assuming the PR requirement of c-lesion at a minimum of 50% enlargement of the affected area. Specifically, the relations between the survival time and the enlargement of the affected area were examined for a total of 8 patients, comparing four defined as MR with an enlargement exceeding 50% under 100% of the affected area in the aforementioned comparative test, and another four who were given the treatment base on exactly the same protocol (data made available by the courtesy of Dr. Shoji Suga and Dr. Hiroaki Iwase in Nagoya National Hospital). As shown in Table 3, this study disclosed that the average enlargement of the affected area was 72.8%, and the average survival time and 50% survival time were 471.8 days and 450.5 days, respectively, though the survival time was shorter for few patients with totally spread gastric cancer. It was considered possible to regard these patients as effective cases because their 50% survival time was longer than that of the patient evaluated by PR criteria for a- and b-lesions.

Table 3. Summary of MR cases (Extension rate of affected area ≥ 50% < 100%) in c lesion
— Tegafur + MMC and UFT + MMC —

Case #	Extension rate of affected area (%)	Survival days		
1	67.4	779	Mean extension rate	72.8%
2	59.1	750	Mean suvival period	471.8 days
3	55.5	314		
4	70.4	474	50% Suvival period	450.5 days
5	77.9	199		
6	89.5	427		
7	77.9	188		
8	87.3	643		

Figure 3 shows the survival time by therapeutic efficacy, as obtained by re-defining PR of c-lesions used in the comparative test as requiring a minimum 50% enlargement of the affected area. 50% survival time based on the existing criteria was 213 days for PR and 198 days for NC, so that no correlation between the efficacy and the survival time can be observed. However, 50% survival time based on the new criteria was 314 days for PR and 211 days for NC, which shows a significant difference and indicates a clear correlation between the efficacy and the survival time.

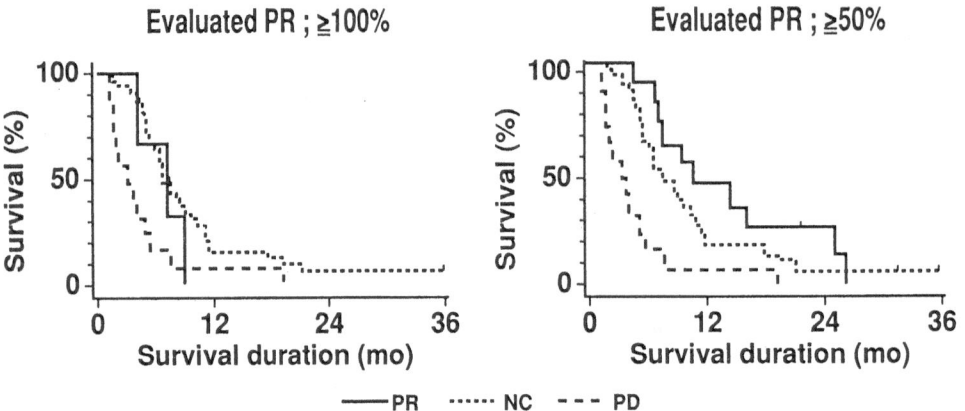

Fig.3 Suvival curves by response in c leision
(Tegafur + MMC and UFT + MMC)

Case Analysis

A case analysis of c-lesion PR (51-year-old male patient) is shown in Figure 5.
The affected area extension rate is obtained by the following formula by measuring the preoperative and postoperative affected area in X-ray films in the barium filled stomach.

$$\text{Extension rate} = \frac{\text{(Postoperative affected area)}-\text{(Preoperative affected area)}}{\text{(Preoperative affected area)}} \times 100\%$$

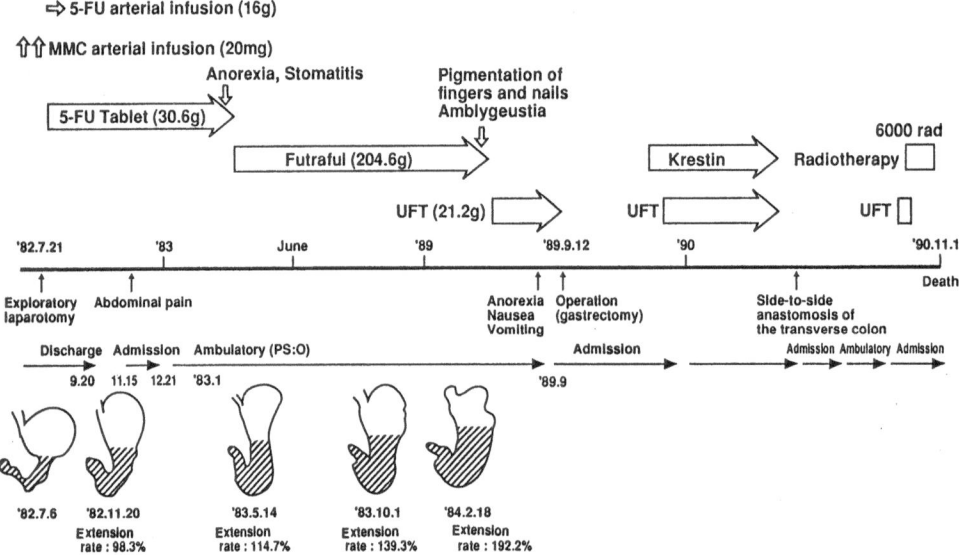

Fig. 4 Treatment course (A case analysis of c-lesion PR)

CONCLUSIONS

On the basis of the above study finding, it is considered appropriate to revise the PR requirement for c-lesion as shown in Table 4.

Table 4. Criteria for evaluating of efficacy of Chemotherapy for gastric cancer in c lesion

	Available Criteria	Revised draft
Evaluating	Extension rate of affected area	Same to the left column
Response		
cCR	not detected	Same to the left column
cPR	≧ 100%	≧ 50%
cNC	< 100%	< 50%
cMR	≧ 100% within 4 wks	≧ 50% within 4 wks
cPD	progression	Same to the left column

The new cPR requirement will be introduced in the 12th Revised Edition of the General Rules for the Gastric Cancer Study.
The aforementioned evaluation scale by type of primary lesion is considered highly useful in making proper evaluation of efficacy of chemotherapy/radiation therapy in the treatment of gastric cancer.

REFERENCES

1. Japanese Research Society for Gastric Cancer, Criteria for Evaluating Efficacy of Chemotherapy/Radiation Therapy in the Treatment of Gastric Cancer (1985) The General Rules for the Gastric Cancer Study, 11th Edition. Kanehara Shuppan, Tokyo, pp 102-105

2. Kurihara M, Izumi T (1991) Evaluation of the Effect of Chemotherapy in Gastric Cancer Patients with an Intact Primary Tumor According to the Criteria of the Japanese Research Society for Gastric Cancer. J. Jpn. Soc. Cancer Ther. 26(3): 644-654

3. Kurihara M, Izumi T, Yoshida S, Ohkubo T, Suga S, Kiyohashi A, Yaosaka T, Takahashi H, Ito T, Sasai T, Akiya T, Akazawa S, Betsuyaku T, Taguchi S (1991) A Cooperative Randomized Study on Tegafur plus Mitomycin C versus Combined Tegafur and Uracil plus Mitomycin C in the Treatment of Advanced Gastric Cancer. Jpn. J. Cancer Res. 82: 613-620

Angiotensin II Induced Hypertension Chemotherapy (IHC) for Advanced Gastric Carcinoma

HARUHIKO SATO, KATSUO SUGIYAMA, KEIICHI ISHIZUKA, MASAHIKO HOSHI, MASANOBU URUSHIYAMA, and MAROH SUZUKI

Department of Clinical Cancer Chemotherapy and Department of Experimental Oncology, The Research Institute for Cancer and Tuberculosis, Tohoku University, Sendai, 980 Japan

ABSTRACT

Under angiotensin II(A II) induced hypertension in which the mean arterial blood pressure did not exceed 150 mmHg, blood flow in tumor tissue increased selectively, while not in normal tissues. A II induced hypertension chemotherapy(IHC) has been carried out since 1978. Two randomized controlled trials, using a combination regimen of ADM,5-FU and MMC for advanced gastric carcinoma, showed significant augmentation of anti-tumor effects without increase of side effects. Surgical and pathological down-staging was observed in stage IV cancer patients. Based on the functional characteristics of tumor microcirculation, IHC which is a system of selective enhancement of drug delivery to tumor, will be useful for patients with any malignant tumors.

KEY WORDS: induced hypertension chemotherapy(IHC), selective enhancement of drug delivery, tumor microcirculation, gastric carcinoma

INTRODUCTION

In cancer chemotherapy, selective enhancement of drug delivery to tumor tissue is essentially important for increase of chemotherapeutic effects, together with selection of sensitive drugs to tumor cells. In some studies on tumor microcirculation[1-3], blood flow in tumor was small and its distribution was much inhomogeneous, as tumor grew, comparing with that in normal tissues. As Gullino PM, et al[2] had described that low and inhomogeneous blood flow within tumor tissues would be a barrier of drug delivery,selective increase of blood flow in tumor has been a purpose for augmentation of effects[1-8].
In 1977, Suzuki M., et al[7,8] found that tumor blood-flow selectively increased under hypertensive state induced by angiotensin II(AII), while blood flow in normal tissues did not increase. AII-induced hypertension chemotherapy (IHC) has been carried out clinically since 1978[9-11], based on the characteristics of tumor microcirculation. In this paper, we deal with the evidences for the difference of microcirculation between tumor and normal tissues, and the results of IHC for advanced gastric carcinoma.

INCREASE OF TUMOR BLOOD FLOW UNDER AII HYPERTENSION

Under AII-induced hypertension state(AII-HT), blood flow of AH109A tumor(a cell line of Yoshida Ascites Hepatomas), the cells of which were subcutaneously transplanted in rats, remarkably increased comparing with that of normotension (NT) (mean increasing rate;5.6 times). However, blood flow in normal tissues such as the brain,liver and bone marrow, unchanged unless the mean arterial blood pressure did exceed 150 mmHg (there is an autoregulation of blood flow)[7,8,12,13]. Moreover, in the kidney and the subcutis, blood flow rather decreased during HT. When AH109A tumors grew in the liver and the muscle, tumor blood flow increased as same as in tumors in the subcutis [12,13]. The increase of blood flow was also observed not only in transplanted tumors, but also in methylcholanthrene induced autochthonous sarcoma[12,13].In various kinds of human tumor cell lines as shown in Table 1, blood flow of subcutaneous xenograftic tumors in nude mice/rats increased with no relation to cell origin or histological types[14,15].In comparison of intensity of tumor area using dynamic CT under AII-HT with that of NT in the same patients, increase of stained regions by contrast media within low density area of tumors was demonstrated under AII-HT.Drug concentration in tumors of rats under AII-HT significantly higher than that under NT[16].

ENHANCEMENT OF CHEMOTHERAPEUTIC EFFECTS

Suzuki et al.[7,8,12,13] had demonstrated that inhibitory effect on tumor growth and prolongation of survival time were significantly enhanced in IHC group than in non-IHC group in which drugs were administrated intravenously by usual manner. In other some experimental systems such as liver and lung metastasis and peritoneal dissemination in rats, augmentation of tumor inhibitory effects by IHC was also seen in a series of experiments [15,17-19].

THE PROCEDURE OF TREATMENT OF IHC

1)Within 2-3 minutes after starting the infusion of AII, the mean arterial blood pressure(BP) was elevated to 150 mmHg level(induction of HT), 2)just after the induction of HT, anti-cancer drugs were injected along with the infusion of AII so as to keep the hypertensive state for 10-15 min (maintenance of HT), 3)BP returned to the previous normotensive state spontaneously within 2-3 min after stopping AII infusion. No any harmful symptom during IHC has been experienced. Patients with active bleeding lesion or heart failure are out of indication for IHC.[9-11,23,24]

Table 1.Change of blood flow of subcutaneously transplanted human cancer cell lines in nude mice/rats

tumor origin	cell line	type of histology	blood flow(ml/min/100g tissue)* normotension	AII-hypertension	mean increase rate (%)
esophagus	TE-8	mod sq	8.8± 7.4	13.3± 9.3	160
stomach	H-111	well ad	6.9±10.6	16.1±13.9	1300
	NS-8	por ad	6.8± 4.5	15.6±10.5	300
	NS-18	pap ad	8.0± 7.8	17.9±18.2	380
colon	FAC	mod ad	10.1± 9.8	18.3±11.2	260
	SCC	por ad	9.2± 5.5	23.8±11.5	330
	KHC	muc ad	6.6± 4.1	16.6±11.4	550
lung	I-87	por ad	12.0± 1.9	68.6±19.1	570

*: mean±SD

THE MECHANISM OF INCREASE OF BLOOD FLOW IN TUMOR

Hori et al[20-22]had reported that newly developed tumor vasculature mainly arose from normal metaarterioles and formed networks of capillaries. The initially branching tumor vessels are named as "starting vessels". Circulatory relation between tumor vessels and normal ones are parallel circuit[22]. According to the experimental observation of Hori et al[21,22], under AII-HT, vascular pressure of the distal sites of normal metaarterioles where starting vessels branched away, elevated so remarkably that blood flow into tumor vascular networks increased. In other words, tumor vasculatures are passive capillary beds that have no regulation for blood flow[12,13,22].

CLINICAL RESULTS(Table 2)

1)Randomized controlled trial(RCT) for advanced gastric carcinoma were conducted. RCT-1 (1981-83)[23] and RCT-2 (1986-89)[24] were performed by cooperative studies of multi-institution attendance. Clinical characteristics between IHC and non-IHC group in which anti-cancer drugs were usually administered under NT were not statistically different in each RCT. In RCTs, a combination schedule of adriamycin, 5-fluorouracil and mitomycin C was used. In RCT-1, 60 patients were entered and 40 were evaluable. One complete(CR) and 8 partial responders(PR) were obtained out of 21 evaluable cases for IHC group. Response rate was 42.9% according to the criteria of Japan Society for Cancer Therapy. Whereas it was 10.5%(2 PR out of 19 evaluable cases) for non-IHC group. Moreover, in RCT-2, among 32 patients in IHC group,4 CR and 8 PR were obtained. Response rate was 31.3%. And then, in non-IHC group, it was 6.7%(2PR out of 30 evaluable cases). Frequency and grade of side effects were not different statistically between both groups in each RCT.

Table 2. Clinical results of randomized controlled trials for advanced gastric
carcinoma(RCT-1:Tohoku IHC Study Group[1981-83] and RCT-2:TY-10721 IHC
Study Group[1986-89])

| | | NO. of patients | | CR | PR | NC(MR) | PD | response | 95% confidence |
		registered	eligible					rate	interval
RCT-1	IHC	33	21	1	8	7(3)	5	42.9*	66.0 -21.8
	non-IHC	27	19	-	2	7(1)	10	10.5*	33.1 - 1.3
RCT-2	IHC	36	32	4	6	10(1)	12	31.3#	47.5 -15.1
	non-IHC	39	30	-	2	14(1)	14	6.7#	18.7 - 0.7

*:$p<0.05$(Wilcoxon test), #:$p<0.05$(chi-square test with Yates'correction)

2) Table 3. shows the results of our phase II trial for stage IV gastric
carcinoma, in which we have carried out using the same regimen of that of
RCTs, since 1978 to 1992. Response rate of non-resectable cases without prior
chemotherapy was 57.7%(5 CR and 10 PR out of 26 evaluable cases). It was
significantly high($p<0.025$) comparing with that of patients who had prior
chemotherapy and recurrence or residual lesions after gastrectomy. Survival in
phase II trial was dependent on clinical response. Median survival for
complete responders after IHC was 25.4 months, and that for PR,NC and PD were
9.0,6.0, and 4.1 months, respectively. Survival time that responders who had
received curative operation after several courses of IHC, tended to be longer
than that of responders who had received prior chemotherapy and no surgery or
recurrent lesions(Table 4).

Table 3. Relation between clinical response and prior chemotherapy in phase II
trial for stage IV gastric carcinoma(1978-1992).

| | prior | NO.of patients | | CR | PR | NC(MR) | PD | response | 95%confidence |
	therapy	eligible	evaluable					rate	interval
non-	-	30	26	5	10	8(3)	3	57.7*	76.7 -36.9
resectable	+	16	14	-	2	9(1)	3	14.3*	42.8 - 1.8
recurrent	-	4	2	-	2	-	-	100	-
or residual	+	24	18	1	2	13(6)	2	16.7*	41.4 - 3.6
total		74	60	6	16	30(10)	8	36.7	50.1 -24.6

*:$p<0.025$(chi-square test with Yates'correction), Fourteen patients were
out of evaluation for reason of secession, ceasing or inadequate follow-up.
Median survival of them was 35 days after start of IHC.

Table 4. Relation between survival time of patients with stage IV gastric
carcinoma and resection for primary lesion after IHC.

| | mean survival time (month) | | |
response	gastrectomy	no resection	recurrence
CR+PR	32.7(n=6)	10.6(n=11)	8.8(n=4)
NC+MR	6.5(n=2)	6.3(n=16)	8.9(n=12)

Among 60 stage-IV-patients treated with IHC, 40 cases had primary lesions.
Ten patients had remarkable responses and 6 out of 10 could receive curative
resection with pathological down staging(15%;6/40). Although it is necessary
to make sure from randomized trial, it may be possible using IHC to increase
the cases with pathological down staging for not only stage IV, but also
other advanced stages. As reported using a model of peritoneal dissemination,
liver and lung metastasis in rats[15,18,19], growth inhibitory effects on

micrometastasis were significantly enhanced by IHC. Hori et al[21] pointed that there are already observed several starting vessels and their newly developed networks which were communicated each other in tumor tissues of 1-2 mm in diameter. Hence, the microcirculation characteristics in tumor tissue are generally observed in any type and size of tumor and moreover, it is able to be applied to enhance drug delivery to tumor, selectively. In stage IV gastric carcinoma, survival of patients was analyzed since 1978 to 1992. When clinical response after IHC was remarkable or when state of disease could be estimated to be better than that without reduction surgery, gastrectomy was performed. Survival of a group with gastrectomy after CR and PR was significantly longer than that of other groups(Table 4). Pathological down staging of the group from stage IV to III and the lower stages in which the depth of infiltration stayed above the proper muscular layers and microscopic metastasis was within the 2nd group of lymphnodes, was observed in 4 cases out of 11 patients who received any curative operation or reduction surgery after more than one course of IHC in phase II trial for advanced gastric carcinoma since 1978. Moreover, in RCT-2, [24] investigating on patients with non-resectable stage IV stomach cancer of our Institutions, 7 cases among 19(36.8%) for IHC group and 4 of 12(33.3%) for non-IHC group had received operation for reduction of tumor burden.
Pathological down staging was observed in 4 of 7 cases(57.1%) for IHC, whereas, none of 4 cases receiving only palliative operation for non-IHC group. Although prospective trial is necessary to confirm, selective enhancement of drug delivery to tumor tissues is essentially important for augmentation of cancer chemotherapy. IHC must be available for any type of cancer, clinically.

REFERENCES

1. Algire GH, Legallais FY, Anderson BF.(1954) Vascular reaction of normal and malignant tissue in vivo. VI.The role of hypotension in the action of components of podophyllin on transplanted sarcoma. J Natl Cancer Inst 14: 879-893.
2. Gullino PM, Grantham FH.(1962) Studies on the exchange of fluids between host and tumor. III. Regulation of blood flow in hepatomas and other rats tumors. J Natl Cancer Inst 28: 211-229.
3. Kjartansson I.(1976) Tumor microcirculation. An experimental study in rat with a comparison of different methods for estimation of tumor blood flow. Acta Chirurg Scand (suppl 471): 5-74.
4. Edlich RF, Rogers W, DeShaso CV Jr, Aust JB.(1966) Effect of vasoactive drugs on tissue blood flow in the hamster melanoma. Cancer Res 26:1420-1424.
5. Burton MA, Gray BN, Self GW, Heggie JC, Townsend PS.(1985) Manipulation of experimental rat and rabbit liver tumor blood flow with angiotensin II. Cancer Res 45: 5390-5393.
6. Chaplin DJ.(1991) The effect of therapy on tumor vascular function. Int J Radiat Biol 60:311-325.
7. Suzuki M, Hori K, Abe I, Saito S.and Sato H.(1978) Characteristic blood circulation in tumor tissue with reference to chemotherapy. Cancer and chemotherapy 5(suppl) :77-80.
8. Suzuki M,Hori K,Abe I,Saito S. and Sato H.(1981) A new approach to cancer chemotherapy : Selective enhancement of tumor blood flow with angiotensin II. J Natl Cancer Inst 67: 663- 669.
9. Sato H, Sato K, Sato Y, Asamura M,Kanamaru R,Sugiyama Z,Kitahara T, Wakui A, Suzuki M, Hori K, Abe I, Saito S. and Sato H.(1981) Induced hypertension chemotherapy of cancer patients by selective enhancement of drug delivery to tumor tissue with angiotensin II. Sci Rep Res Inst,Tokoku Univ Ser-C 28: 32-44.
10. Sato H, Sato K, Sato Y,Mimata Y, Asamura M, Kanamaru R, Wakui A, Suzuki M and Sato H. (1980) Clinical study on selective enhancement of drug delivery by angiotensin II in cancer chemotherapy. In: Metastasis, clinical and experimental aspect. Hellmann K, Hillgard P. and Eccles S.(eds). Martinus Nijhoff Publishers, The Hague, pp388-394.
11. Sato H, Sato K, Sato Y,Asamura M, Kanamaru R, Mimata Y. and Wakui A. (1981) Clinical cancer chemotherapy based on the experimental findings of selective enhancement of drug delivery to tumor tissue by angiotensin II. Jpn J Cancer Chemother 8(suppl) :91-100.
12. Suzuki M,Hori K,Abe I,Saito S. and Sato H.(1984) Functional characteristics of the microcirculation in tumors. Cancer Metastasis Rev 3:115-126.

13. Suzuki M,Hori K,Saito S.Tanda S,Abe I.Sato H. and Sato H.(1989) Functional characteristics of tumor vessels:Selective increase in tumor blood flow. Sci Rep Res Inst,Tokoku Univ Ser-C 36: 37-45.
14. Hoshi M.(1988) Increase of blood flow in human tumors under angiotensin II induced hypertension. Kosankinbyo Kenkyusyo Zasshi 40: 41-52.
15. Ishizuka K.(1993) DDS(in press).
16. Hoshi M,Abe I,Sugiyama K,Ishizuka K,Sato H,Urushiyama M. and Wakui A.(1991) Selective enhancement of the image intensity of contrast media on dynamic CT under angiotensin II human(TY-10721) induced hypertension state. DDS 6: 109-116.
17. Sato H,Hoshi M,Urushiyama M,Sugiyama K. and Wakui A.(1989) Angiotensin II induced hypertension chemotherapy(IHC) and dose intensity(DI).DDS 4:105-110.
18. Urushiyama M.(1990) Growth inhibition of micrometastases in the liver and angiotensin II induced hypertension chemotherapy(IHC).Kosankinbyo Kenkyusho Zasshi 42:133-144.
19. Sugiyama K.(1990) Selective enhancement of drug delivery to the peritoneal tumor and angiotensin II induced hypertension. Kosankinbyo Kenkyusho Zasshi 42: 145-159.
20. Hori K,Suzuki,Tanda S. and Saito S.(1990) In vivo analysis of tumor vascularization in the rat. Jpn J Cancer Res 81:279-288.
21. Hori K,Suzuki M,Tanda S.and Saito S.(1991) Characterization of heterogeneous distribution of tumor blood flow in the rat. Jpn J Cancer Res 82: 109-117.
22. Hori K,Suzuki M,Tanda S,Saito S.and Zang QH.(1993) Functional characterization of   developing tumor vascular system and drug delivery (review). Int J Oncol 2:289-296.
23. Sato H, Hoshi M, Wakui A.(1986) Clinical study on angiotensin induced hypertension chemotherapy(IHC). Jpn J Cancer Chemother 13:1439-1447.
24. Sato H,Wakui A,Hoshi M,Kurihara M,Yokoyama M. and Shimizu H.(1991) Randomized controlled trial of induced hypertension chemotherapy(IHC) using angiotensin II human(TY-10721) in advanced gastric carcinoma.(TY-10721 IHC Study Group Report). Jpn J Cancer Chemother 18:451-460.

Prerequisites of Adjuvant and Neoadjuvant Chemotherapy in Gastric Cancer

TOSHIFUSA NAKAJIMA, KEIICHIRO OTA, SHOU ISHIHARA, HIROHUMI YAMADA, and MITSUMASA NISHI

Division of Gastrointestinal Surgery, Cancer Institute Hospital, Toshima-ku, Tokyo, 170 Japan

ABSTRACT

Prerequisites of adjuvant and neoadjuvant chemotherapy in gastric cancer were elucidated from a review of previous reports and analysis of our own data. Most important factor is the amount of residual tumor after surgery: there were seldom positive reports in terms of survival benefit when the five year survival rate of control group(surgery alone) was less than 40%. Dose intensity was also an influential factor on the outcome. Regional chemotherapy might contribute to increase in the local drug concentration. Rational combination of curative surgery and chemotherapy with high compliance is mandatory for improving the prognosis of advanced gastric cancer.

KEY WORDS: prerequisite of adjuvant chemotherapy, gastric cancer, amount of residual tumor, dose intensity

INTRODUCTION

Although surgical adjuvant chemotherapy in gastric cancer has a long history of clinical trials since late 1950s, its survival benefit is not yet established statistically[1,2]. However, some Japanese trials reported favorable results of subset analysis that a certain survival benefit of 5 to 30% increase in the five year survival rate was observed in the moderately locally advanced cancer(Stage II and III diseases). The present paper aimed to elucidate common conditions from previous reports and our own data which might lead to the successful adjuvant chemotherapy in gastric cancer.

MATERIALS AND METHODS

A review was made with published papers of adjuvant chemotherapy which were carried out in the setting of randomized controlled study in gastric cancer, associated with a retrospective analysis of our data-base of gastric cancer in Cancer Institute Hospital, Tokyo. Chemotherapeutic effect of prolonging life span was evaluated in relation to the five year survival rate of control group, timing of initiation of chemotherapy, and the dose intensity. Neoadjuvant chemotherapy trials of advanced gastric cancer were also referred with a same intent.

RESULTS

Survival Benefit in Relation to the Five Year Survival Rate of Control Groups(Surgery Alone)

Table 1 summarizes the treatment results of adjuvant chemotherapy trials which were carried out in the setting of controlled radomized study, and employed control group treated with surgery alone. Table 1-a shows the results of early day's U.S. clinical trials with Thio-TEPA(triethylene thiophosphoramide) or 5-FudR(5-fluoro-2-deoxyuridine). There was no difference in the survival rate between treated and control groups. The five year survival rate of control group was around 20%. Table 1-b includes the results of regimens in which 5-FU(5-fluorouracil), or combination of 5-FU and nitrosourea compounds was involved. There was no positive results in terms of the

Table 1. Surgical adjuvant chemotherapy in gastric cancer

(a)

Reporters / year	Regimen	Number	5 ysr
Dixon et al (Universy Group) (1971)	TSPA hige dose	82	24
	Control	89	19
	TSPA low dose	177	24
	Control	183	24
Serlin et al (1977)	TSPA hige dose	43	16
	Control	112	16
	TSPA low dose	152	18
	Control	138	24
	FUDR	217	17
	Control	241	15

(b)

Reporters / year	Regimen	Number	5 ysr
Blokhina et al (1972)	5-FU	375	40 *
	Control	402	37
GITSG (1982)	5-FU, MeCCNU	71	45
	Control	71	32
VASOG (1983)	5-FU, MeCCNU	66	38 *
	Control	68	39 *
ECOG (1985)	5-FU, MeCCNU	91	27
	Control	89	34
Hugier at al (1980)	5-FU, VBL, CPA	27	18
	Control	26	19
Schreml et al (1984)	5-FU, BCNU	42	58
	Control	53	42

* 3 year suvival rate

(c)

Reporters / year	Regimen	Number	5 ysr
Imanaga, Nakazato (1977)	MMC, moderate dose	242	68
	Control	283	54
Nakajima et al (1978)	MMC, moderate dose	207	52
	Control	223	44
Hattori et al (1972)	MMC, large dose	146	37
	Control	278	50
Alcobenas et al (1983)	MMC, large dose	33	79
	Control	37	38
Nakajima et al (1980)	MMC, 5-FU, CA	42	67
	Control	38	50
Nakajima et al (1984)	MMC, 5-FU, CA ➔ 5-FU	81	68
	MMC, FT, CA ➔ FT	83	63
	Control	79	51

(d)

Reporters / year	Regimen	Number	5 ysr
Fielding et al (1983)	5-FU, VCR, CPA, MTX ➔ 5-FU, MMC	140	60 *
	5-FU, MMC	141	66
	Control	130	57
Schein et al (1986)	5-FU, ADM, MMC	156	76 **
	Control	155	72
Allum et al (1989)	5-FU, ADM, MMC	145	27
	Radiotherapy	153	20
	Control	145	24
Coombes et al (1990)	5-FU, ADM , MMC	133	46
	Control	148	36

* 12months   ** 30months

life prolongation except one trial(5-FU + MeCCNU vs control) done by the Gastrointestinal Tumor Study Group. Five year survival rate for control groups was around 30% or less (only three year survival rate was available in some papers). Table 1-c lists the treatment results of MMC(mitomycin C) in the adjuvant chemotherapy in gastric cancer, mainly reported from Japan. These trials involved all stages of gastric cancer treated with curative gastrect-omy as their subject, and beneficial results were observed in certain subset of stages(Stage II and III). The five year survival rate was 40 to 50% for stage II or III diseases. Table 1-d shows the treatment results of regimens which commonly include MMC, 5-FU and ADM(adriamycin). There were no survival benefits with these regimens. The five year survival rate was 20 to 30% or less(five year survival rate was not available in some reports). Figure 1 illustrates the treatment results of these clinical trials with plotting five year survival rate of trial groups on the vertical axis and that of control groups on the horizontal axis. Deviated spots above the 45 degree line were observed when the five year survival rate of control group was greater than 40%.

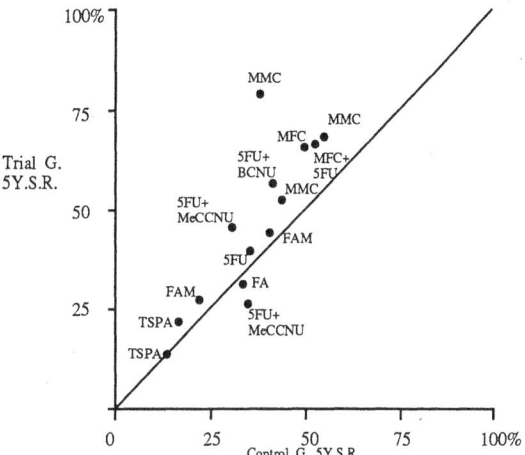

Fig. 1. Treatment results of adjuvant chemotherapy
in gastric cancer

Effect of Dose Intensity on Life Span in Adjuvant Chemotherapy

Postoperative adjuvant chemotherapy was conducted by several cancer hospitals
(including our institute) from 1984 to 1987. Postoperative survivals of
patients treated with curative surgery and adjuvant chemotherapy was analyzed
according to the individual dose intensity of maintenance therapy with 5-FU
or UFT(a compound of Uracil and tegaful, a 5-FU derivative). Individual dose
intensity(IDI) was defined by the following formula[3].

Individual Dose Intensity (I.D.I.)

$$I.D.I. = \frac{\textbf{Total dose given / observed duration}}{\textbf{Total dose proposed / proposed duration}}$$

Group A(n=155) was treated with adjuvant chemotherapy after surgery with a
combination of intravenous MMC, 5-FU and CA(cytosine arabinoside)(MFC),
followed by oral 5-FU. Group B(n=155) was treated with the same intravenous
regimen, followed by UFT. Patients were divided into four subsets according
to IDI fo the maintenance therapy. Subset one was the group with IDI more
than 1.0, subset two was that with IDI from 0.8 to 1.0, subset three was
that with IDI from 0.6 to 0.8, and subset four was that with IDI less than
0.6. Average IDI for intravenous MFC therapy which was common in group A
and B was almost identical in both groups. Postoperative survival curves of
Group A and B were illustrated in Fig.2. There was no difference in the
survival rates among three subsets(1,2 and 3) in Group A. Subset four in
Group A had a poorer prognosis than three subsets. However, there was a
large difference in the survivals among four subsets in Group B, as shown
in the figure. These differences were still observed when the short survivors less than one year were excluded from the calculation.

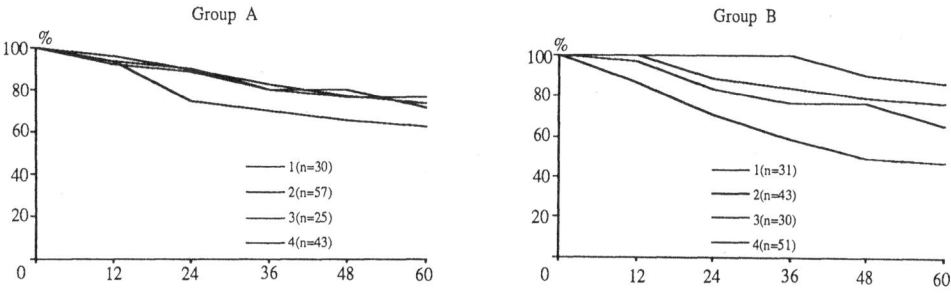

Fig. 2. Effect on the survivals according to the dose intensity(IDI)

Neoadjuvant Chemotherapy for Unresectable Gastric Cancer

Since 1989, a neoadjuvant chemotherapy was carried out for 20 patients with
unresectable primary or metastatic lesions in our hospital[4]. Patients were
subjected to a regimen with five day intravenous infusion of 5-FU(370 mg/m2)
and leucovorin(30 mg/body), followed by intra-aortic delivery of Cisplatinum
(70 mg/m2) and Etoposide(70 mg/m2) on day 6 and 20. This regimen was repeated
two times every five weeks before surgery. Lesions were thoroughly studied
before and after chemotherapy with upper GI series, endoscopy, CT, ultrasonography and MRI. Response rate was 55 % for all cases(Tabel 2). Response rates

Table 2. Response rate according to the sites of tumor lesions

Lesions	Local Response			
	CR+PR	NC	PD	PR(%)
Primary (n=20)	9	6		45.0
Paraaorta node (n=18)	12	3		66.7
Supraclavicular node (n=2)	2			100
Liver (n=7)	3	4		42.8
Peritoneal dissem. (n=5)	1	2	2	20.0
Bone (n=2)		1	1	0
Brain (n=1)			1	0
Total	11	7	2	55.0

by the site of lesions were 66.7% for para-aortic lymph node metastasis,
42.8% for liver metastasis. Patients with supraclavicular node swelling
responded completely to chemotherapy(2/2). Twelve out of 20 patients were
subjected to surgery. Eleven patients were treated with gastrectomy, 8 curative and 3 non-curative. Main toxicity included hematologic and gastrointestinal disturbances,with one toxic death due to bone marrow suppression and
infection. Postoperative survivals were shown in Fig. 3, according to the
type of surgery and type of radicality. Three year survival rate was 23.8%
for all cases, 42.8% for resected cases(responders), and non-resected cases
(non-responders) did not survived more than one year. Three year survival
rate was 62.8% for patients with curative surgery, and 23.0% for palliative
resection.

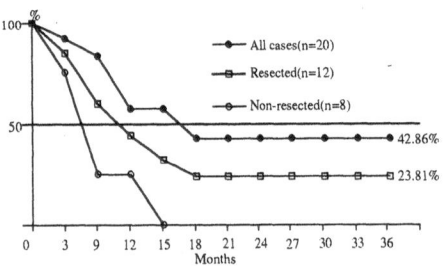

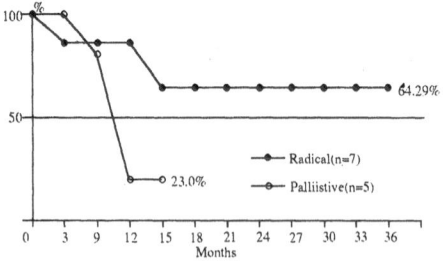

Fig. 3. Survivals of Patients treated with
FLEP Therapy and Surgery

Survivals of Resected Patients
according to Radicality

DISCUSSION

A review of previous adjuvant chemotherapy trials revealed that the effect of
adjuvant chemotherapy was observed in the trials where the five year survival
rate of control group(surgery alone) was more than 40%. If we could assume
that the postoperative survival time is inversely proportional to the amount
of residual tumor left behind surgery, these findings suggest that the pre-

vious postoperative chemotherapy could only control as minimum as residual tumor which produce more than 40% survival rate at five years. Experimental data suggests the inverse relationship between the effect of chemotherapy and tumor burden. Most negative reports from the western world showed that five year survival rates of their control groups were less than 40%, and these findings suggest that the amount of residual tumor after surgery in the western countries is much more than in Japan. Then, the amount of residual tumor seems to be the most important factor which influence the outcome of adjuvant chemotherapy. In order to obtain the positive results in adjuvant chemotherapy in gastric cancer, we should reduce the tumor burden as minimum as to produce more than 40% five year survival rate. It seems reasonable to initiate chemotherapy during or immediately after surgery when the tumor burden is minimum. Almost all western trials initiated chemotherapy more than one month after surgery.

Another important issue is the dose intensity which influence the result of chemotherapy. Dose intensity should be related to both regimens and individuals, or compliance of chemotherapy. Adjuvant chemotherapy in breast cancer had a close correlation between the relative dose intensity and three year survival rate[5], and our recent trial revealed a parallel relationship between the postoperative survival rates and the individual dose intensity of maintenance therapy with UFT, but not with 5-FU. Though the discrepancy is not fully understood, it could be explained by the initial dose setting of UFT, which might barely exceed the minimum effective dose level, and if the compliance is not enough, individual dose intensity fails to reach the minimum effective dose level. The finding that the exclusion of short survivors less than one year did not affect the result suggests the importance of dose intensity per unit time. Poor compliance might be attributed to the toxicity of chemotherapy and poor understanding of patients concerning their disease. Toxicity control and complete information about disease may helpful for decreasing in the number of drop-out from the treatment.

Our recent neoadjuvant chemotherapy suggest the usefulness of regional chemotherapy to control the unresectable lesions. Regional delivery may contribute to increase the local concentration of the drug at the tumor site. Rational combination of regional and systemic chemotherapy, followed by radical surgery would contribute to get the long survivors among patients with primarily unresectable lesions.

REFERENCES

1. Nakajima T, Nishi M (1988) Adjuvant chemotherapy, immunochemotherapy, and neoadjuvant therapy for gastric cancer in Japan. In: Douglass Jr HO (ed) Gastric Cancer(Contemporary Issues in Clinical Oncology 8). Churchill & Livingston, New York, pp125-143
2. Douglass Jr HO (1988) Western surgical adjuvant trials in gastric cancers: Lessons from current trials to be applied to the future. In:Douglass Jr HO (ed) Gastric Cancer(Contemporary Issues in Clinical Concology 8). Churchill & Livingston, New York, pp145-172
3. Coppin CML (1987) The description of chemotherapy delivery: Options and pitfalls. Sem Oncol 14(4 suppl 4):34-42
4. Nakajima T, Ishihara S, Ota K, Yamada H, Nishi M (1992) Down staging of inoperable gastric cancer with biaxial chemotherapy. Proc. of the 45 Annual Meeting of the Society of Surgical Oncology. p130
5. Hryniuk WM, Levin MN (1986) Analysis of dose intensity for adjuvant chemotherapy trials in stage II breast cancer. J Clin Oncol 4: 1162-1170

Adjuvant Therapy of Gastric Cancer in the West

HAROLD O. DOUGLASS, JR.

Department of Surgery, State University of New York at Buffalo and Department of Surgical Oncology, Roswell Park Cancer Institute, Buffalo, NY 14263, USA

ABSTRACT

Results of Western surgical adjuvant gastric cancer trials have been inconsistent. Useful adjuvant therapy has not been identified. The probable cause may be a defect in trial design. Stratification by serosal involvement and lymph node metastases includes a wide range of prognoses that may not be balanced by randomization. Stratification should be by TNM stage and type of resection of the stomach performed, with data collected to permit quality control of the surgical procedure and pathologic examination. Future trials should be largely limited to patients with UICC Stage IIIA cancers and those Stage II cancers of the proximal stomach.

KEY WORDS

Stomach cancer. Surgical adjuvant therapy. TNM stage. Gastrectomy. Quality control.

INTRODUCTION

Twenty years ago, the first of a new series of Western randomized controlled surgical adjuvant chemotherapy trials following potentially curative resection of gastric cancer, was initiated by the Gastrointestinal Tumor Study Group (GITSG). [1] The initial publication of the results of this trial indicated that a significantly increased number of patients who had been randomized to postoperative 5-fluorouracil (5FU) and methyl-CCNU were alive at the end of five years, when compared to patients in the concurrently randomized control group. At ten years, the significant benefit of treatment persisted. [2]

A few years after the initiation of the GITSG trial, the Eastern Cooperative Oncology Group (ECOG) opened a virtually identical study, but in a different population of patients. [3] This study failed to demonstrate any survival advantage in patients randomized to receive chemotherapy. Indeed, the rate of five-year survival of patients in the control arm was better than in the treatment arm, although the difference was not significant. Minor differences in data management appeared too small to explain why this study failed to confirm the GITSG results.

A randomized third trial by the Veterans Administration Surgical Oncology Group (VASOG), used a somewhat less dose-intensive regimen of the chemotherapeutic agents. [4] Although VASAG had enrolled the largest number of patients in its study, many had palliative rather than potentially curative resections for their gastric cancers. In the curatively resected group of patients, survivals in the treatment and in the untreated control arms were equivalent.

The fourth controlled randomized nitrosourea-5-fluorouracil trial substituted BCNU for methyl-CCNU, but in other respects was similar to the methyl-CCNU trials. Survivals of patients in both treatment and control groups in the report from the University of Heidelberg [5] were similar to those noted by GITSG. The marked survival advantage for the treated patients failed tests of statistical significance since the number of patients entered was too small to permit satisfactory application of these tests.

Subsequent controlled trials were generally doxorubicin-5-fluorouracil based, with or without the addition of mitomycin C. [6,7] With a single exception, they also failed to demonstrate any benefit for adjuvant chemotherapy. That exception was a Spanish trial of high-dose mitomycin C administered as a single agent. Five [8] and ten [9] year survivals were reported to be significantly improved among patients who received chemotherapy as compared to the survival of patients in the randomized control group.

MATERIALS AND METHODS OF RECENT AND CURRENT TRIALS

Based on the initial results of its first trial, [1] the GITSG initiated a second randomized trial, this time using 5FU and methyl-CCNU as the "control arm", and adding doxorubicin (Adr) to the combination to produce a three-drug "treatment" arm. [10] When the results of the other 5FU and nitrosourea based treatment programs became known, it was assumed that the discrepancies between the GITSG results [1] and those of other studies [3,4] were merely due to chance, and that 5FU and methyl-CCNU were ineffective adjuvant therapies. Later results from the International [6] and North Central Cancer Treatment Group [7] trials further suggested that adding Adr would little impact on the results of adjuvant therapy with 5FU and methyl-CCNU.

The second GITSG gastric adjuvant study stratified 212 patients patients in a manner similar to its first trial, but more detailed data was obtained prospectively to allow TNM stagings evaluation of the extent of surgery and the type of hospital in which surgery had been performed. Not only were specially designed forms used, but also copies of original pathology reports and operative notes were obtained, with further contact by the reviewing investigator if the materials submitted did not provide all needed information.

Most surgical adjuvant trials had stratified patients on entry in a fashion similar to the Dukes staging system of colon cancer, emphasizing the presence or absence of lymph node metastases and serosal involvement. Because the recognized poor prognosis of patients with cancers of the proximal stomach, patients treated by esophagogastrectomy and by total gastrectomy were stratified separately from those treated by distal subtotal resection. The 5FU-BCNU trial had stratified by Stage (II vs III) but did not define the staging system and modification used. [5] Only the study from Barcelona had used TNM staging, but numbers of patients within each group were very small. [9]

RESULTS

Wide differences in the survival of the randomized control groups suggested that factors other than chance were affecting trial results. A generated trend toward improved proportions of patients surviving five years was not reflected by prolongation of median survivals in these groups of patients.

Median and Long-Term Survival
of Patients Entered into Control Groups

Study	Median Survival	Long-Term Survival
GITSG	33 months	27% at 5 years
VASOG		39% at 4 years
ECOG	33 months	42% at 5 years
Barcelona	16 months	39% at 5 years
International	30 months	52% at 3 years
NCCTG	22 months	51% at 4 years

As predicted, the addition of Adr to 5FU and methyl-CCNU did not alter
patient survival in the second GITSG trial. Essentially, this trial was
an evaluation of the survival of patients following potentially curative
resection of gastric cancer treated with ineffective chemotherapy that
neither significantly shortened nor significantly prolonged survival.
The results would probably closely correlate with post-operative
survivals of patients who had not received adjuvant treatment.

Survivals paralleled TNM stage quite closely, particularly following
distal gastrectomy. The five-year survivals of patients whose cancers
required either esophagogastrectomy (proximal subtotal gastrectomy) or
total gastrectomy were very similar to each other. In contrast,
the survivals of patients treated by total and proximal subtotal
gastrectomy were very different from those of patients whose cancers
could be treated by distal subtotal resection.

Survival of GITSG Patients According to TNM Stage

Stage[a]	TNM	Survival at 5 Years	
		Distal Gastrectomy	Proximal or Total Gastrectomy
IB	T_1N_1	75%	---
II	T_1N_0	70%	25%
	T_2N_1	45%	31%
IIIA	T_2N_0	40%	20%
	T_3N_2	40%	25%
IIIB	T_2N_1	27%	22%
	T_3N_2	19%	6%

[a]UICC and AJC Staging, 1987 revision

Although the initial stratification parameters appeared to be useful
survival discriminants, the stage of the resected cancer overrode all
stratifications except the type of gastrectomy. Median survivals of
patients with and without peritoneal metastases were 33 and 46 months,
respectively. Median survivals with and without serosal involvement or
full thickness invasion were 32 and 43 months respectively. The median
survival of patients who required either proximal or total gastrectomy
was 28 months, 11 months shorter than the survival of those who could be
treated by distal gastrectomy.

When examined by stage of disease, the five-year survival of patients
with lymph node metastases could be as high as 75% in Stage IB, or as
little as 6% in Stage III B. Unlike some other studies, [11] no
correlation between survival and the number or percentage of involved
lymph nodes could be established in the GITSG trial. Survival of
patients with serosal involvement varied from 6% in Stage IIIB to 40% in
Stage II.

Surgeons at two of the participating institutions performed R_2
resections. Thus, R_2 resections were performed on only 15% of the total
patients entered into the GITSG trial. The vast majority of these

patients required proximal or total gastrectomy. Thus, R_2 resections were performed on 26% of patients requiring proximal or total gastrectomy and on only 7% of patients treated by distal subtotal resection. In stages IB and II, the five-year survival of patients treated by R_2 proximal or total gastrectomy was 75%. In Stage IIIA, five-year survival for this group of patients was 36%, with a somewhat greater impact made on the survival of T_3N_1 than T_2N_2 patients. No advantage of R_2 resection was seen in Stage IIIB T_3N_2 patients.

The role of splenectomy was also evaluated. Splenectomy appeared to have no effect on survival of patients when stratified by TNM stage and type of gastric resection.

Although limitations had been placed on the entry of early gastric cancers into the trial, the inclusion of lymph node metastases or muscularis propria invasion allowed one institution to enter 38% of its entries in Stage IB, while other institutions submitted only patients with more advanced disease. At the other end of the spectrum, three institutions entered one third of their patients with Stage IIIB disease while others entered none.

Analysis of the patient contributions to the GITSG trial suggests another reason for variations in overall survivals in various studies. As suggested in the discussion of R_2 resections, wide variation exists in the types of cases submitted from the individual member institutions. Three quarters of patients referred to the study by the two surgical groups performing R_2 resections had carcinomas requiring by proximal or total gastrectomy. Whereas in one institution, 93% of patients referred to the GITSG trial required proximal or total gastric resections, in another only 12% did.

The frequency of patients with metastatic lymph nodes ranged from 57% to 100%, but were generally clustered around 75-87% for most members. Serosal invasion was noted in as few as 44% of patients from one institution and as many as 88% from another. However, for most members, the frequencies of patients with serosal involvement ranged between 71-80%. Thus, the incidences of lymph node metastases and serosal invasion suggested a deceivingly uniform group of patients entered into the trial, a deception only made apparent by TNM staging of the entries.

In general, smaller community hospitals were likely to submit patients with earlier cancers treated by distal subtotal gastrectomy whereas large referral centers tended to enter patients with more advanced cancers treated by esophagogastrectomy or total gastrectomy. Thus, the composition of a cooperative group is likely to be reflected in the composition of patients entered into a gastric adjuvant therapy trial and in the overall results of the trial.

Current and Future Trials

The current Intergroup adjuvant therapy trial in the United States involves a prospectively randomized controlled program which includes treatment with both chemotherapy and irradiation. Excluded are UICC-AJC Stage IA and all patients with M_1 disease. After an initial course of 5FU and leucovorin (CF) patients[1] are treated with 45 Gy of radiation therapy with 5FU-CF, then two more full courses of 5FU-CF. Since there is no convincing evidence that 5FU-CF is effective in gastric cancer, that radiation therapy will prevent local recurrence, nor that 5FU-CF will be as effective in potentiating the effect of radiation therapy as is 5FU alone, one must worry that the results of this trial, drawing on the resources of all of the cooperative groups in the United States, will be no different from the results of past postoperative adjuvant treatment programs in this disease.

Far more interesting, with greater potential to improve the survival of patients with locally advanced gastric cancer, are the trials of neoadjuvant therapy. At M.D. Anderson hospital, Ajani and co-workers have been administering a combination of etoposide, 5FU and cisplatin (cisDDP) preoperatively in 28 day cycles. [12] At the University of Southern California, Leichman and colleagues have administered 5FU-CF and cisDDP preoperatively with an 8% complete pathologic response rate. [13] Postoperatively patients receive intraperitoneal floxuridine (FUDR) and cisDDP, an approach aimed at controlling transperitoneal metastases. At Roswell Park, we have been administering mitomycin C, 5FU and cisDDP intraperitoneally, starting immediately after the final stages of the surgical reconstruction following the gastric resection. However, we are considering the addition of a preoperative non-5FU based chemotherapeutic component to this regimen.

DISCUSSION

The lack of comparability between the several reports of postoperative adjuvant therapy might have been a more significant problem, had any of these studies convincingly shown benefit. Data is often shown graphically without numerical survival data. Effects of stratifications are sometimes (but not always) discussed, but the presentation of data is fragmentary at best. Although chemotherapy quality control is presented as dose intensity and, when appropriate, radiotherapy quality control is closely monitored, surgical and pathology quality control varies from minimal to non-existent, with review of surgical notes and pathology reports often deferred until after the study has been completed.

Of greater concern is the possibility that the failure to report results by TNM stage and type of resection may have obscured potentially useful treatment leads. Proximal gastric tumors, with their varied routes of lymphatic spread, and N_2 celiac and N_3 para aortic lymph nodes located within a few centimeters of the primary tumor, and with the potential to invade the esophagus and diaphragm, require a much more extensive surgical procedure to explore the potential for curative resection than do antral and greater curvature cancers. There are stomach cancers that can be extensively locally invasive (T_4) but do not metastasize to lymph nodes or distant organs until very late in their courses. These might respond to local therapy, whereas lesions with serosal invasion and peritoneal dissemination might be more responsive to intraperitoneal chemotherapy.

After 20 years of gastric cancer adjuvant treatment studies, it is apparent that there should be minimal criteria for protocol design and for the reporting of results. Adequate numbers of patients must be enrolled. Patients should be stratified by TNM classification and only patients in a limited number of TNM categories should be entered. In the absence of truly effective treatment (response rates 80% with at least one third as complete pathologic responses), the patients with the best and the worst prognoses should be restricted from the trial. The best candidates for protocol adjuvant therapy would be those with T_2N_1, T_3N_0, T_3N_1, T_2N_2 and T_3N_2 (all M_0) gastric cancers.

Because prognosis is affected by the type of resection of the stomach, patients should be further stratified as follows:

> Proximal esophagogastrectomy
> Total gastrectomy
> Distal subtotal gastrectomy

This would lead to a total of 15 stratifications. As a result, an absolute minimum of 300 patients would be needed in the treatment arm with an equal number in the concurrently randomized control (no treatment) arm.

Progressive improvement in the survival of patients who receive no adjuvant therapy (see table above) plus the absence of significant multi-institutional data on the survival of patients with these limited TNM classes of disease, mandate a controlled trial with a "no treatment" arm.

Quality control in surgery and pathology is mandatory, with ongoing review at the time of trial entry of surgical and pathology reports to be sure that information for accurate TNM restaging is supplied and that, as a minimum, a European R_0 (no residual disease) resection has been performed. The numbers of lymph nodes examined and numbers with metastatic disease must be recorded for each patient.

Finally, there should be quality control in the reporting of results. The minimum items included in a report in a peer reviewed journal should be:

> Number of patients total and within
>   each stratification
> Survival by TNM class and by type
>   of gastric resection
> Survival reports to include:
>   median survival
>   1 year survival
>   2 year survival
>   5 year survival
>   WITH CONFIDENCE LIMITS!
> Time to relapse
> Sites of recurrence, by TNM class and type
>   of gastric resection.

If all reports contained this information, there would be no difficulty in comparing trials, even across continents.

REFERENCES

1. The Gastrointestinal Tumor Study Group (1982) Cancer 49:1116-1122.
2. Douglass HO Jr, Stablein DM (1990) In: Salmon SE (ed) Adjuvant Therapy of Cancer VI. WB Saunders, Philadelphia, pp. 405-415.
3. Engstrom PF, Lavin PT, Douglass HO Jr, Brunner KW (1985) Cancer 55:1868-1873.
4. Higgins GA, Amadeo JH, Smith DE, Humphrey EW, Keehn RJ (1983) Cancer 52:1105-1112.
5. Schlag P (1987) World J Surg 11:473-477.
6. Combes RC, Schein PS, Chilvers CED, Wils J, Beretta G, Bliss JM, Rutten A, Amadori D, Cortes-Funes H, Villar-Grimalt A, McArdle C, Rauschecker HF, Boven E, Vassilopoulos P, Welvaart K, Pinto Ferreira E, Wiig J, Gisselbrecht C, Rougier P, Woods EMA for the International Collaborative Cancer Group (1990) J Clin Oncol 8:1362-1369.
7. Krook JE, O'Connell MJ, Wieand HS, Beart RW Jr, Leigh JE, Kugler JW, Foley JF, Pfeifle DM, Twito DI (1991) Cancer 67:2454-2458.
8. Alcobendas F, Milla A, Estape J, Curto J, Pera C (1983) Ann Surg 198:13-17.
9. Estape J, Grau JJ, Lcobendas F, Curto J, Daniels M, Vinolas N, Pera C (1991) Ann Surg 213:219-221.
10. Douglass HO Jr, Stablein DM, Marsh J, Benson A, Mayer R, Weaver D, Bruckner H (1991) Proc Amer Soc Clin Oncology 10:143.
11. Soga J, Kobayashi K, Saito J, Fujimaki M, Muto T (1979) World J Surg 3:701-708.
12. Ajani JA, Ota DM, Jessup M, Ames FC, McBride C, Boddie A, Levin B, Jackson DE, Roh M, Hohn D (1991) Cancer 68:1501-1506.
13. Leichman L, Silberman H, Leichman CG, Spears CP, Ray M, Muggia FM, Kiyabu M, Radin R, Laine L, Stain S, Fuerst M, Groshen S, Donovan A (1992) J Clin Oncology 10:1933-1942.

Immunochemosurgery for Advanced Gastric Cancer

JIN-POK KIM

Department of Surgery, College of Medicine, Seoul National University Hospital, Seoul, Korea

ABSTRACT

ImmunoChemoSurgery was proved to be effective in preventing cancer recurrence and improving 5 year survival rate of stage III gastric cancer patients. To evaluate the effect of immunochemosurgery, two randomized trials were studied in 1976 and 1981. In first trial, 5-fluorouracil, mitomycin C, and cytosine arabinoside for chemotherapy and OK 432 for immunotherapy were used. The 5 YSR for surgery alone (n=64) and immunochemosurgery (n=73) were 23.4% and 44.6%, respectively, a significant difference. In the second trial, there were three groups: group I, immunochemosurgery (n=159); group II, surgery and chemotherapy (n=77); and group III, surgery alone (n=94). 5-Fluorouracil and mitomycin C for chemotherapy and OK-432 for immunotherapy were administered for 2 years. The 5 YSR of group I was 45.3%, significantly higher than the 29.8% of group II and than the 24.4% of group III. The postoperative DNCB test, T-lymphocyte percentage, PHA and con-A-stimulated lymphoblastogenesis and the ADCC test showed more favorable values in the immunochemosurgery group. Therefore, immunochemosurgery is the best multimodality treatment for advanced gastric cancer.

KEY WORDS: Advanced stomach cancer, Radical gastrectomy, Immunochemotherapy,
            Cancer recurrence

INTRODUCTION

Why is immunochemosurgery necessary? Most gastric cancer patients are still in stage III or IV when they are first diagnosed. And the 5-year survival rate for stage III gastric cancer was only 30.6%, which is disappointing. Therefore, the question is raised, "Can surgery alone cure gastric cancer patients?" Yes, but only in stage I and II patients. Surgery alone, however radical it is, can not cure patients with gastric cancer in advanced stages. Stomach cancer in stage III is already systemic disease. To improve the prognosis of advanced stomach cancer, we need systemic treatment such as immunotherapy or chemotherapy in the early postoperative period to kill the micrometastatic or remaining cancer cells even after curative resection.

There have been some encouraging reports of prolonged survival and disease-free interval. Taguchi et al. reported improved survival in patients with stage III gastric carcinoma who received mitomycin C and 5-fluorouracil (5-FU) after surgery. Moertel and Mittelman reported a prolonged disease-free interval and survival after curative resection for gastric carcinoma using 5-FU and methyl-CCNU. Although the results of primary chemotherapy in advanced cases are generally poor, combined administration of mitomycin C, 5-FU, cytosine arabinoside (MFC), or 5-FU and methyl-CCNU (FME) was documented to be efficacious.

In the late 1960s, Mathé reported an immunotherapeutic effect of bacillus Calmette-Guérin (BCG) and allogenic tumor cell vaccine, with an increase in remission duration and survival in a child with leukemia, and Morton et al. reported an immunotherapeutic efficacy of intradermal BCG inoculation on metastatic cutaneous malignant melanoma. Since then the interest in immunotherapy has greatly increased. Rosenberg and many others have shown that immunotherapy can be effective against certain malignancies, including gastric cancer. Immunotherapy alone is rarely effective against clinically measurable cancer. It would be an important therapy, however, to attack cancer cells and to improve host immune status in the case of conjunction with other treatment modalities.

Kim and others have shown that both cell-mediated immunity, measured by T-lymphocyte quantitations, and the positivity of 1-chloro-2,4-dinitrobenzene (DNCB) delayed cutaneous hypersensitivity in patients with malignancy are decreased significantly, and the level of immunosuppressive acid protein (IAP) is significantly higher than that of normal individual. The further the clinical stage of gastric cancer progresses, the more depressed is the cell-mediated immunity of the host (Figure 1). In view of this finding, enhancement of the depressed immune status of the host is thought to be an important aspect in the treatment of cancer patients.

The purpose of this study is to evaluate the therapeutic effectiveness of postoperative immunochemotherapy in advanced, but resectable, adenocarcinoma of the stomach. Survival rate and immune status of patients with stage III gastric carcinoma who received postoperative immunochemotherapy were compared with those of patients who received surgery with no adjuvant therapy.

MATERIALS AND METHODS

First Trial

One hundred thirty-eight patients who had received radical subtotal gastrectomy for stage III gastric cancer were enrolled in this study from 1976 to 1978 at the Department of Surgery, Seoul National University Hospital (Table 1). Before surgery, all patients with stomach cancer underwent a complete history and physical examination with measurements of disease, immune parameters as mentioned below, performance status, routine laboratory tests, and liver scan, and two groups were found comparable. After curative surgery as mentioned in curative surgery section, patients, specifically chosen with histologically confirmed LN-positive stage III adenocarcinoma of the stomach, were randomized as to receiving postoperative immunochemotherapy or not after the routine examination including hemogram, liver function test, and renal function test showed normal values. Patients were ineligible for study if they had previous history of chemotherapy or radiation therapy or if their age was older than 70 years. Initial performance status was within the range of the Eastern Cooperative Oncology Group (ECOG): 0 to 2 in all patients.

Immunologic studies. The following immunologic tests were performed before operation and in the third to fourth postoperative month.
DNCB cutaneous hypersensitivity test.
T lymphocytes (percent and count).
Lymphoblastogenesis by phytohemagglutinin and concanavalin-A stimulation.
Antibody-dependent cellular cytotoxicity.

Postoperative immunochemotherapy. Patients in the immunochemosurgery group received the following therapy:

Immunotherapy. OK-432 (Streptococcus pyogenes preparation) was given intramuscularly with a dosage of 1.0 Klinische Einheit every week from the fourth or fifth postoperative day.

Chemotherapy. The MFC (mitomycin C, 5-FU, and cytosine arabinoside) regimen was selected at random for the patients and started at the eighth to tenth postoperative days. The dosage administration schedule was as follows: MFC-mitomycin C, 4 mg/50 kg; 5-FU, 500 mg/50 kg; cytosine arabinoside, 40 mg/50 kg, given intravenously twice a week for the first 2 weeks and then every week for the next 6 weeks. Then oral 5-FU was given daily with the dosage of 600 mg/50 kg for 18 months after surgery, if the patients tolerated it. Just before each chemotherapy cycle, white blood cell and platelet counts were obtained and liver function tests were checked if indicated. Drug dosage was controlled based on the parameters of hematologic toxicity and other adverse reactions.

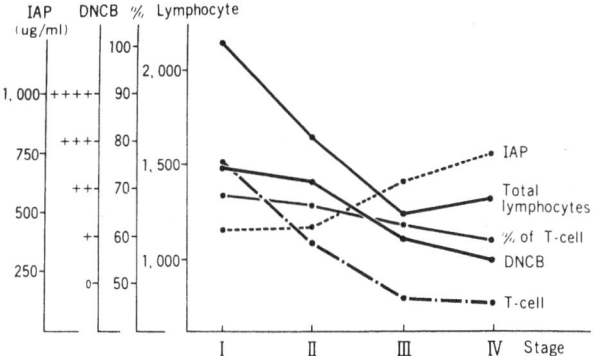

Fig.1. Levels of various immune parameters in each clinical stage of gastric adenocarcinoma. T cell percentage and DNCB positivities were decreased, whereas immunosuppressive acidic proteins were increased according to the advancedment of clinical stage.

TABLE 1. Method (Immunochemosurgery)	
138 Patients With Stomach Cancer, Stage III by TNM Classification	
Group A 64 patients Radical subtotal gastrectomy alone	Group B 74 patients Radical subtotal gastrectomy followed by immunochemotherapy

TABLE 2. Randomization of Gastric Cancer Patients*

Treatment/Patient	No. Entered	No. Evaluated
Immunochemosurgery	170	159†
Postoperative chemotherapy	100	77†
Surgery only	100	94†
Total	370	330 (89%)

* Criteria: age > 30 yr, <70 yr; stage III; performance status 0–2; subtotal gastrectomy with lymph node dissection; Billroth II GJS.
† Discontinued or altered treatment cases were excluded from evaluation.

Second Trial

Postoperative immunochemotherapy. Three hundred seventy histologically proven stage III gastric cancer patients, ranging in age from 30 to 70 years and with performance status between 0 and 2, without systemic disease, were randomly assigned to three groups after curative subtotal gastrectomy as mentioned in curative surgery section from 1981 to 1983: 170 for immunochemosurgery, 100 for postoperative chemotherapy, and 100 for surgery alone (Table 2). Forty patients were excluded because they altered or discontinued treatment.

Before surgery, all patients with stomach cancer underwent a complete physical examination with staging of the disease, immune parameters as mentioned above, performance status, routine laboratory test, and liver scan. Patients were ineligible for the study if they had a previous history of chemotherapy or radiation therapy, or if their age was older than 70. The initial performance status was within the range of the Eastern Cooperative Oncology Group (ECOG): 0 to 2 in all patients.

Postoperative immunotherapy was started from the 4th or 5th postoperative day with OK-432, and chemotherapy was started from the 8th to the 10th postoperative day with mitomycin and 5-FU. Immunotherapy and chemotherapy was continued for 2 years. Three groups were comparable in terms of age, sex, performance status, preoperative immune parameter data, number of LN metastases, and Lauren's classification. The protocol of immunochemotherapy in the second trial was essentially the same as the that of the first trial, except for the omission of cytosine arabinoside in chemotherapy because of toxicity, and the treatment duration is 24 months (Table 3).

Survival rate and immunoparameter studies. Survival rates, calculated from the day of operation, and immune statuses were compared among the three groups. A statistical comparison of patient characteristics and immune parameters was performed, using the chi square test or Student's test. Differences were considered significant at $p < 0.05$. Differences in survival rates among the three groups were determined using the Cox-Mantel test.

TABLE 3. Postoperative Immunochemotherapy Programs

Immunotherapy starts at the 4th or 5th postoperative day, Picibani (*Streptococcus pyogenes* preparation); 1.0 K.E, IM weekly
Chemotherapy starts at the 8th to 10th postoperative day

MF { Mitomycin-C; 4 mg/50 kg / 5-Fluorouracil; 500 mg/50 kg } IV × 2/week for 2 weeks, then weekly 6 times

Duration, 24 months (PMF/2M, PF/22M)

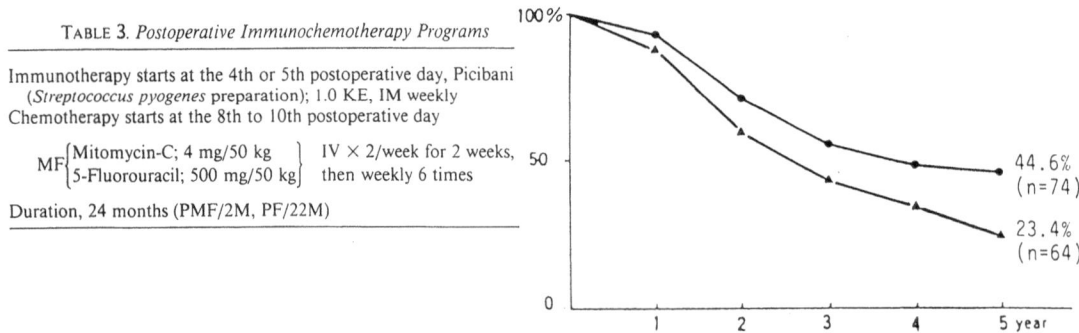

FIG. 2. Survival curve of the immunochemosurgery group and the surgery-alone group in stage II stomach cancer. (●—●) Immunochemosurgery; (▲—▲) surgery alone.

RESULTS

Results of the First Trial

One hundred thirty-eight patients were randomly divided into two groups and followed at least 5 years. Of 138 patients, 74 received postoperative immunochemotherapy, and 64 patients received no further anticancer therapy after surgery. Patient characteristics, preoperative values of immune parameters, and the proportion of histologic type and extent of LN involvement of the two groups of patients were similar.

Curative surgery for gastric cancer performed in this center includes subtotal gastric resection, complete dissection, so-called skeletonization of regional LNs along the celiac axis, hepatic artery, splenic artery, portal vein, and retropancreatic LN, as well as peri-gastric LNs and removal of omentum with adjacent tissues. All the tissues were removed in an en bloc fashion. Frozen biopsy of both resection margins was done in all cases.

Survival rates. Survival curves of the two groups of patients are shown in Figure 2. The 5-year survival rate of the postoperative immunochemotherapy group is 44.6%, and that of the surgery-alone group is 23.4%. The difference in survival rate determined by the Cox-Mantel test is statistically significant (Z=2.09, p<0.05).

Immunoparameter studies. In the DNCB cutaneous hypersensitivity test, preoperative DNCB positivity is 47.4% in the surgery-alone group and 54.8% in the postoperative immuno-chemotherapy group. 1-chloro-2.4-dinitrobenzene positivity at the fourth postoperative month is 73% in the surgery-alone group and 92.9% in the immunochemotherapy group. More patients were converted from negative to positive after postoperative immunochemotherapy.

The T lymphocyte percentage and count in the surgery-alone group were decreased from 58.8±7.8% and 1142±344/mm³ to 56.4±6.9% and 985±495/mm³, respectively, after surgery. In the postoperative immunochemotherapy group, preoperative T cell percentage and count, 55.2±5.6% and 1133±509/mm³, were increased to 58.4±5.9% and 1179±537/mm³, respectively, after therapy.

Postoperative degrees of lymphoblastogenesis by PHA and con-A stimulation are 3653±403 cpm and 4304±463 cpm, respectively, in the surgery-alone group, and 4779±559 cpm and 5412±476 cpm in the immunochemotherapy group. They were much less decreased in the postoperative immunochemotherapy group.

Antibody-dependent cellular cytotoxicity activity at the third postoperative month was 37.7±12.9% in the surgery-alone group and 39.6±11.4% (not significant) in the immunochemo-therapy group. Preoperative and postoperative values of immune parameters are shown in Table 4.

TABLE 4. *Values of Immune Parameters Before and After Surgery*

Immune Parameter	Control		Immunochemotherapy	
	Before Surgery	After Surgery	Before Surgery	After Surgery
DNCB positivity (%)	47.4 (9/18)	73.0 (14/19)	54.8 (24/42)	92.9 (40/42)
T-cell (%)	58.8 ± 7.8	56.4 ± 6.9	55.2 ± 5.6	58.4 ± 5.9
T-cell (count/mm³)	1142 ± 344	985 ± 495	1133 ± 509	1179 ± 537
Blastogenesis (cpm)				
PHA-stimulated	5535 ± 1315	3653 ± 403	5183 ± 852	4779 ± 559
Con A-stimulated	8547 ± 1301	4304 ± 463	8882 ± 1336	5412 ± 476
ADCC activity (%)	36.9 ± 11.6	37.7 ± 12.9	37.2 ± 12.1	39.6 ± 11.4

DNCB, 1-chloro-2.4-dinitrobenzene; ADCC, antibody-dependent cellular cytotoxicity.

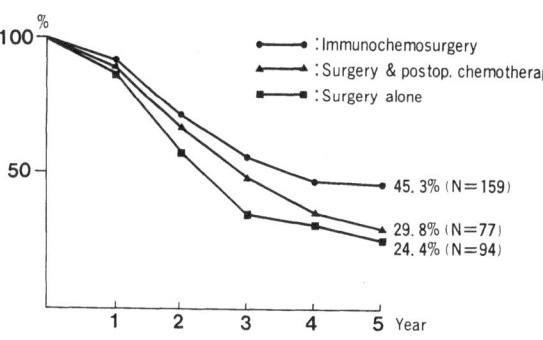

Fig.3. Survival curve of immunochemo-surgery group, surgery and postoper-ative chemotherapy group and surgery -alone group in stage III stomach can-cer (330 cases, 1981-1985). (●) Immun-ochemosurgery, 45.3%(n=159). (▲)Sur-gery and postoperative chemotherapy, 29.8%(n=77). (■)Surgery alone, 24.4% (n=94).

Results of the Second Trial

Follow-up study of the second trial was performed on 330 of 370 (89%) patients for at least 5 years. Of these, 159 patients received postoperative immunochemotherapy; 77, con-ventional adjuvant chemotherapy after operation; and 94, no further therapy. Patient char-acteristics, preoperative values of immune parameters, histologic type, and extent of LN involvement of the three groups of patients were similar (Table 5).

Survival rate. Survival curves of the three groups of patients are shown in Figure 3. The 5-year survival rate of the immunochemosurgery group was 45.3%; of the chemotherapy group, 29.8%; and the surgery-alone group, 24.4%. The difference between the immunochemosurgery group and the other two groups is statistically significant.

Immunoparameter studies. The postoperative T-cell percentage was increased in the immunochemosurgery group after immunochemotherapy, but was decreased in both the postoperative chemotherapy and surgery-alone groups. The positive conversion rate of DNCB-negative patients after treatment was 85.9% in the immunochemosurgery group compared with 72.5% in the postoperative chemotherapy group and 75% in the surgery-alone group. Lymphoblastogenesis and antibody-dependent cellular cytotoxicity activity also was favorable in immunochemosurgery (Table 5).

TABLE 5. *Values of Immune Parameters Before and After Surgery*

Immune Parameter	Immunochemosurgery		Postoperative Chemotherapy		Surgery Alone	
	Before Surgery	After Surgery	Before Surgery	After Surgery	Before Surgery	After Surgery
DNCB positivity (%)	52.5 (41/78)	85.9 (67/78)	48.9 (14/29)	72.5 (21/29)	46.8 (15/32)	75.0 (24/32)
T cell (%)	56.4 ± 6.1	59.7 ± 5.8	59.2 ± 7.4	57.3 ± 6.8	58.7 ± 7.9	56.1 ± 6.8
T cell (count/mm³)	1135 ± 507	1182 ± 541	1146 ± 352	974 ± 496	1154 ± 440	1152 ± 364
Blastogenesis (cpm)						
PHA-stimulated	5279 ± 759	4638 ± 602	5567 ± 1872	2302 ± 290	5536 ± 1321	3654 ± 411
Con A-stimulated	8879 ± 1301	5327 ± 494	8624 ± 1312	2872 ± 340	8502 ± 1321	4409 ± 472
ADCC activity (%)	37.8 ± 11.9	40.2 ± 11.2	36.7 ± 11.0	37.8 ± 11.3	36.8 ± 11.4	37.9 ± 12.8

DISCUSSION

The result of gastric cancer surgery is dependent primarily on clinical stage, the radicality of surgery, and also on patient immunity and other biologic characteristics.
Certainly depth of invasion, presence of LN metastases, especially multiple involvement in more than four LNs, and distant metastases are the most important prognostic factors in gastric carcinoma. The authors analyzed 448 cases of stomach cancer recently to evaluate the prognostic value of Lauren's histologic classification. The 5-year survival rate of the intestinal type (43.7%, n=190) is higher than that of diffuse type (30.4%, n=138)(p<0.05). The distribution of these histologic types are similar among the three groups in this study. Further, the extent of LN metastases as well as presence or absence of metastatic LNs are significant prognostic indicators. It was demonstrated in the author's previous study that 5-year survival rate of patients with one to three metastatic LNs is significantly higher than that of patients with more than four metastatic LN.

Although adjuvant therapy after radical gastric resection has been expected to be the most promising treatment for stomach cancer, there is no long-term follow-up report to demonstrate improvement of survival with use of adjuvant therapy. Several regimens for adjuvant chemotherapy have been suggested and evaluated clinically. The MFC, 5-fluorouracil, adriamycin, and mitomycin-C (FAM), and FME regimens were reported to have good response rate in advanced gastric cancer. The Gastrointestinal Tumor Study Group reported long-term follow-up results of adjuvant chemotherapy with 5-FU and methyl-CCNU after curative resection of gastric cancer. Nissen-Meyer et al. reported decreasing recurrence and death rates when adjuvant chemotherapy was started in the early postoperative period for breast cancer, and no improvement when started 3 weeks after mastectomy. A survival advantage was associated with adjuvant treatment and lasted up to 24 months after surgery. The survival difference between the control and adjuvant therapy groups was nearly 20% after 4 years of follow-up. The survival benefit of the present study is similar to that of the Gastrointestinal Tumor Study Group.

There have been many reports on the effectiveness of immunotherapy for certain malignancies such as acute myeloblastic leukemia, lymphoma, breast cancer, malignant melanoma, ovarian cancer, childhood neuroblastoma, head and neck cancer, esophageal cancer, and stomach cancer. Theoretically, specific immunotherapy should be more beneficial than nonspecific immunotherapy, but is not yet available for clinical use. Non-specific immunotherapy such as various immune potentiators or biologic response modifiers are now commonly in use.

Advantages of postoperative immunochemotherapy have been described in terms of prolonged remission and survival, improved bone marrow tolerance, delayed recurrence, and possible prevention of recurrence. Suga et al. reported prolonged survival for patients treated with MFC and OK-432 (picibanil) compared with those treated with MFC alone for advanced gastric cancer. In these studies, the treatment procedure consisted of two components. Firstly, radical gastrectomy was performed as thoroughly as possible, and regional LNs including adjacent tissues were removed en bloc. Then early postoperative immuno-chemotherapy as a second treatment modality was performed to achieve a destruction of residual tumor cells, including micrometastases, with the body burden of tumor cells minimal.

According to the data presented in this study, it is evident that the 5-year survival rate of patients receiving surgery with early postoperative immunochemotherapy is better than that of the chemotherapy or control group. Immune status data also show improved reactivity in the immunochemotherapy group.

Surgery, as a complete removal of visible tumor mass, is of primary importance for multi-modality therapy. Both types of therapy, however, should be practiced almost simultane-ously to prolong the survival of gastric cancer patients.

Gastric carcinoma probably can be cured with active immunochemosurgery in the near future. To reach this goal, further prospective randomized controlled clinical studies on immunochemosurgery should be initiated. Additionally, measures for local control, such as intraoperative radiation therapy and intraperitoneal chemotherapy, should be considered.

REFERENCES

1. Kim JP, Park JG (1983) The end-results of surgical treatment of gastric cancer. J Korean Med Assoc 26: 637-642
2. The Gastrointestinal Tumor Study Group (1982) A comparative clinical assessment of combination chemotherapy in the management of advanced gastric carcinoma. Cancer 49: 1362-1366
3. Taguchi T, Mattori T, Inoue K (1979) Multihospital randomized study on adjuvant chemo-therapy with mitomycin ± futraful for gastric cancer. In Jones SE, Salmon SE, eds. Adju-vant Therapy of Cancer II. New York: Grune & Stratton, pp581-586
4. Ota K, Kurita S, Nishimura M (1972) Combination therapy with mitomycin-C, 5-fluorouracil and cytosine arabinoside for advanced cancer in man. Jpn J Cancer Chemother 56: 373-385
5. Mathe G (1971) Active immunotherapy. Adv Cancer Res 14: 1-36
6. Morton DL, Eilber FR, Holmes EC (1976) BCG immunotherapy as a systemic adjunct to surgery in malignant melanoma. Med Clin North Am 60: 431-439
7. Rosenberg SA (1985) Lymphokine-activated killer cells: a new approach to immunotherapy of cancer. J Natl Cancer Institute 7: 595-616
8. Gutterman JU, Cardenas JO, Blumenschein GR (1976) Chemoimmunotherapy of advanced breast cancer: prolongation of remission and survival with BCG. Br Med J 2: 1222-1225
9. Hattori T, Mori A, Hirata K, Ito I (1972) Five-year survival rate of gastric cancer pa-tients treated by gastrectomy, large dose of mitomycin-C and/or allogeneic bone marrow transplantation. Gann 63: 517-522
10. Okudaira Y, Sugimachi K, Inokuchi K (1982) Postoperative long-term immunochemother-apy for esophageal carcinoma. Jpn J Surgery 12: 249-268
11. Kim JP, Yoo IH (1978) Relationship between the advance of stomach cancer and the change in immunity. J Korean Surg Soc 20: 195-204
12. Chun SH, Yoo IH, Kim JP (1984) The significance of the measurement of immunosuppre-ssive acid protein (IAP) in various cancer patients. Korean J Immunol 6: 31-42.
13. Orita K, Miwa H, Fukuda H (1976) Preoperative cell-mediated immune status of gastric cancer patient. Cancer 38: 2343-2348
14. Kim JP, Choi WJ (1986) A study on histologic type of gastric carcinoma: analysis of clinico pathologic characterization and its implication as a prognostic factor. 18: 194-213
15. Kim JP, Jung SE (1986) Staging patients with gastric cancer and their prognosis. J Korean Cancer Res Assoc 18: 9-13
16. Nissen-Meyer R, Kjellgren K, Malmio K (1978) Surgical adjuvant chemotherapy: results with one short course with cyclophosphamide after mastectomy for breast cancer. Cancer 41: 2088-2098
17. Suga S, Tsunekawa H, Washino M (1977) Treatment of gastric cancer with special refer-ence to the survivals of the cancer patients treated with multiple combination MFC therapy or immunochemotherapy of MFC plus OK-432 (NSC B116209). Gastroenterol Jpn 12: 20-46
18. Moertel CG, Mittelman JA, Bakemeier RF (1976) Sequential and combination chemotherapy of advanced gastric cancer. Cancer 38: 678-682

Experimental and Clinical Results of Hyperthermo-Chemo-Radiotherapy in Esophageal and Rectal Carcinoma

Keizo Sugimachi, Masaki Mori, Hideo Baba, Masayuki Watanabe, Noriaki Sadanaga, Masahiko Ikebe, and Hiroyuki Kuwano

The Second Department of Surgery, Faculty of Medicine, Kyushu University, Fukuoka, 812 Japan

ABSTRACT

We performed 1) the experimental studies of heat sensitivity of normal and tumor tissues, and the combined effect of heat, radiation and chemotherapy, and 2) the clinical studies of hyperthermo-chemo-radiotherapy (HCR therapy) for patients with esophageal and rectal carcinomas. The experimental studies disclosed that heat sensitivity of tumor tissues was higher than that of normal tissues. The study of the cytocidal effect in multicellular tumor spheroids demonstrated that the inner layer with hypoxic condition was sensitive to heat, while the outer layer with aerobic condition was sensitive to radiation. When treated concomitantly with hyperthermia and radiation, the cells in both layers were similarly and severely damaged. Based on these experimental results, we performed preoperative HCR therapy for patients with esophageal and rectal carcinomas. The survival rates of esophageal cancer patients treated with preoperative HCR therapy were better than those treated with preoperative CR therapy. Concerning the rectal carcinomas, local recurrence was seen in none of 43 patients treated with preoperative HCR therapy. As local hyperthermia had no side effects, HCR therapy is considered to be a hopeful modality to treat patients with malignant lesions of the esophagus and rectum.

KEY WORDS: hyperthermo-chemo-radiotherapy, esophageal cancer, rectal cancer, radiofrequency, endotract electrode

INTRODUCTION

The objective of hyperthermia for cancer patients is to destroy the malignant tissues while minimizing damage to the normal tissues. Biological studies done in many institutes favor the clinical application of hyperthermia in combined modalities. To comprehend the action and mechanisms of hyperthermia and to develop optimal therapy modalities, biological phenomena as well as molecular, metabolic, and physiological events all have to be considered. Several thousands of patients have now been treated with hyperthermia, in various regimens, since the 1970s [1-3]. As the anti-tumor effect of hyperthermia alone will not be sufficient, a combination with radiation and chemotherapy is generally prescribed. In the study, we did 1) the experimental studies of heat sensitivity of normal and tumor tissues, and the combined effect of heart, radiation and chemotherapy, and 2) the clinical studies of hyperthermo-chemo-radiotherapy (HCR therapy) for patients with esophageal and rectal carcinomas.

MATERIALS AND METHODS

1) Experimental studies

a) Heat sensitivity of mouse normal tissues such as esophagus and colon was compared with that of murine sarcoma-180 by using in vitro MTT assay. Changes in % survival were determined following exposure to 43°C heat for 1, 2, 5 and 10 hours.

b) Heat sensitivity of human gastric cancer and adjacent normal tissues was compared by using in vitro MTT assays. Heat-time dependency was examined.

c) The decrease in % survival of 23 human tissues including 15 gastric and 8 colorectal cancers was compared with that of the adjacent normal tissues following exposure to 43°C for 20 hours.

d) To examine the cytocidal effect of hyperthermia alone or in combination with radiation and/or anticancer agents in a more sophisticated model like an in vivo tumor model, multicellular tumor spheroids were used. Cells in the inner layer with hypoxic conditions are sensitive to heat, whereas cells in the outer layer with aerobic conditions are sensitive to radiation.

e) Cytotoxic effects of hyperthermochemoradiotherapy (HCR) on V-79 cells were compared with that of heat alone, heat plus radiation (HR), heat plus chemotherapy (HC), and chemotherapy plus radiation(CR).

2) Clinical studies

a) Cases

Five hundred eighty-five patients with esophageal carcinoma underwent surgical resection in our department. Of these, 136 patients were treated with preoperative HCR therapy. With regard to rectal carcinoma, 43 patients were treated with preoperative HCR therapy.

b) Heating equipment

The Endoradiotherm 100A (Olympus Optical Co., LTD., Japan) is radiofrequency (RF) intraluminal thermal equipment and was developed for treating patients with esophageal cancer (Fig.1) [4,5]. This equipment, which is small and portable with a frequency of 13.56 MHZ and maximum output of 250W, enables bed side treatment. A special treatment room is not needed. The output power, the range of warming temperature and the warming time are set in the control panel, and the on/off control of the RF generator is operated to maintain the temperature range. The intraluminal applicator consists of electrodes, a balloon for the perfusion of cooling water for prevention of overheating of the surface, and two thermocouple sensors for monitoring the temperature of the tumor surface. The extracorporeal applicator is large in size with a perfusion mechanism for cooling the surface, and is usually applied on the anterior chest wall(Fig.2).

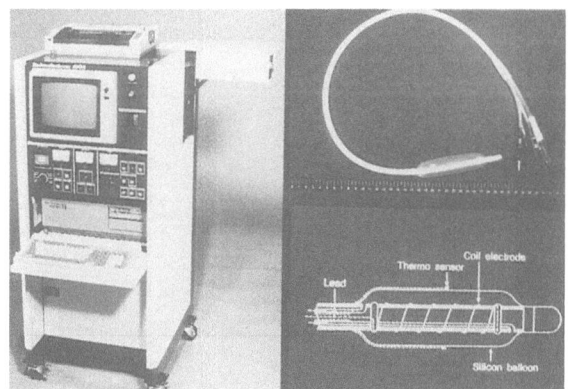

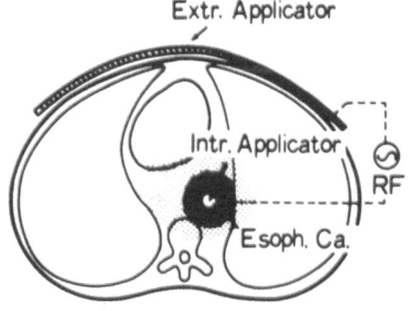

Intraluminal Heating

Fig. 1.Left;Endoradiotherm 100A(Olympus Optical Co., LTD., Japan). Right upper;intraluminal application. Right lower; a schema of the application.

Fig.2.The Achema of intraluminal heating. A thin electrode in the esophagus and a broad counter electrode on the body surface make localization of the electromagnetic field at the esophagus.

c) Treatment regimen of preoperative HCR therapy
These are shown in Figs. 3 and 4.

d) Histologic studies of the resected specimens
The histologic effectiveness of the preoperative therapy was studied in the resected tissues. Patients in whom viable neoplastic cells were completely destroyed were defined as "markedly effective", and patients in whom most of the cancer cells were extensively damaged, despite the presence of a few viable cells, were defined as "moderately effective". All others were categorized as "ineffective".

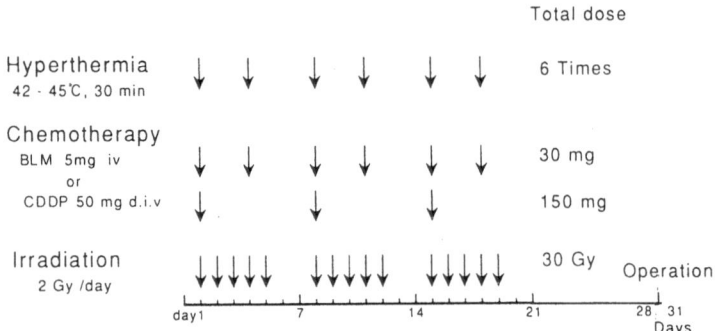

Fig. 3. Regimen of HCR therapy for esophageal carcinoma

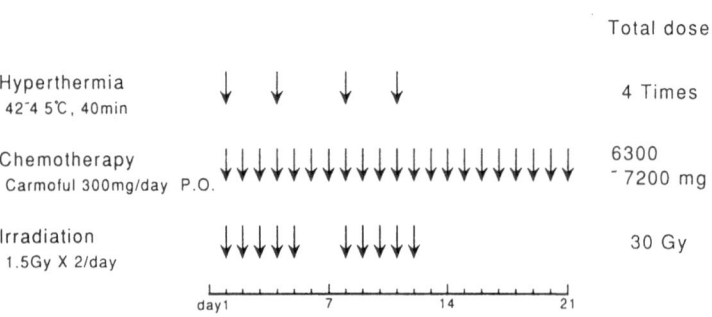

Fig. 4. Regimen of HCR therapy for rectal carcinoma

RESULTS

1) Experimental studies

 a) Percent survival decreased to a greater extent in the S-180 cells than in the normal esophageal or colon tissues, in a time-dependent fashion. At 10 hr of heat treatment, the % survival decreased to 11% for S-180 cells, 21% for colon and 31% for esophagus. Significant differences were noted between the S-180 cells and normal tissues, at all times.
b) Changes in % survival were determined following exposure to 43°C for 5, 10, 15 and 20 hours. The % survival decreased to a greater extent in the gastric cancer tissues than in the adjacent normal tissues, in a time-dependent fashion. Significant differences were noted between the % survival of the tumor and adjacent normal tissues after 10 hours.
c) The succinate dehydrogenase activity decreased to a greater extent in the tumor tissues than in the adjacent normal tissues with significant differences in each organ. The mean succinate dehydrogenase activity was 31 % for the gastric cancer tissues and 53 % for the adjacent normal gastric tissues; 34% for the colorectal cancer tissues and 50%   for the adjacent normal colorectal tissues(Fig. 5).

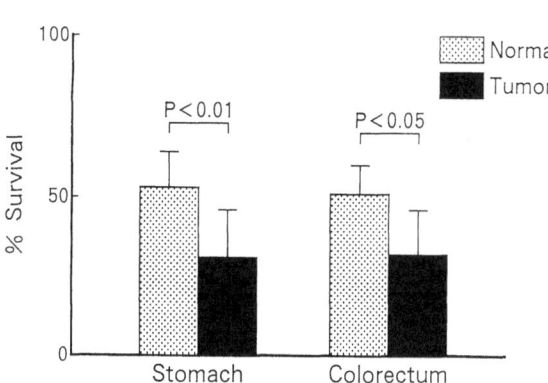

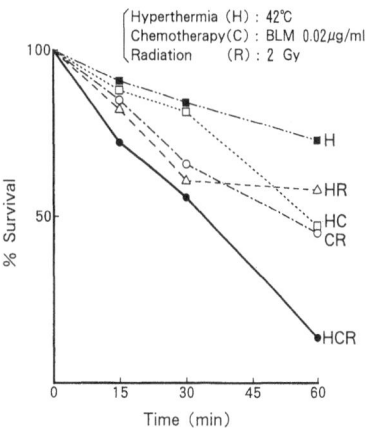

Fig.5. Heat sensitivities of human normal and tumor
tissues of the stomach or colorectum.
Tumor tissues are more sensitive than their
normal counterparts.

Fig.6. Cytotosic effects of each treatment on V-79 cells.
HCR is most effective.

d) The percent survival in the inner layer of the spheroid after treatment with hyperthermia alone was 6.5%, that is
significantly lower than that in the outer (43%). The percent survival in the outer layer after irradiation alone was 3.0%, a value
significantly lower than that in the inner layer (12%). When the multicellular tumor spheroids were treated
concomitantly with hyperthermia and irradiation, the cells in both layers were similarly and severely damaged, with a survival
rate of 0.1% in both layers.
  e) Although percent survival of cells treated with each therapy decreased in a time dependent manner, the cytotoxic effect of
HCR was very significant when compared with other treatments at 60 min exposure(Fig. 6).

2)Clinical studies

a) Esophageal carcinoma
  When comparing HCR with CR, there was no significant difference between the two groups with regard to background
factors, such as age, sex, location, length of the tumor, histology, TNM stage and lymph node metastasis. The detailed
histologic evaluations were made on the resected specimens, and the effect of preoperative therapy was microscopically
classified into the following three grades. Markedly effective (Grade 3): All cancer cells were destroyed
with no evidence of viable cancer cells. Moderately effective (Grade 2): Most of cancer cells were damaged, despite the
presence of viable cancer cells. Ineffective (Grades 0 & 1): No significant changes.   There were 26 patients (19%) and 63
patients (46%) classed as markedly effective and moderately effective in HCR groups, respectively, and 9 patients (8%) and
45 patients (42%) were classed as markedly effective and moderately effective in CR groups, respectively. Effective rates are
65.4% and 50.5% in HCR group and CR group, respectively. Thus, combination of hyperthermia with irradiation and
chemotherapy has a significantly increased anti-tumor effect in patients with esophageal carcinoma.
Figure 7 shows the survival curves for the patients who were treated surgically after preoperative HCR or CR therapy. Five
year survival rates for patients given HCR therapy was 22.3% and that given CR therapy without hyperthermia was 13.7%.
Survival rates of patients given preoperative HCR were significantly better than those of patients given CR therapy (p<0.05).
In cases of TNM stage I and II, there was no significant difference in survival rates in the two groups. In cases of TNM stage III
and IV, however, survival rates were better for patients who received HCR therapy. Thus, preoperative HCR therapy is

useful in patients with rather advanced stage carcinoma of the esophagus. On the other hand, since 1988, we started prospective randomized trials for preoperative HCR therapy and CR therapy. 77 cases were studied. 39 patients received preoperative HCR. There are 9 patients (23%) with markedly efective results in the HCR group, whereas there are only 3 cases with markedly effective results in the CR group. The effective rate of HCR was 66.7% and that of CR was 57.9%. Although there was no significant difference, combination of hypertheria with chemotherapy and irradiation has a tendency to increase anti-tumor effect. Long term survival rates are not yet available, however, survival rates are better in HCR group comparing with CR group over three years.

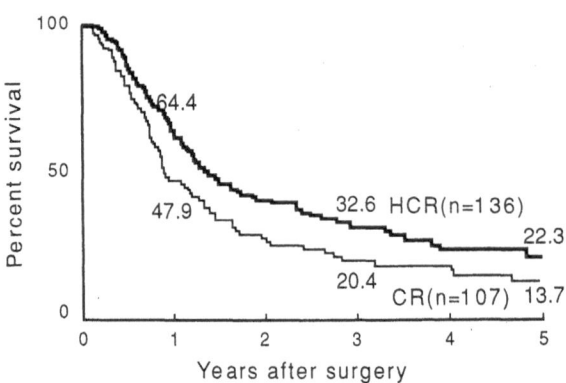

Fig. 7. Survival carves for patients who were treated with HCR or CR
The prognosis is better in HCR than in CR(p<0.05).

b) Rectal carcinoma

43 patients with rectal carcinoma underwent radical surgery after preoperative HCR therapy. Most tumors were seen in the lower rectum. Seven patients underwent low anterior resection, and 36 rectal amputation. The effect of preoperative HCR therapy was evaluated by histopathologic findings of the resected specimen. The criteria is the same as that used in esophageal carcinoma. The summary of effectiveness of preoperative HCR therapy was shown in Fig.   . The effectiveness was recognized in 24 of 43 cases, (56%). To study the effectiveness of preoperative HCR therapy, 23 surgically treated patients with HCR therapy were compared with 48 surgically treated patients without HCR therapy. The recurrence rates within 2 years were compared between the two groups because the follow-up intervals differ. Although there was a difference in time, these two groups were comparable with regard to various prognostic factors. The incidences of local recurrence and that of lung metastasis were very low in those given the HCR therapy. In the control group, however, the incidences were 14.6% and 10.4%, respectively. There were statistical differences with regard to the local recurrence rates between the two groups (p<0.05). The incidence of liver metastasis were much the same between the two groups.

DISCUSSION

Hyperthermia is one additional option for treating clinical malignancies [4-6]. Local hyperthermia has no severe side-effects while providing some benefits. The incidence of a complete response to heat treatment was in the range of 15% and was usually of a short duration [3]. A more recent approach has been to combine irradiation and/or chemotherapy with hyperthermia [4,7]. In both experimental and clinical observations, hyperthermia has an antitumor effect, decreases proliferation of tumor cells and increases the synergistic response to radiotherapy and chemotherapy [2,6]. The long-term survival was significantly improved by preoperative HCR-therapy for patients with carcinoma of the esophagus in a series already reported [4]. We therefore welcomed the addition of hyperthermia in the hope that it would improve not only the long-term survival, but also subjective symptoms and the microscopic responses in the resected specimens in patients judged clinically to have potentially resectable disease. The histopathological effects on esophageal carcinoma show that almost all cancer cells were destroyed in 19% of the patients in the HCR-therapy group, whereas only 8% in those in CR-therapy group were destroyed. Preoperative HCR therapy, as applied in our treatment concept for patients with carcinoma of the esophagus, proved to be a safe and effective modality [9]. The exact mechanism of the anti-tumor effect of hyperthermia is not yet clear, however, circulation failure, hypoxia and acidosis have all been claimed to play an important role in the pathogenesis of these lesions in vivo [8].

Our experience with HCR therapy has revealed favorable results not only for patients with esophageal carcinoma but also for those with rectal carcinoma [5,10]. This treatment protocol was given preoperatively, in an attempt to decrease the likelihood that tumor cells would spread during surgical manipulations. All the patients tolerated this preoperative treatment well. There were no side effects requiring cessation of the HCR therapy. Histopathologic findings of the resected specimens revealed marked or moderate effectiveness in the majority of cases. Control of pelvic local recurrence was feasible and more satisfactory palliation was obtained. Of great interest is the finding that the efficacy of HCR therapy was confirmed not only in cases of local recurrence but also in cases of a lung metastasis.

Finally, great progress has been made in hyperthermia research over the past ten years. Despite some technological advances, there are still many limitations to delivering the optimal amount of heat as well as to monitoring the temperature throughout the treatment volume with regional and even localized techniques. Additional efforts are now being applied to the development of more precise and efficient equipment.

REFERENCES

1. Dewy WC. Interaction of heat with radiation and chemotherapy. Cancer Res (suppl) 44:4714-4720, 1984.
2. Teicher BA, Abrams MJ, Rosbe KW, Herman TS. Cytotoxicisity, radiosensitization, antitumor activity, and interaction with hyperthermia of a Co (III) Mustard complex. Cancer Res 50:6971-6975, 1990.
3. Kim JH, Hahn EW. Clinical and biological studies of localized hyperthermia. Cancer Res 39:2258-2261, 1979.
4. Sugimachi K, Matsuda H, Ohno S, Fukuda A, Matsuoka H, Mori M, Kuwano H. Long term effects of hyperthermia combined with chemotherapy and irradiation for the treatment of patients with carcinoma of the esophagus. Surg Gynecol Obstet 167:319-323,1988.
5. Mori M, Sugimachi K, Matsuda H, Ohno S, Inoue T, Nagamatsu M, Kuwano H. Preoperative hyperthermochemoradiotherapy for patients with rectal cancer. Dis Colon Rectum 32:316-322,1989.
6. Moffat FL, Falk RE, Calhoun K, Langer JC, Dreznik Z, Makowka L, Rotstein LE, Ambus U, Howard V, Campbell A, Laing D, Venturi D, Falk JA. Effect of radiofrequency hyperthermia and chemotheraoy on primary and secondary hepatic malignancies when used with metroidazole. Surgery 94:536-542,1983.
7. Herman TS, Teicher BA, Holden SA, Pfeffer MR, Jones SM. Addition of 2-Nitroimidazole radiosensitizers to cis-Diamminedichloroplatinum (II) with radiation and with or without hyperthermia in the murine ESaIIC fibrosarcoma. Cancer Res 50:2734-2740,1990.
8. Bowers W.JR, Hubbard R, Wagner MA, Chisholm P, Murphy M, Leav I, Hamlet M, Maher J. Integrity of perfuesd rat liver at different heatr loads. Lab Invest 44:99-104,1981.
9. Sugimachi K, Kitamura K, Baba K, Ikebe M, Morita M, Matsuda H, Kuwano H. Hyperthermia combined with chemotherapy and irradiation for patients with carcinoma of the esophagus -A prosepective randomized trial- Int J Hyperthermia 8:289-295, 1992.
10. Mori M, Maehara Y, Inoue T, Shimono R, Kuwano H, Sugimachi K. Sensitivity to heat and radiation of human rectal malignant tissues in vitro. Dis Colon Rectum 33:419-422, 1990.

Esophagus

Immunohistological Evaluation of the Presence of Keratins in Esophageal Cancer

Shinya Tanimura, Masayuki Higashino, Harushi Osugi, and Hiroaki Kinoshita

Second Department of Surgery, Osaka City University Medical School, Osaka, 545 Japan

ABSTRACT

The presence of keratin-subunits in carcinoma tissues was evaluated immunohistologically in 41 patients with esophageal cancer. Molecular weights of keratin polypeptides in carcinoma tissues were investigated by enzyme-labeled antibody technique with four kinds of antikeratin monoclonal antibodies with spectrums of different reacting keratin-subunits. Correlation between staining intensity by each antikeratin antibody and histopathological findings was different from one another. Keratin-subunits of molecular weights of 48 and 56 kilodalton(kd) were frequently found in the carcinoma tissue of high malignancy such as severe lymphatic, venous invasion and intramural metastases. Keratin-subunits of molecular weights of 48 and 56kd were tend to be found in the carcinoma tissue of advanced histological stages with deep infiltration and sever lymphnode metastases.

KEY WORDS: immunohistological staining, enzyme-labeled antibody technique, molecular weights of keratin-subunits

INTRODUCTION

Keratin, one of five intermediate filaments, consists of insoluble fibrous proteins in the cytoplasm of epithelial cells. There are at least 19 keratin-subunits of molecular weights raging from 40 to 70 kd1). Many studies revealed that keratin composition of cells varied in different cell types, in different stages of differentiation and development of carcinoma cells, and in disease states1)2). As far as esophageal cancer is concerned, biochemical technique revealed that the keratin-subunits of low molecular weights appeared at early stage of carcinogenesis and increased accompanied with tumor growth2)3)4). However, few investigators have so far reported definite molecular weights of the keratin-subunits increased in the tissue of esophageal cancer by immunohistological approach. In this study, we investigated the molecular weights of keratin-subunits in the tissue of esophageal cancer by enzyme-labeled antibody technique with four kinds of antikeratin monoclonal antibodies with different spectrums of reacting keratin-subunits. Further more, the corrilation between the molecular weights of keratin-subunits and histopathological findings was evaluated.

MATERIALS AND METHODS

Materials

The forty one esophageal specimens taken from the patients of thoracic esophageal cancer operated from March, 1986 to October, 1990 at our department were studied. All patients (63.3 ± 9.2 years old, 29 males and 12 females) had no anticancer therapy before surgery.

Methods

All of specimens were fixed in formalin, cut into the slices of 5 mm width and stained by hematoxylin-eosin. In each case, histopathological findings, i.e. depth of invasion, histological differentiation, growth pattern, lymphatic invasion, venous invasion, intramural metastses, intraepithelial spread and perineural invasion of the tumor, and multiple carcinomas and atypical epithelium beside the tumor were evaluated. Then, all of adjacent specimens of the cancer lesion were stained for keratin by labeled AB(Avidin-Biotin) method. Antikeratin monoclonal antibodies used in this study and their spectrums of reacting keratin-subunits are as follows: 1)AE-1 (Signet Laboratories); reacts on the acidic (type I) keratin family, the molecular weights of 40,48,50,56.5kd. 2)AE-3 (Signet Laboratories); reacts on the basic (type II) keratin family, the molecular weights of 52,56,58,65-67kd. 3)AE1/AE3 (Lipshaw); reacts on 50,56.5kd keratins in the acidic family and 58,65-67kd keratins in the basic family. 4)Histogen (BioGenex Laboratories); reacts on 40,46,50,56.5kd keratins in the acidic family and 52,58,65-67kd keratins in the basic family. The percentage of the cells stained of all carcinoma cells was calculated in each preparation of keratin staining. The mean value of the percentage of positive cells in all preparations was defined as the intensity of keratin staining. Correlation between the staining intensity and histopathological findings was investigated. The molecular weights of keratin-subunits which increase in the carcinoma tissue of each patient were analized by the difference of staining intensities of four antikeratin antibodies. Correlation between the molecular weights of keratin-subunits in the carcinoma tissues and histopathological findings was also examined.

RESULTS

The tumor cells of 50% or more were stained by AE-1 and AE-3 in 22 and 25 patients (54% and 61%) (Fig.a), while those of 50% or more were stained by AE1/AE3 and Histogen in 17 and 18 patients (41 and 44%). In 8 patients none of the tumor cells were stained by any primary antibody(Fig.b). In stained cells, keratins located in their cytoplasms, not in the nuclei nor cellular membranes. The staining intensity of AE-1 correlated to the severity of lymphatic invasion and that of AE-3 correlated to the severity of lymphatic invasion and the absence of intraepithelial spread. The staining intensity of Histogen correlated to the presence of intamural metastases and multiple carcinomas, although AE1/AE3 did not present any significant findings. Thus, each primary antibody showed different attitude of keratin staining. Then we examined difference among the staining intensities of AE-1, AE1/AE3 and Histogen whose spectrums of reacting keratin-subunits partially overlapped one another, and in the same way compared among AE-3, AE1/AE3 and Histogen. In the tumor tissues of 14 patients, the staining by AE-1 was more intense than AE1/AE3 or Histogen, besides the staining byAE-3 was more intense than AE1/AE3 or Histogen. As only the 48kd keratin did not react to AE1/AE3 and Histogen in the keratin-subunits which reacted to AE-1, the 48kd keratin was thought to increase in these tumor tissues (Table1). In the same way, since only the 56kd keratin did not react to AE1/AE3 and Histogen among the keratins reacted to AE-3, the 56kd keratin was also considered to multiply (Table). In these patients who were considered to have increased 48,56kd keratin-pair in their carcinoma tissues, their histopathological findings were significantly in high malignancy, i.e. with severe lymphatic and venous invasion, or intramural metastases, and in advanced histological stages with deep infiltration and severe lymphnode metastases.

Table. Comparison of Molecular Weights of Kearin-subunits Stained by Four Kinds of Antikeratin Antibodies

Molecular Weights (kd)	Acidic Keratins (pl≦5.7)					Basic Keratins (pl≧6.0)			
	40	46	48	50	56.5	52	56	58	65-67
AE-1	○		◎	○	○				
AE-3						○	☆	○	○
AE1/AE3				○	○			○	○
Histogen	○	○		○	○	○		○	○

◎ : The 48kd keratin is considered to be increased in the carcinoma tissue stained more intensely by AE-1 than by AE1/AE3 or Histogen.

☆ : The 56kd keratin is considered to be increased in the carcinoma tissue stained more intensely by AE-3 than by AE1/AE3 or Histogen.

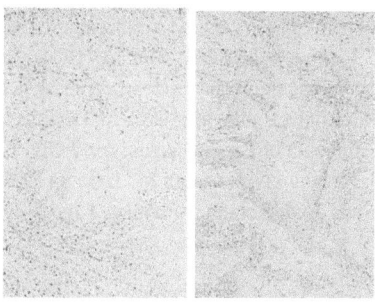

Figure. Keratin Staining
  a : Positive for AE-1 staining.
  b : Negative for Histogen staining.

DISCUSSION

As regards the molecular weights of keratin-subunits in different cell types, in different stages of differentiation and developement and in disease states, Weiss et al5) and Eichner et al6) had investigated in detail by gel electrophoresis and immunoblot analysis. According to their investigations, keratin polypeptides take the form of a pair consisting of each one of acidic keratin subfamily(molecular weights of 40,46,48,50,56.5kd, isoelectric points are less than 5.7) and basic keratin subfamily(molecular weights of 52,56,58,65-67kd, isoelectric points are more than 6.0). Their studies showed that 50 and 58kd keratin-pair existed in all keratinocytes, while 56.5 and 65-67kd keratins were the marker of keratinization. The keratins of 40,46 and 52kd existed in any kinds of cultured epithelial cells. Further they mentioned that 48 and 56kd keratin-pair was the molecular marker for hyperproliferative keratinocytes, e.g. carcinoma cells. In this study the molecular weights of keratin-subunits increased in the tissue of esophageal cancer were detected by the difference of reacting keratin-subunits of four monoclonal antibodies. Althogh there were a few reports that the molecular weights of keratin-subunits in the tissues of esophageal cancer were examined immunohistologically7)8), the keratin-subunits increased in the esophageal cancer have never been detected by the difference in staining intensity of antikeratin antibodies before. It is considered that immunohistological staining by the monoclonal antibody which reacts only on a specified keratin-pair is the best, but under the present situation such specified antikeratin antibodies are very limited. Our result supports earlier reports by biochemical technique2)3)5) that the 48,56kd keratin-pair exists in hyperproliferative keratinocytes, e.g. carcinoma cells and increases accompanied with the tumor growth. Moll et al1) suggested that the 48,56kd keratin-pair normally exists not only in the epidermis but also in the cornea, conjunctiva and esophagus, and it is masked in the normal tissue because of its high turn over rate but appeared accompanied with the cancerous change of keratinocytes because of its hyperproliferation. Since the increase of the 48,56kd keratin-pair in the tissue of esophageal cancer markedly correlated to histopathological malignancy in this study, immunohistological analysis of the molecular weights of keratin-subunits in carcinoma tissues would be useful in evaluation of malignant potential of esophageal cancer.

REFERENCES

1. Moll R, Franke WW, Schiller DL, Geiger B, Klepler R (1982) The catalog of human cytokeratins: patterns of expression in normal epithelia, tumors and cultured cells. Cell 31:11-24
2. Cooper D, Schermer A, Sun TT (1985) Classification of human epithelia and their neoplasm using monoclonal antibodies to keratins: Strategies, applications and limitations. Lab Invest 52:243-256
3. Grace MP, Kim KH, True LD,Fuchs E (1985) Keratin expression of normal esophageal epithelium and squamous cell carcinoma of the esophagus. Cancer Res 45:841-846
4. Banks-Schlegel SP, Harris CC (1984) Aberrant expression of keratin proteins cross-linked envelopes in human esophageal carcinomas. Cancer Res 44:1153-1157
5. Weiss RA, Eichner R, Sun TT (1984) Monoclonal antibody analysis of keratin expression in epidermal disease: a 48 and 56-kdalton keratin as molecular markers for hyperproliferative keratinocytes. J Cell Biol 48:1397-1406
6. Eichner R, Bonitz P, Sun TT (1984) Classification of epidermal keratins according to their immunoreactivity, isoelectric point and mode of expression. J Cell Biol 98:1388-1396
7. Yang K, Lipkin M (1990) AE1 cytokeratin reaction patterns in different differentiation states of squamous cell carcinoma of the esophagus. Am J Clin Pathol 94:261-269
8. Mizutani N, Imamura M, Tobe R (1987) An immunohistochemical study on esophageal carcinomas with various kinds of antikeratin antibodies. J Jpn Surg Soc 88:422-431

Immunohistochemical Evaluation of E-Cadherin and α-Catenin Expression in Human Esophageal Cancer

T. Kadowaki, H. Shiozaki, K. Iihara, M. Inoue, S. Tamura, H. Oka, Y. Doki, S. Matsui, T. Iwazawa, K. Shimaya, A. Nagafuchi, S. Tsukita, and T. Mori

The Second Department of Surgery, Osaka University Medical School, Osaka, 553 and Department of Information Physiology, National Institute for Physiological Science, Okazaki, Aichi, 444 Japan

ABSTRACT

Tumor metastasis is initiated by disaggregation of invasive cells from the primary tumor - a step that requires a breakdown of intercellular adhesion. To investigate the mechanism of dysfunction in cell-cell adhesion of cancerous tissues, we evaluated E-cadherin (E-cad) and α–catenin (α–cat) expression of human esophageal cancer immunohistochemically. Eighty percent of the tumors showed reduced expression of both of the molecules. The frequency of α–cat negative tumors was observed in 47%, but none of them were E-cad negative. These results suggest that esophageal cancers lose α–cat expression more frequently than E-cad, and the loss of α–cat mights cause dysfunction of E-cad-mediated intercellular adhesion.

KEY WORDS: intercellular adhesion molecule, E-cadherin, α–catenin, esophageal cancer.

INTRODUCTION

E-cadherin (E-cad) is a member of the cadherin family, and its expression is restricted to epithelial tissues. They produce the strong intercellular connections, when they are functioning. We demonstrated the existence of impaired E-cad expression in human cancer tissues in previous reports (1). Furthermore, the reduction of E-cad expression was associated with histopathological differentiation, invasiveness and metastasis (2). However, contradictory phenomena were observed; Some undifferentiated carcinomas expressed E-cad but were sparsely invasive. In addition, some differentiated gastric adenocarcinoma metastasized to liver regardless of high amounts of E-cad expression. These observations suggest that these cancer cells might have some mechanism which suppressed cadherin function. Recent studies have demonstrated that cadherins are associated with some cytoplasmic proteins, including catenin α(102kd), β(88kd), and γ(80kd) (3). These proteins bind cytoplasmic domain of E-cad and form a link to the cytoskeleton. Catenins are considered to be key modulators of cadherin action, and their loss or aberrant action may interfere with cadherin-mediated cell-cell adhesion. In this paper we report the expression of E-cad and α–catenin (α–cat) in surgically resected esophageal carcinomas using immunohistochemistry, and we discuss the possible role of cadherin and α–cat responsible for the biological properties of cancer cells.

MATERIALS AND METHODS

Surgical Specimens.

The specimens were surgically obtained from 30 consecutive patients with esophageal squamous cell carcinoma from December 1989 to Augest 1992. There were 25 men and five women with a mean age of 61. 2 years (range, 40-82 years).

Antibodies and Immunohistochemistry.

Two monoclonal antibodies, HECD-1 (4) and α–18, which recognize E-cad and α–cat respectively, were used. The establishment of α–18 will be reported elsewhere. Immunostaining for E-cad and α–cat was performed by the ABC method as described previously (1).

Immunohistochemical Evaluation of E-cad and α–cat Expression.

The intensity of immunostaining for cancer cells was compared with that of normal epithelial cells in the same sample. The cancer cells whose immunostaining was similar to that of normal epithelial cells were defined as positive. The grade of E-cad and α–cat expression of the tumors was semi-quantitatively evaluated according to the proportion of positive cells. When more than 90%, between 10% and 90%, and less than 10% of cancer cells were positively stained, the cases were evaluated as uniformly positive (+), heterogeneous (±), and uniformly negative (-), respectively.

Histopathologic Evaluation and Statistical Analysis.

A consecutive section from each specimen was stained with hematoxylin and eosin for histological evaluation. The pathological classification was based on TNM classification of malignant tumors. The data assessed in this study were primary tumor (T), regional lymph node (N), distant metastasis (M), histological grade of tumor, and invasive pattern of tumor. The chi-square test was used to determine statistical differences between the expression of α–cat and clinicopathological parameters.

RESULTS

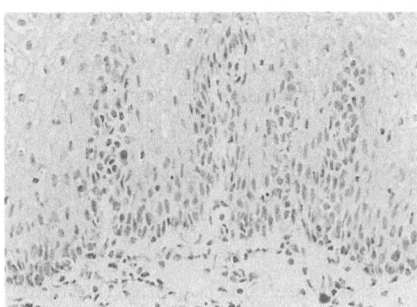

Fig. 1A Immunoreactive α-cat expression in normal esophageal epithelium (ABC method, x66).

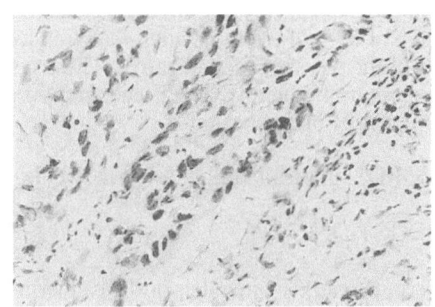

Fig.1B. A moderately differentiated squamous cell carcinoma of esophagus classified into α-cat (±). (ABC method, x66)

α–cat was strongly expressed in all the normal esophageal epithelia at cell-cell boundaries, and weakly detected in fibroblasts and muscle cells (Fig.1A). As for α–cat staining, 30 primary tumors (Fig.1B) were divided into six for (+), 10 for (±) and 14 for (-), respectively. Table 1 shows the relationship between α–cat expression and histological findings. Tumors with negative α–cat expression was more frequent in node-positive cases (63%, 12/19), in poorly differentiated tumors (70%, 7/10) or in infiltrative tumors (67%, 4/6).

Table 2 shows the relationship between the expression of α–cat and that of E-cad. There was a statistically significant correlation between the two immunoreactives (p < 0.01). The frequency of α–cat (-) tumors was 47%, but none was E-cad (-). Considering both α–cat and E-cad simultaneously, 16 of the 30 tumors (53%) had similar expression of both E-cad and α–cat on our criteria. The other 14 tumors (47%) lost α–cat predominantly rather than E-cad and were evaluated as E-cad(±)/α–cat(-). There was no tumor which expressed α–cat but not E-cad.

Table 1 Relationship between clinicopathological findings and α-catenin expression

	No.	(+)		(±)		(-)		p value
Total	30	6	(20%)	10	(33%)	14	(47%)	
T categories								
T1	7	3	(43%)	2	(29%)	2	(29%)	
T2	5	0	(0%)	1	(20%)	4	(80%)	
T3	17	3	(18%)	7	(41%)	7	(41%)	
T4	1	0	(0%)	0	(0%)	1	(100%)	
N categories								
N0	11	5	(45%)	4	(36%)	2	(18%)	p<0.05
N1	19	1	(5%)	6	(32%)	12	(63%)	
M categories								
M0	29	6	(21%)	9	(31%)	14	(48%)	
M1	1	0	(0%)	1	(100%)	0	(0%)	
Differetiation grade								
Well	12	5	(42%)	4	(33%)	3	(25%)	
Moderately	8	1	(13%)	3	(38%)	4	(50%)	
Poorly	10	0	(0%)	3	(30%)	7	(70%)	
Growth pattern								
Expansive	7	4	(57%)	1	(14%)	2	(29%)	
Intermediate	17	2	(12%)	7	(41%)	8	(47%)	
Infiltrative	6	0	(0%)	2	(33%)	4	(67%)	

Table 2 Relationship between α-catenin and E cadherin expression

OK; 30 cases		Expression of α-catenin			
		(+)	(±)	(-)	total
Expression of E-cadherin	(+)	6	0	0	6
	(±)	0	10	14	24
	(-)	0	0	0	0
	total	6	10	14	p<0.01

DISCUSSION

It has been found that E-cad expression was reduced or lost in human carcinomas immunohistochemically, and that its reduction was linked with histopathological differentiation, increased invasiveness, and lymph node metastasis. Of 30 esophageal carcinoma in this study, we found no E-cad-negative tumors, but heterogenous E-cadherin expression in 47% of the tumors. Therefore, E-cad function seemed to be impaired also in esophageal carcinomas. Normal esophageal epithelial cells demonstrated α–cat as well as E-cad strongly at the cell-cell boundaries. On the other hand, only six tumors (20%) showed α–cat as strongly as normal epithelium. Therefore, the reduction of α–cat expression may be one characteristic for esophageal carcinoma.
Twenty-four of 30 tumors (80%) were evaluated as α–cat($\pm$) or (-) according to our criteria. In this immunohistochemical study, 80% of the tumors exhibited reduced-E-cad expression and lost α–cat completely or heterogeneously. Our results were compatible with recent *in vitro* works; Hirano et al. demonstrated by transfection experiments that α–cat rescued the down-regulated cadherin function in human lung cancer cell line, which express cadherin molecules but not α–cat at the protein level (5). The expression of α–cat was correlated with nodal status, histological grade, and infiltrative pattern. Tumor cells with reduced α–cat expression might take advantage of possible dysfunction in E-cad-associated   cell-cell adhesion. It requires further investigations to clarify the biological properties of α–cat in cancer invasion and metastasis.

REFERENCES

1, Shiozaki H., Tahara H., Oka H., Miyata M., Kobayashi K., Tamura S., Iihara K., Doki Y., Hirano S., Takeichi M., and Mori T. (1991) Expression of immuno-reactive E-cadherin adhesion molecules in human cancers. Am. J. Pathol., 139:17-23.
2, Oka H., Shiozaki H., Kobayashi K., Tahara H., Tamura S., Miyata M., Doki Y., Iihara K., Matsuyoshi N., Hirano S., Takeichi M., and Mori T. (1992) Immunohistochemical evaluation of E-cadherin adhesion molecule expression in human gastric cancer. Virchows Arch. [A], 421:149-156.
3, Ozawa M., Baribault H., and Kemler R. (1989) The cytoplasmic domain of the cell adhesion molecule uvomorulin associates with three independent proteins structurally related in different species. EMBO J., 8:1711-1717.
4, Shimoyama, Y., Hirohashi, S., Hirano, S., Noguchi, M., Shimosato, Y., Takeichi, M., and Abe,O. (1989) Cadherin cell adhesion molecules in human epithelial tissues and carcinomas. Cancer Res., 49:2128-2133.
5, Hirano S., Kimoto N., Simoyama Y., Hirohashi S., and Takeichi M. (1992) Identification of a neural α–N-catenin as a key regulator of cadherin function and multicellular organization. Cell, 70:293-301.

A Spectrophotometric Study of DNA Ploidy Patterns of Esophageal Squamous Cell Carcinoma

AMINUR RASHID MINU[1], M. SUNAGAWA[1], T. KAWANO[1], M. ENDO[1], and N. TANAKA[2]

[1]First Department of Surgery, Tokyo Medical and Dental University, Bunkyo-ku, Tokyo, 113 Japan
[2]Sohgo Biomedical Laboratories, Inc., Suginami-ku, Tokyo, 166 Japan

ABSTRACT

DNA ploidy was determined by spectrophotometric analysis of paraffin embedded malignant tissue from 57 patients with squamous cell carcinoma of esophagus. DNA distribution pattern was classified as diploid, low grade aneuploid(LGA) and high grade aneuploid(HGA), according to the location of the peak and degree of dispersion on the DNA histogram. The relationships among DNA distribution patterns, pathologic features, clinical findings and prognosis were investigated. The advanced carcinoma had the higher distribution of HGA pattern(55%). The distributions of diploid pattern were more frequent in early(70%) or superficial(61.5%) esophageal squamous cell carcinoma in comparison with LGA or HGA. In patients with HGA pattern, there was significantly higher frequency of lymph node metastasis(74%), lymphatic and venous invasion as compared with those exhibiting the LGA or diploid pattern. Prognosis in patients with diploidy carcinoma were significantly better than those had HGA pattern (P<0.005). Thus the DNA HGA pattern based on spectrophotometry closely correlates with the factors generally indicative of the aggressive behavior of the malignant tumors. Furthermore the role of the DNA ploidy pattern as a prognostic factor is emphasized.

KEY WORDS: Diploid, Low grade aneuploid, High grade aneuploid, Esophageal squamous cell carcinoma.

INTRODUCTION

Despite improved surgical technique, intensive post-operative care and close look follow-up the prognosis of the advanced esophageal carcinoma remain poor. However, some patients do survive long after surgery. This clinical phenomena suggest that there is variation in the biological malignant potentiality among individual patients with esophageal carcinoma. If tumor with a higher malignant potential could be determined preoperatively from those with a lower one, more accurate treatment could possibly be designed. Prognostically relevant factors based on traditional staging and grading systems are known (1,2). But these factors can not always predict a sufficiently accurate prognosis in individual cases of esophageal cancer. So there is a need for more sophisticated prognostic determinants than clinical staging and morphologic grading system. This study was designed to evaluate the efficacy of nuclear DNA content analysis in determining the prognosis of esophageal squamous cell carcinoma. The DNA ploidy pattern is each was correlated with the histologic grade and other clinicopathologic findings.

MATERIALS AND METHODS

Patients

Fifty-seven patients with squamous cell carcinoma of the esophagus were studied. They were treated in the department of surgery I, Tokyo Medical and Dental University Hospital during the period from 1987 to 1991. There were 51 male and six female ranging in age from 43 to 84 years (mean 61.2). All patients underwent esophageal resection with regional lymph node dissection. None of these 57 patients received preoperative treatment such as radiation or chemotherapy.

specimen preparation

To prepare a specimen for spectrophotometric cellular DNA content measurement, single cell suspension was prepared according to Hedley (3) and colleagues, with some modifications. A thin smear was made on the non-fluorescent glass slides and was fixed by rapid spray (Muto pure chemicals Ltd. Tokyo, Japan) and was dried. The dried slide was passed through a graded series of ethanol and then distilled water. The slide was then transferred from ethanol into HP/DAPI (Hematoporphyrin/ 4´,6-diaminodine-2 phenylindol.2Hcl) staining solution and stained for 15 minutes. Then it was rinsed with distilled water and PBS respectively.

Then the cover slip was applied. The margins of the coverslip were sealed with nail polish. Staining solution was prepared according to Motohide(4).

Nuclear DNA measurement

The fluorescence intensity of the nucleus was measured by a microspectrophotometer (MSPM). We used the specimen slide from measuring the fluorescence intensities of at least 200 nuclei of malignant cells. To obtain a control value of diploid DNA content, the fluorescence intensity of 20 to 25 lymphocytes was measured.

The pattern was determined to be diploid when the peak of histogram was under 2.4c with a dispersion limited to 6c region and as low grade aneuploid pattern when the peak was in-between 2.4c and 3c with a dispersion beyond 3c less than 40% cells. High grade aneuploid was considered when the peak in between 2.4c and 3c with a dispersion beyond 3c more than 40% cells or the peak was beyond 3c.

Statistical analysis

For statistical comparison of the data, the student's t test was used. Survival rate was estimated on the basis of the method of Kaplan and Meier(5). Statistical analysis of the survival rate were carried out using the generalized wilcoxon test. A value of less than 0.05 was considered to be statistically significant.

RESULTS

Table 1 summarizes the DNA ploidy patterns and histopathologic features. The mean length of diploid tumors are slightly smaller than the mean length of LGA or HGA tumors. The incidence in patients with poorly differentiated squamous cell carcinoma was higher in the LGA and HGA tumor than diploid tumors, but the difference was not statistically significant. Marked lymphatic and venous invasion was observed 5/16(31.3%), 4/14(38.6%) and 7/16(43.7%), 6/14(42.8%) in diploid and LGA tumors respectively, whereas in 19/27(70.4%) and 17/27(63%) with HGA tumors, there was a marked lymphatic and venous invasion respectively. This difference was statistically significant. Lymph node metastasis was found in 6/16 (37.5%), 9/14(64.3%) and 20/27 (70.1%) of the patients with diploid, LGA and HGA tumors, respectively and the incidence of lymph node metastasis was significantly higher in LGA and HGA tumors, as compared with diploid(p<0.05).

TABLE 1. Comparison of DNA distribution pattern with histopathologic findings

	DNA ditribution pattern		
	Diploid	LGA	HGA
Tumor size(mean±SDcm)	4.78±2.84	6.5±2.4	5.98±2.79
Total	16	14	27
Histologic types			
Well	3(18.7)	4(28.6)	4(14.8)
Moderately	10(62.5)	5(35.7)	14(51.9)
Poorly	3(18.7)	5(35.7)	9(33.3)
Depth of penetration			
Epithelium	1(6.3)	1(7.1)	0(0)
Mucosa	2(12.5)	0(0)	0(0)
Submucosa	5(31.2)	1(7.1)	3(11.1)
Beyond submucosa	8(50)	12(85.8)	24(88.9)
Lymph node metastasis			
Negative(-)	10(62.5)	5(35.7)	7(25.9)
Positive(+)	6(37.5)	9(64.3)	20(74.1)*
Grade of lymphatic invasion			
Negative(-)	5(31.3)	4(28.6)	1(3.8)
Slight(+)	6(37.6)	6(42.9)	7(25.9)
Marked(++)	5(31.3)	4(28.6)	19(70.4)*
Grade of venous invasion			
Negative(-)	7(43.7)	2(14.3)	2(7.4)
Slight(+)	2(12.5)	6(42.9)	8(29.6)
Marked(++)	7(43.7)	6(42.8)	17(63)*

*There is a statistical difference with Diploid (P<0.05)

Although the number of cases were limited but even it was evident that there was no HGA pattern found among the intraepithelial and the intramucosal tumors. The submucosal tumors had higher incidence (31.2%) of diploid pattern than LGA (7.1%) or HGA (11.1%). But the tumor with beyond submucosal invasion had more frequent incidence of LGA (85.8%) and HGA (88.9%) than diploid (50%) pattern.

Relationship between prognosis and ploidy pattern

Forty-six of 57 patients (11 non cancer death excluded) were analyzed in terms of the post operative prognosis. Figure 1 shows the survival curves of the patients with the different DNA distribution patterns including 13 cases of diploid , 9 of LGA and 24 of HGA tumor. There was a progressive increment in survival rates from HGA to diploid. Patient with diploid tumor had a significantly better(P<0.005) prognosis than those with HGA pattern (fig 1).

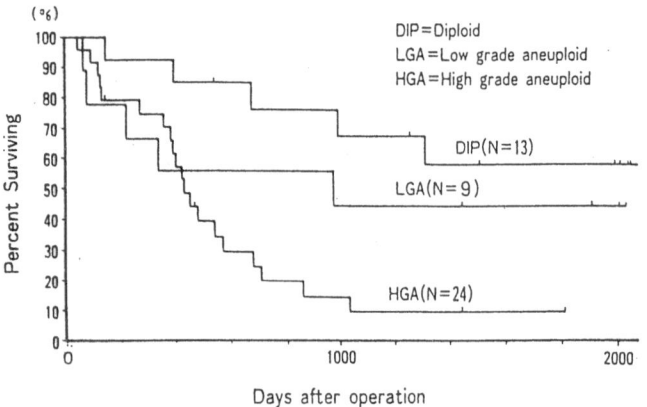

FIG. 1. Survival of patients with diplod, LGA and HGA of DNA distribution pattern. There is a statistical significance between diploid and HGA (P<0.005)

Discussion

The primary purpose of this study was to determine the prognostic significance of DNA ploidy pattern and to investigate the biological behavior of the malignant cells in the esophageal squamous cell carcinoma. During the last several years, a good number of literature have reported the relationship between the nuclear DNA content of a variety of human cancer cells and their malignant potential, measured by FCM or MSPM. We used single cell suspension with cell isolation method. Unlike FCM or MSPM section method this procedure can discriminate well cancer cells from normal cells and allow precise measurement of nuclear DNA content excluding overlapping or destroyed nuclei. In the superficial carcinoma, the distribution was mostly diploid pattern whereas among the cancers having penetration beyond submucosa we found majority of the cases are aneuploid and the degree of aneuploidy increases with deeper penetration. Patient with a diploid or LGA tumor had a more favorable prognosis with a 5 year survival rate of 45% as compared with 9% of patients with HGA tumors. This was statistically significant. Patients with HGA tumors had a worse outcome because they also had, in general, a more advanced histopathological stage. All patients with HGA tumors except one had died within 30 months. Similar results were published by Thomas Böttger et al. (6). Our retrospective study with 57 patients having esophageal squamous cell carcinoma showed a close correlation among HGA pattern , high histologic grade , lymphatic and venous permeation of cancer cells, deeper invasion into the esophageal wall, advanced stages and poor prognosis which mean DNA ploidy pattern is a significant and reliable prognostic factor. These observation suggests that the HGA tumors need close look follow-up and more careful attention for useful therapy. So preoperative determination of ploidy pattern along with other prognostic factors may improve prognostic prediction.

REFERENCES

1. J.R. Siewert, A.H. Hölscher, H.J Dittler. (1990). Preoperative staging and risk analysis in esophageal carcinoma. Hepato-gastroenterol 37:382-387
2. Sugimachi K, Ide H, Okamura T, Matsuura H, Endo M, Inokuchi K. (1984). Cytophotometric DNA analysis of mucosal and submucosal carcinoma of the esophagus. Cancer 53: 2683-2687
3. Hedley DW, Friedlander ML, Taylor IW, et al: (1983) Method for analysis of cellular DNA content in paraffin-embedded pathological material using flow cytometry. J Histochem cytochem 31: 1333-1335
4. Motohide Takahama and Akira Kagaya: (1988). Hematoporphyrin / DAPI Staining: Simplified simultaneous one-step staining of DNA and cell protein and trial application in automated cytological screening by flow cytometry. J Histochem cytochem 36: 1061-1067
5. Kaplan EL, Meier P.(1958). Nonparametric estimation from incomplete observasions. J Am stat Assoc 53: 457-481
6. Thomas Böttger, Stefan Störkel, Michael Stöckle, et al. (1991). DNA Image Cytometry, A prognostic tool in squamous cell carcinoma of the esophagus? cancer 67: 2290-2294

Experimental Radioimmunodetection for Esophageal Carcinoma by Monoclonal Antibody KIS-1 Fragment

Teruhiko Fujii, Hideaki Yamana, Uhi Toh, Sumihiro Ikeda,
Toshiaki Tanaka, Shuichi Nogami, Koji Shinozaki, Genzan Shirouzu,
Hiromasa Fujita, and Teruo Kakegawa

The First Department of Surgery, Kurume University School of Medicine, Kurume, Fukuoka, 830 Japan

ABSTRACT

Monoclonal antibody KIS-1 (IgG$_1$) against human squamous cell carcinoma of the esophagus was digested with papain to yield F(ab')$_2$. The KIS-1 F(ab')$_2$ was labeled with ^{125}I by Iodo-Gen method. %ID/g of the tumor was 0.24 ± 0.10 at 3 days after injection, while that of other organs showed no significant uptakes as much as control IgG$_1$ F(ab')$_2$ injection. Tumor to blood ratio was 2.82 ± 1.46 in KIS-1 F(ab')$_2$ injected group and that was 0.59 ± 0.16 in intact KIS-1 group at 3 days. These results indicate that KIS-1 F(ab')$_2$ may have possibilities in clinical application such as radio-immunodetection for esophageal carcinoma.

KEY WORDS: monoclonal antibody KIS-1, F(ab')$_2$ fragment, biodistribution

INTRODUCTION

Monclonal antibody KIS-1 was produced by immunization by human esophageal cancer cell line KE-2. KIS-1 belongs to the class of IgG$_1$ and reacted with high specificity to esophageal carcinoma in immunostaining experiments using surgically resected human specimens. In clinical application, intact antibody takes long for imaging, or has adverse side effect such as human anti-mouse antibody (HAMA). So we produced F(ab')$_2$ fragment which lack the Fc fragment of antibody to solve these problems. In this study, intact KIS-1 and its F(ab')$_2$ fragment were radioiodinated, and their biodistribution was studied in nude mice bearing a xenograft of a human esophageal carcinoma.

MATERIALS AND METHODS

1. Monoclonal Antibody (MoAb) and Its Purification

MoAb KIS-1 was produced by fusion between mouse myeloma cells (NS-1) and mouse spleen cells immunized with KE-2 cells. KIS-1 was purified from murine ascitic fluid by affinity chromatography.

2. Preparation of F(ab')$_2$ Fragment

The F(ab')$_2$ fragment was produced by digetion with papain. KIS-1(10mg) was dialyzed ag-against the digestion buffer and the activated papain (5%) was added and mixture was incubated for 3 hours at 37℃.

3. Radioiodination

Purified KIS-1 F(ab')$_2$ and the control mouse F(ab')$_2$ were radiolabeled with ^{125}I by using the Iodo-Gen method.

178

4. Biodistribution

The mice bearing human esophageal carcinoma were administered $10\sim20\mu$Ci of either ^{125}I-labeled KIS-1 F(ab')$_2$ or ^{125}I-labeled control F(ab')$_2$ intravenously. At 1, 2, 3 days after the injection, radioactivities of the tumor and every organs were counted.

RESULTS

1. Monoclonal Antibody KIS-1 and Its Fragment

Intact KIS-1 and F(ab')$_2$ fragment analyzed by SDS-PAGE and the molecular weight of F(ab')$_2$ was about 100.000.

2. Biodistribution

After ^{125}I-KIS-1 F(ab')$_2$ injection, %ID/g of the tumor was 0.24 ± 0.10 at day 3, while ^{125}I-control F(ab')$_2$ showed no significant uptakes in the tumor. Tumor to blood ratio were 2.82 ± 1.46 in ^{125}I-KIS-1 F(ab')$_2$ injected group and that was 0.59 ± 0.16 in intact KIS-1 group at 3 days. (Table 1, 2)

Table 1 Distribution of ^{125}I-KIS-1 F(ab')$_2$ in nude mice

(% of injected dose / g tissue)

Organ	Day 1 (n=4)	Day 2 (n=6)	Day 3 (n=7)
Tumor	0.79±0.16	0.42±0.05	0.24±0.11
Blood	2.53±0.45	0.43±0.10	0.09±0.02
Lung	0.92±0.17	0.36±0.10	0.10±0.03
Liver	0.50±0.07	0.10±0.02	0.03±0.01
Spleen	0.56±0.11	0.12±0.04	0.03±0.02
kidney	1.40±0.24	0.24±0.07	0.09±0.04

(* : p <0.01)

Table 2 Distribution of ^{125}I-control F(ab')$_2$ in nude mice

(% of injected dose / g tissue)

Organ	Day 1 (n=3)	Day 2 (n=4)	Day 3 (n=9)
Tumor	1.05±0.75	0.20±0.04	0.05±0.03
Blood	2.17±0.72	0.40±0.06	0.07±0.02
Lung	1.08±0.19	0.26±0.06	0.07±0.03
Liver	0.70±0.21	0.17±0.02	0.05±0.01
Spleen	0.67±0.29	0.20±0.06	0.06±0.02
Kidney	2.43±0.61	0.45±0.18	0.11±0.03

(* : p <0.01)

DISCUSSION

The F(ab')$_2$ fragment was produced by digetion with papain and its molecular weight was about 100KD. In biodistribution, %ID/g of the tumor was 0.24 ± 0.10 at 3 days, after ^{125}I-KIS-1F(ab')$_2$ injection, while other organs examined showed no significant uptakes. Tumor to blood ratio were showed high values more than 2.5 in ^{125}I-KIS-F(ab')$_2$ injected group as compared to 0.6 in intact KIS-1 group. KIS-1 F(ab')$_2$ fragment is cleared more rapidly from the circulation (1)(2) and KIS-1 F(ab')$_2$ fragment was found to give better and more rapid specific tumor localization than intact antibody KIS-1. These results indicate that KIS-1 F(ab')$_2$ fragment may have a possibility in clinical application such as radioimmun-odetection for esophageal carcinoma including lymph node metastasis.

REFERENCES

1. Wahl RL, Parker CW, Philpott GW (1983) Improved radioimaging and tumor localization with monoclonal F(ab')$_2$. J Nucl Med 24: 316-325
2. Kitamura K, Takahashi T, Yamaguchi T, Kitai S, Amagai T and Imanishi J (1990) Monoclonal antibody A7 tumor localization enhancement by its F(ab')$_2$ fragments to colon carcinoma xenografts in nude mice. Jpn J Clin Oncol 20: 139-144

Synergistic Antitumoral Effects of $\triangle^{12}$–Prostaglandin J_2 and Recombinant Human TNF–α on Human Esophageal Cancer Cell Lines

TORU YUNOKI, TOMOHIRO SAITO, MITSUKAZU SAITO, YOSHIAKI KARAKI, KENJI TAZAWA, and MASAO FUJIMAKI

Second Department of Surgery, Toyama Medical and Pharmaceutical University, Toyama, 930-01 Japan

ABSTRACT

In this study, the effects of Δ^{12}-Prostaglandin J_2 (Δ^{12}-PGJ_2) and recombinant human TNF-α (rhTNF-α) were investigated singly and in combination, on cell proliferation in two esophageal cancer cell lines in vitro. Both cell lines showed low sensitivity to either Δ^{12}-PGJ_2 or rhTNF-α alone. However, during combined administration, dose-dependent synergistic effects were observed. these synergistic effects were inhibited by the addition of a reactive oxygen scavenger, dimethyl sulfoxide (DMSO). The results showed that induction of hydroxyl radical production plays an important role in the synergistic antiproliferative effects.

KEY WORDS: Δ^{12}-Prostaglandin J_2, recombinant human TNF-α, esophageal cancer cell lines, hydroxyl radical.

INTRODUCTION

Esophageal cancer has a poor prognosis, even with surgical resection, radiation and adjuvant chemotherapy. Prostaglandins are known to have a variety of pharmacological effects on physiological processes. Prostaglandins (PGs) of the D series were shown to inhibit the growth of various tumor cells. Δ^{12}-PGJ_2 is the ultimate active metabolites of PGD_2. Recently, it was reported that Δ^{12}-PGJ_2 exhibits a potent antitumoral activity against some types of tumor cells in vitro. We investigated the effects of Δ^{12}-PGJ_2 and a monocyte-derived cytokine, rhTNF-α which is cloned and expressed in Escherichia coli, singly and in combination, on esophageal cancer cell lines. We added a radical scavenger to the cell culture to determine whether Δ^{12}-PGJ_2 /rhTNF-α stimulates hydroxyl radical production.

MATERIALS AND METHODS

Materials

As target cell sources, we use two human esophageal cancer cell lines originally established in our labolatory, designated as SGF-7 and SGF-8. These were maintained in monolayer culture in RPMI(Gibco) and Ham's F12(Gibco) mixed in equal proportions with 10% fetal calf serum (Na kashibetsu). Δ^{12}-PGJ_2 was kindly provided by Ono Pharmaceutical Co.,Ltd.(Osaka, Japan). Δ^{12}-PGJ_2 was prepared in absolute ethanol and diluted with culture medium prior to use. The final ethanol concentration was less than 0.1%, it had no effects on the proliferation of two cell lines. The rhTNF-α was kindly provided by Dainippon Pharmaceutical Co.,Ltd. (Osaka,Japan). DMSO, 2,2'-Bipyridine, Cycloheximide were purchased from Wako Pure Chemical Industries , Ltd.(Osaka, Japan).

Methods

1×10^4 cells(100μl) were seeded to 96 well microculture plates. After 24 hours, 100μl complete medium containing various concentrations of Δ^{12}-PGJ_2 and/or rhTNF-α were added and cells were incubated for 72 hours at 37℃, 5% CO_2 environment. Final concentrations were Δ^{12}-PGJ_2: 0, 0.5, 1.0, 2.0 μg/ml and rhTNF-α: 0. 1, 10, 10^2, 10^3 U/ml, respectively. DMSO(40mM), bipyridine(60μM), cycloheximide(0.1μg/ml) were respectively mixed with complete medium. Cytotoxicity was assessed in terms of MTT assay. Briefly, 100μl of 3-(4,5-dimethylthiazol-2 -yl)-2,5-diphenyltetrazolium bromide (MTT) solution (1mg/ml in culture medium) were added to each well. After 4 hours for MTT cleavage, the formazan product was solubilized by the addition of DMSO 150μl.
The optical density (OD) of each well was measured with a microphotometer, using a test wave

length of 540nm and a reference wavelength of 630nm. The relative % viability was calculated by the formula; mean OD (drug treated)/mean OD (control) X100, where mean OD represents the average of quadriplicate results.

Evaluation of synergistic effects

The expected additive effects of two agents were calculated by the formula; $A_1 \times A_2 \div 100$, where A_1 is the relative % viability of cells treated with rhTNF-α, A_2 is that obtained with Δ^{12}-PGJ$_2$. When the combination of rhTNF-α and Δ^{12}-PGJ$_2$ induced 2SD more than the expected additive effects, we defined the interaction of the two agents as synergistic.

RESULTS

Antiproliferative effects of Δ^{12}-PGJ$_2$ and rhTNF-α.

Both cell lines showed low sensitivity to either Δ^{12}-PGJ$_2$ or rhTNF-α alone. However, on combined administration, dose dependent synergistic effects were recognized (Fig.1, 2). In SGF-7, the ID$_{50}$ of rhTNF-α in combination with 0.5μg/ml of Δ^{12}-PGJ$_2$ were less than 1/100 compared with that of rhTNF-α alone. In SGF-8, the ID$_{50}$ of rhTNF-α in combination with 0.5 μg/ml of Δ^{12}-PGJ$_2$ were less than 1/1000 compared with rhTNF-α alone.

Influence of DMSO, a hydroxyl radical scavenger and bipyridine, an iron chelator and cycloheximide, protein synthesis inhibitor on the synergistic effects of Δ^{12}-PGJ$_2$ and rhTNF-α.

With the concurrent addition of DMSO, the antiproliferative effects were inhibited at all concentration of Δ^{12}-PGJ$_2$ and rhTNF-α in both cell lines. The synergistic effects were also inhibited (Fig.3, 4). However, in SGF-8, the synergistic effect of the combination with a high dose of Δ^{12}-PGJ$_2$ (2μg/ml) was not inhibited. After addition of bipyridine, the antiproliferative effects of Δ^{12}-PGJ$_2$ and rhTNF-α were not inhibited. The synergistic effects were not inhibited either. After addition of cycloheximide, the antiproliferative effects of two agents and the synergistic effects were not inhibited.

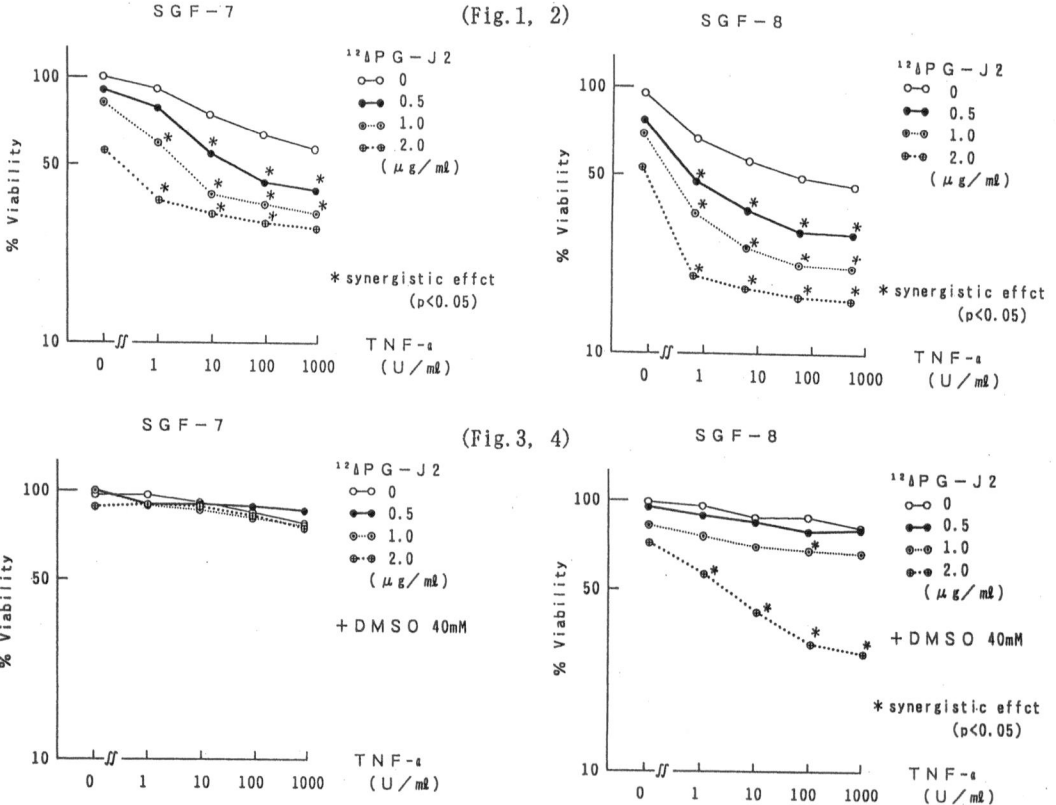

DISCUSSIONS

Prostaglandins are known to have a variety of pharmacological effects on physiological processes. Δ^{12}-PGJ$_2$ is promising as a new class of cytotoxic agents for the treatment of human cancers. In this study, we demonstrated that Δ^{12}-PGJ$_2$ has a potent antiproliferative effect on two esophageal cancer cell lines which were established originally in our labolatory. In combination with rhTNF-α, Δ^{12}-PGJ$_2$ demonstrated synergistic antiproliferative effects. However the mechanism remains unknown. It was reported that when rhTNF-α was bound to cell surface receptor, increases in the hydroxyl radical production may induce cell death. Therefore, we investigated the effect of adding reactive oxygen scavengers to the culture medium. The antiproliferative effects were not inhibited by the addition of bipyridine, although both antiproliferative effects and synergistic effects were inhibited by the addition of DMSO. Hydroxyl radicals may cause cell cytotoxicity from the Δ^{12}-PGJ$_2$ and rhTNF-α. Other researchers reported that the addition of cycloheximide could prevent induction of cytotoxicity by Δ^{12}-PGJ$_2$, suggesting that cell cycle arrest by cycloheximide may be important for protection . However, we did not confirm that findings in this study.
Antiproliferative activity of rhTNF-α was augmented by the addition of Δ^{12}-PGJ$_2$. These results suggest that the combined treatment with Δ^{12}-PGJ$_2$ and rhTNF-α may provide a new approach to obtaining increased responses in clincal trials.

REFERENCES

1. Kato T, Fukushima M, Kurozumi S, Noyori R (1986) Antitumor activity of Δ^7-Prostaglandin A$_1$ and Δ^{12}-Prostaglandin J$_2$ in vitro and in vivo. Cancer Res 46:3538-3542
2. Sakai T, Aoike A, Marui N, Kawai K, Nishino H, Fukushima M (1989) Protection by Cycloheximide against cytotoxicity induced by Vincristine, Colchicine, or Δ^{12}-Prostaglandin J$_2$ on human osteosarcoma cells. Cancer Res 49:1193-1196
3. Mori H, Takada Y, Kondoh H, Tamaya T (1990) Augmentation of antiproliferative activity of recombinant human Tumor Necrosis Factor by Δ^{12}-Prostaglandin J$_2$. Journal of Biological Respponse Modifiers 9:260-263
4. Yamauchi N, Watanabe N, Maeda M, Okamoto T, Sasaki H, Tsuji Y, Umeno H, Akiyama S, Niitsu Y (1992) Mechanism of synergistic cytotoxic effect between Tumor Necrosis Factor and hyperthermia. Jpn.J.Cancer Res 83:540-545
5. Tim Mosmann (1983) Rapid colorimetric assay for cellular growth and survival: Application to proliferation and cytotoxicity assay. J.Immuno.Methods 65:55-63

Esophageal Carcinoma — An Analyses of 502 Cases

İLKER ÖKTEN

Department of Thoracic Surgery, University of Ankara School of Medicine, Ankara, Turkey

ABSTRACT

Five hundred and two cases with esophageal carcinoma, 321 male 191 female, were operated between 1982 and 1992. Median age was 58 years. Localization of the tumors were at cervical and esophagus superior end in 78 (15.53 %), at upper thoracic esophagus in 50 (9.96 %) patients, at middle thoracic esophagus in 145   (28.88 %) patients, at lower thoracic esophagus in 128 (25.49 %) patients, cardia in 101 (20.11 %) patients. Histologic diagnosis were epidermoid carcinoma in 388 (77.28 %) patients, adenocarcinoma in 109 (21.71 %) patients and metastatic or rare type carcinoma in 5 (0.99 %) patients. The operative procedures were performed as fallows; left thoracophrenotomy in 160 patients, laparatomy and right thoracotomy in 108 patients, transhiatal way in 16 patients and right thoracotomy, laparatomy and cervical incision in 10 patients. Resection was performed in 294 patients. In most of the patients stomach was used for reconstruction where as colon and jejunal transposition were performed rarely. Palliative surgical procedures were performed in 119 patients. In 89 patients only exploration was performed. Seven (1.39) patients were at stage I, 13 (2.58 %) patients at stage II, 266 (52.98 %) patients at stage III and 208 (41.13 %) patients at stage IV. Ninety point forty seven percent of the patients who underwent resection were at stage III. Postoperative anastomotic leakage occurred in 16 (4.73 %) patients. Eleven patients died as a result of this anastomotic leakage. Other 14 (4.14 %) patients died of cardiac and pulmonary complications giving a total mortality rate of 4.98 %.

KEY WORDS: esophageal carcinoma, resection, esophageal reconstruction.

INTRODUCTION

In esophageal carcinomas curability problems still exist in spite of advanced surgical techniques and other treatment methods. The surgical indication was necessary in order to provide the gastrointestinal continuity and relieve the symptoms against the decreased curability in the advanced stage of the disease. In this retrospective study covering 10 - year period, the results of 502 surgical operation is reviewed. In this presentation, we discussed our surgical techniques and fallow up results under the light of the literature.

MATERIALS AND METHODS

Between 1982 and 1992 surgical intervention was performed in 502 patients with esophageal carcinomas. Cardia carcinomas invading distal esophagus was also included in this study. Patients were evaluated according to age, sex, site of lesion, histopathologic classification, surgical techniques, staging and postoperative complications. In staging Mannels' method is used(1). Postoperative mortalities were included in survival analysis. Postoperative swallowing function was evaluated in accordance with oral feeding and regurgitation and classified as (1) excellent, able to eat a normal diet and no regurgitation, (2)good, able to eat a normal diet, light dysphagia or mild regurgitation, (3) fair, able to swallow liquids and jell like meals and/or mild regurgitation and (4)poor, severe or total dysphagia and/or severe regurgitation.

RESULTS

Of all the 502 patients (321 (63.94 %) male 181 (36.05 %)female) median age was 58 (range, 27 to 82). In symptom analysis dysphagia is the most common symptom (86.85 % -436 patients), retrosternal pain was the second (35.45 % -178 patients) and weight loss was the third (27.88 % -140 patients). Carcinomas of the cervical and superior end in 78(15.53 %) patients , upper 1/3 thoracic in 50(9.96 %) patients, middle 1/3 thoracic in 145(28.88 %) patients, lower 1/3 thoracic in 128(25.49 %) patients and abdominal esophagus and cardia in 101(20.11 %) patients are diagnosed. Histopathologic examination revealed epidermoid cell carcinoma for 388(77.29 %) patients, adenocarcinoma for 109 (21.71 %) patients, leiomyosarcoma for 2 patients, anaplastic carcinoma for 2 patients and breast carcinoma metastasis for 1 patient.

Surgical technique and reconstruction method was selected according to patients' general condition, localization of lesion and the possibility of whether stomach reconstruction was proper or not. Right thoracotomy was first performed for the patients with thoracic esophageal carcinomas of high possibility of unresectability. In 294 patients resection was performed, resection rate was 58.56 % . Surgical interventions were performed transhiatal in 16 patients, laparatomy and right thoracotomy in 108 patients, left thoracophrenotomy in 160 patients and right thoracotomy, laparatomy and cervical incision in 10 patients. Size of resection was based upon the classical knowledge until 1987 and after 1987 size of resection was based upon the preoperative endoscopic lugol dye. Total laryngopharyngoesophagectomy was performed in 18 patients, total esophagectomy in 8 patients, partial esophagogastrectomy in 268 patients. For reconstruction of gastrointestinal continuity, stomach was used for 281 patients, colon for 8 patients and jejunum for 5 patients. In 208 unresectable patients, gastric bypass was performed in 35 patients with distal esophageal and cardia carcinoma and jejunal bypass in 9 patients. In remaining 164 patients, gastrostomy was performed in 63 patients, jejunostomy in 12 patients and only exploration was performed in 89 patients. Antireflux valve procedure was also performed to avoid postoperative regurgitation in patients with gastric reconstruction. Pyloroplasty was performed only in the patients with partial obstruction in pylorus and antrum or in the patients with high risk factors.

In staging, 7 patients (1.39 %) were classified as stage I, 13 patients (2.58 %) as stage II, 266 patients (52.98 %) as stage III and 208 patients (41.43 %) as Stage IV.

All of the major postoperative complications occurred in 338 patients who underwent anastomosis with or without resection. Anastomotic failure developed in 16(4.73 %) patients and 11(3.25 %) patients died due to sepsis. In this group 14(4.14 %) patients died of cardiac, pulmonary or other associated complications. Total mortality rate was 7.39 % in 338 patients who underwent anastomosis and overall mortality rate was 4.98 % in 502 patients. Functional evaluation after the resection and reconstruction was excellent in 270 patients, good in 9 patients and poor in 2 patients in overall 281 patients with gastric substitution. Severe esophagitis due to regurgitation was determined in 3 patients, mild esophagitis of 5 patients in total 13 patients with jejunal end colon interposition. Two patients with poor swallow were treated with dilatation of anastomosis and medical treatment was performed to all of the patients with esophagitis.

Out of 294 patients with resection and reconstruction 171 patients (130 patients were subjected to 50 Gy radiotherapy) were followed up for long term. Based upon these numbers 3 year survival rate was 28.07 % (48 patients), 5 year survival rate was 17.54 % (30 patients).

DISCUSSION

Between January-1982 and November-1992 surgical intervention was performed in 502 patients with esophageal carcinoma. Pharyngolaryngoesophagectomy was included in this study since 1990. Computerized tomography and endoscopic lugol dye was not used in the preoperative evaluation of the patients for the first half of 10-year period. For this reason, the performed surgical intervention in this period caused a certain drop from 90 % resection rate achievable today(2). Since 1987, all patients had been evaluated with CT and endoscopic lugol dye and as a result of this reliable determination of resection and resectability was achieved.

Laparatomy, right thoracotomy was performed to exclude abdominal metastasis and to provide stomach mobilization in middle and lower 1/3 thoracic esophageal carcinoma. Right thoracotomy was first performed for the patients with thoracic esophageal carcinomas of high possibility of irresectability. Right thoracotomy, laparatomy and cervical incision defined by McKeown was performed if the lesion was at thoracic inlet, at upper 1/3 thoracic esophagus or at middle 1/3 thoracic esophagus with extensive proximal mucosal invasion(3). This technique has certain advantages over transhiatal technique such as increasing possibility of radical resection, easy visualization, decreasing the possibility of sepsis in case of anastomotic insufficiency. Transhiatal technique was preferred because of shorter anesthesia period and easy tolerability in the patients with upper cervical and superior end of the esophageal carcinomas if pathological mediastinal lymph node was not detected(4). In this technique, generally similar to Finneys' definition, we worked as two teams at neck and abdomen at the same time and we saved reasonable time and observed no disadvantages on the contrary of mentioned results (5). Left thoracophrenotomy was preferred mainly for distal end localizations or abdominal esophageal invasions by cardia carcinomas. Radical lymph dissection was performed according to exploratory findings, but no extensive lymph dissection is performed routinely. Gastric transposition was performed for reconstruction in patients with esophagectomy because it has advantages such as reliable vascularization, sufficient length, orientation of a simple isoperistaltism, resectability of the proximal half or lesser curvature and cardia of stomach(6,7,8,9). Colon or jejunal transposition was performed in cases where total-subtotal gastrectomy was required during resection or any gastric operation is performed previously. The stomach was placed in the posterior mediastinum in all cases where gastric reconstruction was performed. Substernal method was used in colon transpositions(10). Antireflux valve procedure which was effective with intragastric pressure was performed to avoid postoperative gastroesophageal reflux and esophagitis in patients who underwent gastric transposition. Side to end anastomosis with 3-0 atraumatic coated silk suture was performed as double layer in the posterior wall and single layer in the anterior wall.

Pyloroplasty was recommended frequently as it could avoid delayed emptying(11). Pyloroplasty was applied only when Olak and Detskys' test factors were positive(12). Postoperative delayed gastric emptying was not detected except in one case where mechanical pressure was exerted on prepyloric area by left lobe of the liver stuck in esophageal hiatus. Medical treatment was required because of bile reflux in 3 patients and Dumping syndrome in 2 patients out of 9 cases where jejunal reconstruction was performed.

Oral feeding was started, as an average, on the 8th day after the reconstructive operation. Total mortality rate was low in overall group and was high if the anastomotic failure developed.

As a conclusion preoperative endoscopic lugol dye and CT of the esophagus are useful for to decide the resectability of the esophageal carcinomas. Gastric transposition is the most preferable surgical technique as it has low morbidity and mortality, also with high curability and survival rates.

REFERENCES

1. Mannell A (1982) Carcinoma of the esophagus. Curr Probl Surg 19:555.
2. Akiyama H (1990) Surgery for cancer of the esophagus; reconstruction of the esophagus. Baltimore: William & Wilkins:55.
3. McKeown KC (1976) Total three-stage oesophagectomy for cancer of the oesophagus. Br J Surg 63:259.
4. Orringer MB(1984)Transhiatal esophagectomy without toracotomy for carcinoma of the thoracic esophagus. Ann Surg 200:282.
5. Finley RJ, Inculet R (1989)The results of esophagogastrectomy without thoracotomy for adenocarcinoma of the esophagogastric junction. Ann Surg 210:535.
6. Finney GG Jr, Montague ACW, Finney DCW (1975) Combined esophagogastrectomy for esophageal carcinoma performed by two surgical teams. Am Surg 41:84.
7. Skinner DB, Dowlatshahi KD, DeMeesterTR(1982) Potentially curable cancer of the esophagus. Cancer 50:2571.
8. Akiyama H(1980) Surgery for carcinoma of the esophagus. Curr Probl Surg 17:50.
9. 9. Wang LS, Huang MH, Huang BS, Chien KY (1992) Gastric substution for resectabl carcinoma of the esophagus. Ann Thorac Surg 53:289.
10. DeMeester TR, Johansson KE, Franze I, Eypasch E, Lu CT, McGill JE, Zaninotto G (1988) Indications, surgical technique, and long-term functional results of colon interposition or bypass. Ann Surg 208:460.
11. Cheung HC, Siu KF, Wong J (1987) Is pyloroplasty necessary in esophageal replacement by stomach? A prospective randomized controlled triad. Surgery 102:19.
12. Olak J, Detsky A (1992) Surgical decision analysis: esophagectomy with or without drainage? Ann Thorac Surg 53:493.

Clinical Study of Superficial Esophageal Carcinoma

AGUSTIN ETCHEGARAY, TATSUYUKI KAWANO, KUNIHIDE YOSHINO, and MITSUO ENDO

The First Department of Surgery, Tokyo Medical and Dental University, Bunkyo-ku, Tokyo, 113 Japan

ABSTRACT

We reviewed 136 consecutive cases of superficial esophageal carcinoma treated at the First Department of Surgery TMDU from 1985 to 1992. There were 122 men and 14 women with a mean age of 61 years. At the time of diagnosis 60.2% were asymptomatic. The incidence of lymph node involvement was 16.1%. We had 26 patients classified as stage 0, 88 patients as stage I, 16 patients as stage IIB, and 6 patients as stage IV. There were 9 patients treated by endoscopic mucosal resection, 26 by transhiatal blunt esophagectomy, and 101 by esophageal resection with lymph node dissection. Until now we have had 11 (8%) patients with cancer recurrence, all of them initially had invasion to the submucosa.

KEY WORDS: superficial esophageal carcinoma, epithelium, muscularis mucosae, submucosa.

INTRODUCTION

The incidence of superficial esophageal carcinoma in Japan has been increasing, and new treatment modalities are now in practice. We undertook the present study to analyze the experience with superficial esophageal carcinoma at TMDU from 1985 to 1992.

MATERIALS AND METHODS

From 1985 to 1992, 136 consecutive patients with superficial esophageal carcinoma were treated at the First Department of Surgery, TMDU. We reviewed the charts and pathological records, all of them having superficial esophageal carcinoma.

Superficial esophageal carcinoma is defined as an esophageal carcinoma in which invasion remains within the submucosa regardless of the lymph node status [1]. The group consisted of 122 (89.7%) men and 14(10.2%) women, with a male to female ratio of 8.7:1. The majority of the patients were in the sixth decade, followed by seventh and eighth decade, with a range of (34-84).

RESULTS

Patient History

On the patient history we found 88(64.7%) patients were smokers, 32 (23.5%) non-smokers, and 16 (11.7%) could not be found. 98 (72.0%) were drinkers, 22 (16.15) non-drinkers, and 16 (11.7%) could not be found.

Symptoms

At the time of diagnosis 82 (60.2%) patients were asymptomatic, 45 (33.0%) when asked, had some kind of complaint or symptom, and 9 (6.6%) could not be found. In the symptomatic group, a feeling of narrowed esophagus, foreign body sensation, and retrosternal pain were the most frequent presenting symptom, followed by "tingling sensation" caused by food intake, and an abnormal feeling. In reviewing the reason for consultation, 42 (30.8%) patients were diagnosed based on symptoms, 68 (50%) patients during a routine health screening, 10 (7.3%) during an examination for other disease, and 6 (4.4%) for other reasons.

Diagnostic Method

The first diagnostic method was endoscopy in 90 (66.1%) patients, radiology in 36 (26.4%) patients, and in 10 (7.3%) the first diagnostic method could not be determined.

Endoscopic Classification

We used the following endoscopic classification of superficial esophageal carcinoma [2].
0:      superficial type.
O-I: superficial and protruding type.
O-II: superficial and flat type
        a) slightly elevated type.
        b) flat type.
        c) slightly depressed type.
O-III: superficial and distinctly depressed type.
According to this classification the majority of the lesions were O-II type, being type O-IIc (slightly depressed) the most frequent (49.2%), followed by combined type (29.4%), of which the most frequent was O-I+IIc (13.2%).

Location of the Tumor

The lesions were located mainly in the middle and lower third, with only one patient with a cervical lesion, and 3 in the abdominal esophagus.

Cervical: 1 (0.7%)
Upper third: 20 (14.7%)
Middle third: 69 (50.7%)
Lower third: 44 (32.3%)
Unknown: 2 (1.4%)

Table 2. Depth of Invasion and Lymph Node Involvement

Depth of invasion	No.(%)	Nodal involvement (%)
ep	26(19.9%)	0
mm	42(30.8%)	1(2.3%)
sm	68(50%)	21(29.4%)

The incidence of carcinoma in situ (Tis) was 19.1%, and tumors classified as (T1) 80.8%, this group was composed of 42 (30.8%) tumors invading the muscularis mucosae, and 68 (50%) involving the submucosa. There was a 16.1% of lymph node metastasis in the whole group, none in the patients with carcinoma in situ, and only 1 (2.3%) patient when the invasion was limited to the muscularis mucosae.

Histologic Type

There was only one case of carcinosarcoma and another of adenocarcinoma, being squamous cell carcinoma the most frequent with an incidence of 98.5%. Moderately differentiated squamous cell carcinoma was the most frequent with 69 (50%) patients, well differentiated with 33 (24.2%), poorly differentiated with 24 (17.6%), and 10 unclassified.

Invasion of Lymphatic and Blood Vessels

There were 49 (36.0%) patients with lymph vessel invasion, only two of them had tumors with invasion within the muscularis mucosae, the rest of them had invaded the submucosa. On blood vessel invasion there were 29 (21.3%) patients with positive blood vessels, only one of them had a tumor invading the muscularis mucosae.

Stage

We classified the patients stage according to the TNM classification for esophageal cancer revised by UICC in 1987 [3]. We had 26 (19.1%) patients classified as stage 0 (Tis,No,Mo), 88 (64.7%) as stage I (T1,No,Mo), 16 (11.7%) as stage IIB (T1,N1,Mo), and 6 (4.4%) as stage IV (T1,N1,M1).

Treatment

There were 9 (6.6%) patients treated by endoscopic mucosal resection, 26 (19.1%) by transhiatal blunt esophagectomy, and the rest 101 (74.2%) by esophageal resection with lymph node dissection, being the most common procedure right thoracotomy, with retrosternal gastric tube reconstruction and a cervical anastomosis, only in four cases we had to use the colon for reconstruction.

Prognosis

We found no recurrence of esophageal carcinoma in patients which tumors had invaded the epithelium or the muscularis mucosae. Until now 22 patients have died, 11 (8%) had cancer recurrence, all of them had invasion to the submucosa, and the other 11 patients died due to other causes.

Table 3. Survival rate in superficial esophageal carcinoma.

Depth of invasion	3 yr	5 yr
ep	92.3%	92.3%
mm	92.8%	85.7%
sm	75.0%	64.7%

DISCUSSION

Here we present our experience with superficial esophageal carcinoma, and describe the importance of an early diagnosis when the patient is asymptomatic. We found that if the invasion is within the muscularis mucosae it is safe to perform a transhiatal blunt esophagectomy, or an endoscopic mucosal resection, because the patients had negative lymph nodes in 97.6% of the cases, compared to 29.4% when the invasion reaches the submucosa.

An early diagnosis is of most importance not only because the prognosis is different but also the opportunity to preserve the esophagus.

REFERENCES

1. Japanese Society for Esophageal Diseases (1976) Guidelines for clinical and pathological studies on carcinoma of the esophagus. Jpn J Surg 6: 69-78.
2. Endo M, Takeshita K, Yoshino K (1988) Oesophagoscopy for the diagnosis of Superficial oesophageal cancer. Surg. Endosc. 2: 205-208.
3. UICC (1987) Classification of Malignant Tumours. Springer Verlag 4th Edition: 40-42.
4. Endo M, Yoshino K, Takeshita K, Kawano T (1991) Analysis of 1.125 cases of early esophageal carcinoma in Japan. Diseases of the Esophagus 2: 71-76.

Clinical Results of Transhiatal Esophagectomy for Carcinoma of the Lower Esophagus

Toshihiro Hirai, Yoshinori Yamashita, Hidenori Mukaida, Takashi Iwata, Akihiro Yoshimoto, and Tetsuya Toge

Department of Surgery, Research Institute for Nuclear Medicine and Biology, Hiroshima University, Hiroshima, 734 Japan

SUMMARY

Thirty three cases with the lower esophageal cancer were submitted to transhiatal esophagectomy. In this procedure, the tumor and lymph node around the middle or lower esophagus could be dissected safely under the direct vision. And, the whole stomach was brought up to the neck through the posterior mediastinal route. As for postoperative complications, Pneumothorax occurred in 8 cases (24%), hoarseness in 4 cases (12%), pneumonia in 3 cases (9%), pyothorax and hemothorax in 2 cases (3%) each. Two cases died within 30 days of operation due to massive bleeding during operation and mediastinitis. Five year survival rate of 31 cases except for 2 cases of postoperative death was 24.8%. First recurrent sites were investigated for 16 cases who recurred. Nine cases recurred to parenchymatous organs, 4 cases to lymph nodes, 2 cases as a dissemination and 1 case to the remnant esophagus. From these results, we concluded that the intensive chemotherapy before or after the operation should be performed rather than extended lymph node dissection of the upper mediastinal area through thoracolaparotomy for the lower esophageal cancer.

KEY WORDS : Esophageal cancer, Transhiatal esophagectomy, Survival rate

INTRODUCTION

Surgical treatment for esophageal cancer is now a safe procedure and most surgeons in Japan are aiming at the superradiacal operation with extended lymph node dissection by numerous deveises to improve the end result of the operation. However, prognosis of the operated esophageal cancer patients is still poor.
We have indicated that excessive operative stress of thoracolaparotomy enhanced tumor growth several times more as compared with that of laparotomy in the experimental studies [1]. From these reasons, if a certain extent of curability would have to be guaranteed, it would be desirable to treat esophageal cancer without opening the chest. Transhiatal esophagectomy (THE) seems to satisfy this purpose for every tumor of the lower esophagus because the tumor and lymph nodes below the tracheal bifurcation can be dissected safely under the direct vision. In this paper, 33 cases of the lower esophageal cancer treated with THE have been presented.

MATERIALS AND METHODS

Thirty three cases of the lower esophageal cancer was submitted to THE from 1982 to 1991. Histological characteristics of them were shown in Table 1.
In the beginning, 10 cases were performed with the longitudinal sternotomy besides dividing the diaphragm. However, the longitudinal sternotomy was of little use to get the wide vision of the mediastinum and the later cases were operated only by dividing the diaphragm. In this procedure, the lymph node dissection around the middle or lower esophagus could be performed safely under the direct vision. The reconstruction was carried out using the whole stomach brought up to the left neck via posterior mediastinal route. Anastomosis was done by the layer to layer fashion.

Table 1 Histological characteristics of 33 cases with carcinoma of the lower esophagus, who underwent transhiatal esophagectomy

stage	cases	curability	cases	Depth of invasion	cases	Degree of Lymph node metastasis	cases
0	4 (12)	curative	21 (64)	ep, mm	4 (12)	n_0	12 (36)
1	2 (6)	non-curative	12 (36)	sm	1 (3)	n_1	2 (6)
2	3 (9)			mp	3 (9)	n_2	10 (30)
3	12 (36)			a_1	9 (27)	n_3	3 (9)
4	12 (36)			a_2	11 (33)	n_4	6 (18)
				a_3	5 (15)		

Abbreviations are according to the guide lines for the clinical and pathologic studies on cavcinoma of the esophagus[2]

( ) : %

RESULTS

Postoperative complications : Pneumothorax occurred in 8 cases (24%), hoarseness in 4 cases (12%), pneumonia in 3 cases (9%), pyothorax and hemothorax in 2 cases (6%) each, hepatitis, pulmonary fibrosis, mediastinitis, atrial fibrillation, subphrenic abscess and massive bleeding during operation in 1 case (3%) each. Generally, postoperative care was remarkably easier to manage as compared with the cases of formal thoracolaparotomy. Since postoperative mechanical ventilation was not necessary, the patient was extubated immediately after surgery. The tracheal tear was not experienced. Cervical esophageal anastomotic leakage occurred in 6 of 33 cases (18%) including 2 (6%) major leakages.

There were 2 cases of the operative death. One died of mediastinitis originated from the remaining tumor ulcerated and invaded to the pericardium and diaphragm on 7th post operative day and the other died of intraoperative massive bleeding due to the accidental injury of azygos vein.

Fig. 1 Actuarial survival curves for patients with carcinoma of the lower esophagus who underwent transhiatal esophagectomy (N = 31)

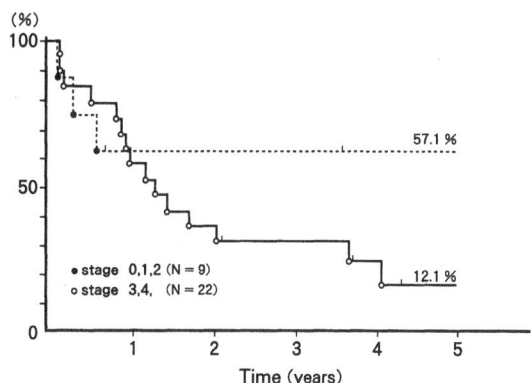

Survival rate by Kaplan-Meier's method : Five year survival rate of 31 cases except for 2 operative mortality cases was 24.8%. That was 57.1% in stage 0.1 and 2 (N = 9) and 12.1% in stage 3 and 4 (N = 22) (Fig. 1).

First recurrent sites : Sixteen recurrent cases hasd been shown in Table 2 ; lung in 4, liver in 4, bone in 1, posterior mediastinal, pulmonary hilar, bifurcation and paraaortic lymph node in 1 each, as dissemination in 2 and the remnant esophagus in 1. No recurrence occurred in the local area.

Table 2. First recurrent sites of carcinoma who underwent transhiatal esophagectomy

	~mp	a1,a2	a3	Total
Reccurence to parenchymatous organs	0	7 (37)	2 (50)	9 (29)
Lung		3	1	4
Liver		3	1	4
Bone		1	0	1
Reccurence to Lymph nodes	0	4 (21)	0	4 (13)
No.112		1		1
No.109		1		1
No.107		1		1
No. 16		1		1
Dissemination	1 (13)	0	1 (25)	2 (6)
Pleural	1		0	1
Peritoneal	0		1	1
Remnant esophagus	0	1 (5)	0	1 (3)
Absolute non-curative resection	1 (13)	1 (5)	1 (25)	3 (10)
No recurrence	6 (75)	5 (26)	0	11 (35)
Unknown	0	1 (5)	0	1 (3)
Total	8	19	4	31

Abbreviation is accordling to the guide lines for the clinical and pathologic studies on carcinoma of the esophagus[6]

DISCUSSION

Superiority of THE are smaller operative stress, easier postoperative management and fewer postoperative complications than transthoracic approach. Opinions of most surgeons regarding above probably be unanimous and our results advocated it except for 2 operative mortality cases. A point at issue of THE for esophageal cancer is curability of the tumor. In fact, there is a problem in curability for large tumor of the middle or upper esophagus. However, for the lower esophageal cancer, curability can be obtained because we can operate under satisfactory vision up to the level of tracheal bifurcation by dividing the diaphragm. From our results, no case recurred to local area. Another point at issue is an impossibility of lymph node dissection of upper mediastinal area. Akiyama et al [3] reported that lymph node metastasis to the upper mediastinal area was positive in 9.8% of the lower esophageal cancer cases. However, our results as for the first recurrence site showed that only 1 case recurred to bifurcation lymph node. On the other hand, 9 cases recurred to the parenchymatous organs. From these results, we concluded that the intensive chemotherapy and radiotherapy before or after THE should be performed as reported [4] rather than extended lymph node dissection through thoracotomy for the lower esophageal cancer to improve their prognosis.

REFERENCES

1. Hattori T, Hamai Y, Takiyama W et al (1980). Gann 71:280-284.
2. Japanese Society for Esophageal Diseases (1976). Jap J Surg 6:69-78.
3. Akiyama H., Tsurumaru M., Kawamura T. et al (1981). Ann Surg 194:438-446.
4. Orringer MB, Forastiere AA, Perez-Tamayo C et al (1990). Ann Thorac Surg 49:348-355.

Esophagectomy in Geriatric Patients

YUTAKA SHIMADA and MASAYUKI IMAMURA

First Department of Surgery, Faculty of Medicine, Kyoto University, Kyoto, 606 Japan

ABSTRACT

From 1979 to September 1992, 260 patients with esophageal cancer were admitted to our department and 33 of these patients (12.7%) were over 75 years of age. Of 33 esophageal cancer cases, 29 patients (87.9%) received curative esophagectomy. The five years survival rate was 39.8% (curative case) with 1 operative death (3.0%) and 3 hospital deaths (9.1%). Minor anastomotic leakage occurred in 3 patients (9.1%) and was cured conservatively. All patients suffered various degrees of delirium. It is our contation that despite advanced aging, curative esophagectomy in those 75 years of age and over can result in long term survival.

Key words: Geriatric Surgery, Esophageal cancer.

INTRODUCTION

Statistics for 1990 showed that the life expectancy of Japanese was 75.86 years in men and 81.81 years in women, and that life expectancy beyond 80 years was 6.91 years in men and 8.67 years in women [1]. There are reports on the outcome of surgery for abdominal disorders in a geriatric age group, however, little is known of the results of resection for esophageal cancer in elderly patients [2-5]. Although due to a combination of improved technology and methodology, radical resection of esophageal cancer has recently become a relatively safe procedure, it is still believed that trasthoracic esophagectomy for cancer of the esophagus is risky over the age of 75. Since 1985 the incidence of patients over 75 years of age, admitted to our department has increased and since 1989 the number of patients over 80 years of age admitted has also increased. This paper describes the surgical procedures and present results to the surgical treatment of geriatirc patients with esophageal cancer.

MATERIAL AND METHODS

From 1979 to September 1992, 260 patients with esophageal cancer were admitted to our department and 235 patients (90.4%) underwent surgical treatment. Of the 235 patients, 223 (95%) patients had squamous cell carcinoma and 194 patients (82.6%) were male. The average age of the patients who received surgical treatment was 63.6 years and 33 patients (14%) were over 75 years of age. The UICC-TNM staging system was used for clinical and pathology-related descriptions. The background data of the patients over 75 years of age is shown in Table 1. The p-TNM stage of these patients was similar to that of other age groups.

Table 1. Background data of esophageal cancer over 75 years old

Age	75-79	80-84	85<
Cases	23	8	2
M : F	19 : 4	6 : 2	1 : 1
Stage I	3	2	0
IIa	2	1	0
IIb	4	2	0
III	9	3	1
IV	5	0	1
Upper thoracic	3	2	1
Middle thoracic	19	4	0
Lower thoracic	1	2	1

Table 2. Strategy of esophagectomy in aged patients

A. Preoperative management
　　1. Cleaning of air way
　　2. Breathing training
　　3. Cessation of smoking
B. Intraoperative management
　　1. Gentle management of tissue
　　2. Preservation of vessel network of greater omentum and resection of left upper side of sternum
　　3. Using highfrequency positive pressure ventilation with double lumen tube
C. Postoperative management
　　1. Respiration by means of bronchoscope
　　2. Deep sleeping by means of medication
　　3. Aided walk
　　4. Mental care surrounded by family

The standard operation methods used have been previously described. In brief, after resectioning the intrathoracic esophagus and the lymphnode dissection, a retrosternal gastric tube was used as an esophageal substitute and esophagogastrostomy was performed by an EEA stapler. In order to avoid a compression of the gastric tube, the left upper part of the sternum was resected [6], and in order to maintain a satisfactory arterial blood supply, the arterial network in the greater omentum was preserved. We used a double lumen tube for intraoperative ventilation. The lung on the operating side was ventilated with HFPPV (high frequency positive pressure ventilation), and the lung on the other side was ventilated with a large tidal volume ventilation [7]. Preoperative and postoperative strategies related to esophagectomy in aged patients are summarized in Table 2. Survival rates were calculated by the Kaplan-Meier method and statistical analyses were carried out using the logrank test. Other statistical analyses were performed using chi-square test.

RESULTS

There were 10 cases (30.3%) of respiratory abnormality, 10 cases (30.3%) of renal abnormality, 17 cases (51.5%) of cardiac abnormality, 7 cases (21.2%) of hepatic abnormality and 9 cases (27.3%) of metabolic abnormality. Forty five point five percent of the patients had two or more organ abnormalities and 21.2% of the patients had three or more organ abnormalities.

Operation methods were as follows;   Thirteen cases uderwent subtotal esophagectomy with cervical esophagogastrostomy, 12 cases underwent intrathoracic esophagogastrostomy (6 cases underwent extensive lymphnode dissection), 1 case underwent jejunal interposition, 2 cases underwent a two step operation with colon interposition, 2 cases underwent subtotal esophagectomy without reconstruction, 2 cases underwent enterostomy and 1 case underwent tube insertion. All resected patients received right or left side thoractomy and there were no cases of blunt dissection.

Twenty cases (60.6%) were extubated the day after surgery. Four cases required subsequent reintubation and 1 of them required long term mechanical ventilation. Tracheotomy was needed in 1 case. Bronchoscopic endothoracheal suction was needed more than 10 times by 7 pateints. Postoperative complications were as follows; Pneumonia occurred in 5 cases and vaious arrythmia occurred in 12 cases. Minor anastomotic leakage occurred in only 3 cases (9.1%) and was cured conservatively. The most common complication encountered in patients more than 75 years of age was postoperative delirium.

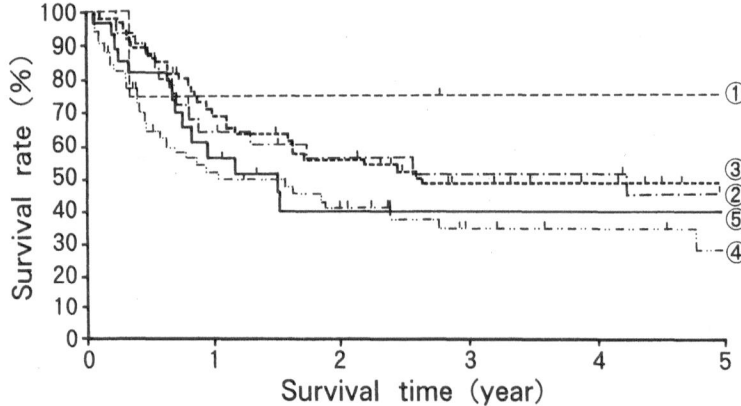

Figure 1. Survival curves of patients of different age groups (Curative cases)
1. 35~44yrs (n=4)   2. 45~54 yrs (n=30)   3. 55~64 yrs (n=70)   4. 65~74 yrs (n=58)
5. 75 yrs< (n=29)   Kaplan-Meier Method

Of 33 cases, 29 (87.9%) were resected curatively with 1 operative death (3.0%) and 3 hospital deaths (9.1%). The five years survival rate (curative case) was 39.8%. Figure 1 shows the postoperative survival curves of patients of different age groups. The survival rate of those over 75 years was comparable with that of patients younger than 75 years.

The treatment of patients over 80 years of age were as follows; Subtotal esophagectomy was performed in 6 cases (60%). Postoperative delirium in those over 80 years of age occurred in 4 cases. One was lost due to a viral infection which occurred three weeks after surgery and led to respiratory failure. We recently performed endoscopic mucosectomy without complication on an 80 years old male patient.

DISCUSSION

Esophageal cancer, with a peak incidence in the sixth decade of life, is a major cancer of the elderly. The choice of treatment for esophageal cancer in the elderly depends mainly on the general clinical state and on the spread of the tumor. Several optional treatments are considered, such as surgical resection, radiotherapy, chemotherapy, laser therapy and palliative intubation therapy. However, long term survival is rare with non surgical therapy. Regarding surgical procedures, transhiatal esophagectomy without thoracotomy, using blunt dissection has been described as a safer and more tolerable procedure [8]. This procedure, however, results in a narrowing of the margins of resection thus giving insufficient access for lymphnode dissection. Transthoracic esophagectomy has a better survival rate than transhiatal resection which is advised only in selective cases [9].

Transthoracic esophagectomy is a standard procedure for esophageal cancer. In our 33 patients over 75 years of age, there were 3 hospital deaths and only 1 operative death. Inspite of the high incidence of preoperative organ abnormalities, our operative results were satisfactory. Preserving the arterial network in the greater omentum of the gastric tube, and decompressing the gastric tube by resectioning the left upper part of the sternum resulted in a low incidence of anastomotic leakage.

It is common for respiratory complications in esophageal cancer patients, particularly the elderly, to lead to fatalities [3]. However, preoperative, intraoperative and postoperative respiratory care in our department, such as; preoperative breath-training and cessation of smoking coupled with intraoperative HFPPV and postoperative bronchoscopic endothoracheal suction, have proved successful in preventing postoperative respiratory complications. The only exceptions to successful postoperative recovery results were as follows; one operative death due to respiratory failure, one case of viral infection indicating a state of immunodeficiency in the patient which resulted in hospital death. The causes of hospital death in the other two cases were advanced stages of the cancer and hepatic failure.

Most recently, endoscopic esophageal mucosectomy was performed on an 80 years old patient. Esophageal cancer was detected in the unstained area of Iodine, and the depth of the cancer cell being limited by mucosa, the tumor could be completely resected using the esophagoscopy [10]. This method is less invasive and therefore more effective for patients with T_{is} cancer. In the case of patients with severe organ dysfunction, this method is recommended.

Since all patients suffered varying degrees of delirium, the importance of postoperative mental care of aged patients should not be undermined. Postoperative care and the mental support of family, aided walking, and deep sleep-inducing medication, all contribute to preventing postoperative delirium.

The surgical approach to carcinoma of the esophagus must be radical, and advanced aging is not of itself a major contraindication to surgery. Despite advanced aging, curative esophagectomy in those 75 years of age and over can result in successful long term survival results.

REFERENCES

1. Health and Welfare Statistics Association (1991) Health and Welfare Statistics in JAPAN.
2. Keppen M (1987) Upper Gastrointestinal Malignancies in the Elderly. Clinics in Geriatric Medicine 3: 637-648.
3. Sugimachi K, Inokuchi K, Ueo H, Matsuura H, Matsuzaki K, and Mori M (1985) Surgical Treatment for Carcinoma of the Esophagus in the Elderly Patients. Surg Gynecol Obstet 160: 317-319.
4. Mohanisingh MP (1976) Mortality of oesophageal surgery in the elderly. Br J Surg 63: 579-580.
5. Peracchia A, Bardini R, Ruol A, Castoro C, Segalin A, Cavazzini F, et al. (1988) Carcinoma of the esophagus in the elderly (70 years of age or older). Indications and results of surgery. Diseases of the Esophagus 1: 147-152.
6. Imamura M, Ohishi K, and Tobe T (1987) Retrosternal Esophagogastrostomy with the EEA stapler. Surg Gynecl Obst 164: 369-371.
7. Imamura M, Yanagibashi K, Tobe T, Shimada Y, Naito M, Arai T, et al. (1988) Transthoracic Resection of Esophageal Cancer in Patients with Pulmonary Dysfunction. Ann Surg 208: 601-605.
8. Orringer M (1984) Transhiatal Esophagectomy without Thoractomy for Carcinoma of the Thoracic Esophagus. Ann Surg 200: 282-288.
9. Fok M, Siu KF and Wong J (1989) A comparison of Transhiatal and Transthoracic Resection for Carcinoma of the Thoracic Esophagus. Am J Surg 158: 414 – 419.
10. Torii A, Kishimoto H, Kajiyama T, Tsukata H, Ueda S, Ohkuma M, et al. (1993) Endoscopic aspiration mucosectomy using an attached cylinder. Jpn J Gastro 90: (in press).

Effect of Postoperative Chemotherapy for Esophageal Carcinoma on Survival

Hirokazu Nagawa, Oichiro Kobori, Yasuyuki Seto, and Tetsuichiro Muto

The First Department of Surgery, University of Tokyo, Bunkyo-ku, Tokyo, 113 Japan

ABSTRACT

We retrospectively analyzed the effect of chemo–radiotherapy. A total of 130 patients with esophageal cancer, diagnosed as stage II or more, were divided into two groups according to the presence (n=45) or absence (n=85) of chemotherapy. Overall survival was better with chemotherapy than without it (p<0.05). There was no statistical difference in survival between patients with (n=58) and without (n=52) radiation therapy. We conclude that postoperative chemotherapy using cisplatin and vindesine may be effective for improving survival in patients with advanced esophageal cancer. Postoperative radiation therapy does not appear to prolong survival.

KEY WORDS: esophageal cancer, postoperative chemotherapy, radiotherapy

INTRODUCTION

Esophageal cancer is a lethal disease and the results of radiation therapy[1] and chemotherapy[2] as single treatment modalities for this disease are often poor. Since the 1981 report of Steiger et al.[3], there has been an increasing interest in combined modality treatment for patients with esophageal cancer. A number of well conducted trials using preoperative chemo–radiotherapy, in which esophageal cancer was regarded as a systemic disease, as well as several autopsy studies have been reported[4]. Nonetheless, only modest improvements in the survival rate of patients with esophageal cancer have been achieved. According to Goldie and Coldman[5], who proposed a possible mechanism of drug resistance based on their study results, the probability of drug resistance may be reduced if tumor burden is low. Therefore, postoperative multimodality treatment including both radiation and chemotherapy has been applied since 1986 in our department for patients with esophageal cancer of stage II or more (based on the TNM system devised by the Japanese Society of Esophageal Diseases[6]). This study was, therefore, retrospectively undertaken to assess the effect of postoperative chemotherapy and/or radiotherapy on survival of patients with esophageal cancer.

PATIENTS AND METHODS

All records of patients with esophageal cancer treated surgically in our department during the period from 1977 through 1991 were reviewed. Since 1986, we have applied postoperative multimodality treatment to all patients below 75 years of age with esophageal cancer of stage II or more. Chemotherapy consisted of cisplatin and vindesine administered by intravenous infusion over six hours at doses of 80 mg/m^2 and 3 mg/m^2, respectively, twice during hospitalization. The radiation regimen consisted of 2.0 Gy daily five days per week up to a total of 50 Gy over five weeks. The treatment volume included mediastinal and supraclavicular nodal regions. One hundred and fifty patients with esophageal cancer of stage II or more underwent esophagectomy. Fifteen patients who died postoperatively during hospitalization were excluded from this review, as were five patients who died of causes other than esophageal cancer. Of the remaining 130 patients, 37 were treated postoperatively with combined radiation and chemotherapy, 21 with radiation therapy alone, five with chemotherapy alone and 47 were treated with surgery alone. Survival was analyzed and compared among these four groups. Background clinicopathological features in these four groups were also evaluated.

One hundred and nineteen patients (91.5%) underwent subtotal esophagectomy through a right thoracotomy with anastomosis in the left neck. In three patients (2.4%), the anastomosis was in the mediastinum. Eight patients(6.1%) underwent blunt esophagectomy, without thoracotomy, with anastomosis in the left neck. The majority of patients also underwent nodal dissection including paraesophageal, paratracheal, subcarinal, cardial, and coeliac nodes. Curability was postoperatively determined according to the relationship between the surgical extent of nodal dissection and pathological findings in dissected lymph nodes (C0: absolute non–curative, CI: relative non–curative, CII: relative curative and CIII: absolute curative resection)[7].

The Wilcoxon test or chi–square test was used to compare the two groups of patients with respect to mean age, incidence of positive lymph nodes, staging and curability. The generalized Wilcoxon test was used to compare the two groups with respect to cumulative survival curves.

RESULTS

Among the 130 patients analyzed in this study, there were 112 males (86.2%) and 18 females (13.8%). The mean age was 62.3 years, with a range of 39 to 79 years. The numbers of patients with stage II, III and IV were 17 (13.1%), 58 (44.6%) and 55 (42.3%), respectively. The numbers of patients with C0, CI, CII and CIII curability were 39 (30.0%), 26 (20.0%), 28 (21.5%) and 37 (28.5%), respectively.

The toxicities of postoperative chemotherapy and/or radiation therapy were tolerated by all patients to whom these treatments were administered. The majority of patients who received chemotherapy experienced nausea and vomiting and myelosuppression was observed in 60%.

Overall survival was better in patients with chemotherapy (n=45) than in those without it (n=85) (p<0.05) (Table 1). In order to examine the effects of chemotherapy alone, fifty–four patients with postoperative radiation therapy were divided into two groups; with (n=37) and without (n=21) chemotherapy. Survival was significantly better with chemotherapy than without it (Table 1). No significant difference was observed between the two groups with respect to clinicopathological features; mean age, incidence of positive regional lymph nodes, stage and curability (Table 2). One–year survival rates with or without chemotherapy according to curability were 46.7% and 11.5% for C0, 53.3% and 45.5% for CI, 66.7% and 67.4% for CII and 80.0 and 76.7 for CIII, respectively. There was a significant difference between with (n=8) and without (n=31) chemotherapy only in patients with C0 esophageal cancer. There was no statistical difference in survival between patients with (n=58) and without (n=52) radiation therapy (Table 1). In order to examine the effects of radiation alone, forty–two patients with chemotherapy were divided into two groups, with (n=37) and without (n=5) radiation therapy. There was no significant difference in survival between the two groups (Table 1). No significant differences were found with respect to the clinicopathological features of the two groups (Table 2).

Table 1. Survival rates of patients with advanced esophageal cancer with or without chemotherapy and radiotherapy

Survival Rate	Overall				RT(+)		RT(−)	
	CT(+)[1] (n= 45)	CT(−)[2] (n= 85)	RT(+) (n= 58)	RT(−) (n= 52)	CT(+)[3] (n= 37)	CT(−)[4] (n= 21)	CT(+) (n= 5)	CT(−) (n=47)
1–year	62.5	47.3	59.6	56.9	64.7	48.6	50.0	56.8
2–year	36.9	26.8	33.9	38.6	41.2	13.9	25.0	37.9
3–year	31.9	21.3	25.9	30.5	34.8	13.9	25.0	30.8

CT:postoperative chemotherapy, RT:postoperative radiotherapy.
There are significant differences between 1 and 2, and between 3 and 4 (p<0.05).

Table 2. Clinicopathologic features of groups with or without chemotherapy and radiotherapy

Factor	RT(+)(n=58)		P	CT(+)(n=42)		P
	CT(+)(n=37)	CT(−)(n=21)		RT(+)(n=37)	RT(−)(n=5)	
Age	59.7± 7.6	59.7± 9.7	0.4	59.7± 7.6	56.4± 11.9	0.3
Node positive	84%(31/37)	82%(14/17)	1.0	84%(31/37)	80%(4/5)	1.0
Stage II	6	1		6	1	
III	15	8	0.5	15	0	0.2
IV	16	8		16	4	
C0	5	7		5	2	
I	12	2	0.1	12	2	0.4
II	5	3		5	0	
III	15	5		15	1	

CT:postoperative chemotherapy, RT:postoperative radiotherapy.

DISCUSSION

Although esophageal cancer treatment is still the subject of considerable debate, over the past 10 years combined therapy including surgery, chemotherapy and radiation therapy has produced improvement in overall survival[8,9]. Chemotherapy with cisplatin and vindesine, in particular, produces a high response rate[10]. There is, however, controversy as to when chemotherapy and radiotherapy should be performed. The advantages of preoperative chemotherapy and radiotherapy are as follows. (1) Preoperative chemo- and radiation therapy may be better tolerated, in terms of performance status, than postoperative treatments. (2) A favorable subset of patients can be identified as "responders" because the effects of chemo-radiotherapy can be evaluated preoperatively. The response to chemotherapy is, however, only in the 50% range for loco-regional disease[8,11]. Therefore, a large group of patients will not only be subject to drug toxicity but also suffer disease progression during chemotherapy. The concept of preoperative chemotherapy is based on the viewpoint that esophageal cancer is a systemic disease. According to Anderson's autopsy study on esophageal squamous cell carcinoma[4], lymph nodes, especially thoracic nodes, are the most common metastatic site. Surgical procedures in which esophagectomy includes thoracic and abdominal lymph node dissection can, however, reduce recurrence in these nodes. According to Goldie's hypothesis[5], removing the tumor burden as extensively as possible minimizes the probability of drug resistance. Furthermore, we found that moderate doses of cisplatin and vindesine administered postoperatively were well tolerated. Thus, esophagectomy should be performed as the treatment of first choice to enhance the possibility of cure, except in unresectable cases, and postoperative adjuvant therapy should also be done for patients with advanced esophageal cancer because the recurrence rate in these patients remains high even when curative resection has been performed. In light of these observations, since 1986, we have postoperatively applied cisplatin and vindesine for all patients below 75 years of age with esophageal cancer of stage II or more. To our knowledge, no prospective controlled study has been conducted in which the survival of patients with postoperative chemo-radiotherapy was compared with that of patients who did not receive adjuvant therapy. Only one study has reported encouraging results of postoperative adjuvant chemotherapy for operable esophageal cancer[12]. In this study, however, the survival of patients with postoperative adjuvant therapy was not compared with that of those without adjuvant therapy. Although our study was conducted retrospectively, postoperative chemotherapy produced an observable improvement in the survival curve. Furthermore, clinicopathologic features did not differ between patients with and those without chemotherapy. No remarkable effects of postoperative radiation therapy were observed in this study. Nonetheless, we can not definitely rule out the possible effectiveness of postoperative radiation therapy because the number of patients was too small for adequate analysis of survival curves. The results of this study demonstrate the feasibility of postoperative adjuvant chemo-radiotherapy, providing encouraging results for patients with advanced esophageal cancer.

REFERENCES

1. Richmond J, Seydel HG, Bae Y, Lewis J, Burdakin J and Jacobsen G (1987) Comparison of three treatment strategies for esophageal cancer within a single institution. Int J Radiation Oncology Biol Phys 13:1617–1620
2. Rosenberg J, Lichter A, Leichman L (1989) Cancer of the esophagus. In: De Vita V, Hellman S, Rosenberg S (eds) Cancer: Principles and Practice of Oncology. JB Lippincott, Philadelphia, pp 725–764
3. Steiger Z, Franklin R, Wilson RF Leichman L, Seydel H, Loh JJK, Vaishamapayan G, Knechtges T, Asfaw I, Miller P, Pietruk T, Vaitkevicius V (1981) Eradication and palliation of squamous cell carcinoma of the esophagus with chemotherapy, radiotherapy, and surgical therapy. J Thorac Cardiovasc Surg 82:713–719
4. Anderson LL, Lad TH (1982) Autopsy findings in squamous-cell carcinoma of the esophagus. Cancer 50:1587–1590
5. Goldie JH, Coldman AJ (1984) The genetic origin of drug resistance in neoplasms: Implications for systemic therapy. Cancer Res 44:3643–3653
6. Japanese Society of Oesophageal Diseases (1976) Guideline of clinical and pathological studies for carcinoma of oesophagus. Jap J Surg, 6:64
7. Japanese Society for Esophageal Diseases (1992) Guide lines for the clinical and pathologic studies on carcinoma of the esophagus(8th Edition). Kanehara and Co. Tokyo, p 26
8. Roth JA, Pass HI, Flanagan MM, Graeber GM, Rosenberg JC, Steinberg S (1988) Randomized clinical trial of preoperative and postoperative adjuvant chemotherapy with cisplatin, vindesine, and bleomycin for carcinoma of the esophagus. J Thorac Cardiovasc Surg 96:242–248
9. Mountain CF (1988) Combined therapy for carcinoma of oesophagus: Panacea or Puzzle. Ann Thorac Surg 45:353–354
10. Kelsen DP, Bains M, Chapman R, Golbey R (1981) Cisplatin, vindesine, and bleomycin (DVB) combination chemotherapy for esophageal carcinoma. Cancer Treat Rep 65:781–785
11. Kelsen DP (1988) Chemotherapy for loco-regional and advanced oesophageal cancer. Cancer principles and practice. Oncol Updates 2:10
12. Sharma S, D'Cruz AK, Kannan R, Vyas J (1992) Postoperative adjuvant chemotherapy for operable esophageal cancer: A pilot clinical study. J Surg Oncol 50:101–104

Clinicopathological Evaluation of the Three-Field Lymph Node Dissection for Thoracic Esophageal Cancer

Akihiro Toyosaka, Eizo Okamoto, Yoshiyuki Nakai, Hideaki Ishikawa, and Yoshifumi Tomimoto

First Department of Surgery, Hyogo College of Medicine, Nishinomiya, Hyogo, 663 Japan

ABSTRACT

Twenty-six patients receiving radical three-field lymph node dissections for thoracic esophageal cancer were investigated clinicopathologically for comparison with patients undergoing two-field lymph node dissection. There was no significant difference in the postoperative complications between the two groups. Nineteen (73.1%) out of 26 cases with the three-field dissection and 25 (44.6%) out of 56 cases with the two-field dissection had metastatic lymph nodes. In the three-field dissection, the metastatic rates in the cervical, mediastinal and abdominal nodes were 34.6%, 57.6% and 34.6%, respectively. The three-field dissection showed a high rate of metastases to the cervicothoracic transitional area. The 5-year survival rate in the three-field dissection group was 55%, and 22% in the two-field dissection group (P<0.05). We think that an increasingly enhanced prognosis can be expected with greater improvement in the operative technique.

KEY WORDS: esophageal cancer, lymph node dissection, lymph node metastases

INTRODUCTION

In thoracic esophageal cancer, the postoperative relapse rate is high, especially at the cervical lymph nodes, and this has been a great obstacle to the improvement of long-term survival of the patients.[1,2] In Japan, radical three-field lymph node dissection of the cervical, mediastinal, and abdominal regions has recently been employed in several institutions.[1-5] However, there are various problems in the evaluation of this extended dissection, as it seems to involve an increase in postoperative complications.[3-5] We have performed the radical three-field lymph node dissection as the standard operation for thoracic esophageal cancer since 1987. The purpose of this paper is to clinicopathologically evaluate the patients who underwent three-field lymph node dissection for thoracic esophageal cancer.

MATERIALS AND METHODS

Since 1987, three-field lymph node dissection for thoracic esophageal cancer has been systematically employed as a standard operation. A total of 26 patients underwent this type of surgery. The criteria indicating the three-field lymph node dissection were as follows (1) Age: patients under the age of 75 years (2) Location: all cases of thoracic esophageal cancer (3) Depth of cancer invasion: all resectable cases with some degree of radicality (4) Cases with no high risks such as cardiopulmonary or hepatorenal disorders. Fifty-six cases of thoracic esophageal cancer with two-field lymph node dissection were investigated as historical control between 1980 and 1987. The two-field lymph node dissection implies the usual lymph node dissection of the mediastinum and abdomen, but with the lymph node dissection along the bilateral reccurrent laryngeal nerves not being sufficiently performed. In these cases, the rates of lymph node metastases, mortality and morbidity, postoperative complications, as well as the survival rate were investigated. In the operative procedure involving a three-field lymph node dissection, we protect the recurrent nerves bilaterally in both the thoracic and cervical regions, looking directly at their continuity from both

Table 1. Lymph node metastatic rate in relation to lymph node location

Location of dissected lymph nodes	Neck	Mediastinum	Abdomen	Total
Three-field lymph node dissection (n=26)	9/26 (34.6%)	15/26** (57.6%)	9/26 (34.6%)	19/26* (73.1%)
Two-field lymph node dissection (n=56)		20/56 (35.7%)	15/56 (26.8%)	25/56 (44.6%)

* $P < 0.05$, ** $P < 0.05$ when compared with two-field dissection

regions in the cervicothoracic transitional area.   Specifically, they are encircled with tapes on both sides to avoid any possible damage to them, after which sufficient dissection in the cervicothoracic area can be performed systematically.

RESULTS

Mortality, morbidity and postoperative complications

There was no significant difference between the two groups in background factors such as age of the patients, the location of the primary tumor and the depth of cancer invasion. Direct operative death within 30 days after surgery involved one case (3.8%) among the 26 cases of the three-field dissection and 3 cases (5.4%) among the 56 cases of the two-field dissection.   The death of the one patient following the three-field dissection was from severe pulmonary congestion accompanied by chronic pancreatitis.   The postoperative complications were analyzed in the two- and three-lymph node dissection. Pneumonia occurred in 15.3% and 19.2% in the three- and two-field dissections, respectively, showing no significant difference between the two groups.   In the periods of postoperative intubations, however, the patients with three-field dissections required significantly more prolonged tracheal intubation than those who had two-field dissections ($P < 0.01$).   Recurrent nerve paralysis was found in 7 cases (25%) of the 26 with three-field dissections, and there was accidental cutting of the left recurrent nerve in the mediastinum in 3 cases during the early trials of performing this type of surgery, and transient paralysis in the other 4 cases. No permanent paralysis has occurred since we implemented the technique of encircling the recurrent nerve with tape.   Permanent paralysis was significantly lower in the patients undergoing the three-field dissection ($P < 0.05$).

Lymph node metastases

Nineteen (73.1%) out of 26 cases of three-field lymph node dissections and 25 (44.6%) out of 56 cases of two-field lymph node dissections had metastatic lymph nodes.   The rate in cervical nodes (supraclavicular and deep cervical) was 34.6% of the 26 patients in whom a three-field lymph node dissection was performed. Among them, 19.2% were on the right and 19.2% on the left, showing no difference in laterality of the metastasis.   The rate of metastases in the mediastinum was 57.6% in the three-field dissection group and 35.7% in the two-field dissection group, indicating a significantly higher rate of metastasis in the former. The metastatic rate in the abdominal lymph nodes was 34.6% in the three-field group and 26.8% in the two-field group (Table 1). For the cervical nodes, the metastatic rate was as high as 30-60% in the Iu and Im cases of three-field lymph node dissections. For the mediastinum, the rates of metastases were 34.6% for the nodes along the right recurrent nerve and 38.4% for those along the left recurrent nerve.   The rate of metastasis for the paratracheal nodes along both recurrent nerves was higher in relation to other mediastinal nodes.

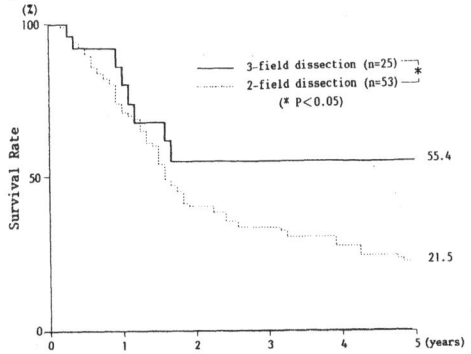

Figure 1. Patients survival rates of three-
or two-field lymph node dissection

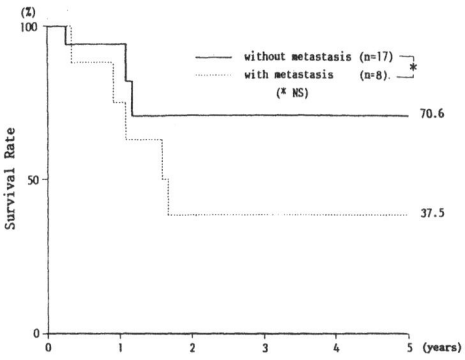

Figure 2. Cervical node metastases and
patient survival

Survival rate

Patient survival curves of the two- or three-field lymph node dissections are shown in
figure 1. The operative death occurring within 30 days was excluded. The 5-year survival
rate of 25 patients who underwent three-field lymph node dissections was 55%, whereas that
of the 53 patients undergoing two-field lymph node dissections was 21.5% (P<0.05). Survival
rate curves were compared between cases with positive or negative cervical lymph nodes. The
survival rate was superior in patients without cervical node metastases (NS) (Fig. 2).

DISCUSSION

There have been discussions on both the merits and shortcomings of three-field lymph node
dissections.[3-5] The three-field dissection showed a high rate of metastases to the
cervicothoracic transitional area, especially paratracheal nodes or nodes along both the
recurrent nerves.[1-5] This indicates the necessity of extended lymph node dissection of the
cervicothoracic region for thoracic esophageal cancer. Certainly our operative results in
the three-field lymph node dissection group showed significantly better prognosis in 5-year
survival compared with the usual two-field lymph node dissection group. However, the three-
field lymph node dissection has been reported to involve higher postoperative risks.[3-5] In
our series, the three-field lymph node dissection group showed no significant difference in
the postoperative complications compared with the two-field dissection group, except for a
more prolonged intubation after surgery. We think that an increasingly enhanced prognosis
and fewer postoperative risks will accompany greater improvement of the surgical technique
having the means for the best preservation of tracheopulmonary branches of the vagal nerve,
although there is a limit to improving the curative results by means of surgery alone.

REFERENCES

1. Isono K, Onoda S, Okuyama K, Sato H (1985) Recurrence of intrathoracic esophageal cancer.
   Jpn J Clin Oncol 15: 49-60
2. Sugimachi K, Inokuchi K, Kuwano H, Kai H, Okamura T, Okudaira Y (1983) Patterns of
   recurrence after curative resection for carcinoma of the thoracic part of the esophagus.
   Surg Gynecol Obstet 157: 568-571
3. Isono K, Ochiai T, Okuyama K, Onoda S (1990) The treatment of lymph node metastatis from
   esophageal cancer by extensive lymphadenectomy. Jpn J Surg 20:151-157
4. Tsurumaru M, Akiyama H, Udagawa H (1990) Evaluation of the colo-thoraco-abdominal
   dissection for intrathoracic esophageal carcinoma (in Japanese). J Jpn Surg Soc 90: 1612-
   1615
5. Isono K, Sato H, Nakayama K (1991) Results of a nationwide study on the three-field lymph
   node dissection of esophageal cancer. Oncology 48: 411-420

The Surgical Significance of Proper Nodes Along the Right Laryngeal Nerve Chain Situated in the Supreme Portion of the Thorax, Designated as "Top Nodes"

TETSURO NISHIHIRA, JUNZO SAYAMA, HARUMASA UEDA, KOU SUGAWARA, RYUZABURO SHINEHA, and SHOZO MORI

The Second Department of Surgery, Tohoku University School of Medicine, Sendai, 980 Japan

ABSTRACT

This paper presents the significance of "top nodes" as a relay point of afferent lymph flow from the mediastinum and the point of efferent flow to the cervical area. These nodes belong to the laryngeal nerve chain and are anatomically situated along the trachea, right subclavian artery and esophagus. By precise microscopic examination of all dissected lymph nodes, lymph was determined to principally flow from the superior mediastinal field to the cervical region in Iu cases. In Im cases, lymph flow was broadly distributed from the superior, middle and inferior mediastinal regions to the cervical and abdominal regions. In Ei cases, lymph tended to flow from the inferior mediastinal region to the abdominal region.

KEYWORDS: esophageal cancer, node metastasis, top nodes, recurrent nerve chain, mediastinal lymph flow

INTRODUCTION

Mediastinal lymph flow remains obscure in many respects. Malignant tumors arising in the mediastinum may present with diverse metastases. For example, superficial cancer (sm, involving the submucosa) may occasionally be accompanied by massive metastases in the thorax or abdomen. On the contrary, about one-third of esophageal carcinomas are negative for lymph node metastases, or only a few lymph nodes may be positive, making prolonged survival after successful surgical resection possible. Consequently, the choice of the sites and extent of lymph node dissection is a problem which frequently confronts the surgeon when designing a strategy to treat carcinomas of the esophagus.

To cope with this situation, extensive dissection of the superior mediastinum has been advocated in the surgical treatment of carcinomas of the intrathoracic esophagus. Some authorities recommend that this procedure be accompanied by modified radical neck dissection or by median sternotomy to permit thorough dissection of the region extending from the neck to the superior mediastinum. However, despite the active development and trial of new surgical approaches, results in terms of patient survival have not necessarily been satisfactory. Fortunately, compilation and analysis of the results of extensive lymph node dissection have helped elucidate which sites of primary tumors have the highest risk of metastasis. These data help us to specify important groups of lymph nodes which should be surgically dissected to significantly reduce the possibility of recurrence. In our department, prime importance is assigned to the lymph nodes lying along the right recurrent laryngeal nerve situated in the supreme portion of the thorax, as these nodes mark the point at which beyond lymph does not flow from the mediastinum to the neck. This group of lymph nodes has been designated as "top nodes." The anatomical and surgical significance of these nodes, first described in our department about 15 years ago, is presented.

MATERIALS AND METHODS

Patients

From Jan. 1986 to June 1992, a total of 262 patients with carcinomas of the intrathoracic esophagus were treated. Surgical resection was performed in 221 (84.0%) of these patients. Curative surgery was attempted in 171 of these latter cases (average age, 62.9 years; 144 males, 27 females).

Macroscopic and Microscopic Findings of the Tumors

The mean longitudinal size of the tumors was radiographically estimated to be 5.5 cm, while that of the resected tumors was 4.5 cm. Histologically, 161 lesions were diagnosed to be squamous cell carcinomas, 4 were anaplastic carcinomas, 2 were adenocarcinomas, and 4 lesions could not be classified. The histopathologic depth of tumor invasion was classified using the pT component of the TNM classification. The average number of dissected lymph nodes was 46.3. The rate of node metastasis was calculated by dividing the total number of dissected proper nodes by the number of positive lymph nodes. The preoperative stage of the carcinomas was assessed, on the basis of the patients' records, using the TNM classification of the Union Internationale Contre le Cancer.

Operative Procedures and Field of Lymph Node Dissection[1]

The lymph nodes in the upper mediastium and the top nodes along the laryngeal nerve chain are dissected. The reconstructed esophagus is pulled up into the neck for anastomosis through the posterior mediastinal route.

Analysis of Esophageal Lymph Flow Using OK-432 and Anti-Su-Ps Antibody

Before surgery, with the informed consent of the patients and their families, 5 KE of OK-432 was injected into the submucosal layer of the oral side of the tumor under endoscopic guidance in 12 cases. Regional lymph nodes were dissected intraoperatively, 5-7 hours after OK-432 injection. Each lymph node was immediately lyophilized at -80°C and stored until immunostaining. For the detection of OK-432 by immunostaining, frozen lymph nodes were thawed and fixed in 10% buffered formalin. The nodes were then embedded in paraffin and cut to include the largest cross-sectional area. The specimens were immunostained with rabbit anti-Su-Ps antiserum from a rabbit immunized with OK-432, using the peroxide-antiperoxidase (PAP) complex method to localize OK-432. Finally, the specimens were counterstained with hematoxylin and mounted for light microscopic examination. To confirm the specificity of the immunostaining, normal rabbit serum was used as a negative control. Based on the results obtained for the above studies on lymph node metastases and immunohistochemical properties, the direction of lymph flow was postulated for each of the principal sites of cancer.

RESULTS

Rate of Lymph Node Metastasis

The total rate of lymph node metastasis was 58.5% (100 out of 171 cases). The overall rate of metastasis in the upper third of the thoracic esophagus was 75.0% (9 out of 12 cases). A metastatic rate of over 20% was noted in the top, left thoracic paratracheal and right para-espopageal lymph nodes. The metastatic rate was over 10% in the right and left cervical paraesophageal, left tracheobronchial and subaortic lymph nodes, and over 5% in the right and left deep cervical, right thoracic paratracheal, retrotracheal and left pulmonal hilar lymph nodes. In the middle third of the thoracic esophagus, the overall metastatic rate was 58.8%. A metastatic rate of over 20% was detected in the top lymph nodes, and a rate of over 10% was seen in the upper thoracic paraesophageal, bifurcation, middle thoracic para-esophageal, right cardiac, left cardiac, lesser curvature and left gastric artery lymph nodes. The rate was over 5% in the left thoracic paratracheal, lower thoracic paraesophageal and posterior mediastinal lymph nodes. In the lower third of the thoracic esophagus, the overall metastatic rate was 55.4%. Metastatic rates of over 10% were noted in the lower thoracic paraesophageal, posterior mediastinal, right cardiac, left cardiac, left gastric and lesser curvature lymph nodes. Rates of over 10% were found in top, bifurcation, middle thoracic paraesophageal and celiac artery lymph nodes.

Immunohistochemically Positive Nodes with Anti-Su-Ps Monoclonal Antibody after Intratumoral Injection of OK-432

In Iu cases, OK-432 was present in the cervical and superior mediastinal lymph nodes as well as in the bifurcation lymph nodes, which did not show clinical signs of metastasis.

Metastatic Rates of Top Nodes

Among the 171 patients studied, 30 (17.5%) had metastases in the top nodes. Of the 42 patients undergoing neck dissection in this study, 16 presented with cervical lymph node metastases. Nine (56%) of these latter patients also had positive signs of metastases in the top lymph nodes. Therefore, in about 40% of these cases, metastases occurred in the cervical lymph nodes without passing through the top nodes. In cases where metastases occurred in the cervical lymph nodes via the top nodes (positive metastases in both the top nodes and cervical lymph nodes), the site of lymph node metastasis in the neck was predominantly the cervical paraesophageal lymph nodes.

DISCUSSION

The authors use the term "top nodes" to designate the lymph nodes on the right side of the paratracheal lymph nodes, also referred to as the right recurrent nerve lymph nodes, a principal subgroup of the cervical esophageal lymph nodes. The efferent ducts of these nodes are generally thought to empty into the deep cervical lymph nodes. Top nodes thus constitute an important group of cervical esophageal lymph nodes which are also paratracheal lymph nodes. As top nodes naturally bear an intimate relationship with mediastinal paratracheal lymph nodes or paraesophageal lymph nodes and intercommunicate with the mediastinal and deep cervical lymph nodes, their status is considered to reflect lymph node metastases in the mediastinum and neck.

Having defined the position of the top nodes, we would like to address several interesting findings of the present investigation. The first concerns the relationship between top nodes and other lymph nodes, i.e., the route of metastasis. As top nodes are considered to be the lymph nodes situated at the inferior part of the right recurrent nerve lymph node chain, cancer cells entering the paratracheal region may go beyond the top nodes and metastasize to the superiorly situated paratracheal lymph nodes. The lymphatic system at the cervicothoracic junction may involve a number of routes which convey lymph: (a) to the cervical paraesophageal lymph nodes via the top nodes (possibly also from the top nodes to the deep cervical lymph nodes and/or the supraclavicular lymph nodes); or by other routes not involving the top nodes, (b) to the deep cervical lymph nodes or supraclavicular lymph nodes by ascending the inside of the esophageal wall; or, (c) to the deep cervical lymph nodes or supraclavicular lymph nodes by ascending the left side of the trachea. The present investigation indicated that (a) was the predominant pattern in about 30% of the cases, while (b) and (c) accounted for the remaining 70% of cases. Metastatic routes taken by esophageal carcinomas to the top nodes are therefore diverse, reflecting the complex patterns of mediastinal lymph flow and the spread of cancer.

Next, the prognosis of patients with positive signs of top node metastases also warrants discussion. Although the prognosis of these cases was initially considered to be poor, recent reports indicate the outlook for patients with top node metastases is not necessarily unfavorable, particularly when metastasis is evident only in top nodes. However, currently available evidence does not allow for definitive statements to be made on the prognosis of these patients at present. Studies suggest that there is no significant difference between the prognosis of patients with positive top node metastases and those with metatases in lymph nodes other than top nodes.

Finally, the therapeutic significance of top node dissection should be discussed. The top node metastatic rate was high (17.5%), and among the 30 cases with top node metastases, excluding absolute noncuratively resected cases, the 1-year survival rate was 67.8% (19 out of 28 cases), the 3-year survival rate was 50% (8 out of 16 cases), and the 5-year survival rate was 50% (4 out of 8 cases). The prognosis of patients with top node metastases did not differ from that of patients with metastases in other lymph nodes. Furthermore, as surgical dissection of the top nodes can be performed easily and safely, we believe that this procedure can significantly contribute to improved patient prognosis.

REFERENCES

1. Nishihira T, Mori S, Hirayama K (1992) Extensive lymph node dissection for thoracic esophageal carcinoma. Dis esophagus V(2):79-87

Total Pharyngolaryngoesophagectomy for Hypopharyngeal, Laryngeal, and Cervical Esophageal Carcinoma

İLKER ÖKTEN and ADEM GÜNGÖR

Department of Thoracic Surgery, University of Ankara School of Medicine, Ankara, Turkey

ABSTRACT

Eighteen cases, 11 male 7 female, with esophagus superior end, hypopharynx and invasive larynx carcinoma were operated between 1990- 1992. Median age was 49 years. Localization of the tumors were 16 cases at esophageal superior end and hypopharynx, 2 cases at larynx. Lesion located at between 14 and 19 cm from upper teeth arcus. While transhiatal approach was used in ten patients, thoracotomy and laparatomy and cervical approach in 8 patients. Bilateral cervical lymph dissection was performed in 12 patients. A mediastinal lymph dissection added to bilateral cervical dissection in 8 (44.4 %) patients. Gastric transposition was used for reconstruction in 17 patients. Oropharyngokologastrostomy was performed for one patient who previously underwent intrathoracic anastomosis. All of the patients had epidermoid cell carcinoma . Minimal anastomotic leakage devoloped in 4 (22.2 %) patients which healed spontaneously. The cause of perioperative mortality was postoperative mediastinitis in the first case, cerebral infarct in the second case and myocardial infarction was in the third case. Two patients died because of tumor recurrence 3 and 6 months after the operation. We have not detected any recurrence or metastasis of the tumor in the surviving group although our longest fallow up period 28 months.

Key Words: Pharyngolaryngoesophagectomy, gastric reconstruction.

INTRODUCTION

The expected 1 year survival rate for the esophageal and hypopharynx carcinomas after the diagnosis mentioned 20 % and 40 % recpectively, if surgical intervention did not perform (1).
For this reason the only way to increase the survival and the possibility of curability rate is the surgical treatment .

MATERIALS AND METHODS

Between September-1990 and December-1992 surgical intervention is performed for 18 patients with esophagus superior end carcinoma, hypopharynx carcinoma and larynx carcinoma with esophageal invasion. All patients are evaluated in age, sex, lesion origin and location, surgical technique and reconstruction method, staging, postoperative complications and survival rate. Because the number of the patients were limited statistical study is not performed. As a staging method Mannels ' 1982 method is used.

RESULTS

Of all the 18 cases, 11 (61.11 %) were male and 7 (38.88 %) were female. Median age was 49 (range, 27 to 68). Lesion origin was larynx in 2 (11.11 %) cases and esophagus superior end and hypopharynx in 16 (88.88 %)cases. Site of lesions were between 14 and 19 cm from upper teeth arcus. Surgical interventions performed were transhiatal technique for 10 patients and rigth thoracotomy, laparatomy and cervical incision for 8 patients. Based upon the explorative findings total thyroidectomy is performed for 5 patients (27.77 %) and hemithyroidectomy is performed for 13 (72.22 %) patients. Bilateral cervical lymph dissection is performed for 12 (66.6 %) patients and unilateral for 6 (33.33 %) patients. In 8 of the 12 bilateral cases thoracic esophageal dissection and mediastinal lymph dissection is performed by right thoracotomy. For reconstruction, gastric transposition is performed for 17 patients and left colon transposition is performed for one patient who underwent intrathoracic anastomosis previously. Histopathologic examination for all cases revealed epidermoid cell carcinoma. Postoperation anastomotic minimal leakage occurred for 4 (22.22 %) patients and all of these 4 patients recovered spontaneously with in 3-8 days. One patient died due to preoperative mediastinitis, one another due to tracheal rupture as a result of cerebral heamorhagic infarct, and third one due to myocardial infarction on the 5th, 7th, and 8th day after the operation respectively. One of the patient died in the 3rd month after the operation as a result of nasopharynx and cerebral metastasis and one another who had oropharyngocologastrostomy died 6.5 months later the operation due to intrathoracic residual tumor. As of December-1992 the longest survival is 28 months and metastasis, relapse and residual tumor is not detected in the surviving group.

DISCUSSIONS

Between September-1990 and December-1992 surgical intervention is performed for 18 patients with esophagus superior end carcinoma, hypopharynx carcinoma and larynx carcinoma with esophageal invasion . In the selection of the surgical procedure, length and the localization of the lesion, preoperative tracheobroncoscopy, mediastinal computerized tomography (CT) and previously performed the operations were the major factors. In 8 patients with the lesions extending to the thoracic inlet or having mediastinal lymphadenopathy with pathological size, right thoracotomy, laparatomy and cervical incision is performed. In the remaining 10 patient transhiatal technique is performed.

In 8 patients who underwent transthoracic operation and in 4 of 10 patients who are exposed to transhiatal operation , bilateral cervical lymph dissection was performed. For the remaining 6 patients unilateral lymph dissections was performed in accordance with explorative findings. Recent studies suggests that extended lymph dissections improves the survival rate , and for this reason we performed bilateral lymph dissection and we believed that lymph nodes which may seem as normal may have tumor cells in it. Based upon the degree of invasion of the gland by tumor total thyroidectomy was performed for 5 patients and hemithyroidectomy was performed in 13 patients. In patients who were exposed to total thyroidectomy, parathyroid glands are dissected and inoculated subcuteneously.

There are four surgical techniques for postresection reconstruction in laryngopharyngoesophageal area. (1) free cuteneal grafts, (2) local or regional cuteneal, myocuteneal grafts, (3) transposition of distal organs in gastrointestinal system, and (4) free jejunal or colon grafts(2).

Although the free cuteneal grafts are the first applied technique it is not recommended because of long hospitalization time, 70 %-90 % morbidity rate, 7 %-16 % mortality rate, high postoperative dysfunction and requirement for multiple operations, applicability in only limited resection(3,4)

Although local or regional myocuteneal grafts provide high curability and survival rate after limited resection, it is recommended more often because of anastomotic insufficiently and postoperative dysfunction, for revision of recurrent cases.

Superiority of the latter two techniques of the stomach and colon transposition over the colon and jejunal free graft or vice versa is still discussed. Although the colon transposition is recommended for reconstruction because of its advantages, gastric transposition can be performed where applicable because colon transposition has disadvantages of the number of the anastomosis, the sterility difficulties and anastomotic leakage(5) . Similar disadvantages exist in free vascularized colon grafts. Gastric transposition and free vascularized jejunal graft are highly recommended and applied because of their high operative success rate, low postoperative morbidity and mortality rate, high anastomotic function and high curability and survival rate. Free vascularized jejunal graft has disadvantage of applicability only after limited resection and hence increased postoperative relapse possibility and increased operation time and morbidity as a result of additional vascular and intestinal anastomosis requirement. Gastric transposition is recommended by many authors because it has advantages of reliable vascularisation, low suture tension due to long graft length, one operation and anastomosis, low possibility of residual tumor (1,10,12,20,21). Gastric transposition is performed for all patients except one who had previous transhiatally esophagogastrectomy and extensive tumor invasion in mediastinum. In this patient substernal colon transposition is performed.

In all the patients for whom gastric transposition is performed, no routine pyloroplasty performed.

All patients were staged as having stage III except one who had residual tumor. One of the patients was operated on after preoperative 50 Gy radiotherapy.

Two patients died because of postoperative extreme reasons. For one of these who had mediastinitis after previous emergency tracheotomy, mediastinal drainage was planned and resection was performed at the operation. This patient died of sepsis after 5 days later the operation. In one another case the patient had ischemic cerebral infarct due to tracheal rupture because of hiperinflation of endotracheal tube cuff. This leaded to hemorrhagic cerebral infarct and herniation on the 7th day after operation. We lost this patient. In another patient died of myocardial infarction on the 8th day after operation. In 4 patients minimal anastomotic leakage occurred. In all four of these patients leakage stopped spontaneously in 3-8 days after the diagnosis of leakage. No postoperative reflux was detected as a result of application of antireflux valve procedure in gastric transposition cases. Postoperative average 40 Gy cervical and mediastinal radiotherapy was performed for all patients except one who had preoperative radiotherapy.

The patient who had preoperative radiotherapy had relapsed in nasopharynx 3 months after the operation and died in 15 days. Another patient who is exposed to colon transposition had multiple metastasis 6 months after operation and died. The remaining 13 patients are still alive. No relapse and residual tumor is detected.

Total mortality rate is 16.66 % (3 patients), anastomotic leakage 22.22 % (4 patients),and relapse rate 5.55 % (1 patient). As of December -1992 the longest survival rate is 28 months and the shortest survival is 2 months, average survival is 15.11 months.

REFERENCES

1. Bains S M, Spiro R H(1979)Pharyngolaryngectomy, total extrathoracic esophagectomy and gastric transposition. Gyn & Obst 149:693.
2. Bafitis H, Stalling J O, Ban J(1989) A reliable method for monitoring microvascular patency of free jejunal transfers in reconstructing the pharynx and cervical esophagus. Plastic and Reconstructive Surg 83:896.
3. Kato H, Watanabe H, Tachimori Y, Iuzuka T(1991)Evaluation of lymph node dissection for thoracic esophageal carcinoma. Ann Thorac Surg 51:931.
4. Biel M, Maisel R H (1987) Free jejunal outograft reconstruction of the pharyngoesophagus:Review of a 10-year experience. Otolaryngo Head Neck Surg 97:369.
5. Flyn M B, Banis J, Acland R(1989)Reconstruction free bowel outografts after pharyngoesophageal or laryngopharyngoesophageal resection.Am J Surg 158:333.
6. Goldberg M, Freeman J, Gullane P J, Patterson G A, Todd T R J, McShane D(1989)Transhiatal esophagectomy with gastric transposition for pharyngolaryngeal malignant disease. J Thorac Cardiovasc Surg 97:327.
7. Schecter G L, Baker J W, Gilbert D A(1987) Functional evaluation of pharyngolaryngeal reconstructive techniques. Arch Otolaryngol Head Nect Surg 113:40.

Reconstruction with Free Jejunal Autograft for Cervical Esophageal Stenosis

Hiroto Hayashi, Takuo Murakami, Akira Tangoku, Hiroshi Kusanagi, Toshihiro Saeki, and Takashi Suzuki

Department of Surgery II, Yamaguchi University School of Medicine, Ube, Yamaguchi, 755 Japan

ABSTRACT

Since 1986, reconstruction with free jejunal autograft has been conducted on 8 patients for cervical esophageal stenosis caused by malignant tumor. There were 2 cases each of carcinoma of the hypopharynx, of the cervical esophagus and of the residual esophagus and 1 case of recurrent carcinoma of the pharynx and of the thyroid respectively. In all cases, we used the jejunum with the second jejunal artery and vein as the pedicle. Postoperative complications included only one case of minor leakage of pharyngo-jejunostomy. There was no necrosis of the graft or hemorrhage. The patients were able to begin taking food two weeks after surgery and thereafter continued smooth food-intake, except for one patient with a passage disorder due to early recurrence. These results suggest that this technique is an effective and safe reconstruction method for stenosis of the cervical esophagus due to malignant tumor.

KEY WORDS: reconstruction of the cervical esophagus, free jejunal autograft, microvascular surgery

INTRODUCTION

Reconstruction for stenosis of the esophagus conventionally uses the stomach or colon. However, there are an increasing number of cases in which surgical stress and/or complication were minimized by other techniques. The free jejunal autograft, introduced by Seidenberg et al. [1] in 1959, is highly recommended as a safer technique and is supported by recent developments in microvascular surgery. Since 1986 we have performed reconstruction of the cervical esophagus using the free jejunal graft technique, with successful results.

MATERIALS AND METHODS

Eight patients who underwent reconstruction with free jejunal autograft, between 1986 and 1992 at Yamaguchi University Hospital, were studied. The eight cases included 2 cases each of reconstruction for carcinoma of the hypopharynx, of the cervical part of the esophagus and of the residual esophagus, and 1 case each of recurrent carcinoma of the pharynx and of the thyroid gland. Moreover, 4 (50%) of 8 cases were subsequent surgeries due to multiple cancer and/or recurrent cancer. The patients, 3 males and 5 females, were aged 49 to 77 with an average age of 60. This technique was indicated for patients with malignant cancer limited to the cervical region and without lymph node or remote metastasis in the thoracic and abdominal regions. For cancer of the hypopharynx and of the cervical part of the esophagus in particular, the existence of multiple lesions needed to be confirmed with endoscopy before surgery, and when stenosis was so serious that the endoscope could not be inserted, indication to proceed was defined by intraoperative endoscopy. In the graft, anastomoses of the vessels were performed first to shorten the duration of ischemia. In all cases, after resecting about 20 cm of the jejunum including the 2nd jejunal artery and vein as the pedicle and after anastomosis of the vessels, reconstruction of the digestive tract was performed, without cooling or perfusion with special liquid. The recipient vessels included the superior thyroid artery in 7 cases, transverse cervical artery in 1, superior thyroid vein in 3, external jugular vein in 2, internal jugular vein in 1, anterior jugular vein in 1 and the facial vein in 1. Anastomosis of the vessels was performed using 9-0 or 10-0 monofilament nylon under a microscope at 20x magnification. In 6 of 8 cases, arterial reconstruction was conducted first, while venous reconstruction was first in 2 cases. In 2 cases in which the arterial reconstruction was conducted first, replantation of the jejunum was performed due to profound congestion in the graft. In one case, due to thrombus in the anastomosis, re-anastomosis of the artery was performed during surgery. The average time of ischemia in the graft was 2 hours and 30 minutes (range : 1 hour and 30 minutes - 4 hours and 20 minutes).

RESULTS

1. Postoperative Course
The length of postoperative follow-up was 5 years and 7 months in the longest case and 2 months in the shortest case, with an average of 18.1 months. In 8 patients, 3 survived and 5 died from cachexia.
2. Graft Survival Rate
The graft survival rate was 100%, without necrosis of the intestinal tract and hemorrhage.

Table 1. Summary of eight patients reconstructed with free jejunal graft

Patient	Sex/Age	Site of Tumor	Intraoperative Complication (Treatment)	Postoperative Complication	Swallowing Mechanism	Warm Ischemia (Hours)
1	M/72	Pharynx	-	-	Good	1.5
2	M/52	Residual esophagus	-	-	Good	3.4
3	F/53	Cervical esophagus	-	-	Good	2.0
4	M/52	Residual esophagus	Congestion of the graft(Replantation)	-	Good	2.4
5	F/57	Pharynx	Congestion of the graft(Replantation)	Minor Leakage	Good	1.7
6	F/66	Recurrence of pharyngeal cancer	-	-	Poor(due to recurrence)	2.6
7	F/49	Cervical esophagus	-	-	Good	2.7
8	F/77	Thyroid gland	Arterial thrombus (Re-anastomosis of artery)	-	Good	4.3

3. Postoperative Complication
There was only one postoperative complication, minor leakage of the pharyngo-jejunostomy. There was no serious complication of the respiratory system.
4. Oral Intake
The patients, except the one with minor leakage, were able to begin taking food two weeks after surgery and thereafter continued smooth food intake except one case of a passage disorder due to early recurrence (Table 1).

DISCUSSION

As reconstructive surgery for cervical esophageal stenosis caused by malignant tumor, the stomach tubes have been conventionally used via the posterior mediastinal route [2]. For recurrent cancer of the esophagus or with gastrectomy, however, the stomach tube cannot be used for reconstruction and, in aged or poor risk patients, surgical stress must be minimized. In recent years, supported by microvascular surgery under a microscope [3], very safe procedures using a free jejunal autograft have been made possible with minimal surgical stress. In our experience, serious postoperative complications such as respiratory problems have not occurred so far. This technique was safely performed on patients more than 70 years of age and in patients undergoing preoperative radiotherapy. It was reported by Kato et al. [4] that the start of digestion in patients who underwent the free graft of the jejunum can be permitted 10 days or three weeks after surgery. Our experience also showed that, except for one patient with minor leakage from the digestive tract, 7 patients could start oral intake about 2 weeks after surgery. For a while after the start of digestion, due to edema of the graft or surrounding tissue or due to peristalsis of the graft itself, the patients could not take food smoothly, however, they gradually begun to eat more food, resulting in the desired digestion in the end. This tendency was more apparent in patients with a loosened intestinal tract to be grafted. Therefore, special care was given to such patients so that the reconstruction could be performed in a straight line, making the graft as short as possible without inducing flexion. After taking a slightly longer intestinal tract segment, anastomosis of the vessels is performed first. Such procedures as heparinization, cooling and perfusion for the intestinal tract were not done. In 2 cases in which the artery was anastomosed and declamped due to congestion in the graft, replantation was carried out during surgery. For this reason, in our recent cases, we anastomose the artery and vein and let the blood in the vein flow first and in the artery second. Immediately after the resumption of blood flow, the color of the graft improved and peristalsis occurred. The duration of ischemia in the graft ranged from 1 hour and 30 minutes to 4 hours and 20 minutes and even in the case of re-anastomosis of the artery due to arterial thrombus, which resulted in the longest duration of ischemia in the graft, necrosis of the graft did not occur. The digestive reconstruction should be anastomosed so carefully that the anastomosed part of the vessels is not damaged by surgical procedures. It is important to reconstruct the graft in a position that does not cause flexion or kinking of the vessels, in particular, the vein. The rate of success achieved by our technique is 100% at present because of the small series.

CONCLUSION

1. The reconstruction with free jejunal autograft was performed on 8 patients with cervical esophageal stenosis caused by malignant tumor.
2. No necrosis of the grafted jejunum occurred and patients took food smoothly except one with a passage disorder due to recurrence of tumor.
3. Reconstruction using free jejunal autograft was found to be effective and safe for stenosis of the digestive tract caused by cervical malignant tumor.

REFERENCES

1. Seidenberg B, Rosenak SS, Hurwitt ES (1959) Immediate reconstruction of the cervical esophagus by a revascularized isolated jejunal segment. Ann Surg 149 : 162-171
2. Skinner DB (1980) Esophageal reconstruction. Am J Surg 139 : 810-814
3. Flynn MB, Acland RD (1979) Free intestinal autografts for reconstruction following pharyngolaryngoesophagectomy. Surg Gynecol Obstet 149 : 858-862
4. Kato H, Iizuka T, Watanabe H, Terui S, Ono I, Ebihara S, Harii K (1984) Free jejunal grafts for reconstruction following pharyngolaryngoesophagectomy. Jpn Gastroenterol Surg 17 : 837-843

Stomach

Evaluation of E-Cadherins in Growth Patterns of Gastric Cancer and Its Degree of Cell Differentiation

ZHI-PING CHEN, JIAN-CHUN CHAI, YAO-LING KUANG, SHAO-JI JIANG,
SHU-DONG XIO, and SHI YAO

Ren Ji Hospital Affiliated to Shanghai Second Medical University,
Shanghai Institute of Digestive Disease, Shanghai 200001, China

ABSTRACT

The growth pattern in gastric cancer(GC) classified into expanding and
infiltrative type proposed by professor Ming. This study examined the
expression of E-Cadherins(E-Cad), an intercellular adhesion molecules,
in 46 resected specimens of GC(expanding in22 and infiltrativein 24) by
using immunohistochemical staining method. The results showed: (1)Reduction
or absence of E-Cad expression in 61% of GC. (2) Expanding type of GC
retaining E-Cad expression in 77.3% while infiltrative type lossing the
expression in 100%. (3) E-Cad expression with cell differentiation, both
well and poorly differentiated cancer cells were 80% and 16.1% respectively.
It is concluded that E-Cad might be helpful to explain the underlying
mechanism of ming's classification of growth pattern in GC.

KEY WORDS: E-Cadherin, growth pattern, degree of cell differentiation
           gastric cancer.

INTRODUCTION

According to growth pattern, professor Ming(1977)proposed a classification
of gastric cancer(GC) into two types: 1. Expanding type 2. Infiltrative type.
It has been widely accepted but underlying mechanism has not been studied.
This study used E-Cadherin(E-Cad), an intercellular adhesion molecules, to
see any help in explaining the growth pattern and degree of differentiation
of GC.

MATERIALS AND METHOD

Forty six surgical resected specimens of GC were collected at Ren Ji Hospital
from November 1990 to February 1992. They included expanding type in 22,
infiltrative type in 24, and between them mixed type in 13. Fresh specimens
performed serial cryostatic section at 5 um thickness, using anti-E-Cadherin
McAbs and extravidin peroxidase kit to E-Cadherin molecules. Immunohistochemical staining method used ABC method, and brown color stained granules
as positive. The expression was graded according to the method of Shiozaki.

RESULTS

1. Gastric mucosa adjacent to the tumor mass had E-Cad expression all preserved homogenously in the gastric faveolar epithelia, whereas 61%(28/46)
   of GC specimens showed reduction or even absence of E-Cad expression.
2. Expanding type of Ming's classification in GC retained expression as high
   as 77.3%(17/22), while infiltrative type completely lost the expression in
   100%(24/24).
3. Correlating the E-Cad expression with cell differentiation of GC, both well
   and poorly differentiated cancer cells were 80%(12/15) and 16.1%(5/31)
   respectively.

DISCUSSION

E-Cadherin is a calcium dependent homophilic CAM widely distributed in epithelium. It regulates epithelial intercellular recognition, adhesion between
the same type tissue cells, and maintains integrity and polarity. E-Cad might
be helpful to explain the underlying mechanism of Ming's classification of
growth pattern in GC.

REFERENCES

1. Ming SC(1977): Gastric carcinoma-a pathobiological classification.
   Cancer 39: 2475
2. Liotta LA(1986): Tumor invasion and metastasis-role of the extracellular matrix. Cancer Research 46: 1
3. Shiozaki H(1991): Expression of immunoreactive E-Cadherin adhesion
   molecules in human cancer. American J. Pathology 139: 17
4. Shioyama Y, Hirohashi S(1991); Expression of E-and P-Cadherin in
   gastric carcinoma. Cancer Research 51: 2185
5. Liotta LA(1992): Cancer cell invasion and metastasis.
   Scientific American 2: 34

Ornithine Decarboxylase Activity in Human Stomach Cancer

SINYA TERASHIMA, YASUSHI TERANISHI, YUTAKA HOSHINO, MITUMASA OGATA,
HITOSHI INOUE, and RYOICHI MOTOKI

First Department of Surgery, Fukushima Medical College, Fukushima, 960-12 Japan

ABSTRACT

Ornithine decarboxylase (ODC) activity was measured in 70 gastric and 20 non-gastric cancer patients. Mean ODC activity of cancer tissue, normal mucosa from cancer-bearing stomach and normal mucosa from non-gastric cancer patients was 475.7 ± 47.7, 270.0 ± 32.4, and 80.5 ± 7.5 nmol/hour/mg protein, respectively ($P < 0.05$). Among gastric cancer patients, ODC activity in cancer tissue was significantly higher in those with lymph node metastasis, serosal invasion and peritoneal dissemination than in those without these features. High ODC activity was correlated with poor short-term survival (1 year). These results suggest that mucosal ODC activity may be a useful marker for assessing biological activity in gastric cancer patients.

KEY WORDS: ornithine decarboxylase activity, stomach cancer, biological marker

INTRODUCTION

Recently, polyamines have attracted the attention of many investigators, because cell growth is related to polyamine synthesis. Among the enzymes involved polyamine synthesis, special attention has been paid to ornithine decarboxylase (ODC), which is first metabolizing, rate-limiting and sensitive to various stimuli[1]. ODC activity is generally elevated in tumor tissue compared with normal tissue in both experimental and human cancers[2]. However, few reports are available concerning ODC activity in human gastric cancer[3,4,5]. In this study, we examined the ODC activity in human gastric cancer tissue using biopsy specimens. We also examined the relationship of ODC activity in the cancer tissue to clinicopathological factors and 1 year follow up, to determine whether ODC activity can be a useful biological marker for stomach cancer.

PATIENTS AND METHODS

All tissue samples were obtained by endoscopic biopsies in 70 patients with gastric cancer and 20 without gastric cancer as controls. Cancer patients consisted of 49 men and 21 women, ranging from 27 to 84 years old with a mean age of 60.4. The control patients were 13 men and 7 women, ranging from 37 to 74 years old with a mean age of 55.6. All cancer patients underwent elective surgery.
Specimens were frozen immediately in liquid nitrogen. In all cases, tissues were obtained with the informed consent of the patients. Tissue samples were stored at -80℃ and assayed for ODC activity within 2 weeks. ODC activity was determined by double measurement of $^{14}CO_2$ as described by Russel and Snyder[6]. Specimens were homogenized using a polytron tissue homogenizer (Brinkman Instruments, Westbury, NY) in 3 ml sodium phosphate buffer (50 mmol, pH 7.2) containing 0.1 mmol EDTA and 0.1 mmol pyridoxal phosphate. Tissue homogenates were then centrifuged for 15 min at 30,000 G at 2 ℃. An aliquot of the supernatant was incubated in a shaking bath for 1 hour at 37℃ in a reaction mixture containing 0.5μ Ci of DL-[1-^{14}C] ornithine (Amersham Corporation, Arlington Heights, IL). After 60 min, the reaction was stopped by the addition of 0.4 ml of citric acid (2.0 mmol) and liberated $^{14}CO_2$ was trapped for 30 min. Then 200 ml of Sintilamine (Wako Jyunyaku, Osaka) was poured into each vial for scintillation counting of ^{14}C. Values are expressed as nanomoles carbon dioxide (CO_2) released/hour/mg protein. Protein concentration of the enzyme preparation was determined using the Lowry method[7].

RESULTS

Mean ODC activity± SE in the gastric cancer tissue and normal-appearing mucosa from gastric cancer patients was 475.5±47.7 and 270.0±32.4 respectively. Thus, cancer tissue had significantly higher ODC activity than the normal appearing mucosa with gastric cancer (P<0.05). Mean ODC activity in the mucosa of non-gastric cancer patients was 80.5±7.5 (Fig.1).

Correlation between the clinicopathological findings and ODC activity in the gastric cancer tissue is summarized in Table 1. Among 70 stomach cancer cases, there were 32 early (tumor limited to the mucosa and submucosa) cancers and 38 advanced (tumor with invasion below muscularis propria) cases. Mean ODC activity in the early gastric cancer patients was 370.2±55.4, while that in the advanced cancer patients was 564.6±72.6. Size of the gastric cancers ranged from 0.5 to 15.7 cm with a mean value of 5.3 cm. Mean ODC activity in the tumors less than 4.9 cm in size was 337.8 ±44.1, while that in tumors over more than 5.0 cm in size was 630.4±81.6. Mean ODC activity in the cases with lymph node metastasis was 635.9±84.0, while in those with no lymph node metastasis it was 348.4 ±45.6. Mean ODC activity in patients with peritoneal dissemination was 751.3± 173.2, compared with in those without dissemination was 435± 47.3. ODC activity was also compared with the degree of adenocarcinoma differentiation. Stomach adenocarcinomas were divided into two groups according to the WHO classification. Low grade (well or moderately-differentiated) cancer was associated with a mean ODC activity of 413.6±40.5 and high grade (poorly differentiated) cancer with a mean of 544.3± 76.2. There was no correlation between the differentiation and ODC levels. Among stage IV patients, ODC activity in those who survived less than 1 year was 1101.3 ±202.2, ODC in those who survived at least 1 year was 604.5±130.4 (Fig.2).

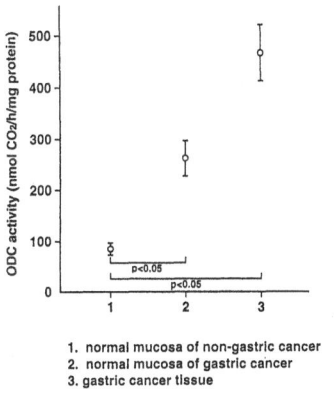

Fig. 1 Individual value of ODC activity

(mean± SE)

1. normal mucosa of non-gastric cancer
2. normal mucosa of gastric cancer
3. gastric cancer tissue

Table 1. Correlation between ODC activity in cancer tissue and clinicopathological factors

Characteristic		Mean ODC activity ± SE (nmol CO_2/h/mg protein)	
1) Size of tumor			
less than 4.9 cm	(n=37)	337.8±44.1	$p<0.05$
more than 5.0 cm	(n=33)	630.4±81.6	
2) Depth of tumor			
early cancer	(n=32)	370.2±55.4	$p<0.05$
advanced cancer	(n=38)	564.6±72.6	
3) Lymphnode metastasis			
negative	(n=39)	348.4±45.6	$p<0.05$
positive	(n=31)	635.9±84.0	
4) Peritoneal dissemination			
negative	(n=61)	435.0±47.3	$p<0.05$
positive	(n= 9)	751.3±173.2	
5) Liver metastasis			
negative	(n=66)	474.6±55.8	N.S.
positive	(n= 4)	677.8±89.2	
6) Histology			
well of moderately	(n=34)	413.6±40.5	N.S.
poorly	(n=34)	544.3±76.2	

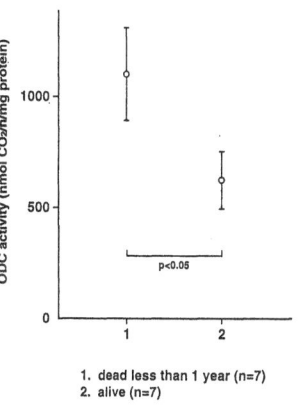

1. dead less than 1 year (n=7)
2. alive (n=7)

Fig. 2 ODC activity in the tumor tissue in relation to 1 year follow-up of stage IV patients

DISCUSSION

Polyamines are essential for cell proliferation, and ornithine decarboxylase is the first and rate-limiting enzyme in the synthesis of polyamines[1]. This enzyme is thought to play an important role in the regulation of cell growth and also has been studied in connection with tumor promotion and the development of cancer. Marked induction of ODC activity has been reported in experimental intestinal carcinogenesis[8,9,10]. In humans, ODC activity associated with cancer of the skin[11], large bowel[12,13], head and neck[2] has been described. ODC activity is generally elevated in tumor tissue compared with normal tissue in both experimental and human cancers. But there are few reports concerning ODC activity in human stomach cancer[3,4,5].

As ODC has a half life on the order of 10 minutes, which is the shortest half life of known enzymes, we compared ODC activity in endoscopic biopsy specimens with that in surgical samples from the same 5 patients. ODC activity in biopsy specimens was approximately two to ten fold higher than that in operative specimens (data not shown). Porter et al.[12] reported similar results with a comparison of biopsy and surgical specimens, and recommended that ODC activity be measured using biopsy samples.

The time required for resection of tissue by surgery may be sufficient to account for a substantial loss in enzyme activity. In this study, we measured ODC activity using biopsy samples.

Our results indicate that gastric cancer tissue had approximately six fold higher ODC activity than the normal mucosa from non-gastric cancer patients, and even the normal appearing mucosa in those with gastric cancer had three fold higher ODC activity than that of patients without gastric cancer. These data confirm earlier findings by Berdinskikh et al.[4] and by Okuzumi et al.[5]. These differences in ODC activity may be related to differences in proliferative activity.

When ODC activity in the cancer tissue was correlated with clinicopathological factors, ODC activity was significantly higher in patients with lymph node metastasis, serosal invasion and peritoneal dissemination than in those without these features. There was no correlation between ODC activity and liver metastasis or adenocarcinoma differentiation. Okuzumi et al.[5] reported no correlation between ODC activity in the mucosa of gastric cancer and histophathological factors. Berdinskikh et al.[4] and Westin et al.[2] mentioned an inverse relationship between ODC activity in adenocarcinomas and differentiation of the cancers of the stomach, large intestine, head and neck, respectively. A more detailed investigation is recommended.

We could not evaluate cumulative five year survival rates because of the short duration of follow-up. However, among stage IV patients, there was a significant increase in mortality within 1 year in contrast to that in cancer patients with a high level of ODC activity in tumor tissue. This suggests that high ODC activity in tumor tissue is associated with aggressive cancer. Sensitive methods are needed to assess tumor biology on the molecular level in order to obtain good results with the treatment of malignant tumors. Determination of ODC activity in tumor tissue may be a marker of tumor activity and may have prognostic significance for survival.

REFERENCES

1. Tabor C and Tabor H.: Polyamines. Ann Rev Biochem 53: 749-790, 1984

2. Westin T, Edstrom S, Lundholm K, and Gustafsson B. Evaluation of ornithine decarboxylase activity as a marker for tumor growth rate in malignant tumors. Am J Surg 162: 288-293, 1991

3. Lundell L, Rosengren E: Polyamine levels in human gastric carcinoma. Scand J Gastroenterol 21: 829-832, 1986

4. Berdinskikh NK, Ignatenko NA, Ganina KP, Chorniy VA. Ornithine decarboxylase activity and polyamine content in adenocarcinomas of human stomach and large intestine. Int J Cancer 47: 496-498, 1881

5. Okuzumi J, Yamane T, Kitao Y, Tokiwa K, Yamaguchi T, Fujita Y, Nishino H, Iwashima A, Takahashi T. Increased mucosl ornithine decarbosylase activity in human gastric cancer. Cancer Res. 51: 1448-1451, 1991

6. Russel D, and Synder S. Amine synthesis in rapidly growing tissue: ornithine decarboxylase activity in regenerating rat liver, chick embryo and various tumor. Proc Nat Acad Sci 60: 1420-1427, 1968

7. Lowry OH, Rosebrough NJ, Farr Al et al. Protein measurement with the folin phenol reagent. J Biol Chem 193: 265-275, 1951

8. Takano S, Matushima M, Erturk E et al. Early induction of rat colonic ornithine and S-adenosyl-L-methionine decarboxykase activities by N-methyl-N'-nitro-N-nitrosoguanidine or bile salts. Cancer Res 41: 624-628, 1981

9. Furihata C, Yoshida S, Sato Y, and Matsushima T. Induction of ornithine decarboxylase and DNA synthesis in rat stomach mucosa by glandular stomach carcinogens. Jpn J Cancer Res 78: 1363-1369, 1987

10. Furihata C, Tamazawa R, Matsushima T, and Tatematsu T. Potential tumor-promoting activity of bile acids in rat glandular stomach. Jpn J Cancer Res 78: 32-39, 1987.

11. Scalabrino G, Ferioli M, Modera D et al. Levels of activity of polyamine biosynthetic decarboxylases as indicators of the degree of malignancy of human neoplastic tissues. Advanc Polyamine Res 3: 451-462, 1981

12. Porter CW, Herrera-Ornelas L, Pera MS, Petrelli NF, Mittelman A. Polyamine biosynthetic activity in normal and neoplastic human colorectal tissues. Cancer 60: 1275-1281, 1987

13. La Muraglia G, Lacaine F, and Malt R. High ornithine decarboxylase activity and polyamine levels in human colorectal neoplasia. Ann Surg 204: 89-93, 1986

Significance of *Helicobacter Pylori* in Gastrocarcinogenesis: Special Reference to Tissue IgA Antibody in Chronic Gastritis and Intestinal Metaplasia

NORIO MATSUKURA[1], MASAHIKO ONDA[1], AKIRA TOKUNAGA[1], TAKESHI OKUDA[1], ITSURO FUJITA[1] TADASHI TERAMOTO[1], KIYOHIKO YAMASHITA[1], and NOBUTAKA YAMADA[2]

[1]First Department of Surgery, [2]Division of Pathology, Nippon Medical School, Bunkyo-ku, Tokyo, 113 Japa

ABSTRACT

Epidemiological reports have indicated that infection with *Helicobacter pylori* in the stomach induces chronic gastritis and is closely correlated with intestinal metaplasia and gastric cancer. In this study, we investigated *H.pylori* infection by detection of tissue IgA antibody (Ab) against *H.pylori* in the mucosae of patients with chronic gastritis, intestinal metaplasia and gastric cancer. Tissue IgA Ab was assayed by ELISA and expressed semi-quantitatively as an index (sample O.D./cut-off O.D.;1.2<, positive; <0.8, negative). The results showed that 1) indices of tissue IgA Ab against H.pylori were correlated with the severity of chronic gastritis/ intestinal metaplasia, and 2) tissue IgA Ab against *H.pylori* was negative in cancerous tissue, in contrast high positivity in the surrounding mucosa. These results show that H.pylori infection is closely correlated with precursory lesions of gastric cancer such as chronic gastritis and intestinal metaplasia.

KEY WORDS: *Helicobacter pylori*, tissue IgA antibody, chronic gastritis,   intestinal metaplasia, gastric cancer

INTRODUCTION

Chronic gastritis and intestinal metaplasia had been investigated as precursory lesions of gastric cancer[1,2] and epidemiological reports indicate that food habits are important factors associated with these diseases. Since the discovery of *Helicobacter pylori* in the stomach , extensive investigation has clarified that *H.pylori* infection is an important etiological factor of chronic active gastritis. However, it is still open to question whether *H.pylori* infection causes chronic atrophic gastritis and intestinal metaplasia. Recently, close correlation between seropositivity for IgG antibody (Ab) against *H.pylori* and the incidence of gastric cancer in the USA was reported[3,4]. Our previous study showed that the positivity rate for serum IgG Ab against *H.pylori* in 260 non-symptomatic Japanese controls was 41% in those less than 1 year old, 9% in those aged 1-2 yr, about 15% at 3-14 yr, 35% at 15-19 yr, 70% at 20-24 yr, increasing gradually thereafter to 89% in individuals in their 40s[5]. Therefore, it is difficult to distinguish cancer patients from the non-symptomatic population by serum IgG Ab in Japan. To clarify the correlation between chronic gastritis and/or intestinal metaplasia and gastric cancer, we investigated tissue IgA Ab. Since IgA is a major local antigen in the gastric mucosa, and the severity of chronic gastritis and/or intestinal metaplasia differs in different parts of the stomach, IgA Ab against *H.pylori* may reflect a more direct correlation between these diseases and *H.pylori* infection than serum IgG Ab[6].

PATIENTS AND METHODS

Seventy-nine patients were examined endoscopically in our department between April 1992 and March 1993, and diagnosed as having of chronic gastritis with various degrees of intestinal metaplasia. Chronic gastritis was further diagnosed as 27 cases of superficial gastritis, 27 cases of erosive gastritis and 25 cases of chronic atrophic gastritis. Thirty-eight cases of gastric cancer were diagnosed by X-ray and endoscopy; 18 cases were early and 20 were advanced. Two biopsies were taken from the same spot for examinatin of histology and tissue IgA Ab against *H.pylori* and 442 samples were biopsied from tissue of chronic gastritis and gastric cancer. Tissue IgA Ab against *H.pylori* was determined by ELISA (SERION;MBC). Details of the assay method are given briefly as follows: 1) About 5 mg of biopsied tissue was homogenized with 1 ml of dilution buffer, 2) centrifuged at 3000 rpm for 10 min, and the supernatant was assayed with an ELISA kit. The results were expressed semi-quantitatively as an index: tissue sample O.D./ cut-off serum O.D. Less than 1.0 were regarded as negative, more than 1.2 as positive, and 1.0-1.2 as inconclusive. Statistical significance was calculated by Student's-*t* test.

RESULTS

Indices of tissue IgA Ab against *H.pylori* in chronic gastritis are summarized in Figure 1. The stomach was divided into 3 parts; namely the antrum, angulus and corpus (body). Severity of gastritis was classified by the degree of small round cell infiltration : namely, mild, moderate or severe. There were statistically significant differences between mild and severe chronic gastritis (p<0.02) in the antrum and corpus. The antrum and angulus showed slightly higher indices than the corpus. Fig.2 shows the index of tissue IgA Ab against *H.pylori* in intestinal metaplasia. The severity of intestinal metaplasia were classified as slight, moderate or severe according to the frequency of appearance of metaplastic glands. Severe intestinal metaplasia showed a significantly higher (p<0.03) index of tissue IgA against *H.pylori* than slight cases. Index of tissue IgA against *H.pylori* in gastric cancer is shown in Fig.3. Biopsied tissues from ulcerative lesions of cancer had no IgA Ab against *H.pylori* ,in contrast to a high index of tissue IgA against H.pylori in the surrounding non-cancerous mucosa.

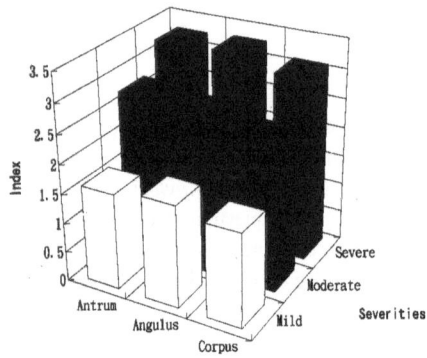

Fig.1 : Index of tissue IgA antibody against *H.pylori* in chronic gastritis: The stomch was classified into 3 parts from the anal to the oral side: antrum, angulus, corpus (body). Chronic gastritis was classified into 3 classes by severity: mild (white column), moderate (gray column), severe (black column).

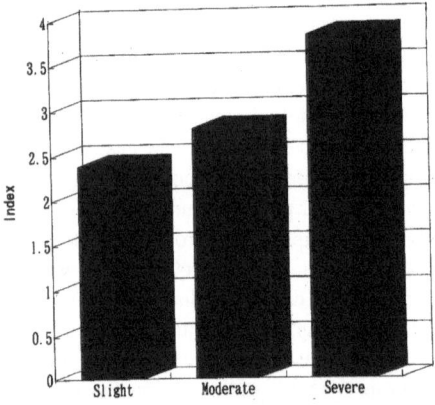

Fig.2 : Index of tissue IgA antibody against *H.pylori* in intestinal metaplasia: Intestinal metaplasia was classified into 3 classes by severity: slight, moderate, severe.

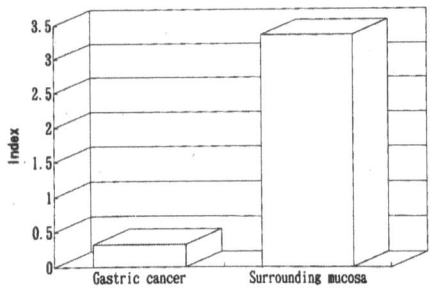

Fig.3 : Index of tissue IgA antibody against *H.pylori* in gastric cancer: gastric cancer means ulcerated part of gastric cancer. Surrounding mucosa means non-cancerous surrounding mucosa.

DISCUSSION

The etiology of chronic gastritis has not yet been clarified and intestinal metaplasia in the stomach, which is accompanies chronic gastritis, has been suggested to be a precancerous change[1]. We have reported that intestinal metaplasia can be classified into 2 types, namely complete and incomplete types, the former having enzymatic and mucin characteristics similar to those of the small intestine, and the latter being similar to the colon[2]. Moreover, intestinal metaplasia has been induced in rats using the gastric mutagen and carcinogen, N-methyl-N'-nitro-N-nitrosoguanidine[7]. Recently, *H.pylori* infection in the stomach has been focused on in relationton to the etiology of chronic gastritis, and reports from the USA have indicated that infection with *H.pylori is* a risk factor for gastric cancer[3,4]. Our investigation[5] along with another paper[8] have indicated that *H.pylori* infection is common in the non-symptomatic adult population in Japan, in contrast with a low incidence in the USA. Thus serological assay of IgG Ab against *H.pylori* is insufficient for clarifying the etiological correlation of *H.pylori* infection and gastrocarcinogenesis in Japan. To our knowlege, the present report is the first on tissue IgA Ab assay. The results shows that the index of tissue IgA Ab is correlated with the severity of chronic gastritis, and that the gastric antrum showes a higher index than the body. The index was also correlated with the severity of intestinal metaplasia. Since microscopically few *H.pylori* organisms were detected in metaplastic mucosa but many were present in the gastric pits of chronic gastritis (data not shown), a high index of tissue IgA Ab against *H.pylori* in metaplastic mucosa may indicate the etiological importance of local immunity to *H.pylori* in the induction of intestinal metaplasia. Interestingly, no IgA Ab against *H.pylori* was detected in ulcerated areas of gastric cancer, in contrast with high positivity in the surrounding mucosa. These results indicate that *H.pylori* is closely correlated with the severity of chronic gastritis and intestinal metaplasia. However, more studies are required in order to clarify the etiological correlation between *H.pylori* infection and gastric cancer.

REFERENCES

1.Correa P (1988) A human model of gastric carcinogenesis. Cancer Res 48:3554-3560
2.Matsukura N, Suzuki K, Kawachi T, Aoyagi M, Sugimura T, Kitaoka H, Numajiri H, Shirota A, Itabashi M, Hirota T (1980) Distribution of marker enzymes and mucin in intestinal metaplasia in human stomach and relation of complete and incomplete types of intestinal metaplasia to minute gastric carcinoma. J Natl Cancer Inst 65:231-240
3.Parsonnet J, Friedman GD, Vandersteen DP, Chang Y, Vogelman JH, Orentreich N, Sibley RK (1991) *Helicobacter pylori* infection and the risk of gastric carcinoma. N Engl J Med 325:1127-1131
4.Nomura A, Stemmermann GN, Chyou P-H, Kato I, Perez-Perez GI, Blaser MJ (1991) *Helicobacter pylori* infection and gastric carcinoma among Japanese Americans in Hawaii. N Engl J Med 325:1132-1136
5.Matsukura N (1993) in preparation.
6.Craanen ME, Dekker W, Blok P, Ferwerda J, Tytgat GNJ (1992) Intestinal metaplasia and *Helicobacter pylori*: an endoscopical bioptic study of the gastric antrum. Gut 33:16-20
7.Matsukura N, Kawachi T, Sasajima K, Sano T, Sugimura T, Hirota T (1978) Induction of intestinal metaplasi a in the stomach of rats by N-metyl-N'-nitro-N-nitrosoguanidine. J Natl Cancer Inst 61:141-144
8.Asaka M, Kimura T, kudo M, Takeda H, Mitani S, Miyazaki T, Miki K, Graham DY (1992) Relationship of *Helicobacter pylori* to serum pepsinogens in an asymptomatic Japanese population. Gastroenterology 102:760-766

Risk of Cancer Development in the Gastric Remnant by B-II Resection

KEN KONDO[1], SEIJI AKIYAMA[1], KATUKI ITO[1], YASUHISA YOKOYAMA[2], and HIROSI TAKAGI[1]

[1]Department of Surgery II, Nagoya University School of Medicine, Nagoya, 467 Japan
[2]Yokoyama Gastrointestinal Hospital, Nagoya, 466 Japan

ABSTRACT

In a long term follow up study of 2613 patients undergoing partial gastrectomy for benign gastroduodenal diseases between 1960 to 1964, the risk of cancdr development was studied. The incidence of the gastric stump cancer was evaluated in756 patients alive more than 20 years after Billroth I (B-I) gastrectomy and 299 patients after Billroth II (B-II) gastrectomy. Four cases of cancers were observed in the patients after B-II gastrectomy and two cases after B-I gastrectomy. The incidence of cancer (0.539/1000population) of male patients who had undergone B-II gastrectomy at less than 40 years old, was 4 times higher than that of B-I resected patients. Resected thirty-one cancers of gastric remnant after partial gastrectomy for benign disease were examined. Significantly more cancers(16/21) developed at the anastomotic site by B-II than by B-I (3/10) (p<0.05). Those findings suggested that the patients who had undergone B-II gastrectomy more than 20 years before had a higher cancer risk at the anastomotic site than the patients with B-I gastrectomy.

KEY WORDS: gastric stump cancer, Billroth II gastrectomy

INTRODUCTION

European reports indicate that the incidence of gastric stump carcinoma following ulcer surgery is higher than that in unoperated persons (1-4). But the increased risk has not been shown clealy in Japan (5-6). In order to clarify the risk of gastric stump carcinoma after B-ll resection, we have done statistical and clinicopathological study in patients who had undergone partial gastrectomy for benign disease.

MATERIALS AND METHODS

Statistical Analysis

Our study popuration was a total of 2613 patients who had undergone partial gastrectomy for benign gastroduodenal disease between 1960-1964 in Yokoyama Gastrointestinal hospital for the observation period of 20 years and more after the operation. Finally, 50.5% of all patients could be followed up the mail-questionnaire. The incidence of gastric stump carcinoma in 756 patients alive more than 20 years after the B-II gastrectomy and in 299 patients after the B-I gastrectomy was determined. X^2 test was used to compare the incidences between the two types of operation.

Analysis of Operated Cases

Twenty-nine patients were operated for gastric stump carcinoma in department of surgery II, Nagoya University and Yokoyama gastrointestinal hospital. These carcinomas were analyzed clinicopathologically in detail.

RESULTS

Table 1 shows the incidence of gastric stump carcinoma in patients alive 20 years and more after gastrectomy for benign disease. Four cases of cancers were observed in the patients after B-II gastrectomy and two cases after B-I gastrectomy. The incidence of cancer (0.539/1000population) of male patients who had undergone B-II gastrectomy at less than 40 years old, was 4 times higher than that of B-I resected patients. As shown in Fig.1, 16 of 21 (76%) carcinomas in the patients received B-II gastrectomy were anastomotic carcinomas compared with only 3 of 10 (30%) carcinomas in B-I gastrectomy (p<0.05). Table 2 compares the clinical features of anastomotic and cardiac carcinomas in the 25 patients. The mean age at the first operation was higher in the patients with cardiac cancers than in those with anastomotic cancers. The mean interval between ulcer surgery and the diagnosis of gastric stump carcinoma was slightly longer than in the patients with anastomotic carcinomas (19.9 years) than in those with cardiac carcinoma (15.4 years).

Table 1. Incidence of gastric stump carcinoma in patients 20years after gastrectomy for benign disease

Age*	male					female		
	Method of Operation	Number of patients	Cases of cancer	Observed person-year	Incidence rate**	Method of Operation	Number of patients	Cases of cancer
40year~	B-I	399	1	1131	0.088	B-I	91	0
	B-II	126	1	396	0.253	B-II	11	0
~39year	B-I	230	1	746	0.134	B-I	36	0
	B-II	156	3	557	0.539	B-II	6	0

* at first operation
** per 1000 population
B-I : Billroth I
B-II : Billroth II

Table 2. Comparison of Anastomotic and Cardiac Gastric Cancer

	Anastomotic (n=18)	Cardiac (n=7)	Total
Mean age (yr)	38.4 ± 8.1	45.6 ± 13.6	40.4 ± 10.2
Male/Female	14/4	6/1	20/5
Location of original ulcer			
Duodenal	8	3	11
Gastric	5	3	8
Combined	5	1	6
Other	1	0	1
Method of primary operation			
Billroth I	3	6	9
Billroth II	15	1	16
Interval after primary operation (yr)	19.9 ± 6.1	15.4 ± 7.4	18.6 ± 6.7

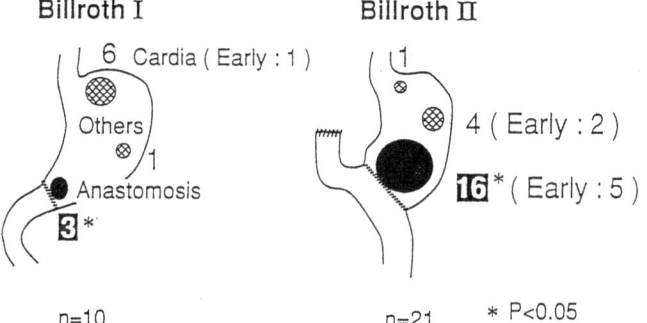

Billroth I

6 Cardia (Early : 1)
Others
1
Anastomosis
3 *

n=10

Billroth II

1
4 (Early : 2)
16 * (Early : 5)

n=21   * P<0.05

Fig. 1 Site of gastric stump carcinoma

DISCUSSION

This paper discribes the risk of development of carcinoma in the gastric remnant by B-II resection. Our data indicates a close relationship between B-II gastrectomy and the development of anastomotic carcinoma 20 years after the operation (7). In the anastomotic cancer, duodenogastric reflux was considered as main causal factors in carcinogenesis (8). The mechanism of postoperative carcinogenesis was thought to be different between B-I gastrectomy and B-II gastrectomy.

REFERENCES

1. Domellof L, Janunger KG (1977) The risk for gastric carcinoma after partcial gastrectomy . Am. J. Surg 134: 581-584
2. Fischer AB, Graem N, Jensen OM (1983) Risk of gastric cancer after Billroth II resecti on for duodenal ulcer. BR.J.Surg 70: 552-554
3. C.Toftgaard (1989) Gastric cancer after pept ic ulcer surgery. Ann. Surg 210: 159-164
4. Caygill CP, Hill MJ, Kirkham JS (1986) Mortality from gastric cancer following gastric surgery for peptic ulcer. Lancet,1: 929-931
5. Tokudome S, Kono S, Ikeda M (1984) A prospective study on primary gastric stump cancer following partial gastrectomy for benign gastroduodenal disease. Cancer Res 44: 2208-2212
6. Asano A, Mizuno S, Sasaki R, Aoki K (1987) The long term prognosis of patients gastrectomized for benign gastroduodenal diseases. Jpn J Cancer Res(Gann) 78: 337-348
7. Kondo K, Yamauchi M, Sasaki R, Yokoyama Y, Takagi H (1991) Statistical and pathological study of carcinoma in the gastric remnant. Jpn J Gastroenterol Surg 24: 2105-2112
8. Kondo K, Suzuki H, Nagayo T (1984) The influence of gastro-jejunal anastomosis on gastric carcinogenesis in rats. Jpn J Cancer Res (Gann) 75 : 362-369

Study on Cancer of the Gastric Remnant by the Type of Reconstruction at Previous Gastrectomy

Takashi Sakamoto, Tetsuro Shimizu, Naoki Nomura, Iwao Yamashita, Masaru Sawataishi, Akira Yamada, Yoshiaki Karaki, Kenji Tazawa, and Masao Fujimaki

The Second Department of Surgery, Toyama Medical and Pharmaceutical University, Toyama, 930-01 Japan

ABSTRACT

In our study on carcinoma of the remnant stomach which detected more than 10 years after the initial gastrectomy, there was a difference in the period from the initial operation to the detection of carcinoma of the remnant stomach and the main site of occupancy by the carcinoma on detection according to reconstruction method employed in the initial gastrectomy. Periodical endoscopic screening of the gastric remnant after distal partial gastrectomy is essential, and careful attention should be paid for the findings in the region of gastric suture line particularly in the cases of Billroth I reconstruction.

KEY WORDS: remnant gastric carcinoma, distal partial gastrectomy, Billroth I method, Billroth II method

INTRODUCTION

With recent improvement in prognosis of the resected cases of gastric cancer in addition to the patients who underwent gastrectomy because of peptic ulcer, the cases of long-term observations after gastrectomy have increased in number and interest in carcinoma of the remnant stomach has been on the increase. However, the definition of carcinoma of the remnant stomach has not yet to be established; and there has been no established view about the incidence, etiology [1] and treatment of it. In the present report, carcinoma of the remnant stomach is defined as the cases where carcinoma was detected in the gastric remnant more than 10 years after gastrectomy irrespective of whether the initial disease is benign or malignant [2]; characteristics of carcinoma of the remnant stomach as viewed by the method of reconstruction at the initial operation in the cases of distal partial gastrectomy are studied with an aim to contributing to improvement in the therapeutic results of carcinoma of the remnant stomach in the future.

PATIENTS AND METHODS

From among the cases of carcinoma of the remnant stomach subjected to the surgical operation at 2nd Department of Surgery, Toyama Medical and Pharmaceutical University Hospital, Toyama, Japan, from October 1979 to February 1993, 20 cases underwent the initial gastrectomy more than 10 years earlier as mentioned above. The method of the initial operation is broken down to 1 case after proximal gastrectomy - esophagogastrostomy, 1 case after segmental gastrectomy and 18 cases after distal partial gastrectomy. In this report, the cases after distal partial gastrectomy were used as the subjects and studied by the methods of reconstruction.

RESULTS

The reconstruction method after distal partial gastrectomy consisted of Billroth I method (hereinafter abbreviated to B-I) 10 cases (6 male cases; 4 female cases) and the Billroth II method (hereinafter abbreviated to B-II) 8 cases (7 male cases; 1 female case).

In B-I there were gastric ulcer 7 cases, duodenal ulcer 1 case and gastric cancer 2 cases, while in B-II there were gastric ulcer 5 cases, duodenal ulcer 2 cases and gastroduodenal ulcer 1 case.

The interval between initial gastrectomy and detection of carcinoma of the remnant stomach was significantly long in B-II, with the period being 10 to 25 years (15.5±5.3years) in B-I and 19 to 40 years (24.5±6.9 years) in B-II.

Twelve out of 18 cases were resected: B-I 6 cases; B-II 6 cases. A clinicopathological study was done for each case.

The main site of location of cancer in the remnant stomach was divided into the region of anastomosis line (region of anastomosis between the remnant stomach and duodenum or jejunum), region of suture line (region of suture extending from the lesser curvature to antero-posterior wall that is created when the stomach was dissected) and non-cut end region (where the main portion of cancer does not extend to either the region of anastomosis or region of suture) for study as illustrated in Fig. 1. Difference according to the method of reconstruction were noted, with the suture line 4 cases, non-cut end region 2 cases and no region of anastomosis line in B-I and the region of anastomosis line 4 cases and region of suture line 2 cases in B-II (Fig.1).

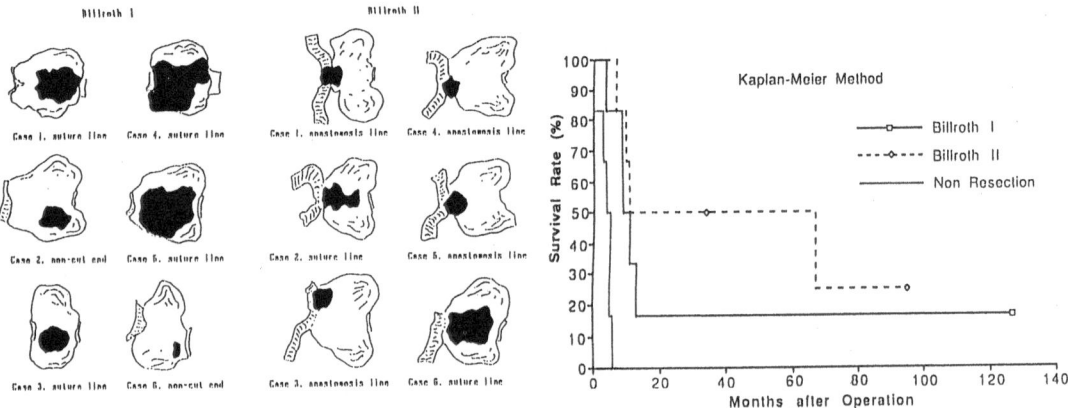

Fig.1 Location of carcinoma of the remnant stomach in the resected cases

Fig.2 Survival curves of remnant gastric cancer after surgical treatment (initial operation: distal partial gastrectomy)

Table 1 Operative and pathological findings of the resected cases

[Billroth I]

	Age·Sex	Location of the lesion[1]	Operative findings	Histologic stage	Histologic type	Curability[2]	Outcome[3]
1	59·M	A	P2 HO n4(+) ssγ	stage IV	por	n-b	13months·D
2	69·F	C	PO HO n2(+) se	stage III	tub2	c-b	127months·A
3	68·M	A	P2 HO n4(+) sei	stage IV	por	n-b	9months·D
4	57·M	A	PO HO n2(+) se	stage III	por	n-a	9months·D
5	60·M	A	P2 HO n4(+) si	stage IV	por	n-b	11months·D
6	75·M	C	PO HO n(-) sm	stage I	tub1	c-a	4months·D[4]

[Billroth II]

	Age·Sex	Location of the lesion[1]	Operative findings	Histologic stage	Histologic type	Curability[2]	Outcome[3]
1	42·M	B	PO HO n4(+) se	stage IV	por	n-b	7months·D
2	58·M	A	P3 HO n(-) ssγ	stage IV	por	n-b	10months·D
3	65·M	B	PO HO n(-) ssβ	stage I	por	c-a	11months·D[4]
4	52·M	B	PO HO n(-) ssα	stage I	pap	c-a	95months·A
5	70·M	B	PO HO n(-) ssγ	stage II	por	c-a	67months·D
6	72·M	A	PO HO n4(+) se	stage IV	tub1	n-a	34months·A

[1];A: suture line; B:anastomosis line; C:non-cut end, [2]; c-a:absolute curative resection; c-b: relative curative resection; n-a:relative non-curative resection; n-b:absolute non-curative resection, [3]; A:alive; D:dead, [4]:died of another disease

Operative findings and pathological findings [3] are presented in Table 1. Regarding the degree of histologic stage, there were many advanced cases in B-I, with stage I 1 case, stage III 1 case and stage IV 4 cases in B-I and stage I 2 cases, Stage II 1 case and stage IV 3 cases in B-II.

The survival curve after operation of carcinoma of the remnant stomach is illustrated in Fig. 2. In both group B-I and group B-II, the outcome was very poor because there were many ceases which were already advanced when carcinoma was detected. As of February 1993, there are only three survival cases: 1 case in B-I and 2 cases in B-II. They were all resected cases.

DISCUSSION

At present when long-term survival after gastrectomy has become possible irrespective of the etiologic disease, studying the characteristics of carcinoma of the remnant stomach and making efforts for prevention or early detection of it are important.

In the cases we encountered, though not mentioned as data, there were many cases in which the initial disease was malignant in cases of carcinoma of the remnant stomach which underwent the initial operation within 10 years. This indicates that the range of resection should be determined carefully by taking the predilection region left unremoved and possibility of multiple cancer into consideration in performing partial gastrectomy for gastric cancer.

In the cases which underwent the first operation more than 10 years earlier, there were many cases of peptic ulcer, but difference in the number of cases according to the method of reconstruction were not observed. Small as the number of cases is, the interval from the initial operation to detection of carcinoma of the remnant stomach was shorter in the cases after B-I than in the cases after B-II, and the cancer was characteristically found more often in region of gastric suture line in B-I; after B-II, on the other hand, the cancer was founded more frequently in the region of anastomosis line. As to the etiology and incidence of carcinoma of the remnant stomach, some have reported that the backward flowing of duodenal juice is concerned with development of carcinoma of the remnant stomach and that the incidence is higher after B-II than after B-I [4], while others have reported that there is no difference between the two [5].

It appears that the B-I reconstruction has been employed by preference recently, so careful attention should be paid to carcinoma of the remnant stomach after B-I. As matters to be marked in following up, special attention should be paid to the findings of the sutured region of the gastric remnant formed on gastrectomy in the cases of B-I reconstruction, although it is a region difficult to observe in the remnant stomach, of which inner space is small.

Even in the carcinoma of the remnant stomach, good prognosis can be expected, if it is detected early; so, there is a need to make a careful follow-up mainly by endoscopic examination over a long period of time.

REFERENCES

1. Tersmette AC, Giardiello FM, Offerhaus JA, Tersmette KWF, Ohara K, Vandenbroucke JP, Tytgat GNJ (1991) Geographical variance in the risk of gastric stump cancer: No increased risk in Japan? Jpn. J. Cancer Res. 82:266-272
2. Kidokoro T, Hayashida Y, Urabe M (1985) Long-term surgical results of carcinoma of the gastric remnant: A statistical analysis of 613 patients from 98 institutions. World J. Surg. 9:966-971
3. Japanese Research Society for Gastric Cancer (1981) The general rules for the gastric cancer study in surgery and pathology. Jpn. J. Surg. 11:127-139
4. Miwa K, Kamata T, Hasegawa H, Fujimura T, Segawa M, Matsumoto H, Miyata R, Kozaka T, Yonemura Y, Miyazaki I, Hattori T (1990) Gastric surgery and cancer risk. Gastroenterological Surgery 13:1505-1512
5. Pointner R, Schwab G, Konigsrainer A, Bodner E, Schmid KW (1989) Gastric stump cancer: Etiopathologocal and clinical aspects. Endoscopy 21:115-119

Tumor Markers (AFP, CEA, CA19-9, CA125) for Detecting Recurrence of Gastric Cancer

WANSIK YU, SEUNG DU MOON, and ILWOO WHANG

Department of Surgery, Kyungpook National University, Taegu 700-412, Korea

ABSTRACT

The presence of serum markers was evaluated in 58 patients with recurrent gastric cancer. Of 32 patients with peritoneal recurrence, the percentage of patients whose serum samples were positive for AFP, CEA, CA19-9, and CA125 was 18.8, 37.5, 50, and 50%, respectively. Positive serum levels of these markers correlated with recurrence at lymph nodes (n=11) in 45.5, 54.5, 27.3, and 36.4%, respectively. Positive AFP, CEA, CA19-9, and CA125 in serum were detected in 30, 60, 30, and 70% of hepatic recurrence (n=10), respectively. Positive rate of serum CA19-9 and CA125 was 40 and 20% of patients with recurrent cancer at remnant stomach (n=5), respectively. Combined analysis of these serum markers revealed that 87.5% was positive in peritoneal recurrence, 90.9% in recurrence at lymph nodes, 100% in hepatic recurrence, and 60% in recurrence at remnant stomach.

KEY WORDS: recurred gastric cancer, tumor marker, diagnosis

INTRODUCTION

The gastric cancer is diagnosed by radiographic studies and endoscopic biopsy. The efficient and noninvasive diagnostic procedures such as the identification of serum tumor markers specifically associated with a high percentage of patients with gastric cancer have been developed. The tumor markers currently available are carcinoembryonic antigen (CEA), alpha-fetoprotein (AFP), CA19-9, and CA125, and many other markers are also under clinical evaluation.
AFP can be produced by gastric cancer cells [1]. CEA, which was initially described as a tumor and organ specific colorectal antigen, can be detected in other tumors such as stomach, pancreas, lung, and breast as well as in inflammatory normal adult and fetal organs of the gastrointestinal tract [2]. In patients with stage IV gastric cancer, positive rate of serum CEA levels is reported to be 37% [3]. CA19-9 is the sialylated Lewis(a) blood group antigen. Elevated serum levels of this marker can be found in as high as 72% of the patients with gastric cancer [4]. The sensitivity of CA125 in detecting gastric cancer is 53% [5]. The highest sensitivity can be achieved using a combination of these antigens, such as CEA and CA 19-9 [6]. These serum tumor markers are used in early detection of cancer recurrence [7].
We designed this study to evaluate the efficieny of these tumor markers in detecting the recurrence of gastric cancer and found that combined assay of the serum AFP, CEA, CA19-9, and CA125 was a useful diagnostic procedure for detecting the recurrence of gastric cancer.

MATERIALS AND METHODS

We measured the serum AFP, CEA, CA19-9, and CA125 in sera of 58 patients (male 47, female 11) with recurred gastric cancer who underwent curative surgery previously. Mean age was 54 years ranging from 22 to 76 years. Recurrence was identified by reoperation or computerized tomography. Of these, 32 patients had local or peritoneal recurrence, 11 had recurrence in distant lymph nodes such as Virchow's node or retroperitoneal nodes, 10 in liver, and

5 in remnant stomach after subtotal gastrectomy.
Serum AFP and CEA were determined by using microparticle enzyme immunoassay (MEIA) kits of Abbott Laboratories. Immunoradiometric assay kits of CIS biointernational were used for the quantitative determination of CA19-9 and CA125. We followed suggested cutoff limit by Choi et al. [5]; 10 ng/ml for AFP, 5 ng/ml for CEA, 37 units/ml for CA19-9, 32 units/ml for CA125.

RESULTS

Positive rate of serum AFP was 24.1% (14/58), CEA 41.4% (24/58), CA19-9 32.8% (19/58), and CA125 48.3% (28/58).
Of the 32 patients with local or peritoneal recurrence, AFP was positive in 6 (18.8%), CEA in 12 (37.5%), CA19-9 in 16 (50%), and CA125 in 16 (50%). Positive serum AFP, CEA, CA19-9, and CA125 levels were found in 5 (45.5%), 6 (54.5%), 3 (27.3%), and 4 (36.4%) of 11 patients with recurrences at distant lymph nodes respectively. Among the 10 patients with hepatic recurrence, 3 had positive serum for AFP (30%), 6 for CEA (60%), 3 for CA19-9 (30%), and 7 for CA125 (70%). Positive rate of serum CA19-9 was 40% (2/5) while CA125 was positive in 20% (1/5) of the patients with recurrent cancer at remnant stomach. AFP and CEA were negative in these patients.
Combination assays using CA19-9 and CA125 increased the positive rate to 75% in local or peritoneal recurrence and to 60% in recurrence at remnant stomach. AFP and CEA increased the positive rate to 72.2% in nodal recurrence, CEA and CA125 to 90% in hepatic recurrence. Positive rate of combination assays using CEA, CA19-9, CA125 was 93.1%. Combined analysis of these four markers correlated with local or peritoneal recurrence in 87.5%, with recurrence at distant lymph nodes in 90.9%, with hepatic recurrence in 100%, and with recurrence at remnant stomach in 60%.

DISCUSSION

The value of tumor markers in the gastric cancer can be summarized as 1) diagnosis of the disease including the screening programm [6], 2) early detection of recurrent cancer [7], 3) determining the prognosis [8], 4) monitoring the response to adjuvant treatment [9-10]. CEA level measured in the peritoneal washing [11] as well as in serum can be an adjunctive tool for predicting the postsurgical prognosis in gastric cancer. The CEA doubling time by the analysis of serial CEA level measurement was used to predict the period of survival of the patients with gastric cancer [12].
In the report of Kim et al. [13], CEA is positive in 46%, CA19-9 in 62%, CA125 in 31% of 17 recurred gastric cancer patients. Of 10 recurred patients, 2 patients had positive serum for CEA and 5 had positive serum for CA 19-9 [14]. Six of 11 patients (54.5%) had elevated serum level of CEA [15].
Takahashi et al. [16] reported that 72.2% of 36 cases of peritoneal recurrence revealed positive CA125. This figure is somewhat higher than our result of 50%, but the sample size is limited in both studies.
Guadagni et al. [15] reported in their study of TAG-72 and CEA, the elevation of one or both markers correlated with recurrence in 10 of 11 patients. Simultaneous measurements of two tumor markers result in a better diagnostic sensitivity. According to our data CA19-9 and CA125 could detect peritoneal recurrence in 75% of cases and 60% of remnant stomach recurrence. AFP and CEA had positive rate of 72.2% of nodal recurrence. Positive rate for either CEA or CA125 in hepatic recurrence was 90%. Combination assay for these four tumor markers revealed the highest sensitivity for detecting recurrence. These findings suggest that the combined use of serum tumor markers might be an effective noninvasive diagnostic method for detection of recurrence in patients with gastric cancer.

REFERENCES

1. Ooi A, Nakanishi I, Sakamoto N, Tsukada Y, Takahashi Y, Minamoto T, Mai M (1990) Alpha-fetoprotein (AFP)-producing gastric carcinoma. Is it hepa-

toid differentiation? Cancer 65:1741-1747

2. Lamerz R (1992) CEA determination in the follow-up of extracolorectal neoplasms. Int J Biol Markers 7:171-178

3. Koga T, Kano T, Souda K, Oka N, Inoguchi K (1987) The clinical usefukness of preoperative CEA determination in gastric cancer. Jpn J Surg 17:342-347

4. Ritts RE Jr, Del Villano BC, Go VL, Herberman RB, Klug TL, Zurawski VR Jr (1984) Initial clinical evaluation of an immunoradiometric assay for CA19-9 using the NCI serum bank. Int J Cancer 33:339-345

5. Choi JR, Kang PJ, Lee KU, Cha KS, Yang US, Huh Y, Moon HK (1990) Diagnostic significance of the tumor markers; CA19-9, CEA, CA125 and AFP, in patients with gastrointestinal and hepatobiliary disease. Kor J Gastroenterol 22:301-309

6. Harrison JD, Stanley J, Morris DL (1989) CEA and CA 19.9 in gastric juice and serum: an aid in the diagnosis of gastric carcinoma? Eur J Surg Oncol 15:253-257

7. Bates SE, Longo DL (1987) Use of serum tumor markers in cancer diagnosis and management. Semin Oncol 14:102-138

8. Maehara Y, Sugimachi K, Akagi M, Kakegawa T, Shimazu H, Tomita M (1990) Serum carcinoembryonic antigen level increases correlate with tumor progression in patients with differentiated gastric carcinoma following noncurative resection. Cancer Res 50:3952-3955

9. Ogoshi K, Mitomi T (1989) Clinical effects of PSK on esophageal and gastric cancer patients and usefulness of serum levels of glycoproteins and HLA antigens as prognostic indicators. J Jpn Surg Societ 90:1443-1446

10. Imamura Y, Yasutake K, Yoshimura Y, Oya M, Matsushita K, Tokisue M, Ohno S, Masuda T (1990) The changes in tumor markers such as serum CEA, CA 19-9, TPA and CA 125 in the chemotherapy of patients with advanced gastric cancer. Jpn J Cancer Chemother 17:1501-1507

11. Asao T, Fukuda T, Yazawa S, Nagamachi Y (1989) CEA levels in peritoneal washings from gastric cancer patients as a prognostic guide. Cancer Lett 47:79-81

12. Umehara Y, Miyahara T, Yoshida M, Isobe S, Oba N, Harada Y (1990) A study of growth and malignancy grading of stomach and colorectal cancers by serial serum carcinoembryonic antigen levels analysis. J Jpn Surg Societ 91:661-666

13. Kim HT, Sohn SS, Kang JS (1992) CEA, CA19-9 and CA125 in patients with gastrointestinal carcinoma. J Kor Cancer Assoc 24:647-655

14. Guadagni F, Roselli M, Amato T, Cosimelli M, Perri P, Casale V, Carlini M, Santoro E, Cavaliere R, Greiner JW, Schlom J (1992) CA 72-4 measurement of tumor-associated glycoprotein 72 (TAG-72) as a serum marker in the management of gastric carcinoma. Cancer Res 52:1222-1227

15. Guadagni F, Roselli M, Amato T, Cosimelli M, Mannella E, Perri P, Abbolito MR, Cavaliere R, Colcher D, Greiner JW, Schlom J (1991) Tumor-associated glycoprotein-72 serum levels complement carcinoembryonic antigen levels in monitoring patients with gastrointestinal carcinoma: A longitudinal study. Cancer 68:2443-2450

16. Takahashi Y, Suga T, Mai M (1992) Clinical significance of serum CA125 values in patients with gastric cancers - especially correlation with peritonitis carcinomatosa. Jpn J Cancer Chemother 19:975-979

Non-Anatomical Prognostic Factors for Gastric Cancer Patients: Significance of Tumor Markers

Augusta Onorato[1], Hisanao Ohkura[2], Kazuo Okajima[1], Mitsuru Sasako[1], Taira Kinoshita[1], and Keiichi Maruyama[1]

[1]Gastric Surgery Division, [2]Department of Medical Oncology, National Cancer Center Hospital, Chuo-ku, Tokyo, 104 Japan

ABSTRACTS

Prognostic significance of non-anatomical factors was studied using data of primary gastric cancer patients treated surgically at National Cancer Center in 10 years period (1976 - 1985). It was notable that Pre-operative CEA level showed strong correlation to Stage, curability, and five year survival rate in 1,612 patients, and pre-operative AFP level showed the same correlation in 1,933 patients. By multi-variate analysis of prognostic factors including tumor markers, depth of invasion was the most significant factor, followed by lymph node metastasis, distant metastasis, pre-operative CA 19-9, and lymph node dissection. Tumor marker is one of the important prognostic factors, and can be regarded as M1 in the TNM Classification.

KEY WORDS: Gastric cancer, Tumor markers, Prognostic factors, TNM Classification

INTRODUCTION

The aim of this study is to clarify possibility of non-anatomical prognostic factors as a new component for TNM Classification of gastric cancer. It is well known that gastric cancer patients with high serum level of carcinoembryonic antigen (CEA), alpha-fetoprotein (AFP), CA-19-9, CA-125, ST-439 show poor prognosis. Furthermore, bone marrow metastasis should be considered in cases with abnormally increased fibrin degenerate product (FDP). Prognostic significance of those non-anatomical prognostic factors were statistically studied together with anatomical prognostic factors by univariate and multi-variate analyses.

MATERIALS AND METHODS

Tumor markers were examined pre-operatively and post-operatively in primary gastric cancer patients treated surgically at the National Cancer Center Hospital in 10 years period from 1976 to 1985. Serum level of CEA (n=1,612), AFP (n=1,933), CA19-9 (n=852), CA 125 (n=21), ST 439 (n=210), and FDP (n=1,029) were periodically checked and recorded. Correlations of those markers and the Stage, curability, and prognosis were studied. Survivals were calculated by Kaplan-Mayer method. And the prognostic significance of tumor markers was studied by multi-variate analysis using the SAS software.

RESULTS

Patients with higher pre-operative tumor marker level belonged to the advanced Stages (Table 1). Tumor markers were positive in large proportion of Stage IV patients; 52.2% in CEA, 66.7% in CA 19-9, 30.7% in ST 439, and 75.5% in CA 125. When the series were divided in normal level group, slight high group, and remarkably high group, strong correlation was observed between the groups and 4 years survival rates in the CEA, AFP, CA 19-9, and FDP (Table 2). Additionally the higher pre-operative serum CEA groups had lower proportion of curative resection, and poorer 5 year survival rate (Table 3). Patients with higher CEA level (more than 30 ng/ml) showed lower proportion of Stage I and II (9.8%), lower curative resection rate (26.8%), and lower 5 year survival rate (30.5%). The quite same trend was observed in the pre-operative serum AFP (Table 4). The AFP highest group (>200 ng/ml) showed low proportion of Stage I and II (14.3%), a few curative resection (19.0%), and low 5 year survival rate (9.5%). These data suggested that the CEA and AFP would be one of the important prognostic factor for gastric cancer patients.

Table 1. Incidence of positive tumor markers by Stages

Tumor markers		No. of patients	Stage-I	Stage-II	Stage-III	Stage-IV
CEA	(>5ng/ml)	1,612	5.0%	7.4%	17.8%	52.2%
CA19-9	(>37U/ml)	210	2.9	11.3	36.7	66.7
ST 439	(>7U/ml)	210	4.8	10.0	30.2	30.7
CA 125	(>35U/ml)	21	0.0	0.0	0.0	75.5

Table 2. Pre-operative tumor marker level and prognosis

		Normal	Slight high	Remark. high
CEA	Serum level (ng/ml)	0 - 5	6 - 20	21 -
	No. of patients	912	113	42
	4 year surv. rate	79.4	60.7	39.5
AFP	Serum level (ng/ml)	0 - 20	21 - 100	101 -
	No. of patients	852	8	9
	4 year surv. rate	76.3	37.5	0.0
CA 19-9	Serum level (U/ml)	0 - 37	38 - 100	101 -
	No. of patients	742	110	67
	4 year surv. rate	80.8	65.8	0.0
FDP	Serum level (micro-g/ml)	0 - 5	6 - 10	11 -
	No. of patients	1,010	19	6
	4 year surv. rate	76.9	0.0	0.0

Table 3. Pre-operative serum CEA level and prognosis

CEA level (ng/ml)	No. of patients	Proportion of patients	Stage I + II	Curative resection	5 year surv. rate
0.1-4.9	1,320	82.0%	61.2%	78.7%	71.0%
5.0-7.4	107	6.7	46.7	72.0	73.8
7.5-29.9	100	6.2	32.0	48.0	53.0
30.0-	82	5.1	9.8	26.8	30.5

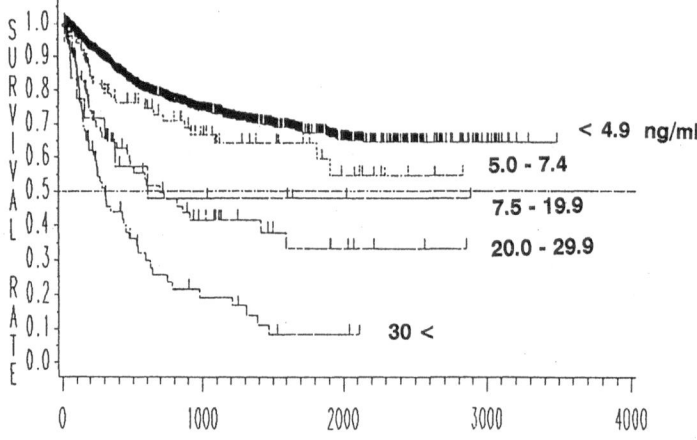

Fig. 1 Survivals of primary gastric cancer patients grouped by pre-operative serum CEA level

Table 4. Pre-operative serum AFP level and prognosis

AFP level (ng/ml)	No. of patients	Proportion of patients	Stage I + II	Curative resection	5 year surv. rate
0.1-19.9	1,874	96.9%	52.5%	74.1%	77.8%
20-199	38	2.0	21.1	44.7	23.7
200-	21	1.1	14.3	19.0	9.5

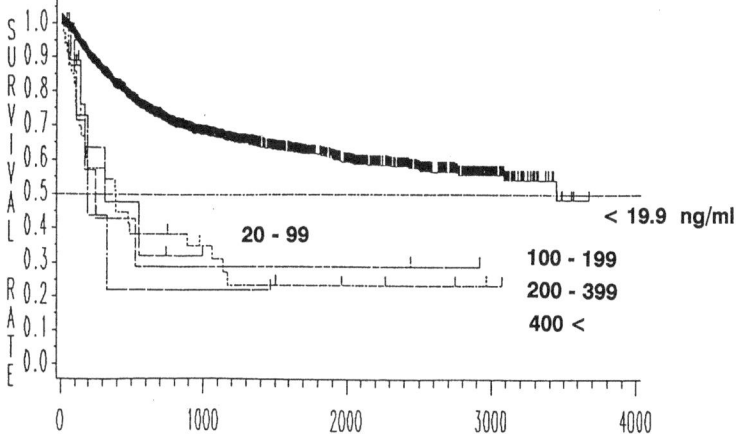

Fig. 2 Survivals of primary gastric cancer patients grouped by pre-operative serum AFP level

To know the most significant prognostic factors for gastric cancer patients, data of the series including CEA, AFP, CA 19-9, CA 125, and FDP were studied by multivariate analysis using Cox's hazard model (SAS software). The most important prognostic factor was the depth of invasion (Ratio of risk: 9.57) followed by lymph node metastasis (3.50), distant metastasis (2.92), CA 19-9 level (2.19), and degree of lymph node dissection (1.64) (Table 5). It is notable that the CA 19-9 was more significant than CEA or AFP in the multi-variate analysis.

5. The most important prognostic factors studied by multi-variate analysis

Prognostic factor	Ratio of risk	X-square	Beta	SE
1. Depth of invasion	9.57	33.54	0.752	0.130
2. Lymph node metastasis	3.50	13.82	0.418	0.112
3. Distant metastasis	2.92	21.01	1.073	0.234
4. CA 19-9 level	2.19	10.05	0.393	0.124
5. Lymph node dissection	1.64	4.85	2.033	0.223

In conclusion, this study clarified the significance of several non-anatomical prognostic factors for gastric cancer patients. We would like to propose that the high level of tumor marker should be regarded as M1 in the coming TNM Classification.

REFERENCES

1. Ohkura H, Saitoh D, Moriya Y, Maruyama K (1989) Karkinos 2: 1273-1279
2. Hermanek P, Maruyama K (1992) Report to UICC General Meeting for TNM Classification

Gastric Acid Secretion and Serum Gastrin Levels in Gastric Cancer

MASAO MIYAJI, KYOJI OGOSHI, KENJI NAKAMURA, KUNIHIRO IWATA, YASUMASA KONDOH, TOMOO TAJIMA, and TOSHIO MITOMI

Department of Surgery, School of Medicine, Tokai University, Isehara, Kanagawa, 259-11 Japan

ABSTRACT

We investigated the association between gastric acid secretion, serum gastrin levels, and the differentiation of tumor cells in gastric cancer .Gastric acid output after stimulation by tetragastrin, and serum gastrin levels after stimulation by a test meal were, examined in 128 primary gastric cancer patients, in whom the tumor had invaded the mucosa. After tumors were histologically confirmed as adenocarcinomas, the patients underwent gastrectomy. Gastric ulcer patients showed decreases in both integrated gastrin response (T-IGR) after a test meal, and in gastric acid secretion related to their age. On the other hand, early gastric cancer patients showed decrease in acid secretion but an increase in T-IGR.
There was a significantly positive correlation between age and serum gastrin level, and a significantly negative correlation between age and gastric acid secretion, in patients with well differentiated adenocarcinomas. However, patients with poorly differentiated adenocarcinomas did not show any correlation between age and either serum gastrin level or gastric acid secretion. We suggest that low acid secretion and endogenous hypergastrinemia, related to aging, may play an important role in developing cancer cells in well differentiated gastric cancers especially in the elderly.

Key Words:gastric acid secretion, gastric cancer, gastrin, aging

INTRODUCTION

It is well known that older people have physiologically decreased gastric acid secretion due to mucosal atrophy, and that decreased acid secretion also is frequently observed in patients with gastric cancer. It is also known that the release of gastrin stimulates gastric acid secretion by the trophic action on parietal cells. In recent years, gastrin has been found to be a trophic factor for some stomach and colorectal cancer cells as well[1]. However, the role of gastrin in tumor initiation and promotion remains unclear. In this study, we evaluated the possible association between gastric acid secretion, serum gastrin levels, and the differentiation of tumor cells.

MATERIALS AND METHODS

This study consisted of 128 patients with resected gastric cancer and 97 gastric ulcer patients as controls. We examined basal acid output (BAO) and maximal acid output (MAO) after stimulation by tetragastrin, and the fasting serum gastrin level and integrated gastrin response (T-IGR) after administration of a test meal (200 cal. including 10 g protein). All resected tissues underwent a detailed pathological examination, and the patients were classified into two groups as follows:1) differentiated type (papillary and tubular adenocarcinomas), and 2) undifferentiated type (poorly differentiated adenocarcinoma and signet-ring cell carcinoma). Blood samples were collected and serum gastrin levels were determined with a RIA kit (Dainabot CO., LTD.)

RESULTS

Fig. 1 shows the MAO levels in the gastric ulcer and cancer patients

according to age. Both patients showed a decreased acid output with aging.
On the other hand, although the gastric ulcer patients showed a decreased T-
IGR, the gastric cancer patients showed an increased T-IGR, with aging(Fig 2).
Fig 3 shows the acid output in patients with the differentiated and
undifferentiated types of gastric cancers.
Patients with the differentiated type of cancer showed a significantly lower
acid output.
Fig 4 shows the serum gastrin levels after administration of the test meal.
Patients with the differentiated type of gastric cancer showed significantly
higher serum gastrin levels.

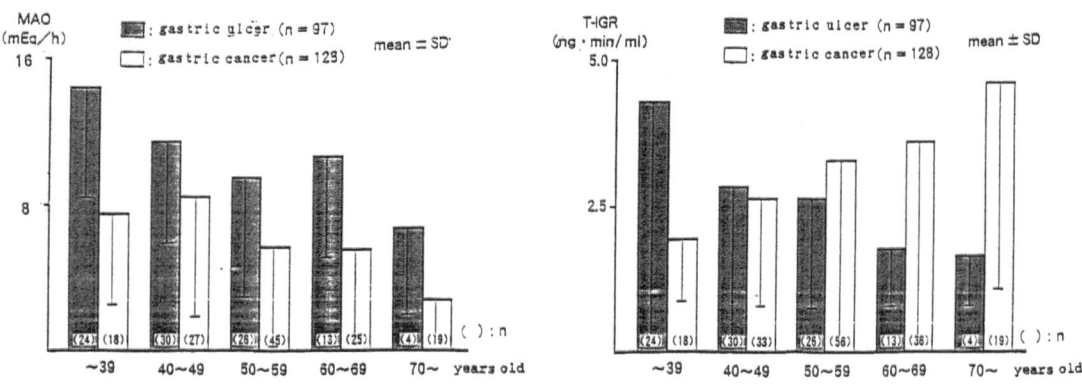

Fig.1 Maximal acid output(MAO) in the
gastric ulcer and cancer patients
according to age.

Fig. 2 Integrated gastrin response in
the gastric ulcer and cancer
patients according to age.

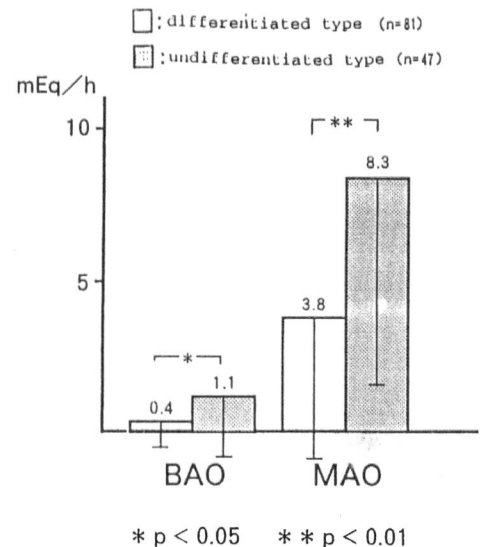

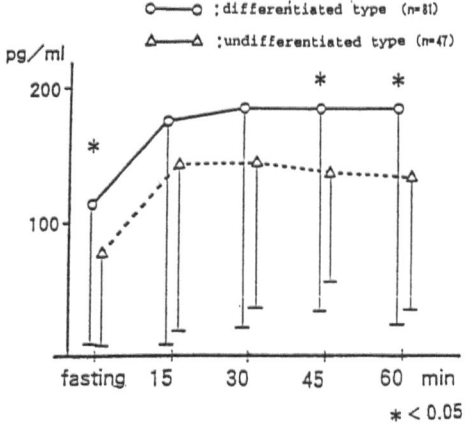

Fig 3 Acid output in patients with the
differentiated and undifferentiated types of gastric cancers.

Fig 4 Serum gastrin levels after
administration of the
test meal.

DISCUSSION

It is generally recognized that gastric cancer and atrophy of the gastric mucosa are relatively common in older people, and that hypo- and a-chlorhydria in the clinical setting are a consequence of aging. An increased in the gastric juice nitrite concentration is paralleled by an elevation of the pH value. The increase in nitrosamines found in the gastric juice of atrophic gastritis patients[2]. Moreover, it is reported that gastric cancer occurs with increased frequency in patients with pernicious anemia who are common achlorhydria[3.4].
These results speculate that there may be a close relationship between the presence of gastric cancer and gastric acid secretion.
On the other hand pentagastrin exerts a specific trophic effect on the gastric mucosa[5]. Gastric carcinogenesis and hypergastrinemia have been discussed. However, the effect of endogenous hypergastrinemia on gastric carcinogenesis is still unclear.
We reported that gastric secretion showed a significant correlation with the PHA skin test and that patients with depressed or excavated types of cancer; with superficial carcinoma; with signet ring cell carcinomas; and youngers individuals showed a higher acid output than did other groups[6]. We also reported that gastric cancer patients with normal acid secretion had normal immunity and better survival rates than those with decreased acid secretion[7,8]. We thought that these results were a phenomenon of a neuro-immune effects on cancer behavior.
In this investigation, patients with gastric cancers and gastric ulcers showed decreased acid secretion related to aging. However, their serum gastrin levels were different; gastric cancer patients had an increased integrated gastrin response, in contrast to the gastric ulcer patients, whose response was decreased.
From these results, we speculate that low acid secretion and endogenous hypergastrinemia may play important roles in developing cancer in well-differentiated types of gastric cancer.

REFERENCES

1. Watson SA, Durrant LG, Crosbie JD, Morris DJ (1989) The in vitro growth response of primary human colorectal and gastric cancer cells to gastrin. Int J Cancer 43:692-696
2. Dolby JM, Webster ADB, Borriello SP,Barclay FE, Bartholomew BA, Hill MJ (1984) Bacterial colonization and nitrite concentration in achlorhydric stomachs of patients of patients with primary hypogammaglobulinemia or classical pernicious anemia. Scand J Gastroenterol 19:105-110
3. Zamchek N, Grable E, Ley A, Norman L (1955) Occurrence of gastric cancer among patients with pernicious anaemia at the Boston City Hospital. New Eng J Med 252:1103-1110
4. Blakburn EK, Callender ST, Dacie, Doll R, Girdwood RH, Mollin DL, Saracci R, Stafford L, Thompson RB, Varadi S, Whetherley-Mein G (1968) Possible association between pernicious anaemia and leukaemia:a prospective study of 1,625 patients with a note on the very high incidence of stomach cancer. Int J Cancer 3:163-170
5. Johnson LR. (1977) New aspects of the trophic action of gastrointestinal hormones. Gastroenterology 72:788-792
6. Ogoshi K, Miyaji M, Iwata S, Hara S, Kondoh Y, Mitomi T, Harasawa S,Tani N (1989) Gastric acid secretions and serum gastrin levels in patients with mucosal and submucosal gastric cancer. Jpn J Cancer Clin 35:999-1003
7. Ogoshi K, Iwata S, Hara S, Kondoh Y, Hanaue H, Mitomi T, Harasawa S, Tani N (1989) Gastric acid secretion and cellular immunity in patients with gastric cancer. Jpn J Cancer Clin 35:450-454
8. Ogoshi K, Iwata K, Hara S, Kondoh Y, Mitomi T (1990) Preoperative gastric acid secretion of the gastric cancer patients and their prognosis. Jpn J Surg 91:47-51

Early Detection of α-Fetoprotein Producing Gastric Cancer by Reverse Transcriptase-Polymerase Chain Reaction

Y. Yamada[1], H. Sawada[1], A. Watanabe[1], H. Nakano[1], and M. Terada[2]

[1]First Department of Surgery, Nara Medical University, Kashihara, Nara, 634 Japan
[2]Genetics Division, National Cancer Center Research Institute, Chuo-ku, Tokyo, 104 Japan

ABSTRACT

Expression of α-fetoprotein (AFP) mRNA was detected in surgical specimens of gastric cancers by reverse transcriptase-polymerase chain reaction (RT-PCR). The specificity of the PCR products was confirmed by hybridization with an AFP cDNA probe. With this method, AFP mRNA was detected in three of 14 surgical specimens of gastric cancers . However, elevation of serum AFP was found in only one of these three patients. The rapid and sensitive detection by RT-PCR of AFP mRNA in tissue specimens of gastric cancers is expected to provide essential information for the diagnosis and treatment of AFP producing gastric cancer.

KEY WORDS: Gastric cancer, α-fetoprotein (AFP) , mRNA, Reverse transcriptase-polymerase chain reaction (RT-PCR)

INTRODUCTION

α-fetoprotein (AFP) is an oncofetal protein that appears in the fetal stage. Reappearance of AFP in adult serum has been identified as a marker of malignant tumors such as hepatocellular carcinoma and teratocarcinoma. However, elevation of serum AFP has been found not only in connection with hepatocellular and embryonal carcinomas but also with malignant tumors of the gastrointestinal tract (1,2). Such an elevated serum AFP level in a gastric cancer patient was first described by Bourreille et al. in 1970 (3). The actual localization of AFP in gastric cancer cells was found by immunohistochemical stain method (4). However diagnosis is usually successful only in advanced cases frequently accompanied by liver metastasis (5), while the prognosis of AFP producing gastric cancers appears poor (6). It is also reported that AFP producing early gastric cancers have the same tendency to metastasize to the liver as do AFP producing advanced gastric cancers (7).

We previously succeeded in establishing a serially transplantable AFP producing gastric cancer line in nude mice which showed a correlation between elevated serum AFP level and tumor growth (8). In another report, we demonstrated that AFP producing gastric cancers possess a higher potential for liver metastasis than non-AFP producing gastric cancers, a distinguishing feature which reflects a poor prognosis (9).

However, chemotherapy is reportedly beneficial for AFP producing gastric cancer (10). Therefore, early diagnosis of AFP producing gastric cancer before elevation of serum AFP occurs may be important to prevent recurrence and improve the prognosis.

In this study, we investigated the detection of AFP mRNA in surgical specimens of gastric cancers by Reverse transcriptase-polymerase chain reaction (RT-PCR) analysis, and found it to be a rapid and sensitive method.

MATERIALS AND METHODS

Tissues and RNA Extraction

Fourteen surgical specimens of gastric cancers were obtained at the National Cancer Center Hospital. All tissues were quickly frozen in liquid nitrogen and stored at -80°C until analysis. Total RNA was extracted with

CsCl/guanidinumisothiocyanate as described (11).

RT-PCR Analysis

The method for RT-PCR was essentially as described (12). Briefly, cDNA was synthesized from 1μg of total RNA by murine leukemia virus reverse transcriptase (Bethesda Research Laboratories) using random hexamer as a primer. The RNA·cDNA hybrid was subsequently amplified by PCR using a GeneAmp kit (Perkin-Elmer/Cetus) with AFP-specific oligonucleotide primers. Primers were synthesized with an Applied Biosystems model 381A DNA synthesizer. According to the published sequence (13), the following sequences were used for primers: PAF1, GCTGACATTATTATCGGACA; and PAF2, CTCTTCAGCAAAGCAGACTT. PCR was performed with 30-cycle amplification for 1min at 94ºC (denaturation), 1min at 55ºC (annealing) and 2min at 72ºC (extension). After 30 cycles, a 10min extension at 72ºC was added.

Agarose Gel Electrophoresis

PCR products were electrophoresed on a 3% agarose gel, stained with ethidium bromide and visualized by ultraviolet illumination.

RESULTS

We designed a set of primers that would allow us to distinguish between amplified cDNA and chromosomal DNA.

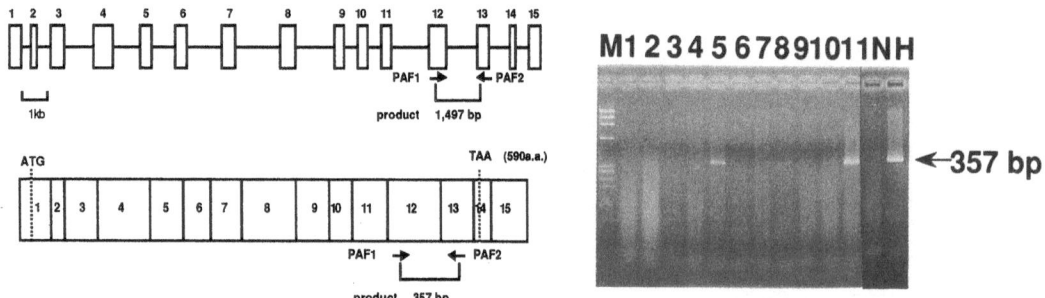

Fig. 1. AFP gene and cDNA structure and positions of PCR primers, PAF1 and PAF2. Upper part: amplification of chromosomal DNA. Lower part: amplification of cDNA.

Fig. 2. Analysis of RT-PCR products. The length of the product is indicated on the right. Lane M, molecular size marker (øX174 digested with HaeIII); lanes 1 to 11, surgical specimens of gastric cancers; lane N, noncancerous gastric mucosa as a negative control; lane H, hepatocellurar carcinoma as a positive control.

AS outlined in Fig. 1, the PCR primers PAF1 and PAF2 amplify a 357-base pair (bp) fragment extending from exon 12 to exon 13 of the AFP cDNA when cDNA is amplified and a 1,497-bp fragment when chromosomal DNA is amplified (13,14). This difference in size is based on containing intron 12. RT-PCR analysis identified the expected 357 bp band in three out of 14 samples (Fig. 2). Under these conditions, the 1,497 bp band was not detectable in this study. The specificity of the RT-PCR products was confirmed by Southern blot analysis and hybridization to a human AFP cDNA probe (data not shown). The serum AFP level of one of these three cases was elevated to 1,045ng/ml but no elevation was detected in the other two cases before surgery.

DISCUSSION

We analyzed the expression of AFP mRNA detected by the RT-PCR method in surgical specimens of gastric cancers. The specificity of the RT-PCR products was confirmed by hybridization with a human AFP cDNA probe. Expression of AFP mRNA was found in three out of 14 specimens. However, elevation of serum AFP before surgery was not found in two of these three patients. All three patient died of recurrence of gastric cancers in less than 2 years and 3 months. Unfortunately, the serum AFP of these patients was not measured after surgery, so, it could not be determined whether the serum AFP levels of these cases were elevated at recurrence. It will be necessary for further investigation of latent AFP producing gastric cancers such as elevation of serum AFP at recurrence in cases where no such elevation was found before surgery. The rapid and sensitive detection by RT-PCR of AFP mRNA in tissue specimens of gastric cancers is expected to provide essential information for the diagnosis and treatment of AFP producing gastric cancer.

REFERENCES

1. Abelev GI, Assecritova IV, Kraevsky NA, Perova SD, Pervodchikova NI (1967) Embryonal serum alphaglobulin in cancer patients. Int J Cancer 2: 551-558
2. Tatarinov JS (1961) Prsence of embryonal alphaglobulin in the serum of patients with primary hepatocarcinoma. Vopr Med Khim 10: 90-91
3. Bourreille J, Metayer P, Sauger F, Matray F, Foudimare A (1970) Existence d'α-fetoprotein au cours d'un cancer secondarie du foie d'origine gastrique. Presse Med 78: 1277-1278
4. Kodama T, Kameya T, Hirota T, Shimosato Y, Ohkura H, Mukojima T, Kitaoka H (1981) Production of alpha-fetoprotein, normal serum proteins, and human chorionic gonadotropin in stomach cancer: histologic and immunohistovhemical analyses of 35 cases. Cancer 48: 1647-1655
5. Kato K, Akai S, Tobita Y, Tsutsui K, Tsunoda H, Suzuki M (1974) α-fetoprotein-positive cases in cancers except for hepatoma and malignant teratoma; mainly on the sum up data in Japan. Gan No Rinsho 20: 376-382 (in japanese)
6. Chang Y-C, Nagasue N, Kohno H, Ohiwa K, Yamanoi Y, Nakamura T (1992) Xenotransplantation of alpha-fetoprotein-producing gastric cancers into nude mice. Cancer 69: 872-877
7. Change Y-C, Nagasue N, Abe S, Kohno H, Yamanoi A, Uchida M, Nakamura T (1990) The Characters of AFP-Producing Early Gastric Cancer. J Jpn Surg Soc 91: 1574-1580 (in japanese)
8. Ezaki T, Nakatani K, Miyagi N, Sakamoto K, Takahashi S, Emi Y, Shiratori T, Konishi Y (1983) Establishment of an alpha-fetoprotein-producing human gastric carcinoma in nude mice. Gann 74: 870-877
9. Sawada H, Nakatani K, Watanabe A, Nishiwada T, Okumura T, Yamada Y, Yano T, Shino Y, Ymada T, Tanase M, Nakano M, Tsutsumi M, Nakae D, Konishi Y (1992) The Potential for the Development of Liver Metastasis from Alpha-fetoprotein-producing Human Gastric Carcinomas in Nude Mice. Jpn J Clin Oncol 22: 303-307
10. Kato M, Kinoshita K, Sawa T, Yoshimitu S, Yonemura Y, Miwa K, Miyazaki I, Matsui Y (1990) Early Gastric Cancer of Type IIa + IIc Producing α-fetoprotein with Liver Metastasis. Jpn J Gastroenterol Surg 23: 2624-2628 (in japanese)
11. Maniatis T, Fritsch EF, Sambrook J (1982) Molecular Cloning: A Laboratory Manual. Cold Spring Harbor Laboratory, Cold Spring Harbor, NY.
12. Saiki R, Gelfand DH, Stoffel S, Scharf SJ, Higuchi R, Horn GT, Mullis KB, Erlich HA (1988) Primer-Directed Enzymatic Amplification of DNA with a Thermostable DNA Polymerase. Science 239: 487-491
13. Morinaga T, Sakai M, Thomas GW, Tamaoki T (1983) Primary structures of α-fetoprotein and its mRNA. Proc Natl Acad Sci USA 80: 4604-4608
14. Peter EMG, Rita Z, Carol B, Achilles D (1987) Structure, Polymorphism, and novel Repeated DNA Elements Revealed by a Complete Sequence of the Human α-Fetoprotein Gene. Biochemistry 26: 1332-1343

Preoperative Prediction of Gastric Cancer Extension by in Vitro Labelling Index of Bromodeoxyuridine

Kazuo Sugiyama, Yutaka Yonemura, Toru Kamata, Shigekazu Ooyama, Takasi Fujimura, Hisasi Matumoto, Koichiro Tugawa, Itasu Ninomiya, Hiroyuki Sahara, Yasuo Hirono, Hiroyuki Takamura, Koichi Miwa, and Ituo Miyazaki

Department of Surgery II, School of Medicine, Kanazawa University, Kanazawa, 920 Japan

ABSTRACT

In vitro labelling index(L.I.) of BrdU was evaluated as a preoperaitve predictor of gastric cancer extension. Biopsy specimens were obtained preoperatively and labelled by BrdU. BrdU were stained immunohistochemically and labelling index was calculated. Patients with L.I. more than 10% had a significantly higher risk of node involvement and venous invasion. Patients with L.I. omre than 20% had a significantly higher risk of liver metastasis. Patients with L.I. more than 25% had a significantly higher risk of submucosal invasion. In conclusion, in vitro BrdU labelling is an available technique as a preoperative predictor of node involvement, venous invasion, submucosal invasion and prognosis in gastric cancer.

KEY WORDS: iv vitro BrdU labelling, preoperative prediction, gastric cancer

INTRODUCTON

Bromodeoxyuridine(BrdU)is taken up into nuclear DNA at S phase of cell cycle(1). BrdU labeling index is thoght to reflect tumor proliferative activity. Sasaki(2) developed in vitro BrdU labeling technique. In this study, we determined in vitro BrdU labeling index of gastric cancer preoperatively using biopsy specimens and demonstrate its clinical value.

Patients and Methods

Patients
Consequent 187 patients histologically diagnosed as gastric cancer were included in this study.

In vitro labeling of BrdU
Before operation, 3 or 4 pieces of biopsy specimens were obtained and labeled by BrdU in vitro according to the method of Sasaki as the following(2). Specimens were immediately put into a vial that contained RPMI-1640 culture medium (GIBCO, Grand Island, NY) including BrdU (Sigma Chemical Co., London, England) at a concentration of 400 μM. Bials were stoppered, filled with carbogen gas (oxygen with 5% carbon dioxide) at three times atomspheric pressure, and incubated at 37℃ for an hour. Then the specimens were fixed with 70% ethanol enbedded in paraffine.

Immunohistochemical staining
Materials were cut into thick sections and dewaxed. They were denatured with hydrochloric acid (2N,30min) at room temperature, neutralized by sodium tetraborate (0.1M,10min), treated with protease (0.05%,10min) and blocked by hydrogen peroxide (0.3% in methanol, 30min). Then they were pretreated with normal gout serum and incubated in monoclonal antibody anti BrdU (Becton Dickinson, Mountain View, CA) at a dilution of 1:100 overnight at 4℃. They were incubated in biotinylated gout anti-mouse IgG (TAGO, Bullingame,CA) at a dilution of 1:30 for an hour at room temperature and incubated in avidine biotin peroxidase complex (Vector, Burlingame, CA) for 30 minutes at room temperature. Finally they were treated with 3,3'-diaminobenzidine and counterstained with hematoxylin for light microscopy.

Labeling index of BrdU was defined as the percentage of the cancer cells positive for BrdU against more than 300 cancer cells.

Results

The mean BrdU labelling index of total cases was $16.0 \pm 8.4\%$. BrdU labelling indices according to each pathological parameter were shown in Table 1. The mean BrdU labelling index of patients with microscopic involvement of nodes was significantly higher than that of patients without microscopic involvement ($p<0.01$). The mean BrdU labelling index of patients with venous invasion was significantly higher than that of patients without venous invasion($p<0.01$). Moreover, the mean BrdU labelling index of patients with liver metastasis was significantly higher than that of patients without liver matastasis ($p<0.05$). There were no significant differences in the BrdU labelling indices of patients according to peritoneal dissemination, lymph vessel invasion and histological classification. BrdU labelling indices according to the gastric wall depth of tumor invasion were shown in Table 2. The mean BrdU labelling index in mucosa(13.2%) was significantly less than that of submucosa(17.3%), proper muscle(18.7%), and subserosa(16.1%) ($p<0.02$, $p<0.05$, and $p<0.01$ respectively).

Incidence of tumor invasion and metastasis in the view of BrdU labelling index was shown in Table 3. Incidence of node involvement in tumors with BrdU labelling index less than 10% was significantly lower than that with BrdU labelling index 10% and more (24% vs. 52%, $p<0.001$). Incidence of venous invasion in tumors with BrdU labelling index less than 10% was significantly lower than that with BrdU labelling index 10% and more (24% vs. 40%). Furhermore, incidence of liver metastasis in tumors with BrdU labelling index less than 20% was significantly lower than that with BrdU labelling index 20% and more (1% vs. 14%, $p<0.01$). Confined to early gastric cancers, incidence of submucosal carcinoma in the patients with BrdU labelling index 25% and more was significantly greater(100%) than that with BrdU labelling index less than 25% (46%, $p<0.01$) and that with BrdU labelling index less than 10% (30%, $p<0.01$) (Table 4).

Kaplan-Meier calculations showed that survival rates became smaller according to the degree of BrdU labelling index (Figure 1). Five year survival rates were 92% (BrdU L.I. less than 5%), 83% (BrdU L.I. more than 5% and less than 10%), 68%(BrdU L.I. more than 10% and less than 15%) and 58% (BrdU L.I. more than 15%). The differences were significant between BrdU L.I. more than 15% and BrdU L.I. less than 5% ($p=0.025$). And so was between BrdU L.I. more than 15% and BrdU L.I. more than 5% and less than 10% ($p=0.024$).

Table 1. BrdU Labelling Indices of Each Pathological Finding

	BrdU labelling Index (%)	
n (-)	14.5 ± 8.7	] p<0.01
n (+)	17.7 ± 7.5	
H (-)	15.5 ± 8.4	] p<0.05
H (+)	21.1 ± 6.3	
v (-)	14.7 ± 8.5	] p<0.01
v (+)	18.1 ± 7.9	

Table2. BrdU Labelling Indices in Each Depth of Tumor Invasion

Tumor Depth	BrdU Labelling Index(%)		
m	13.2 ± 6.6%	] p<0.02	
sm	17.3 ± 9.2%		] p<0.05
pm	18.7 ± 11.9%		] p<0.01
ss ≤	16.1 ± 7.7%		

Table 3. Rate of Metastases and Invasion under / above Cutoff Levels of BrdU Laballing Indices

BrdU Labelling Index	Node Involvement		Venous Invasion	
<10%	24%	] P<0.001	24%	] P<0.05
10% ≤	52%		40%	

BrdU Labelling Index	Liver Metastasis	
<20%	1%	] P<0.01
20% ≤	14%	

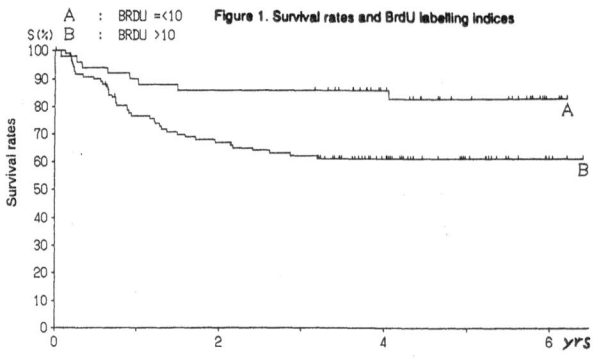

Figure 1. Survival rates and BrdU labelling indices

Table 4. BrdU Labelling Indices and Incidence of Mucosal or Submucosal Invasion in Early Gastric Cancer

BrdU labelling index	m	sm		
<10%	70%	30%		
10 ~ 25%	54%	46%	] p<0.01	] P<0.01
25%<	0%	100%		

Discussion

The incidence of node involvement increases more in submucosal carcinoma than in mucosal carcinoma. In this study BrdU labelling index of mucosal carcinoma is significantly lower than carcinomas which invaded deeper than submucosa. Practically, high risk level of BrdU labbeling index was assumed to be more than 10% for node involvement and venous invasion, and more than 20% for liver metastasis. In early gastric cancer, BrdU labelling indiecs less than 10% represented relatively high incidence(70%) of mucosal tumor. On the other hands, all of early gastric cancers with BrdU labelling index 25% and more represented submucosal invasion. These values gave us the most significant difference between above the value and under the value. Though these values are not necessarily an absolute indicator for metastases and stomach wall invasion, the possibility is significantly high. Even according to the depth of tumor invasion in stomach wall, node involvements were almost correlated with BrdU labelling indices in order. These results means that BrdU labelling index express malignancy independent on the depth of tumor invasion, which influences node involvement extremly.

BrdU labelling index reflected survival rates. It is suggested that these results were caused by two effects, first: node involvement or liver metastasis which is related labelling index as described previously, second: malignant potential, which was independent on pathological parameters as observed in stage 3.

In conclusion, preoperative calculations of BrdU labelling index have a predictive value for node involvement, liver metastasis and venous invasion, and a prognostic value. This method will help surgeons in a choice of operative procedure for gastric cancer, including node dissection and additional chemotherapy. Furthermore, its accuracy will be more increased in combination with other imaging technique or tumor markers which have ever established.

RERERENCES

1. Gratzner HG (1982) Monoclonal antiboby to 5-bromo and 5-iododeoxyuridine: a new agent for detection of DNA replication. Science 218:474-475
2. Sasaki K, Takahashi M (1980) Preservation of cell cycle characteristics in solid tumor in vitro. Cancer Rec 40: 4810-4812
3. Christov K, Vassilev N (1987) Flow cytometric analysis of DNA and cell proliferation in ovarian tumors. Cancer 60:121-124
4. Volm M, Mattern J, Sonka J (1985) DNA distribution in non small cell lung carcinomas and its relationship to clinical behavior. Cytometry 6: 348-351

Immunohistochemical Study of PCNA (Proliferating Cell Nuclear Antigen) in Gastric Cancer with Special Reference to Progression and Prognosis

Kiyoshi Maeda, Yong-Suk Chung, Naoyoshi Onoda, Nobuya Yamada, Yuichi Arimoto, Atsunori Nitta, Yasuyuki Kato, and Michio Sowa

First Department of Surgery, Osaka City University Medical School, Osaka, 545 Japan

ABSTRACT

We investigated the correlation between tumor's proliferative activity and progression of gastric carcinoma using immunohistochemical staining with PC10 monoclonal antibody recognizing Proliferating Cell Nuclear Antigen (PCNA). PCNA labeling index became higher as the histologic stage increased. Also, in patients with lymph node metastasis and peritoneal metastasis, labeling index was significantly higher. Moreover in patients with high PCNA labeling index ($\geq$50%), prognosis was significantly poorer than in those with low index (<50%). These result suggested PCNA labeling index is associated with tumor stage and is useful as one of the prognostic factors.

KEY WORDS: Proliferating Cell Nuclear Antigen, Gastric Carcinoma, Proliferation Kinetics

INTRODUCTION

Proliferating Cell Nuclear Antigen (PCNA), also called DNA polymerase δ-associated protein, is found in the cells of the proliferative compartment and is essential for DNA replication [1,2]. Recently, many studies have reported on the correlation between malignant potential of various carcinomas and cell proliferation kinetics [3,4]. In this study, we investigated the correlation between the expression of PCNA and prognosis of gastric cancer, by immunohistochemical study using anti-PCNA monoclonal antibody.

MATERIALS AND METHODS

Clinical Materials

Eighty patients with gastric carcinoma were studied. These patients were pathlogically staged according to the general rules for gastric cancer [5]. According to histologic stage, 31 cases belonging to stage I, 10 to stage II, 19 to stage III and 20 to stage IV. Sixty-six patients had curative and 14 patients had non-curative surgical procedures. These patients were examined endoscopically before operation, then tissue specimens were sampled from the tumor. After fixing these specimens with 10% formalin for less than 2 hours, specimens were embedded in paraffin. Sections were cut at 4 μm, mounted on glass slides overnight at room temperature.

Methods

As primary antibody, PC10 (Novocastra Lab. Ltd.) was diluted 100 times and reacted with specimens at room temperature for 1 hour. Immunohistochemical staining was performed by streptoavidine - biotin method. More than 500 tumor cells were microscopically counted in each samples. The PCNA labeling index was calculated as the percentage of positive cell nuclei.

Statistical Methods

Student's t-test were used for statistical analyses. Survival curves were calculated using the Kaplan-Meier method any analyzed by the general Wilcoxon test.

RESULT

PCNA staining was confined to the nuclei, while the cytoplasm and cell membrane remained
unstained. PCNA labeling index varied within the range of 6-84% with a mean (±SD; standard
deviation) value of 39.8±19.5%.
Table 1 shows the correlation between PCNA labeling index and various clinicopathologic
factors. There was no statistically significant association between PCNA labeling index
and histologic type. However significant differences were existed with respect to depth of
invasion, lymph node metastasis and peritoneal metastasis.
The mean PCNA labeling index in cases with lymph node metastasis, peritoneal metastasis was
significantly higher than that in those without metastasis. Regarding the relationship
with depth of invasion, the PCNA index was higher as depth of invasion became more serious.
Also, the same tendency was seen between PCNA labeling index and histologic stage.
Prognosis was studied about 66 curative cases. We devided 66 curative cases into a high
PCNA grade group where the PCNA index was more than 50% and a low PCNA grade group where
the index was less than 50%. The survival rate of these 66 curative cases was calculated
using Kaplan-Meier method. As a result, as shown in Figure 1, we found the prognosis of
the high PCNA grade group to be significantly poorer than that of the low PCNA grade group.

Table 1. Correlation between
clinicopathologic factors and
PCNA labeling index

Variable	PCNA labeling index	P value
Histologic type		
well (n=39)	37.4±19.4	N S
low (n=41)	45.9±15.9	
Lymph node metastasis		
negative (n=36)	30.0±15.3	<0.005
positive (n=44)	51.5±14.1	
Depth of invasion		
m (n=12)	16.0± 9.2 *	
sm (n=13)	31.2±13.8 **	
pm (n=19)	46.1±10.7	
ss (n= 8)	52.0± 5.2	
se (n=18)	49.7±15.6	
sei (n=10)	55.9±12.6	
Liver metastasis		
negative (n=76)	41.1±18.0	N S
positive (n=4)	54.3±16.6	
Peritoneal metastasis		
negative (n=70)	36.4±17.7	<0.01
positive (n=10)	56.8±13.5	
Stage		
I (n=31)	26.8±13.7	
II (n=10)	45.6±12.8	
III (n=19)	47.3±10.1	
IV (n=20)	57.9±14.8 ***	

* : significantly lower (p<0.01) than other groups.
** : significantly lower (p<0.01) than cases with pm,ss,se and sei.
*** : significantly higher (p<0.01) than stage I.

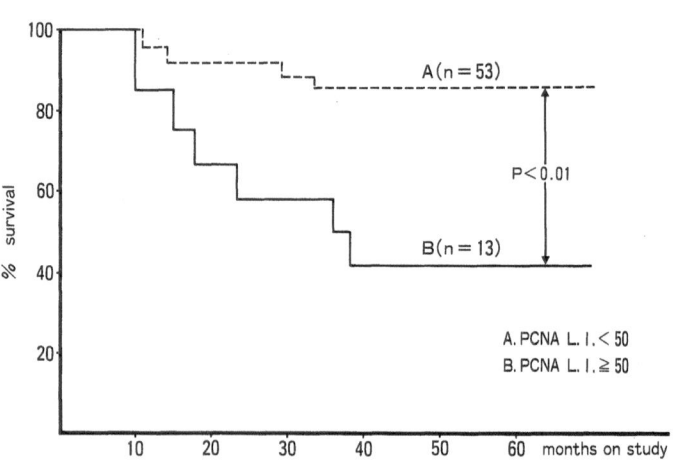

Fig.1 Survival rate after curative resection

DISCUSSION

Recently, many studies have reported that cell kinetic information may be useful in judging
the malignant potential of various carcinomas [3,4] and Cell proliferation has been
measured by means of DNA ploidy analysis [3] or bromodeoxyuridine (BrdU) immunostaining [4].
PCNA has been known as an auxiliary protein of DNA polymerase δ and is thought to be
expressed in the nuclei particularly in late G1 and S-phases [1,2]. And so, PCNA has drawn
attention as one of the parameters for cell proliferation kinetics. Also, the relationship of PCNA with malignant potential of various cancers has been reported [6,7].
Hall et al studied the expression of PCNA in some neoplasms and reported that PCNA immunostaining may be useful as an indicator of malignant potential [6]. In our study, it was
revealed that the PCNA labeling index shows higher values in histologically advanced stages
and that for clinicopathologic factors, higher grade of PCNA expression was observed among
cases with lymph node metastasis and peritoneal metastasis. As for the correlation between
depth of invasion and the expression of PCNA, the deeper the tumor invasion, the higher the
PCNA labeling index. Yonemura et al reported that higher levels of PCNA expression was
seen in patients with advanced stage and with lymph node metastasis [7]. And our result

also suggested that PCNA may be useful as an indicator of proliferative activity and progression of gastric carcinoma.

In relation to prognosis, Yonemura et al reported that among 120 cases with gastric cancer, the high PCNA grade group where the labeling index was more than 40% had significantly poorer prognosis than the low PCNA grade group where the index was less than 40% [7]. Our study, too, showed significantly poorer prognosis in the high PCNA grade group and the PCNA labeling index was considered useful as a prognostic factor.

As a result of this study, PCNA labeling index is associated to tumor stage and may be a good prognostic factor in patients with gastric carcinoma.

REFERENCE

1. Bravo R, Frank R, Blundell PA, Macdonald-Bravo H. (1987) Cyclin/PCNA is the auxiliary protein of DNA polymerase δ. Nature 326:515-517
2. Garcia RL, Coltrera MD, Gown AM. (1989) Analysis of proliferative grade using anti-PCNA/cyclin in fixed, embedded tissues. Am J Pathol 134:733-739
3. Sowa M, Yoshino H, Kato Y, Nishimura M, Kamino K, Umeyama K. (1988) An analysis of the DNA ploidy patterns of gastric cancer. Cancer 62:1325-30
4. Gratznen HG. (1982) Monoclonal antibody to 5-bromo- and 5-iodo-deoxyuridine; a new reagent for detection of DNA replication. Science 218:474-5
5. Japanese Research Society for Gastric Cancer. (1985) The general rules for gastric cancer study 11
6. Hall PA, Levison DA, Woods AC, Yu CC-W, Kellock DB, Watkins JA. (1990) Proliferating cell nuclear antigen (PCNA) immunolocalization in paraffin sections - an index of cell proliferation with evidence of peregulated expression in some neoplasms. J Pathol 16:285-94
7. Yonemura Y, Yamaguchi A, Kaji M, Fusida Y, Tsugawa K, Luis F. (1992) Correlation of proliferating cell nuclear antigen (PCNA) labeling rate and malignancy in gastric cancer. Jpn J Surg 93:661

c-myc Gene Expression in Primary Gastric Cancer

Naoyoshi Onoda, Kiyoshi Maeda, Itsuo Nakanishi, Yasuyuki Kondo, Nobuya Yamada, Yoshito Yamashita, Yong-Suk Chung, and Michio Sowa

First Department of Surgery, Osaka City University Medical School, Osaka, 545 Japan

ABSTRACT

In this study, we investigated the expression of c-myc mRNA in 48 patients with primary gastric cancer (51 lesions) and 11 metastatic lymph node lesions. Thirty-five (68.6%) of the primary lesions demonstrated c-myc mRNA overexpression, including 18 of 20 (90%) early stage lesions and 17 of 31 (54.8%) of lesions of advanced cancer. C-myc mRNA overexpression was detected in all metastatic lymph node lesions. Overexpression of c-myc mRNA appeared to be frequent in gastric cancer even in early stage lesions. No relationship was found between c-myc mRNA overexpression in primary lesions and tumor progression, including lymph node metastasis.

KEY WORDS: primary gastric cancer, c-myc gene, messenger RNA, lymph node metastasis

INTRODUCTION

C-myc is a cellular oncogene, and the human homologue to the v-myc gene of avian myelo-cytomasis virus MC29 [1]. The c-myc oncogene has been reported to play an important role in cell proliferation [2]. Messenger RNA expression is reported to be excessive in proliferating cells. Some studies have reported that c-myc protein accumulation or DNA amplification correlates with the clinical stages and prognosis of gastric cancer, and have suggested that the c-myc gene plays an important role in cancer progression [3,4]. These studies, however, provide no explanation how gene overexpression occurs. The frequency of c-myc protein expression in gastric cancer has been reported to be between 20 to 50%, while c-myc DNA amplification is thought to appear in only a few cases of this type of cancer. The findings of these studies suggest that overexpression of c-myc mRNA occurs in many cases of gastric cancer. However, only a few studies of mRNA expression in gastric cancer have been made, and, furthermore, those cases studies have been limited to those of advanced stage [5,6]. In this study, we investigated the expression of c-myc mRNA in cases of primary gastric cancer in an effort to determine the relationship between c-myc mRNA expression in tissue and clinico-pathological findings.

PATIENTS & METHODS

PATIENTS

Forty-eight patients with primary gastric cancer (51 lesions) were studied, including 20 with early disease (without invasion to the muscle layer) and 31 with advanced disease (invasion deeper than the muscle layer). Cancerous lesions and normal mucosal tissues were sampled from surgical specimens. Metastatic lesions in lymph nodes were also sampled from 11 patients.

PROBE

C-myc cDNA was a 1,400 bp EcoRI/CH4A-restricted fragment of human Burkitt's lymphoma genomic c-myc 3rd exon sequence (Oncor, Inc., MD) and was labeled using the random priming method (Multiprime DNA Labelling System, Amersham International plc, UK) with ^{32}P.

RNA ISOLATION & NORTHERN BLOT HYBRIDIZATION

Total RNA was isolated using the acid guandium thiocyanate-phenol chroloform method [7]. Twenty µg of total RNA were electrophoresed on a 1% agarose gel containing formaldehyde and then transferred to nylon membrane (Hybond-N, Amersham International plc.). The membranes were hybridized with ^{32}P-labeled c-myc cDNA probe. Autoradiography and densitometric quantitation were subsequently performed.

Clinical and histopathological findings were classified according to "The General Rules for the Gastric Cancer Study in Surgery and Pathology" [8]. The statistical significances of findings was calculated using Student's t-test for mean values and the χ2-test for frequencies.

RESULTS

C-myc mRNA was detected as a single band of 2.3 kb transcript in all samples examined, including normal mucosa. No band other than the 2.3 kb transcript was recognized (Fig.). The densitometric level (level) of c-myc mRNA expression was almost constant in normal mucosal tissues. In cancer tissues, however, this level varied. The latter had levels 0.2 - 18.9 (avg. 3.88±4.47) times those of normal mucosal tissues of the same patient. Thirty-five of 51 cancer lesions (68.6%) studied had an "excess" level (more than 1.1 times that in normal mucosa) of c-myc mRNA expression (overexpression).

No significant relationship was found between histological type of tumor and c-myc mRNA expression, and no relationship was found between c-myc mRNA level and presence or absence of liver metastasis, peritoneal dissemination or lymph node metastasis. Overexpression of c-myc mRNA was more commonly observed in patients with early stage disease. In early cancers, the frequency of c-myc mRNA overexpression was as high as 90% and was significantly higher than that in advanced cancers (Table). When lesions were divided into two groups based on style of growth, the infiltrating type of lesion was found to be associated significantly less frequently with c-myc mRNA overexpression than was the expanding type. The level of the infiltrating type was also significantly lower (Table). All metastatic lesions in lymph nodes showed c-myc mRNA overexpression, which ranged between 1.2 and 20 (avg. 6.64±5.81) times that in normal mucosa. These levels were even higher than those for primary cancer lesions (Fig).

Case　　44

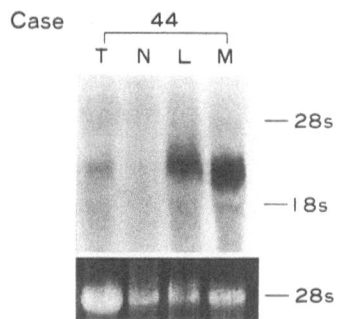

— 28s

— 18s

— 28s

Fig. Result of Northern Hybridization
C: Control RNA extracted from HL60 cells.
T: Cancer tissue N: Normal mucosa
L: Metastatic lesion of lymph node
M: Metastatic lesion of liver

C-myc mRNA was detected as single band of 2.3 kb.

Table C-myc m RNA expression in gastric cancer Relationship between mRNA expression and cancer progression

	n	overexpression	fold
Depth of invasion			
Early	20	18 (90.0%)	6.15±5.63
m	6	6 (100%)	8.51±5.59
sm	14	12 (85.7%)	4.96±5.26
Advanced	31	17 (54.8%)	2.42±2.66
pm	7	4 (57.1%)	2.40±1.49
ss	5	2 (40.0%)	2.26±1.92
>se	19	11 (57.9%)	2.47±3.06
Growth style			
Expansive	36	29 (80.6%)	4.99±5.05
Infiltrative	15	6 (40.0%)	1.85±1.77

* p<0.05

DISCUSSION

C-myc is one of the important oncogenes whose function is closely related to cell proliferation [2]. C-myc mRNA expression is thought to be high in frequency in gastric cancer tissues, but only a few studies concerning this hypothesis have been reported [5,6]. Moreover, in those studies, investigation was limited to advanced cases of gastric cancer, and the status of c-myc mRNA expression in early gastric cancer is not yet known. Previous studies of advanced gastric cancer reported almost the same frequency (39, 54%) of c-myc mRNA overexpression as in our patients with advanced disease. However, the frequency of overexpression in advanced cases was lower than that in early cases. Moreover, no relationship was found between clinical stage and level of mRNA expression. These findings suggest that c-myc mRNA overexpression in primary lesions may play a role in the formation of those lesions in the early stage of gastric cancer, and have little relationship to progression of cancer.

On the other hand, some studies of c-myc gene product expression using immunohistochemical staining techniques have shown that the c-myc gene product accumulates more frequently in advanced cancers [3]. On patients with advanced disease, the frequency of c-myc protein accumulation, reported in former studies, was only, slightly lower than the rate of mRNA overexpression, shown in this study. While c-myc protein was reported to accumulate in only 17% of patients with early disease. Discrepancies in frequencies observed may exist between c-myc mRNA overexpression and protein expression, especially for early cancers. Why this discrepancy exists is unclear, but it may bear some relationship to cancer progression.

Regression of c-myc mRNA transcription may explain the decreased level of c-myc mRNA in advanced gastric cancer tissues. C-myc gene transcription has been reported to be repressed by some factors such as TGF-β1 [9]. This point is of interest in regard to the regulation of c-myc gene expression in gastric cancer and cancer progression.

Metastatic lesions were found to have a higher level of c-myc mRNA than were primary lesion. Metastatic lesion had a high density of cancer cells and lacked the rich connective tissue observed in primary lesions. This histological difference may provide the reason why higher mRNA levels was seen in metastatic lesion. However, possibility that c-myc mRNA expression may have been uncontrollable and unsuppressed in metastatic lesions was also suggested by these findings. Further study will be required to clarify the significance to clearize the meaning of c-myc mRNA expression in gastric cancer tissues.

REFERENCES

1. Sheiness D, Bishop JM (1979) DNA and RNA from uninfected vertebrate cells contain nucleotide sequence related to the putative transforming gene of avian myelocytomatosis virus. J Virol 31: 514-521
2. Kelly K, Cochran BH, Stiles CD, Leder P (1983) Cell specific regulation of the c-myc gene by lymphocyte mitogens and platelet-delived growth factor. Cell 35: 603-610
3. Ninomiya I, Yonemura Y, Matsuo H, Sugiyama K, Miwa K, Miyazaki I, Shuku H (1991) Expression of c-myc gene product in gastric carcinoma. Oncology 48: 149-153
4. Ranzani GN, Pellegata NS, Previdere C, Saragoni A, Vio A, Maltoni M, Amadori D (1990) Heterogeneous protooncogene amplification correlates with tumor progression and presence of metastases in gastric cancer patients. Cancer Res 50: 7811-7814
5. Tsuboi K, Hirayoshi K, Takeuchi K, Shimada Y, Ohshio G, Tobe T, Hatanaka M (1987) Expression of the c-myc gene in human gastrointestinal malignancies. Biochem Biophys Res Commum 146: 699-704
6. Zborovskaya IB, Spitkovsky DD, Kisseljv FL (1988) C-myc expression as a possible prognostic factor in some forms of human cancer. The cancer journal 2: 134-138
7. Chomczynski P, Sacchi N (1987) Single-step Method of RNA Isolation by Acid Guanidinium Thiocyanate-Phenol-Chloroform Extraction. Anal Biochem 162: 156-159
8. Japanese Reserch Society for Gastric Cancer (1981) The General Rules for the Gastric Cancer Study in Surgery and Pathology. Jpn J Surg 11: 127-145
9. Pietenpol JA, Stein RW, Moran E, Yaciuk P, Shlegel R, Lyons RM, Pittelkow MR, Munger K, Howley PM, Moses HL (1990) TGF-β1 inhibition of c-myc transcription and growth in keratinocytes is abrogated by viral transforming proteins with pRB binding domains. Cell 61: 777-785

Expression of CD44 Molecule in Gastric Cancer

MASAFUMI MARUIWA, HIROSHI KUMEGAWA, TETSU SUEMATSU, SHINJI KAWABATA, JUNJI OHTA, ISSEI KODAMA, KIKUO KOUFUJI, JINRYO TAKEDA, and TERUO KAKEGAWA

The First Department of Surgery, Kurume University, School of Medicine, Kurume, Fukuoka, 830 Japan

ABSTRACT

The expression of the CD44 molecule was investigated in 111 cases of a resected gastric cancer, and also in 5 gastric cancer cell lines. An immunohistochemical study using frozen sections revealed that the mucosal lymphocytes and the pyloric glands deep in the normal mucosa reacted to the anti-CD44 monoclonal antibody. 54 cases (48.6%) were stained on the cell surface involving the intercellular aspect. Well-differentiated cancer showed the highest frequency of CD44 expression, among the various histological types. Moreover, cases with extensive vascular invasion frequently expressed CD44 (75%) and CD44-positive cases had a significantly higher rate of metastasis to the liver than did negative cases. Flowcytometric analysis revealed expression of CD44 on the cell surface in one of 5 examined cell lines.

KEY WORDS: gastric cancer, CD44, liver metastasis

INTRODUCTION

CD44 is a cell surface glycoprotein expressed by various types of cell, such as hematopoietic cells, cells from mesenchymal origin, and epithelial cells. This adhesive molecule plays a role in lymphocyte migration, cell-cell adhesion, and cell-substrate interaction. Recent investigations have revealed the expression of this molecule by various tumor cells [1], the correlation with tumor aggressiveness [2], and its metastatic potential [3,4]. The present study examined the expression and the localization of CD44 in gastric cancer and compared the clinicopathological features of the CD44-positive cases with those of the CD44-negative cases to investigate the biological role of CD44.

MATERIALS AND METHODS

Materials

A total of 111 cases of gastric cancer including 16 early and 95 advanced were examined immunohistochemically. Their histological distribution was papillary adenocarcinoma 7 cases, well-differentiated adenocarcinoma 23 cases, moderately-differentiated adenocarcinoma 19 cases, poorly-differentiated adenocarcinoma 41 cases, signet-ring cell carcinoma 14 cases, and mucinous adenocarcinoma 7 cases. The tissues of the primary tumor, as well as the metastatic lymph nodes from 27 cases, the tissue of the metastatic liver tumors in 2 cases, and peritoneum in 10 cases were snap frozen in OCT compound (Lab-Tek products, USA) for the immunohistochemical study. Five gastric cancer cell lines (MKN-28, KATO-III, AGS, AZ-521, and SBL-HSC-1802) were prepared for flowcytometric analysis. SBL-HSC-1802 was provided by Dr Ueda (Research Institute of Life Sciences, Snow Brand Milk Products Co., Tochigi).

Immunohistochemistry

Frozen tissue sections, 4-to-6 μm thick, were fixed in acetone for 10 minutes and then stained with anti-CD44 monoclonal antibody (Becton Dickinson, USA) by the avidin-biotin complex (ABC) method using the Vector ABC kit (Vector Laboratories, USA) as previously described [5].
In brief, sections were first incubated with normal horse serum, followed by incubation of an appropriate dilution of the primary antibody. Then the sections were incubated with biotinylated horse anti-mouse antibody, and with avidin-biotinylated peroxidase complexes. Each incubation was followed by 3 washes using phosphate-buffered saline (PBS), and the endogenous peroxidase activity was blocked by incubating with hydrogen peroxidase. 3-amino-9-ethylcarbasole was used as the chromogen.

Flowcytometric analysis

Approximately half-a-million cultured gastric cancer cells were washed using FACS buffer (0.2% Bovine serum albumin and 0.1% NaN3 in PBS) and incubated with anti-CD44 monoclonal antibody. After washing, the cells were incubated with FITC-conjugated goat anti-mouse IgG (TAGO, USA). The cells were then fixed with 4% paraformaldehyde and analyzed by an Ortho cytoron (Ortho Diagnostic Systems, USA).

Statistical analysis

The chi-square test was used for the statistical analysis of the values obtained.

RESULTS

CD44 was expressed on the mucosal lymphocytes and on the cell surface of the pyloric glands deep in the normal gastric mucosa (Fig 1). CD44 was localized on the whole cell surface involving the intercellular aspect. In the lymphoid follicles, lymphocytes around the germinal center reacted to anti-CD44 monoclonal antibody. The cell surface of the lower part of the squamous epithelium in the esophagus was also stained by the antibody (Fig 1). The fibrous and muscular tissues were also weakly stained.

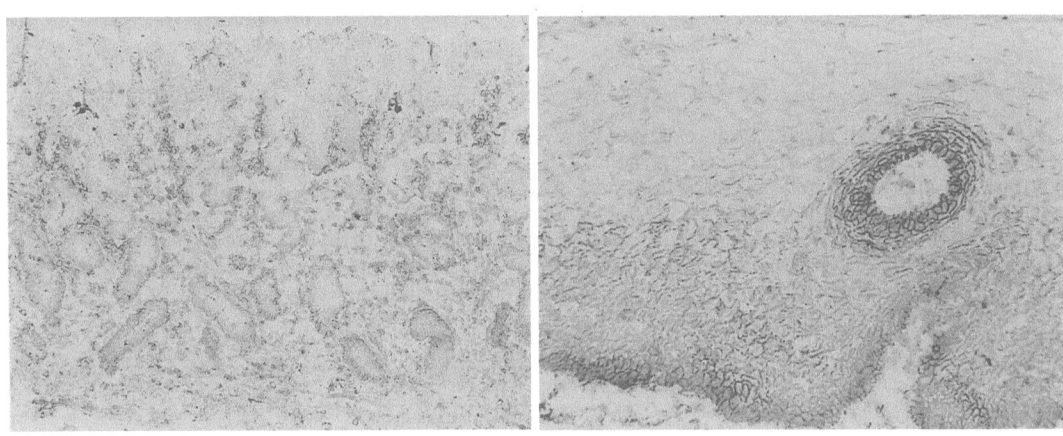

Fig. 1 Distribution of the CD44 in the normal gastric mucosa (left), and in the esophageal epithelium (right). The mucosal lymphocytes as well as the deep pyrolic glands and the deeper layer of the squamous epithelium were CD44-positive.

54 cases (48.6%) of gastric cancer cases were focally or diffusely stained. The CD44-positive gastric cancer cases involved all histological types, and the well-differentiated type represented the highest reactivity (60.9%) among them. CD44 was strongly stained on the cell surface involving the intercellular aspect (Fig. 2). The fibrous stroma also reacted to anti-CD44 antibody in 19% of the CD44-positive cases and in 3.5% of the CD44-negative cases. No correlation was found between the CD44 expression in the primary cancer and its following clinicopathological features; stage, histological depth of cancer invasion, degree of cancer cell invasion into lymph vessels, level of lymph nodes metastasis, gross feature, presence of peritoneal dissemination, degree of fibrous stroma and lymphoid infiltration. However, the cases with extensive vascular invasion frequently expressed CD44 (75%). Furthermore, the incidence of CD44-positive reaction in the primary site was significantly higher in cases with metastasis to the liver than in cases without metastasis (Table 1). Tissues from metastatic cancer in the liver were CD44-positive. One gastric cancer cell line (SBL-HSC-1802) expressed CD44 on the cell surface, out of 5 cell lines examined by flowcytometry (Fig. 3).

Table 1 Positivity of CD44 in gastric cancer with or without liver metastasis

Liver metastasis (+)	9/10	(90%)	$p<0.05$
Liver metastasis (-)	46/101	(46%)	

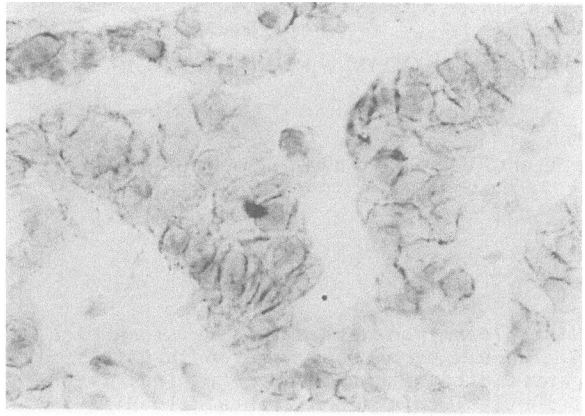

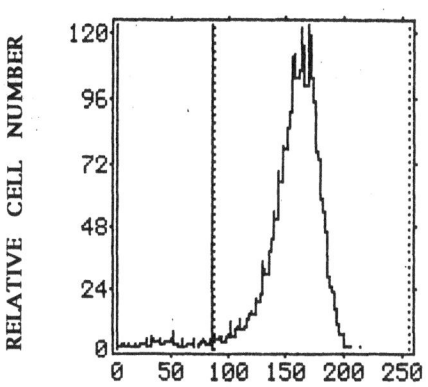

FLUORESCENCE INTENSITY

Fig. 2 CD44 was positive on the cell surface involving the intercellular aspect in resected gastric cancer.

Fig. 3 A representative histogram of gastric cancer cells examined by flowcytometry.

DISCUSSION

The purpose of this study was to investigate the biological role of the CD44 molecule in cases of a resected gastric cancer and in cell lines by immunohistochemical staining and flowcytometric analysis. CD44 has been shown to contribute to cell-cell adhesion in the in vitro experiment by transfecting the CD44 cDNA into mouse fibroblasts [6]. The present study supports the role of CD44 in cell-cell adhesion. As demonstrated by the immunohistochemical observations, CD44 was expressed on those cells considered to adhere strongly to each other in the normal gastric mucosa and in the squamous epithelium. A high incidence of CD44 expression in well-differentiated gastric cancer also supports its role in adhesion. However, although with relatively low incidence, some cases of scattered type that may involved reduced adhesion were also CD44-positive. Possible heterogeneity of the molecule may exist as well as various amounts of the molecule in cancer. CD44 may play a vital role in determining the outcome of hematogenously disseminating melanoma cells [4]. Also the CD44-immunoglobulin fusion protein inhibits tumor growth in vivo [2]. It is known that CD44H regulates tumor cell migration on hyaluronate-coated substrates [7], and CD44 variants confer metastatic behavior to rat pancreatic carcinoma cells [3]. Our findings that CD44-positive cases occurred frequently in cases with metastasis to the liver also suggests a correlation between CD44 and the malignant attitude of cancer cells. In conclusion, CD44 is probably related to cell attachment and to the malignant behavior of cancer cells. However, isoforms and variants of CD44 that have different functions have been described [3,8] . Further investigation is required using panels of monoclonal antibodies distinguishing between different epitopes of CD44, and the in vitro and/or in vivo study using CD44-positive gastric cancer cell lines may provide further useful data.

REFERENCES

1. Kuppner MC, Meir EV, Gauthier Th, Hamou M-F, Tribolet N (1992) Differential expression of the CD44 molecule in human brain tumors. Int J Cancer 50: 572-577
2. Sy MS, Guo YJ, Stamenkovic I (1992) Inhibition of tumor growth in vivo with a soluble CD44-immunoglobulin fusion protein. J Exp Med 176: 623-627
3. Hofmann M, Rudy W, Zoller M, Tolg C, Ponta H, Herrlich P, Gunthert U (1991) CD44 splice variants confer Metastatic behavior in rats: homologous sequences are expressed in human tumor cell lines. Cancer Res 51: 5292-5297
4. Birch M, Mitchell S, Hart IR (1991) Isolation and characterization of human melanoma cell variants expressing high and low levels of CD44. Cancer Res 51: 6660-6667
5. Sugihara S, Martin SR, Hsuing CK, Maruiwa M, Bloch KJ, Moscicki RA, Bhan AK (1990) Monoclonal antibodies to rat Kupffer cells; anti-KCA-1 distinguishes Kupffer cells from other macrophages. Am J Pathol 136: 345-355
6. John TS, Meyer J, Idzerda R, Gallatin WM (1990) Expression of CD44 confers a new adhesive phenotype on transfected cells. Cell 60: 45-52
7. Thomas L, Byers RH, Vink J, Stamenkovic I (1992) CD44H regulates tumor cell migration on hyaluronate-coated substrate. J Cell Biol 118: 971-977
8. Stamenkovic I, Aruffo A, Amiot M, Seed B (1991) The hematopoietic and epithelial forms of CD44 are distinct polypeptides with different adhesion potentials for hyaluronate-bearing cells. EMBO J 10: 343-348

Sialyl-Tn Antigen as a Predictor of Survival Time for Patients with Gastric Carcinoma

Xiao Chun Ma[1], Nobukuni Terata[1], Masashi Kodama[1], and Takanori Hattori[2]

[1]The First Department of Surgery, [2]The First Department of Pathology, Shiga University of Medical Science, Otsu, 520-21 Japan

ABSTRACT

Expression of sialyl-Tn antigen (STN) was examined by a immunohistochemical method in 85 primary gastric carcinomas. The STN expression occured in 53(62.3%) cancers, and the positive staining was correlated with tumor penetration, lymph nodes metastasis, and stages. Five-year survival rate for patients with STN-positive cancers(47.2%) were significantly lower than those with STN-negative cancers(84.4%,P<0.01),and patients with STN-positive cancers at stage III and stage IV had a worse prognosis. Therefore, it is suggested that a careful follow-up study and intensive post-operative therapy are needed for patients with advanced gastric carcers with positive STN expression.

KEY WORDS: gastric carcinoma, sialyl-Tn antigen, prognosis

INTRODUCTION

Oncogenic transformation is often associated with changes in glycosylation in either glycolipids or glycoproteins in cell membranes. Recently, a novel monoclonal antibody recognizing a core structure of mucin type carbohydrate chain has been made by Kjelden et al(1). This antibody(TKH2) directed to the tumor-associated O-linked sialyl Tn 2-6-α-N-acetylgalactosaminyl (sialyl-Tn(STN)) epitope was generated by immunization with ovine submaxillary mucin. Immunohistochemical studies have demonstrated that STN is expressed in human cancer cells (1-3), whereas its expression in normal adult tissues is highly restricted (1,3). In this study, we examined the expression of STN in gastric cancers of different stages,and determine whether the expression of STN might influence the prognosis of patients with gastric carcinoma.

MATERIALS AND METHODS

Patients
Eighty five patiens with gastric carcinomas were used. They had undergone gastrectomy in the Department of Surgery, Shiga University of Medical Science Hospital, from 1981 to 1986. Histologic classification was made according to the criteria of the Japanese Research Society for Gastric Cancer(4).

Immunoperoxidase Staining

The expression and localizaton of STN in the tissues was determined immunohistochemically by the avidin-biotin-peroxidase complex (ABC) method using 10% formalin-fixed and paraffin-embedded sections. The primary monoclonal antibody TKH2 (Otsuka Assay Labs, Tokushima, Japan) were used. Negative controls were prepared by substituting normal mouse serum or PBS for primary antibody which resulted in no detectable staining. A tumor was considered negative if it expressed STN in fewer than 5% of the fields.

Statistical Analysis

Statistical comparisons between groups were performed on actual case numbers using the chi-square test or Students't test. Overall survival curves of each group was calculated with the Kaplan-Meier method and the generalized Wilcoxon tests.

RESULTS

Of 85 patients with gastric carcinoma, 51 were male, and 34 were female (Tab.1). There were 53 cases(62.3%) who had STN positive tumors and 32(37.7%) STN negative tumors. No obvious relation was found between STN positivety and age or sex of patients. Of 85 patients with gastric cancer, seven of 19(37%)with stage I, nine of 17(53%) with stage II, 23 of 33(70%) with stage III, and 14(87%) with stage IV showed expressed positive stainig of STN. Stage I and stage II cases

Table 1. Clinicopathologic Characteristics of Patients with
Positive and Negative Sialyl-Tn Stained Gastric Cancers (n=85)

	STN staining	
	Negative(%)	Positive(%)
Sex		
Male	19(37)	32(63)
Female	13(38)	21(62)
Mean age(yr)	55.55	57.64
Stage		*
I	12(63)	7(37)
II	8(47)	9(53)
III	10(30)	23(70)
IV	2(12)	14(87)
Histologic type		
Differentiated	18(41)	26(59)
Undifferentiated	14(34)	27(66)
Depth of invasion		**
Mucosa+Submucosa	14(61)	9(39)
Muscularis propria	7(54)	6(46)
Serosa	11(19)	38(81)
Metastases to the lymph nodes		**
Negative	20(54)	17(46)
Positive	12(25)	36(75)
Total	32(37.7)	53(62.3)

*:P<0.05,**:P<0.01. P value based on the chi-square test or Students't test.

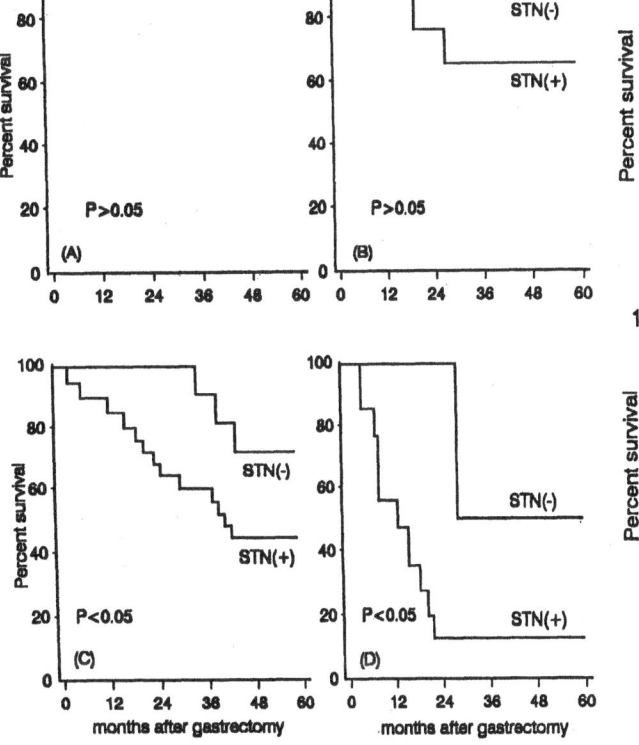

Fig 1. Five-year survival of patients by stage and STN status
(A) StageI,(B) StageII,(C) StageIII,(D) StageIV.

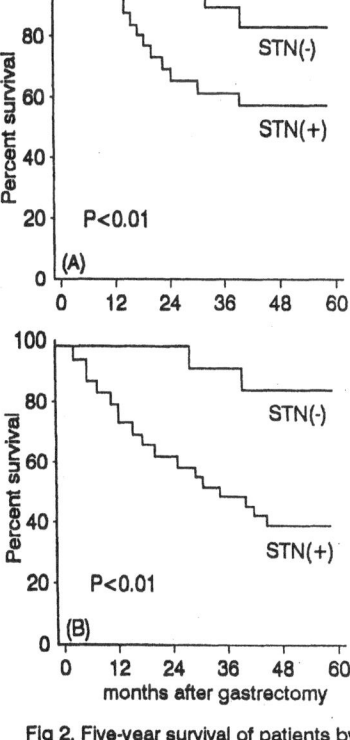

Fig 2. Five-year survival of patients by histologic category and STN status
(A) Differentiated adenocarcinoma
(B) Undifferentiated adenocarcinoma

showed a signficantlly low frequent expression of STN compared with more advanced cases(P<0.05). STN positive tumors were observed in nine of 23 patients in tumor invasion was limited to the mucosa or submucosa. This rate increased in proportion to invasion deeper layers(P<0.01). STN positive tumors were associated with a higher incidence of lymph node metastasis(P<0.01). When 5-year survival was analyzed according to both stages and STN status (Fig.1), patients with STN positive tumor had a worse prognosis in stage III (70% versus 43.5%; P<0.05) and stage IV (50% versus 11.4%; P<0.05). Fig 2 demonstrate the influence of tumor histologic type on overall survival. Within each histologic group, the 5-year survival was worse in patients with STN positive tumors(P<0.01).

DISCUSSION

Tumorigenic transformation is almost invariablly associated with altered glycosylation of glycoproteins or glycolipids in cell membranes(5). These changes are thought to be associated with altered cell adhesion and development of invasive and metastatic properties (6). Since the first observation of STN expression on tumor tissues by Kjelden et al, several histochemical and serologic studies have revealed correlation between the expression of STN and histologic grade, tumor size and advancing stage (7-9). In present study, we demonstrated 53 out 0f 85 patients (62%) expressed positive STN in gastric cancers. The stage I and stage II disease showed a significantlly low frequence of STN expression compared with more advanced cases, and the highly positive expression was observed following advanced of the disease. Thus, the STN expression may be a marker of invasion, possibly reflecting the cancer cells aggresiveness. We have demonstrate that patients with positive expression of STN in gastric cancer had a shorter survival time than patients with negatives. The similar results have been shown in colon and ovarian carcinomas, respectively (8,10). The lower survival rate of patients with higher STN expression may reflect their higher tumor burden. The apparently better prognosis of patients with early gastric cancers can simply interpreted to be due to the less tumor burden, but it is difficult to expain a reason why the STN negative, advanced cancers showed a relatively longer survival time. This cannot be simply attributed to the sizes or histological types of tumor. Patients with STN positive cancers in stage III and stage IV, mostly died during the early postoperative period. This antigen may be of considerable importance in deciding whether postresection patients require further therapy or not.

REFERENCES

1. Kjeldsen t, Clausen H, Hirohashi S. Preparation and characterization of monoclonal antibodies directed to the tumor-associated O-linked sialosyl-2-6 -N-acetylgalactosaminyl(sialosyl-Tn)epitope. Cancer Res 48:4361-4367
2. Inoue M, Ton SM, Ogawa H, Tanizawa O. Expression of Tn and sialyl-Tn antigens in tumor tissues of the ovary. Am J Clin Pathol 96:711-716
3. Itzkowitz SH, Yuan M, Montgomery CK. Expression of Tn, sialosyl-Tn, and T antigen in colon cancer. Cancer Res 49:197-204
4. Japannese Research Society for Gastric Cancer. The general rules for the gastric cancer study in surgery and pathology. Jpn J Surg 11:127-145
5. Smets LA, Van Beek WP. Carbohydrates of the tumor cell surface. Biochim Bio phys Acta 783:237-249
6. Altevogt P, Fogel M, Cheingsong PR, Dennis J, Robinson P,Schirrmacher V. Different patterns of lectin binding cell surface sialylation detected on related high and low metastatic tumor cell lines. Cancer Res 43:5138-5144
7. Kobayashi H, Terao T, Kawashima Y. Clinical evaluation of circulating serum sialyl Tn antigen level in patients with epithelial ovarian cancer. J Clin Oncol 9:983-987
8. Kobayashi H, Terao T, Kawashima Y. Circulating serum STN antigen as a prognostic marker in epithlial ovarian cancer. Jpn J Cancer Chemother 18:1651-1655
9. Motoo Y, Kawakami H, Watanabe H. Serum sialyl-Tn antigen level in patients with digestive cancers. Oncology 48:321-326
10. Itzkowitz SH, Bloom EJ, Kokal WA, Modin G, Hakomari SI, Kim YS. Sialosyl-Tn. A novel mucin antigen associated with prognosis in colorectal cancer patients. Cancer 66:1960-1966

Expression of Sialosyl Tn Antigen in Gastric Cancer

Takashi Yamada, Akihiko Watanabe, Hidetomo Sawada, Yukishige Yamada, Tomoaki Yano, Naoto Ueyama, Yoshihide Shino, Masahiro Tanase, and Hiroshige Nakano

The First Department of Surgery, Nara Medical University, Kashihara, Nara, 634 Japan

ABSTRACT

Expression of sialosyl Tn antigen (STN) of surgically resected spesimens in human gastric cancers, using the monoclonal antibody (TKH-2), was evaluated immunohistochemically in 42 patients measured serum STN level and in 45 patients with advanced cancer followed over five years after gastrectomy. Staining intensity was graded as follows: (-), less than 5% of cancer lesion; (+), 5-50%; (++), more than 50%. STN was mainly stained in cell membranes and cytoplasm, and the positive rate was 57.2%, which was higher than that of serum STN level. The positive rate of STN in differentiated adenocarcinoma was higher than in undifferentiated adenocarcinoma. Advanced cases indicated a tendency to express in more cancer lesion than did early cases. The estimate 5-year survival in advanced cases was better in negative cases than in positive cases. These results suggest that STN is available for a useful tumor marker in advanced case of gastric cancer.

KEY WORDS: Sialosyl Tn antigen, Gastric cancer, immunohistochemistry

INTRODUCTION

Many tumor assosiated antigens, especially carbohydrate antigens, are clinically used as an index for the diagnosis and prognosis of patients with cancer. A new carbohydrate antigen, Sialosyl Tn antigen, has undergone a change in core structure and therefore has a different structure from other carbohydrate antigens. The structure of sialosyl Tn antigen has the sialylated form of a glycoprotein with N-acetyl galactose linked O-glycosdically to serin or threonin(1). Recently, MoAb TKH-2 directed to sialosyl Tn antigen was generated by immunization with bovine submaxillary mucin. With this MoAb, immunodetective studies for gynecologic and colorectal cancer have been conducted, some of which have demonstrated its usefullness as a marker for monitoring of cancer and the correlation with prognosis.(2-4) However, little information on the characteristics of sialosyl Tn antigen for the detection of gastric cancer is available, and little is known about its clinical value and its relevance for the prognosis of patients with gastric cancer. In this study, we examined the immunohistochemical reactivity for sialosyl Tn antigen, using this antibody, compared with clinical factors and prognosis.

MATERIALS AND METHODS

We obtained 42 tissues of primary gastric cancer resected surgically between October 1990 and July 1991 at the First department of Surgery, Nara medical University Hospital, and preoperative serum STN antigen level were measured for all of these cases. The clinicopathological data of 42 patients with primary gastric cancer follows as; Stage I: 19 cases; Stage II: 4; Stage III: 13; Stage IV: 6. These were classified according to the general rules for gastric cancer studies proposed by the Japanese Research Society for Gastric Cancer. These stages were classified according to four factors; peritoneal dissemination, liver metastasis, lymphnode involvement, and serosal invasion(5). Circulating serum STN antigen concentration(U/ml) was determined with a competitive radioimmunoassay Kit (Otsuka Laboratories,Tokushima,Japan),and we defined more than 45U/ml as elevation. In addition, we also obtained tissues from 45 cases followed over 5years after curative operation between May 1979 and March 1987. These tissue sample were fixed in 10% formalin, embedded in paraffin and cut into 5μm thick serial sections.

ANTIBODY

Monoclonal antibody TKH-2 (mouse IgG1) used in this study was generalized as an antibody for detection of sialosyl Tn antigen. This antibody was raised against ovine submaxillary mucin.

IMMUNOHISTOCHEMISTRY

Localization of sialosyl Tn antigen was determined immunohistochemically with the avidin-viotin peroxidase method (ABC) (6). Briefly, the tissue sections were deparaffinized with xylene, and washed in 0.05mol/l phosphate buffer saline (PBS) PH7.4 for 10 min. To block endogenous peroxidase, the tissue sections were immersed in a 0.3% H_2O_2/methanol solution for 30 min, and washed for 20 min. Then 5% normal rabbit serum was applied to inhibit nonspecific binding for 20 min, and TKH-2 as primary monoclonal antibody was applied for 2 hours at room temperature. After washing in PBS, the sections were incubated for 20 min with biotinylated anti-mouse IgG. They were then treated with avidin peroxidase complex for 2 hours, further washed for 10 min and incubated with 3-3 diaminobenzidine. Finally, after counterstaining with meyer Hematoxylin, they were dehydrated in graded ethanol and xylene, and mounted.
The localization of the antigen was investigated without knowledge of clinico pathological information of each cases. Staining intesty was graded as follows: (-), less than 5% of cancer lesion ; (+), 5-50% ; (++), more than 50%.

RESULTS

Expression of STN in gastric cancer tissues was recognized in 24 of the 42 cases (57.2%), and in seven cases of these (16.7%) was expressed in over 50% of the cancer lesions. Expression in non-cancerous lesions was localized in intestinal metaplasia but absent in other normal tissues. In cancer tissues, STN was mainly expressed on cell membranes and in cytoplasma, and also on extracellular mucin . Expression in signet-ring cells and cancer cells with lymphatic vessels invasion could be occasionally found in undifferentiated carcinomas. The relationship between expression of STN antigen and histological cancer type is shown in Table 1.The positive rate of expression in differentiated adenocarcinomas was higher than in undifferentiated ones($p<0.05$). Two of three cases with mucinous carcinoma showed strong staining. There was no statistically significant correlation among individual stages, but advanced cases indicated a tendency to express in more cancer lesion than did early cases. All cases showing strong staining were advanced cases with lymphnode metastasis or serosal invasion. (table 2 3)

Table 1. Expression of STN according to histological type

Histological type	No. of cases	Expression of STN (%) (-)	(+)	(++)
Differentiated	23	7 (30.4)	11 (47.8)	5 (21.7)
			69.6 *	
Undifferentiated	16	10 (62.5)	6 (37.5)	0 (0)
			37.5 *	
Others	3	1 (0.0)	0 (0)	2(66.7)

* : p<0.05

Table 2. Expression of STN according to stage in gastric cancer

stage	No. of cases	Expression of STN (%) (-)	(+)	(++)
I	19	8 (42.1)	11 (57.9)	0 (0)
II	4	2 (50.0)	2 (50.0)	0 (0)
III	13	6 (46.2)	2 (15.4)	5 (38.5)
IV	6	2 (33.3)	2 (33.3)	2 (33.3)

The positive case in serum level was one of 18 cases (5.6%) with (-) immunohistochemically, one of 17 cases (5.9%) with (+) and six of 7 cases (85.7%) with (++). The average of serum antigen level was 27.1±11.5U/ml ,24.5±15.4U/ml and 413.7±796.9U/ml for (-), (+) and (++), and (++) case was significantly higher than (-) case ($p<o.o 5$). Overall 5-year survival of patients with STN positive tumor was 35.4%, whereas that with negative was 59.2%. STN positive case was poor prognosis compared with negative case($0.05<p<0.1$). (Fig1)

Table 3. Expression of STN according to depth of invasion , lymphnode metastasis

	No. of cases	Expression of STN (%)		
		(-)	(+)	(++)
depth of invasion				
m,sm	21	10 (47.6)	11 (52.4)	0 (0)
pm<	21	8 (38.1)	6 (28.6)	7 (33.3)
lymphnode metastasis				
n(-)	21	11 (52.4)	10 (47.6)	0 (0)
n(+)	21	7 (33.3)	7 (33.3)	7 (33.3)

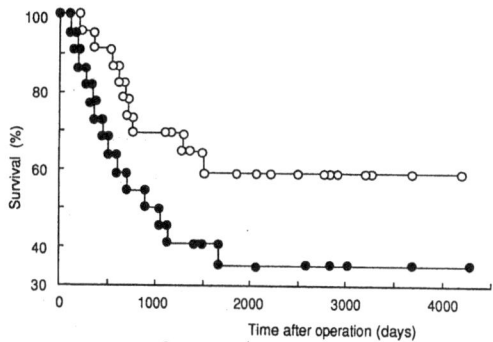

O : STN negative. ● : STN positive.

fig 1.Postoperative survival of patients with gastric cancer (stage III) in relation to the expression of STN

DISCUSSION

STN is considered to be a tumor associated antigen with cancer specificity with little expression in normal tissues, and in this study we observed the expression of STN only in the intestinal metaplasia in noncancerous tissue. The staining pattern for gastric cancer tissue was in the cell membrane and cytoplasm, similar to that for colon cancer as reported(3). Previous report indicated that the expression of STN presented in the transitional mucosa in colon cancer, suggesting the expression of carbohydrate antigens such as STN is associated with the precancerous state(3). STN is expected to be useful as a marker for carcinomatous peritonitis and to be strongly associated with undifferentiated carcinoma. However, there may also be an association between STN and differentiated carcinoma, because in this study the expression rate of differentiated carcinomas is higher than that of undifferentiated ones and STN is expressed in almost all of the intestinal metaplasia. Furthermore, we investigated the relation between the immunohistochemical expression of STN and prognosis for the cases with the same advanced stage, stage III. Our study indicats that the expression of STN in gastric cancer is related to poor prognosis. The expression of STN was not associated with other factors, such as age, sex or tumor location. These observations suggest that the expression of STN may reflect malignant potential and prognosis for gastric cancer. In conclusion, We expected that sialosyl Tn antigen will be useful as an index of malignancy and for predicting poor prognosis in patients with gastric cancer.

REFERENCES

1. Kjeldsen T, Clausen H, Hirohashi S, Ogawa T, Iijima H, Hakomori S. (1988) Preparation and characterization of monoclonal antibodies directed to the tumor-associated O-linked sialosyl-2-6 -N-acetylgalactosaminyl (sialosyl-Tn) epitope. Cancer Res 48:2214-2220.
2. Inoue M, Ogawa H, Nakanishi K(1990) Clinical value of sialosyl Tn antigen in patients with gynecologic tumors. Obstet Gynecol 75:1032-1036.
3. Itzkowitz SH, Yuan M, Montgomery CK, Kjeldsen T, Takahashi HK, Bigbee WL, Kim YS (1989) Expression of Tn, sialosyl-Tn, and T antigens in human colon cancer. Cancer Res 49:197-204.
4. Itzkowitz SH, Bloom EJ, Kokal W, Modin G, Hakomori S, Kim YS (1990) Sialosyl Tn: a novel mucin antigen associated with prognosis in colorectal cancer patients. Cancer (Phila.), 66:1960-1966.
5. Japanese Reseach Society for Gastric Cancer.(1981) The general rules for the gastric cancer study. Jpn J Surg 11:127-145
6. Hsu SM, Raine L, Fanger H.(1981) Use of avidin-biotin-peroxidase complex(ABC) in immunoperoxidase techniques: a comparison between ABC and unlabeled antibody PAP procedures. J Histochem Cytochem 29: 577-580.

Immunohistochemical Evaluation of α-Catenin, Cadherin-Associated Intercellular Protein, Expression in Human Gastric Cancer

S. MATSUI[1], H. SHIOZAKI[1], M. INOUE[1], S. TAMURA[1], H. OKA[1], Y. DOKI[1], K. IIHARA[1], T. KADOWAKI[1], T. IWAZAWA[1], K. SHIMAYA[1], A. NAGAFUCHI[2], S. TSUKITA[2], and T. MORI[1]

[1]Department of Surgery II, Osaka University Medical School, Osaka, 553 Japan
[2]Department of Information Physiology, National Institute for Physiological Sciences, Okazaki, Aichi, 444 Japan

ABSTRACT

Immunohistochemical study of α-catenin, cadherin associated intercellular protein, was performed in 36 human gastric cancer tissues. All normal epithelium strongly expressed α-catenin as well as E-cadherin, while 67% of the tumor had reduced expression of α-catenin. Compared to E-cadherin expression, α-catenin expression was similar in 26 cases (72%), but weaker in 9 cases (25%). The reduction of α-catenin expression was associated with dedifferentiation, and infiltrative growth. These results indicated that the reduction of α-catenin expression may play a crucial role for cancer invasion through down-regulation of E-cadherin function.

KEY WORDS: α-catenin, immunohistochemistry, gastric cancer

INTRODUCTION

In epithelial tissues, E-cadherin (E-cad) plays a major role in intercellular physical adhesion [1]. Recent studies suggest that cadherins require anchoring to the actin-based cytoskelton via catenins through its cytoplasmic domain, for exhibiting the cell-cell binding function [2-4]. Therefore, catenins are considered to modulate the function of cadherin, and the loss of catenins may induce impairing of cadherin-mediated cell-cell adhesion [5,6]. In order to clarify the correlation of α-catenin (α-cat) molecule with invasion of human cancer cells in vivo, we evaluated the expression using immunohistochemical technique, and analyzed the relationship between its staining and clinicopathological factors. Furthermore, we investigated the relationship between α-cat and E-cad expression in surgically resected human gastric cancer tissue.

PATIENTS AND METHODS.

Patients

Frozen tumor samples were obtained from consecutive 36 patients with gastric cancer in department of Surgery-II, Osaka University Medical School . The age of the patients ranged from 28 to 82 years (mean, 59.8). All patients had not received anticancer therapy prior to the operation.

Antibodies and Immunohistochemical Procedure.

Immunostaining for E-cad and α-cat was performed by the avidin-biotin-perioxidase complex method as described previously [7]. The sections were fixed with 3.6% paraformaldehyde. Anti-human E-cad mAb (HECD-1) diluted 1:1000 and anti-human α-cat mAb (α18) diluted 1: 5 were used for primary antibodies.

Evaluation of E-cad and α-cat Staining.

The intensity of E-cad and α-cat staining for cancer cells was compared with that for normal epithelium. The cancer cells whose E-cad and α-cat staining were strong as normal epithelial cells were defined as positive. The cancer cells which show much weaker or negative staining were defined as negative. The grade of E-cad and α-cat expression of the tumor was semiquantitatively evaluated according to the proportion of positive cells. When more than 90%, between 10% to 90%, and less than 10% of the cancer cells were positive, the tumors were evaluated as positive (+), heterogeneous (+-), and negative (-), respectively.

Histopathological Findings and Statistical Analysis.

A consecutive section from each specimen was stained with haematoxylin and eosin for histological evaluation. The statistical analysis was performed comparing (+), (+-) and (-) by chi-square test.

RESULTS

Immunohistochemical Reactivity of α-cat.

α-cat and E-cad were strongly expressed in all the noncancerous epithelium at cell-cell boundaries, but α-cat was weakly detected in fibrobrasts and smooth muscle cells. Thirty-six gastric cancers showed various expressions of α-cat, and 12 tumors were classified into uniformly positive (+), 9 heterogeneous (+-) and 15 uniformly negative (-) according to our criteria.

Correlation of α-cat Immunostaining with Clinicopathological Factors.

Table1 shows the relationship of α-cat expression to histological findings. Histological type was divided into well, moderately or poorly differentiated carcinoma. The frequency of (+) tumor was higher in well differentiated carcinoma (82%, 9/11), whereas low in moderately (8%, 1/12) or poorly differentiated tumours (15%, 2/13). On the other hand, (-) tumor was not observed in well differentiated carcinoma, but 33% (4/12) of moderately differentiated carcinoma and 85% (11/13) of poorly differentiated carcinoma were assessed as negative. Thus, the reduction of the α-cat staining was significantly associated with dedifferentiation (p < 0.01). Moreover, α-cat expression was also associated with the invasion pattern (INF) of cancer cells, but not with depth of invasion.

Correlation between α-cat and E-cad Immunostaining.

Table 2 shows the correlation between the two molecules. On our criteria, α-cat expression was similar to E-cad in 26 cases (72%). All the other tumors with one exception (9 cases ; 25%) lost α-cat predominantely, compared to E-cad (Fig. 1A B).

Table 1.
Relationship between α-cat and clinicopathological factors

	α-cat expression					
	preserved	reduced				
	(+)	(±)	(-)	subtotal		
histological type						
well	9 (82%)	2	0	2	(18%)	
mod	1 (8%)	7	4	11	(92%)	※
por	2 (15%)	0	11	11	(85%)	
INF α	3 (75%)	0	1	1	(25%)	
β	9 (41%)	6	7	13	(59%)	※ ※
γ	0 (0%)	3	7	10	(100%)	
depth of invasion						
m, sm	7 (64%)	2	2	4	(36%)	
pm	3 (33%)	1	5	6	(67%)	
ss, se, si	2 (13%)	6	8	14	(87%)	

※ p < 0.01
※ ※ p < 0.05

Table 2.
Relationship between α-cat and E-cad expression

		α-cat expression		
		(+)	(±)	(-)
E-cad	(+)	11	2	2
expression	(±)	-	7	5
	(-)	1	-	8

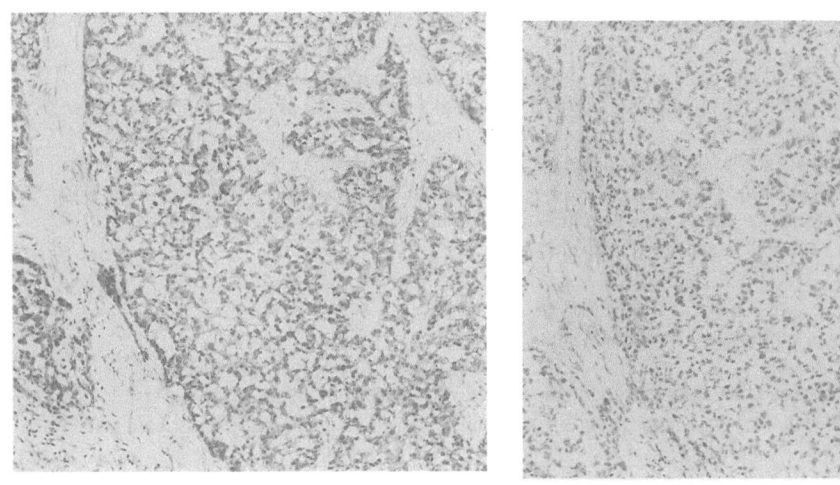

(A) E-cad expression (+)   (B) α-cat expression (-)

Fig.1A B poorly differentiated adenocarcinoma.

DISCUSSION

Our results suggest that down-regulation of α-cat expression as well as E-cad was a characteristic for gastric carcinoma. However, further investigations are required to determine whether α–cat expression may modify the invasive / metastatic potential of cancer cells.

REFERENCES

1. Takeichi M (1988) The cadherins : cell-cell adhesion molecules controling animal morphogenesis. Development 102 : 639-655
2. Hirano S , Nose A , Hatta K , Kawakami A , Takeichi M (1987) Calcium-dependent cell-cell adhesion molecule (cadherins) subclass specificities and possible involvement of actin bundles. J Cell Biol 106 : 2501-2510
3. Nagafuchi A and Takeichi M (1988) Cell binding function of E-cadherin is regulated by the cytoplasmic domain. EMBO J 7 : 3679-3684
4. Ozawa M , Baribault H , Kemler R (1989) The cytoplasmic domain of the cell adhesion molecule uvomorulin associated with three independent proteins structurally related in different species. EMBO J 8 : 1711-1717
5. Shimoyama Y, Nagafuchi A, Fujita S, Gotoh M, Takeichi M, Tsukita S, Hirohashi S (1992) Cadherin dysfunction in human cancer cell line : possible involvement of loss of α-catenin expression in reduced cell-cell adhesiveness. Cancer Res 52 : 5770-5774
6. Nagafuchi A, Takeichi M, Tsukita S (1991) The 102 kd cadherin-associated protein : similarity to vinculin and posttranscriptional regulation of expression. Cell 65 : 849-857
7. Hsu SM, Raine L, Fanger H (1981) Use of avidin-biotin-peroxidase complex (ABC) in immunoperioxidase techniques : a comparison between ABC and unlabeled antibody (PAP) procedures. J. Histochem Cytochem 29: 577-580

Expression of Tenascin in Gastric Cancers and Their Clinicopathological Features

SHIGEO OKAMURA, YOSHINORI HAMADA, KANJI TANAKA, YASUSHI NAKANE, and KOSHIRO HIOKI

The Second Department of Surgery, Kansai Medical University, Moriguchi, Osaka, 570 Japan

ABSTRACT

We investigated the relationship between tenascin (TN) expression and clinicopathological features in 185 patients with gastric cancers. Histological sections of resected tissues were immunostained using the indirect immunoperoxidase method with mouse monoclonal antibody to TN, and cases with more than 50% of the tumor stroma demonstrating binding were classified as positive. TN was positive in 37 cases (20%). In this positive group 81.1% were found to be of differentiated type and the mean age was 64.9 years old, these values being significantly higher as compared with the negative group. These results suggest that TN expression may be related to intestinal metaplasia.

KEY WORDS: tenascin, extracellular matrix, gastric cancer

INTRODUCTION

TN, an extracellular matrix glycoprotein, was first described as myotendinous antigen by Chiquet and Fambrough [1] in 1984. Although its biological function is unclear at present, TN is considered to play an important role in cancer growth [2] and invasion [3]. Recently, a number of reports have suggested its potential as an useful marker for predicting the prognosis of patients with colonic [4] and breast cancers [5]. However, TN expression in gastric cancers has only attracted limited attention, prompting the present investigation of possible relationships with clinicopathological features.

MATERIALS AND METHODS

Surgical materials from 185 patients with gastric cancers undergoing operation in our Department from 1982 to 1991 was investigated. Pathologic diagnoses were made according to the General Rules for Gastric Cancer Study (11th Edition), the Japanese Research Society for Gastric Cancer. The removed tumor tissues were fixed in 10% formalin for paraffin sections. After being deparaffinized, sections were stained by routine preparation of the indirect immunoperoxidase method using mouse monoclonal antibody to TN (BIOHIT, Finland). The cases where more than 50% of the tumor stroma was immunostained by TN were classified as positive. The data were analyzed using the chi-square test and Student's t test.

RESULTS

Localization of TN

Positive TN staining was generally recognized in the muscularis mucosae, muscularis propria and blood vessel walls, and as to be delicate bands in lymphoid follicles. The lamina propria mucosae was negative and areas of ulceration intensely positive. In cancerous lesions TN was distributed chiefly in the extracellular matrix of the differentiated carcinomas (Fig.1) and was only rarely present in that of the undifferentiated carcinomas (Fig.2).

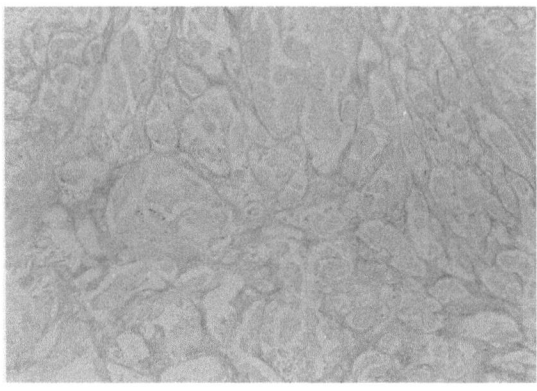 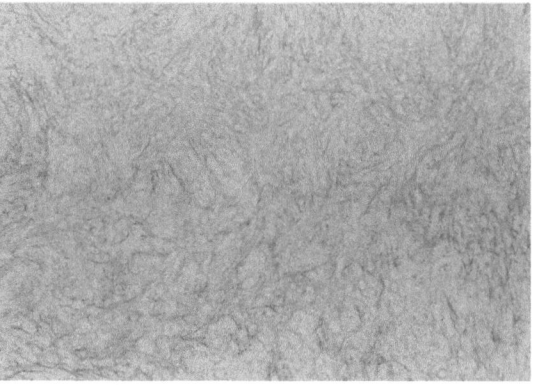

Fig.1 TN expression in papillary adenocarcinoma

Fig.2 TN expression in poorly differentiated adenocarcinoma

Correlation between TN expression and clinicopathological features

TN was positive in 37 cases (20%) and negative in 148 cases (80%) as shown in Table 1. The mean age was 64.9 years old in the positive group and 59.0 years old in the negative group, the difference being significant for total and male patients. With regard to the location of primary cancers antral tumors were found at a significantly higher rate than in other location (Table 2).

Table 1. Relationship between average age and sex of patients and tenascin expression

Patient data	Negative	Positive
number of patients	148 (80%)	37 (20%)
male	93 (80.1%)	22 (19.9%)
female	55 (78.6%)	15 (11.4%)
age	59.0 ± 11.8	64.9 ± 10.9*
male	60.0 ± 11.1	65.9 ± 12.0**
female	57.3 ± 12.6	63.5 ± 9.1

* $P < 0.01$, ** $P < 0.05$

Table 2. Relationship between tumor location and tenascin expression

Location	Negative	Positive	Positive rate
A	62 (41.8%)	24 (64.8%)	27.9% ⎤
M	57 (38.5%)	8 (21.6%)	12.3% ⎥ *
C	26 (17.5%)	5 (13.5%)	16.1% ⎦

* $P < 0.05$

TN expression rate was highest in papillary adenocarcinomas and was higher in differentiated as compared with undifferentiated type gastric cancers (Table 3). TN expression rate tended to be higher according to the degree of cancer infiltration. Borrmann 1 and Borrmann 2 type gastric cancers predominated in the positive group and Borrmann 3 and Borrmann 4 type in the negative group. Serum carcinoembryonic antigen (CEA) level (normal range, 0 - 5 ng/ml) was significantly higher in the positive group (Table 4), but no relationship was observed between CEA staining and TN staining by immunohistochemistry. No relationship was observed for lymph node involvement, tumor size, invasion into lymph vessels, invasion into veins , stage grouping and survival rate.

Table 3. Relationship between histological type and tenascin expression

Histology	Negative	Positive	Positive rate	
pap	12 (8.1%)	10 (27.0%)	45.4%	
tub1	64 (43.2%)	2 (5.4%)	13.3%	
tub2	4 (2.7%)	16 (43.2%)	20.0%	*
muc	44 (29.7%)	3 (8.1%)	42.8%	
por	11 (7.4%)	4 (10.8%)	8.3%	
sig		1 (2.7%)	8.3%	

* P < 0.05

Table 4. Relationship between serum CEA level and tenascin expression

	Negative	Positive
CEA values (ng/ml)	3.6 ± 6.9	23.7 ± 91.1 *
CEA positive rate	12.8%	29.7%

* P < 0.05

DISCUSSION

In the present study, investigation of the relationship between TN expression and clinicopathological features of gastric cancers revealed a significantly higher proportion of differentiated gastric carcinomas than in negative cases. Earlier a high rate in squamous cell carcinomas was reported [6]. In addition, TN expression was found to be significantly associated with an antral location and greater patient age. These results suggest that TN may be related to intestinal metaplasia. Sugawara et al. [4] reported that they observed very strong TN expression in all cases of non–metastatic colonic carcinoma studied and noted the presence of a dense TN accumulation to correlate well with a good prognoses. However, in our study, no differences were observed with regard to survival rate or degree of lymphatic involvement rate between TN positive and negative groups. Thus, TN can not be recommended as a marker to predict the prognosis of gastric cancer patients. While we found the serum CEA levels to be significantly higher in the TN positive group, as compared with the TN negative group, no relationship was evident between CEA and TN expression by immunohistochemical staining. The reason for this is unclear but it is well known that a high incidence of differentiated gastric cancers produce CEA. One further finding of interest in the present study was the TN expression in the lymphoid follicles. This result suggests that TN might play some role in immunoreactions. Further investigations are closely required, to clarify the biological functions of TN.

REFERENCES

1. Chiquet M, Fambrough MC (1984) Chick myotendinous antigen. 1. A monoclonal antibody as a marker for tendon and muscle morphogenesis. J Cell Biol 98 : 1926 – 1936
2. Chiquet – Ehrismann R, Mackie EJ, Pearson CA, Sakakura T (1986) Tenascin : an extracellular matrix protein involved in tissue interactions during fetal development and oncogenesis. Cell 47 : 131 – 139
3. Chiquet – Ehrismann R, Kalla P, Pearson CA, Beck K, Chiquet M (1988) Tenascin interferes with fibronectin action. Cell 53 : 383 – 390
4. Sugawara I, Hirakoshi J, Masunaga A, Itoyama S, Sakakura T (1991) Reduced tenascin expression in colonic carcinoma with lymphogenous metastasis. Invasion Metastasis 11 : 325 – 331
5. Shoji T, Kamiya T, Tsubura A, Hamada Y, Hatana T, Hioki K, Morii S (in press) Tenascin staining possibility and the survival of patients with invasive breast carcinoma. J Surg Research
6. Anbazhagan R, Sakakura T, Gusterson BA (1990) The distribution of immuno – reactive tenascin in the epithelial – mesenchymal areas of benign and malignant squamous epithelia. Virchows Archiv B Cell Pathol 59 : 59 – 63

Study of a Synthesized New Carbohydrate Antigen in Gastro-Intestinal Cancers

Yoshito Yamashita[1], Yong-Suk Chung[1], Tetsuji Sawada[1], Yasuyuki Kondo[1], Kwang Sa Kim[1], Akimasa Inui[1], Masahiro Okuno[1], Ryuichi Horie[2], Takashi Saito[2], Keiichi Murayama[2], and Michio Sowa[1]

[1]The First Department of Surgery, Osaka City University Medical School, Osaka, 545 Japan
[2]Biotechnology Research Laboratory, TOSOH Corporation, Kanagawa, Japan

ABSTRACT

In this study, a novel monoclonal antibody (F1α-75) directed to a carbohydrate antigen (F1α), which was chemically synthesized, was raised and the expression of F1α was evaluated in gastric and colon cancers. The core structure of F1α is a mucin-type carbohydrate chain which has never been reported before (Galβ1→4GlcNAcβ1→6GalNAcα1→Cer). As a matter of fact, F1α was found in human cancerous tissues of stomach and colon, but not in normal tissues thereof. The positive rate of F1α was 79.0% in 81 gastric cancers and 38.4% in 73 colon cancers. Among histologic types of gastric cancer, the positive rate of F1α was highest for poorly differentiated adenocarcinoma and low for well differentiated tubular adenocarcinoma. The results suggested that F1α may be a novel type of tumor marker which has a high specificity for gastric cancers and that additional cancer-associated antigens can possibly be found by using this approach.

KEY WORDS: synthesized antigen, monoclonal antibody, gastric cancer

INTRODUCTION

Recently, many monoclonal antibodies have been produced against various kinds of cancer cells and many cancer-associated carbohydrate antigens on cancer cell membrane were found. But few of these carbohydrate chains have been chemically defined, moreover, they have ill-defined or even questionable cancer-specificity. Therefore, novel monoclonal antibodies directed to the chemically synthesized carbohydrate antigens were raised in order to find novel carbohydrate antigens, which structures have been defined [1]. The structure of the synthesized carbohydrate antigen (F1α) which was used in this study has been predicted from previously defined cancer-associated antigens, being unique and not known before. By using a monoclonal antibody (F1α-75) directed to F1α, the expression of F1α was immunohistochemically evaluated in human cancerous and normal tissues of stomach and colon.

MATERIALS AND METHODS

Synthesized antigen

The core structure of the chemically synthesized antigen (F1α) is a mucin-type carbohydrate chain, which has been predicted from previously defined cancer-associated antigens and never been reported (Fig.1). BALB/C mice were immunized with this antigen, spleen cells of the mice were fused with mouse myeloma cells and a hybridoma which produces the antibody (F1α-75) directed to F1α was obtained. The immunogloblin class of F1α-75 is IgM.

Tissues

Eighty-one formalin-fixed and paraffin-embedded gastric cancer and 73 colon cancer specimens were obtained from the First Department of Surgery, Osaka City University Medical School, Osaka, Japan. The gastric cancers comprised 38 poorly differentiated adenocarcinomas, 17 moderately differentiated tubular adenocarcinomas, 7 well differentiated tubular adenocarcinomas, 11 papillary adenocarcinomas, 2 signet ring cell carcinomas, 5 mucinous carcinomas, and 1 undifferentiated carcinoma.

Immunohistochemical staining

Sections (3μm) of paraffin-embedded tissue were deparaffinized with xylene and ethanol and sequentially incubated for 90 minutes with the primary antibody, F1α-75. Following this, immunohistochemistry was performed by using the reagents for streptavidin-biotin immuno-peroxidase, Maxitags (Shandon/Lipshow). After completion of the entire immune reaction, the slides were counterstained with hematoxylin, dehydrate, cleared, and mounted.
The intensity of immunostaining was graded as follows: -, no cancer cells immunostained; +, less than 10% of cancer cells immunostained; ++, 10~50% of cancer cells immunostained; +++, more than 50% of cancer cells immunostained.

Gal β1 → 4GlcNAc β1 → 6GalNAc1 α → Cer

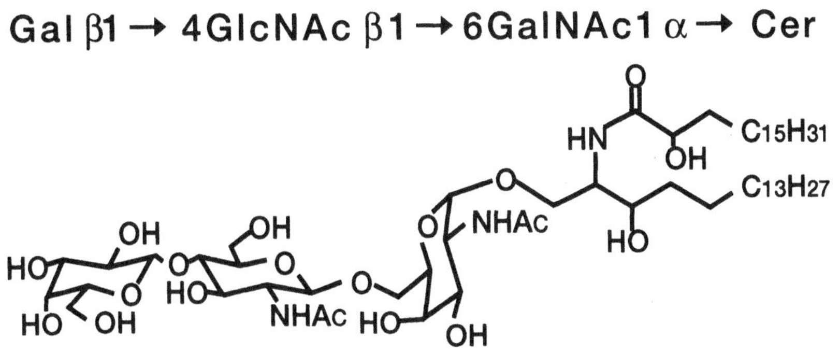

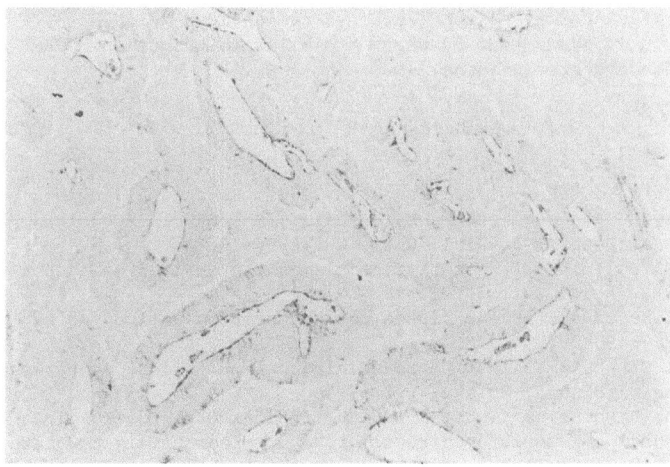

Fig.1 Structure of the chemically synthesized carbohydrate antigen (F1α)

Fig.2 Microphotography of the resected specimen showing the expression of F1α

RESULT

F1α was found in human cancerous tissues of stomach and colon (Fig.2). The immunohisto-chemical expression rate of F1α was 79.0% in 81 gastric cancers and 38.4% in 73 colon cancers. F1α-75 was very strongly positive (+++) in 24.8% gastric cancer and 1.4% colon cancers and was strongly positive (++) in 25.6% gastric cancers and 16.4% colon cancers and weakly positive (+) in 28.6% gastric cancers and 20.5% colon cancers (Table 1). There was a variation in the localization of F1α, thus, F1α was present in the luminal surface of the malignant tubules or in the cytoplasm of the tumor cells and was also found in the stroma or luminal exudate. This antigen was absent in normal tissues of stomach and colon. When relating to the histological types of gastric cancer, the expression rate of F1α was highest for poorly differentiated adenocarcinoma and low for well differentiated tubular adenocarcinoma (Table 2).

Table 1. Expression of F1α in gastric and colon cancers

	+	++	+++	total
Gastric cancer	28.6	25.6	24.8	79.0
Colon cancer	20.5	16.5	1.4	38.4

(%)

Table 2. Expression of F1α in relation to the histological types of gastric cancer

	+	++	+++	total
poorly dif. ad.	31.6	21.8	31.6	85.0
moderately dif. ad.	22.2	38.9	16.7	77.8
well dif. ad.	27.7	16.7	16.7	61.1
papillary ad.	25.0	33.3	16.7	75.0

dif. differentiated (%)
ad. adenocarcinoma

DISCUSSION

Incomplete synthesis of the cabohydrate chains during the course of a malignant transformation has been reported by Hakomori [2]. A method to obtain monoclonal antibodies using cancer cells as an immunogen was established [3] and many cancer-associated carbohydrate antigens have been found. However, the structures of few of these antigens have been determined to date [4-6] because the monoclonal antibodies were raised against cancer cells but not well predefined target antigen. In the light of defined cancer-associated carbohydrate antigens, several novel structures of cancer-associated carbohydrate antigens which have never been reported yet can be imaged. In this study, a novel antigen of the same structure as predicted (F1α) was chemically synthesized and the monoclonal antibody directed to the antigen (F1α-75) was raised. As a matter of fact, F1α was found in human cancerous tissues of stomach and colon and especially, the immunohistochemical expression rate of F1α was high for gastric cancers. This antigen was absent in normal tissues of stomach and colon and it was surmised that F1α might be synthesized during the course of malignant transformation. F1α is a new type of cancer associated carbohydrate antigen which has a high specificity for gastric cancer. It seems that by using a similar technique one can discover other cancer-associated carbohydrate antigens.

REFERENCE

1. Shigeta K, Ito Y, Ogawa T, Kirihata Y, Hakomori S, Kannagi R (1987) Monoclonal antibodies directed to chemically synthesized lactogangliotetraosylceramide, a leukemia-associated antigen having a novel branching structure. J. Biol. Chem. 262:1358-1362
2. Hakomori S, Murakami WT (1968) Glycolipids of hamster fibroblasts and derived malignant-transformed cell lines. Proc. Natl. Acad. Sci. 59:254-261
3. Kohler G, Milstein C (1975) Continuous cultures of fused cells secreting antibody of predifined specificity. Nature 256:495-497
4. Magnani J, Brockhaus M, Smith D, Ginsburg V (1981) A monosialoganglioside is a monoclonal antibody-defined antigen of colon carcinoma, Science 212:55-56
5. Kannagi R, Nudelman E, Levery SB, Hakomori S (1982) A series of human erythrocyte glycosphingolipids reacting to the monoclonal antibody directed to a developmentally regulated antigen, SSEA-1, J. Biol. Chem. 257:14865-14873
6. Kjeldsen T, Clausen H, Hirohashi S, Ogawa T, Iijima H, Hakomori S (1988) Preparation and characterization of monoclonal antibodies directed to the tumor-associated O-linked sialosyl-2→6 α-N-acetylgalactosaminyl (Sialosyl-Tn) epitope. Cancer Res. 48:2214-2220

Histochemical Study of the Extra-Cellular Stroma in Gastric Cancer

T. Noguchi, Y. Uchida, M. Oya, N. Kubo, and S. Murakami

Second Department of Surgery, Oita Medical University, Hasama-machi, Oita-gun, Oita, 879-55 Japan

ABSTRACT

To elucidate the stromal characteristics in gastric carcinoma, we investigated the localization of some types of collagen fibers which are main fibrous comporments in the interstitial connective tissue and various proteoglicans such as hyaluronic acid (HS) and chondroitin sulfate (CS) using the immunohistochemical and enzymatic histochemical techniques.

INTRODUCTION

We have recently had more opportunities for early detections and treatments of gastric cancers with the development of diagnostic techniques, while progressive gastric cancers to which radical surgery is not applicable are still present. Among them, gastric scirrhous carcinoma show rapid progression and are difficult to be detected in early stage, consequently leading to extremely unfavorable therapeutic results [1] . The proliferation of scirrhous carcinoma is characterized by complication of hyperplasia of the connective tissue abundant in the interstitial tissue [2] , and it is of importance to identify the distribution of components in the connective tissue in order to elucidate the condition. In this study, we performed immunohistochemical and enzymatic histochemical investigations on distributions of collagen, as a main fibrous component in the interstitial connective tissue as well as various proteoglicans such as hyaluronic acid and chondroitin sulfate in the tissue of scirrhous carcinoma. Although conventionallysclerosing gastric cancer has been used as subject, non sclerosing gastric cancer (whose tissue type was signet ring cell carcinoma) was also studied for comparison in this study.

In general, proteoglycans in the tissue are recognized to be undetectable by routine enzyme-antibody method because of their trace amount. Therefore, we used IgG-gold-silver method to amplify immune responses [3] .

Table. 1
Alcian Blue Staining and Enzymatic Digestion Method

		pH 2.5	pH 1.0
Tumor cells		+++ → +++ Hyaluronidase	++ → ++ Chondroitinase
Interstitial tissus	Scirrhous	++ → +	++ → +
	normal	+ → +	± → ±

Table. 2
The Distribution of Chondroitin Sulfate Isomers

	Increased connective tissue	Infiltrated area by tumor cells
Dermatan sulfate	+++	++ (undifferentiated) + (differentiated)
6S-chondroitin sulfate	− ∼ ±	++ (undifferentiated) ± (differentiated)
4S-chondroitin sulfate	± ∼ +	+

MATERIALS AND METHOD

Fifteen cases with scirrhous carcinoma and five cases with the other types who had had operations at our department were emploved. Specimens were fixed in 10% formalin added 2% calcium acetate and PLP solution. Alcian blue-pH 1.0 and 2.5 staining and enzymatic digestion method (methods by actinomycotic hyaluronidase digestion, and by chondroitinase ABC and AC digestion) were combined to investigate the distribution of mucopolysaccharides [Table.1] .
The distribution of the chondroitin sulfate isomers such as 4S-CS, 6S-CS and DS were investigated immunohistochemically after enzymatic digestion of chondroitinase ABC. Different types of collagen fibers were stained by anti-collagen I, II, and IV antibody.

263

RESULTS

The immunohistochemistry for different types of collagen demonstrated marked hyperplasia of type I collagen especially in scirrhous carcinoma [Fig.1] . Promotion of moderate staining property of type II collagen was obserbed at the most infiltrative site of the undifferenciated carcinoma. Type IV collagen showed mainly staining property in proliferetive region of the tunica muscularis propriae. As for proteoglycan, both of hyaruronic acid and chondroitin sulfate were increased, and yet the latter was more marked. Regarding chondroitin sulfate isomers, 4S-CS and DS were present in dense connective tissue and 6S-CS in relatively coarse connective tissue of the region where cancer cells infiltrated [Table.2] [Fig.2.3.4] .

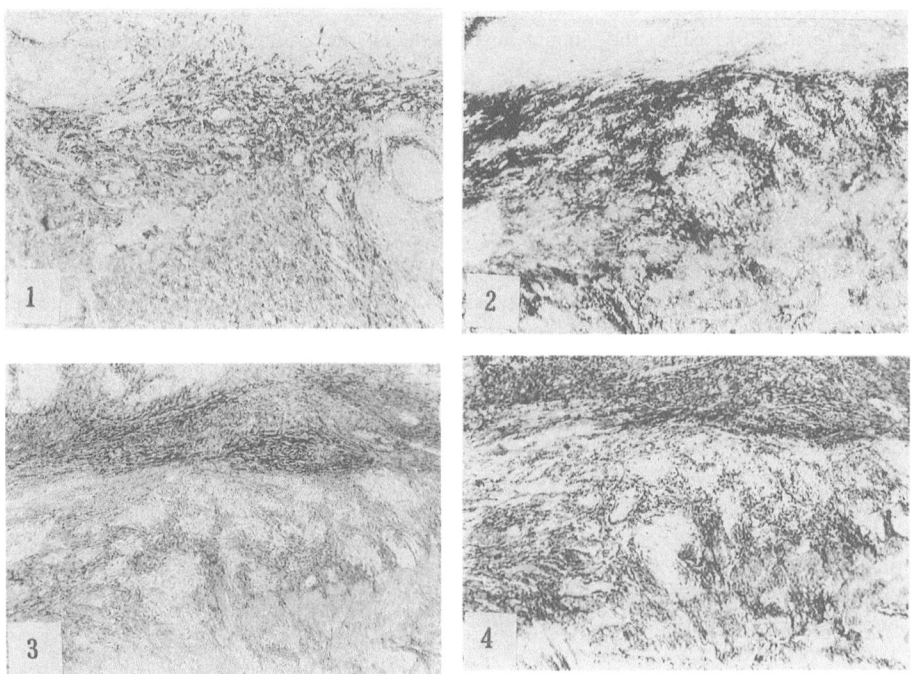

Fig.1 Type I collagen. We can see marked hyperplasia in scirrhous carcinoma
Fig.2 6s-chondroitin sulfate   Fig.3 4s-chondroitin sulfate
Fig.4 Dermatan sulfate
4s-CS and DS were present in dense connective tissue and 6s-CS in relatively coarse connective tissue of the region where cancer cells infiltrated.

DISCUSSION

Alcian blue staining method followed by enzymatic digestion was conventionally used for the histological demonstration of proteoglycans. Application of this method to scirrhous carcinoma revealed the presence of hyaluronic acid and chondroitin sulfate isomers, however, latter was not be characterized in detail. Therefore, enzyme-antibody method using monoclonal antibody was utilized [4,5] . Although acetic acid alcohol fixation is recommended for this method, IgG-gold-silver method used in this study produced less non specific and highly sensitive reactions in routine formalin-fixed tissue sections. The amount of chondroitin sulfate increased in the interstitial connective tissue of scirrhous carcinoma in comparison with normal gastric wall. Chondroitin sulfate has been reported to participate in the mechanism promoting growth and development of tumor cells mainly in the results of biochemical researches [6,7] , and histochemical results of this study might support one of the characteristics for growth and progression of scirrhous carcinoma. It is of note that the amount of chondroitin sulfate increased in scirrhous carcinoma which shows more rapid tumordevelopment than other types of cancers. Moreover, an increase in the amount of hyaluronic acid was obserbed in the interstitium of scirrhous carcinoma, suggesting that increases in hyaluronic acid and chondroitin sulfate in the interstitium may be the main cause of hardening of the gastric wall because hyaluronic acid is known to closely participate in tissue4 elasticity and hardness. Concerning tissue distribution of chondroitin sulfate isomers, chondroitin 6 sulfate was present in relatively coarse fibrosing layer surrounding the tumor cells, and chondroitin 4 sulfate mainly distributed in the region where close connective tissues were regularly arranged a little apart from there.Dermatan sulfate was widely distributed in the both layers. From this, it was presumed that L-aduronic acid as a component of dermatan sulfate participates in the regular arrangement of collagen fibrils, whereas dermatan sulfate may be relatively decreased and disorders arrangement of the fibrils with an increase in chondroitin sulfafte, which is to facilitate the infiltration of the tumor cells [8] .

There is a report on the typing immunohistology of collagen fibers that the collagens type I and III increase equally in amount [9] . Our results showed that collagens type I and III are the main components in the interstitium of scirrhous carcinoma, and that, an increase in collagen type I is specific.   Some have reported that the region where collagen type I is present contains dermatan sulfate by nearly 100 % and the region where collagen type III is present contains chondroitin 4 sulfate, chondroitin 6 sulfate, dermatan sulfate and heparan sulfate [10] . It is very interesting to suggest the possible coexistence of collagen type I and dermatan sulfate when addressing our result that both collage type I and dermatan sulfate increased in the interstitium of scirrhous carcinoma. Type IV collagen were located more broadly in the stroma of undifferentiated carcinoma, particulary in scirrhous carcinoma than differentiated carcinoma.

We histochemically studied collagen fibers and proteoglicans in the cellular interstitium of scirrhous carcinoma and reported slight specificity as compared with non-sclerosing gastric cancers. It is still remained to be solved whether environmental changes in the interstitial tissue were caused by the cancer cells or were secondary of were primary ones in the interstitium still remains to be solved, but it is supposed that these changes may participate in the specificity of proliferation and the progression of scirrhous carcinoma.

These results suggest that specific stromal change in gastric carcinoma may be related with the histrogical types and the growth patterns.

REFERENCES

1.Kaibara N, Maeta M, Hamazoe R, Koga S (1989)Multimodality treatment of scirrhous carcinoma of the stomach. Gastroenterological Surgery 12:1317-1321

2.Nakamura K, Saitoh Y (1986) Clinicopathological aspects of scirrhous carcinoma of the stomach. Saishin-Igaku 41:951-959

3 Takita T, Shimada T, Kitamura H, et al (1990) Studies on the physical developer for use in immunohistochemistry. Acta Histochem cytochem 23:647-662

4. Sobue M, Fukatsu T, Nakashima N, Takeuchi J, Kato T, Ogura T, Nakagaki S (1987) Immunohistichemical localization of chondroitin sulfate and dermatan sulfate proteoglycan in human connective tissues. Connective Tissue 19;117-126

5. Takahashi N (1989) Immunohistochemical study on the relationship between cancer cell growth and storoma changes of gastric carcinoma.

6. Ozzello L, Lasfargues EY, Murray MR (1960) Growth promoting activity of acid mucopolysaccharides on a strain of human mammary carcinoma cells. Cancer Res 20:600

7. Takeuchi J (1965) Growth-promoting effect of chondroitin sulfate on solid Ehrlich ascites tumor. Nature 207;537

8. Iozzo RV (1985) Neoplastic modulation of extracellular matrix: Colon carcinoma cells release polypeptides that alter proteoglycan metabolism in colon fibroblasts. J. Biol. Chem. 260:7464

9.Minamoto T, Mai M, Ooi A (1990) Biochemical Immunohistochemical Profiles of collagen types and plasminogen activators in desmoplastic reaction of gastric carcinoma. Prceedings of Japanese Research Society for Gastroenterological Carcinogenesis 2:267-271

10. Junqueria LCU, Toledo OMS, MOntes GS (1981) Correlation of specific sulfated glycosasminoglycans with collagen types I , II and III. Cell Tissue Res 217:171-175

The Value of Microvessels in the Tumor of Gastric Carcinoma

FUMIO SEKI, HIROYUKI YAMAOKA, JUNICHI WAKASUGI, YASUHIRO KOIZUMI, KUNIYA TANAKA, and HIROSHI SHIMADA

Second Department of Surgery, Yokohama City University, Yokohama, 236 Japan

ABSTRACT

33 patients with gasric carcinoma were studied to examine the relationship between the micrvessel count and their histological findings or prognosis.Microvessels were identified by staining their endotherial cells for factor VIII-related antigen with use of a standard immunoperoxidase technique and counted per 200x field.The mean microvessel count was 39.1±28.6. The microvessel count was being higher according to tumor growth and occurence of lymphnode metastasis.Borrmann4 type and poorly differentiated adenocarcinoma had high microvessel count.But themicrovessel count was not correlated with the site of recurrence or prognosis of gastric carcinoma.

KEY WORDS: tumor angiogenesis,microvessel count,factor VIII-related antigen,gastric carcinoma

INTRODUCTION

Angiogenesis is necessary for tumor growth in every carcinoma.And according to the increase of tumor vessels,the chance of metastasis might increase(1,2).The grade of angiogenesis can be measured by counting the microvessels in the tumor(3).The aim of this study is to examine the relationship between the number of microvessels in histological study of gastric carcinoma and biological malignancy.We want to know the patients who undergo curative operation but recur in the future.If we can predict prognostic factors,treating them more intensively after the operation we might decrease recurrence rate.Various parameters are studied to answer this question.We expect that the microvessel count might be the parameter for prospecting the prognosis of gastric carcinoma.

MATERIALS AND METHODS

33 patients with gastric carcinoma were studied.Their characters are showed at Table-1.Early and extremely advanced gastric carcinoma was excluded from the materials.Curative operations were performed for all cases at Second Department of Surgery,Yokohama City University between 1983 and 1985.They were all followed at this hospital.The site of recurrence and survival time were recorded.

Microvessel Staining and Counting

According to the previous study(1),the microvessels by staining their endotherial cells for factor VIII-related antigen with use of a standard immunoperoxidase technique were identified using paraffin enbedded specimens.Using light microscopy,microvessels were seen as fragment about 10 micrometer in diameter.The individual numbers of microvessel were counted per 200x field(0.7386mm2) at three points that had most high density of microvessels in the tumor.The average count of the three points was defined as the microvessel count of the tumor

Statistical Analysis

The microvessel count was compared with the age,sex,tumor size,Borrmann classification,depth of tumor invasion, lymphnode metastasis,lymphovascular invasion,histological pattern,histological stage,site of recurrence and survival time.The lymphnode metastasis, lymphovascular invasion and histological stage were based on Japanese Reseach Society for Gastric Cancer.Student's t tset was used to determine statistical significance.Genarallized Wilcoxon test was used to determine statistical significance of survival curves.They were all performed by Fisher software using

NEC PC-9801personal computer.

RESULTS

Microvessel Count

Mean microvessel count of the tumor($\pm$SD) was 39.1$\pm$28.6 per 200x field.The relationship between the microvessel count and histoclinical findings are showed at Table-2.

Clinical Findings and Microvessel Count

There was no difference in microvessel count between men(30.1$\pm$23.9) and women(51.0$\pm$33.4).There was no statistical significance between age and microvessel count.

Histological Findings and Microvessel Count

The microvessel count was compared with maximum size of tumor.Mean tumor size($\pm$SD) was 60.1$\pm$30.8mm.Tumor size was divided into two groups.The maximum size of one group was samaller than 50mm.The maximum size of the other group was larger than 50mm.Microvessel count of the former(31.2$\pm$20.2) was significantly lower than that of the latter(46.0$\pm$31.5)(p<0.05).Looking the relationship between Borrmann classification and microvessel count, Borrmann4 type had high microvessel count(68.5$\pm$31.5) compared with other Borrmann type.There was statistical significance between Borrmann4 type and Borrmann1 type(23.5$\pm$10.6),Borrmann4 type and Borrmann3 type(23.0$\pm$17.0)(p<0.05).Looking the depth of tumor invasion,it was proper muscle layer to serosal layer.The patients whose umor invasion were up to proper muscle or reaching to other structure were excluded from the materials.There was no statistical significance among depth of tumor invasion such as proper muscle(51.0$\pm$25.5),subserosa(40.2$\pm$31.4) and whole layer(37.1$\pm$28.5).Lympnode metastasis was graded 0 to 4.Grade0 had no lymphnode metastasis histologically. Grade1 had lymphnode metastasis near the region of tumor existance.Grade2 had farer lymphnode metastasis.The patients that had external lymphnode metastasis(Grade3 or 4) were excluded from the materials.The microvessel count was being higher according to the grade of lymphnode metastasis.There was the statistical significance between grade0(23.1$\pm$14.9)and grade2(45.7$\pm$30.0)(p<0.05).Another point of view,every patient whose microvessel count was higher than 50 per 200x field had lymphnode metastasis.Lymphovascular invasion was graded 0 to 3.Grade0 had no lymphovascular invasion and grade3 had severe one.There was no statistical significance in microvessel count among grade of lymphovascular invasion.The microvessel count whose histological pattern was well differentiated adenocarcinoma was 20.0$\pm$9.7.This count was significantly lower than that of moderately differentiated adenocarcinoma(52.8$\pm$28.1) or poorly differentiated adenocarcinoma(51.3$\pm$31.1)(p<0.01). But there was no statistical significance between the differentiated type and the undifferentiated type.Looking histological stage,the all cases were stage2 or stage3.Stage2 included the cases whose depth of tumor invasion were proper muscle or subseroa or had grade1lymphnode metastasis.Stage3 included the cases whose tumor invasion were whole layer or had grade2 lymphnode metastasis.These two groups had no liver metastasis and no peritoneal dissemination at the operation.The microvessel count of stage3(43.5$\pm$16.1) was significantly higher than that of stage2(25.8$\pm$16.1) (p<0.05).

Site of Recurrence and Prognosis

In 33 patients,15 patients did not recur and lived.15 patients died of recurrence of gastric carcinoma.The sites of recurrence was lymphnode(n=6),liver(n=3) and peritoneal dissemination(n=6).3 patients died caused by another disease.There was no statistical significance in microvessel count between recurrence group(42.8$\pm$23.3) and no recurrence group(43.1$\pm$33.1).And microvessel count had no difference among the site of recurrence such as lymphnode(36.8$\pm$13.3),liver(51.0$\pm$31.8) and peritoneal dissemination(43.5$\pm$41.6).The mean survival time of all patients($\pm$SD) was 1249$\pm$1028 days.The 5-year survival rate of all patients was 37.5%.We compared high microvessel count group with low microvessel count group.The survival rate whose microvessel count was higher than 40 per 200x field was 53.5%.The survival rate whose microvessel count was lower than 40 per 200x field was 21.1%. There was no statistical significance in two groups.

Table-1 Characters of Materials

```
Age(years old)    57.7±12.7              Sex        Men   : 21
Operation    Subtotal gastrectomy : 24              Women : 12
             Total gastrectomy    : 9    Borrmann classification  0 : 5
Maximum size of tumor(mm)  60.1±30.8                              1 : 2
Histological pattern       tub1 : 5                               2 : 10
                           tub2 : 8                               3 : 6
                           por  : 10                              4 : 4
                           sig  : 5                               5 : 6
Depth of tumor invasion    pm : 4     Lymphnode metastasis   0 : 6
                           ss : 9                            1 : 11
                           se : 19                           2 : 16
Site of recurrence  No recurrence : 15  Lymphovascular invasion  0 : 7
                    Lymphnode     : 6                            1 : 9
                    Liver         : 3                            2 : 0
                    Dissemination : 6                            3 : 6
Survival time(days)    1249±1028      Histological stage     2 : 6
                                                             3 : 27
```

Table-2 Relationship Between Microvessel Count and Histoclinical Findings

	Sex	Histological Stage	Maximum Size of Tumor	Depth of Tumor Invasion	Lymphnode Metastasis
Men	30.1±23.9	stage2 25.8±16.1 ⌐ *	<50mm 31.2±20.2 ⌐ *	pm 51.0±25.5	grade0 23.1±14.9 ⌐
Women	51.0±33.4	stage3 43.5±29.5 ⌐	>=50mm 46.0±31.5 ⌐	ss 40.2±31.4	grade1 41.4±30.0 ⌐ *
				se 37.1±28.5	grsde2 45.7±30.0 ⌐

Lymphovascular Invasion	Histological Pattern	Borrmann Classification	Site of Recurrence
grade0 29.1±15.2	tub1 20.0±9.7 ⌐ **	1 type 23.5±10.6 ⌐	No Recurrence 42.8±23.3
grade1 50.4±32.8	tub2 52.8±28.1 ⌐	2 type 40.0±31.5 ⌐ *	Lymphnode 36.8±13.3
grade2 no patient	por 51.3±31.1 ⌐	3 type 23.0±17.0 ⌐ *	Liver 51.0±31.8
grade3 26.5±20.3	sig 37.2±30.5	4 type 68.5±31.5 ⌐	Dissemination 45.3±41.6

student's t test   * : p<0.05   ** : p<0.01

DISCUSSION

Previous study descrived that micrvessel count of the tumor was correlated to the biological malignancy(1,2).In breast carcinoma,microvessel count could prospect its prognosis(4,5).We specurate the microvessel count of gastric carcinoma might prospect its progosis.In this study,we can not discover the relationship between the micrvessel count and site of recurrence or prognosis.In the histological study,microvessel count of gastric carcinoma was correlated to the tumor size,Borrmann classification,lymphnode metastasis,histlogical pattern and histological stage.Microvessel count was being higher according to the tumor growth and the occurence of lymphnode metastasis.And Borrmann4 type and poorly differentiated adenocarcinoma had high microvessel count.In a process of tomor growth, angiogenesis does not occur uniformly.Some tumor has a lot of tumor vessels,and some has a little.The difference is unclear.Various angiogenetic factors secreted from the tumor might be the reason.In the future we must study in this point.In this study microvessel count was not useful parameter for prospecting the site of recurrence or prognosis of gastric carcinoma.

REFERRENCES

1.Folkman J.,Klagsbrun M. Angiogenic factors. Science 235:442-447;1987

2.Folkman J. What is the evidence that tumors are angiogenesis dependent? J.Nat.Can.Inst.82:4-6;1990

3.Weidner N.,Semple J.P.,Welch W.R.,Folkman J. Tumor angiogenesis and metastasis-correlation in invasive breast carcinoma. N.Engl.J.Med.324:1-8;1991

4.Weidner N.,Folkman J.,Pozza F.,Be lacqua P.,Allred E.N.,Moore D.H.,Meli S.,Gasparino G. Tumor angiogenesis:A new significant and independent prognostic indicator in early-stage breast carcinoma. J.Nat.Can.Inst. 84:1875-1887;1992

5.Kato T.,Kimura T.,Murai H.,Kamio T.,Fujii A.,Yamamoto K.,Hamano K. A study of angiogenesis in breast cancer with factor VIII-related antigen staining. J.Jpn.Soc.Cancer Ther. 27:1819-1828;1992

Diagnosis of Lymph Nodes with Metastasis from Stomach Cancer Using Ultrasonography

YOUICHI KITAMURA, HIROYOSHI SUZUKI, TSUYOSHI SASAGAWA, and KIYOTAKA YAMAMOTO

The Institute of Gastro Enterology, Tokyo Women's Medical College, Shinjuku-ku, Tokyo, Japan

ABSTRACT

Diagnosis of Lymph nodes metastasis has not been studied thoroughly. Thus, the diagnosis of lymph nodes metastasis using ultrasonography were examined. The following 3 items are defined as the criteria of metastasis (1) the major axis is more than 5mm, (2) the shape is spherical, (3) uniformly low internal echo is observed. Cases for which the extent of occupation by cancer was small were, how ever, not consistent with the above criteria. This is a future problem.

KEY WORKDS: Diagnosis of Lymph Nodes Ultrasonography

INTRODUCTION

As a result of advances in imaging modalities and endoscopy it has become easier to detect gastric cancer. Moreover, as the cancer conciousness(understanding)of the general public has increased, various forms of screening examination have come to be performed more widely, and the percentage of early cancers detected has been continually. However, advanced gastric cancer is still a common problem. In early gastric cancer, a thorough preoperative examination consists simply of clearly localizing the cancer within the stomach. However, in patients with advanced cancer, there is also a need for preoperative staging(preoperative determination of the degree of tumor progression). Thus, it must be determined whether liver metastases are present, whether peritoneal dissemination has occurred, what the depth of invasion is, and whether lymph node metastasis has occured. The greatest therapeutic advantage that can be expected of surgical treatment is the resection of lymph node metastases. Thus, from this standpoint as well, the preoperative diagnosis of lymph node metastases is also important. In this study, we investigated the ultrasound criteria for a diagnosis of lymph node metastasis.

METHODS

The information obtained by ultrasonography was classified into 3 parameters, i.e., size, shape, and internal echo. We then compared lymph node metastasis-positive and -negative patients with regard to each of these 3 parameters, and determined the diagnositic criteria for lymph node metastasis.

RESULTS

1. Assessment of lymph node size: Lymph nodes related to the stomach were classified into groups No.1-16 (Fig.1) according to Japanese Research Society for Gastric Caner. Since the size of these lymph nodes varies according to their site, we compared metastasis-negative lymph nodes with the longest diameter of metastasis-positive lymph nodes of the same group, and with the diameters at right angles of the longest diameter. The size of the normal lymph nodes varied according to site, and Nos. 4d, 8, 11 and 12 were larger. In the patients with lymph node metastases, all of the nodes were larger than the corresponding normal ones, and Nos. 6, 8, 13, and 16 showed the greatest increase in size. (Fig.-2)

Fig-1

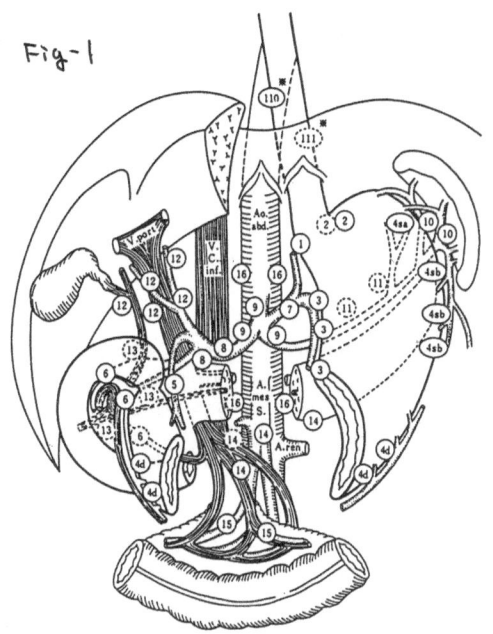

Mean size of lymph nodes removed from a given site derived from formaline fixed samples (n=100)　Fig-2

No.	Metastase(−)	Metastase(+)
1	3.9×4.0 mm	44.3×6.7 mm
2	3.4×3.6	5.1×7.0
3	4.0×4.6	7.8×7.0
4sa	2.7×3.0	4.2×5.2
4sb	2.8×2.9	3.2×3.4
4d	4.4×5.0	5.3×6.5
5	4.1×4.2	4.9×6.1
6	4.2×5.3	7.0×9.1
7	4.3×4.5	6.4×6.6
8	5.4×5.5	6.7×8.0
9	3.0×3.0	5.1×7.1
10	3.9×4.4	5.2×7.1
11	3.8×5.0	3.6×6.0
12	5.3×5.2	⟨7.0×12.0⟩
13	4.8×4.8	11.0×12.0⟩
14	2.0×2.0	5.0×9.7
15	⟨4.0×5.0⟩	⟨5.0×10.0⟩
16	4.2×4.9	7.8×8.0

2. Assessment of shape: The shape of the normal lymph nodes was oval and flat. Metastasis-positive lymph nodes with a longest diameter < 5mm were spherical, while those with a longest diameter < 10mm were slightly oval and those with a maximum diameter ≥ 10mm were oval. Although normal lymph nodes exhibited the same differences according to size, the metastatic lymph nodes were clearly rounder at all sizes. (Fig.-3)

The ratio of maximum to minimum diameter of lymph nodes in relation to the presence or absence of metastasis　Fig-3

	absence n=100	presence n=100
5 mm≧	1.61	1.33
5～10mm≦	1.87	1.54
10mm>	2.13	1.71

3. Lymph node internal echo: There were differences in the extent of metastatic involvement of the individual lymph nodes, i.e., there was a complete spectrum from nodes 100% occupied by cancer to nodes with cancer cells only at the periphery or with cancer cells scattered internally. When the lymph nodes were completely occupied by cancer, they showed a uniform low echogenicity. In contrast, lymph nodes with 50-70% replacement by cancer cells had an uneven echo pattern with some areas of high echogenicity. When under 30% of the lymph node was replaced by cancer and when cancercells were only present at the margin of the node, internal high echogenicity became more common and it was difficult to distinguish these nodes from normal one.

4. Diagnostic accuracy: We investigated 3 types of ultrasonography, i.e., external ultrasonography (US), endoscopic ultrasonography (EUS), and intraoperative ultrasonography (IOUS). Since imaging varied depending on the anatomical location of each lymph node group, the diagnostic accuracy also changed. The results are summarized in the table (Fig.-4)

Detection of Lymph-node metastasis by
ultra sonograph-es (n=38) Fig- 4

No.	US	EUS	IOUS	Total accuracy
1	14.3%	57.1%	57.1%	57.1%
2	0	50.0	50.0	50.0
3	37.5	62.5	87.5	93.7
4	26.7	40.0	73.3	86.7
5	33.3	66.7	66.7	100.0
6	27.3	9.1	66.6	90.9
7	50.0	12.5	87.5	87.5
8	60.0	20.0	100.0	100.0
9	0	0	100.0	100.0
10	0	20.0	40.0	40.0
11	33.3	33.3	33.3	66.7
12	0	0	100.0	100.0
13	50.0	0	100.0	100.0
14				
15			100.0	100.0
16				
17			50.0	50.0

DISCUSSION

We devised diagnostic criteria for lymph node metastases and performed 3 types of
ultrasonography on the basis of these criteria. It was possible to achieve a high diagnostic
accuracy for metastatic lymph nodes ≥ 10 mm in size. However, when the nodes were < 5 mm and
had few cancer cells, there was little change in the internal echo. Moreover, many of the
nodes < 5 mm were normal, making it more difficult to identify those with metastases.
Accordingly, the detection of lymph nodes without many cancer cells was unsatisfactory. This
problem may be solved in the future by the development of substances which can highlight
metastases and make ultrasonographic diagnosis easier.

CONCLUSION

We defined the 3 parameters listed below as ultrasonographic diagnostic criteria for lymph
node metastasis:
1. Longest diameter ≥ 5 mm
2. Spherical
3. Uniform low echogenicity

REFERENCES

1. Gastric Cancer Research Society Ed.: Rules for Managing Gastric Cancer, Kanehara Shuppan,
   1985
2. Katayama Kouji et al.: Assessment of gastric lymph low by the double isotope method, Nihon
   Shokaki Geka Gakkai Shi, 8: 1414-1419, 1985
3. Kitamura Yoichi et al.: Diagnosis of gastric cancer lymph node metastases, Gaka Shindan,
   18: 12, 1464-1471, 1988

Prognostic Factors for Gastric Cancer Patients — Alternation of the Significance in 6,540 Patients Treated Over a 30-Year Period

Kazuo Okajima, Mitsuru Sasako, Taira Kinoshita, and Keiichi Maruyama

Gastric Surgery Division, National Cancer Center Hospital, Chuo-ku, Tokyo, 104 Japan

ABSTRACT

In the 30 years from 1962 to 1991, we treated 6,540 patients with primary gastric cancer, in the National Cancer Center Hospital. We evaluated the most important prognostic factor using multi-valuate analysis (Cox's proportional hazard model). The highest significance is Depth of invasion (RR;4.31), and LN metastasis (RR;3.72), Distant metastasis (RR;2.34), Age(RR;2.25), LN dissection (RR;1.75), Macroscopic type (RR;1.04) were followed.

KEY WORDS: gastric cancer, prognostic factor,

INTRODUCTION

Many prognostic factors were studied for gastric cancer patient. It is well known that significance of factors can not be evaluated by uni-variate analysis.The purpose of this study is to know the prognostic factors of gastric cancer patients using uni-variate and multi-variate analysis, and to demonstrate the alternation of the significance caused by increase of early stage cancer and improvement of treatment method.

MATERIAL

6,540 patients with primary gastric cancer were treated surgically in the National Cancer Center Hospital Tokyo in the 30 years period from 1962 to 1991. Detailed data of host, tumor, and treatment factors were recorded in a computer. Follow-up data were also collected,and the number of lost in follow up was 20 (0.3%). We follow up the patients closely by out patient clinic and letter.

METHOD

After the check of independence and significance of the factors, following 12 factors were analyzed prognostic significance was analyzed by multi-variate analysis (Cox's proportional hazard model, SAS soft ware, PHGLM produced).

PROGNOSTIC FACTORS ANALYZED

Host : Sex = male or female
      Age = -50, 51-60, 61-70, 71- years old
Tumor : Location = Upper, Middle and Lower part of the stomach
      Macroscopic type = early gastric cancer, Borr.type 1, Borr.type2, Borr.type 3, Borr.type4 and type5 (unclassified)
      Maximal diameter = -30, 31-60, 61-90, 91- mm
      Depth of invasion = intramucosal, submucosal, proper muscle layer, subserosal layer and S1, S2, S3
      Lymph node metastasis = N0, N1, N2 and N3,4 evaluated by histological findings
      Histological type = well or moderately differentiated tubular adenocarcinoma and papillary adenocarcinoma, and
           other.

Treatment : Resection extent = distal gastrectomy or total gastrectomy
            Combined resection = combined resection was performed or not
            LN dissection = R0, R1, R2 and R3,4
            Chemotherapy = chemotherapy was performed or not

Host	Tumor	Treatment
Sex	Location	Resection extent
Age	Macroscopic type	Combine resection
	Maximal diameter	Lymph node dissection
	Depth of invasion	Chemotherapy
	Lymph node metastasis	
	Histological type	

Fig.1 ANALYZED FACTORS

RESULT

Treatment result of primary gastric cancer in the 30 years period from 1962 to 1991. 6,865 patients with primary cancer were treated surgically. 6,540 cases were resected (resectability is 95.3%) and 5 years survival rate was 57.7%. 5,416 cases were curatively resected (78.9%), and 69.2% of the group survived more than 5 years. To know the trend, 30 years were equally divided in three period each 10 years. It was notable that (1) early stage cancer increased, (2) 5 years survival rate was elevated from 45% to 71%, (3) improvement of treatment results were dominant in Stage II (61% to 76%), and Stage IIIa (39% to 63%). (4) instead of increasing early Stage cancer, surgical treatment became more extensive but more safe (operative mortality decreased form 2.3% to 0.4%). Patients with N0 had increased 788 to 1427 cases, and the 5 years survival rate elevated from 77% to 89%. 5 years survival also elevated from 42% to 66% in the N1, and from 18% to 36% in the N2. These improvement were produced by progress of systematic lymph node dissection. 30 years trend of survivals by lymph node dissection was the R2 operation (complete removal of N1 and N2 lymph nodes) was standard procedure in our hospital, and the 5 years survival rate elevated from 53% to 73%. Fig 2 shows the trend of prognostic factors for gastric cancer patient. The first 10 years, the highest ratio of risk is observed in Depth of invasion. Next is LN metastasis and Distant metastasis is followed. This tendency is same as next 10 years and last 10 years. But last 10 years, Age factor become more important factor than Distant metastasis.

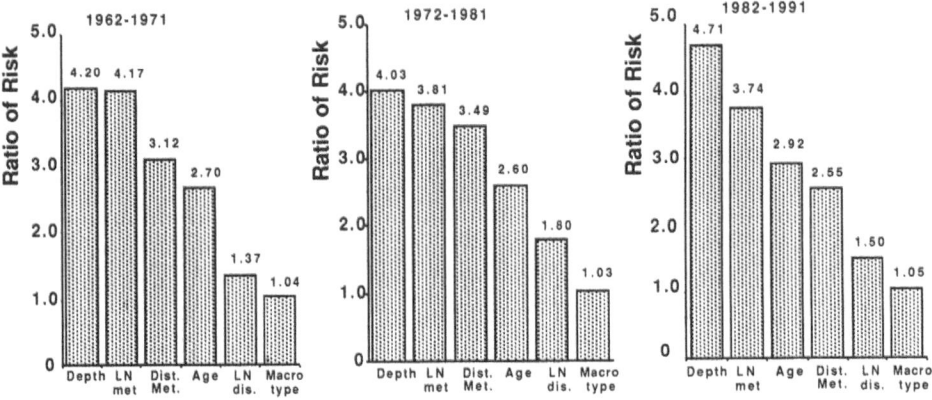

Fig 2 TREND OF PROGNOSTIC FACTOR FOR GASTRIC CANCER PATIENT

Fig. 2 shows the important prognostic factors for gastric cancer patient in these 30 years period. Through the 30 years, the most significant factor is observed in Depth of invasion, the ratio of risk is 4.31. And next is LN metastasis (RR;3.72),

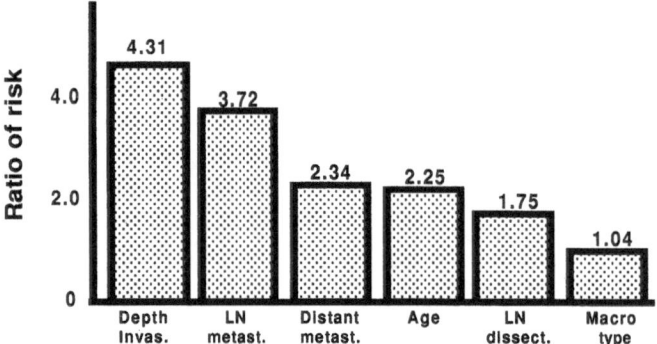

Distant metastasis (RR;2.34), Age (RR;2.34), LN dissection (RR;1.75) and Macroscopic type is followed(RR;1.0)

Fig. 3 IMPORTANT PROGNOSTIC FACTORS FOR GASTRIC CANCER PATIENT

Fig. 3 shows, among the 12 prognostic factors, the most significant factor was depth of invasion (Ratio of risk : 4.31), followed by lympt node metastasis (3.72), distant metastasis (2.34), age (2.25), and extent of lymph node dissection (1.75). It was notable that lymph node dissection, a treatment factor, was one of the most important prognostic factor or gastric cancer ptients.

DISCUSSION

Prognostic factors of gastric cancer patients were studied using data of 6,540 patients with primary gastric cancer treated surgically in the 30 years period. 12 prognostic factors were investigated by multi-variate analysis, using Cox' proportional hazard model. The most significant factor was depth of invasion, Ratio of risk 4.31, LN metastasis, distant metastasis, age and LN dissection were followed. In the 30 years period, prognostic significance of LN metastasis was decreased from 4.17 to 3.74 in the Ratio of risk. It means that patients associate with N2 metastasis cloud be cured in the last period. The other data also demonstrated the important role of lymph node dissection in gastric cancer surgery.

Clinicopathological Characteristics of Cases with Metastasis to Lower Mediastinal Lymph Nodes and Treatment in Gastric Cancer with Esophageal Invasion

MASATSUGU KITAMURA, KUNIYOSHI ARAI, and KAORU MIYASHITA

Department of Surgery, Tokyo Metropolitan Komagome Hospital, Bunkyo-ku, Tokyo, 113 Japan

ABSTRACT

In 118 gastric cancer patients with esophageal invasion who had undergone lymphadenectomy in the lower mediastinum, a study was conducted to explore characteristics of positive lymph node metastasis. The patients with positive lymph node metastasis in the lower mediastinal area (29 cases) had larger tumor, a higher rate of peritoneal dissemination, and had more cases of type 3 and 4 than the negative group (89 cases). The former group also had more non curative resections and more undifferentiated tumors (p<0.01). The rate of mediastinal lymph node metastasis was 24.6%. The outcome was significantly worse in patients with positive mediastinal lymph node metastasis than in those without it.

KEY WORDS: prognosis of gastric cancer with esophageal invasion, metastatic rate of lower mediastinal lymph node

INTRODUCTION

Most of the cases of gastric cancer with esophageal invasion are cases of advanced gastric cancer, in which the outcome of therapy is known to be rather poor. In order to improve the outcome, it is necessary to perform an extensive resection and thorough lymphadenectomy, and select a proper approach to a safe reconstruction. Although the rate of lymph node metastasis in the lower mediastinum is reported to be 10-25% [1, 2, 3], few detailed studies have been made. Here we report the actual state and prognosis of lymph node metastasis in the lower mediastinum.

MATERIALS AND METHODS

Out of 2595 cases of resection of gastric cancer performed between 1975 and 1992, 196 cases with esophageal invasion were selected as the subjects in the present study. One hundred and 5 cases recieved laparosternophrenotomy and 91 cases recieved the thoracoabdominal approach. Of these, 118 cases in which a thorough examination of lymph node in the lower mediastinum was performed, were selected and classified into either a positive mediastinal lymph node group (29 cases) and a negative lymph node group (89 cases) to comparatively explore their clinicopathological characteristics. Concerning the approach, if the tumor invades the esophagus within 4 cm from the esophago-gastric junction in localized type and within 3 cm in invasive type, laparosternophrenotomy approach was performed, while in those with esophageal invasion exceeding the above limits, the thoracoabdominal approach was utilized.

RESULTS

The comparison between the positive and negative lymph node groups revealed that the diameter of tumor was significantly larger, with a significantly higher peritoneal dissemination (p<0.01) in the positive metastasis group than in the negative group. The number of cases of type 3 and 4 was also high in the positive group. In the positive metastatic group, the rate of noncurative resections was significantly high, with an advanced stage of lymph node metastasis. In this group, the ratio of undifferentiated type was significantly high, with a significantly high ow(+) rate as compared with the

negative group. Histologically, the length of esophageal invasion was 3.4 cm
in the positive group and 1.7 cm in the negative group, with a significantly
longer distance in the former group. As for the relationship between tumor
diameters and the rates of mediastinal lymph node metastasis, no metastasis
was observed in the length less than 5 cm but the rate of metastasis was 38%
in the length more than 10.1 cm. As for the relationship of macroscopic
lengths of invasion, the rate of metastasis was 14% in the length less than 1
cm and 56% in the length more than 4.1 cm. As for the relationship of the
depth, the rate of metastasis was 7% in ss and 36% in se or deeper. As for
the relationship of lymph nodes in the abdominal and thoracic cavities,
mediastinal lymph node metastasis increased as the extent of metastasis in
the abdominal cavity increased. Table 1 shows the rate of metastasis in the
lower mediastinal lymph node. The rate of lymph node metastasis in the lower
mediastinum was 20.6% for No.110 (paraesophageal lymph node), 13.5% for No.111
(diaphragmatic lymph node), 6.3% for No.112 (posterior mediastinal lymph node)
and 24.6% overall. Of the cases of gastric cancer with esophageal invasion,
the 5 year survival was 44% in those without metastasis of the lymph node, and
as poor as 0% in those with the metastasis.

Table 1. Metastatic rate of lower mediastinal lymph nodes

		Approach		Total
		Laparosternophrenotomy	Thoracoabdominal	
No. of cases		61	57	118
L.Node Number	No.110	5/45 (11.1)%	15/52 (28.8)%	20/97 (20.6)%
	No.111	2/42 (4.8)	8/32 (25.0)	10/74 (13.5)
	No.112	3/40 (7.5)	1/23 (4.3)	4/63 (6.3)
Metastatic Rate		9/61 (14.8)	20/57 (35.1)	29/118 (24.6)

DISCUSSION

Our findings indicated that of gastric cancer with esophageal invasion,
prognosis of the cases with mediastinal lymph node metastasis was very poor.
These cases would consist mostly of a highly advanced invasive type cancer, of
which prognosis might be determined by noncurative factors in the abdominal
cavity. If the intra-abdominal procedure is curative, it is necessary to
perform mediastinal lymphadenectomy in combination with an additional
chemotherapy to achieve a satisfactory clinical outcome.

REFERENCES

1. Awane Y, Kitamura M, Konishi T (1984) Lower mediastinal lymph node
   dissection for the tumor of the gastric cardia. Surgery 38, 1047-1052
   (in Japanese)
2. Oohashi I, Toyoda S, Oota H (1978) Treatment of tumor of esophago gastric
   junction--method of lymph node dissection--Surgery 32, 835-842 (in Japanese)
3. Kitamura M, Arai K, Miyashita K (1992) Clinicopathological characteristics
   of cases with metastasis to lower mediastinal lymph node and treatment in
   gastric cancer with esophageal invasion Jp. Gastroenterological Surgery
   25(10) 1992 (in Japanese)

Surgical Approach for Gastric Cancer Extended to the Esophagus

TAKASHI AIKOU, SHOUJI NATSUGOE, TETUSHI SAIHARA, SHUITI HOKITA,
MASAMICHI BABA, and HISAAKI SHIMAZU

The First Department of Surgery, Kagoshima University of Medicine, Kagoshima, 890 Japan

ABSTRACT

In a total of 179 patients with gastric cancer invading the esophagus, the authors retrospectively assessed the surgical approach. These patients were divided into two groups according to the tumor location ; 88 cardiac cancer and 91 non-cardiac cancer. Clinicopathologic characteristics, such as gross appearance, cell type, serosal invasion, and peritoneal dissemination were significantly different between cardiac and non-cardiac cancer.   A thoracoabdominal approach was performed in 95 and a abdominal approach in 84. Since 1986, the incidence of thoracotomy has decreased because of using endoscopic ultrasonography (EUS) and device of automatic suture. EUS imaging of the boundary between liver and heart was useful in assessing the esophageal invasion. In cases of esophageal invasion longer than 20 mm in localized type, 10 mm in diffuse type, and/or nodal involvement in the medistinum was detected, thoracoabdominal approach should be performed toobtain tumor-free margin at the proximal stump and a better prognosis.

KEY WORDS : cardiac cancer, thoracoabdominal approach, esophageal invasion

INTRODUCTION

The surgical treatment for gastric cancer extended to the esophagus remains a subject of controversy [1-2]. The debate centers around the surgical approach, the extent of resection and the benefit of a complete lymphadenectomy. In this study we attempted to answer some question. Firstly, what are the characteristic features of gastric cancer with esophageal invasion ? Secondly, how should be assessed the extent of the tumor and lymph node metastasis ? Finally, what is the optimal approach for cure of this tumor ?

MATERIALS AND METHODS

One hundred seventy-nine patients with gastric cancer invading the esophagus underwent esophago-gastrectomy between 1973 and 1990. These patients were divided into two groups according to the tumor location. One was tumors centered within 2 cm from Esophago-Gastric (EG) junction, namely, cardiac cancer, the number of patients was 88, and the other is tumor arisen in the upper-third of the stomach (68) or diffuse infiltrative carcinoma (23), namely non-cardiac cancer, it was 91 patients. The demographic data, the operative records were carefully reviewed to determine the type of resection performed,the extent of lymphadenectomy for each case and whether a complete resection of gross disease was deemed accomplished by the operating surgeon. Pathology reports were scrutinized to determine the degree of transmural invasion, the size and location of the tumor, the total number of lymph nodes excised with specimen as well as the number and location of all lymph nodes involved with carcinoma. Final staging was based on the General rules of the Gastric Cancer Study, the Japanese Research Society for Gastric Cancer [3].
Statistical analysis of the data was performed using the generalized Wilcoxon test.

RESULT

All 179 patients were referred with diagnosis of gastric cancer invading the esophagus. There were 143 males and 36 females for a male to female ratio of 4:1. Cardiac and non-cardiac cancer groups differed significantly with respect to gross appearance, cell type, serosal invasion and peritoneal dissemination (Table 1). However, there were no statistically significant difference with regard to age, sex, nodal involvement, and liver metastasis. In the cardiac cancer group, Borrmann type 2 or 3, and well differentiated cell type were common. In non-cardiac cancer group, serosal invasion was prominent. Sixty-one, or 69 %, of 88 patients with cardiac cancer underwent resection by thoracoabdominal approach. On the other hand, 40, or 44%, of 91 patients with non-cardiac cancer was done through thoracoabdominal approach. Total gastrectomy was done in 84% of non-cardiac cancer group, whereas in half of the patients of cardiac cancer group. The tumor was palliatively resected in 63% of patients with non-cardiac cancer, and in 36% of those with cardiac cancer (Table 2).

Table 1. Clinicopathologic Features

	Cardiac Ca.	Non-Cardiac Ca.	
Cell type			$p < 0.01$
well diff.	61	40	
poorly diff.	27	51	
Serosal Invasion			$p < 0.01$
negative	50	25	
positive	38	66	
Peritoneal Dissemination			$p < 0.01$
negative	79	64	
positive	9	27	

well diff.: well differentiated

Table 2. Surgical Procedure

	Cardiac Ca.	Non-Cardiac Ca.	
Approach			$p < 0.01$
TAA	61	40	
AA	27	51	
Gastrectomy			$p < 0.01$
total	41	76	
proximal	47	15	
Radicality			$p < 0.01$
curative	56	34	
palliative	52	57	

TAA: thoracoabdominal approach

We selected the thoracoabodominal approach based on the following criteria, i.e., esophageal invasion more than 20 mm in tumor of localized type, more than 10 mm in tumor of diffuse type. The endoscopic ultrasonography and the device of automatic suture have been employed since 1986, the incidence of thoracoabdominal approach decreased in 43% from 56%. Ultrasonographic imaging of the boundary between liver and heart, being 3 cm distant from EG junction, was helpful in assessing the esophageal invasion. And we also could identified the EG junction by the difference of layer structure between the the stomach and esophagus. Table 3 shows the difference between expected and actual distance of esophageal invasion from EG junction. Twenty-two of 27 tumors, or 82 %, were proved to be within 10 mm difference. Before 1986, positive rate of cancer infiltration at the resection margin was 7.6%, however after 1986, it was confirmed in only one patient who was aged person with chronic obstructive lung disease. Thus the endoscopic ultrasonography provided accurate detection of esophageal invasion.

Table 3. Difference of Esophageal Invasion between Expected and Actual Distance

	Cardiac Cancer (n=14)	Non-Cardiac Cancer (n=13)	Total (n=27)
Greater than 10 mm		2	2
Within 10 mm	13 (93%)	9 (69%)	22 (82%)
Less than 10 mm	1	2	3

(Endoscopic Ultrasonography, 1986-1990)

Metastasis to the regional lymph nodes was present in 141 patients (79%).
Lymph nodemetastasis in the mediastinum was found in 5, or 15 % of 34 patients with cardiac cancer underwent thoracoabdominal approach, whereas 9 (32%) out of 26 patients with non-cardiac cancer had positive nodes. Among 14 patients with nodal involvement in the mediastinum, two thirds of those had abdominal para-aortic lymph node metastasis.

DISCUSSION

The carcinoma with invading the esophagus consists mainly of 3 tumors, i.e.,tumor arisen in cardiac region, tumor in the upper-third of the stomach, and diffuse infiltrative tumor. The definition of cardiac portion is, however, not unequivocal. In the present study, we defined tumor arisen in the portion within 3 cm distant from EG junction as cardiac cancer. We also defined tumor in the upper third of the stomach, and diffuse infiltrative carcinoma as non-cardiac cancer. Cardiac and non-cardiac cancer differed significantly with respect to gross appearance, cell type, serosal invasion, and peritoneal invasion. For patients with non-cardiac cancer invading the esophagus, therewas high rate of poorly differentiated cell type and serosal invasion. Okamura et al.[4] reported that the main risk factors for esophageal invasion are anatomic location, advanced disease, gross appearance, serosal invasion, and lymph node metastasis.
Husenmann [5] pointed out that, to minimize local recurrence, the histologic type should be given attention because diffuse tumors tend to infiltrate, extensive esophageal invasion. The choice of an operative approach, particularly whether it need thoracotomy or not, is most important for surgical treatment of patients with gastric carcinoma invading the esophagus. The crucial factors in selecting surgical approach were to obtain a tumor-free margin at the proximal stump and to remove regional lymph nodes that are likely to be involved by metastasis. In order to obtain the information about esophageal invasion, we have employed the EUS since 1986 which provided accurate detection of it. Ultrasonographic imaging of the boundary between liver and heart, and of layer structure was very helpful in assessing the extent of tumor invasion. As to the difference between expected and actual distance of esophageal invasion from EG junction, 82 % of cases were proved to be within 10 mm difference. We have selected the thoracoabdominal approach based on the esophageal invasion more than 20 mm in case with localized type, more than 10 mm in cases with diffuse type. As the result, positive rate of cancer infiltration at the resection margin has decreased. The thoracoabdominal approach also has the advantage of simultaneous exposure of the distal esophagus and stomach, and in this type of surgical approach, a more precise anastomosis can be performed with greater ease under direct vision. An another important issue is lymph node metastasis in the mediastinum. In the literature, there has been reported that patients with adenocarcinoma of the cardia commonly had nodal involvement in the abdomen and the mediastinum. This is because of the extensive anastomosis of lymphatic draining between the gastric cardia and distal esophagus. We reported previously [6] the stereoscopic finding of lymphatic communication in this region. When the dye was injected into the submucosa of gastric cardia, lymphocapillaries extended across EG junction were seen. This evidence suggest that mediastinal nodal involvement may occur in cases with carcinoma invading esophagus. In conclusion, in cases of esophageal invasion longer than 20 mm in localized type, 10 mm in diffuse type was detected by endoscopic ultrasonography, thoracoabdominal approach should be performed to obtain tumor-free margin at the proximal stump and a better prognosis.

REFERENCES

1. Akiyama H, Miyazono H, Tsurumaru M, Hashimoto C, Kawamura T (1979) Thoracoabdominal approach for carcinoma of the cardia. Am J Surg 137:345-349
2. Aikou T, Shimazu H (1989) Difference in main lymphatic pathways from the lower esophagus and gastric cardia. Jpn J Surg 19:290-295
3. Japanese Research Society for Gastric Cancer (1981) The general rules for the gastric cancer study in surgery and pathology. Jpn J Surg 11:127-39
4. Okamura T, Korenaga D, Baba H (1989) Thoracoabdominal approach for cure of patients with an adenocarcinoma in the upper third of the stomach. Am Surg 55:248-251
5. Husemann B (1989) Cardia carcinoma considered as a distinct clinical entity. Br J Surg 76:136-139
6. Aikou T, Natsugoe S, Tanabe G, Shimazu H (1987) Lymph drainage originating from the lower esophagus and gastric cardia as measured by radioisotope uptake in the regional lymph nodes following lymphoscintigraphy. Lymphology 20:145-151

A New Surgical Approach for Resection of Cancer of Gastric Cardia

Nobuhiko Tanigawa, Takumi Shimomatsuya, Tetsuya Horiuchi, Masaru Uchinami, Yasuhiko Masuda, and Ryusuke Muraoka

The Second Department of Surgery, Fukui Medical University, Matsuoka-cho, Yoshida-gun, Fukui, 910-11 Japan

ABSTRACT

Thirty-five consecutive patients with adenocarcinoma of the gastric cardia were operated with a new technique which involved wide resection of the peri-hiatal diaphragm, dissection of the upper abdominal and lower mediastinal lymph nodes, and resection of the stomach including a portion of the lower esophagus without thoracotomy. The mediastinal node stations were affected in 25 % of patients, whose tumor invaded to the serosa. Hhypotension with or without atrial arrythmias and pleural tears occurred during surgery in 20 patients (57 %), and in 18 (51 %), respectively. Postoperatively, hypoxia requiring reintubation developed in 7 patients (19 %), pleural effusions needed tube drainage in 16 (46 %), atelectasis in 5 (14 %) and anastomotic leaks in 3 (9 %). The cumulative 5 year survival rate for 21 patients was 62 %, whereas none of the patients with stage IV disease lived for more than 2 years after surgery. We believe this technique is a reasonable and safe alternative to the left thoracotomy approach for resection of cancer of the gastric cardia.

KEY WORDS: cancer of the gastric cardia, wide resection of diaphragm, mediastinal dissection, avoiding thoracotomy

INTRODUCTION

The surgical management of patients with cancer of the cardia is controversial, not only with regard to the surgical approach, but also to the extent of resection (1). A thoracoabdominal incision (2), left thoracotomy (3), the Ivor Lewis approach (4), and transhiatal resection (5) have their supporters. The problems inherent to this disease include not only tumor spreading to the lower esophagus and/or to adjacent structures close to the esophageal hiatus, but also prevalence of metastases to lower mediastinal lymph nodes as well as to upper abdominal nodes. With the aim of resolving these problems and reducing operative morbidity, we have treated this disease for the past 5 years with a newly developed technique which involves wide resection of the peri-hiatal diaphragm. The resection area of the diaphragm includes not only the diaphragmatic crura as other methods (6,7), but also the tissue surrounding the esophageal hiatus. Our clinical experiences of 35 patients subjected consecutively to this method are reported here.

MATERIALS AND METHODS

Thirty-five consecutive patients underwent en bloc resection of cardia cancer without thoracotomy between January 1987 and June 1992 at the Fukui Medical University. All tumors were adenocarcinoma. The male to female ratio was 22:13, with an average age of 61.1 years (40 to 85 years). All patients were pathologically staged according to the TNM classification (17): 2 (6 %) were in stage I, 9 (26 %) in stage II, 10 (29 %) in stage III, and 14 (40 %) in stage IV.

Surgical Procedure

The abdomen was entered through an upper midline incision extending toward the lower abdomen. Dissection of perigastric and nonperigastric upper abdominal lymph nodes was performed along the left gastric, common hepatic, splenic and celiac arteries and abdominal aorta. The diaphragmatic tissue around the hiatus (about 6-7 cm in width) was resected in continuity with the esophagus as follow. Firstly the left triangular ligament was cut to mobilize the left lobe of the liver inward, so that the left lateral wall of the inferior vena cava was visible. The left phrenic vein was ligated and cut at the level

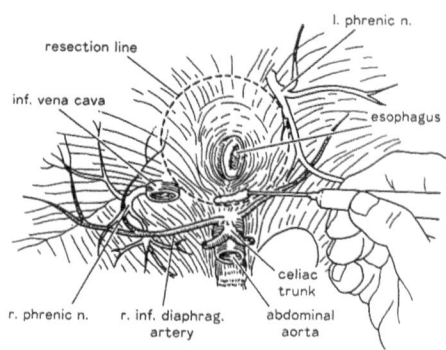

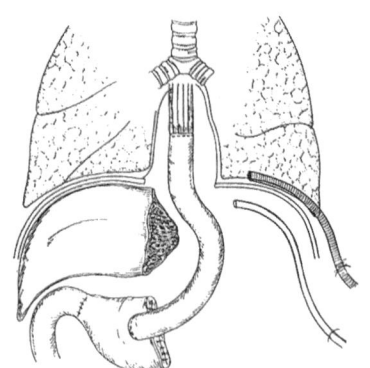

Fig.2 Reconstruction is completed.
Jejunal loop interposition is shown.

where the right edge of the resection line would be. Next, the resection line was marked with an eclectrocautery. The peri-hiatal diaphragm was cut in a counterclockwise direction along the marked resection line, which was close to the inferior vena cava on the right side, the abdominal aorta on the posterior side, the left phrenic nerve on the left side, and the central tendon on the anterior side (Fig. 1). The resected tissue in this procedure included not only the crural muscle but also the diaphragmatic tissue surrounding the hiatus.

In the opened mediastinal space, the posterior mediastinal tissue containing the lymph nodes along the lower part of the thoracic esophagus was dissected under direct vision toward the carina. Then the continuity of the gastro-intestinal tract was restored by a Roux-Y procedure in the patients who underwent total gastrectomy and by jejunal loop interposition in ones who were subjected to proximal gastrectomy (Fig. 2). Numbering of the upper abdominal and lower mediastinal lymph node stations has been defined by the Japanese classification. When the location of cancer is in the upper third, N1 is defined as node stations 1 to 4, N2 5 to 11, N3 12 to 14, N4 15,16 and the lower mediastinal node stations 110-112 are denoted as N3. All those lymph nodes were removed en bloc or partially to achieve at least a so-called R2 resection (dissection of N1 and N2 nodes) in all patients. To determine the significance for dissection of the lower mediastinal lymph nodes, the incidence of nodal involvement were microscopically investigated according to the depth of tumor invasion in the stomach wall.

RESULTS

The mean duration of the procedure was 4.8 hours (range: 3.5 to 9 hours). Mean blood loss was 824 mL (range: 320 to 1,467). Total gastrectomy was performed in 23 patients and proximal gastrectomy in the other 12 patients with a T1 or T2 tumor. The most common histologic type was poorly differentiated adenocarcinoma (34 %). The differentiated papillary and tubular cancers comprised 52 %.The continuity of the gastrointestinal tract was restored by a Roux-Y procedure in 23 patients who underwent total gastrectomy and by jujunal loop interposition in 12 patients who were subjected to proximal gastrectomy.

Proximal gastrectomy was performed for the patients with a T1 or T2 tumor; 2 patients (100 %) with stage I disease, 5 (55 %) with stage II, and 5 (50 %) with stage III. Complications associated with this operation was as follow. Intraoperatively, hypotension with or without atrial arrythmias occurred in 19 patients (58%). Tears of the pleural membrane occurred in 18 patients (51%). Reintubation was required in seven patients (19%) within 72 hours of extubation in whom hypoxia developed. Pleural effusions, which were observed in most patients, required tube drainage in 16 patients (46%). Atelectasis and anastomotic leaks were experienced in 5 (14%) and in 3 (9%), respectively. The depth of tumor invasion into the stomach wall correlated strongly with the incidence of nodal involvement, which significantly increased when the tumor penetrated to the serosa. The lower mediastinal node stations were involved in a quater of the patients whose tumors peneterated to the serosa (Table 1). The cumulative 5 year survival rates for 2 patients with stage I disease, for 9 with stage II, and for 10 with stage III were 100 %, 73 %, and 38 %, respectively.

In contrast, none of the patients with stage IV disease lived for more than 2 years after surgery. The average duration of survival in these patients was only 9.1 months.

Table 1. Incidence of tumor involvement stratified by the depth of tumor invasion

Depth of invasion	N1 Station number 1 - 4	N2 Station number 5 - 11	Lower mediastinal Station number 110, 111, 112	N3 included 16 Station number 12 - 16
s (-)[a]	6/15 (40 %)[b]	3/15 (20 %)	0/15 (0 %)	1/12 (8 %)
s (+)	17/20 (85 %)	11/20 (55 %)	5/20 (25 %)	5/18 (28 %)

[a] s(-): the tumor did not invade to the serosa, s(+): the tumor invaded to the serosa.
[b] number of patients with nodal involvement/number of patients underwent node dissection.

DISCUSSION

The wide resection of the peri-hiatal diaphragm provides for adequate removal of tumorous invasion into the peri-hiatal stuructures. A second advantage is the possibility of the mediastinal dissection up to the carina from the abdominal cavity. In addition, there is no post-thoracotomy incisional pain by avoiding thoracotomy. No serious complications associated with such wide resection of the diaphgragm were experienced. Dissection of the mediastinum is possible up to the carina from the abdominal cavity. The lower mediastinum can be reached much more easily than when following the transthoracic approach. This new technique, therefore, presents no drawbacks compared with the left thoracotomy in terms of an adequate resection of the cancer. The extent of lymph node metastases and the depth of invasion are the two most important prognostic factors in gastric cancer without distant metastases. Node metastases can be resected with subsequent long term survival, but opinions differ as to the desirable extent of node dissection. The lymphatic spread of the gastric cancer to the mediastinal node stations has not clearly defined. But, those stations were affected in one fourth of patients with tumor invading to the serosa in this study. This high incidence of node involvement seems to indicate the significance of the dissection of lower mediastinal nodes in patients with an advanced stage of cardia cancer. Some reports indicated that surgical treatment of adenocarcinoma of the cardia is curative only if the disease is in stage I or II, but not in case of stage III or IV disease (8). Nevertheless, the current study suggests that some patients with stage III disease can also be cured when the surgical technique decribed here is used. Our survival data compares favorably with the 22.5 percent of 5 year survival in case of stage III disease reported by Ellis et al., who followed the left thoracotomy approach (3). Since a thoracotomy is avoided, the procedure is better tolerated by debilita ted patients or those with chronic pulmonary disease. Thus, we believe that this technique is a reasonable alternative to the left thoracotomy approach for neoplasms in the gastric cardia.

REFERENCES

1. Paolini A, Tosato F, Cassese M, Marchi CD, Grande M, Paoletti P, Gherardini P, Fegiz G (1986) Total gastrectomy in the treatment of adenocarcinoma of the cardia. Am J Surg 151:238-243
2. Akiyama H, Miyazono H, Tsurumaru T, Hashimoto C, Kawamura T (1979) Thoracoabdominal approach for carcinoma of the cardia of the stomach. Am J Surg 137:345-352
3. Ellis HF, Gibb PS, Watkins EJr (1988) Limited esophagogastrectomy for carcinoma of the cardia. Indications, Technique, and Results. Ann Surg 208:354-361
4. King MR, Pairolero PC, Trastek VF, Payne WS, Bernatz PE (1987) Ivor Lewis esophago-gastrectomy for carcinoma of the esophagus: early and late functional results. Ann Thorac Surg 44:119-122
5. Orringer MB (1984) Transhiatal esophagectomy without thoracotomy for carcinoma of the thoracic esophagus. Ann Surg 200:282-288
6. Finely RJ, Grace M, Duff JH (1985) Esophagectomy without thoracotomy for carcinoma of the cardia and lower part of the esophagus. Surg Gynecol Obstet 160:49-56
7. DeMeester TR, Zaninotto G, Johansson K-E (1988) Selective therapeutic approach to cancer of the lower esophagus and cardia. J Thorac Cardiovasc Surg 95:42-54
8. Hölscher AH, Siewert JR (1985) Surgical treatment of adenocarcinoma of the gastro-esophageal junction: results of a European questionnaire (GEEMO). Dig Surg 2:1-8

A Study on the Status of Lymph Node Motastasis in Cancer of the Upper Third Stomach

Yoshio Kitamura, Kota Okinaga, Tokuyuki Yokohata, and Tatuo Jibu

The Second Department of Surgery, Teikyo University School of Medicine, Itabashi-ku, Tokyo, 173 Japan

ABSTRACT

We studied the status of lymph node metastasis in cancer of the upper third stomach (55 cases) in which cancer invasion was limited in the subserosal layer. As lymph node metastasis was negative for No.3, No.4d, No.5 and No.6 in patients with cancer invasion limited in the submucosal layer (22 cases), these cases can be candidates for proximal gastrectomy. As lymph node metastasis was positive for No.3 in patients with gastric cancer located in C and involved the proper muscle layer, further study is necessary to get conclusion for proximal gastrectomy in these cases. Proximal gastrectomy should not be indicated for patients with cancer invasion extends beyond the proper muscle layer because of metastasis for No.4d, No.5 and No.6 lymph nodes.

key ward: gastric cancer, lymph node metastasis, proximal gastrectomy

INTRODUCTION

In terms of quality of life, more conservative surgery is advocated for less advanced stage of gastric cancer. The extent of gastric resection depends on not only extension of tumor, but also the status of lymph node metastasis. The purpose of this study is to determining of indication for proximal gastrectomy.

PATIENTS AND METHODS

Five hundred and one patients underwent partial or total gastrectomy for gastric cancer from January of 1980 to December of 1992 at the Second Department of Surgery, Teikyo University Hospital. In 65 patients (13.0%) the main location of gastric cancer was the upper third of stomach. 55 of 65 patients who had cancer invasion limited within the subserosal layer were included in this study ; 45 male and 10 famale patients. Total gastrectomy was performed in all these patients. Extended lymphadenectomy were perfomed in 48 cases. Preoperative endoscopic injection of activated charcoal was performed in 16 patients. 37 cases were localized in the upper third of the stomach (C), 7 cases were located in both the upper third of the stomach and the lower esophagus (CE), 6 cases were mainly in the upper third of the stomach with extension to the middle third of the stomach (CM), and 5 cases were located in the upper third of stomach with extension to both middle third and the esophargus (CME) (Table 1).

RESULTS

24 cases (43.6%) were early cancer and 32 cases (56.4%) were advanced cancer. Advanced cancer included 12 cases of Borrmann II type and 20 of Borrmann III type. 23 (41.8%) of 55 patients had lymph node metastases, three had peritoneal dissemination, and two had hepatic metastases. 27 patients were classified to Stage I, 11 to stage II, to stage III, and 9 to stage IV according to classification by Japanese Research Association of Gastric Cancer. Histologically, 45 cases were differentiated type and 8 were undifferetiated type. Curative surgery was performed in 47 patients, while non-curative surgery was performed in 8 patients.

Table 1. Location and depth in upper third gastric cancer

	m	sm	pm	ss	se~	Total
C	9	11	5	12	5	42
CE	0	2	0	5	5	10
CM	0	0	2	4	2	8
CME	0	0	0	5	0	5
Total	9	13	7	26	10	65

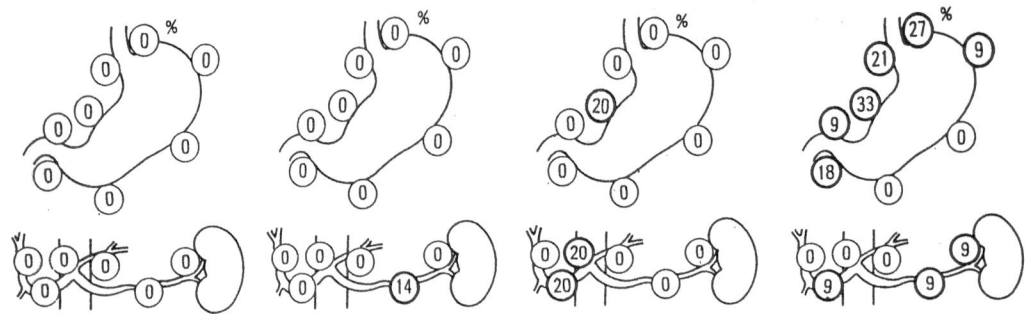

depth m (9 cases)　　depth sm (11 cases)　　depth pm (5 cases)　　depth ss (12 cases)

Fig. 1　Lymph node metastasis of gastric cancer in area C (%)

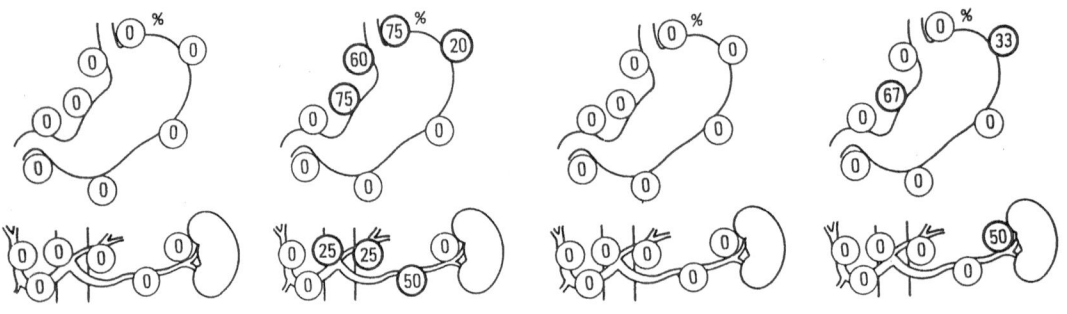

depth pm (2 cases)　　depth ss (5 cases)　　　depth pm (2 cases)　　depth ss (4 cases)

Fig. 2　Lymph node metastasis of gastric　　　　Fig. 3 Lymph node metastasis of gastric
　　　　cancer in area CE (%)　　　　　　　　　　　cancer in area CM (%)

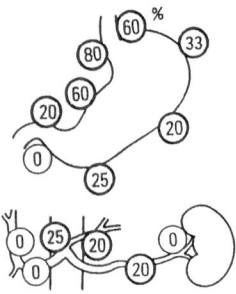

depth ss (5 cases)

Fig. 4　Lymph node metastasis of gastric cancer in area CME (%)

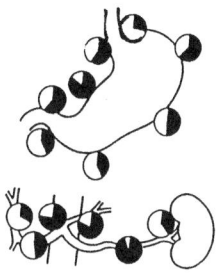

Fig. 5 Staining of lymph nodes with activated charcoal
injection into the area C (16 cases)

There was no metastasis for No.3, No.4d, No.5, and No.6 lymph node in patients with gastric cancer located in C and
its cancer invasion limited within submucosal layer. However, there were positive metastases for No.3 lymph node
if cancer invasion extended to the proper muscle layer though metastasis was negative in No.5, and No.6 lymph nodes.
High percentage of metastases in most of regional lymph nodes were observed in patients with cancer invasion
extended to the serosa. More than 50% of the regional lymph nodes of the stomach were stained with endoscopically
injected charcoal around the cancer lesion in the wall of the upper third stomach.

DISCUSSION
Recent trend of consideration on quality of life has made some changes in selection of procedures for gastric
cancer. Total gastrectomy has been a standard procedure for cancer of the upper third stomach for complete
dissection of regional lymph nodes. However, total removal of the stomach causes loss of reservoir function of the
stomach, nutritional problems, and may result in anemia. If there is no chance of metastasis to those regional
lymph nodes, total gastrectomy is not essential as far as the cancer lesion can be removed with proper non-cancerous
margin. The present study showed that no metastasis in No.3, No.4d, No.5, and No.6 lymph nodes was found in early
gastric cancer located in C and CE. Althogh number of our studied cases were small, no metastases in these regional
lymph nodes except No.3 lymph nodes were reported in the larger series. [1][2] Therefore, proximal gastrectomy can be
indicated for early gastric cancer in C and CE. On the other hand, there were positive metastases in No.3 lymph
nodes when cancer invation involved the proper muscle layer though No.5 and No.6 lymph nodes were negative for
metastasis. Although proximal gastrectomy can be performed if all of the metastatic No.3 lymph nodes can be removed,
further study is necessary to get conclusion on indication for proximal gastrectomy in these cases.

CONCLUSION

1. There was no metastasis in No.3, No.4d, No.5, and No.6 lymph nodes in early gastric cancer located in C and CE.
   Proximal gastrectomy can be performed for early gastric cancer in C and CE.

2. Lymph node metastasis was positive for No.3. in patients with gastric cancer located in C and involved the proper
   muscle layer, further study is necessary to get conclusion for proximal gastrectomy in these cases.

REFERENCES

1) Maruyama K, Kitaoka K, Hirata K. (1983) Surgical treatment for cardiac gastric cancer : Total gastrectomy or
   proximal gastrectomy ? Gastroenterological Surgery 6:1425-1431

2) Kitamura M, Arai K, Miyasita K. (1991) Indication and clinical results of proximal gastrectomy with special
   referance to lymph node metastases in upper gastric cancer. Journal of Japanese Society for Clinical Surgery
   52:1454-1460

Role of MMC-Adsorbed Activated Carbon (MMC-CH$_{40}$) in Guiding Resection of the Lymph Nodes in Patients with Gastric Cancer

XIAO-DONG QI ET AL.

Department of Oncology, The First Affiliated Hospital, China Medical University, Shenyang 110001, China

Key words: Stomach Carcinoma, Lymph node metastasis, Gastric endoscopy, MMC–CH40

INTRODUCTION

In cases of radical surgery for gastric cancer, lymph node metastasis accounts for 70.8% of the carcinomas. As such, it is very important to remove as much lymph nodes as possible to prevent cancer recurrence as well as to increase the survival rate of the patients. We injected MMC–CH40 (MMC adsorbed activated carbon) into the gastric wall preoperatively to guide lymph node dissection during surgery. Lymph nodes stained black were dissected and the results were compared with the unstained control group. This paper comprises a summary of this study and discussion of the clinical value of MMC–CH40.

MATERIALS AND METHODS

1.1 Patients

Eighty–nine patients with gastric cancer were hospitalized in our institute between July, 1991 and July, 1992. Of these, 58 cases underwent radical surgey. These 58 cases were randomly divided into two groups. R_2 or R_3 radical surgery were performed in 22 cases after preoperative injection of CH40 under endoscopy. R_2 or R_3 radical operation was performed in 26 cases without CH40 (the control group) (Table 1).

1.2 Preparation of MMC–CH40,

A suspension of 5% CH40 (minute particle diameter of 21nm, produced by Mitsubishi Chemicals Co., Ltd., Tokyo, Japan) was mixed with stabilizer (polyvinylpyrrolidone), which was donated by Professor Toshio Takahashi and Lecturer Akeo Hagiwara. Before injection, ml of a 0.154M saline solution and 2 mg of mitomycin C (MMC) were added. Two ml of 5% CH40 suspension was then injected into the MMC solution, producing a MMC–CH40 suspension with a total volume of 4 ml.

Table 1 Operation Model and Cases

Model	MMC–CH40	Control
Total Gastrectomy	4	6
Proximal Gastrectomy	2	1
Distal Gastrectomy	16	19
R_2	9	12
R_3	13	14

1.3 Method of injection of MMC–CH40

MMC–CH40 (0.5–1.0ml injection, 3–4 injections for each case) was injected into the submucosa in a 1cm zone near the foci of the gastric cancer 15 days before the operation.

1.4 Examination of the lymph nodes

Resected lymph nodes were carefully examined following surgery. The numbers of black stained and non stained lymph nodes were counted. Black–stained and non–stained lymph nodes were prepared for histological examination and then, observed using a microscope, and compared with the control group.

RESULTS

2.1 Average number of resected lymph nodes for each case

1033 lymph nodes were resected from 22 patients in the MMC–CH40 group. The average number of lymph nodes resected for each case was 47.0. In the control group, the average number resected was 28.1, which was significantly less than in the MMC–CH40 group ($P < 0.05$). Furthermore, more lymph nodes were compartment one and two in the MMC–CH40 group than in the control group (Table 2).

Table 2 Average Number of Resected Lymph Nodes

Compartment	Group	MMC–CH40	Control
	1	4.46(102/22)	2.69(70/26)
	2	0.74(16/22)	1.42(32/26)
	3	6.59(145/22)	4.72(123/26)
	4sa	0.59(13/22)	0.38(10/26)
N_1	4sb	2.50(55/22)	1.58(41/26)
	4d	5.18(114/22)	4.00(104/26)
	5	2.86(63/22)	0.88(23/26)
	6	9.18(202/22)	3.33(86/26)
		32.3(710/22)	19.0(494/26)
	7	5.23(115/22)	3.65(95/26)
	8	3.33(73/22)	1.65(43/26)
N_2	9	1.27(28/22)	0.54(14/26)
	10	0.55(12/22)	0.46(12/26)
	11	1.95(43/22)	1.19(31/26)
		12.3(271/22)	7.50(195/26)
	12	1.17(28/22)	0.77(20/26)
N_3	13	0.68(15/22)	0.27(7/26)
	14	0.23(5/22)	0.19(5/26)
	15	0.18(4/22)	0.35(9/26)
		2.36(52/22)	1.58(41/26)
Total		47.0(1033/22)	28.1(730/26)

2.2 The metastatic rate of resected nodes

The metastatic rate of resected lymph nodes was 68% in the MMC–CH40 group and 77% in the control group. While the latter rate of metastasis was somewhat higher than the former, there was no statistically significant difference between the two.

2.3 The metastatic frequency of resected lymph nodes

The metastatic frequency of resected lymph nodes in the MMC–CH40 group was 16% compared to 32% in he

4control group. This difference was significant (P<0.01). As the number of resected lymph nodes in the MMC–CH40 group was higher than in the control group, the metastatic frequency in the MMC–CH group was relatively low. The average number of resected metastatic lymph nodes in the MMC–CH40 group was 7.55 (166/22), which was higher than the number in the control group (6.23, 162/26). In patients with lymph node metastasis, the average number of resected metastatic lymph nodes in the MMC–CH40 group (11.07, 166/22) was higher than in the control group (7.36, 162/22). This suggests that lymph nodes which were not resected during conventional surgey were resected using this method. Moreover, lymph nodes which previously could not be examined were were detectable using MMC–CH40. (Table 3)

2.4 Black stained resected lymph nodes in the MMC–CH40 group.
Of the 1033 lymph nodes in the MMC–CH40 group 693 (67%) were stained black. In compartment 1 (N_1), 67.5% were stained black. In N_2 and N_3, 67.2% and 61.5% respectively were stained. There was no significant difference in staining rates among these three compartments.

Table 3 Comparison of the Average Number of Resected Metastatic Lymph Nodes in Patients with Lymph Node Metastases

MMC–CH40	11.07	(166/15)
Control	7.36	(162/26)

2.5 Metastatic frequency of resected lymph nodes stained black versus non stained lymph nodes in the MMC–CH40 group.
The metastatic frequency of black stained lymph nodes in the MMC–CH40 group was 12.8% (89/693), compared to 22.3% (76/340) for non–stained lymph nodes. This difference was statistically significant (P<0.01) (Table 4).
The following factors are related to these observations :
(1) When there is lymph node metastasis, the lymph sinus and lymphatic plexus are obstructed by the cancer embolus and diffusion of activated carbon is impaired.
(2) More small lymph nodes than large nodes are stained black, so that the proportion of metastatic lymph node tissue is smaller than the proportion of metastatic nodes.

2.6 Relation between the timing of MMC–CH40 injection and the metastatic frequency of black stained lymph nodes.
MMC–CH40 was injected 1–5 days, 6–10 days or 11–15 days before surgery. The

Table 4 Comparison of the Metastatic Frequency of Resected Lymph Nodes between Black Stained and Non Stained Lymph Nodes

	Resected LN	Metastatic LN	Metastatic Frequency
Black Stained LN	693	89	12.8%
Non Stained LN	340	76	22.3%

frequency of metastasis of black stained lymph nodes was 67%, 62%, and 77% respectively for these 3 time periods. There was no significant difference among these groups.

CONCLUSION
(1) Immediately after celiotomy, most of the lymph nodes around the cancer were stained black. This finding suggests that MMC–CH40 is potentially very useful for delineating the resection area. The average number of resected lymph nodes was 47 in the MMC–CH40 group, which was higher than in the control group (28.1).
(2) The proportion of total resected lymph nodes which were stained black was 67%.
(3) When lymph node metastasis was confined, the average number of resected lymph nodes was greater in the MMC–CH40 group than in the control group.
(4) A satisfactory number of black–stained lymph nodes could be obtained during surgery when activated carbon was injected under endoscopy 15 days before surgery.
(5) No complications nor side effects emerged in any of the 22 cases in this series.
(6) Further evaluation of MMC–CH40 for this purpose is necessary. Most notably, R_4 superextensive dissection, observation of the pattern of lymph node metastasis with gastric cancer, the relation between staining lymph node size, and the effect of intralymphnodal injection of MMC–CH40 all require subsequent study. Furthermore, emulsion and oil dosage forms which can be adsorbed easily by lymphatic tissue should be tested and compared with MMC–CH40.
(7) This method should prove useful in guiding lymph nodes dissection and in examining the lymph nodes following surgery.

MMC-CH$_{40}$ Staining the Regional Lymphnodes in the Use of Radical Operation for Gastric Cancer

Gu-Xiang Ye[1], Xin-Chang Jiang[2], Wei-Que Lu[3], Wei Shen[4],
Xiao-Wei Huang[1], and Lian Zhang[1]

[1]The Department of Surgery, The Departments of [2]Pathology, [3]Pharmacy, [4]Clinical Laboratory, The Central Hospital in Yang-Pu District, Shanghai 200090, China

ABSTRACT

In the present study, 1-2 ml MMC-CH$_{40}$ have been injected directly into the lymphnodes (LNs) around the cancer during the operation. LN clearing number (23$\pm$11 LNs/case) was 1.13 times higher after the injection compared with the control group (10$\pm$5 LNs/ case). The LN black-staining rate was 83.9%. No-staining LNs were located mostly at the 1st station, half of which were metastated. When the lymphadenectomy was performed, there was no interfere with the thoroughness of LNs clearance, even if the LNs were not stained black. Meanwhile, the satisfaction of 2nd and 3rd station of LNs staining black will be helpful in lymphadenectomy.

KEY WORDS: Gastric Cancer, Lymphnode, Staining Agent.

INTRODUCTION

The role of radical lymphadenectomy in the operative treatment of gastric cancer remains controversial [1]. Japanese authors considered that the survival rate was markedly increased after radical lymphadenectomy, and emphasized that the clearing regional lymphnodes (LNs) thoroughly was one of the important factors directly affecting the prognosis of the gastric cancer patients [2]. Many researchers is looking for a staining method of LNs, attempt to help to clear regional LNs [3]. Since December 1989, MMC-CH$_{40}$ have been used in the radical operation on the gastric cancer patients and reported as below.

MATERIALS AND METHODS

Ultrafine carbon particles which is 0.1um in diameter (made in China), 10 mg, poly-vinylpyrrolidone (pvp) 4 mg, were mixed with 1 ml saline and made up a suspension, as discribed by Hagiwara [4]. The suspension were sterilized and sealed in a glass tube. Before administration, the suspension was mixed with 4 mg MMC and shaken for two minutes, so that the MMC was adsorbed to ultrafine carbon particles (MMC-CH$_{40}$). Since December 1989, 24 patients of progressing gastric cancer either at the corpus or the antrum, at an average age of 60 years (range 38-72 years), 16 men and 8 women, were included in the study. The patients were randomly divided into 2 groups, each composed of 12 cases. In the injection group (group I), after an exploratory examina-tion, a swelling LN was found around the greater and/or lesser curature of the stomach near cancer. MMC-CH$_{40}$ 1-2ml was injected directly through a thin-needle into the LN, following the injection, radical operation was performed. In the control group (group C), nothing was injected and the radical operation was only performed. After the operation, the standard pathological inspection were performed on all removed samples. Number of LNs were carefully counted, and checked out if the LNs was stained black. The data were statistically analysised. Accouding to standard, the LNs which were stained black were sliced as usual. After H.E. staining, the slice was carefully examined on the light microscope to see whether the stained LNs was metastatic and any reaction of LNs against MMC-CH$_{40}$.

RESULTS

In group I, if radical operation can be performed, MMC-CH$_{40}$ was directly injected into LNs. It can be observed with the naked-eye that ultrafine carbon particles more rapidly flowed through the efferent lymphduct into regional LNs, which were stained black. There were 23 ± 11 LNs have been cleared in group I and 10 ± 5 LNs, in group C. Difference between two groups was very significance (p<0.01). LN clearing rate in group I was 1.13 times higher than that in group C. In group I total 237 LNs were cleared, among them there were 28 metastatic LNs (11.8%); In group C 111 LNs was cleared, among them there were 38 metastatic LNs (34.2%). Difference between two groups was very significance (p<0.01). Number and percentage of cleared LNs of both groups at different station were listed in table 1. It was suggested that only first station of LNs was cleared in group C. Few LNs at 2nd and 3rd station were cleared. In group I, more LNs at 2nd and 3rd station were cleared. Although the clearance rate at 1st station was decreased, the absolute number was one time increased.

Table 1: Comparison of clearance rate of LNs between two groups

No. of station	group I			group c		
	clearing No.	(%)	metastating No.	clearing No.	(%)	metastating No.
I	202	85.2	25	106	95.5	37
II	27	11.4	3	5	4.5	1
III	8	3.4	0	0	0	0
at all	237	100	28 (11.8%)	111	100	38 (34.2%)

* metastating LNs / clearing LNs

Staining rates of LNs at each station in group I were listed in table 2. It indicated that black-staining (BS) rate of 2nd and 3rd station LNs was much higher than of 1st station LNs. Non-BS LNs were 38, 16%(38/237). They were mostly situated at group ③.④. ⑤.⑥ of the 1st station and group ①.⑦ of the 2nd station. Half of the non-BS LNs in the 1st station were metastatic. It was suggested that non-BS LNs were mostly situated around the cancer lesion, and part of them was metastatic.
There were 28 metastatic LNs in the group I. Among them BS LNs were 11 (39.3%), non-BS LNs were 17 (60.7%). Non-metastatic LNs were 188 (90.0%), non-BS 21 (10.0%). The difference of BS rate between metastatic LNs and non-metastatic LNs was very significant (p<0.01). It indicated that BS rate in metastatic LNs were much lower than that in non-metastatic LNs, and non-BS metastatic LNs were mostly situated in 1st station around the cancer lesion.

Table 2: Staining rate of LNs at each station in group I

LNs station No.	removed LNs	staining LNs	(%)
I	202	167	82.7
II	27	24	88.9
III	8	8	100.0
at all	237	199	83.9

⟩ (91.4) *

* p<0.01

Microscopic inspection indicated that in BS normal LNs carbon particles was mostly situated in sinus of LNs, and had a slight reaction of foreign body. Sinus cells were poliferated and phagocyted carbon particles. There were little carbon particles in lymph medulla and follicles. In BS metastatic LNs, most of carbon particles were situated in the normal residual lymph tissue and the others were situated in the area around or the centre of the cancer.

DISCUSSION

MMC-CH_{40} injected directly in the LNs during operation was a simple procedure. LNs around the stomach were black stained immediately. It helped surgeon to recognize and clean the regional LNs. LNs clearance rate was 1.13 times higher than the one in the group C. The naked-eye distinguishing rate of BS was 83.9%. Sawai et al have reported that when MMC-CH_{40} was injected into submucosa through an endoscopy two days before operation, naked-eye distinguishing rate of BS was 68.8% [5]. The reasons why the BS rate was high in this series were because: MMC-CH_{40} was injected directly into LNs and MMC-CH_{40} flowed into LNs through lymphducts and stained rapidly and satisfactorily. While in Sawai's report, MMC-CH_{40} was injected indirectly through an endoscopy two days before the operation. Carbon particles must be absorbed into LNs and then flowed into regional LNs. The partial MMC-CH_{40} which have been flowed into LNs might flow into remote LNs from regional LNs. So the BS rate was low. The amount of LNs clearing in this series was lower than that of Sawai's. The reasons for this were following: (1)The most of the cases in this series were performed R_1 operation. While in the latter R_2 or R_3 operation were performed. (2)The detection methods of the removed LNs were different. LNs were detected by palpation in this series and the detected rate of LNs was low. High detecting rate of LNs was achieved with a fat-dissolve method [6]. Furthermore, indirect injection preoperatively was complicated, need an endoscopy and patients felt heartburn after the procedure. Therefore direct injection deserved to be recommended, because it was simple and safe, stained rapidly and satisfactorily.

This study indicated that LNs BS rate in group I was 83.9%, but BS rate of metastatic LNs was only 11.8%. BS rate of metastatic LNs in group I was 39.3%. Non-BS rate was 60.7%. Non-BS metastatic LNs were mostly situated in group ③.④.⑤.⑥, around the cancer lesion. It indicated that MMC-CH_{40} was lymphilia and not tumor-philia. The reasons why some normal and metastatic LNs were not stained were listed as below: LNs around the tumor were easily invasived by the tumor cells. If the afferent lymphducts were obstructed by tumor cells, carbon particles can't penetrate to stain. The normal LNs between the metastatic LNs were not stained may be that the efferent lymphducts of metastatic LNs were obstructed by cancer embolus. Carbon particles can't flow into next normal LN through the efferent duct. 2nd and 3rd station LNs were stained satisfactorily because the metastatic LNs were mostly situated in 1st station. When the radical operation of gastric cancer was performed, the metastatic LNs around the cancer can be cleaned thoroughly even if they were not stained and it didn't interfere with the thoroughness of LNs clearing. The 2nd and 3rd station LNs were stained black, and can improve the effect of R_2 and R_3 operation. Carbon particles had an adhesion function. They will progressively release the anti-carcinoma agents into the unresected LNs, and play an important role in the regional chemical treatment.

REFERENCES

1. Behrns KE, Dalton RR, van Heerden JA, Sarr MG (1992) Extended lymph node dissection for gastric cancer; Is it of value? Surg Clin N Am 72:433-444.
2. Mishima Y, Hirayama R (1987) The role of lymph node surgery in gastric cancer. World J Surg 11:406-411.
3. Maruyama K, Okabayashi K, Kiroshita T (1987) Progress in gastric cancer Surgery and its limits of radicality. World J Surg 11:418-425.
4. Hagiwara A, Takahashi T, Lee R, Ueda T, Takeda M (1984) In vitro examination of Mitomycin C. adsorbed to small sized activated carbon particle. Akita J Med 10:419-422.
5. Sawai K, Takahashi S, Kato G, Takenaka A, Tokuda H, Hagiwara A, Takahashi T (1985) Endoscopic injection of activated carbon particle (CH_{44}) for extended lymphadenectomy of gastric cancer. Jpn J Gastroenterol Surg 18:912-917.
6. Zhang QF, Zhao JH, Zhao TZ, Ding L (1987) The inspecting method of lymphnodes after the specimen have been resected. Chinese J oncology 9:223.

The Evaluation of Intraoperative Injection of Microcarbon Particles to Extended Lymph Nodes Dissection for Gastric Cancer

ZHI-PING CHEN, ZHEN-MING GAO, and RAO SHI

Department of Surgery, Ren Ji Hospital, Shanghai Second Medical University, Shanghai 200001, China

ABSTRACT

This study is to evaluate the results of local injection with microcarbon particles to gastric wall and 1st group of regional draining lymph nodes during surgery for gastric cancer, 10 cases with injection and other 10 cases as control. The radical gastrectomy was performed. All specimens with nodes collected for pathological study, the number of both stained and un- stained ndes were statistically counted. Results: (1) The average amount of nodes dissected in injection group was more than in control (P<0.01) (2) More stained nodes was in group I and Ⅱ of regional nodes. (3) In injection group, 8.8% of stained nodes were proved to be metastatic, but unstained node proved to be metastatic were 75%. Conclusion: This method is beneficial to extended radical lymphadenectomy for gastric cancer but no special selec- tiveness to lymph nodes metastasis.

KEY WORDS: Injection of microcarbon particles, lymph nodes dissection, gastric csncer

INTRODUCTION

It is very important to obtain result that the regional lymph nodes should be dissected completely during surgery for advanced gastric cancer. Sawai and Takahashi proposed that endoscopic injection of microcarbon particlec (CH44) into gastric wall should be performed two days before surgical proce- dure, and Maruyama modified the method by injection of Indian ink into lymph node along greater culvature of stomach during surgery, thus the stained lymph nodes could be removed easily. This paper deals with the results of injection of microcarbon particle (25 mu in diameter supplied by Shanghai Carbon Works) into gastric wall and the 1st group of draining lymph nodes during surgery for gastric cancer from April 1990 to March 1991 at our hospital, to evaluate this method in radical dissection of the staining nodes.

MATERIALS AND METHODS

Twenty patients with advanced gastric cancer located at antrum were chosen for study. The ratio of male to female was 1.5:1, age ranged from 42 to 65. According to the Japanese staging of SNPH, there were 14 cases of stage II and 6 cases of stage III respectively, Borrmann's classification were type II in 5 and type III in 15. Patients were divided into two groups: 10 cases with injection of microcarbon suspension were performed with R2 in 18 and R3 in 2 cases. In the injection group, the carbon suspension in 0.5-1.0ml dose was injected into gastric intramural layer 1cm outside of tumor mass for 3 points and also a lymph node along the greater culvature of the stomach. All the specimens including lymph nodes were collected for pathological study. The number of both stained and unstained regional nodes were carefully counted, and the data were calculated statistically.

RESULTS

The average amount of nodes dissected was 21.5 in the injection group,
which was more than average number of 13.7 in the control group (P<0.01).
The percentage of staining nodes in the injection group was 54.8%(102/186).
More staining nodes were noticed in the group I and II of the regional
draining lymph nodes, especially in nodes along left gastric artery(No.7),
nodes along common hepatic artery (No.8), nodes along celiac artery (No.9),
and right cardial node (No.1). In two cases, group III nodes were stained
instead of only group II, one to nodes along hepatoduodenal ligament(No.12)
and one in para-aortic artery (No.16). In the injection group, 8.8% (9/102)
of the stained lymph nodes were proved to be metastaic, as confirmed by
pathological section, while only 25%(6/24) of the stained lymph nodes which
were suspected to be metastatic by its gross appearence during surgery were
confirmed by histological study. The unstained nodes in this group proved
to be metastatic were 75%.

DISCUSSION

Regional draining lymph nodes can be stained by the injection of microcarbon
to gastric wall. The result of this study reveals that stained nodes are found
more in number in group II of the regional lymph nodes than group I.   It is
the fact that the method is beneficial to the extended radical lymphadenectomy
in R2 procedure which is indicated for major part of the patients with gastric
cancer. As to the phenomenon of staining of group III lymph nodes without
involvement of group II, it might be the result of local metastasis blocking
lymph channels. The fact that metastatic lymph nodes were not stained and the
stained nodes were not metastatic, denotes that this method provides no special selectiveness to lymph metastasis.

REFERENCES

1. Sawai K, Takahashi, S, Kato, G, Takenaka A, Tokuda H, Hagiwara A,
   Takahashi T (1985): Endoscopic injection of activated carbon particle
   (CH44) for extented radical lymphadenectomy of gastric cancer. Japanese J.
   gastroenterological Surgery 18: 912-917
2. Hagiwara A, Takahashi T, Ueda T, Iwamoto A, Yamashida H (1988):Enhanced
   therapeutic efficacy on lymph node metastasis by use of Peplomycin adsorbed
   on small activated carbon particles. Anticancer Research 8: 287-290
3. Maruyama K, Okabayashi K, Kinoshita T (1987):Progress in gastric cancer
   surgery in Japan and its limits of radicalyity. World J. Surgery 11: 418-425
4. Japanese Research Society for gastric cancer(1985):The general rules for
   gastric cancer study, 1th ed.

Is It Correct Whether Pancreato-Splenectomy Is Essential for Dissection and Removal of Lymph Nodes Along the Splenic Artery?

Yoshitaka Yamamura, Tsuyoshi Kito, Junichi Sakamoto, and Hiroaki Nakazato

Department of Gastroenterological Surgery, Aichi Cancer Center Hospital, Nagoya, 464 Japan

ABSTRACT

Eighty two patients with pathological metastasis to the lymph nodes along the splenic artery (L_{11}) were divided into two groups (pancreato-splenectomy(PS)(+):19 cases, PS(-):63 cases). Their backgrounds were not different. Five year survival rate of PS(+) group was 10.5%, and that of PS(-) group was 12.8%. Residual lymph nodes were microscopically detected in the previously dissected pancreas specimen in three out of eight cases studied. Those lymph nodes were few in number, small in size and all of them were cancer negative. From these results, we concluded that dissection of L_{11} without PS might be a clinically satisfactory procedure against advanced gastric carcinoma.

KEY WORDS: pancreato-splenectomy, dissection of lymph nodes along the splenic artery, metastasis to the lymph nodes along the splenic artery

INTRODUCTION

Pancreato-splenectomy(PS) is usually performed in Japan in cases of total or proximal gastrectomy against advanced gastric carcinoma. However, we speculated that the removal of the lymph nodes along the splenic artery(L_{11}) without PS might also be satisfactory for prognosis. Therefore, clinical and pathological studies were carried out to prove our hypothesis.

MATERIALS AND METHODS

Clinical Study

Of 1,849 patients who underwent gastric resection in our institute from 1981 to 1990, eighty two patients (4.4%) had pathological metastasis to L_{11}. They were divided into two groups (PS(+):19 patients, PS(-):63 patients) respectively, and cumulative survival rates were compared. This study was not a randomized controlled study. The chi-square(χ^2) test was used to evaluate the patients' background factors. At the end of 1991, the survival rate was calculated by the Kaplan and Meier method, and its statistical significance was evaluated by the Logrank method.

Pathological Study

Eight patients who underwent total gastric resection from 1990 to 1992 were registered in this study. L_{11} was dissected by meticulous removal of tissues surrounding the splenic artery (Fig. 1). After satisfactory dissection seemed to have been carried out, PS was performed, and the resected specimen was microscopically examined at every four or five millimeters for the residual lymph nodes.

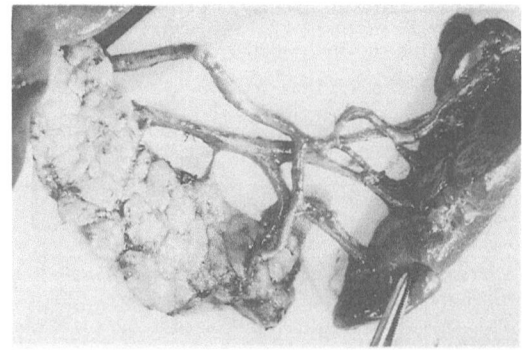

Fig.1 L_{11} was dissected by meticulous removal of tissues surrounding the splenic artery.

RESULTS

Clinical Study

Table 1 shows the background factors of PS(+) group (19 patients) and PS(-) group (63 patients). There was a significant difference in the depth of cancer invasion (p<0.05). However, there was no significant difference between the two groups in the distribution of prognostic factors such as age, sex, classification of lymph node metastasis, liver and peritoneal metastasis and curability of operation. As shown in Fig. 2, the one, two, three, four and five year survival rates of PS(+) group were 47.4%, 15.8%, 15.8%, 10.5%, 10.5%, and those of PS(-) group were 57.1%, 31.2%, 21.3%, 17.1%, 12.8% respectively. The survival rates of PS(-) group were higher than those of PS(+) group, but there was no significant difference between the two groups.

Table 1. Background factors of patients with or without pancreatico-splenectomy

	pancreatico-splenectomy(+) (n=19)	pancreatico-splenectomy(-) (n=63)	
Age			
-49	8	16	
50-59	3	18	N.S
60-69	7	20	
70-	1	9	
Sex			
male	11	35	N.S
female	8	28	
Lymph node meta.			
n2	10	37	
n3	1	12	N.S
n4	8	14	
Depth of invasion			
m	0	0	
sm	0	1	
pm	1	5	p<0.05
ss	2	8	
se	10	48	
si	6	1	
Liver meta.			
(−)	18	59	N.S
(+)	1	4	
Peritoneal meta.			
(−)	12	45	N.S
(+)	7	18	
Curability			
curative	5	22	N.S
non-curative	14	41	

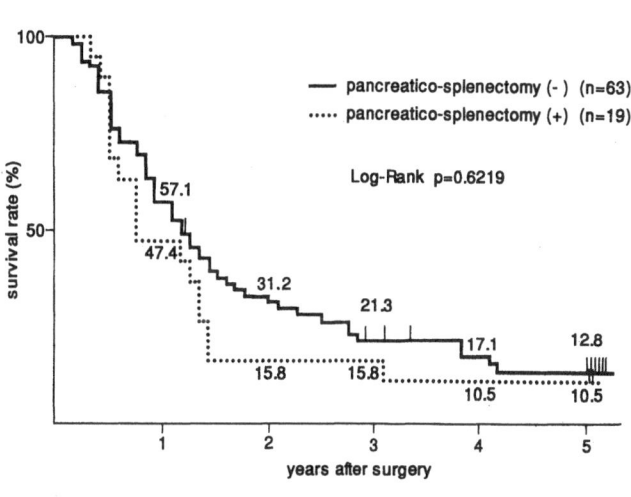

Fig. 2 Comparison of survival rates of patients who had pathological metastasis to L_{11}

Pathological study

Eight patients with advanced gastric carcinoma were registered in this study. Table 2 shows these eight patients and their results of the study. Residual lymph nodes of L_{11} were detected in three (case 2, 4 and 7) out of eight cases. However, they were very few in number and small in size (0.5~1.0mm in diameter) and cancer metastasis was not observed in any of these residual lymph node specimens.

DISCUSSION

For the purpose of the complete dissection of L_{10} (lymph node at the splenic hilus) and L_{11}, PS is usually performed in Japan in cases of total or proximal gastric resection against advanced gastric cancer. The frequency of pathological metastasis to L_{11} was 4.4% in all our cases of gastric cancer, and 18% in cases with cancer in the upper third of the stomach [2]. Okano et al recommended total gastrectomy with distal pancreato-splenectomy for complete removal of L_{11} lymph nodes because of high frequency of metastasis to L_{11} in the patients with cancer in the upper or middle third of the stomach with lymph node metastasis to the right cardial lymph nodes, the lymph nodes along the short gastric artery, along the left gastroepiploic artery, along the left gastric artery or along the common hepatic artery [3]. Kamata et al also advocated that the pancreatosplenectomy had to be carried out in advanced gastric cancer[2]. However, Ishizaki reported that the reduction of glucose tolerance was noted on patients undergoing pancreato-spleno-total gastrectomy [4]. Yonemura et al also described that the insulin secretion was significantly lowered after resection of 50 to 65 percent of pancreas below the preoperative level [5].

Table 2. Registered cases in the pathological study (1990~1992)

| Case | Gross finding | | | | Histological type | Histological finding | | | Residual lymph node of L_{11}(size) |
	Location	Size(cm)	Gross type	H P S N		Depth of invadion	Lymph node meta. (n)	Meta. to L_{11}	
1. N.N. 39 F	C	8 x 5	IIc adv.	0 0 2 1	sig	ss 7	0	no	no
2. R.I. 56 M	C	3.5 x 3.5	Borr. 2	0 0 2 2	por	ss 7	0	no	yes (0.5mm x 1)
3. K.H. 44 M	Ce	8 x 5	Borr. 2	0 0 2 1	tub2	se	1	no	no
4. M.Y. 60 M	C	11 x 8	Borr. 3	0 0 2 1	tub2	pm	2	no	yes (1.0mm x 1)
5. T.I. 63 M	C	4.5 x 4.5	Borr. 3	0 0 1 1	por	ss 7	2	no	no
6. M.S. 37 F	Cm	18 x 14	Borr. 4	0 0 2 1	por	ss 7	1	no	no
7. Y.M. 67 F	Ce	7 x 4	Borr. 2	0 0 0 1	por	se	2	no	yes (0.5mm x 1)
8. M.I. 54 M	MAc	14 x 10	Borr. 4	0 0 2 2	sig	ss 7	2	no	no

We have asserted that the lymph node dissection of L_{11} is possible without PS. In our pathological study, the lymph nodes along the splenic artery (L_{11}) were dissected by meticulous removal of tissues surrounding the splenic artery. Macroscopically there seemed to be no lymph nodes along the splenic artery after dissection. However, residual lymph nodes of L_{11} were detected microscopically in three out of eight cases. They were very few, small (0.5 ~ 1.0mm in diameter) and cancer negative. In other five cases all lymph nodes of L_{11} were completely dissected. On the other hand, in our clinical study against the patients who had lymph node metastasis to L_{11} the survival rates of PS(-) group were higher than those of PS(+) group, although the difference did not reach to a statistically significant level. Prognostic variables such as age, sex, classification of lymph node metastasis, liver metastasis, peritoneal metastasis and curability of operation revealed no statistical differences. This study was not a randomized controlled trial, and more deeply invaded cases were significantly observed in PS(+) group. However, although there are some problems in our study, these results might support our speculation. Kinoshita et al also reported that the five year survival rate of pancreas-preserving operation (PP) group was better than those of distal pancreatectomy (DP) group, and the incidence of hospital death and complications were higher in the DP group [6].
From these results, we concluded that the pancreatico-splenectomy was not always essential for prophylactic dissection of lymph nodes along the splenic artery.

REFERENCES

1. Japanese Research Society for Gastric Cancer (1981) The General Rules for the Gastric Cancer Study in Surgery and Pathology. Jpn J Surg 11:127-139
2. Kamata T, Yonemura Y, Ooyama S, Takegawa S, Kimura H, Matsumoto H, Tsugawa K, Kosaka T, Miwa K, Miyazaki I (1990) Indication of pancreatosplenectomy for gastric cancer on the upper part of the stomach. Jpn J Gastroenterol Surg 23:7-11
3. Okano S, Sawai K, Yamaguchi M, Seiki K, Taniguchi H, Hagiwara A, Yamaguchi T, Takahashi T (1992) A study on lymph nodes metastases along the splenic artery of gastric cancer. Jpn J Gastroenterol Surg 25:2110-2117
4. Ishizaki E (1992) A study of postoperative glycometabolism after pancreato-spleno-total gastrectomy with refference to changes in glucose tolerance followed in termes of intravenous glucose tolerance test and glycosylated hemoglobin. J Jpn Soc Clin Surg 53:7-18
5. Yonemura Y, Miyazaki I, Miwa K, Hagino S (1981) The endocrine function of the pancreas after partial pancreatectomy. J Jpn Surg Soc 82:671-680
6. Kinoshita T, Maruyama K, Sasako M, Ooyama S (1992) A comparison of distal pancreatectomy and the pancreas-preserving operation for advanced gastric cancer in regard to the quality of life of the patients and the treatment results. Jpn J Gastroenterol Surg 25:2618-2623

Evaluation of Super Extensive Lymph Node Dissection (R4) for Advanced Gastric Cancer

SHIGERU TAKAHASHI, HAJIME TOKUDA, HIROSHI MATSUSHIGE, ATSUSHI TAKENAKA, MAKOTO KATO, and NORIMASA WATANABE

The Department of Surgery, Kyoto Second Red Cross Hospital, Kyoto, 602 Japan

ABSTRACT

Our super extensive lymph node dissection (SELD (R4)) was designed to remove the nodes as thoroughly as possible from the para-aortic area. In our previous studies, cases of exposed scrosa presented high rates of n4 metastasis. However, when the positive rate in n4 was low, R4 dissection significantly increased the 5 year survival rate compared to the rate in highly positive cases. Five hundred forty three patients who underwent curative resection for primary gastric cancer between 1979 and 1988 were reviewed. In stage I, any resection (R) produced good prognosis. In stage II, III or IV, the prognosis of the patients treated by the R4 dissection was better than that of those with R2 or R3 dissections, although the survival curves of R2 or R3 dissections were nearly equal. SELD (R4), however, required a longer duration of surgery, with greater loss of blood and had a higher rate of complications than conventional R2, R3 dissection.

KEY WORDS: super extensive lymph node dissection (R4), para-aortic lymph node, gastric cancer

INTRODUCTION

One of the most significant prognostic factors of gastric cancer is lymph node metastasis. In Japan, for the surgical cure of the gastric cancer, R2 or R3 lymph node dissection is usually employed. However, in our previous studies, the para-aortic lymph nodes (n4) were confirmed as the terminal destination of the lymphatic flow in the upper abdominal cavity. Accordingly, since 1983, for progressive gastric cancer, we have dissected n4 from the diaphragm to around the inferior mesenteric artery. We designated this procedure "super extensive lymph node dissection (R4)".

PRINCIPAL STEPS OF SUPER EXTENSIVE LYMPH NODE DISSECTION (R4)

Pre-operative EUS findings and super selective angiogram suggest that the tumor is exposed to the serosa. Laparotomy is performed by transverse chevron incision with the xyphoid process at its peak to allow the easier manipulation during surgery.
Serosal invasion and/or parastomach lymph nodes metastasis are inspected grossly, and if there were no factors inhibiting radical resection, R4 dissection is initiated.

1) Separation is made along the fusion fascia to shift the left kidney and the descending colon, and the posterior para-aortic nodes are dissected. 2) The pancreato-renal fusion is then split, and the left, anterior para-aortic nodes are dissected. 3) The lymph nodes along the left inferior-phrenic artery and vein are dissected distally en bloc. 4) The para-aortic lymph nodes is made on the caudal side down to the level of the inferior mesentric trunk. The left testicular or ovarian vein is ligated and resected. 5) The para celiac trunk and superior mesenteric artery nodes are dissected. 6) Lifting the inferior edge of the pancreas, the lymph nodes along the superior mesenteric artery and vein are dissected to the distally. The venous trunk of Henle is ligated and resected. 7) Kocher's mobilization is used, and the lymph nodes between the aorta and vena cava are dissected. 8) Then the dissection is continued to the R3 level.

PATIENTS AND METHODS

To evaluate the 5 year survival rate after R4 surgery, cumulative survival rates for each stage of gastric cancer were compared according to the extent of lymph node dissection (R) for 543 patients treated surgically in our department between 1979 and 1988. Clinical follow up was possible in 540 of 543 patients. Nineteen patients died of other diseases. Nine patients died of unknown causes. There were two hospital deaths from pneumonia and hepatic failure, respectively. Three patients were lost to clinical follow up. Survival curves were calculated by the Kaplan-Meier method, and the differences between the curves were measured by a generalized Wilcoxon test. One hundred and ninety seven patients treated by R4 dissection were analyzed according to the depth of gastric cancer to determine the frequency of n4 metastasis in the gastric cancer with serosal invasion.

RESULTS

1) Table 1 summarizes patient information according to the stage and mode of dissection (R). Of 543 curative surgeries performed in our department between 1979 and 1988, 197 patients received with R4 dissection. As the stage deteriorated, the percentage receiving R4 dissection increased from 22.6% in stage I to 52.0% in stage IV.

Table 1. Number of patients according to the stage and mode of dissection (R)

stage	R0	R1+7	R2	R3	SELD (R4)
I (n=261)	6	29	125	42	59
II (n=84)	0	7	22	17	38
III (n=112)	0	7	34	20	51
IV (n=86)	0	10	15	12	49
	6	53	196	91	197

2) Lymph node metastasis in 198 patients with gastric cancer who have undergone the super extensive lymph node dissection (R4) are shown in table 2.
While metastasis were almost limited to n2 lymph nodes in patients with intramural cancer, in the patients with serosal invasion, n4 metastasis occurred at a high rate of 27.3% (30/110), comparable to n1 or n2 cases.

Table 2. Nodal status according to cancer location in the SELD (R4) cases (n=197)

serosal invasion	location	n0	n1	n2	n3	n4	
negative (n=87)	upper third	12	2	0	0	2	(12.5%)
	middle third	22	3	3	0	1	(3.4%)
	lower third	27	8	4	1	1	(2.4%)
	entire stomach	1	0	0	0	0	(0.0%)
positive (n=110)	upper third	3	4	7	0	7	(33.3%)
	middle third	4	7	6	0	4	(19.0%)
	lower third	9	11	6	5	11	(26.2%)
	entire stomach	5	3	10	0	8	(30.8%)

3) Cumulative 5-year survival rate at each stage of gastric cancer treated at our department between 1979 and 1988 are summarized in table 3. In advanced gastric cancer patients (stage II, III, IV), prognosis after R4 dissection were better than R2 or R3 dissection.

Table 3. 5-year survival rate (%) in each stage according to the method of dissection

stage	R1	R2	R3	R4	
I	97.2	100.0	100.0	97.8	
II	85.7	74.3	63.7	90.9	$p < 0.05$
III	26.7	46.7	39.0	58.0	
IV	0.0	6.7	9.1	21.5	

COMPLICATION

Table 4 shows complications in 197 patients with R4 dissection. Leakage (5.6%) and left pleural effusion (5.1%) occurred more often than in R1, R2 or R3 cases. Only 6 deaths were seen in R4 cases (3.1%), although no deaths occurred among R2 cases.
Table 5 shows blood loss and length of surgery according to the mode of dissection (R). R4 dissection had a longer duration of surgery, with greater loss of blood and by the higher rate of complications than conventional R2, R3 dissection.

Table 4. complications of the R4 patients

complication	SELD (R4) n=197	R3 n=91	R2 or R1 n=249
leakage	11	1	5
left pleural effusion	10	1	3
stenosis of the anastomosis	8	2	1
intraabdominal abscess	5	1	3
(bleeding)	(3)	(0)	(1)
fistula of the pancreas	3	1	2
hepatic failure	3	0	0
ileus .surgery	2	1	3
total complications	42 (21.3%)	7 (7.7%)	17 (6.8%)
mortality	6 (3.1%)	1 (1.1%)	0 (0.0%)

Table 5. Blood loss and duration according to the mode of resection (R)

mode of dissection	blood loss (gr)	duration (min)
SELD (R4)	1116.7 (150-3700)	321.4 (108-570)
R3	723.1 (90-3000)	219.2 (85-480)
R2	518.9 (30-3200)	184.3 (45-370)
R1+7	355.3 (30-1480)	147.5 (30-310)

COMMENTS
We found that even patients with stage II, III or IV advanced gastric cancer who underwent R4 dissection had better a outcome than those who underwent R1, R2, or R3 dissection.
In conclusion, our results suggest that R4 dissection has considerable benefits in terms of the prognosis for advanced gastric cancer. Although complications are frequent, they can be managed, and mortality can be limited.

REFERENCES

1. Japanese Research Society for Gastric Cancer (1981) The general Rules for Gastric Cancer Study in Surgery and Pathology. Japanese Journal of Surgery Vol.11, No.2: 127-139
2. Takahashi S, Takahashi T, Sawai K, Hagiwara A, Tokuda H, Kato G, Takenaka A (1987) Studies on Para-aortic Metastic Lymph Nodes of Gastric Cancer after Endoscopic Injection of Activated Carbon Particle. Journal of Japan Surgical Society 35-40.
3. Takahashi S (1990) Study of Para-aortic Lymph Node Metastasis of Gastric Cancer Subjected to SuperExtensive Lymph Node Dissection. Journal of Japan Surgical Society 91 (1): 29-35

Metastasis to Minute Lymph Node in Gastric Cancer, Its Significance for Indication of Endoscopic or Local Surgical Treatments

SUNG-JOON KWON[1], KEIICHI MARUYAMA[2], MITSURU SASAKO[2], and TAIRA KINOSHITA[2]

[1]Department of General Surgery, Hanyang University Hospital, Seoul 133-792, Korea
[2]Gastric Surgery Division, National Cancer Center Hospital, Chuo-ku, Tokyo, 104 Japan

ABSTRACT

In a recent case of limited gastric resection for early gastric cancer with submucosal invasion, we found metastatic carcinoma in a minute lymph node at the gastric serosa. In a prospective study to determine the incidence of such metastases, we studied 200 consecutive patients. Our data showed that minute gastric serosal lymph nodes occurred in 43 cases(22%). However metastatic carcinoma in early gastric cancer to these nodes was uncommon, occurring in 1 case(2.3%). It is concluded that even if metastasis to minute lymph nodes at the gastric serosa had been previously missed,they would not have affected the data base for the management of early gastric cancer, particularly for endoscopic or local surgical treatment, because of the rarity of metastasis to these lymph nodes. Nevertheless it should be noted that metastasis to minute gastric serosal lymph nodes can sometimes occur.

KEY WORDS : minute gastric serosal lymph node, gastric cancer, endoscopic or local surgical treatment

INTRODUCTION

Now so many interests are focused to detect metastatic lesion more accurately. including about the status of very small sized lymph node. Most surgeons consider lymph node dissection an essential part of gastrectomy for cancer in that possible metastasis are removable and a more radical resection results. But in some cases, endoscopic treatment is tried under the guideline of indications about which type can be free from the lymph node metastasis. Such an indications were determined by a retrospective analysis of many operated cases. In that analysis, the status of such minute lymph node was not considered and ignored. But if metastasis exists in such minute lymph node, the patient could be upstaged, for example from no to n1 and may have worse prognosis if treated endoscopically without operative resection. According to our experience, we analysed the status of such minute lymph nodes.

MATERIALS AND METHODS

Materials

In 71 year old female patient, macroscopically type I shaped gastric mass located at the posterior wall of the mid-body was confirmed as papillo-tubular adenocarcinoma by endoscopic biopsy and the expected depth of invasion as mucosa layer, measured as 1.5-2.0cm in diameter. So a limited partial gastrectomy was performed. But during that operation, the result of frozen examination of one minute lymph node(1mm in diameter) attached to the gastric serosal wall along the lesser curvature(Fig.1) was metastatic lymph node. The operation was extended as distal subtotal gastrectomy(Fig.2) combined with level 2 lymphadenectomy, as absolute curative resection. The pathologic examination showed one another metastatic perigastric lymph node(among 17 perigastric lymph node) which was located along the lesser curvature near from the metastatic minute lymph node. The tumor was measured as 1.5x1.3x1.0 cm and the depth of invasion was submucosa. The lymphatic permeation and the vascular invasion were grade 1. Five years after the operation, the patient was dead from pneumonia. From this experience, we started to analyze the importance of the minute lymph nodes.

Methods

The minute lymph nodes were carefully picked up from the gastric serosal wall during and after the operation in all cases of resected gastric carcinoma excluding absolute noncurative resection cases. In 43 cases(43/200, 22%), such a minute lymph node was found and all of them were pathologically examined. For these minute lymph nodes, we nominated as Range I lymph node which located within 2cm from the margin of the main tumor and those located more than 2cm as Range II lymph node. Total number of Range I lymph node in 43 cases was 68 and 2 out of 7 Range I lymph node in one case showed metastasis. Among 70 Range II lymph nodes in 43 cases, metastasis was not found. The case with metastatic Range I lymph node was double primary gastric cancer. Main tumor was located at the posterior wall of cardia,

3.2cm x3.3cm in size, moderately differentiated adenocarcinoma with subserosal invasion. And the minor tumor was at the anterior wall of body, 1.0cmx1.0cm in size, well differentiated adenocarcinoma with mucosal invasion. For this patient, a total gastrectomy and R3 lymphadenectomy was performed. The final pathology of the perigastric and extraperigastric lymph node was n1 state(1/109). The pathologic examination of the lymph node was performed using conventional method(not using fat clearing method), fixed in formalin followed H&E stain.

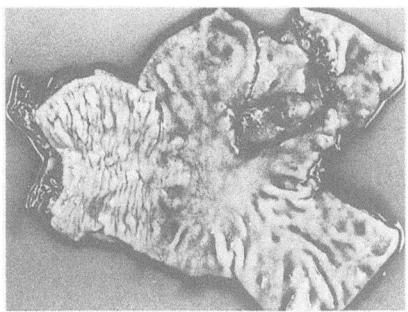

Fig.1 Minute lymph node attached to the gastric serosal wall

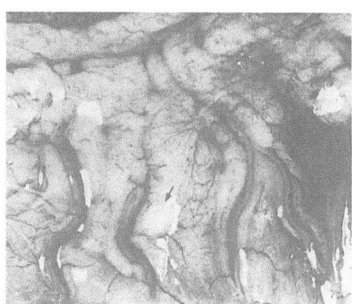

Fig.2 Distal subtotal gastrectomy after limited partial gastrectomy

RESULTS

Existence of minute lymph nodes and its metastasis according to lymph node metastasis ;
The minute lymph nodes was found in 43 cases among 200 patients, and its percentage was 22%. Of 43 cases having minute lymph node, 2 cases showed metastasis as 5%. It was noteworthy that the percentage of existence did not increase by the elevation in the N-stage. And metastasis at the minute nodes was observed only in "n1 group"(Table 1).

Table 1. Existence of minute lymph nodes and its metastasis according to lymph node metastasis

	Existence	Metastasis
Total	43/200=22%	2/43= 5%
n0	26/122=21%	0/26= 0%
n1	10/ 38=26%	2/10=20%
n2	3/ 23=13%	0/ 3= 0%
n3	1/ 3=33%	0/ 1= 0%
n4	3/ 14=21%	0/ 3= 0%

Table 2. Existence of minute lymph nodes and its metastasis according to macroscopic type

		Existence	Metastasis
EGC type	I	1/ 6=17%	1/ 1=100%
	IIa	2/13=15%	0/ 2= 0%
	IIc	15/77=19%	0/15= 0%
	III	1/ 2=50%	0/ 1= 0%
Borrmann's type	I	0/ 2= 0%	0/ 0= 0%
	II	4/23=17%	0/ 4= 0%
	III	13/49=27%	0/13= 0%
	IV	0/13= 0%	0/ 0= 0%
	V	7/13=54%	1/ 7=14%

Table 3. Existence of minute lymph nodes and its metastasis according to macroscopic type

	Existence	Metastasis
m	10/51=20%	0/10= 0%
sm	8/48=17%	1/ 8=13%
pm	6/22=27%	0/ 6= 0%
ss	9/14=64%	1/ 9=11%
se	10/48=21%	0/10= 0%
si	0/17= 0%	0/ 0= 0%

Table 4. Existence of minute lymph nodes and its metastasis according to histological type

	Existence	Metastasis
Papillary	3/ 6=50%	1/ 3=33%
Well Diff.	7/51=14%	0/ 7= 0%
Mod. Diff.	7/45=16%	1/ 7=14%
Poor Diff.	15/52=29%	0/15= 0%
Sig. Ring	10/43=23%	0/10= 0%
Mucinous	1/ 3=33%	0/ 1= 0%

Table 5. Existence of minute lymph nodes and its metastasis according to lymphatic invasion

	Existence	Metastasis
ly 0	17/85=20%	0/17= 0%
ly 1	10/52=19%	1/10=10%
ly 2	7/28=25%	1/ 7=14%
ly 3	9/29=31%	0/ 9= 0%

Existence of minute lymph nodes and its metastasis according to macroscopic type ;
According to macroscopic type, there was also no difference in the percentage of the existence and its metastasis(Table 2).
Existence of minute lymph nodes and its metastasis according to depth of invasion ;
There was no difference according to the depth of invasion(Table 3).
Existence of minute lymph nodes and its metastasis according to histological type ;
The histologic type also showed no difference(Table 4).
Existence of minute lymph nodes and its metastasis according to lymphatic invasion ;
We expected that the lymphatic invasion would have an influence on the minute lymph node metastasis. However, it had no significance in the existence and metastasis(Table 5).

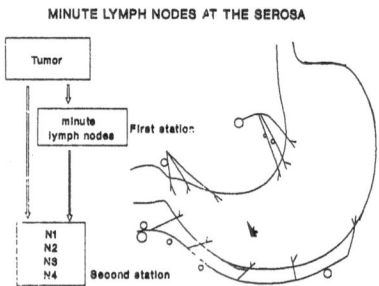

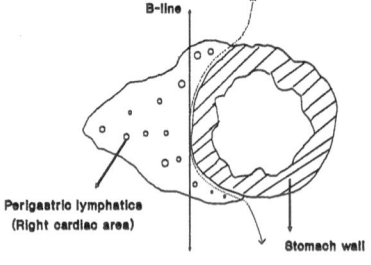

Fig.3 Lymphatic flows of the Stomach

Fig.4 Schematic draw of removal of the lymphatics around right cardiac area.

DISCUSSION

Endoscopic treatment for early gastric cancer has recently become the treatment of choice for lesions, even in patients without surgical risks, because of the decreased quality of life which may follow after surgery. The ratio of endoscopic treatment to surgery for early gastric cancer has been increasing yearly. For the successful endoscopic treatment of early gastric cancer, the existence of lymph node metastasis is the most important problem. To find out the indications of endoscopic treatment for early gastric cancer, many operated cases from multi-institute were collected and analysed. During such an analysis, the minute lymph nodes attached to the gastric serosal wall were not considered yet. In one operation planned to perform a limited partial gastrectomy for the elevated type early gastric cancer measured endoscopically as 1.5-2.0 cm in diameter, one minute lymph node attached to the gastric serosal wall was proved to be metastatic lymph node by frozen examination. Previously, such a minute lymph node (about 1mm in diameter) was ignored during lymph node dissection and about its analysis. Such finding became a motivation for us to start to search for these minute lymph node and include them into pathologic examination with usual perigastric and extraperigastric lymph nodes. Among 200 cases of resected gastric cancer(except absolute noncurative resection cases), minute lymph nodes were found in 43 cases(Detection ratio ; 22%). From these 43 cases, only two cases showed metastasis(Ratio of metastasis in detected cases ; 5%). The existence of minute lymph nodes and its metastasis were analyzed according to macroscopic type,depth of invasion,histological type and lymphatic invasion. But none of these factors showed significant difference. The results suggest that whether we had missed these minute lymph nodes or not before this study, the data base used for the indications of local treatment(endoscopic treatment or limited local surgical treatment without any lymph node dissection) has no need to be changed. We consider the minute lymph node as the first station at the lymphatic channels from the primary tumor(Fig.3). Lymphatic flows from the tumor will pass through the minute nodes at the serosa, but the other flows will directly pour into the conventional perigastric lymph nodes. We tried to know the percentage of existence and incidence of metastasis at the nodes. Although the percentage of the existence of the minute lymph nodes was 22% and its metastasis was 5%, surgeons should pay attention to the existence of such nodes and its possibility of metastasis during operation of gastric cancer. Especially when we perform a distal subtotal gastrectomy, the lymphatics located at the right cardiac area should be removed meticulously just like drawn as A-line in Fig.4. If the lymphatics were removed just as B-line in Fig.4, there exist a possibility to remain metastatic minute lymph node. Additionally we would like to stress the importance of the metastatic minute nodes when we consider the indications of endoscopic treatment for early gastric cancer.

Roux-en-Y End-to-Side Esophagojejunostomy with Stapler After Total Gastrectomy

Choong Bai Kim, Kwang Wook Suh, and Jin Sik Min

Department of Surgery, Yonsei University College of Medicine, Seoul, Korea

ABSTRACT

100 gastric cancer patients who underwent total gastrectomy and Roux-en-Y, End-to-Side esophagojejunostomy by using stapler were analysed with regard to operative result and complication. In addition, whether a routine use of Levin tube after total gastrectomy is necessary, 20 patients were randomly divided into 2 and were compared by postoperative course; for 10 patients Levin tube was removed at recovery room and for another 10, tube was indwelled until peristalsis returned. Median time for anastomosis was 18 minutes(15 to 45 minutes). 25-mm-cartridges were prefered, 85% of 25 mm vs 15% of 28 mm. In 92 patients, procedures were uneventful. Intraoperative problems happened in 8: 2 misfirings of stapler due to mechanical error, 6 incomplete doughnut tissues. Anastomotic leakage occurred in 2 patients and during follow up period 2 cases of anastomotic stricture were found. They were successfully treated by endoscopic dilatations. There was no operative mortality, nor other complication. Timing of removal of Levin tube did not affect duration of hospital stay and starting day of oral intake.

KEY WORDS: total gastrectomy, esophagojejunostomy, stapler

INTRODUCTION

Esophagojejunostomy after total gastrectomy is a time-consuming procedure and has a risk of several dreadful complications. Stapled anastomosis has facilitated the procedure and is now regarded as a standard technique for reconstruction of digestive tract after total gastrectomy. Since 1988, we have also performed nearly all cases of esophagojejunostomy by using the EEA stapler and manipulating the stapler is now considered as an ordinary procedure in our institution. In the present study, we present the result of experience of stapled esophagojejunostomy after total gastrectomy.

MATERIALS AND METHODS

From January 1987 to June 1992, 520 patients underwent total gastrectomy for gastric cancer in Yonsei University Hospital. Among them, 100 patients who underwent esophagojejunostomy by one surgeon(CBK) were evaluated for their operative results and complications. For mechanical suturing, EEA and TA devices(United States Surgical Co.,Norwalk, Conn.) were used. Males were 57 and females were 43. Median age was 55(34 to 71). The techniques employed were similar to those described by Walther(Fig.1,2)(1).For evaluation whether the routine use of Levin tube after total gastrectomy is necessary, 20 patients were randomy divided into 2 groups; Levin tube was removed at recovery room in 10 patients and Levin tube was indwelled until peristalsis returned in 10 patients. Both groups were compared according to postoperative course. Anastomosis was checked before starting oral intake with swallowing test dye(25mL of Gentian violet). If no leakage was observed through drain, patient started to drink fluid. If the procedure of anastomosis had been eventful, upper GI series with water-soluble contrast medium were performed in addition to test dye swallowing. Patients were regularly followed by endoscopy and barium meal study. Studies were performed 3,6,9,12 months after operation and every 6 months thereafter. Fig.3 showes barium meal study performed 1 year after operation.

RESULTS

The median time required for anastomosis was 18 minutes(range of 15 to 45 minutes). In 85 patients, 25-mm cartridges were used. In 92 patients, the procedures were uneventful. Table 1 shows intraoperative problems and postoperative complications. 2 misfirings of stapler resulted from mechanical errors and were treated by restaplings. In 6 cases, doughnut tissues were incomplete and unless the esophageal ring was incomplete(4 cases), only reinforcement of outer coat was made but if the esophageal ring was incomplete(2 cases), reanastomosis by restapling was performed. There were 2 leakages revealed by upper GI series and leakages were closed 7 to 10 days after total parenteral nutrition therapy. During follow up, anastomotic stricture was found in 2 patients. In both cases, a pediatric endoscope(12 mm in diameter) could not be passed the anastomosis. They were successfully treated by endoscopic dilatations. Median hospital stay was 12 days(range of 10 to 19 days)and there was no operative mortality. Table 2 shows comparison of two groups by postoperative course. Timing of removal of Levin tube did not affect the hospital stay and starding day of oral intake of both groups.

Table 1. Intraoperative problem and posoperative complication

Intraoperative problem	
Misfiring of stapler	2
Incomplete doughnut tissue	6
Postoperative complication	
Stricture	2
Leakage	2

Table 2. Comparison of two groups by postoperative course

	Group I	Group II	p
Nausea	2	0	
Fever	6	2	
Sore throat	3	0	
Hospital stay	15.1±3.3 days	13.1±1.4 days	NS
Starting day of oral intake	4.0±0.8	4.3±0.7	NS

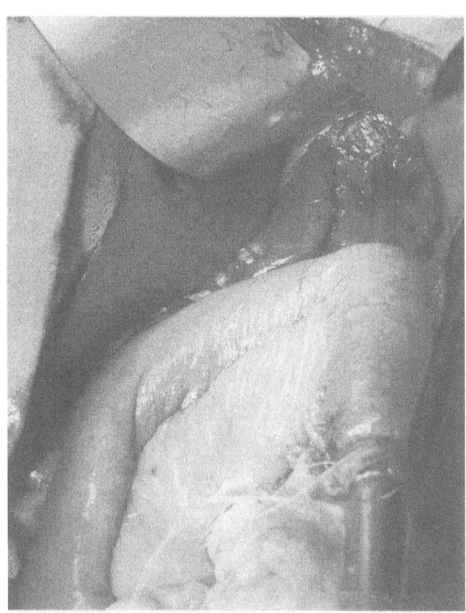

Fig 1. Operative feature that esophagojeju-no stomy is prepared. Esophageal purse string suture with 2-0 Prolene was securely tied. There is no problem during advancing the anvil into the esophageal lumen.

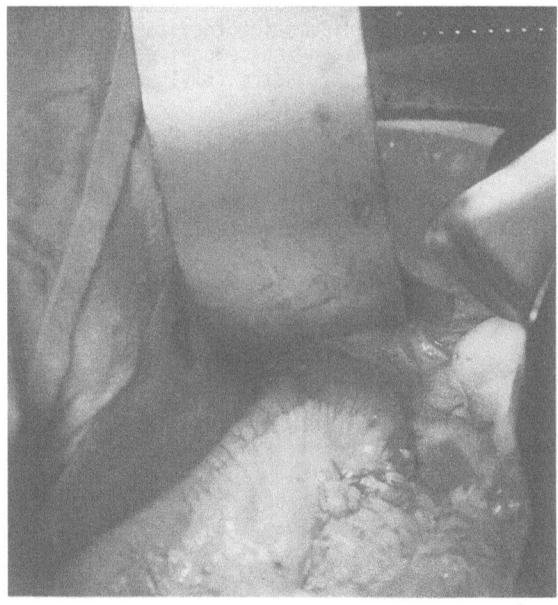

Fig 2. Operative feature of completion of esophagojejunostomy. Jejunal Roux-en-Y loop is ascended via antecolic route and there is no tension.

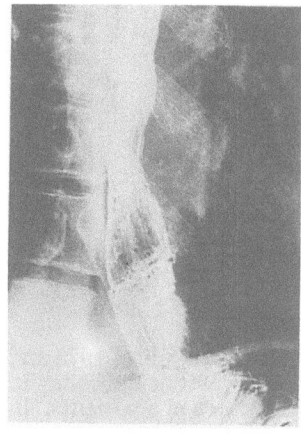

Fig.3 Barium meal study, 1
year after operation. There
is no stricture of anastomosis.

DISCUSSION

In spite of several advantages of stapler, a numerous study failed to prove that caomplication
rate after stapled anastomosis was definitely lower than sutured one (1-6). Rate of anastomotic leakage after stapled esophagojejunostomy still ranges 3 -10% (1-6). We think this was
probably due to misunderstanding and underestimation of the pitfalls of stapling procedures.
First, surgical principles of anastomosis; adequate blood supply, absence of sepsis, freedom
from tension and adequately cleared serosal surface is more importanat than in sutured anastomosis. Second correct and tight tying of purse string suture around the esophageal end is
indispensible condition. If too loose, doughnut tissue may be incomplete (4) and if too much
tissues is incorporated into the purse string suture, they may protrude outwards making anastomosis insecure. This pitfall is thought to be closely related to intraoperative problems
in our series. Third, the choice of adequate size of cartridge is important. With stapled anastomosis, anastomotic narrowing due to a stricture is a more common complication than leakage.
An inverse relationship has been reported between the incidence of stricture and the size of
stapled head (6). But it is dangerous to think that the larger the better because oversized
staple head can make more serious problems such as mucosal tearing and subsequent leakages.
Thus, choice of the largest cartridge that will not tear the esophageal mucosa is important.
Only minimal amount of intestinal contents were decompressed after total gastrectomy. Levin
tube merely cause some postoperative problems such as sore throat and fever and did not affect entire postoperative courses. So routine use of Levin tube after total gastrectomy may be
omitted with careful observations. In summary, we performed 100 esophagojejunostomy with stapler without any serious complication and could save total operating time significantly. We
think that the stapler, when properly used, can facilitate the esophagojejunostomy safely and
routine use of Levin tube after total gastrectomy may be unnecessary.

REFERENCES

1. Walther BS, Oscarson JEA, Graffner HOL, Vallgren S, Evander A (1986) Esophagojejunostomy
   with the EEA stapler. Surgery 99:598-603
2. Chassin JL, Rifkind KM, Turner JW (1984) Errors and pitfalls in stapling gastrointestinal
   tract anastomoses. Surg Clin North Am 64:441-459
3. Hedberg SE, Helmy AH (1984) Experience with gastrointestinal stapling at the Massachusetts
   General Hospital. Surg Clin North Am 64:511-528
4. Roberts P, Williamson WA, Sanders LB (1991) Pitfalls in use of stapler in gastrointestinal
   tract surgery. Surg Clin North Am 71:1247-1257
5. Campion JP, Grossetti D, Launoid B (1984) Circular anastomosis stapler. An alternative to
   purse-string suture. Arch Surg 119:232-233
6. Muehrcke DD, Kaplan DK, Donnelly RJ (1989) Anastomotic narrowing after esophagogastrectomy
   with EEA stapling device. J Thorac Cardiovasc Surg 97:434-438

The Role of Absolute Noncurative Gastrectomy for Primary Gastric Cancer

Tetsuji Fujita, Kazuo Matai, and Kenji Sakurai

First Department of Surgery, The Jikei University, School of Medicine, Minato-ku, Tokyo, 105 Japan

ABSTRACT

One hundred patients underwent a palliative procedure for primary gastric cancer between 1975 and 1984. Palliative partial resection of the stomach was performed in 59 patients, gastrojejunostomy in 17 patients, laparotomy and closure in 21 patients, and other palliative procedures in 3 patients. In cases without a distant metastasis to the peritoneum, the mean survival time after noncurative gastrectomy was significantly longer than that after other palliative procedures (16.4 versus 10.6 months, respectively). Similarly, in the absence of metastases to both liver lobes, there was a significant difference between the two groups with regard to the mean survival time.

KEY WORDS: gastric cancer, palliative partial gastrectomy, survival

INTRODUCTION

With refinements in diagnostic methods, the frequency of early gastric cancer has steadily increased, reaching 50% at the end of 1980s in Japan [1]. However, we know that advanced gastric cancer will never vanish. When curative resection is not possible, the election or rejection of palliative procedures depends on the surgeon's judgement and attitude. Additionally, this intraoperative decision may affect the quality of life and survival after surgery. The aim of this study is to evaluate the therapeutic significance of palliative gastrectomy in patients with advanced gastric cancer.

MATERIALS AND METHODS

Postoperative chemotherapy has been routinely used in patients with advanced gastric cancer since 1985. Adjuvant chemotherapy may affect the survival and the quality of life after surgery. Therefore, we studied retrospectively 546 patients treated for primary gastric cancer between 1975 and 1984. Of 546 patients 100 underwent a palliative procedure. The resection was classified as palliative if metastatic disease was left behind in the abdominal cavity, or if microscopic examination revealed tumor tissue in the resection lines. Palliative resection was performed in 59 patients, gastrojejunostomy in 17 patients, laparotomy and closure in 21 patients, and other procedures in 3 patients (Table 1). Palliative total gastrectomy was not performed during this period. Eighty-eight of 100 patients could be followed up until death. The mean survival times were compared between patients who underwent palliative resection and those who received other palliative procedures. Intergroup significance was tested by Students' t-test and then we considered significant at $p < 0.05$.

RESULTS

Direct cancer invasion to other organs and peritoneal metastasis were less frequently encountered in patients who underwent resection of the stomach than in patients who received other palliative procedures. However, there was no difference in the frequency of liver metastasis between the two groups. The mean survival time after noncurative gastrectomy was 12.8 months, that was significantly ($p < 0.01$) longer than 7.1 months in patients who underwent gastrojejunostomy. However, there was no difference in the mean survival time between patients who underwent noncurative gastrectomy and patients subjected to exploratory laparotomy (12.8 versus 9.7 months, respectively) (Fig. 1). Unless there was a distant peritoneal metastasis, the mean survival time after noncurative gastrectomy was 16.4 months and it was 10.6 months after other palliative procedures, a significant difference ($p < 0.05$). However, in patients with scattered or diffuse peitoneal metastases (each grade of metastasis is expressed as P_2 or P_3 according to the General Rules for the Gastric Cancer Study in Japan [2]), there was no difference in the mean survival time between the two groups (Fig. 2). In cases without liver metastasis (H_0) or with metastases limited to one lobe (H_1), the mean survival time after noncurative gastrectomy was 17.0 months, and it was 9.1 months after other palliative procedures, a significant difference ($p < 0.01$). However, in patients with scattered metastases to both lobes (H_2 or H_3), there was no difference in the mean survival time between the two groups. (Fig. 3)

Table 1. Palliative Operations for Gastric Cancer

Surgery	Number
Laparotomy and closure	21[*](2)
Gastroenterostomy	17 (5)
Gastrostomy	2
LeVeen shunt	1
Noncurative gastrectomy	59 (5)
Total	100 (12)

* Figures in parenthesis show number of patients in whom follow-up data were lost

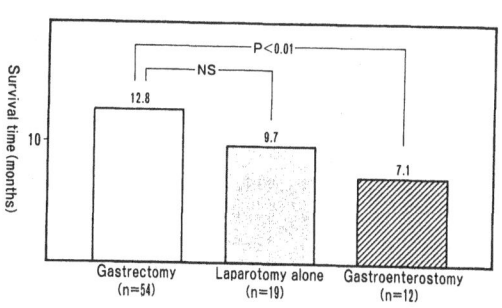

Fig. 1 Mean Survival Time and Operative Procedures

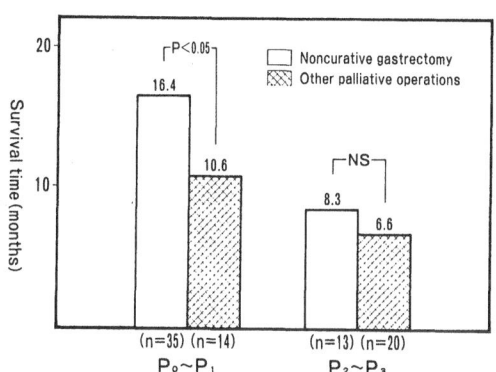

Fig. 2 Mean Survival Time According to Grade of Peritoneal Metastasis (Deaths within 30 days after surgery are excluded)

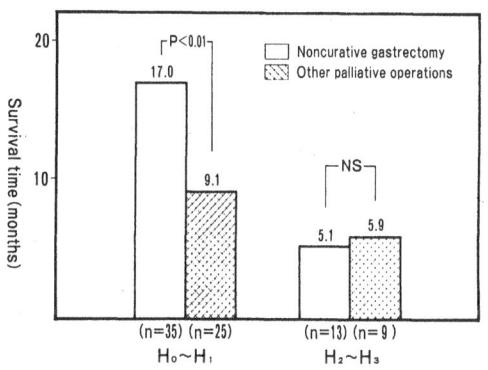

Fig. 3 Mean Survival Time According to Grade of Liver Metastasis (Deaths within 30 days after surgery are excluded)

DISCUSSION

It has been reported that the postoperative survival time of patients subjected to noncurative gastrectomy exceeds that of patients receiving other palliative procedures [3,4]. In this study the mean survival time of patients who underwent noncurative gastrectomy was significantly longer than that of patients subjected to gastrojejunostomy. However, there was no difference in the mean survival time between patients who underwent noncurative gastrectomy and patients subjected to laparotomy alone. A subpopulation that may benefit from palliative resection should be defined. Koga et al. [5] reported that the mean survival time after noncurative gastrectomy was significantly longer than that after laparotomy alone in patients with metastasis limited to one liver lobe (H_1) or with a few scattered metastases to both lobes (H_2). However, according to their report, there was no significant difference in the mean survival time between the two groups in patients with numerous scattered metastases to both lobes (H_3). Results of our study are almost consistent with those of their study. Meijer et al. [6] stated that palliative resection should be avoided in patients with peritoneal carcinomatosis. We agree with their policy, because it was shown that the mean survival time after noncurative gastrectomy was similar to that after other palliative procedures when massive peritoneal metastases were present. Although the goal for paliative resection is prolongation of the survival time, the quality of life should also be concerned. Many agree that noncurative gastrectomy provides the satisfactory palliation more often than does the other palliative procedure [6,7]. Regrettably, we could not describe the effect of palliative resection on postoperative quality of life, because it was hard to evaluate the quality of life precisely by hospital records. Although data were not shown, the operative morbidity and mortality for noncurative gastrectomy were similar to those for other palliative procedures. We suggest that palliative resection prolongs the survival of patients with noncurable gastric cancer when both peritoneal and hepatic metastases are absent or limited.

REFERENCES

1.   Nabeya K (1989) Analysis of recurrent early gastric cancer based on questionaries (in Japanese). Japanese Research Society for Gastric Cancer. Tokyo, pp 1-6
2.   Japanese Research Society for Gastric Cancer (1985) The General Rules for the Gastric Cancer Study (in Japanese). Kanehara Shuppan. Tokyo, pp 2-9
3.   Shanhon DB, Horowitz S, Kelly WD (1956) Cancer of the stomach, an analysis of 1152 cases. Surgery 39: 204-221
4.   Inberg M, Heinonen R, Rantakokko V, Viikari SJ (1975) Surgical treatment of gastric carcinoma. Arch Surg 110: 703-707
5.   Koga S, Kawaguchi H, Kishimoto H, Tanaka K, Miyano Y, Kimura O, Takeda R, Nishidoi H (1980) Therapeutic significance of noncurative gastrectomy for gastric cancer with liver metastasis. Am J Surg 140: 356-359
6.   Meijer S, De Bakker OJGB, Hoitsma HFW (1985) Palliative resection in gastric cancer. J Surg Oncol 23: 77-80
7.   Ekbom GA, Glevsteen JJ (1980) Gastric malignancy: Resection for palliation. Surgery 88: 476-481

Proper Indication of Gastrectomy for the Gastric Carcinomas with Liver Metastasis

Kazuo Hirose, Atsushi Iida, Akio Yamaguchi, and Gizo Nakagawara

The First Department of Surgery, Fukui Medical School, Matsuoka-cho, Yoshida-gun, Fukui, 910-11 Japan

ABSTRUCT

In 36 gastric carcinomas with synchronous liver metastasis, the influence of the degrees of liver metastasis and gastrectomy with lymphnode dissection upon the survival, was studied. In nine gastrectomy-patients who had less than seven metastatic liver tumors and underwent radical lymphadenectomy, more favorable median survival time and 1-year survival were obtained, 456 days and 67%, than in other 20 gastrectomy-patients who received palliative lympadenectomy regardless of the numbers of liver metastasis, as well as than in the seven patients who were not resectable.

KEY WORDS:gastric carcinoma, liver metastasis, hepatic arterial infusion chemotherapy

INTRODUCTION

Gastric carcinomas with liver metastasis are often accompanied with peritoneal metastasis and locally extensive lesions, such as lymphnode metastasis and direct tumor invasion to the neighbouring organs. Therefore, it remains still unknown in the surgical treatment of the gastric cancer patients with liver metastasis, whether or not gastrectomy and regional lymphadenectomy combined with perioperative chemotherapy are really effective to prolong the postoperative survival. In this paper, clinical results in the gastric carcinomas with liver metastasis, treated in our institute during the past ten years, were retrospectively studied. And the proper indication for surgical resection of the primary gastric tumor and the regional lymphnodes were considered.

PATIENTS AND METHODS

From October 1983 to December 1992, 36 patients of the gastric carcinomas with liver metastasis were admitted and treated in the First Department of Surgery, Fukui Medical School Hospital. Liver metastasis was diagnosed by abdominal ultrasound examinations, CT scans and and the operative findings. The degrees of liver metastasis in the patients were subdivided into the following three types;(1)one or two metastatic tumors in the unilateral left or right lobe of the liver(H_1, n=7), (2)less than seven metastatic tumors in the both lobes (H_2, n=10), and (3)seven or more metastatic tumors in the boths lobes (H_3, n=19).
Among these 36 patients, 29 patients, who consisted of all of seven H_1-, nine of the H_2- and 13 of the H_3-patients underwent gastrectomy and perioperative anticancer chemotherapy. The other only one H_2- and six H_3- patients were not resectable and treated only by chemotherapy. The methods of gastrectomy were subdivided into the two categolies, according to "local curability", that is, the presence or absence of the extrahepatic remnant lesions in the other site, such as the peritoneum, lymphnodes and adjacent organs;The first was gastrectomy with "radical" regional lymphnode dissection and combined resection of the invaded adjacent organs, resulted in no macroscopic cancer remnance("curative" gastrectomy group, n=9). The second was gastrectomy without complete lymphnode dissection and combined resection, resulted in the overt tumor remnance("palliative" gastrectomy group, n=20). Table 1 shows the relation of degrees of liver metastasis and local curability in the 29 gastrectomy patients. Curative gastrectomy could be perfomed only in three H_1- and six H_2-patients.
Resection of the metastatic liver tumors, was possible only in four of the 29 gastrectomy-patients;three H_1- and one H_2-patients. The operative procedure consisted of three partial resections and one segmental resection.
In 13 of the 29 gastrectomy-patients, hepatic arterial infusion chemotherapy(HAIC) was additionally done with Mitomycin C(10 to 20 mg/body), Adriamycin(20-30 mg/body) and 5-FU(500mg/body), several times in the perioperative periods. In seven patients, arterial catheter was inserted into the hepatic artery via the femoral artery by the Seldinger's technique. In the other six patients, implantable drug delivery device, INFUSE-A-PORT[R] (Shiley INFUSAID INC., USA) was implanted during the gastrectomy operation, and catheter was placed in the proper hepatic artery via the gastroduodenal artery.

Table 1. Degrees of liver metastasis and local curability of
gastrectomy in the 29 patients who received gastrectomy

Degrees of liver metastasis	No.of patients	Local curability of gastrectomy	
		curative☆	palliative★
H_1	7	3	4
H_2	9	6	3
H_3	13	0	13
Total	29	9	20

☆:Gastrectomy with "radical" lymphnode dissection, resulted
in no macroscopic cancer remnance except in the liver
★:Gastrectomy without complete lymphnode dissection, resulted
in the overt tumor remnance in the other sites

In order to evaluate the clinical outcomes after the therapy with or without gastrectomy, the
36 patients were classified into the four groups, as shown in Table 2, according to the
degrees of the liver metastasis and local curability of gastrectomy;H_1- or H_2-patients with
curative gastrectomy(group A, n=9), H_1- or H_2-patients with palliuative gastrectomy(group B,
n=7), H_3-patients with palliative gastrectomy(gouup C, n=13) and H_3-patients without
gastrectomy(group D, n=7).

Table 2. Four clinical groups according to the degrees of liver metastasis
and the "local curability" of gastrectomy

Clinical group	No. of patients	Degrees of liver metastasis and "local curability" gastrectomy
A	9	H_1- or H_2-patients who underwent curative gastrectomy
B	7	H_1- or H_2-patients who underwent palliative gastrectomy
C	13	H_3-patients who underwent palliative gastrectomy
D	7	H_3-patients who were not resectable

Results of the treatments were estimated by calculating the postoperative survival rate with
the method of Kaplan and Meier [1].

RESULTS

Fig.1 shows the survival of the four clinical groups shown in Table 2. Survivals for group A
were more favorble than those for the other three groups; The median survival times for

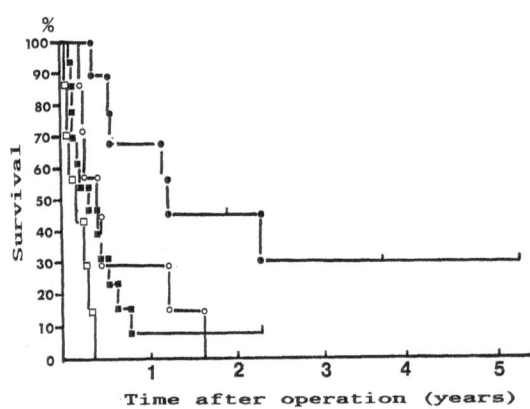

Fig.1 Survival of the four clinical groups
according to the degree of liver metastasis
and the "local curability" of gastrectomy
 ●-●:group A (n=9),   O-O:group B (n=7)
 ■-■:group C (n=13),   □-□:group D (n=7)

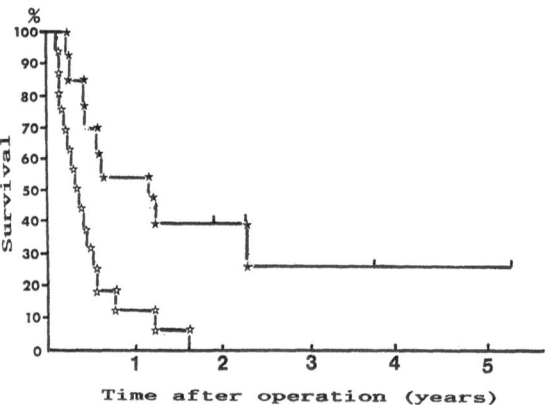

Fig.2 Survival of the patients who underwent
gastrectomy with or without hepatic arterial
infusion chemotherapy(HAIC)
 ★-★:HAIC(+), n=13
 ☆-☆:HAIC(-), n=16

group A, B, C and D at the time of analysis(March 31, 1993) were 456, 155, 157 and 67 days, respectively. Three patients in the group A and one patients are still alive 662 to 1908 days after operation. While the 1-year and 2-years survival rates for group A were 67 and 44%, the 1-year survival for group B, C and D were 29, 7.7 and 0%,respectively. The difference in the 180-days survivals between group A and B and that in the 1-year survivals between group A and C were statisically significant(p<0.01 and p<0.001, respectively).

Fig.2 shows the survival of the 29 gastrectomy-patients with or without HAIC. Survivals for the patients with HAIC were more favorable than those without HIAC(p<0.05);the median survival times and the 1-year survival rate were 429 days and 54%, and 114 days and 13%, respectively. Four of 13 patients with HAIC are still alive.

Four patients who lived more than two years, 1940 to 838 days, after gastrectomy are shown in Table 3. Three patients are still alive. All four patients were treated with HAIC using INFUSE-A-PORT. Three patients had H_2-metastasis and underwent curative gastrectomy, that is, belonged to group A.

Among four patients who underwent both curative gastrectomy and hepatic resection, two patients treated with HAIC using INFUSE-A-PORT, are still alive, 1360 days without recurrence and 693 days with hepatic recerrence, respectively. Another one patient with HAIC died 456 days due to the hepatic recurrence. The other patient without HAIC died 136 days.

Table 3. Four longterm survivors of gastric cancers with synchronous liver metastasis, who lived more than two years after gastrectomy

Patient No. (age, sex)	Tumor location, Borrmann's type	Operative findings	Curability of gastrectomy	Hepatic arterial infusion	Prognosis
1.(58, M)	A, type 2	$H_2P_0S_3N_3$	curative	+	1940 days, alive
2.(72, M)	C, type 3	$H_2P_0S_2N_4$	curative★	+	1360 days, alive
3.(82, M)	A, type 3	$H_2P_0S_3N_2$	curative	+	842 days, dead
4.(55, M)	A, unclassified☆	$H_3P_0S_2N_3$	palliative	+	838 days, alive

★:Partial resection of two hepatic metastatic tumors was perfomed.
☆:Carcinoid tumor

DISCUSSION

Prognosis of gastric carcers with liver metastasis is generally extremely poor. Bengmark et al. reported that a mean survival was six months for the untreated patients with liver metastasis [2]. According to Okuyama et al., prognosis depended on the presense of the peritoneal dissemination:when the patients had simultanuous peritoneal metastasis, there was no significant difference in the survivals between gastrectomy-cases and nonresectable cases [3]. But, previous reports rarely described cocerning the efficacy of the appropriate regional lymphadenectomy.

This paper desclibes the influence of the degrees of liver metastasis and local curability of the gastrectomy, upon the survival of the gastric carcinomas with liver metastasis. When the numbers of the metastatic liver tumors were seven or more, the patients who underwent gastrectomy survived not so longer than nonresectable patients. However, When the numbers were relatively small, less than seven, surgical results depended on the curability of gastrectomy and regional lymphadenectomy:curative gastrectomy resulted in significantly favorable survivals than palliative gastrectomy. This results mean the some important influence of the extrahepatic metastatic lesions upon the patient's survival.

We also studied the effect of the hepatic arterial infusion chemotherapy(HAIC) on the survivals of the gastrectomy patients. The patients treated with HAIC showed favorable survivals than those without HAIC. All four longterm survivors underwent both curative gastrectomy and HAIC. These results in this study imply that favorable clinical results are expexted only in gastric cancers with several metastatic liver tumors, if both curative gastrectomy and HAIC can be perfomed.

REFERENCES

1. Kaplan EL, Meier P (1958) Nonparametric estimation from incomplete observations. J Am Stat Assoc 53:459-481
2. Bengmark S, Hafstrom L (1978) The natural course of liver cancers. Prog Clic Cancer 7:195-200
3. Okuyama K, Onoda S, Tohnosu N, yamamoto Y, Koide Y, Hanaoka A, Seki Y, Hara T, Nishijima H, Isono K (1988) The prognosticsignificance of resection of primary tumor in gastric and colorectal cancer patients with synchronous liver metastasis. Jpn J Surg 18:7-17

Gastric Cancer Developing 40 Years After Simple Gastrojejunostomy

Katsutoshi Taniguchi, Hiroshi Tanimura, Takehiro Nakai, and Mizobata Shizuma

Department of Gastroenterological Surgery, Wakayama Medical College, Wakayama, 640 Japan

ABSTRACT

Two patients with gastric cancer developing over 40 years after gastrojejunostomy without gastric resection were operated on. These rare cases were reported and the literature was reviewed. The first case was a 72-year-old male with a chief complaint of heart burn. He had gastrojejunostomy for a perforation of duodenal ulcer 42 years ago. He was diagnosed as gastric cancer by endoscopy. A subtotal gastrectomy was performed. Histological diagnosis was papillary adenocarcinoma. The second case was a 85-year-old female who had gastrojejunostomy for gastric ulcer 40 years ago. She was examined for abdominal fullness and diagnosed as anastomotic cancer. She received subtotal gastrectomy. Histological diagnosis was moderately differentiated adenocarcinoma. The patients recovered. The good prognosis was obtained by radical operation.

KEY WORD: cancer, stomach, gastrojejunostomy

INTRODUCTION

Gastric remnant carcinoma has been well known as a cancer developing over ten years after gastrectomy for treatment of benign or malignant diseases, though gastric cancer occurring many years after simple gastrojejunostomy without gastrectomy for benign gastric diseases is very rare. Last year we operated on two cases with gastric carcinoma developing over 40 years after gastrectomy for treatment of peptic ulcer.

CASE REPORT

Case 1.

A 72-year-old man had been having heart burn for the past three years. He received gastrojejunostomy for treatment of perforated duodenal ulcer forty-two years ago. He had radiological examination of the stomach and was diagnosed reflux esophagitis. Two months ago he was diagnosed as gastric cancer by endoscopy. A double-contrast upper gastrointestinal (GI) study shows an abnormal shadow around a gastrojejunostomy at the greater curvature of the antrum (Fig. 1). Endoscopy demonstrated severe reflux esophagitis and a protruding tumor around the anastomotic region of the stomach (Fig. 2). The histopathological diagnosis of biopsy was group V (gastric carcinoma). Before gastric surgery, the chest X-ray showed a tumor shadow in the right lung and he had undergone right lobectomy in the Department of Thoracic Surgery, Wakayama Medical College before gastric surgery. The resected lung tumor was large cell carcinoma microscopically. Two months later he received a subtotal gastrectomy, partial jejunal resection, and Roux-en-Y anastomosis. The resected specimen showed firm circumferential tumor as an advanced gastric cancer of Borrmann type 3 around the anastomotic region of the stomach. Histology revealed papillary adenocarcinoma without metastases of lymph nodes. The cancer involved from mucosa to propria muscle (pm). His postoperative course was not eventful and he was discharged on the postoperative twentieth day.

Case 2

An 85-year-old female presented with a four-months history of abdominal fullness. She received gastrojejunostomy for gastric ulcer 40 years ago. She was diagnosed as early gastric cancer by endoscopy. Biopsy indicated Group V (signet ring cell carcinoma). Her general condition was good and no abnormal laboratory data could be found. A double-contrast upper GI series showed a rigidity and mucosal fold convergence in the gastrojejunostomy region of the antrum (Fig. 3). Endoscopy revealed a redness and superficial ulcerative lesion as IIc type of early gastric cancer at the edge of anastomosis (Fig. 4). At operation the tumor was not detected by palpation of the stomach. Subtotal gastrectomy, partial jejunal resection, and Billroth I reconstruction were performed. A small superficial ulcer (IIc type) was found at the anastomotic region of the specimen. The histological diagnosis was moderately differentiated tubular adenocarcinoma, early cancer, which reached through mucosal layer but not to proprietary muscle (sm). She recovered and was discharged one month after the operation.

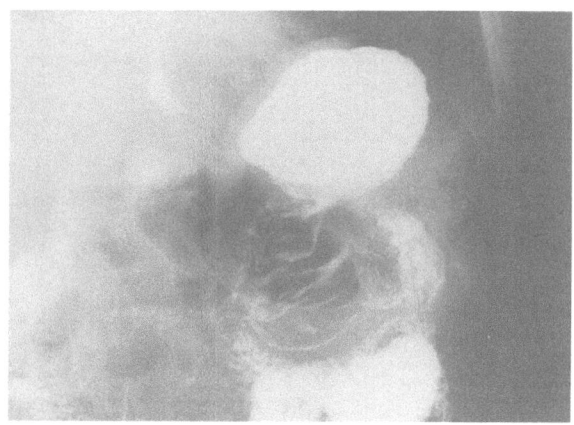

Fig. 1 Double-contrast upper GI series demonstrating a tumor shadow around the anastomosis

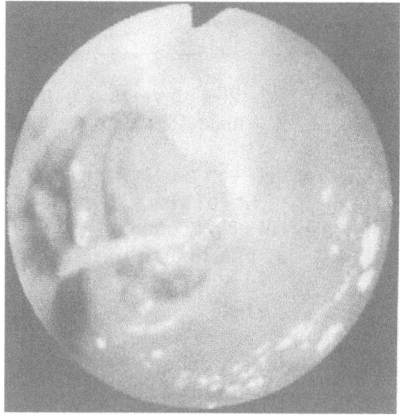

Fig. 2 Endoscopic picture showing gastric cancer at the anastomosis

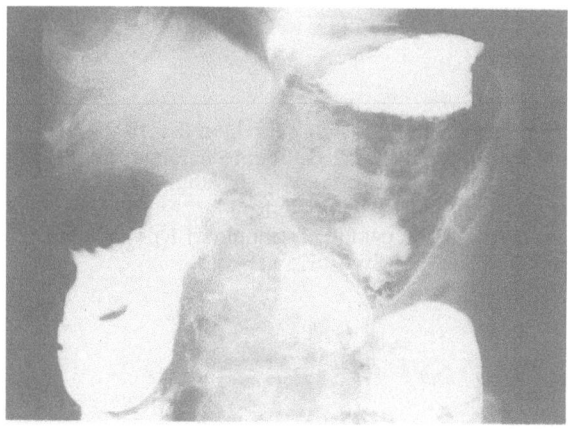

Fig. 3 Double-contrast upper GI series demonstrating rigidity at anastomotic region of the antrum

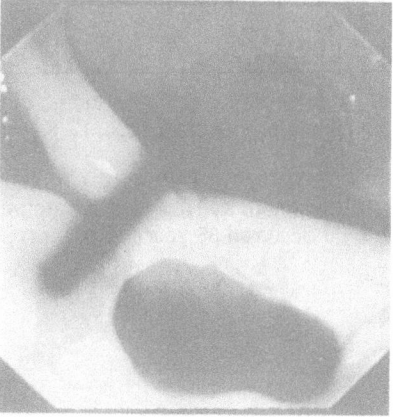

Fig. 4 Endoscopic picture showing small superficial ulceration, type IIc early cancer

DISCUSSION

The incidence of gastric cancer after gastrectomy is lower than that of gastric remnant or stump cancer [1,2]. We treated 25 patients with gastric remnat carcinoma occurring over ten years after gastrectomy, but only two patients with gastric carcinoma after simple gasrectomy. We collected 25 cases with gastric cancer after gastrectomy reported in Japan (Table 1) [1]. In characteristics of the patients, the age distribution was from 25 to 85 years old with the mean age of 61 years old. Twenty-two patients were male and three female. The male was dominant. The interval between primary operation and detection of gastric cancer was 12 to 51 years. The gastric cancers were located in anastomotic region in 14 cases (61%), antrum in 6 cases (24%) and whole stomach in 2 cases (8%). Nine patients had early cancer and ten patients advanced cancer.

Table 1. Review of the literature; 25 cases with gastric cancer
after gastrojejunostomy reported in Japan
(1960–1993)

Age : 25 - 85 years old, mean ; 61 years old	
Sex : male 22 cases, female 3 cases	
Interval between primary operation and detecting gastric cancer:	
12 - 51 years, mean; 25 years	
Location of gastric cancer:	
anastomotic region	14 cases (61%)
antrum	6 cases (24%)
whole	2 cases (8%)
Stage of cancer	
early cancer	9 cases (36%)
advanced cancer	10 cases (40%)

For the treatment total or partial gastrectomy were performed in 21 cases (84%) and unresectable cases were only two. In our patients, gastric cancers were detected over 40 years later after primary operation, and radical operation was performed successfully. Early diagnosis by endoscopy and radical operation for treatment of these patients led to their good prognosis and recovery.

REFERENCES

1. Beatson GT (1926) Carcinoma of the stomach after gastro-jejunostomy. Br Med J 1:15
2. Demirkol VK, Cilingiroglu K, Kecer M (1988) Magenkarzinom nach Gatroenterostomie. Zent bl Chir 113: 1472-1475
3. Fujii T, Umezu T, Tanaka T, Kohfuji K, Hirai Y, Tsuji Y, Iwai H, Yasumoto K, Hashimoto K, Takeda J, Kakegawa T (1991) A case of early gastric carcinoma of type IIc occurred 36 years after gasrojejunostomy. J Jpn Soc Clin Surg 52: 115-120

A Rare Case of Huge Gastric Carcinoma with Extramural Growth

Yasuo Hosouchi, Yukio Nagamachi, Seiichi Takenoshita, Ryoji Katoh, Tanji Suzuki, Hiroshi Koitabashi, Katuhiko Tukada, Masahito Iizuka, and Erito Mochiki

First Department of Surgery, Gunma University School of Medicine, Maebashi, 371 Japan

ABSTRACT

A rare case of gastric carcinoma which grew extramurally and invaded into the transverse mesocolon and pancreas is reported. The patient was a 67-year-old female, complaining of anorexia, weight loss and abdominal distension. She was diagnosed as gastric carcinoma with extramural growth. Intraoperative findings included a fist-sized, elastic hard tumor on the greater curvature that infiltrated into the transverse mesocolon and pancreas head($S_3P_0H_0N_1$ stage 4). Histopathologically, it was diagnosed as a poorly differentiated adenocarcinoma. The main tumor invaded deeply into the subserosal soft tissue($10 \times 8.5 \times 6.5$ cm). However upper part of the tumor appeared on the mucosal surface as a small erosion(1.2×0.9 cm in diameter).

KEY WORDS: gastric carcinoma, extramural growth

INTRODUCTION

There are generally two types of progress in the development of gastric cancer; one growing into the gastric wall and the other growing into the lumen. A recently observed case reported here is a comparatively rare case of an extramurally growing type cancer of the stomach. This case is described here in detail and discussed with reference to the cases published in the literature.

CASE

Patient : a 67-year-old woman
Chief Complaint : loss of appetite, weight loss, epigastralgia
Past History : cerebral infarction
Family History : non-contributory
Present Illness : She began to have an epigastralgia in May, 1992 and noted a loss of appetite since September, 1992. As she lost 8 kg for 5 months, she was admitted into the previous hospital. On October 7, 1992, she was referred here for medical workup.
Illness at Admission : She was 142 cm in height and 38 kg in weight. Physical examination revealed no abnormality in regions of the neck and the chest. Any enlargement of Virchow's lymph node was not detected on palpation. An elastic hard tumor was revealed in the area ranging from epigastrium to right hypochondrium by palpatic exploration of the abdominal region. The tumor was immovable and its size was as large as the palm. Digital examination disclosed no Schnitzler's metastasis.
Data of the physical examination carried at admission : Slight anemia, leakocytosis and increase of LDH(726 IU/L), and serum amylase(421 IU/L) were noticed. The tumor markers; CEA and CA19-9 were 83.6 ng/ml and 91 U/ml, both of which are abnormally high.
X-ray findings of the stomach (Fig. 1) : A comparatively moderate rising of the area ranging from the lower body to the pyloric part was noticed in her electopositioning filling picture. There was a filling defect apparently, being an exclusion from outer gastric wall.

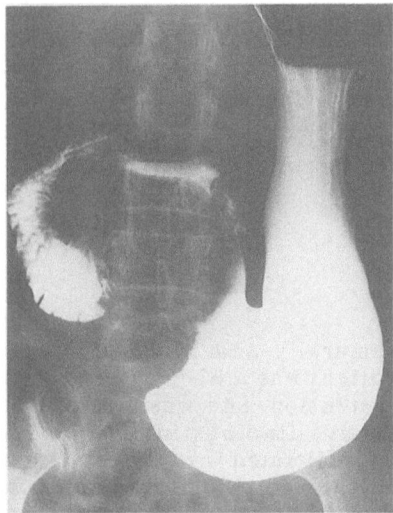

Fig. 1 X-ray findings of the stomach

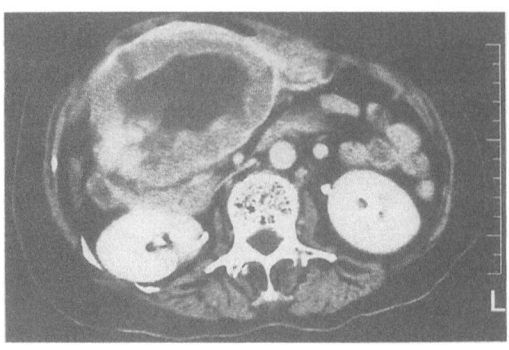

Fig. 2 CT findings

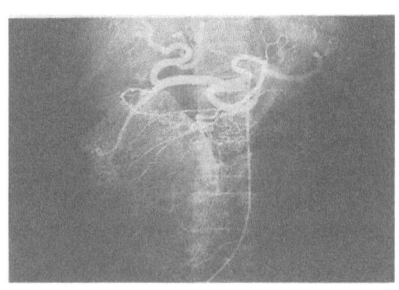

Fig. 3 Celiac arteriography findings

CT findings (Fig 2) : There was a central necrosis adjacent to the greater curvature side of pyloric part. A clear image of tumor showing capsular formation was detected in its peripheral region.

Celiac Arteriography (Fig. 3) : The tumor was revealed as a hypervascular tumor by celiac arteriography. The main feeder was left gastric artery and right gastroepiploic artery.

Preoperative diagnosis : Gastro-endoscope revealed an erosion, approximately 1 cm in diameter in the lower part of the great curvature. The biopsy specimen demonstrated to be an adenocarcinoma. Any marked change except for an exclusion was not observed in the other part of the gastric mucosa. It was diagnosed as an extramural growing type gastric cancer, but the possibility that it might be a complicated tumor due to gastric cancer and leiomyosarcoma originating from the stomach, still remains.

Operative findings : There was a palm-sized elastic hard tumor in the area ranging from the lower body to pylorus along the greater curvature. This tumor had a flat surface covered with serous membrane and some part of the tumor invaded directly into the transverse-mesocolon and the pancreas head was noticed. Subtotal gastrectomy with partial resection of the transverse colon and the pancreas was performed. The operative diagnosis was $S_3P_0H_0N_1(+)$ stage 4.

Excised specimen findings(Fig. 4) : There was an erosion 12×9 mm in diameter on the mucosal surface of the lower great curvature (indicated by an arrow), whereas the other region did not show abnormality.

Gross description of surgical specimen (Fig. 5) : The specimen consisted of grayish white clustered nodules accompanied with degeneration and necrosis in the central part. The growing region of the tumor was mainly found in the area from muscularis propria to subserosal soft tissue. The size of the tumor was $10 \times 8.5 \times 6.5$ cm.

Histopathological findings : The tumor is composed of poorly differentiated malignant cells. Mallory's staining revealed a formation of cell nest (Fig. 6). It was diagnosed as poorly differentiated adenocarcinoma of the stomach. Microscopic observation at low powerfield revealed that a poorly differentiated adenocarcinoma infiltrating into the mucosa was localized only in the erosive region, whereas the other part of the mucosa appeared intact (Fig. 7). It was diagnosed as poorly differentiated adenocarcinoma, $INF\gamma$, ly_2, v_2, ow(-), aw(-), $n_1(+)$(No6), sei(mesocolon, pancreas).

Clinical course; the patient was diagnosed as an extramural growing type gastric cancer and discharged on the 48th day after the operation. She is still under postoperative observation.

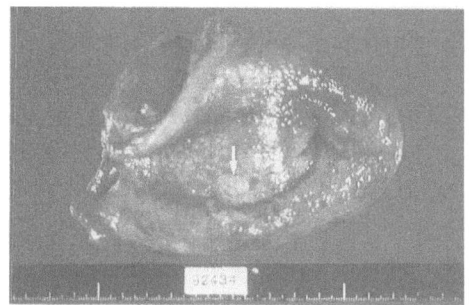

Fig. 4 Excised specimen findings

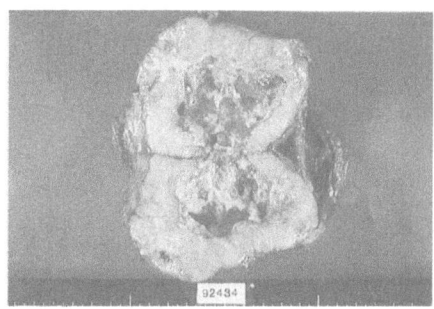

Fig. 5 Gross description of the tumor

Fig. 6 HIstopathological findings
(Mallory's staining)

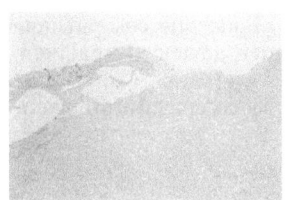

Fig. 7 Microscopic findings at low
powerfield of the erosive lesion

DISCUSSION

There are 46 cases of extramural growing gastric cancer including our case, reported in Japan since Ubukata and Nagai's report in 1928[1]. The parcentage of this type of cancer shows approximately 0.1 % in all types of gastric cancer. The sex ratio was about 1:1 among 45 cases excluding one case without its description; 22 male cases and 23 female cases. The average age was 55.2 years old. The most frequent chief complaint was abdominal tumor, found 26cases out of 41 (63.4%). The cases preoperatively diagnosed to be gastric cancer were 25 out of 39 cases reported with its clear description, (64.1%). Only 11 cases of them (28.2%) had been diagnosed to be an extramurally growing type, including misdiagnosed as omental sarcoma, gastric leiomyosarcoma and so on. This type occurred highly in the greater curvature side in the lower part of stomach. Since it is difficult to detect the symptoms until the tumor grows up to a large-sized, infiltrations to other organs, such as the transverse-mesocolon, the pancreas and the abdominal wall, the prognosis is generally unsatisfactory. Matsuda et al.[2] proposed two types of the progress in developing pattern of extramurally growing type gastric cancer. The first is a gastric cancer, infiltrating and proliferating, specifically into the lower part of the stomach wall, originating from gastric mucosa. The second type is, originating from aberrant gland present below the lamina propria and growing to form a submucosal tumor and stick out from the stomach. Since the lumen was covered with normal mucosa except for the erosive lesion in our case, it is assumed that the tumor might be the second type originating from some ectopic gland in the stomach. However, it is difficult to identify the developing process when the tumor has grown extensively, as well as in the most of the previous reports.

REFERENCES

1) Ubukata M, NAGAI H: So called extramurally growing gastric cancer- A case report. Pathology and Therapy 1 : 361-363, 1928
2) Matsuda Y, Sakakibara N, Suzuki H, et al.: Two cases of huge gastric carcinoma with extramural growth : Jpn J Gastroenterol Surg 9 : 134-137, 1976

Multidisciplinary Treatment of Gastric Endocrine Cell Carcinoma and Large Liver Metastasis

KATSUTOSHI TANIGUCHI, HIROSHI TANIMURA, and YOSHIA UMEMOTO

Department of Gastroenterological Surgery, Wakayama Medical College, Wakayama, 640 Japan

ABSTRACT

Gastric endocrine cell carcinoma is rare. The multidisciplinary treatment of a 52-year-old man with endocrine cell carcinoma and liver metastasis was reported. A total gastrectomy and left hepatectomy were performed. After the operation he had adjuvant plus maintenance chemotherapy of UFT, 5-FU, ADM, and MMC. MMC, 5-FU, ADM, and CDDP had high chemosensitivity and were used for intra-arterial infusion chemotherapy. Furthermore they were periodically injected into the hepatic artery from a vascular access device. Nine months later he died of liver metastases in spite of aggressive treatments. Endocrine cell carcinoma with liver metastasis is one of the most serious diseases and we need a more advanced treatment.

KEY WORD: endocrine cell carcinoma. stomach, multidisciplinary treatment, chemotherapy, liver metastasis

INTRODUCTION

Endocrine cell carcinoma is rare in the stomach. It should be distinguished from carcinoid as a new concept, because it is more malignant in pathological and clinical courses than carcinoid. We will report one case of gastric endocrine cell carcinoma with liver metastasis and its multidisciplinary treatment.

CASE REPORT

A 52-year-old man had been suffering from upper abdominal pain and anorexia for the past year. He received a regular physical examination twice a year. He had an upper gastrointestinal series for continuous abdominal pain and loss of appetite in September, 1992. He was diagnosed as gastric cancer by a general physician and referred to our institution for an operation. His present condition was not abnormal. An abdominal mass and the liver were not palpable. Examination of the blood disclosed 3,350,000 red blood cells and 6,900 white blood cells. The liver function was within normal range as GOT was 21 U/l, GPT 9 U/l, ALP 294 U/l, and LDH 294 U/l. The tumor markers (CEA, AFT, and CA19-9) were not elevated. The upper gastrointestinal series demonstrated a big tumor, Schattendefekt at the antrum and angle (Fig 1). The tumor was clear-cutting elevated with a large crater. The endoscopy showed an elevated tumor at the angle as an advanced gastric cancer of Borrmann type 2 (Fig. 2). The histological diagnosis of biopsies from the tumor was endocrine cell carcinoma. An ultrasound and CT scan demonstrated a liver metastatic tumor, 3 cm in diameter, near the gallbladder.

A radical total gastrectomy with removal of lymph nodes, splenectomy, partial pancreatectomy, cholecystectomy, and left hepatectomy were performed. Roux-en-Y esophagojejunostomy and jejunojejunostomy were done by EEA and TA auto-suture. The operation time was 7 hours. The gastric tumor was 5 x 5 x 2 cm in length and had a large crater with invasion to the pancreas. The metastatic liver tumor was located in the S4 region of the liver.

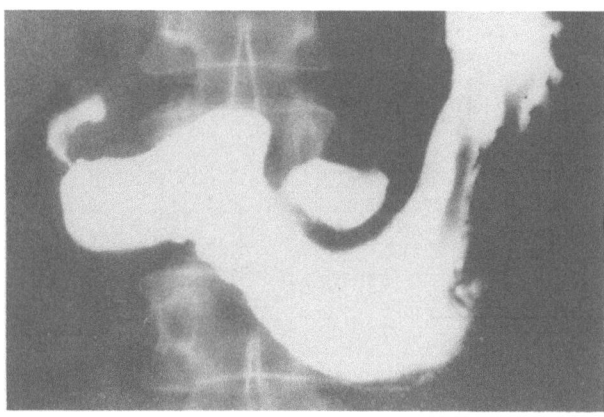

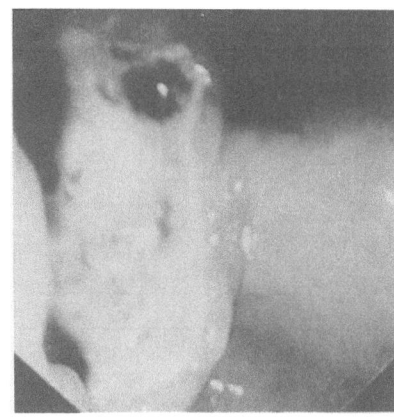

Fig.1 An upper GI series showing a big defect
and crater in the antrum and angle

Fig.2 Endoscopic picture showing as an
advanced gastric cancer of Borrmann type 2

Microscopically the tumor was composed of small uniformed cells which were arranged in irregular nets and infiltration strands. The nuclei were round, oval, spindle and various shaped in hematoxylin eosin stain (Fig. 3). In the immunohistochemical stain by the avidinbiotinin-perioxidase complex method, NSE (neuro specific enolase), synaptophysin, chromogranin and glucagon were positive. Serotonin, calcitonin, somatomedine, gastorin, and insulin were negative stains. We measured serotonin, glucagon, carcitonin in the blood, and 5-HIAA in the urine before and after the operation. Serotonin was higher than normal levels before the operation (table 1).

Table 1. Biochemical Mediator in blood and urine

		Before operation	Two weeks after operation
Serotonin in blood	(under 0.14 µg/ml)	0.34 µg/ml	0.16µg/ml
5-HIAA in urine	(1.6-4.4 mg/ml)	4.0 mg/ml	
Glucagon in blood	(10.1-145.3 pg/ml BG)	84 pg/ml BG	150 pg/ml BG
Carcitonin in blood	(under 80 pg/ml)	35 pg/ml	55 pg/ml

For chemotherapy, we used mitomycin C (MMC) 10 mg intraperitoneally at the end of operation. A chemosensitivity (succinic dehydrogenase inhibition-SDI) test was done in the resected gastric tumor. Cisdichlorodiamine platinum (CDDP), Adreamycine (ADM), 5-Fluorouracil (5-FU) had high sensitivity as 98, 97, 91, and 90% SDI inhibition rate respectively. ADM (20 mg), MMC (10 mg), 5-FU (500 mg) were administered intravenously from two weeks to four weeks after the operation. Three months later the small liver metastasis was found in CT. Immediately, ADM, MMC, CDDP (50 mg) were used from the hepatic artery by Seldinger technic and angiography was carried out. The tumor size was slightly decreasing. ADM and MMC were periodically injected into the hepatic artery from a vascular access device (reservoir) embedded in the femoral region. Moreover UFT was administered orally for maintenance chemotherapy for 6 months (Fig. 3).

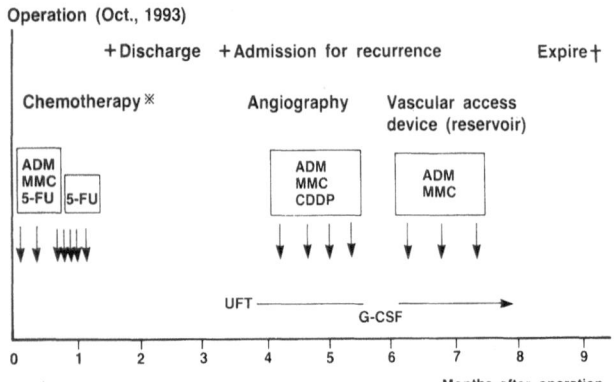

※ CDDP, ADM, 5-FU, and MMC had high chemosensitivity (SDI).

Fig. 3 The postoperative course and chemotherapy

For a while his white blood cells decreased to 1,600 and increased to the normal levels by granulocyte colony stimulating factor (G-CSF). The patient endured the aggressive chemotherapy. Eight months after the operation the hepatic tumor was increased with a threatening rupture (Fig. 4). Unfortunately he expired in spite of the aggressive surgery and multidisciplinary treatment nine months after the operation.

DISCUSSION

Endocrine cell carcinoma is distinguished from carcinoid in histological and clinical courses as a new concept [1]. The case reports of endocrine cell carcinoma were few, because it might be confused with malignant carcinoid and endocrine cell carcinoid [2-5]. The overall five-year survival rates have been quoted 60 per cent as carcinoid, and 20 to 40 per cent as malignant carcinoid [6]. The prognosis of gastric endocrine cell carcinoma with liver metastasis was very poor. So, we performed a radical operation and aggressive chemotherapy according to our chemosensitivity test. The patient presented, had a rapid growth of gastric endocrine carcinoma, liver metastasis, and recurrence. The prognosis was poor. From our experience and literature, endocrine cell carcinoma with liver metastasis is one of the most serious diseases and we need an more advanced form of treatment.

REFERENCES

1. Iwafuchi M, Watanabe H, Ishihara N (1987) Neoplastic endocrine cells in carcinoma of the small intestine. Hum Pathol 18: 185-194
2. Ito S, Ohta Y, Hiromatsu A, Maruyama M, Kawano Y, Irie K (1985) A case report of gastric endocrine cell carcinoma with psammomatous carcification. J Jpn Soc Clin Cytol 24: 507-512
3. Okabe N, Kubo J, Kono S, Yasuda Y, Sukegawa S, Kushida N, Sakurai K. Narimiya N, Tadokoro M (1990) Gastric carcinoid tumor -a case report, review of the literature and histopathological findings-. Jikeikai Med J 37: 179-185
4. Hamada H. Yasuda T, Katsuki Y, Kudou K, Yamaguchi H, Tsuji T, Nishimura A (1991) Three cases of carcinoid of the stomach - two with liver metastasis and one accompanied with sigmoid colon cancer- . Jpn J Gastroenterol Surg 24: 2758-2762
5. Hayashi J, Ohashi N, Sanda M, Imai T, Hidaka N (1992) A case of carcinoid tumor of the stomach with multiple liver metastases. J Jpn Soc Clin Surg 53: 1144-1147
6. Taison M D (1974) Carcinoid syndrome. Surg Clin North Am 54: 409

Limited Surgery for the Early Gastric Cancer

Akira Kurita, Shigemitsu Takashima, Ryuichirou Ohashi,
Takahiro Takayama, Hiroyuki Soga, and Wataru Takiyama

Department of Surgery, Shikoku Cancer Center Hospital, Matsuyama, 790 Japan

ABSTRACT

To establish the indication of the limitted surgery for the early gastric cancer, we
analised 520 cases of the gastric cancer patiants who had gastrectomy in our hospital from
1976 to 1988.Two hundreds ninety one cases of 520 patients had in situ carcinoma(mucosal
cancer),whereas the rest had further invasion into the submucosa(submucosal cancer).All
the mucosal cancers,less than 10 mm in maximum diameter,were free for histological lymph
vessel permiation.Moreover they had no nodal metastasis in the regional lymph nodes. We
histologically found nodal metastasis in 6 cases(2.1%),which were larger than 20 mm in
maximum diameter.As for the mucosal cancers less than 10 mm,the endoscopic mucosal resection might be employed.For the mucosal cancers less than 20 mm,the limited operation(wedge
resection) dispensing with lymph adenectomy could be available.

KEY WORDS:early gastric cancer,mucosal cancer,limited surgery,endoscopic mucosal resection,
wedge resection

INTRODUCTION

The prognosis of the surgically resected early gastric cancer generally is very good,
especially of cancers limited to the mucosa[1,2].In addition,preoperative assessment of
the cancer progression in view of superficial extent and gastric wall invasion has been
promoted.In Japan,the surgery of the early gastric cancer generally is subtotal gastrectomy combined with R2-lymph adenectomy.But,some cases are free of nodal metastasis,and
might be cured without its dissection. We analized resected early gastric cancers clinicopathologically, and assessed what cancers we could do the limited operation without impairing curability.

MATERIALS AND METHODS

From 1976 to 1988,a total of 591 early gastric cancers was resected.There were 520 cases
of solitary cancers.They consisted of 291 cases of the cancers limited to the mucosa
(mucosal cancer) and 229 cases of the cancers invading submucosa(submucosal cancer).They
were studied clinicopathologically,especially in terms of nodal matastasis,lymph vessel
permiation,depth of gastric wall invasion,maximum diameter,macroscopical appearance,and
prognosis.
In this article,the terms were categorized according to the Japanese Research Society for
Gastric Cancer[3].

RESULTS

Table 1 shows the numbers of the cancers in view of the macroscopical findings.There were
small numbers of cases of which diameter were larger than 100 mm.So called minute cancer,
less than 10 mm, predominated in the mucosal cancer. Others were evenly distributed in
various size.In the mucosal cancers,superficial depressed type(IIc) cancers were superior
in numbers;200 cases (68.7%) followed by superficial minimally elevated type(IIa);41 cases
(14.1%).In the submucosal cancers,IIc type cancers also were predominant;132 cases (57.6%),
followed by superficial elevation with central depressed type(IIa+IIc);39 cases (17.0%).
Table 2 shows the pathological findings.Nodal metastasis developped in 6 cases (2.1%) in
the mucosal cancers,on the other hand in the submucosal cancers,there were 36 (15.7%) node

positive cases. Lymph vessel permiation was proved in 15 cases (5.2%) and 184 cases(82.1%) respectively.In the mucosal cancers,lymph vessel permiation nagative cases were also node negative except one.But, this tendency did not apply in the submucosal cancers.

Table 1.Macroscopical findings

1. Location

	A	M	C	AMC	Total
m	124	150	15	2	291
sm	98	101	28	2	229

m : mucosal cancer, sm : submucosal cancer
A : distal third of stomach
M : middle third of stomach
C : proximal third of stomach

2. Maximum Diameter

mm	≦10	10<≦20	20<≦30	30<≦50	50<≦100	100<	Total
m	41	79	67	83	38	3	291
sm	6	39	50	71	57	6	229

3. Macroscopic Type

	I	IIa	IIb	IIa+IIc	IIa+IIb	IIc	IIc+III	III	others	Total
m	12	41	5	15	5	200	2	2	9	291
sm	12	18	0	39	2	132	9	1	16	229

I : protruded lesions, IIa : superficial minimally elevated lesions,
IIb : superficial flat lesions, IIc : superficial minimally depressed lesions,
III : excavated or depressed lesions

Table 2.Microscopical findings

1. Histological Differentiation

	pap	tub₁	tub₂	por	muc	sig	unknown	Total
m	27	138	50	64	0	11	1	291
sm	17	76	77	53	2	3	1	229

pap : papillary, tub₁ : well differentiated tubular, tub₂ : moderately differentiated tubular,
por : poorly differentiated tubular, muc : mucinous, sig : signet ring cell

2. Nodal Metastasis and Lymph Vessel Permiation (ly)

a. mucosal cancer

	n₀	n₁	n₂
ly₀	273	1	0
ly₁	10	3	2

b. submucosal cancer

	n₀	n₁	n₂	n₃,₄
ly₀	39	1	0	0
ly₁	123	15	3	0
ly₂	26	8	4	1
ly₃	1	1	1	1

n₀ : no nodal metastasis, n₁ : metastasis to the first-echelon nodes
n₂ : metastasis to the second-echelon nodes, n₃,₄ : metastasis to the third and/ or fourth-echelon nodes

The correlation between tumor size and lymph vessel permiation was shown in Table 3 and 4. In the depressed type mucosal cancers,tumors less than 10 mm appeared free of lymph vessel permiation. Though, once the tumor was exceeding 10 mm,lymph vessel permiation positive cases appeared.On the contrary,submucosal cancers developped high rate of lymph vessel permiation even less than 10 mm.In the elevated type mucosal cancers, there were no instances with lymph vessel permiation up to 50 mm in greatest diameter.Conversely,submucosel cancers had a possibility of lymph vessel permiation at any size,as was seen in the depressed cases.

Table 3.Correlation between tumor size and lymph vessel permiaton
-depression predominant type (including IIc, IIc+III, III+IIc, III)-

1. Mucosal Cancer

mm	≦10	10<≦20	20<≦30	30<≦50
ly₀	31	52	49	39
ly₁	0	2	4	3

2. Submucosal Cancer

mm	≦10	10<≦20	20<≦30	30<≦50
ly₀	2	4	7	5
ly₁	2	14	24	37
ly₂	0	2	3	9
ly₃	0	0	1	0

Table 4.Correlation between tumor size and lymph vessel permiation
-elevation predominant type (including I, IIa, IIb, IIa+IIc, IIa+IIb)-

1. Mucosal Cancer

mm	<10	10<≦20	20<≦30	30<≦50	50<≦70
ly₀	10	25	14	19	6
ly₁	0	0	0	0	1

2. Submucosal Cancer

mm	<10	10<≦20	20<≦30	30<≦50	50<≦70
ly₀	0	3	3	4	2
ly₁	1	14	9	8	7
ly₂	0	1	3	6	0
ly₃	0	0	0	0	1

Table 5.Cases of node positive mucosal cancers

1. n₁ ; metastasis to the first-echelon nodes

case	location	macroscopic type	maximum diameter(mm)	histological differentiation	site of positive nodes	prognosis
1	AM	Borrmann III	65	por	No.4	A. NED.
2	A	IIc	60	por	No.4	A. NED.
3	M	IIc	20	por	No.4 & No.6	A. NED.
4	M	IIc	23	por	No.4	A. NED.

A ; alive, NED ; no evidence of disease

2. n₂ ; metastasis to the second-echelon nodes

case	location	macroscopic type	maximum diameter(mm)	histological differentiation	site of positive nodes	prognosis
5	A	IIc	70	por	No. 1.3.4.5.6.8	DOD
6	M	IIc	23	por+sig	No. 1.3.4.5.6.8	DOD

DOD : died of disease

Table 5 shows node positive mucosal cancers resected in our institute.All the cases appeared macroscopically depressed type. Maximum diameter were in excess of 20 mm.Histologically, all the cases developped poorly differentiated adenocacinoma.The two cases metastatic to the second-echelon lymph nodes died of gastric cancer,whereas four cases,metastatic to the first-echelon nodes,are alive and well without any recurrent signs.

DISCUSSION

In Japan,node positive gastric cancers occupied 3.0 to 5.2% of the mucosal cancer,whereas of the submucosal node positive cancers accounted for 14.5 to 22.4%[4].These facts were not exceptional in our institute. Lymph vessel permiation suggests the potential of nodal metastasis.In mucosal cancers,tumors less than 10 mm in diameter had no lymph vessel permiations or nodal matastasis. In other words,we could ignor both two factors in the mucosal cancers less than 10 mm.These factors above mentioned applied in the depressed type cancer.In the elevated one,there were no node positive cases, although lymph vessel permiation appeared positive when the tumor grew up to 50 mm in diameter.As for the depressed type mucosal cancer less than 10 mm,endoscopic mucosal resection might be available regardless of the histological differentiation[5].For the elevated one,upper limit of the size might be postulated at 50 mm.As the analized numbers were too small about the elevated lesions,we considered that the indication should be the same as the depressed case. Some authors estimated the upper limit at 20 mm in the case of elevated lesions[6]. And, some authors stated that poorly and undifferentiated type mucosal cancers should be excluded[7].Mucosal cancers less than 20 mm did not have any nodal matastasis.So,these mucosal cancers could be cured by local resection,namely wedge resection. But,close endoscopic follow up should be needed for investigation of the second primary gastric cancers [8].
Conversely,submucosal cancers had not only lymph vessel permiations but nodal metastasis even in the case of minute stage.So,limitted surgery should not be proceeded in submucosal cancers.
In conclusion,as for the mucosal cancers less than 10 mm in diameter,the endoscopic resection might be available.And for the mucosal cancers less than 20 mm,the local resection, namely wedge resection should be proceeded.

REFERENCES

1.Iwanaga T,Furukawa H,Kousaki G (1975) Relapse of early gastric cancer and its prevention. Rinshougeka,31:29-35
2.Kitou T,Yamamura Y,Hirai T,Sakamoto J,Yasui K,Morimoto T,Kato T,Yasue M,Miyaishi S, Nakazato H (1989) Surgical treatment for early gastric cancer. Jpn J Gastroenterol Surg 22 :24-31
3.Japsnese Research Society for Gastric Cancer.(1981) The general rules for the gastric cancer study in surgery and pathology. Jpn J Surg 11:127-139
4.Sakita T (1983) Study on early gastric cancer throughout Japan. Gastrointest Endosc 25: 317-343
5.Tada M,Shimada M,Yanai H,Arima K,Kanda M,Okazaki Y,Takemoto T,Kinoshita Y,Kinoshita K, Iida Y,Watanabe H (1984) New technique of gastric biopsy. Stomach and Intestine 19:1107- 1116
6.Nashimoto A,Tanaka S,Miyashita K,Sasaki K,Muto T,Soga J (1988) Clinicopathological study for early gastric cancer -indication of conservative surgery and radical endoscopic treatment for early gastric cancer-. J Jpn Surg Soc 89:1780-1788
7.Karita M,Tada M,Okita K,Andou M,Takemoto T,Nagasaki S,Shimada Y,Iida Y (1989) Definition of the adaptation of endoscopic surgery for early gastric cancer -special examination the relationship between the histological differentiation of the intramucosal gastric cancer and the lymph node metastasis-. J Jpn Soc Cancer Ther 24:1572-1584
8.Kurita A,Takashima S,Funakoshi M,Kawashima K,Kino K,Yokoyama N,Soga H (1992) A study of multiple early gastric carcinoma -assessment of proper gastrectomy- Japanese Journal of Cancer of the Digestive Organs 2:371-375

Pylorus Preserving Gastrectomy (PPG) with Lymph Node Dissection for Early Gastric Cancer in the Middle Third of the Stomach

Hiroshi Minato, Kiyoshi Sawai, Tsuguo Fujioka, Masahide Yamaguchi, Keisuke Kanemitsu, Shinji Okano, Hiroki Taniguchi, Akio Hagiwara, Tetsurou Yamane, Toshiharu Yamaguchi, and Toshio Takahashi

The First Department of Surgery, Kyoto Prefectural University of Medicine, Kyoto, 602 Japan

ABSTRACT

We carried out pylorus preserving gastrectomy (PPG) on sixteen patients with early gastric cancer in the middle third of the stomach. PPG is used to prevent dumping syndrome and to protect against secondary carcinogenesis due to bile juice reflex. The oral resection line was the same as in subtotal gastrectomy and the anal resection line was 1.5 centimeter to the oral side of the pyloric ring. We carried out R_1 or R_1+No.7 lymph node dissection when cancer invasion was limited to the mucosa, and R_2 lymph node dissection when cancer invasion was limited to the submucosa. We preserved the pyloric artery to maintain blood flow in the pylorus.

ADVANTAGES of PPG (1) Curability : The lymph nodes in compartments one and two (R_2) can be completely removed as well as in conventional subtotal gastrectomy. (2) Safety : There was no significant difference in blood flow at the anastomosis site between the two types of operation. (3) Gastritis of the remnant stomach : An endoscopical biopsy of the remnant stomach showed fewer pathological findings of atrophy and gastritis in PPG patients when compared with conventional subtotal gastrectomy patients.

DISADVANTAGES of PPG (1) Stagnation of the stomach: Discharges of gastric juice from the naso-gastric tube continued for three days after the operation, and the patients' first meal was delayed for one or two days compared to the typical course after conventional subtotal gastrectomy.

KEY WORDS : pylorus preserving gastrectomy (PPG), early gastric cancer, lymph node dissection

INTRODUCTION

Pylorus preserving gastrectomy (PPG) is a procedure for benign gastric disease which was performed by Maki and associates in 1964 [1]. This procedure has been evaluated highly with respect to postoperative condition, because the preserved pylorus continues to function. Recently, some authors reported this procedure adapted for early gastric cancer located in the middle third of the stomach [2-4]. The procedure caused the following questions " Can you dissect the suprapyloric lymph node and the subpyloric lymph node perfectly? " and " Does PPG cause blood flow disturbance of the anastomosis site? ". To answer these two questions, we carried out a vascular anatomical study by angiography which was performed on 181 patients with gastric cancer. Our clinical experience of 16 patients subjected to PPG is reported in this manuscript.

PATIENTS and MATERIAL

We established the indication for pylorus preserving gastrectomy (PPG) as being single early gastric cancer in the middle third of the stomach. PPG was performed on sixteen patients with this indication during 1991 and 1992. During this same period, eleven patients with early gastric cancer in the lower third of the stomach received conventional subtotal gastrectomy (SG).

Branching patterns of the pyloric branch

Angiography was performed on 181 patients with gastric cancer to determine the origin of the pyloric branch.

PPG procedure

The oral resection line is the same as in subtotal gastrectomy. The anal resection line is 1.5cm to the oral side of the pyloric ring. R_1 or R_1+No.7 lymph node dissection was performed when cancer invasion was limited to the mucosa, and R_2 lymph node dissection was carried out when cancer invasion was limited to the submucosa. We preserved the pyloric artery. Layer to layer anastomosis was used. We performed conventional subtotal gastrectomy when cancer seemed to invade to the muscle layer or there was obvious lymph node metastasis at laparotomy.

Blood flow measurement

We measured blood flow at the mid–stomach region, at the prepyloric area and at the first part of the duodenum using a lazor–doppler blood flowmeter before gastrectomy and after anastomosis.

Postoperative course

The postoperative courses of the patients receiving PPG and SG were compared while they remained in the hospital.

Gastritis of the remnant stomach

We performed endoscopy and biopsy of the remnant stomach more than three months postoperatively. The degree of gastritis of the remnant stomach was compared between the two procedures.

The clinicopathological findings were analyzed according to The General Rules for the Gastric Cancer Study in Surgery and Pathology by The Japanese Research Society for Gastric Cancer [5]. The statistical significance of differences between the two groups was determined by χ^2 test.

RESULTS

The original point of the pyloric branch is shown in table 1. Twenty four patients (13.3%) had the pyloric artery originating from the right gastroepiploic artery. The remainder (except unknown) of 86.1% patients had the pyloric artery originating from the proximal side of the right gastroepiploic artery. When the patients had the pyloric artery branching from proximal side of the right gastroepiploic artery, the gastroepiploic artery could be ligated at its root without blood flow disturbance of the pylorus. When the patients had the pyloric artery branching from the right gastroepiploic artery, the gastroepiploic artery had to be ligated at the peripheral side of the branching point of the pyloric artery. In either case by taking care of the branching pattern of the pyloric artery, the subpyloric lymph nodes can be dissected while preserving the blood flow of the pylorus.

The details of the 16 patients are represented in table 2. 13 patients had cancer invasion limited to the mucosa, 3 patients had cancer invasion limited to the submucosa. Only one patient had lymph nodal involvement limited to the perigastric nodes.

Table 1. The origin of the pyloric artery

Artery	Number(%)
same location as the ASPD	87(48.1)
ASPD	41(22.7)
gastroduodenal artery	24(13.3)
PSPD	4(2.2)
right gastroepiploic artery	24(13.3)
unknown	1(0.6)

ASPD: anterior superior pancreaticoduodenal artery
PSPD: posterior superior pancreaticoduodenal artery

The origin of the pyloric branch is shown. The pyloric artery were branching from the right gastroepiploic artery in 13.3% patients. In these cases, the gastroepiploic artery had to be ligated at the peripheral side of the branching point of the pyloric artery. In the remaining cases, the gastroepiploic artery could be ligated at its root without causing blood flow disturbance of the pylorus.

Table 2. Patient characteristics

Gender		Lymph node dissection	
male	12	R1	4
female	4	R1+No.7	8
		R2	4
Age			
mean	58.6	Depth of invasion	
range	45–86	mucosa	13
		submucosa	3
Morphological type			
IIa	5	Nodal involvement	
IIc	9	n0	15
III	2	n1	1

Change of blood flow between before and after gastrectomy as measured by lazor–doppler blood flowmeter is shown in table 3. Change of blood flow in the anastomosis site after PPG is less than after conventional subtotal gastrectomy, however, there is no significant difference between the two groups.

The comparison of the postoperative courses between PPG and subtotal gastrectomy is shown in table 4. The period before removal of the naso–gastric tube after PPG and the admission period of PPG were longer than those of subtotal gastrectomy. Difference between the two groups were significant.

The endoscopic biopsies of the remnant stomach showed fewer pathological findings of atrophy and gastritis in patients treated by PPG as compared to the patients treated by conventional subtotal gastrectomy.

Table 3. Change in blood flow after gastrectomy

Procedure	Site	At laparotomy	After anastomosis	Change
PPG	Upper body	1960.1±858.1mV	2128.7±221.4mV	+8.6%
	Anastomosis	2939.5±1433.8mV	2695.6±665.9mV	−8.3%
Subtotal gastrectomy	Upper body	2692.5±1173.8mV	2645.1±936.8mV	−1.7%
	Anastomosis	4012.2±2316.1mV	3286.9±1410.2mV	−18.1%

Table 4. Comparison of the postoperative courses

Procedure	Removal of naso−gastric tube	First meal	Admission period
PPG(n=16)	3.7 days	5.4 days	27.7 days
	P<0.001	N.S	P<0.05
Subtotal gastrectomy(n=11)	1.1 days	4.5 days	19.5 days

DISCUSSION

Pylorus preserving gastrectomy (PPG) is one of the limited operations that has been tried recently in Japan for early gastric cancer in the middle third of the stomach. The majority of the patients (86.1%) had the pyloric artery originating from the proximal side of the right gastroepiploic artery. In these patients, we could easily dissect the suprapyloric lymph node and the subpyloric lymph node perfectly without causing blood flow disturbance at the pylorus. The pyloric artery branched from right gastroepiploic artery in 13.3% patients. In these cases, we had to ligate at the peripheral side of the branching point of the pyloric artery and dissect the subpyloric lymph node carefully. Blood flow at the anastomosis site of subtotal gastrectomy was higher than that of PPG. But there was no significant difference in the reduction in the rate of blood flow between PPG and subtotal gastrectomy. Therefore, it was proved that blood flow of the pylorus was maintained when PPG with R_1 or R_2 lymph nodes dissection preserving the pyloric artery was performed. In our small experience, blood flow at the anastomosis site was not significantly different between R_1 and R_2 lymph node dissection in PPG preserved pyloric artery. According to these results, we suggest that indication of PPG could be extended to advanced gastric cancer in the middle third of the stomach. A disadvantage of PPG with lymph nodes dissection is stagnation of the stomach. Discharges of gastric juice from the naso−gastric tube continued for three days after PPG and admission period was prolonged in PPG patients. Stagnation seems to be caused by amputation of pyloric branch of the vagal nerve. But there was no significant difference in taking a meal after leaving hospital between the two groups. Although we have no long−term follow up study of this procedure for malignant disease, long−term observation after PPG for benign gastric disease proved that the amount of food taken after PPG was more than after that of SG, and body weight loss was less than after that of SG. Gastritis of the remnant stomach were fewer in patients performed PPG as compared to the patients performed SG. We expect that the long−term condition after PPG for malignant disease would be more comfortable than that of SG. We plan to carry out pylorus preserving gastrectomy for malignant gastric disease actively, continue long−term observation and reevaluate PPG for gastric cancer.

REFERENCES

1. Maki T, Shiratori T, Hatafuku T, Sugawara K (1967) Pylorus−preserving gastrectomy as an improved operation for gastric ulcer.Surgery 61:838
2. Nakatani K, Watanabe A, Nakano H, Shiratori T (1991) Pylorus preserving gastrectomy for early gastric cancer. Operation 45:1825−1829 (in Japanese)
3. Matsuno S, Sasaki I, Naitou H, Shiiba K, Saitou Y, Oouchi A, Miyagawa H (1991) Pylorus preserving gastrectomy for early gastric cancer. Operation 45:1975−1981 (in Japanese)
4. Sasaki I, Naitou H, Funayama H, Kouyama Y, Shiiba K, Matsuno S (1993) Pylorus−preserving gastrectomy for gastric ulcer and early gastric cancer. Journal of Clinical Surgery. 48:161−167 (in Japanese)
5. Japanese Research Society for Gastric Cancer (1981) The general rules for the gastric cancer study in surgery and pathology. Parts 1&2. Jap. J. Surg. 11:127−139

Pylorus-Preserving Gastrectomy for Gastric Cancer

Hidetomo Sawada, Kastunori Nakatani, Akihiko Watanabe,
Yukishige Yamada, Tomoaki Yano, Yoshihide Shino, Naoto Ueyama,
Takashi Yamada, Masahiro Tanase, and Hiroshige Nakano

First Department of Surgery, Nara Medical University, Kashihara, Nara, 634 Japan

ABSTRACT

We applied Pylorus-preserving gastrectomy(PPG) to cases of early gastric cancer at the middle third of the stomach. The patients were operated on between 1989 and 1992 and reconstructed with the following procedures: 24 cases with PPG and 23 cases with Billroth I(B-I). In comparison with B-I, PPG involved fewer incidences of the dumping syndrome, reflux esophagitis and gastritis of the residual stomach , and showed a more normal pattern on oral glucose tolerance test(OGTT) and gastrin secretion test. Thus PPG should be considered a physiologically advantageous procedure for early gastric cancer at the middle third of the stomach.

KEY WORDS: Pylorus-preserving gastrectomy, early gastric cancer

INTRODUCTION

The detection of early gastric cancer cases has been improving chiefly due to the better diagnostic techniques [1,2]. Since the prognosis of these early gastric cancer case is excellent, it is essential to improve the operating procedure so that the patients can be assured of a satisfactory quality of life. Pylorus preserving gastrectomy(PPG) was developed by Maki, Shiratori, et al in 1967 to avoid the bile reflux and dumping syndrome by preserving the sphincteric function of the pyloric ring [3]. Digestion can also be facilitated by a rhythmical emptying of food into the duodenum from the stomach. Since 1989, we have been applying this PPG to cases of early gastric cancer at the middle third of the stomach. These cases were diagnosed endoscopic ultrasonographycally as cancer invasion limited to the submucosal layer. For the present study, we compared and assessed the PPG and Billroth-I(B-I) procedures from the point of view of the postoperative quality of the patients' life.

MATERIALS AND METHOD

A total of 47 cases with early gastric cancer at the middle third of the stomach, who underwent radical gastrectomy with lymph node dissection at the First Department of Surgery, Nara Medical University between 1989 and 1992, were studied. There were 24 cases with PPG and 23 cases with B-I. The only technical difference between PPG and conventional distal gastrectomy is that for PPG the stomach is resected at 1.5cm proximal to the pyloric ring. The usual lymph node dissection is performed in the conventional manner. The critical point of this procedure is that the first branch of the supraduodenal artery should be retained for the blood supply to the remaining pyloric region. The incidence of the dumping syndrome by personal interview, endoscopic observation of inflammatory changes of the esophagus and residual stomach , 75g oral glucose torelance test and gastrin secretion test, was for 13 PPG cases and 14 B-I cases who had undergone gastrectomy more than six months before this assessment.

RESULTS

Clinical Data for Patients

Macroscopic type, depth of cancer invasion, histological type and lymphnode metastasis assessed according to the General Rules for Gastric Cancer Study in Surgery and Pathology established by the Japanese Research Society for Gastric Cancer [4,5] are shown in Table 1. Except for histological type, there were no significant differences between the two groups.

Table 1. Clinical data for patients

Operative method	PPG	B-I
No. of cases	24	23
Macroscopic type		
Elevated	4	7
Flat	0	1
Depressed	20	15
Depth of invasion		
m	17	15
sm	6	7
pm	1	1
Histological type		
Differentiated	13	20
Undifferentiated	11	3
Lymphnode metastasis		
n (-)	23	23
n (+)	1	0

Table 2. Endoscopic Findings for Residual Stomach and Esophagus

	PPG		B-I	
No. of cases	13		14	
Esophagus				
Discoloring type (%)	2	(15.3)	3	(21.4)
Erosive and/or ulcerative type (%)	0	(0)	1	(7.1)
Uneven type (%)	0	(0)	0	(0)
Total (%)	2	(15.3)	4	(28.6)
Residual stomach				
Ulcer (%)	0	(0)	0	(0)
Erosion (%)	0	(0)	0	(0)
Redness (%)	2	(15.3)	9	(64.3)

Operation Time ,Admission Period and Number of Dissected Lymph Nodes in the Pyloric Region

The operation time (mean+s.d.) was 216.4+40.3 min. for the PPG group and 204.7+32.6 min. for the B-I group. The average admission period (mean+s.d.) was 34.3 +14.3 days for the PPG group and 29.7+11.2 days for the B-I group. The number of dissected suprapyloric (No. 5) and subpyloric (No.6) lymph nodes was 0.7 and 3.0 for the PPG group, and 1.1 and 3.9 for the B-I group, respectively. These findings show no significant differences between the two groups.

Changes in Postoperative Body Weight and Incidence of the Dumping Syndrome Established by Interview six Months Postoperatively

Postoperative changes in body weight were observed in 17 PPG cases and 16 B-I cases six months after the operation. The mean change for the PPG group was a 0.3 kg gain, in contrast to a 1.3 kg loss for the B-I group. The incidence of dumping syndrome was also established for 13 PPG patients and 14 B-I patients by personal interview. Whereas none of thePPG patients complained of the dumping syndrome, 2 cases of the B-I group did.

Postoperative Endoscopic Findings for Esophagus and Residual Stomach

The postoperative mucosal condition of the esophagus and residual stomach was observed endoscopically in 13 PPG and 14 B-I cases. The results are shown in Table 2. Reflux esophagitis was classified into the following three types according to the diagnostic classification established by the Japanese Society for Esophageal Diseases: 1. Discoloring type; 2. Erosive and/or ulcerative type;3. Uneven type. The incidence of reflux esophagitis was15.3% of PPG patients and 28.6% of B-I patients. Wheareas PPG cases had only the discoloring type, B-I cases had both the discoloring and erosive and/or ulcerative type. Regarding gastritis of residual stomach, the incidence of redness was 15.3% for PPG cases, significantly lower than the 64.3% for B-I cases (p<0.01, chi square test). There were no cases with ulcer or erosion in either group.

75g Oral Glucose Tolerance Test and Gastrin Secretion Test

The results of the75g oral glucose tolerance test (OGTT) are shown in Fig 1. In B-I patients, blood sugar levels increased during the first 30 minutes after the oral trial with 75g glucose to reach a peak of approximately double the 0 time value and gradually decreased after there. On the other hand, no such increase was seen in PPG patients. For the gastrin secretion test, serum gastrin levels were monitored in a time-dependent manner after the patients had taken a test meal within 120 minutes. PPG patients showed a better response to the test meal trial than the B-I patients(Fig 2). The serum gastrin level of PPG patients was significantly higher than that of B-I patients.

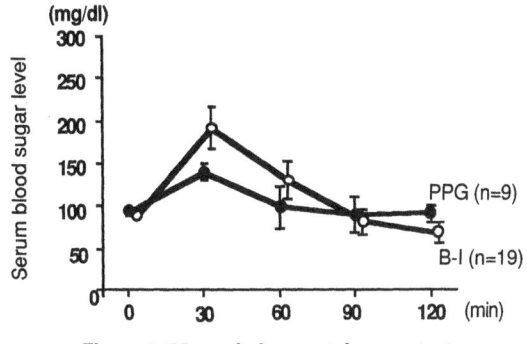

Figure 1. 75g oral glucose tolerance test

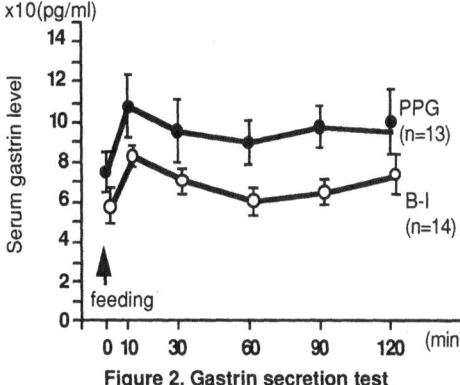

Figure 2. Gastrin secretion test

DISCUSSION

Many cases operated on with conventional distal gastrectomy followed by B-I reconstruction show malnutrition and body weight loss. In addition to malnutrition, dumping syndrome, reflux esophagitis and gastritis of the residual stomach are the major unfavorable sequelae that bother patients after conventional gastrectomy. As early gastric cancer cases appear to have a better prognosis than advanced cases, any operative procedure that dose not interfere with the quality of life in the long run should be applied to early cases. PPG was developed in order to prevent postoperative unfavorable sequelae for gastric ulcer patients by preserving the pyloric function [3]. We applied PPG to cases of early gastric cancer located in the middle third of the stomach and evaluated the safety and radicality of this procedure. Our results show that operation time and hospitalixation period after operation are substantially the same for PPG and B-I cases. The number of dissected lymphnodes in the pyloric region was also almost same for both groups. Thus we conclude that PPG is a safe radical procedure.

We used personal interviews and endoscopic examination to study the post operative condition, especially dumping syndrome , reflux esophagitis and gastritis of the residual stomach in PPG and B-I cases. The PPG group had lower incidences for all these disorders than the B-I group. Results of the postoperative OGTT and gastrin secretion tests showed a more normal pattern for PPG than for B-I.

In conclusion, PPG is surgically advantageous for early gastric cancer occuring at the middle third of the stomach because of the findings described in this study. Moreover, PPG allows for a complete dissection of the lymphnode in the pyloric region. We hope to apply this PPG not only to early gastric cancer cases but also to advanced cases whose prepyloric region can be preserved to a length of at least 1.5cm.

REFERENCES

1. Sakita T, Oguro Y, Takasu S (1971) The development of endoscopic diagnosis of early carcinoma of the stomach. Jpn J Clin Oncol 1:113-128
2. Lawrence M, Shiu MH (1991) Early gastric cancer. Twenty-eight-year experience. Ann Surg 213:327-334
3. Maki T, Shiratori T, Hatafuku T, Sugawara K (1967) Pylorus-preserving gastrectomy as an improved operation for gastric ulcer. Surgery 61:838
4. The Japanese Research Society for Gastric Cancer(1981) The general rules for the gastric cancer study in surgery and pathology. Part I. clinical classification. Jpn J Surg 11: 127-139
5. The Japanese Research Society Committee on Histological Classification of Gastric Cancer(1981) The general rules for the gastric cancer study in surgery and pathology. Part II. histological classification of gastric cancer. Jpn J Surg 11: 140-145

Indication and Postoperative Evaluation of Pylorus Preserving Gastrectomy for Early Gastric Cancer

SHINICHI YAMADA, KUNIO OKAJIMA, HIROSHI ISOZAKI, EIJI NAKATA,
JUNKO NISHIMURA, MASAKAZU TANIMURA, and TADASHI ICHINONA

Department of Surgery, Osaka Medical College, Takatsuki, Osaka, 569 Japan

ABSTRACT

Pylorus preserving gastrectomy(PPG) should be indicated for early gastric cancer as follows;
  1. In the case of Type I or IIa, PPG is indicated for histologically differentiated type,
     15 to 30 mm in tumor size with mucosal invasion and less than 15 mm in tumor size with
     submucosal invasion.
  2. In the case of Type IIa + IIc, IIc + IIa, IIc or IIc + III, PPG is indicated for less
     than 10 mm in tumor size with peptic ulcer in cancer focus regardless to hitological
     type.
  3. Cancer focus is at least 3.5 cm away from the pyloric ring. In the case of PPG serum
     acetaminophen level after oral administration increased grdually and contractility
     of gallbladder was kept as same as pre-operative conditon.

KEY WORDS: pylorus preserving gastrectomy, early gastric cancer, serum acetaminophen level

INTRODUCTION

In recent years, with advances in the daignosis of gastric cancer, especially smaller sized
one.
With the purpose of exactly difining the indication of studies of Clinico-Pathological analysis of early gastric cacner, functional evaluation of residual stomach and preserved pyloric
ring, and of contraction of gallbladder.

SUBJECTS AND METHOD

The subject of clinico-pathological analysis were 577 cases with early, single gastric cancer
treated at our department during past 14 years.
Postoperative function was evaluated as follows.
  1. Function of residual stomach and preserved pyloric ring was examined by Acetaminophen
     method.
  2. Capability of contraction of gallbladder stimulated with test meal.
Histological type of cancer was divided into two groups;
  1. Differentiated type (papillary adenocarcinoma, well differentiated tubular adenocar-
     cinoma, moderately differentiated tubular adenocarcinoma and mucinous carcinoma)
  2. Poorly differentiated type (poorly differentiated adenocarcinoma and signet ring cell
     carcinoma)

RESULTS

In the case of mucosal cancer, the peak of tumor size was 20 to 24 mm. Lymph node metastasis
was confirmed in the case of 15 mm or greater in tumor size. The rate of lymph node metastasis reached 20% of the cases of 45 to 49 mm in tumor size (Table 1).
In the case of submucosal cancer, the peak of tumor size was 30 to 34 mm. Lymph node metastasis was confirmed in the case of 10 mm or greater in tumor size. The rate of lymph node
metastasis reached 37.5% of the cases of 50 to 54 mm in tumor size (Table 2).
For macroscopic type of I or IIa, invasion to the submucosal layer was observed with tumor
size of over 5 to 9 mm in the case of histologically differentiated type of tumors. Lymph
node metastasis was detected in only the case of 30 mm or greater in tumor size (Fig. 1).
For macroscopic type of IIa + IIc or IIc + IIa, the submucosal invasion was observed in the
case of 10 mm in tumor size regardless histological type. Lymph node metastasis was positive
already when the tumor size reached 15 mm to 19 mm (Fig. 2)

Table 1 Tumor size and Lymph node metastatic rate in mucosal cancer of stomach

Tumor size (mm)	Number of cases	Cases of Lymph node metastasis	Rate of Lymph node metastasis
1~ 4	11	0	
5~ 9	30	0	
10~14	47	0	
15~19	46	2	4.3
20~24	52	2	3.8
25~29	34	0	
30~34	23	0	
35~39	19	0	
40~44	13	1	7.7
45~49	10	2	20.0
50~54	5	1	20.0
55~59	4		
60≦	20	1	5.0

Table 2 Tumor size and Lymph node metastatic rate in submucosal cancer of stomach

Tumor size (mm)	Number of cases	Cases of Lymph node metastasis	Rate of Lymph node metastasis
1~ 4	1	0	
5~ 9	10	0	
10~14	20	2	10.0
15~19	33	4	12.1
20~24	35	1	2.9
25~29	32	5	15.6
30~34	44	7	15.9
35~39	17	5	29.4
40~44	11	3	27.3
45~49	21	4	19.0
50~54	8	3	37.5
55~59	7	1	14.3
60≦	24	8	33.3

Fig. 1 Tumor size, Histological type and rate of submucosal invasion of type I or IIa cancer

Differentiated type	Tumor size (mm)	Poorly differentiated type.
	1~4	
25.0	5~9	
	10~14	
22.2	15~19	
41.7	20~24	100
66.7	25~29	
26.8	30≦	100

● Case of lymph node metastasis

Fig. 2 Tumor size, Histological type and rate of submucosal invasion of type IIa+IIc or IIc+IIa cancer

Differentiated type	Tumor size (mm)	Poorly differentiated type.
	1~4	
0/3	5~9	
37.5	10~14	100
60.0	15~19	100
60.0	20~24	100
37.5	25~29	33.3
64.7	30≦	28.6

● Case of lymph node metastasis

For macroscopic type of IIc or IIc + III, even smaller tumor size invasion to submucosal layer was observed whether the histological was differentiated or poorly differentiated type. Lymph node metastasis was confirmed in the group of 10 to 14 mm or greater (Fig. 3).

Fig. 3 Tumor size, Histological type and rate of submucosal invasion of type IIc or IIc+III cancer

Differentiated type	Tumor size (mm)	Poorly differentiated type.
12.5	1~4	0/3
20.0	5~9	28.6
36.0	10~14	20.0
33.3	15~19	30.8
40.8	20~24	26.1
45.0	25~29	31.3
44.2	30≦	50.0

● Case of lymph node metastasis

In the case of distal gastrectomy serum Acetaminophen level was high as soon as oral administration. But in the case of pylorus preserving gastrectomy serum Acetaminophesn level increased slowly similar to the pre-operative one (Fig. 4).

Fig. 4 Serum Acetaminophen level associated with operative method

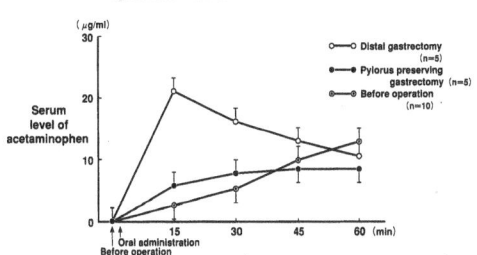

In the case of pylorus preserving gastrectomy gallbladder contractility test stimulating by test meal examined using by ultrasonography revealed the similar pattern to pre-opertive one (Fig. 5).

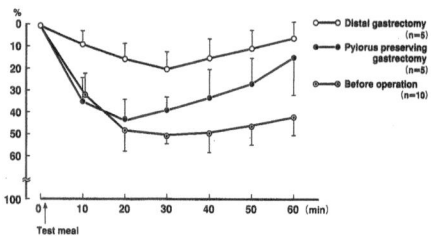

Fig. 5 Contractility of gallbladder associated with operative method

CONCLUSIONS

1. Indication of Pylorus preserving gastrectomy addition to condition of Table 3 cancer focus was at least 3.5 cm away from the pyloric ring.
2. Pattern of discharge examined by Acetaminophen method in cases treated by pylorus preserving gastrectomy was similar to pre-operative pattern.
3. Contractility of gallbladder in cases treated by pylorus preserving gastrectomy was kept as same as condition of before operation.

Table 3 Indication of pylorus preserving gastrectomy based on clinico-pathological analysis

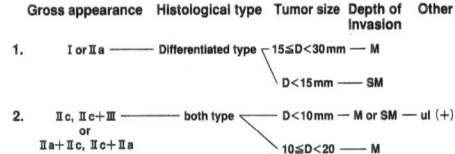

REFERENCES

1. Yamada S., Okajima K. (1991) Rational lymph node dissection for gastric cancer. J. Clinical Surgery 46:1067-1074
2. Nakano H., Watanabe A., Sawada H., Yamada Y., Nakatani K. (1993) Inidcation and Results of pylorus preserving gastrectomy for gastric cancer. Surgical Therapy 68:131-135
3. Nakatani K., Watanabe A., Sawada H., Okumura T., Yamada Y., Nakano H., Siratori T. (1991) Pylorus preserving gastrectomy for early gastric cancer. J. Japan Surgical Society 92:783

Gallbladder Function After Pylorus Preserving Gastrectomy for Gastric Cancer

MASASHI KODAMA, KENJI KOYAMA, TEISAO CHIDA, and AKIRA ARAKAWA

The First Department of Surgery, Akita University School of Medicine, Akita, 010 Japan

ABSTRACT

Gallbladder functions were evaluated in patients who had undergone pylorus preserving gastrectomy for early gastric cancer using ultrasonography, comparing with those in patients undergone conventional distal gastrectomy. The resting gallbladder area showed no dilatation after pylorus preserving gastrectomy. The deterioration of the contractile function after pylorus preserving gastrectomy was slight, compared with that after conventional distal gastrectomy. It suggested that pylorus preserving gastrectomy had advantage to decrease the incidence of postgastrectomy cholecystolithiasis.

KEY WORDS: pylorus preserving gastrectomy, preservation of the hepatic branch of vagal nerve, early gastric cancer, gallbladder function

INTRODUCTION

The postgastrectomy cholecystolithiasis is one of the complications which deteriorate the quality of life in patients with gastric cancer. Since vagotomy is one of causes for developing gallstone[1], we have attempted to preserve hepatic and pyloric branches of the vagal nerve uninjured in the operative procedure of pylorus preserving gastrectomy (PPG) to prevent gallbladder dysfunction after surgery. In this present study, we studied the advantage of PPG on postoperative gallbladder function by evaluating the resting gallbladder area and the gallbladder contractile function in patients with early gastric cancer received PPG, comparing with that received conventional distal gastrectomy(CDG).

PATIENTS AND METHODS

The indication for PPG for early gastric cancer located in themiddle third of the stomach was as wa had already reported[2], (1) any case with tumors smaller than 2.0 cm in maximum length, and (2) cases with a tumor of 2.0 to 4.0 cm if it is a mucosal cancer if it is located at the greater curvature, or if it is an elevated type IIa cancer. In 23 patients with above mentioned conditions, admitted in our department between 1989 and 1991, PPG was performed for 13 patients and CDG with gastroduodenostomy was performed for 10 patients randomly. In the operative procedure, PPG is different from CDG in that it retains a 1.5 cm length of the pyloric cuff and it neglects to dissect the suprapyloric lymph node with the remaining hepatic and pyloric branches of the vagal nerve being preserved as shown in Fig. 1. The resting gallbladder area and gallbladder contractile function were prospectively studied using ultrasonography before operation, at 2 weeks, 6 months and 1 year after operation. The gallbladder area was measured by planimeter equipped in the ultrasonographic apparatus. The gallbladder contractile function was determined by calculating the ratio of the gallbladder area at 20 minutes after intramuscular injection of cerulein (20 ug) to the original gallbladder area. Each value was expressed as mean+standard error of the mean. Student's t test was used for statistical analysis. Values of p smaller than 0.05 were considered significant.

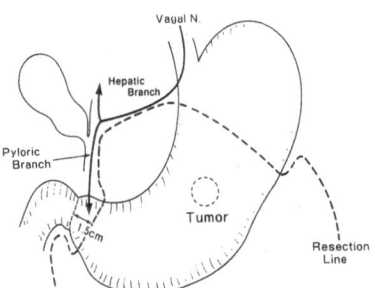

Fig 1. Preservation of Hepatic Branch
of Vagal Nerve in PPG

RESULTS

Changes in resting gallbladder area

In PPG patients, the resting gallbladder area showed no significant changes
throughout the observation period as shown in Fig 2. However, in CDG patients,
it was significantly enlarged from $11.3+1.2cm^2$ to $15.8+1.5cm^2$ (2 weeks) and to
$15.0+1.1cm^2$ (6 months) after surgery. The resting gallbladder area after CDG
did not return to the preoperative levels in 1 year and it was significantly
enlarged at 2 weeks and 6 months comparing with that after PPG .

Changes in gallblader contractile function

In PPG patients, the percentage of the original resting gallbladder area at 20
minuts after injection of cerulein increased from $37.5+5.1$% to
$53.1+6.6$%(2weeks) but recovered thereafter as shown in closed squares in Fig 2.
In CDG patients, it showed similar change and the values were higher than those
of PPG at any observation period. But there was no significant difference. The
results indicated that the gallbladder contracile function was suppressed in
both PPG and CDG, but the extent was slight in PPG.

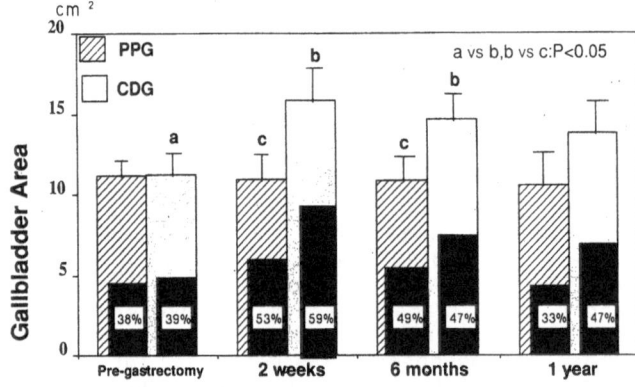

Fig. 2 Resting Gallbladder Area and Contractile Rate(%)
after Administration of Cerulein

DISCUSSION

The postgastrectomy cholecystolithiasis has been considered tobe associated
with dilatation and deterioration of contractile function of the gallbladder,
causative factors of which are probably the removal of hepatic branch of the
vagal nerve[1], the disorder of gut hormone by the gastrointestinal reconstruction [3], the long-term total parenteral nutrition and the adhesion of gallbladder to the surrounding organs. In those factors described above, the denervation of the vagal nerve can play an important role for the stone formation[4,5]. Our recent investigation of the postgastrectomy state in the gastric cancer patients[6] revealed that the stone formatiopn was detected in 27%

of the patients after total gastrectomy with truncal vagotomy at the level of abdominal esophagus, which supports the significance of vagal nerve factor. The present study disclosed that resting gallbladder area was not affected and that gallbladder contractile function was less suppressed after PPG which preserved the hepatic branch of vagal nerve, comparing with CDG which removed it. These results indicated that the preservation of hepatic branch of the vagal nerve plays a very important role on the retention of postgastrectomy gallbladder function. It also suggested that PPG has advantage to decrease the incidence of postgastrectomy cholecystolthiasis.

REFERENCES

1. Fletcher, D.M., Clark, C.G. (1986) Gallstones and gastric Surgery a review. Br. J. Surg. 55:895-899
2. Koadama, M., Koyama, K. (1991) Indication for pylorus preserving gastrectomy for early gastric cancer located in the middle third of the stomach. World J. Surg. 15:628-634
3. Horwitz, A., Kirson, S.M. :Cholecystitis and cholelithiasis as a sequel to gastric surgery: A clinical impression. (1965) Am. J. Surg. 109:760-762
4. Johnson, F.E., Boyden, E.A. (1952) The effect of double vagotomy on the motor activity of the human gallbladder. Surgery 32:591-602
5. Inoue, K., Fuchigami, A., Higashide, S., Sumi, S., Kogire, M., Suzuki, T., Tobe, T. (1992) Gallbladder sludge and stone formation in relation to contrac tile function after gastrectomy : A prospective study. Ann. Surg. 215: 19-26
6. Kodama, M., Koyama, H., Sone, S., Sakusabe, M., Narisawa, T, Koyama, K. (1990) Quality of life after resection of stomach by Questionaire. . Jpn. Soc. Clin. Surg. 51:466-471

Adverse Effects of Regurgitant Duodenal Content on the Mucosa of the Residual Stomach After Partial Gastrectomy

RYUKICHI HADA[1], YASUNORI MIKAMI[1], DAI SEITO[1], YUZURU SUGIYAMA[1], HIDETOSHI SUZUKI[1], MITSURU KONN[1], and MASANORI OZAWA[2]

[1]Department of Surgery, Hirosaki University School of Medicine, Hirosaki, 036 Japan
[2]Department of Surgery, Hakodate Municipal Hospital, Hakodate, Hokkaido, 040 Japan

ABSTRACT

Three groups of patients partially gastrectomized by Billroth II, Billroth I or pylorus-preserving procedure were evaluated for amount of bile acids in the gastric aspirate and histologic changes in the remnant gastric mucosa. The amount of bile acids was the highest and glandular dysplasia of the mucosa most predominant in the B-II group. Rats with either gastrojejunostomy or simple gastrotomy were maintained with an usual laboratory diet. Intestinal type adenoma and carcinoma developed exclusively in the gastrojejunostomized rats. Prolonged exposure of the gastric mucosa to bilious content may result in its histological changes that possibly lead to development of carcinoma.

INTRODUCTION

Adverse effects of regurgitant duodenal content on the mucosa of the residual stomach after partial gastrectomy have long been postulated in connection with the possibility of developing carcinoma[1,2,3]. Employment of pylorus-preserving gastrectomy for cancer, if it does not jeopardize the curativity, may partly be verified on this reason. We attempted to correlate bile acids levels in the gastric aspirate and histological changes occurring at the mucosa of the residual stomach of partially gastrectomized patients. We also conducted an animal experiment utilizing rats to examine whether the gastric mucosa persistently exposed to duodenal content exhibits any histological change which can be related to development of carcinoma.

MATERIALS AND METHODS

Clinical Study

Three comparable groups, each consisting of 7 patients (mean age: 60-64 yrs, male to female ratio: 5 vs. 2 or 6 vs. 1) gastrectomized for more than 18 months by Billroth II (B-II), Billroth I (B-I) or pylorus-preserving gastrectomy (PPG) were randomly extracted. Gastric aspirate was obtained after a 12 h overnight fast. Concentrations of total bile acid and bile acid fractions in the gastric aspirate were determined by GLC. Biopsy specimens were obtained from four sites of the residual stomach: the anastomotic region, the lesser curvature near the anastomosis, the mid portion of the anterior or posterior wall. The specimens were stained with hematoxylin-eosin and were microscopically examined for histological features.

Experimental Study

Sixty-five male Wister rats (280-350g) undergoing gastrojejunostomy (G-J rats) and 10 rats with simple gastrotomy (control) were maintained with pelleted stock laboratory diet. Thirty-six out of the 65 G-J rats and all of the control rats survived more than 56 weeks. These were sacrificed at the 56th to 70th postoperative week. The removed stomach was examined macroscopically, and then, it was fixed with formalin. Sections were stained with hematoxylin-eosin for histological analysis.

RESULTS

Clinical Study

The total bile acid (TBA) as well as each individual fractional bile acid level (LCA, DCA, CDCA, UDCA, CA) and the amount of the gastric aspirate were significantly higher in the B-II group (P<0.05) than in other two groups (Fig 1). The mean amount of total bile acid in the gastric aspirate collected for 60 min under the fasted condition was 1.7×10^5 for the B-II, 2.94×10^4 for the B-I and 5.70 mg/h for the PPG group.

Histologic features of the gastric mucosa related to site of biopsy are detailed in Table 1. Foci of glandular dysplasia (neoplastic change) were most frequently observed at the anastomotic region: 5/7 for the B-II and 2/7 for the B-I group (Fig 2). Such precancerous change was also seen in the specimens from the lesser curvature and anterior/posterior wall of 2 B-II patients. No neoplastic change was observed in the PPG group.

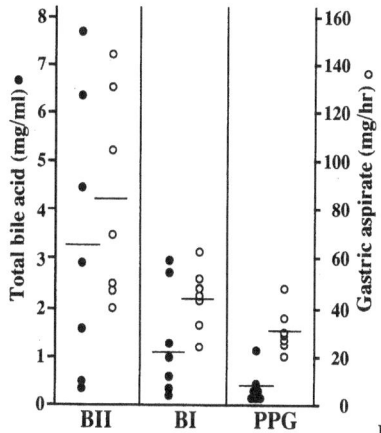

Fig 1. Total bile acid in the gastric aspirate.

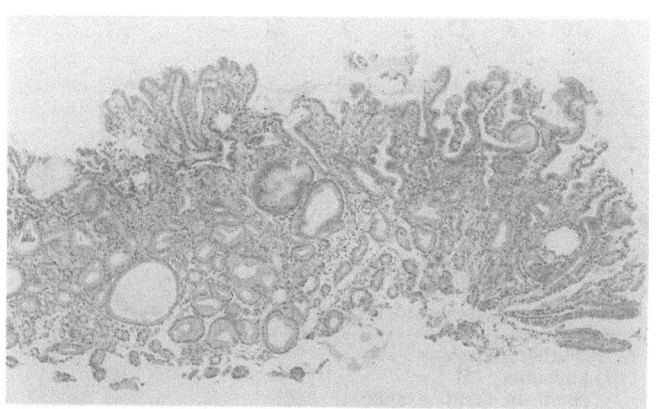

Fig 2. A biopsy specimen from the residual stomach after B-II resection. A 60 year-old man gastrectomized for 9 years. Glandular atypism, pseudopyloric glands and cystic dilatations are observed.

Table 1. Histological features of biopsy specimen from partially gastrectomized patients

	Anastomotic Region			Lesser Curvature Near Anastomosis			Anterior or Posterior Wall			Greater Curvature		
	BII	BI	PPG	BII	BI	PPG	BII	BI	PPG	BII	BI	PPG
Inflammatory change Acute gastritis	0	2	3	0	1	2	0	1	2	1	1	3
Chronic gastritis Atrophic non-metaplasic change	6	3	5	5	3	4	4	4	6	6	4	4
Intestinal meta-plastic change	1	1	2	0	2	3	0	1	2	0	1	2
Neoplastic change*	5	2	0	1	0	0	1	0	0	0	0	0
No remarks	0	0	0	1	1	1	1	1	1	0	1	1

* Glandular dysplasia more than <u>moderate</u> in Morson's classification [4] was defined as neoplastic change.

Experimental Study

In each of the 36 G-J rats, grossly protuberant mucosal lesions, small or large, were seen at the glandular part of the stomach exclusively along the anastomotic suture line (Fig 3). When those larger than 3 mm in diameter were counted, a total of 48 lesions were identified in 32 rats. Distribution of these lesions related to size and configuration were shown in Table 2. No such lesions were seen in the control rats.

Three-hundred and eight sections from the 36 G-J rats were histologically examined. There were

47 protuberant, 1 flat and 2 depressed lesions (Table 3). Of the 47 protuberant lesions, 31 were adenomas and 10 were carcinomas. As the glandular epithelial cells of the adenomas were with brush-borders, positive PAS and positive Alcianbue stains, the adenomas were diagnosed as *intestinal type adenomas*. All of the 10 adenocarcinomas were papillary or moderate to well differentiated tubular adenocarcinomas (Fig 4). They were always accompanied by intestinal type adenomas around them.

Table 2. Size and configuration of protuberant lesions at the glandular stomach of gastrojejunostomied rats

Diameter (mm)	Gross type*				Total
	I	II	III	IV	
≤ 5	3	10	0	0	13
≤10	3	17	4	0	24
≤15	2	0	3	0	5
15<	1	0	5	0	6
Total	9	27	12	0	48

* Yamada's classification

Table 3. Histology of mucosal lesions at the glandular stomach of gastrojejunostomied rats

A. Protuberant lesions   47
  1) adenoma   31
    slight~moderate dysplasia**   23
    moderate~severe dysplasia**   8
  2) adenocarcinoma   10
  3) granuloma   4
  4) cyst   2
B. Flat lesion   1
  1) extramural cyst   1
C. Depressed lesion   2
  1) adenocarcinoma   2

** The grade of dysplasia based on Morson's classification[4]

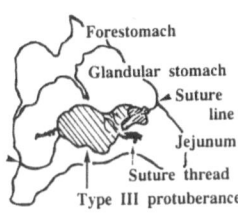

Fig 3. Resected stomach from a gastrojejunostomied rat. A type III protuberant lesion at the anastomotic line. The black spots are the suture thread exposed.

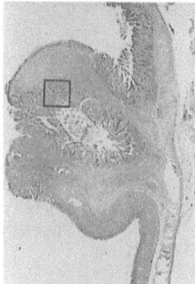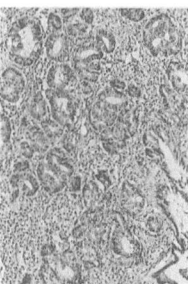

Fig 4. Histological appearance of a protuberant lesion. Severe glandular atypism seen near at the top of the protuberance (□). The magnified view shows moderately differentiated tubular adenocarcinoma.

DISCUSSION

In our series, glandular dysplasia, which has been considered to be important as a precancerous condition[4], was more frequently observed in the B-II group than in other two groups. This histological change could at least partly be correlated to the amount of regurgitant duodenal (bilious) content. Our animal experiment exemplified the effect of duodenal content on the gastric mucosa to develop carcinoma.

REFERENCES

1) Domellof L, Eriksson S, Jaunger KG (1975) Late occurrence of precancerous changes and carcinoma of the gastric stump after Billroth II resection. Acta Chir Scand 141:292-297.
2) Morgernstern L, Yamakawa T, Seltzer D (1973) Carcinoma of the gastric stump. Am J Surg 125:29-38.
3) Meister H, Schlag P, Weber E, Bockler R, Merkle P (1981) Frequency of cancerous and precancerous epithelial lesions in the stomach in different models for enterogastric reflux. Scand J Gastroenterol 16 (Suppl 67):165-168.
4) Morson BC, Sobin LH, Grundmann E, Johansen A, Nagayo T, Serck-Hanssen A (1980) Precancerous conditions and epithelial dysplasia in the stomach. J Clin Pathol 33:711-721.

Early Stomach Cancer in Turkey

NECATI ÖRMECI, SALIM DEMIRCI, ÖZDEN TULUNAY, IŞINSU KUZU, HIKMET AKGÜL, ÖZDEN UZUNALIMOĞLU, and SERDAR YOL

Departments of Gastroenterology, Oncologic Surgery and Pathology, Ankara University School of Medicine, Ankara, Turkey

ABSTRACT

The Stomach cancer has been encountered as the most common tumor in gastrointestinal system in Turkey.We have periodically performed the upper gastrointestinal endoscopy for the patients with precancerous lesions such as intestinal metaplasia, atrophic gastritis and polyps.We have used dyes such as metilen blue, indigocarmin during the examination in selective cases.We have preoperatively diagnosed forty one cases ,31 male and 10 female, in early stage of the cancer since 1987 up to now.In order to diagnose the early stomach cancer, it is necessary to perform periodically endoscopic examinations and dye endoscopy in high risk groups for gastric cancer.

KEY WORDS:Early Stomach Cancer, Dye Scattering.

INTRODUCTION

Early gastric cancer (EGC) was first defined by the Japanese as carcinoma of the stomach in which the depth of invasion is limited the mucosa and submucosa, regardless of the presence or absence of lymph node metastases.Allthough the incidence of gastric cancer has decreased in the world over the past 50 years.This disease still remains the highest cause of cancer death in men among the gastrointestinal malignancies in Turkey. In Japan where the incidence of gastric cancer is encountered the highest in the world ,mass screening programs have resulted in a significant reduction of the gastric cancer death rate. Although prognosis of the stomach cancer has been improved all due to the advences in surgical techniques, adjuvant chemotherapy, and radiotherapy imposed in Turkey, the disease still seems to challange us concerning early stage diagnosis of the disease.

We rewiew herein the experiences of our department in the detection of patients with EGC.

MATERIAL AND METHOD

The patients who admitted to our endoscopy laboratory with the complaints of gastrointestinal symptoms were routinely performed esophagogastroduodenoscopy. The patients with precancerous lesions such as intestinal metaplasia ,severe atrophic gastritis and polyp were periodically followed up and dye scatterig method such as indigocarmine or metilen blue were used when necessary.

We have preoperatively diagnosed fourty one cases, 31 male and 10 female,in early stage of the cancer since 1987 up to now. Mean age was 51.96 year (range 26-75).

RESULTS

We have classified fourty one cases as shown in Table I according to endoscopic classification for early stomach cancer of Japanese Endoscopy Society in 1962.

Table I:Macroscopic Classification of the EGC cases.

Type I   : 5 cases
Type IIa   : 2 cases
Type IIb   : 1 case
Type IIc   : 28 cases (Figure 1,2)
Type III   : 1 case
Type IIa +IIc : 1 case
Type IIc +IIb   : 3 cases

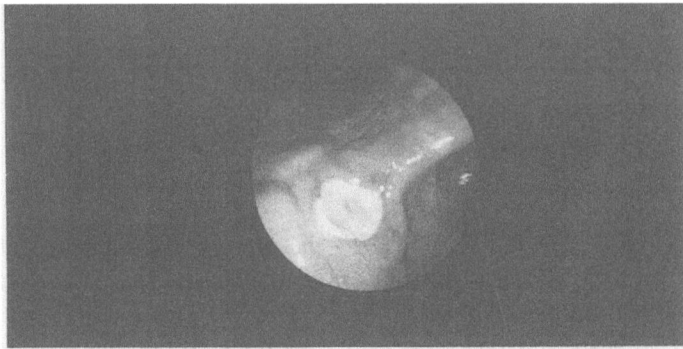

Figure 1: Type II-c carcinoma with mucosal fold convergence, abrubt disruption of the fold, ulcer in the center.

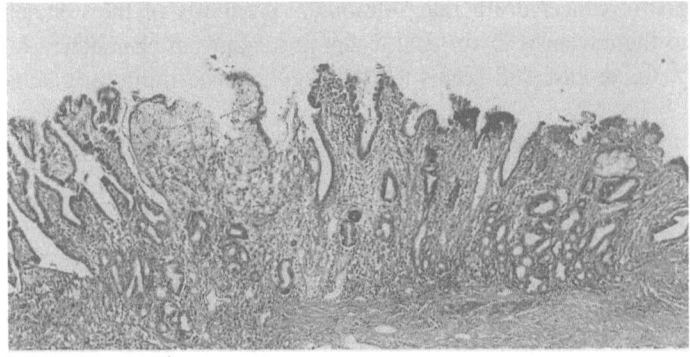

Figure II: Early gastric carcinoma, arising at the peripheral mucosal area (framed, of the benign looking ulcer (arrow) [x 40, H.E.].

All except one patients had been operated on the General Rules for the Gastric Cancer Study in Surgery and Pathology (1).One patient with severe congestive heart failure could not have a operation and died two months after the diagnosis. Five cases with early type I first have undergone polypectomy and then gastrectomy, and no evidence of methastasis to the lymph node or wessels was detected. Lesions were located at corpus with a rate of 48.80 %, at antrum 46.34 %, at angulus 2.43 % and at stoma 2.43 % .Histopathological diagnosis was the diffuse type in 11 cases (26.82 %) and intestinal type in 30 cases (73.18 %).Vertical invasion of the lesion was in mucosa in 17 cases (42.5 %) and in submucosa in 23 cases (57.5 %).There were methastasis to the lymph nodes in two cases with diffuse type carsinomas.

DISCUSSION

In 1962, The Japanese Endoscopic Society adopted the term early gastric carcinoma to discribe those lesions in which tumor invasion was limited to either the mucosal or submucosal layer ,with or without regional lymph node methastasis.

The researchers in western world have claimed that biologic behavior of the stomach cancer differs in Japan and Western Countries .From the data obtained it is concluded that it takes many years for the precancerous state to develop into microscopically recognisable cancer, and many years from this state to grow to a clinically detectable EGC ,and, than often more than five years again for EGC to progress into advanced gastric cancer .

In our series ,two suspected cases who could not be diagnosed histopathologically were proved to developed manifest cancer after 15 months aproximately.

In contrast to Japan the incidence of gastric carcinoma is approximately eight times lower in the western world and has been slowly declining during recent years.In addition ,the average proportion of cancers diagnosed at an early stage is only one third of the figures reported from Japan, however, the five year survival rates do not reach those of Japenese patients (2).

Conserning the age, sex distribution, localisation of the tumor ,histopathologic pattern of the tumor, the clinical and biological behavior of our cases are similar to those reported in the Japanese and European literature.

Since 1970, fiberoptic endoscopy has become widely accepted for the diagnostic purposes in Turkey, however, the use of double contrast radiology is not being used widespread yet.We have been using the dye scattering methods when necessary since 1986.

The most important factors influacing the prognosis of patients with gastric cancer are depth of invasion and lymph node methastasis where these factors are remarcably more significant than other variables, such as type of cancer location and histologic type (3). For this reason the best treatment of the stomach cancer is to diagnose it in early stage.

REFERENCES

1. Japanese Research Society for Gastric Cancer.The General Rules for the Gastric Cancer Study in Surgery and Pathology.Japanese Journal of Surgery 11(2):127_139,1991.
2. Eckardt FV,Giebler W,Kanzler G,Remmele W,and Bernhard G.Clinical and Morphological Characteristics of Early Gastric Cancer.Gastroenterology 98:708_714,1990.
3. Maruyama K.The most important Prognostic Factors for Gastric Cancer Patients. Scan J Gastroenterol 22(Suppl 133):63_68,1987

Multiple Early Cancer of the Stomach

KUNIYOSHI ARAI, MASATSUGU KITAMURA, and KAORU MIYASHITA

Department of Surgery, Tokyo Metropolitan Komagome Hospital, Bunkyo-ku, Tokyo, 113 Japan

ABSTRACT

During the past fifteen years, resections were performed in 744 patients with early gastric cancer, leading to the discovery of synchronous multiple early cancer (MC) in 151 cases (20%). The frequency of old-aged patients and differentiated carcinoma was statistically higher (p<0.01) in MC than in solitary early cancer (SC). When this period was subdivided into five three-year periods, the prevalence of MC gradually increased showing a correlation with the mean age : 8% in the Ist period vs 31% in the Vth period. On the contrary, no differences were found in the diagnostic rate of MC through the periods.

KEY WORDS: early gastric cancer, synchronous multiple cancer,
            old-aged patient with gastric cancer

INTRODUCTION

Although the incidence of cases of synchronous multiple early cancer (MC) of the stomach has been increasing recently [1,2], the reason has not been clarified In this paper, the cause was examined from the clinicopathological characteristics of MC as compared with solitary early cancer (SC).

MATERIALS AND METHODS

During the fifteen years from 1975 to 1989, 744 cases of early gastric cancer were resected in our hospital. They consisted of 151 cases (20%) of MC based on the criteria of Moertel et al [3] and 593 cases (80%) of SC. Regarding the number of MC lesions, 98 were double, 25 triple and 28 quadruple or more (maximum; 16 lesions). The clinicopathological findings of the MC group were compared with those of the SC group. Transition in the prevalence of MC, and also the accuracy of diagnosis in the preoperative examination and with the fresh specimen were studied in five three-year periods as follows. Ist period : 1975-1977, IInd : 1978-1980, IIIrd : 1981-1983, IVth : 1984-1986, Vth : 1987-1989. Quantitative data were analyzed for statistical significance using Student's t test and the chi-squared test.

RESULTS

The number of early gastric cancer cases was 75 in the Ist period, 91 in the IInd period, 152 in the IIIrd period, 197 in the IVth period and 229 in the Vth period. The prevalence of MC cases, which gradually increased, was 8% (6 cases) in the Ist period, 13% (12 cases) in the IInd period, 18% (27 cases) in the IIIrd period, 21% (34 cases) in the IVth period and 31% (72 cases) in the Vth period, respectively (Fig.1).
The mean age (57.9 yrs vs 65.1 yrs) and the rate of the differentiated carcinoma

342

(57% vs 73%) were statistically higher in the MC group than in the SC group (p<0 .01), whereas no differences were seen with regard to the sex ratio, and the location, the macroscopic classification and the depth of the main lesion (Table 1).

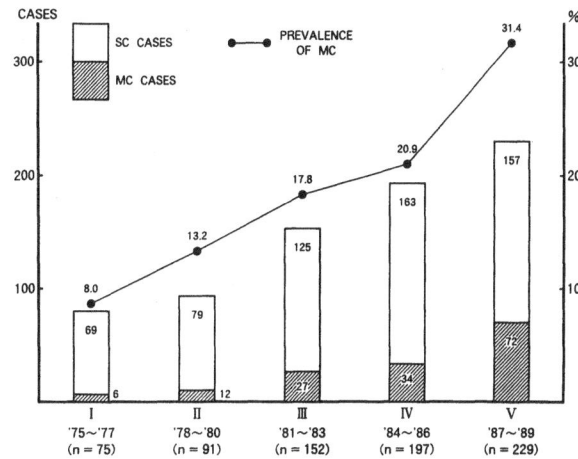

Fig.1 Transition in periodic prevalence of MC

Table 1. Comparison of clinicopathological backgrounds between SC and MC.

	Solitary (n=593)	Multiple (n=151)	analysis
Age (yrs)	57.9	65.1	p<0.01
Sex ratio (M/F)	365/228	103/48	ns
Location			
upper	56(9)	10(7)	
middle	317(54)	78(52)	ns
lower	220(37)	68(42)	
Macroscopic classification			
elevated	67(11)	26(17)	
flat	7(1)	2(1)	ns
depressed	334(56)	77(51)	
mixed	185(31)	46(31)	
Microscopic type			
differentiated	337(57)	110(73)	p<0.01
undifferentiated	256(43)	41(27)	
Depth			
mucosal	316(53)	84(56)	ns
submucosal	277(47)	67(44)	
Tumor size (cm)	3.5	3.1	p<0.05

Numbers in parentheses: % values.

The mean age became higher with the transition through the periods, which was 54.1 yrs in the Ist period, 57.2 yrs in the IInd period, 58.8 yrs in the IIIrd period, 60.2 yrs in the IVth period and 61.7 yrs in the Vth period (Fig.2). The prevalence of MC cases stratified by age was 8% in patients less than 50 years of age, 14% in 50 year-olds, 24% in 60 year-olds and 34% in patients more than 70 years of age. This result revealed taht older patients had a higher incidence of MC.
On the contrary, no improvement was seen in the diagnostic rate of MC through the periods; preoperative diagnostic rate ranged from 35% to 50% and 44% to 67% in fresh specimens. Preoperative misdiagnosis of MC as SC was 91 (60%) out of

151 cases and the rate of corrected diagnosis of all lesions was no more than
21% (Table 2).

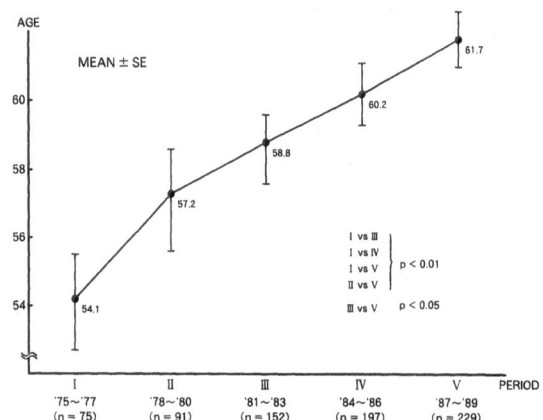

Fig.2 Transition in periodical mean age

Table 2. Number of detected MC lesions

	Single	Multiple		Overall
		Several	All	MC cases
Preoperative	91(60)	28(19)	32(21)	151
In specimen	73(48)	27(18)	52(34)	151

Numbers in parentheses: % values.

DISCUSSION

The prevalence of MC, which has been increasing of late, was reported to be over
10%[1,2] of early gastric cancer around 1990. Although these authors attributed
this increase to the improvement of diagnostic examination, no supporting data
was found. On the other hand it was a fact that MC cases were more frequent
among old-aged patients and were more differentiated compared with SC cases.
Here we analyze the cause of the increase from the standpoint of transition in
age and the preoperative diagnosis. The findings showed that the prevalence of
MC steadily increased in correlation the mean age, whereas no relation was found
with the rate of diagnosis. Consequently we concluded that the cause of the
recent higher frequency of MC was mainly attributable to increase in old-aged
patients and not to the improvement of detection of the lesions. About one-third
of the early gastric cancer cases, with the limitation of those over 60 years
and differentiated type, were MC cases, of which the rate of diagnosable cases
for MC was no more than 50% preoperatively nor in the fresh specimen.
These findings point to the need for careful examination and treatment in these
high risk groups.

REFERENCES

1. Brandt D, Muramatsu Y, Ushio K, et al (1989) Synchronous early gastric
   cancer. Radiology 173:649-652
2. Yoshikawa T, Kitamura M, Arai K, et al (1989) Clinicopathological study of
   multiple early gastric cancer. Jpn J Gastroenterol Surg 22:1062-1066
3. Moertel CG, Bargen A, Soule EH (1957) Multiple gastric cancers. - Review of
   the literature and study of 42 cases - Gastroenteroloy 32:1095-1103.

Are There Any Pathologic Differences Between Mucosal and Submucosal Cancer of the Stomach?

Cho Hyun Park, Jong Seo Lee, and In Chul Kim

Department of Surgery, Catholic University Medical College, Seoul 137-040, Korea

ABSTRACT

In a retrospective study of 312 of early gastric cancer, we analyzed the pathologic differences in relation to the depth of invasion. The differences were significant between mucosal and submucosal cancers in regard to lymph node metastasis(2.8% vs 21.5%), lymphatic/venous invasion(0% vs 20.5%/7.3%), gross appearance and histologic type. No significant differences were found between the groups concerning clinical features, location and tumor size. All nine cases with a recurrence were exclusively the patients with submucosal cancer. Kaplan-Meier estimate 5-year survival was 98% in mucosal cancer and 79% in submucosal cancer.

KEY WORDS: early gastric cancer, pathologic difference

INTRODUCTION

It is widely accepted that the prognosis of early gastric cancer after curative resection is very favorable, ranging between 80% and 95% of a 5-year survival rate. However, varying degrees of lymph node metastasis and 3% -10% of recurrence[1-2] has been reported in early gastric cancer and the prognosis of submucosal cancer is worse than mucosal cancer. Therefore, from the viewpoint of surgery and endoscopic treatment as well as preoperative diagnosis of early gastric cancer it is required to define the different pathologic features between mucosal and submucosal cancer. In this study, we analyzed the clinicopathologic profiles of early gastric cancer in relation to the depth of tumor invasion.

PATIENTS AND METHODS

From 1980 through 1991, 1729 patients underwent operation for gastric adenocarcinoma at Department of Surgery, Catholic University Medical College in Seoul, Korea. Three hundred and twelve cases(18.0%) were histologically confirmed as early gastric cancer. One hundred and seven (34.3%) patients had tumor confined to the mucosa, while the tumor extended into the submucosa in 205 (65.7%). There has been an increasing tendency of annual incidence of early gastric cancer(12.6% in the first half vs 21.0% in the second half). Medical records of these patients were reviewed and data regarding clinicopathologic profiles including recurrence and survival were collected. The clinicopathological findings were analyzed according to the General Rules for Japan Gastric Cancer Study.

RESULTS

Gross Type, Location and Depth of Invasion

The incidence of protruded type was higher in submucosal cancer(24.4%) than in mucosal cancer(9.3%) and the type IIb cancers were mostly confined to the mucosa. On the other hand the type I cancers almostly invaded the submucosal layer. Although there was no significant difference in tumor distribution between mucosal and submucosal cancer, deep invasion was predominant in C region(upper portion of stomach). Multiplicity occurred in 13 (4.2%) patients, 4(3.7%) in mucosal cancer and 9(4.4%) in submucosal cancer.

Lymph Node Metastasis and Venous/Lymphatic Invasion

Of the 312 cases of early gastric cancer, there were 47 cases(15.1%) with lymph node metastasis. The incidence of lymph node metastasis was 2.8% in mucosal cancer and 21.5% in those with submucosal cancer(Table 1). All three cases of lymph node

Table 1. Lymph node metastasis and venous/lymphatic invasion in early gastric cancer

Depth of invasion	No. of cases	Lymph node metastasis N1(%)	N2(%)	Venous invasion(%)	Lymphatic invasion(%)
Mucosa	107	3(2.8)	0(0)	0(0)	0(0)
Submucosa	205	34(16.6)	10(4.9)	42(20.5)	15(7.3)
Total	312	37(11.9)	10(3.2)	42(13.5)	15(4.8)

metastasis in mucosal cancer involved the group 1 perigastric nodes. In submucosal cancer metastatic rate of group 1 node was 16.6% and 4.9% in group 2. No nodes of group 3 or group 4 were involved. Of the 3 cases of mucosal cancer with lymph node metastasis, 2 were with the elevated type(IIa and IIa + IIc) and remaining one with the depressed type(IIc). In submucosal cancer, the incidence of the lymph node metastasis of the elevated type was higher than that of the depressed : 36.0% and 16.8%, respectively. In terms of tumor size, submucosal cancers were slightly larger than mucosal cancers(average 3.4 cm vs 2.3 cm) and the larger the cancer the higher the metastatic rate of lymph node. Histologically, differentiated type was more common in submucosal cancer(61.0%) than in mucosal cancer(42.1%). However, lymph node metastasis occurred frequently in undifferentiated type of submucosal cancer. Niether lymphatic nor venous invasion was noted in mucosal cancer(Table 1). In submucosal cancer, venous and lymphatic invasion rates were 7.3% and 20.5%, respectively.

Recurrence

Nine patients developed either local or systemic recurrence of disease(Table 2). All of them were patients with submucosal cancer. Mean interval from surgery to recurrence was 30.4 months. Differentiated carcinoma(7 cases), macroscopically

Table 2. Pathologic findings of nine patients with recurrent early gastric cancer

Case	Location	Gross type	size	Depth	LN status	Histo- logy	Lymph. invasion	Venous invasion	Recur site	Survival
1	M	IIa	1.0x1.0	sm	N0	Diff.	+	-	Peritoneum	34mo
2	A	I	3.7x2.9	sm	N0	Diff.	-	-	Gastric stump	48mo
3	A	I	6.5x5.4	sm	N0	Diff.	-	+	Liver	36mo
4	A	I	2.5x2.0	sm	N2	Diff.	-	-	Lymph node	12mo(alive)
5	A	IIc	1.3x1.0	sm	N1	Diff.	-	-	Liver	56mo
6	A	IIc	3.0x1.5	sm	N1	Undiff.	-	-	Bone	34mo
7	A	IIa	6.0x2.0	sm	N1	Diff.	-	-	Lung	49mo(alive)
8	M	IIc	4.0x3.0	sm	N2	Undiff.	-	-	Lymph node	23mo
9	M	I	2.7x2.0	sm	N0	Diff.	+	-	Bone	46mo

elevated type(6cases) and lymph node metastasis(5 cases) were frequently associated with recurrence. The mean survival of this group was 7.1 months after detection of recurrence.

Survival

Kaplan-Meier estimate 5-year survival was 98% for patients with mucosal cancer and 79% for those with submucosal cancer(overall 5-year survival rate : 86.3%). The

5-year survival rate in patients of submucosal cancer with lymph node metastasis was only 60%, which is much lower than those without lymph node involve ment(88.5%)(Fig.1).

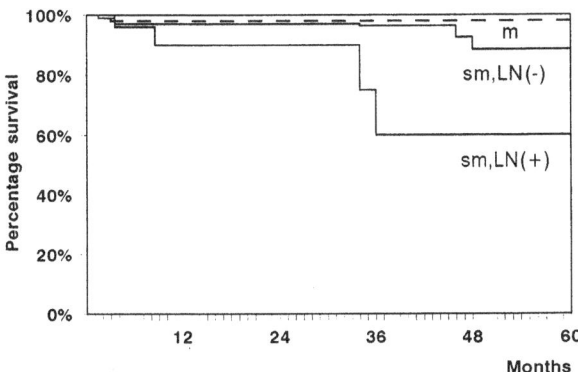

Fig.1 Kaplan-Meier survival curves for early gastric cancer according to the depth of invasion(m:mucosal cancer, sm: submucosal cancer, LN:lymph node)

DISCUSSION

In this study, we found that nearly eight-fold increase in the incidence of lymph node metastasis in submucosal cancer compared with mucosal cancer. Furthermore, 4.9% of lymph node metastasis in submucosal cancer reached to the group 2 nodes. This fact suggests that R2 resection with complete excision of groups 1 and 2 lymph nodes is the principle surgical procedure for early gastric cancer. Another major difference between mucosal and submucosal cancer was the degree of lymphatic and venous invasion. A morphologic basis for these differences has been observed earlier using transmission electron microscopy[3]. In this study, all nine cases with a recurrence were exclusively the patients with submucosal cancer which clearly indicates that the depth of cancer invasion strongly affects the prognosis. Submucosal cancers with a macroscopically elevated type, differentiated carcinoma and lymph node metastasis were the high-risk cancers for recurrence. Accordingly, the survival rate of submucosal cancer was lower than those with mucosal cancer. Moreover, the survival rate for submucosal cancer with lymph node involvement was unexpectedly low(60% of 5-year survival rate). The similar result has also been reported by Inoue et al[4]. Concerning the clinicopathological differences between mucosal and submucosal cancer, therapeutic approach of submucosal cancer should be different from mucosal cancer.

REFERRENCES

1. Kodama Y, Inokuchi K, Soejima K, Matsusaka T, Okamura T (1981) Growth patterns and prognosis in early gastric carcinoma. Cancer 51:320-326
2. Matsusaka T, Kodama Y, Soejima K, Miyazaki M, Yoshimura K, Sugimachi Y, Inokuchi K (1980) Recurrence in early gastric cancer. A morphologic evaluation. Cancer 46:168-172
3. Lehnert T, Erlandson RA, Decosse JJ (1985) Lymph and blood capillaries of the human gastric mucosa. A morphologic basis for metastasis in early gastric carcinoma. Gastroenterology 89:939-950
4. Inoue K, Tobe T, Kan N, Nio Y, Sakai M, Takeuchi E, Sugiyama T (1991) Problems in the definition and treatment of early gastric cancer. Br J Surg 78:818-821

Recurrence of Early Gastric Cancer

Tsutomu Namieno[1], Tsunemi Higashi[1], Yukifumi Kondo[1],
Masatoshi Takahashi[1], Akihiko Gotoda[1], Akihiko Kataoka[1],
Akifumi Yamashita[1], Norihiko Takahashi[1], Kazumitsu Koito[2],
Akimichi Imamura[2], Toshihiro Suga[2], Yoshio Murashima[2], and
Jun-ichi Uchino[3]

Departments of [1]Surgery and [2]Gastroenterology, Sapporo-Kosei, General Hospital, Sapporo, 060 Japan
[3]Department of First Surgery, Hokkaido University Hospital, Sapporo, 060 Japan

ABSTRACT

We have reviewed 1,585 cases of early of gastric cancer to investigate recurrent cases following a curative resection. Sixteen of these patients experienced a recurrence: 14 highly-graded and 2 low-graded differentiated adenocarcinomas. Of the recurrences observed 14 were submucosal (87.5%) and 2 were mucosal (12.5%) cancers. According to the macroscopic appearance of the primary lesions, 12 primaries were composed of some elevated component. In particular, the mixed type, elevated and depressed, was significantly frequent in lymph node metastases and microvessel invasions ($p < 0.02 - 0.001$). In conclusion highly-graded adenocarcinomas of the stomach invading a submucosal layer with its surface being elevated and depressed has a high potential of recurrence.

KEY WORDS : gastric cancer, recurrence

INTRODUCTION

Development of the radiological double contrast method and advances in endoscopy has enabled the detection of a lot of early gastric cancers in Japan. The postoperative outcome in early gastric cancers is much better than in advanced cases. The 5-year survival rate exceed 90% (1-4). However, we sometimes encountered recurrences of early gastric cancers after a curative resection. This seemed to suggest that there might be some pathological problems, so we reviewed our experience with early gastric cancers in order to investigate pathological differences concerning the recurrence of early gastric cancers.

PATIENTS AND METHODS

We studied 1,585 primary, early gastric cancers during a 27-year period. These cancers were resected with curative surgery performed at the department of surgery, Sapporo-Kosei General Hospital.The shortest follow-up period was 4 years. Clinicopathological descriptions including both macroscopic and microscopic findings were presented by The General Rules for the Gastric Study in Surgery and Pathology in Japan (5). All histopathologic specimens were examined to determine the depth of gastric wall invasion, the histologic type and the extent of lymphatic and vascular vessel invasion of the cancer cells. With respect to lymph node dissection, the nomenclature was described in the above (5) and summarized in Figure 1 and Table 1. The recurrent cases were found by reviewing medical records including laboratory data,ultrasonography, computed tomography, peritoneal punctures or laparotomy. The X^2- test was used for statistical analysis.

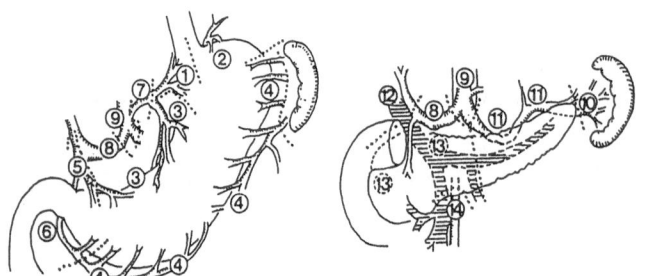

Figure 1. Designating number of regional lymph nodes (5)

①: right cardial,②: left cardial,③: lesser curvature,④: greater curvature,
⑤: suprapyrolic,⑥: infrapyrolic,⑦: left gastric artery,⑧: common hepatic artery,
⑨: celiac artery,⑩: splenic hilus,
⑪: splenic artery,⑫: hepatoduodenal ligament,⑬: retropancreatic,⑭: mesenteric root.

Table 1. Grouping of regional lymph nodes according to the location of tumor (5)

Location of tumor	Group1 (n_1)	Group2 (n_2)	Group3 (n_3)
Lower third	3.4.5.6	1.7.8.9	2.10.11.12 13.14
Middle third	1.3.4.5.6	2.7.8.9 10.11	12.13.14
Upper third	1.2.3.4	5.6.7.8 9.10.11	12.13.14

Operation method

R_1 : Gastrectomy with complete dissection of the group 1 lymph modes.

R_2 : Gestrectomy with complete dissection of the group 1 and 2 lymph nodes.

R_3 : Gestrectomy with complete dissection of the group 1, 2 and 3 lymph nodes.

RESULTS

Incidence of Recurrence

The incidence of recurrence in these 1,585 cases was 16 (1.0%) : 13 males (mean age: 61yr 5mo) and 3 females (mean age: 62yr 7mo).Although the rates of mucosal cancer (m-Ca) and submucosal cancer (sm-Ca) were not significantly different, the sm-Cas were present in 14 (87.5%) of the 16 recurrences with significant difference compared with the m-Cas. The histologic types of these recurrences were 7 papillary, 7 tubular, one poorly differentiated adenocarcinomas and one signet ring cell.

Pathology of submucosal cancers

We have analyzed the pathological factors of a total of 802 cases of sm-Ca according to the macroscopic appearances of the primary lesions: elevated, depressed and mixed types, as shown in Table 2.

Table 2. Pathology of sm-Cas according to the macroscopic appearance of the primary lesions

Type	No.	Lymph node metastasis	Lymph vessel invasion	Vascular vessel invasion
Elevated	93	7.5%	25.8%	7.5%
Depressed	667	14.1% ⎤a ⎤b	21.4% ⎤b	5.4% ⎤b ⎤c
Mixed	124	25.8% ⎦ ⎦	36.3% ⎦	18.5% ⎦ ⎦

ap < 0.01 , bp < 0.001, cp <0.02

The respective percentages of lymph node metastasis, lymph or vascular vessel invasions are described in Table 2. The data indicates that the mixed type was most frequently microinvasive with significance compared with the other types, and that a primary with some elevated component tended to invade microvessels.

DISCUSSION

The postoperative prognosis for early gastric cancer is generally favorable, however, recurrent cases are sometimes encountered, and their pathological features are not completely clear. The present data revealed that some well-differentiated sm-adenocarcinomas were frequently recurrent compared with m-Cas and that their macroscopic surface was related to their incidence recurrence; the elevated and depressed, uneven, type had a high incidence of recurrence as well as the of other reports (1, 4, 6) and its pathological features were significantly prominent compared with those of the other types.

REFERENCES

1. Ohta H, Noguchi Y, Takagi K, Nishi M, Kajitani T, Kato Y (1987) Early gastric carcinoma with special reference to macroscopic classification. Cancer. 60: 1099-1106.
2. Kito T, Yamamura Y, Kobayashi S (1988) Surgical treatment of early gastric cancer. Anticancer Res. 8: 335-338.

3. Koga S, Kaibara N, Tamura H, Nishidoi H, Kimura O (1984) Cause of late postoperative death in patients with early gastric cancer with special reference to recurrence and the incidence of metachronous primary cancer in other organs. Surgery. 6: 511-516.

4. Kitaoka Y, Yoshikawa K, Hirota T, Itabashi M, (1984) Surgical treatment of early gastric cancer. Jpn J Clin Oncol. 14: 283-293.

5. Japanese Research Society for Gastric Cancer. (1981) The general rules for the gastric cancer study in surgery and pathology. Jpn J Surg. 11:127-139.

6. Gentsch HH, Groitl H, Giedle J (1981) Results of surgical treatment of early gastric cancer in 113 patients. World J Surg. 5: 103-107.

A Study of Rational Dissection of Regional Lymph Node in Early Gastric Cancer

XIANG HU, KUNIO OKAJIMA, SHINICHI YAMADA, EIJI NAKATA, JUNKO NISHIMURA, and TADASHI ICHINONA

Department of Surgery, Osaka Medical College, Takatsuki, Osaka, 569 Japan

ABSTRACT

In the present study covering a total of 577 patients with single early gastric cancer treated by us during the past 14 years, we examined the possibility of rational operation. Where the cancers were of elevated type of I or IIa, in macroscopic observation and where the histological type was differentiated type, no metastasis to lymph node was observed with the tumor size being less than 30 mm. However, where the cancers were of depressed type of IIc or IIc+III, metastasis to lymph node was observed with the tumor size being 10-14 mm or larger, regardless of histological type. Therefore, the indication of rational operation for early gastric cancer should be determined, considering macroscopic findings, histological type and the tumor size.

KEY WORDS: early gastric cancer, rational dessection, lymph node metastasis.

INTRODUCTION

Recently rational operation for gastric cancer have been proposed with the increase of incidence of early gastric cancer. With the purpose of establishing the indication of rational operation for early gastric cancer, we conducted a study of clinicopathological analysis on regional lymph node metastasis.

SUBJECTS AND METHODS

We investigated the following items in 577 patients with single early gastric cancer in our department during the past 14 years from August 1978 to July 1992 : 1) correlation between depth of invasion and lymph node metastasis, 2) correlation of tumor size, depth of invasion and lymph node metastasis, 3) lymph node metastasis related to gross type and tumor size.

RESULTS

Of the 577 cases of early gastric cancer invasion to the mucosal layer (m-cancer) was found in 314 cases and invasion to the submucosal layer (sm-cancer) was found in 263 cases. There were 53 cases with lymph node metastasis, among the cases of early gastric cacner. Of the 314 cases with m-cancer, lymph node metastasis was noted in 9 cases(3.1%). There were 5 cases (1.7%) with metastasis to lymph node of group 1 [$n_1(+)$], 2 cases (0.7%) with $n_2(+)$ and $n_3(+)$, respectively. There were 44 cases (16.8%) with lymph node metastasis in sm-cancer, rate of $n_1(+)$, $n_2(+)$, $n_3(+)$ and $n_4(+)$ were 13.3%(35/263), 2.3%(6/263), 0.4%(1/263), 0.8%(2/263), respectively (Fig. 1).

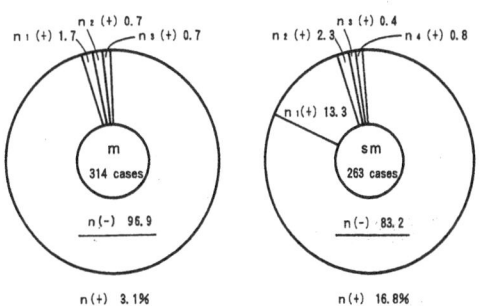

n(-): no lymph node metastasis, $n_1(+)$: metastasis to lymph nodes of group 1, $n_2(-)$: metastasis to lymph nodes of group 2, $n_3(+)$: metastasis to lymph nodes of group 3, $n_4(+)$: metastasis to lymph nodes of group4.

Fig. 1. Degree of lymph node metastasis according to depth of invasion in early gastric cancer

Fig. 2, 3 shows the rate of lymph node metastasis related to tumor size, histological type and depth of invasion. In m-cancer lymph node metastasis was observed in 5 cases with more than 15 mm, among the differentiated type. Lymph node metastasis was observed in 4 cases of sm-1 cancer with tumor size more than 25 mm, and 20 cases of sm-2 cancer more than 10 mm. In poorly differentiated type, lymph node metastasis were 3 cases, of m-cancer more than 15 mm, and 12 cases of sm-2 cancer more than 10 mm. But, regardless of depth of invasion or histological type, no lymph node metastasis was observed in all the early gastric cancer with tumor size less than 10 mm, and in m-cancer or sm-1 cancer with tumor size less than 15 mm.

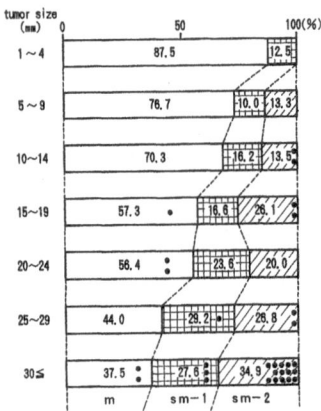

• case with lymph node metastasis

sm-1: depth of invasion confined to upper half of submucosal layer.
sm-2: depth of invasion confined to lower half of submucosal layer.

Fig. 2. Lymph node metastasis related to tumor size and depth of invasion in early gastric cancer
— differentiated type of cancer —

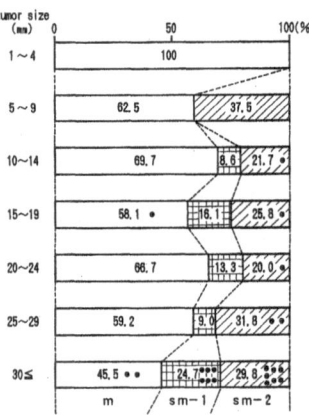

• case with lymph node metastasis

Differentiated type of cancer: papillary and tublar adenocarcinoma
Poorly differentiated type of cancer: poorly differentiated adenocarcinoma and signet-ring cell carcinoma.

Fig. 3. Lymph node metastasis related to tumor size and depth of invasion in early gastric cancer
— poorly differentiated type of cancer —

Fig. 4, 5 shows the lymph node metastasis related to tumor size, gross type and histological type. In elevated type (I, IIa) lymph node metastasis was observed in 7.1%(1/14) of differentiated type with tumor size more than 30 mm. But, in the cancer less than 30 mm, no lymph node metastasis was seen, and lymph node metastatic rate was noted in 9.8%(4/41) of the mixed type (IIa+IIc, IIc+IIa) more than 15 mm, among differentiated type. In cancer less than 15 mm, there was no lymph node metastasis. In depressed gross type (IIc or IIc+III), regardless of histological type, lymph node metastasis was not observed in cancer less than 10 mm.

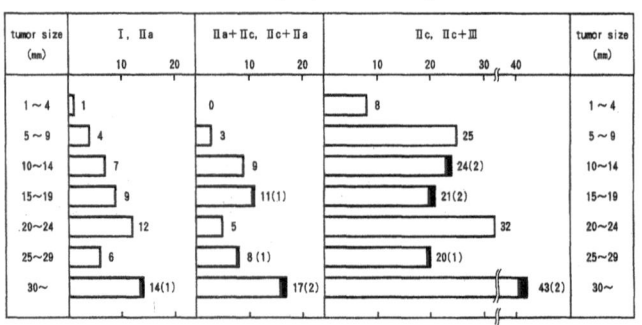

■ case with lymph node metastasis
( )number of case with lymph node metastasis

Type I : protrusion into the gastric lumen is eminent.
Type IIa: the surface is slightly elevated.
Type IIc: the surface is slightly depressed.
Type III: an excavation in the gastric wall is prominent.
Elevated type (I, IIa), depressed type (IIc, IIc+III), mixed type (IIa+IIc, IIc+IIa)

Fig. 4. Lymph node metastasis related to tumor size and gross type in early gastric cancer
— differentiated type —

tumor size (mm)	I, IIa		IIa+IIc, IIc+IIa		IIc, IIc+III				tumor size (mm)
	10		10		10	20	30	60	
1~4					3				1~4
5~9					7				5~9
10~14			2			20(1)			10~14
15~19			2			26(1)			15~19
20~24	1(1)		2			23			20~24
25~29			3			16			25~29
30~	1(1)		7					60(10)	30~

■ case with lymph node metastasis
( )number of case with lymph node metastasis

Fig. 5. Lymph node metastasis related to tumor size and gross type in early gastric cancer
— poorly differentiated type —

DISCUSSION

Early gastric cancer is defined as cancer which is confined to the mucosa or submucosa, regardless of the presence of lymph node metastasis. But, lymph node metastasis is an important factor in considering surgical treatment and prognosis. There were 53 cases (9.2%) with lymph node metastasis. Lymph node metastasis was observed in 2.9% with m-cancer, and in 16.8% with sm-cancer. Without reference to depth of invasion to mucosa or submucosa, lymph node metastasis was recognized in group 3 or group 4. In m-cancer, rate of $n_3(+)$ was 0.7%. In sm-cancer rate of $n_3(+)$ and $n_4(+)$ was 0.4%, 0.8%, respectivly. In order to obtain radical cure, in such patients, the R_2 or R_3 operation would be advised. For that reason, in principle, R_2 operation should be performed(1) as surgical procedure for early gastric cancer. As metastatic route of perigastric lymph node and actual status of lymph node metastasis has been clarified, rational operation for early gastric cancer has been proposed recently (2). In order to establish the criteria for selecting rational operation on early gastric cancer, we conducted a study of clinicopathological analysis on regional lymph node metastasis. In the present study, lymph node metastasis was not observed in the cases as followings : 1) cancer less than 10 mm in tumor size, 2) cancer with elevated type (I or IIa) less than 30 mm among differentiated type, 3) in the case of type(IIa+IIc) or (IIc+IIa) less than 15 mm, 4) in the case of type IIc or IIc+III, with m or sm-1 cancer less than 15 mm. This result suggested the possibility that rational limited operation can be performed, with curability for early gastric cancer. By analysis of the relationship between lymph node metastasis and clinicopathological findings, led to our new policy of surgical treatment for early gastric cancer (Fig. 6) :

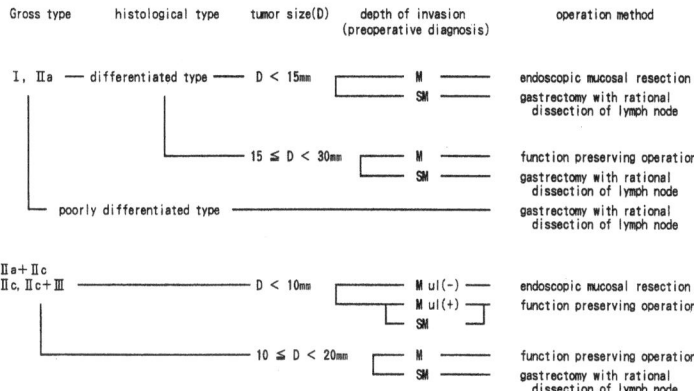

Fig. 6. Flow chart of rational operation for early gastric cancer

1) Endoscopic mucosal rsection should be applied to the cases as follows : (1) the mixed or depressed type of m-cancer less than 10 mm without ulceration, (2) the elevated type (I, IIa) of m-cancer among differentiated type less than 15 mm.
2) Function preserving operation should be applied to the cases as follows : (1) the mixed type or depressed type of m-cancer, less than 20 mm without ulceration or less than 10 mm with uleration, (2) sm-cancer less than 10 mm, (3) the elevated type of m-cancer less than 30 mm among differentiated type.
3) Limited operation with rational dissection of lymph node should be applied to the cases as follows : (1) among the differentiated type, elevated type of sm-cancer less than 30 mm, (2) elevated type of poorly differentiated type cancer, (3) the mixed or depressed type of sm-cancer less than 20 mm in tumor size.
Thus, in selecting limited operation, decision should be made, taking into consideration macroscopic findings, histological type and the tumor size.

REFERENCES

1. Yamada S, Okajima K (1991) Rational lymph node dissection for gastric cancer. J Clin Surg 46:1067-1074
2. Okajima K, Yamada S (1991) Some considerations on endoscopic radical resection of early gastric cancer. Stomach and Intestine 26:371-377

Study of Distribution of Minute Gastric Cancerous Foci in Multiple Early Gastric Cancer Cases — In Order to Decide the Extent of Gastric Resection

Motomichi Urabe, Shing-Han Liu, Noboru Mizobuchi, Kazuhiko Yasuda, Hitoshi Funabiki, and Noburu Sakakibara

First Department of Surgery, Juntendo University School of Medicine, Bunkyo-ku, Tokyo, 113 Japan

ABSTRACT

In this study, we analyzed the relationship between the distribution of cancerous foci and the condition of the surrounding mucosa on the 28 cases of multiple early gastric cancer having the co-existence of minute cancerous focus. The macroscopic types of the minute foci were the IIb or IIc type, and only one focus was diagnosed by the preoperative examination. The main foci and the minute foci were mainly in the same surrounding gastric mucosa, and mainly showed the same histologic type. In cases that had cancerous focus located in the intermediate zone, the foci showed the tendency of multiplicity and the minute foci distributed widely in the intermediate zone.

KEY WORDS: multiple early gastric cancer, minute cancerous focus, extent of gastrectomy

INTRODUCTION

The reasonable radical operation for early gastric cancer includes the suitable extent of lymph node dissection and the adequate limits of gastrectomy. It must be noted whether any cancerous tissue remains in the gastric remnant or not, especially the co-existence of the minute cancerous foci as it usually cannot be diagnosed before the operation[1-3]. The study was carried out to see the relationship between the distribution of the cancerous lesions and the condition of the mucosa surrounding the lesions on the cases with multiple early gastric cancer containing the minute foci.

MATERIALS AND METHODS

In the study, the cancerous focus of less than 5 mm in maximal dimension was defined as minute cancerous focus[1-3]. From January 1971 to December 1992, resections for early gastric cancer were performed on 1092 patients at our department, and synchronous multiple early cancer were found in 91 cases(8.3%). Among these multiple cases, 30 cases(33.0%) had the minute cancerous foci. For each resected specimen, the atrophic pattern of fundic gland mucosae was detected histologically. The boundary line can be defined as follows:(1) f boundary line; the point where a nest-like group of parietal cells or fundic gland mucosae start to appear.(2) F boundary line;the point where fundic gland mucosae become continuous without intestinal metaplasia. Then, the gastric mucosa can be divided into 3 parts ; pyloric gland zone, intermediate zone, and fundic gland zone[4]. As shown in Fig.1, these cases were divided into 4 types. But, the"

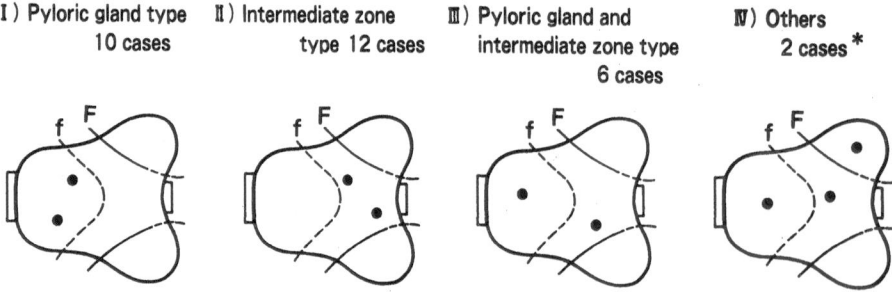

Fig.1 Types of multiple gastric cancer classified by the surrounding gastric mucosa

others"type of 2 cases(*)had numerous minute foci over the whole part of the stomach. Because of the special distribution, these 2 cases were excluded from the subjects. The clinicopathological details of the study was according to the general rules for gastric cancer in Japan[5].

RESULTS

Although the subjects were multiple gastric cancer cases, the majority were double early cancer cases. But, in cases of the intermediate zone type, and the pyloric gland and intermediate zone type, one third had more than 2 foci(Table 1). As for the proportion of minute focus in the overall cancerous foci, there was 60.0% in the pyloric gland and intermediate zone type, higher than in the other 2 types(Table 2). So, In cases that had cancerous focus located in the intermediate zone, the cancerous foci showed the tendency of multiplicity.

Table 1. Type of surrounding mucosa and number of cancerous focus

Type of surrounding mucosa	No. of cases	Cases with 2 foci	Cases with more than 2 foci
I) Pyloric gland type	10	9	1 (10.0%)
II) Intermediate zone type	12	8	4 (33.3%)
III) Pyloric gland and intermediate zone type	6	4	2 (33.3%)

Table 2. Type of surrounding mucosa and proportion of minute focus

Type of surrounding mucosa	No. of cases	No. of cancerous foci	No. of minute foci
I) Pyloric gland type	10	21	10 (47.6%)
II) Intermediate zone type	12	27	12 (44.4%)
III) Pyloric gland and intermediate zone type	6	15	9 (60.0%)

Concerning the macroscopic type of the minute foci, the majority of the pyloric gland type were the IIc type, and conversely, the majority of the pyloric gland and intermediate zone type were the IIb type. As shown in Table 3, only one focus of IIc type accompaning an ulcer scar in the intermediate zone was diagnosed before the operation. Table 4 shows the histologic type of the minute foci, the majority of all types were differentiated adenocarcinoma.

Table 3. Macroscopic classification of minute cancerous focus

Type of surrounding mucosa	No. of minute foci	Macroscopic classification IIb	IIc
I)Pyloric gland type	10	3	7
II)Intermediate zone type	12	5	7 (1)
III)Pyloric gland and intermediate zone type	9	7	2

( ): focus found by preoperative diagnosis

Table 4. Macroscopic classification and histologic type of minute cancerous focus

Type of surrounding mucosa	No. of minute foci	Histologic type diff.	undiff.
I)Pyloric gland type	10	8	2
II)Intermediate zone type	12	10	2
III)Pyloric gland and intermediate zone type	9	8	1

diff. : differentiated adenocarcinoma   undiff. : poorly or undifferentiated adenocarcinoma

Comparing the histologic type between the main focus and the minute focus, which both foci were located in the same surrounding mucosa as the intermediate zone type and the pyloric gland type, almost all cases showed the same histologic type. But, among the cases of the pyloric gland and intermediate zone type, one third showed a different histologic type(Table 5).

Table 5. Histologic type of main cancerous focus and minute cancerous focus

Type of surrounding mucosa	No. of cases	diff./diff.	undiff./undiff.	diff./undiff.
I) Pyloric gland type	10	8	2	0
II) Intermediate zone type	12	9	2	1
III) Pyloric gland and intermediate zone type	6	3	1	2

diff. : differentiated adenocarcinoma   undiff. : poorly or undifferentiated adenocarcinoma

Fig. 2 shows the distancé and the relationship of situation between main focus and minute focus. In the pyloric gland type, the minute foci were usually found around the main focus, and the average distance was only 17.9mm. In the intermediate zone type, the minute foci were located vertically apart from the main focus with the average distance of 35.6mm. In the pyloric gland and intermediate zone type, the minute foci lie scattered over the oral and anal side with the longest average distance of 46.8mm. So, in the cases having a cancerous focus in the intermediate zone, the distribution of minute focus may be spread widely over the intermediate zone.

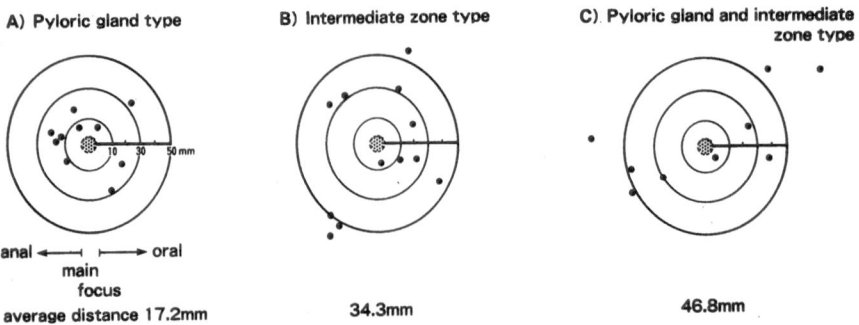

Fig. 2 Distance and relation of situation between main focus and minute focus

Fig. 3 demonstrates the location of minute foci in the multiple early cancer cases. The stomach is divided into 3 parts (upper, middle, and lower third indicated as C, M, and A). Almost all minute foci were located in the middle and lower third of the stomach. Only one focus was located in the lesser curvature of the upper third of the stomach.

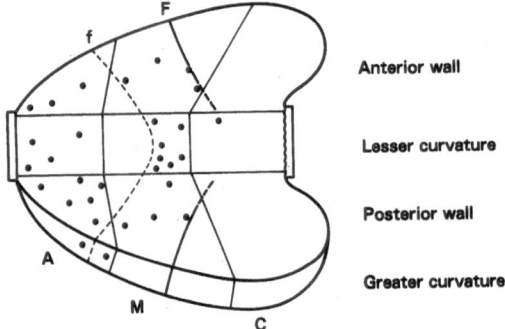

Fig. 3 The location of minute foci in the multiple early gastric cancer cases

DISCUSSION

The operative method for gastric cancer was discussed recently, in which either the extensive radical or reduced procedure would be indicated. In a previous report, for preserving the immunity reaction of the neighboring normal lymph node, reduced lymph node dissection is suggested for early gastric cancer[6]. In the present study, the co-existence of minute cancerous focus in early gastric cancer cases was analyzed for understanding the risk of the cancerous focus remaining during the subtotal gastrectomy. However, the minute cancerous foci in multiple early gastric cancer cases almost could not be diagnosed before the operation, and the minute foci in the cases, in which the main cancerous focus were located in the intermediate zone of gastric mucosae, would distribute widely over the intermediate zone. So, in the preoperative examination for early gastric cancer, the stomach must be observed in detail. It is not only for the extention of the main cancerous lesion but also for the existence of the minute focus, especially in the intermediate zone. According to our results, it is emphasized that even for early gastric cancer in the lower and middle third of the stomach, resection of the oral side must be done as near as possible to the cardia in order to remove the intermediate zone.

REFERENCES

1. Oohara T, Tohma H, Takezoe K, Ukawa S, Johjima Y, Asakura R, Aono G, Kurosaka H (1982) Minute gastric cancers less than 5 mm in diameter. Cancer 50:801-810
2. Iishi H, Tatsuta M, Okuda S (1985) Endoscopic diagnosis of minute gastric cancer of less than 5 mm in diameter. Cancer 56:655-659
3. Noguchi Y, Ohta H, Takagi K, Ike H, Takahashi T, Ohashi I, Kuno K, Kajitani T, Kato Y (1985) Synchronous multiple early gastric cancinoma: a study of 178 cases. World J Surg 9: 786-793
4. Nakamura k, Sugano H, Tagagi K (1968) Carcinoma of the stomach in incipient phase. Gann 59: 251-258
5. Japanese Research Society for Gastric Cancer(1981) The general rules for the gastric cancer study in surgery and pathology. Jpn J Surg 11:127-139
6. Sakakibara N, Urabe M, Liu SH (1988) Rational standard operation for early gastric cancer. Gast-enterol Surg 11:195-200

Indication for Curative Endoscopic Mucosal Resection for Early Gastric Cancer: Analysis of 290 Surgical Cases

ATSUNOBU MISUMI, AKITOSHI MURAKAMI, TOSHIHIKO HIRATA, HIROFUMI KAKO, KOICHI ARIMA, UBEHIKO HONMYO, SEIICHI MIZUMOTO, ICHIRO YOSHINAKA, SIGEKI OHSHIMA, and MICHIO OGAWA

Second Department of Surgery, Kumamoto University School of Medicine, Kumamoto, 860 Japan

ABSTRACT

In the present study, lymph node metastasis and incontinuous invasion were evaluated in 290 gastrectomy cases of early gastric cancer. All mucosal cancers (m-cancers) were free of lymph node metastasis whereas 24.4% of submucosal cancers (sm-cancers) showed the metastasis. Grossly, lymph node metastasis was absent in elevated lesions of 20 mm or less in size, depressed lesions of 10 mm or less, and all flat lesions; histologically, well differentiated lesions of 20 mm or less and moderately or poorly differentiated lesions of 10 mm or less. Among 34 cases with the main lesion of 20 mm or less, regardless of the gross and histologic types, incontinuous invasion was located within 2 mm from the main lesion in 97.1%.

KEY WORDS: endoscopic mucosal resection, indication for endoscopic therapy, early gastric cancer.

INTRODUCTION

Recently, for patients with small or minute gastric cancer (1) endoscopic therapy has been aggressively performed as an alternative of surgical operation (2-7). When endoscopic therapy, including endoscopic mucosal resection (EMR), is performed as a curative treatment of gastric cancer, its indication should be assessed strictly.

MATERIALS AND METHODS

Two hundred and ninety resected stomachs with early gastric cancer were serially sectioned into blocks of 0.5 cm x 4 cm in size for histological examination. In these cases, lymph node metastasis was investigated, with respect to the depth of invasion and size of cancer, based on the general rules for gastric cancer study for surgery and pathology established by Japanese Research Society for Gastric Cancer (8). Invasion index in the submucosa was measured by multiplication of the following three dimensional factors: the number of sections showing submucosal invasion, the maximum diameter of the invasion, and the depth of the invasion. The index was then classified into the following three: α sm-invasion with index being 50 or less, β sm-invasion with index being from 50 to 100, and γ sm-invasion with the index being more than 100. Incontinuous invasion near the main lesion was also investigated. An invasion that was distant 0.1 mm or greater from the margin of main lesion on the histological section was regarded as incontinuous. Incontinuous invasion was examined dividing the size of the main lesion into the following three groups: S-size group of 20 mm or less, M-size group of 21 through 40 mm, and L-size group of 41 mm or greater.

RESULTS.

All m-cancers were free of the metastasis whereas 24.4% of sm-cancers showed the metastasis. Regarding invasion index, the rate of lymph node metastasis for α, β, and γ sm-invasions were 15.5%, 30.4%, and 47.6%, respectively, showing a close correlation between the degree of the invasion and the rate of the metastasis (Table 1). Grossly, lymph nodes were negative for metastasis in lesions 20 mm or less in size in elevated type, those 10 mm or less in depressed type, and all those in flat type (Fig. 1A). Histologically, lymph nodes were negative for metastasis in those 20 mm or less in well differentiated type, those of 10 mm or less in moderately and poorly differentiated types (Fig. 1B). The rate of incontinuous invasion was 5.4% for elevated type, 4.0% for flat type, and 12.2% for depressed type; the last rate was significantly higher than the formers (P<0.01) (Table 1). Histologically, the rate was 7.1% for well

Table 1. Rate of Lymph Node Metastasis in Relation to the Depth of Invasion

Depth of invasion	Rate of lymph node metastasis
m (n=109)	0.0% (0)
sm (n=150)	24.0% (36)
α-invasion	15.5%*
β-invasion	30.4%
γ-invasion	47.6%*
Total (n=259)	13.9% (36)

Parentheses express the number of cases.
*Significantly different (P <0.01)

357

differentiated type, 8.9% for moderately differentiated type, and 14.1% for poorly differentiated type, showing a significant difference between well and poorly differentiated cancers (P<0.01) (Table 2).

Location of incontinuous invasion from the main lesion was 3.7 mm in maximum with the average being 0.9±0.5 mm for elevated type, 0.9±0.2 mm for flat type, and 1.1± 0.7 mm for depressed type. Histologically, the location was 0.8±0.6 mm for well differentiated type, 0.9±0.5 mm for moderately differentiated type, and 1.2±0.8 mm for poorly differentiated type; showing a significant difference between well and poorly differentiated types (P <0.005) (Table 2). Regarding the size of the main lesion, the location of incontinuous invasion was 0.9±0.7 mm for S-size group, 0.8+0.3 mm for M-size group, and 1.3+0.8 mm for L-size group; showing significant differences between the S- and L-size groups (P< 0.01), and between the M- and L-size groups (P<0.05) (Table 2). Based on the previous reports that the maximum excisable size of the lesion was 20 mm (6), we concentrated on 34 cases of S-size group that were associated with incontinuous invasion. In these cases, regardless of gross and histologic types, incontinuous invasion located within 2 mm from the main lesion in 97.1% as a whole (Fig. 2). These results indicate that in EMR, the resection stump with a clearance 2 mm or greater from margins of main lesion is well regarded as complete resection of cancer, or negative for stump involvement.

Table 2. Incidence of Incontinuous Invasion and Its Location from the Main Tumor

	Incidence (%)	Location (mm)
Macroscopic type		
Elevated	5.4*	0.9±0.5
Flat	4.0	0.9±0.2
Depressed	12.2	1.1±0.7
Histologic type		
Well	7.1**	0.8±0.6***
Moderate	8.9	0.9±0.5
Poor	14.1	1.2±0.8
Size of tumor		
S (≤ 20 mm)		0.9±0.7****
M (21-40 mm)		0.8±0.3
L (≥41 mm)		1.3±0.8

*P<0.01 between elevated and depressed types, and between flat and depressed types; **P<0.01 between well and poorly differentiated types; ***P<0.005 between well and poorly differentiated types; ****P<0.01 between the S- and L-size groups, and P<0.05 between the M- and L-size groups.

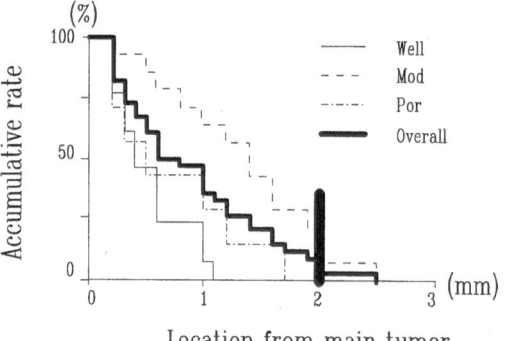

Fig. 1. in relation to macroscopic type / B: in relation to histologic type
○: lymph node metastasis (−)
✳: lymph node metastasis (+)

Fig. 1. Lymph node metastasis in early gastric carcinoma.

Fig. 2. Accumulative rate and location of incontinuous invasion.

DISCUSSION

As indication for radical endoscopic therapy, including EMR, the following two are inevitable presumptions: one that the lesion is free of lymph node metastasis, and the other that the lesion is able to be completely eradicated. This study suggests that mucosal early gastric cancers confined to the mucosa are almost always free of lymph node metastasis whereas those penetrating into the submucosa have some risk for the metastasis. Consequently, sm-cancers are not indicated for curative EMR. In this study, grossly, all flat cancers, elevated cancers measuring 20 mm or smaller, and depressed cancers measuring 10 mm or smaller were free of lymph node metastasis. Histologically, well differentiated cancers 20 mm or smaller and moderately and poorly differentiated cancers 10 mm or smaller were free of the metastasis. Therefore, these lesions are candidates for curative EMR on the basis of lymph node metastasis. In this study, when confined to cases 20 mm or less, incontinuous invasion located within 2 mm from the main lesion in 97.1% as a whole (Fig. 2), regardless of gross and histologic types. In additional or piece-meal EMR, it is almost impossible to reconstitute the lesion with specimens, and in turn to judge completeness of the resection. Therefore, curative EMR should be performed by single collection, from the viewpoint of evaluation of complete resection. In conclusions, the choice of procedure for curative endoscopic therapy for gastric cancer is EMR, and it should be performed by single collection. Indicated gastric cancers for curative EMR are those 20 mm or less in elevated type, those 10 mm or less in depressed type, and all those in flat type, grossly; those 20 mm or less in well differentiated type, those of 10 mm or less in moderately and poorly differentiated types, histologically. When histological examination after EMR reveals a clearance 2 mm or greater from the main lesion and without submucosal invasion, the treatment is judged as curative.

REFERENCES

1. Nakamura K, Sugano H, Takagi K (1968) Carcinoma of the stomach in incipient phase:its histogenesis and histological appearances. GANN 59:251-258.
2. Takekoshi T, Takagi K, Kato Y (1990) Radical endoscopic treatment of early gastric cancer. Gann Monograph on Cancer Research 37:111-126.
3. Takemoto T, Tada M, Yanai H, Karita M, Okita K (1989) Significance of strip biopsy, with particular reference to endoscopic "mucosectomy". Dig Endosc 1:4-9.
4. Hirao M, Asanuma T, Masuda K, Miyazaki A (1988) Endoscopic resection of early gastric cancer following locally injecting hypertonic saline-epinephrine. Stomach and Intestine. 23:399-409 (English abstract).
5. Fujimori T, Nakamura T, Hirayama D, Satonaka K, Ajiki T, Kitazawa S et al. (1992) Endoscopic mucosectomy for early gastric cancer using modified strip biopsy. Endoscopy 24:187-189.
6. Takechi K, Mihara M, Saito Y, Endo J, Maekawa H, Usui T et al. (1992) A modified technique for endoscopic mucosal resection of small early gastric carcinomas. Endoscopy 24:215-217.
7. Tanaka K,Shibue T, Takasaki Y, Sameshima Y, Matsumoto J, Yamashita Y et al. (1990) Clinical evaluation of endoscopic gastric mucosal resection. Dig Endosc 2:19-27.
8. Japanese Research Society for Gastric Cancer (1981) The general rules for the gastric cancer study in surgery and pathology. Jpn J Surg 11:127-145.

Lymph Node — Targeting Delivery of Adriamycin by Liposomal Administration into Gastric Submucosa in Rabbits

Yoshimi Akamo[1], Isamu Mizuno[1], Toshihisa Yotsuyanagi[2], Tatsuo Ichino[1], Noritaka Tanimoto[1], Tetsuya Yamamoto[1], Tamotsu Yasui[1], Mariko Nagata[2], Nagao Shinagawa[1], and Jiro Yura[1]

[1]First Department of Surgery, Nagoya City University Medical School, Nagoya, 467 Japan
[2]Faculty of Pharmaceutical Sciences, Nagoya City University, Nagoya, 467 Japan

ABSTRACT

We studied tissue distribution of adriamycin for up to 7 days after gastric submucosal injection of Liposomal adriamycin (Lipo-ADR) (0.4 mg/kg) and i.v. of an equal dose of free adriamycin (F-ADR) in rabbits. The AUC of the regional lymph nodes was 85.4 μg·day/g after the submucosal injection and 8.44 μg·day/g after the i.v. The targeting index of the regional lymph nodes, defined as the ratio of the AUC after the submucosal injection to the i.v., was 10.1, and of the bone marrow was 0.25. Gastric submucosal injection of Lipo-ADR enhanced lymph node-specific delivery of ADR.

KEY WORDS : lymph node-targeting delivery, gastric submucosal injection, adriamycin, liposomes, tissue distribution

INTRODUCTION

Preoperative regional chemotherapy targeting lymph nodes is a promising approach for prevention of lymph node recurrence of gastric cancer following surgery [1]. ADR is commonly used to treat patients with gastric cancer. Its anticancer efficacy may depend on the dose administered; in vitro studies have demonstrated that the cytocidal efficacy of ADR depends on its concentration and duration of exposure. Despite its clinical efficacy, high-dose ADR administered intravenously is associated with severe manifestations of acute toxicity, such as bone marrow suppression and immunosuppression, as well as cumulative dose-limiting cardiotoxicity. The ability to deliver ADR to regional lymph nodes via an appropriate route, thus increasing its therapeutic index would enhance the drug's therapeutic efficacy and reduce the risk of toxic side effects. The gastric submucosal injection of F-ADR makes it possible to selectively target the regional lymph nodes [2]. However, injection of F-ADR into the gastric submucosa causes a severe ulceration because of local toxicity. An appropriate drug carrier is needed to minimized ADR's local toxicity before gastric submucosal injection can be an effective approach. Liposomes have been studied extensively as a vehicle for improving the delivery of various therapeutic agents to a targeted organ. Liposomal ADR has been found to attenuate direct tissue toxicity. Furthermore, regional administration provided more efficient drug delivery to the targeted organ. We investigated the ability of gastric submucosal injection of Lipo-ADR to provide efficient and selective delivery of drug to the regional lymph nodes in a rabbit model [3] and the potential clinical usefulness of this route of administration in preoperative adjuvant chemotherapy for prevention of recurrence of gastric cancer in lymph nodes [1].

MATERIALS AND METHODS

Preparation of Lyophilized Lipo-ADR.

Adriamycin-containing liposomes were prepared by the reverse-phase evaporation method. Lipo-ADR contained 10 mg of ADR, 100 mg of egg lecithin, 24 mg of cholesterol, and 100 mg of lactose. This products was stored at -20 ˙ C.

Reconstitution of Lipo-ADR.

To reconstitute Lipo-ADR, 9.7 ml of sterile saline was added to each vial. Lipo-ADR was adjusted to a concentration of 1 mg/ml of ADR potency. This reconstitution produced multi-lamellar vesicles (MLVs) with particle sizes ranging from approximately 1 to 10 μm. The median diameter of particles was 3.85 μm and the mode diameter was 4.41 μm. The entrapment efficacy, defined as the ratio of the total amount of ADR associated with the MLVs to the total amount of ADR in the sample, was 41.7 $\pm$ 3.2%(mean of 4 independent experiments $\pm$ SD).

Tissue distribution studies.

Rabbits weighing 2.0 to 3.0 kg were anesthetized and underwent gastrotomy. 0.4 ml/kg Lipo-ADR (total ADR potency of 0.4 mg/kg) was injected into the gastric submucosa of the posterior wall in the antrum. An equal dose of F-ADR (1 mg/ml) was injected into the gastric submucosa or administered intravenously in control animals. For tissue distribution studies, eighty-four rabbits were anesthetized and sacrificed at 1 h, 6 h, 12 h, 1 day, 2 days, 4 days, and 7 days after drug administrations. Various organs, including the regional lymph nodes of the stomach surrounding the portal vein, the bone marrow of the right femur, the heart, the spleen, and the liver, were excised immediately, rinsed in saline, weighed, and stored at -40 °C. The ADR concentration of these tissues was measured by HPLC. Drug distribution to the various organs was estimated by the AUC of ADR concentrations from 1h to 7 days after drug administration. In addition, the targeting index of the various organs, defined as the ratio of the AUC after the gastric submucosal administration of Lipo-ADR or F-ADR to the AUC after i.v. administration of F-ADR, was determined.

RESULTS

ADR Levels in the Regional Lymph Nodes of the Stomach.

After the gastric submucosal injection of Lipo-ADR or F-ADR, ADR concentrations in the regional lymph nodes of the stomach were significantly higher than after i.v. administration of F-ADR and remained high for up to 1 days (Fig. 1). The maximum ADR concentration in the regional lymph nodes after gastric submucosal injection of Lipo-ADR was 87.0 μg/g at 6 h, which was 24.8 times higher than the maximum concentration 6 h after i.v. administration of F-ADR. The maximum concentration of F-ADR after gastric submucosal injection was 52.1 μg/g at 1 h; ADR concentrations gradually decreased thereafter (Fig. 1). The difference between the gastric submucosal injection groups was significant only at 6 h. The area under the ADR concentration-time curve (AUC) was 85.4 μg/g·day after gastric submucosal injection of Lipo-ADR, 69.2 μg/g·day after gastric submucosal injection of F-ADR, and 8.44 μg/g·day after i.v. administration of F-ADR. The targeting index was 10.1 for gastric submucosal injection of Lipo-ADR, and 8.20 for gastric submucosal injection of F-ADR. Gastric submucosal administration enhanced delivery of drug to the regional lymph nodes compared with i.v. administration (Fig. 1, Table I).

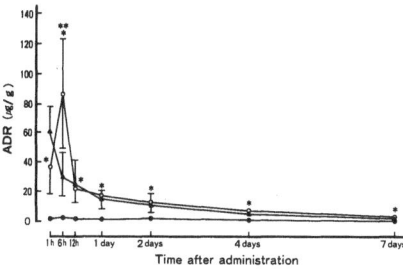

Fig. 1.   Adriamycin levels in regional lymph nodes of the stomach.   Lipo-ADR (O) or F-ADR (▲) (ADR potency of 0.4 mg/kg) was injected into the gastric submucosa. An equal dose of F-ADR was administered i.v. (●).   Circles and triangles represent the mean of 4 independent experiments; bars are SD (where no bar appears, SD is smaller than the symbol); * P<0.05 Lipo-ADR gastric submucosal injection group vs F-ADR i.v. group and ** P<0.05 Lipo-ADR gastric submucosal injection group vs F-ADR gastric submucosal injection group. Reprinted from Akamo et al. [3] with the permission of the publisher.

AUC values of ADR and Targeting Indices in the Bone Marrow, Heart, Spleen, and Liver.

AUC values in the bone marrow, heart, and spleen were low after the gastric submucosal injection of Lipo-ADR compared with values after i.v. administration of F-ADR (Table I).

Table I. AUC Values of ADR and the Targeting Indices

| Organ | AUC (μg/g·day)[a] | | | Targeting index[c] |
| | Gastric submucosal injection[b] | | i.v.[b] | |
	Lipo-ADR	F-ADR	F-ADR	
Lymph nodes	85.4		8.44	10.1
		69.2		8.20
Bone marrow	1.11		4.51	0.25
Heart	0.45		0.96	0.47
Spleen	2.60		6.27	0.41
Liver	1.04		1.19	0.87

a) AUC was estimated from data from 7 days of observation.
b) The dose of ADR was 0.4 mg/kg.
c) Targeting index was defined as the ratio of the AUC after gastric submucosal injection to the AUC after i.v. administration.
Reprinted from Akamo et al. [3] with the permission of the publisher.

DISCUSSION

Regional lymph nodes are common sites of gastric cancer recurrence after surgery. To improve the prognosis, several investigators have attempted to target regional chemotherapy to the lymph nodes [1]. The endoscopic injection of Lipo-ADR into the gastric submucosa adjacent to the main tumor could reduce the risk of lymph node recurrence and improve prognosis. Gastric submucosal injection of F-ADR is an effective method for specific delivery of ADR to the regional lymph nodes [2]. However, this type of regional chemotherapy is associated with local toxicity to the gastric wall, which manifests as an ulcer. This toxicity may be attenuated by encapsulating of ADR in liposomes [3]. The use of liposomes has been shown to enhance the selective delivery of various anticancer drugs, increase their anticancer efficacy, and reduce various toxic side effects. However, liposomes cannot be routinely used in clinical practice because of the need for multi-step preparation and their physicochemical properties. The Lipo-ADR used in this study was prepared as a freeze-dried mixture. This ready-to-use freeze-dried form made long-term preservation of the lyophilized Lipo-ADR possible and ensures an accurate dose of ADR in the Lipo-ADR preparation. Thus, this form may facilitate clinical use of the drug. Our Lipo-ADR preparation contained 41.7% of liposome-entrapped ADR and 58.3% of free ADR. The entrapment efficacy was stable 24 hours after the preparation of the liposome form because of the equilibrium between liposome-entrapped ADR and free ADR. To explore the feasibility of this method of targeting regional chemotherapy to the lymph nodes, we investigated ADR delivery to various organs in a rabbit model after gastric submucosal injection of Lipo-ADR, gastric submucosal injection of F-ADR, and i.v. administration of F-ADR. Tissue ADR levels were measured 1 h, 6 h, 12 h, 1 day, 2 days, 4 days, and 7 days after drug administration. ADR delivery was expressed as the area under the tissue ADR concentration-time curve (Table I). The AUC of tissue ADR concentration has been shown to correlate well with anticancer efficacy and toxic side effects. The AUC of the regional lymph nodes of the stomach after gastric submucosal injection of ADR was significantly higher than after i.v. administration of F-ADR. In addition, the AUC of the regional lymph nodes was significantly higher than that of other tissues after gastric submucosal injection. The targeting index for the regional lymph nodes was 10.1 after gastric submucosal injection of Lipo-ADR and 8.20 after gastric submucosal injection of F-ADR. Gastric submucosal injection of ADR significantly enhanced drug delivery to the regional lymph nodes as compared with i.v. administration. However, the injection of F-ADR into the gastric submucosa caused severe ulceration and is not appropriate for clinical use. Injection of Lipo-ADR reduced the local toxicity and enhanced lymph node-specific delivery of drug [3]. The targeting indices for the bone marrow, heart, and spleen after gastric submucosal injection of Lipo-ADR were very low, indicating that the unfavorable ADR delivery to these organs was reduced. These data demonstrate that the gastric submucosal injection of Lipo-ADR is an effective means of targeting the regional lymph nodes. Therefore, the gastric submucosal injection of Lipo-ADR may reduce the risk of lymph node recurrence and improve prognosis of patients with gastric cancer.

REFERENCES

1. Akamo Y, Mizuno I, Yotsuyanagi T, Ichino T, Yamamoto T, Yasui T, Itabashi Y, Tanimoto N, Shinagawa N, Yura J (1992) Gastric submucosal injection of liposomal adriamycin targeting regional lymph nodes in patients with gastric cancer. Proc. AACR 33:255
2. Akamo Y, Mizuno I, Yotsuyanagi T, Ichino T, Tanimoto N (1992) Gastric submucosal administration of adriamycin for lymph node-targeting in rabbits. Nagoya Med. J. 36: 233-242
3. Akamo Y, Yotsuyanagi T, Mizuno I, Ichino T, Tanimoto N, Kurahashi S, Saito T, Yamamoto T, Yasui T, Itabashi Y, Yura J (1993) Delivery of lymph node-targeted adriamycin by gastric submucosal liposomal injection in rabbits. Jpn. J. Cancer Res. 84:208-213

Anti-Cancer Effects of Preoperative Chemotherapy for Gastric Carcinoma — The Relationship Between Histopathological Effects and Thymidilate Synthetase Inhibition Rate (TSIR)

KAZUHIDE KUMAGAI, AKIRA YASUI, YOSHIAKI NISHIDA, KOJI SHIMIZU, KOKI MASUO, and KENICHI YAMAGATA

Department of Surgery, Showa University, Toyosu Hospital, Koto-ku, Tokyo, 135 Japan

ABSTRACT

In a previous study, the prognosis of positive histopathological effect cases with pre-operative chemotherapy was significantly better than negative histopathological effect cases in advanced gastric cancer. This time, we investigated the relationship between the histopathological effects and Thymidilate Synthetase Inhibition Rate (TSIR). Object were 14 resected gastric cancer with preoperative chemotherapy of 5-Fu 300 mg/day for 14 days by oral administration. FdUMP, TS-free and TS-total were measured by the tumor sample and TSIR value was calculated. TSIR value were distributed from 0% to 90.7%, averaged 46.9%. TSIR value of the cases with positive histopathological effect indicated 70.5%, TSIR value without histopathological effect was 23.5%.

KEY WORDS : thymidilate synthetase inhibition rate, histopathological effect, preoperative chemotherapy, gastric carcinoma

INTRODUCTION

In Japan, gastric carcinoma remains the most common cause of death from cancer [1]. To decrease the recurrent rates of curative operation for advanced gastric carcinoma, postoperative adjuvant chemotherapy was introduced [2], but the effect of adjuvant chemotherapy for prognosis has not been attained [3]. Since 1982, we tried to undertake preoperative chemotherapy, especially administering slight toxicity without negative response. With the histopathological effect of the resected stomach, 46 out of 62 patients showed a positive histopathological effect. The prognosis of positive histopathological effect cases was significantly better than negative histopathological effect cases in advanced gastric carcinoma.
This time, we investigated the relationship between the histopathological effects and thymidilate synthetase inhibition rate (TSIR).

PATIENTS AND METHOD

Patients Characteristics

Our series consisted of 14 patients.
All patients were diagnosed with carcinoma by an endoscopic biopsy specimen. The averaged age was 59 y.o (42 - 74). The male to female ratio was 8:6. The gross type were 5 in type 0, 2 in type 2, 4 in type 3, 2 in type 4 and 1 in type 5. Histologically, 3 cases included either well or moderately differentiated tubular adenocarcinoma, while 11 were undifferentiated carcinoma as signet ring cell carcinoma or poorly differentiated carcinoma. There were 7 positive lymphnode involvement cases and 7 negative lymphnode metastatic cases. Concerning the stage due to Japanese classification, 5 were in stage I, 2 in stage II, 6 in stage III and 1 in stage IV.

Chemotherapy

We used 5-fluorouracil (5-Fu) for preoperative chemotherapy for oral administration. The method of administration was 300 mg/day daily for 2 weeks.

Histological Effects

The histological effect by chemotherapy was based on the "General Rules for Gastric Cancer of the Japanese Research Society for Gastric Cancer" [4]. The evaluation of the chemotherapy treatment was shown as the extent of the cancer tissue damaged area of the cancerous lesion. The evaluation of the histopathological effect of chemotherapy was divided into 4 main grades, Grade 0 showed no effect, Grade 1a showed a slight effect, cancer tissue damaged under 1/3rd, Grade 1b, slight effect which had cancer tissue damaged over 1/3 but under 2/3, Grade 2 showed a fair effect, cancer tissue damaged over 2/3 and Grade 3 showed an excellent effect, no cancer remaining.

Thymidilate Synthetase Inhibition Rate

Solid tissues from gastric cancerous lesions were placed immediately on dry ice and were maintained at -80°C until processed. TS assays were done by the modified spears' method [5]. The results were calculated as percentage inhibition of TS, which was (1-TS-free/TS-total) × 100.

RESULTS

Histopathological Response

There were 7 cases of Grade 0, 5 cases of Grade 1a and 2 cases of Grade 1b. There were no cases of Grade 2 and no cases of complete response, histopathologically. Over-all, the cases with any cancer tissue damaged area in the cancerous lesion were 7 out of 14.

Thymidilate Synthetase Inhibition Rate (TSIR)

The value of TSIR were distributed from 0% to 90.7%. The average TSIR value was 46.9±32.2%. TSIR value of the cases with positive histopathological effect indicated 70.5±12.9%. On the other hand, TSIR value with negative histopathological effect was 23.5±25.3% (fig. 1). There was significant differences between them (P<0.05).
Concerning the relationship between the histopathological effect and the TSIR value, all of the 6 cases which indicated the TSIR value under 50% showed Grade 0. 7 cases out of 8 which indicated the TSIR value over 50% showed Grade 1a or Grade 1b. TSIR value with Grade 1a were distributed from 51.1% to 83.9%. 2 cases with Grade 1b indicated TSIR value over 70% (fig. 2).

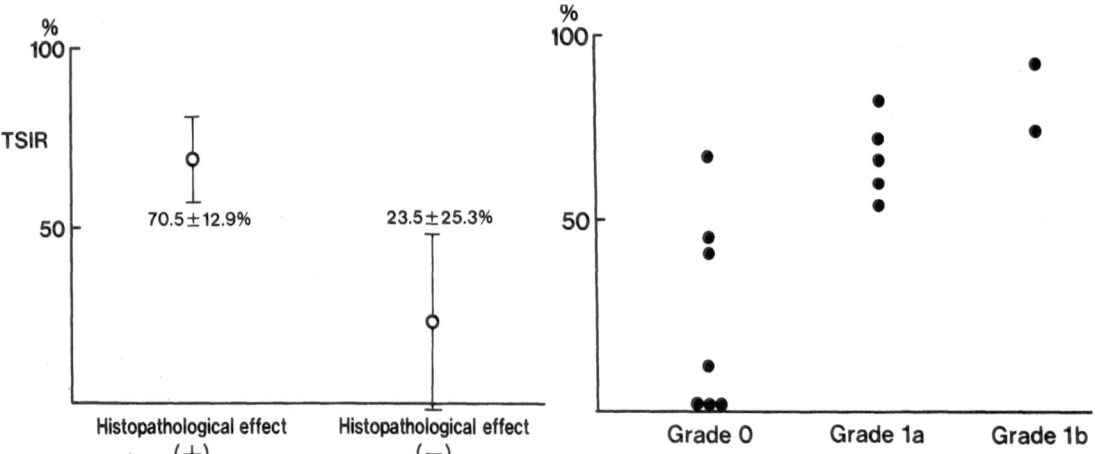

Fig. 1 Histopathological effects and Thymidilate Synthetase Inhibition Rate (TSIR) (1)

Fig. 2 Histopathological effects and Thymidilate Synthetase Inhibition Rate (TSIR) (2)

DISCUSSION

Our purpose of preoperative adjuvant chemotherapy is in the prevention of cancer cells scattered in operation, elimination of established micrometastasis or microcancer foci and decreasing cancer cell activity. Furthermore, we have undertaken to investigate the chemosensitivity with histopathological studies of the resected stomach. Our previous study of preoperative chemotherapy showed that the five year survival rate of positive histopathological effect cases were significantly better than negative histopathological effect cases [6]. Especially, such a tendency could be recognized in stage II and III cases (TNM classification). These data supports the existence of chemosensitivity for positive histopathological effect cases.

The mechanism of cytotoxic action of 5-Fu that is best understood is inhibition of TS, the final enzyme of the de novo pathway that converts dUMP to thymidilate by reductive methylation. Intensive studies in recent years have greatly detailed the chemistry and biochemical kinetics of inhibition of TS by FdUMP. FdUMP competes with dUMP for initial binding to TS, and then from a frozen transition state analogue of the normal reaction in the presence of CH_2FH_4.

That is to say, a research of TSIR for cancerous tissue is the extent of chemosensitivity of 5-Fu. In our series, the averaged value of TSIR shows 46.9±32.2. Futami et al described TS inhibition rates in tumor tissue as 45.5±13.3% in tegafur group and 56.1±13.0% in UFT group [7].

There was a strong relationship between the prognosis of gastric cancer and the existence of histopathological effects in our previous study of preoperative chemotherapy. This time, there is also a strong relation between the TSIR value and the extent of the histopathological effect. The measurement of TSIR indicates the chemosensitivity of 5-Fu and it is useful for a guide to therapeutic planning.

REFERENCES

1. Kurihara M, Aoki K. (1986) Mortality of cancer of the digestive organs. The past, present and future. GANN Monograph on Cancer Research, 31:3-17.
2. Inokuchi K, Hattori T, Taguchi T, Abe O, Ogawa N. (1984) Postoperative adjuvant chemotherapy for gastric cancer. Analysis of data on 1805 patients followed for 5 years. Cancer, 53: 2393-2397.
3. Lise M, Nitti D, Marchet A, Fornasiero A. (1991) Adjuvant treatment for gastric cancer. Anti-Cancer Drugs. 2:433-445.
4. Japanese Research Society for Gastric Cancer. (1985) The general rules for the gastric cancer study. Tokyo. Kanehara Shuppan, (in Japanese).
5. Spears CP, Shahinian AH, Moran RG, Heidelberger C, Corbett TH. (1982) In viro kinetics of thymidylate synthetase inhibition in 5-fluorouracil-sensitive and - resistant murine colon adenocarcinomas. Cancer Res 42:450-456.
6. Kumagai K, Yasui A, Nishida Y, Masuo K. (1993) Estimation of adjuvant preoperative chemotherapy for gastric carcinoma. Jpn J Gastroenterol Surg. 26:703.
7. Futami K, Arima S, Yoshimura S, Okamoto T, Yamasaki K, Koto T, Yamasaki S, Kawahara K, Ikuno T. (1991) Drug concentration in cancerous large bowel tissue and thymidylate synthase inhibition rate after administration of tegafur and UFT. Jpn J Cancer Chemother 18:215-220.

Neoadjuvant Chemotherapy for Far Advanced Scirrhous Carcinoma (Linitis Plastica) of the Stomach and Its Significance

MASAYOSHI MAI, YUTAKA TAKAHASHI, TOSHIHIRO FUJIMOTO, TOHRU ITOH, YASUSHI DEGUCHI, and CHENG-DONG HUANG

The Department of Surgery, Cancer Research Institute, Kanazawa University, Kanazawa, 921 Japan

ABSTRACT

Considering high potential for biological malignancies of far advanced scirrhous type carcinoma of the stomach, we attempted preoperative induction chemotherapy(neoadjuvant chemotherapy) against far advanced scirrhous carcinoma associated with distant metastases. Anti-cancer drugs used in this study were a combination of FAM or sequential administration of MTX/5-Fu. Preoperative chemotherapy was carried out on 24 patients prior to surgery. The response to chemotherapy showed shrinking shrinking of massive nodal involvement in 50%(5/10), complete disappearance of malignant ascites in 77.8%(7/9).The morphological improvement of primary gastric lesions were obtained in 9 out of 24 cases (37.5%). All toxicities occurred in less than 10% of the patients except for nausea and leucopenia, which occurred to a mild or moderate. In 15 cases(68.2%) total gastrectomy was done with extended lymph node dissection. In one of 9 cases showing marked improvement, no viable cancer cells were seen in whole stomach associated with multiple foci of fibrogranulomatous lesions of regional nodes after giving MTX/5Fu of three cycles. Disease-free survival of neoadjuvant group showed a significant prolongation of its median survival of 14 months, compared to that of 4 months in surgery alone group. Our result lead to the conclusion that the patients whose tumor was effectively destroyed by neoadjuvant chemotherapy had a good prognosis.

KEY WORDS: scirrhous carcinoma of the stomach, neoadjuvant chemotherapy, sequential methotrexate and 5-fluouracil therapy

INTRODUCTION

Scirrhous carcinoma of the stomach is a common form of far advanced scirrhous gastric cancer that carries a particularly gloomy prognosis. Despite recent progress achieved with various therapy in Japan, so far advanced gastric carcinoma remains lethal disease with an extremely poor prognosis. Overall five-year survival of far advanced scirrhous carcinoma demonstrated a disappointing 10% or less, even if curative resection might be done, mostly affecting the paraaortic nodes, pancreas or peritoneum. It would be more disastrous for these patients to allow carcinomatous peritonitis even on the first visit to our clinic. Considering high potential for biological malignancies of far advanced scirrhous carcinoma patients, we attempted preoperative induction chemotherapy, namely, neoadjuvant chemotherapy In this report the response of neoadjuvant chemotherapy and follow-up evaluation were documented herein, and several modifications and refinement to the protocol were also described.

PATIENTS AND METHODS

The term of far advanced scirrhous carcinoma used here is synonymous with linitis plastica or Borrmann IV type carcinoma. Between Feb.1985 and Apr.1990 24 patients with far advanced scirrhous carcinoma of Stage IV were first managed with basal chemotherapy prior to subsequent resection. The mean age was 53.4 years(range 28-73), with 7 patients being less than 50 years of age. There were 13 male and 11 female. All patients had distant metastatic indicator lesions including primary gastric lesions(Table 1), of whom eleven patients had carcinomatous peritonitis associated with malignant ascites or carcinomatous pleural effusion. Nearly half of patients had had massive lymphadenopathy as indicator lesions in cervical nodes and paraaortic nodes in abdominal CT scan. Three female had metastatic carcinoma in ovaries. The treatment plan was shown in Fig.1.

(1) FAM-OK432

5-FU | 500mg × 5 | 500mg

IHC* | ADR 30mg (one shot) | MMC 10mg (one shot) | OP.

OK432 | 0   1   2   3

(2) sequential MTX·5-FU

MTX(IHC*) | 30mg/m² I.V. | 30mg/m² | 30mg/m² | 30mg/m²

5-FU** | 750mg I.V. | 750mg | 750mg | 750mg | OP.

OK432 | 0   1   2   3

Fig.1 Protocol of neoadjuvant chemotherapy for so far advanced scirrhous type of gastric carcinoma

Table 1 Pretreatment patients characteristis

Clinical Presentation	
Number of patients	24 cases
Age (Years), Median	53.4 (28~73)
$\leq$ 50	17 cases
> 50	7 cases
Sex Male	13 cases
Female	11 cases
Metastatic sites	
Malignant ascites	9 cases
Carcinomatous peritonitis	11 cases
Massive nodal involvement on CT	10 cases
Ovaries	3 cases
Others (liver, bone, CBD)	3 cases
★Elevation of tumor marker (CEA, CA 19·9, CA 125)	15 cases

Anti-cancer drugs used in this study were a combination chemotherapy consisting of 5-fluorouracil, Adriamycin and mitomycinC (FAM)[1] of 9 cases at the beginning of this trial trial and mainly employed a low-dose methotrexate and high-dose 5-fluorouracil(MTX/5FU) of 16 cases as sequential combination[2].

RESULTS

We indicated the preoperative chemotherapy against 24 inoperable patients with scirrhous carcinoma of the stomach. Table 2 showed response rates of primary and metastatic sites. The morphological improvement of primary gastric lesions was obtained in 9 out of 24 cases(35.7%), but it is noteworthy that metastatic sites showed high response, that is, shrinking of nodal involvement in 50 %(5/10), complete disappearance of malignant ascites in 77.8%(7/9) and marked decrease of tumor marker levels such as CEA, CA19-9 or CA125 in 86.6%(13/15). Regarding objective tumor responses among two protocols.MTX/5FU regimen had an improved response rates(61.5%) compared with FAM(50%) including metastatic sites. All toxicities occurred in less than 10% of the patients except for mild nausea and leucopenia,both of which was reversible by discontinuation of drug therapy.

Table 2 The response rates of neoadjuvant chemotherapy

The morphological improvement of primary gastric lesion	9/24 (35.7%)
The shrinking or disappearance of nodal invoement	5/10 (50.0%)
Disappearance of pleural or peritoneal fluid due to carcinomatosa	7/9 (77.8%)
Marked decrease of tumor marker (CEA, Ca19-9, CA125)	13/15 (86.6%)

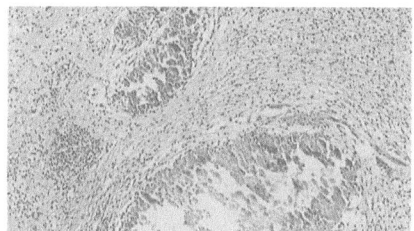

Fig.2 Most of dissected metastatic nodes showing the replacement into granulofibromatous tissue,mingled with necrotic cancer cells

Consequently, we succeeded to obtain downstaging of tumor spread in approximately in approximately 80%, and total gastrectomy could be carried out in 15 cases(68.2%). There was no increase in surgical complications as a result of utilizing chemotherapy. One of 9 cases showing marked improvement of primary gastric lesions showed complete response(CR). One patient showing CR was a 33-year old male who was poorly nourished associated with a large mass in the mid-abdomen on the first visit to our hospital. A single dose of MTX 30mg and thirty minute drip infusion of 5-Fu 750mg were started at seven days intervals. After giving three cycles abdominal mass disappeared with a fairly good recovery. Thereafter, total gastrectomy was done with an extended lymphadenectomy. In the detailed investigation of histology,surprisingly, viable cancer cell disappeared completely in whole stomach despite serial sectioning of primary gastric tumor site and most of dissected metastatic nodes were replaced into fibromatous tissue, mingled with necrotic and regenerative cancer cells (Fig.3). However, microresidual| cancer cell nests were seen in two lymph nodes along hepatoduodenal ligament and splenic hilus. The patient had a disease-free survival of 15 months until he recurred with carcinomatous peritonitis. The primary endpoint to evaluate therapeutic activity in this study is patient survival. There was a significant superiority for neoadjuvant chemotherapy group of 15 cases (p<0.01) compared with surgery or chemotherapy alone. While the median survival time(MST) of surgery or chemotherapy groups were 4-6 months, MST of neoadjuvant chemotherapy group showed 14 months with a fairly good survival.

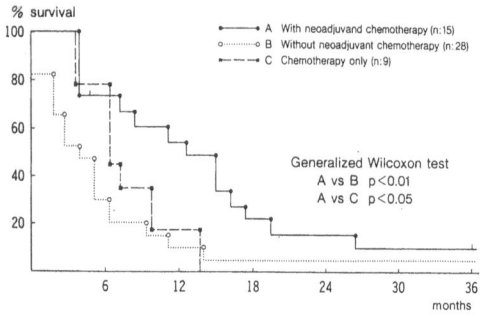

Fig.3   The disease-free survival with or without neoadjuvant chemotherapy

DISCUSSION

The overall chemotherapy results described in this series of patients with untreated systemic advanced disease of so far advanced scirrhous carcinoma was quite encouraging[3]. The relatively infrequent and mild toxicities revealed that the resimen was well tolerated. The overall response also significantly (p<0.01) correlates with the response to the initial treatment. In 1982 neoadjuvant neoadjuvant chemotherapy was proposedby Frei III[4]. He stressed a new strategy that majority neoadjuvant therapy not only provides substantial regression of the primary in the majority of patients with osteogenic sarcoma but also results in a substantially improved disease-free and overall survival, particularly in patients with systemically responsive disease.

The standard chemotherapy for inoperable gastric carcinoma such as so far advanced scirrhous type is 5-fluorouracil(5FU) and many agents have been combined with with 5-FU to improve its e fficacy with variable success. Our trial employing FAM and MTX/5-FU succeed ed to obtain high response rates of nearly 80%, especially in metastatic lesions. The treatment of MTX/5-FU also demonstrated a remarkable effects agai nst the patients with pleural or peritoneal effusion caused by carcinomatous dissemination. The mechanism of interaction of MTX/5-FU is of particular in terest. MTX antagonizes dihydrofolate reductase causing the depletion of intracellular reduced folate and de novo pyrimidine synthesis is blocked. Consequently, de novo purine synthesis als o inhibited resulting in an expanded intracellular PRPP pool and the increased PRPP is utilized to promote the co nversion of 5-FU to 5-FdUMP[2][5]. The ultimate ability of cure surgical resection to reduce tumor spread and recurrence, prolong survival and perhaps in far advanced carcinoma of the stomach awaits future prospective randomized studies.

REFERENCES

1.Macdonald JS,Wooley PV,Smythe T,Ueno W,Hoth D and Schein(1979) 5-fluorouracil,Adriamycin and mitomycin-C(FAM) combination chemotherapy in the treatment of advanced gastric cancer. Cancer44:44-47.

2.Cadman E,Heimer P and Davis(1979)Enhanced 5-fluorouracil nucleotide formation after methotrexate adminis tration:explanation for drug synnergism. Science 205:1135-1137.

3.Mai M,Ogino T,Takahashi Y et al(1990) Study on neoadjuvant chemotherapy for Borrmann 4 type carcinoma of the stomach and its significance(1990) J Jpn Soc Cancer Ther 25:586-597

4.Frei F III(1982) Clinical cancer research:an embattled species.Cancer 30:224-229.

5.Abe T,Yashige H,Inazawa et al:The use of Diamox in the sequential methotrexate-5-fluorouracil therapy of advanced gastrointestinal cancer(1988) Eur.J Cancer Clin Oncol 24:799-800.

Neoadjuvant Chemotherapy (UFT·CDDP Therapy) for Borrmann 4 Type Gastric Carcinoma

Nobuhiko Tadaoka, Sumio Takayama, Chiaki Sekine, Tsutomu Fujimori, Hiroshi Nimura, Jun Tsutsumi, Hirotaka Kashimura, Yoshifumi Sano, Katsuya Hirai, and Teruaki Aoki

Department of Surgery, Jikei University School of Medicine, Minato-ku, Tokyo, 105 Japan

ABSTRACT

We conducted neoadjuvant chemotherapy with CDDP-UFT for Borrmann 4 type gastric carcinoma and report here our findings on its usefulness. The study included an investigation of the association between measured DNA ploidy pattern and chemotherapeutic efficacy. We administered two three-week course of CDDP 100mg/m^2 (day1) UFT400g/m^2 (on consecutive days) preoperatively to 13 cases of Borrmann 4 type gastric carcinoma judged to be curatively unresectable. In addition, the DNA contents in the cancer tissue cell nuclei was mesured by flow cytometry before and after the chemotherapy. The response rate was 53.8%(7/13) and there was no difference found in therpeutic efficacy with difference in the DNA ploidy pattern. Ten cases were resectable. Cases exhibiting more marked histological efficacy were those an accumulation of S phase fraction among the diploid cases and thosewith a tendency toward flattening of the aneuploid peak among aneuploid cases.

KEY WORDS: neoadjuvant chemotherapy, gastric cancer, CDDP, UFT, DNA ploidy

INTRODUCTION

The outcome of therapy for advanced cancer still remains unsatisfactory despite numeruos attempts at treatment with avariety of approaches. In the present study, we investigated the efficasy of CDDP-UFT-based neoadjuvant chemotherapy in patients with Borrmann 4 type gastric carcinoma. In principle, the efficacy of chemothrapy for is evaluated from morphological changes seen from X-ray and endoscopic findings. However, in some cases with diffuse infiltrative gastric carcinoma lesions, the efficacy of treatment cannot be evaluated easily by these methods. We attempted to evaluate the efficacy of chemotherapy by analyzing differences in the DNA ploidy pattern before and after the administration of chemotherapy.

PATIENTS AND METHODS

Thirteen curatively unresectable patients with Borrmann 4 type gastric carcinoma were treated with neoadjuvant chemotherapy consisting of CDDP 100mg/m^2 (day1) and UFT 400g/m^2 (on consecutive days). These cases were given two three-week courses of the therapy preoperatively. Cancer tissue specimen were sampled under endoscopic observation from the same site before chemotherapy, after one course of chemotherapy and immediately after surgery. Cells were isolated using a Triton X-100, subjected to PI staining, then their contents of nuclear DNA measured by flow cytometry (FACS-CAN).

RESULTS

1. Results of therapy

Among the 13 patients in whom evaluation was possible, PR was obtained in 7
cases, therby giving a response rate of 53.8%. However, if the results are limited to the primary lesion, most of the cases were NC or MR. Side effects
were relatively mild. The primary lesion was resectable in 10 cases. Histological findings revealed that 2/3rds of the cancer cells disappeared in 5 of
the 10 cases.

2. Results of nuclear DNA measurement

Nine (69.2%) of the 13 cases exhibited an aneuplpoid pattern. With a CV value
of 6.0 or less as the evaluation control, the mean CV value was 3.66±1.70. No
corrlation was found between differences in the ploidy pattern and the response rate. However, among the diploid cases there was a tendency for increase
of the %S phase fraction among cases showing greater histological efficacy.
Fig. 1 shows the diploid cases (cases 2, 3). The X-ray findings disclosed that
the chemotherapeutic response in both of these cases was NC. Increase in the
%S phase fraction among the 3 cases showing high histlogical efficacy. Among
the aneuploid cases, a tendency was seen for flattening of the aneuploid peak
in cases showing higher histological efficacy. Cases 4 and 6 shown in Fig. 2
were aneuploid. The efficacy of chemotherapy in both of these cases was NC,
but one (case 6) showed histological efficacy and the other (case 4) did not.
Change in the histograms revealed that the histologically inefficacious case
(case 4) showed an increase in the proportion of aneuploid cells, whereas the
histologically efficacious case showed a decrease in the proportion of aneuploid cells after one course of chemotherapy, and the pattern changed to
diploid after the second course of chemotherapy.

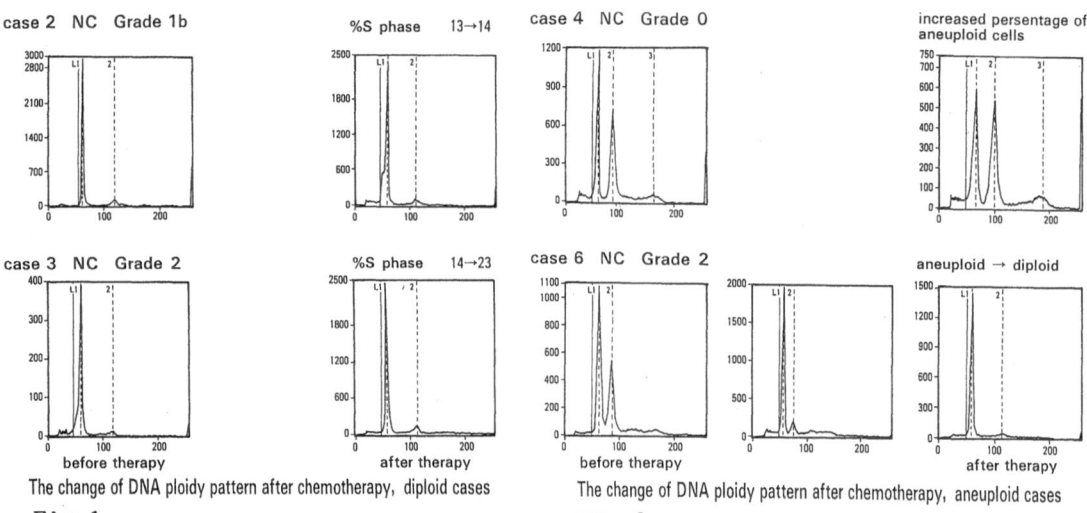

The change of DNA ploidy pattern after chemotherapy, diploid cases

Fig. 1

The change of DNA ploidy pattern after chemotherapy, aneuploid cases

Fig. 2

DISCUSSION

With the measure of prehydration to overcome the problem of renal disorders and the emergence of antiemetics that act antagonistically on 5-HT3 recepter the side effects attributable to CDDP have been appreciably lightened, thereby allowing the use of FP therapy as a safe regimen of preoperative neoadjuvant chemotherapy. In Japan there are several pyrimidine fluoride-based drugs for oral administration, which are the subject of various attempts at modifing this chemotherapy. UFT is a compound drug consisting of Tegaful and uracil, and has been demonstrated to raise the intratumor concentration of 5-FU in a highly specific manner when administered orally. However, non-compliance is a major problem of oral administration. With the exception of patients in whom oral administration is physically impossible because of stenosis or obstruction of the gastrointestinal tract, we believe that the use of an enteric coated UFT granules with few side effects in combination with a 5-HT3- receptor-antagonizing antiemetic can resolve the noncompliance problem. In the present study, we obtained compliance with the chemothrapeutic regime in every case. Side effects consisted largely of gastrointestinal disorders and leukopenia, but most were Grade 2 or below and manageble. The mild level of side effects in contrast to the high level of response rate was a characteristic feature of this treatment and indicated that neoadjuvant chemotherapy is both safe and effective. The use of imaging alone to diagnse the response of chemotherapy for gasric carcinoma is inadequate in some patients, particulalry in cases of diffuse infiltrative gastric carcinoma. In the patients examined in the present study, the X ray findings were not adequate to assess the efficacy of chemotherapy on the primary gastric lesion. By contrast, the histological findings , which should more accurately reflect the therapeutic efficacy, revealed differences in the quantity of residual cancer cells among the cases classed as NC. Consequently, the accuracy of commonly practiced methods of evaluating response is limited and a more accurate marker is needed. The number of clinical cases used to investigate the correlation between DNA ploidy pattern and the efficacy of chemothrapy is still small since the existence of numerous modifing factors in the body impedes observation of the time course of changes. However, the results of this study indicate that analysis of the DNA ploidy pattern may serve as an objective marker of chemotherapeutic efficacy.

REFERENCES

1. Suga S, (1990) Chemotherapy of advanced gastric cancer with special reference to Borrmann type 4 (scirrhous) cancer ── its principles and practic ── Maruzen, Nagoya
2. Wilke H, Preusser P, Fink U, Gunzer U, Meyer H-J, Meyer J, Siewert J R, Achterrath W, Leanz L, Knipp H, Schmoll H J (1989) Preoperative chemotherapy in locally advanced and nonresectable gastric cancer:a phase II study with etoposide , doxorubicin , and cisplatin. J Clin Oncol 7:1318-1326

Effects of Neoadjuvant Chemotherapy on High-Grade Advanced Gastric Cancers

Yutaka Yonemura[1], Toshiharu Sawa[1], Kazuo Kinoshita[1], Nobuo Matsuki[1], Sigehiro Tanaka[1], Tooru Takashima[1], Hironobu Kimura[1], Toru Kamata[1], Takashi Fujimura[1], Kazuo Sugiyama[1], Itsuo Miyazaki[1], Motohiro Tanaka[2], Yoshio Endou[2], and Takuma Sasaki[2]

[1]The Second Department of Surgery, School of Medicine, [2]Department of Experimental Therapeutics, Cancer Research Institute, Kanazawa University, Kanazawa, Japan

Abstract

Twenty-nine cases with high-grade advanced gastric cancer were preoperatively treated with PMUE therapy by a combined use of CDDP 75mg/m^2, MMC10mg/body, Etopocide 150mg/body and UFT 400mg/day. The mean number of courses administered was 2.9 (1-9 courses). The patients received a mean of 1.6 courses (1-4 courses) preoperatively and 1.3 courses postoperatively. The response rate was 62% (18/29), and all the responders were judged as partial response. The resectability rate was 79% and the potentially curable cases were found in 11 cases. The one year survival rate and median survival from initial therapy were 66% and 19.5 months. However, patients with nonresectable tumor showed no survival advantage by the neoadjuvant chemotherapy. These results indicate that the neoadjuvant chemotherapy induces the down staging for the patients with high-grade advanced gastric cancer. In these patients, neoadjuvant chemotherapy and then surgery should be considered.

Key words: neoadjuvant chemotherapy, cisplatin, gastric cancer

Introduction

Despite the introduction of a variety of multidisciprinary therapies, the therapeutic results in advanced gastric cancer remain extremely poor. Recently, favorable results have been reported with the preoperative chemotherapy (neoadjuvant cemotherapy) for the treatment of patients with cancers of the head-and neck or ovary. However, for gastric cancer, the effectiveness of conventional chemotherapy was too limited in the past to have promise in the neoadjuvant setting. In this article, we report the effects of neoadjuvant chemotherapy on high-grade advanced gastric cancer.

Materials and Methods

Twenty-nine consecutive patients with primary gastric cancer in whom the presence of Stage IV was confirmed by preoperative diagnostic imaging using CT scan, ultrasonography, or laparoscopy between 1988 and 1991 were enrolled in this study. All patients had histologically confirmed cancer of the stomach. Each patients preoperatively received one to four courses of PMUE therapy, and then underwent operation 4-8 weeks later. PMUE was administered at three weeks intervals with one course consisting of intravenous infused CDDP 75mg/m^2 and MMC 10 mg/body on the first day followed by etoposide 50 mg/body on the 3rd, 4th, and 5th days. UFT (Tegaful+Uracil) 400 mg/body was daily administered orally from the first day. Patients were evaluated every 2 to 4 weeks with measurement of indicator lesions by CT scan, sonography, and endoscopy. Survival was estimated according to the Kaplan-Meier method.

Results

As shown in Table-1, every patients had Stage IV factors. The invasion to contiguous orgens, peritoneal dissemination, liver metastasis, and para-aortic lymph node metastasis was observed in 16, 13, 14, and 25 patients, respectively. The mean preoperative course of neoadjuvant chemotherapy was 1.6 courses (1-4 courses) and 15 cases postoperatively received a mean of 1.3 course (0-9 courses). Fourteen cases did not receive PMUE therapy after surgery. We could not get any complete response (CR), but partial response was observed in 62% (18/29) of the cases (Table-2). Regarding the relation between the response rate and number of courses, only 6 cases (46%) showed an effect with one course, while an effect was achieved in 12 cases (75%) with 2 courses or more. Operation was performed but revealed nonresectability in six cases. The resection of the primary tumors was performed in 79% (23 cases) of cases, and the potentially curable resection was done in 11 cases (38%). Potentially curable intent means that the surgeon found no evidence of residual tumor and resected all grossly visible tumor. However, two of the patients died within one month after surgery. The cause of death were anastomotic leakage in one case and cahexia in one case, respectively. Survival after the initiation of therapy is shown in Figure-1. The one year survival rate and median survival from initial treatment were 66% and 19.5 months, respectively. The survival in the resected cases was significantly better than that in nonresected cases (Figure-2). Figure-3 shows the survival difference between responders and nonresponderes. The survival of responders was better than that of nonresponders, but there was no significant diffence in survival between these two groups. Side effect are listed in Table-3. The most frequently observed side effect was leukopenia, following thrombocytopenia, alopecia, and nausea. However, all the patients tolerated well with this regimen, and no chemotherapy death was observed.

Discussion

The aims of neoadjuvant chemotherapy include: 1)enhancement of the effect of local therapy such as surgery by reducing the tumor burden (down staging), 2)eradication of micrometastatic foci outside of the operative field, and 3) facilitation of organ conservation by making possible a reductionin the scope of the operation[1]. However, the role of the neoadjuvant chemotherapy in gastric cancer remains unsettled. In the present study, the increase in the number of cases in which potentially curable resection was made possible was demonstrated by the neoadjuvant chemotherapy. As the results, a improved survival rate was found in the resected cases. However, in nonresected cases, no survival-enhancing effect was observed by the neoadjuvant chemotherapy. These results support the conviction that the effect of chemotherapy and the extent of the tumor burden are inversely related[2], with the postoperative prognosis determined by the volume of malignant cells remaining in the body. Accordingly, to achieve a survival-enhancing effect, it is imperative that adequate preoperative cytoreduction with neoadjuvant chemotherapy be performed and that primary tumor and metastatic foci be vigorously dissected surgically. In this sense, it is important that regimens using as neoadjuvant chemotherapy must have a very high response rate. PMUE therapy, which we developed in 1987[3], shows a high response rate, comparable to that of EAP therapy, which is known to have the highest response rate for gastric cancer.

Regarding the neoadjuvant-chemotherapy courses, two courses may be optimal especially in views of the response rate and the fact that the preoperative hospital stay must be prolonged when more than two courses are used.

These results suggest that the neoadjuvant chemotherapy improve the incidence of curable resection in patients with highly advanced gastric cancer. This is attributed to the preoperative cytoreduction at the sites of distant metastases achieved by neoadjuvant chemotherapy, resulting in a reduction in the postoperative burden of residual cancer.

Table-1:Patients characteristics

	Neoadjuvant
Total number	29
Male/Female	20/9
Median age (range)	64.5(38-74)
Median performance status (range)	2(1-3)
Histology	
Differentiated type	17
Poorly differentiated type	12
Invasion to contiguous structures (S₁)	
Negative	13
Positive	16
Peritoneal dissemination	
Negative	16
Positive	13
Liver metastasis	
Negative	15
Positive	14
Lymph node metastasis to Group 3 or 4.	
Negative	4
Positive	25
Macroscopic type	
Localized	6
Infiltrating	23

Table-2:Response to treatment

CR	PR	NC	PD	CR+PR
0	18	11	0	18 (62%)

Table-3:Incidence of grade 3 or 4 side effect

Side effects	Neoadjuvant
Gastro-intestinal	2 (11%)
Leukopenia	6 (33%)
Thrombocytopenia	3 (17%)
Renal disfunction	1 (6%)
Alopecia	2 (11%)

Figure-1: **Survival from chemotherapy**

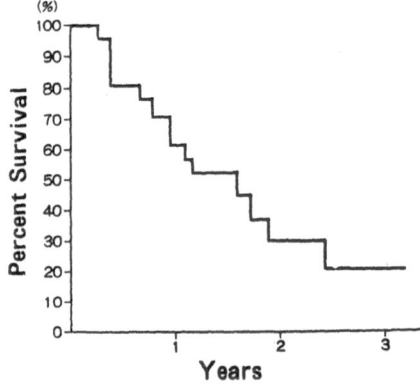

Figure-2: **Survival from treatment**

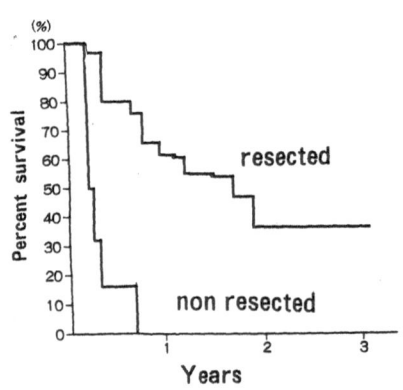

Figure-3: Survival from treatment of patients,who underwent neoadjuvant chemotherapy, according to response to treatment

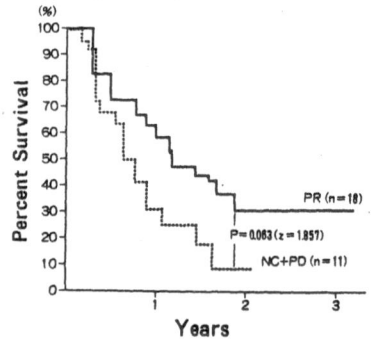

References

1)Frei Ⅲ、E (1982) Clinical cancer research: an embattled species. Cancer. 50:1979-1992

2)Frei Ⅲ, E, Miller D, Clark JR, et al (1986) Clinical and scientific consideration in preoperative (neoadjuvant) chemotherapy. Recent results in cancer research. vol 103. Springer-Verlag. Berlin, Heiderberg. pp1-5

3)Sawa T, Kinoshita K, Takegawa S, et al (1990) Effect of PMUE (CDDP, MMC, UFT, and Etopocide) for terminal gastric cancer. Jpn J Cancer Chemother. 17:2381-2386

Pharmacological Study of Continuously Infused Tegafur or 5-Fluorouracil in Treatments of Patients with Gastric Adenocarcinoma

H. Suzuki and S. Matsumoto

Department of Surgery, Second Teaching Hospital, Fujita Health University of Medicine, Nagoya, 454 Japan

ABSTRACT

The continuous intravenous infusions of 800 mg/body/day of tegafur in 4 patients and 500 mg/body/day of 5-Fu in 3 patients undergoing gastrectomy were carried out for 3 days before operation. The mean concentration of 5-Fu in the regions of gastric cancer after continuous infusions of tegafur was 3.8 times higher than that in the normal regions and 8.4 times higher than that in the sera. In the cases of continuous infusion of 5-Fu, the significant difference was not admitted. Continuous intravenous infusion of tegafur could introduce selective high concentration of 5-Fu in cancer tissues.

KEY WORDS: tegafur, 5-fluorouracil, gastric cancer, continuous intravenous infusion, tissue concentration

INTRODUCTION

We have examined two fluorinated pyrimidines, 5-Fu and tegafur, as chemotherapeutic agents for gastric cancer patients.

After continuous infusion of 5-Fu or tegafur, the concentrations of 5-Fu in the regions of gastric cancer were compared to those in the regions of normal gastric tissues, lymphnodes, and sera.

MATERIALS AND METHODS

Patient and therapy

7 patients with gastric adenocarcinoma, aged 51-80, who were undergoing therapeutic surgery, were destined to 5-Fu group or tegafur group randomly (Table 1).

The continuous intravenous infusions of 800 mg/body/day of tegafur in 4 patients and 500 mg/body/day of 5-Fu in 3 patients undergoing resectable gastrectomy were carried out from 3 days before operation to 7 days after operation. 20 mg of mitomycin C was administered to patients on the first postoperative day (Fig. 1).

Table 1   Cases

case	age	stage	histology	drug	prognosis	
K.I.	65	IV	Por	5-Fu	17M	dead
I.K.	80	III	Por	5-Fu	54M	alive
S.M.	67	IV	Tub 2	5-Fu	16M	dead
N.Y.	51	IV	Tub 2	Tegafur	9M	dead
O.H.	76	II	Tub 1	Tegafur	18M	dead
H.M.	55	III	Tub 1	Tegafur	53M	alive
K.H.	71	III	Tub 2	Tegafur	56M	alive

Fig. 1   Protocols

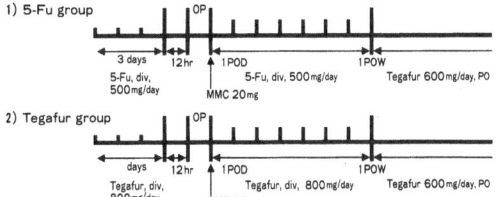

Plasma concentration of 5-Fu and tegafur

Plasma concentrations of 5-Fu or tegafur were measured at fixed times. 5-Fu was measured by the method of GC-MF (Marunaka et al). Tegafur was measured by HPLC.

Tissue concentration of 5-Fu or tegafur

Fresh cancer tissues, normal gastric tissues, metastatic or normal regional lymphnodes, and plasma were obtained, and stored at −80°C. The concentrations of 5-Fu or tegafur were measured as described above.

RESULT

Plasma concentration

1) Plasma concentrations of 5-Fu or tegafur were measured at fixed times after infusion of each drug. Mean plasma concentration of 5-Fu after continuous infusion of 5-Fu was higher than that after continuous infusion of tegafur (5-Fu group: 0.08−0.28 µg/ml, tegafur group: 0.01−0.03 µg/ml) (Fig. 2).

2) Mean plasma concentration of tegafur increased rapidly and reached a plateau after 24 hrs. Although the plasma concentration of tegafur was 13.4±2.7 μg/ml at 72 hrs, the plasma concentration of 5-Fu was only 0.03 μg/ml. These results could introduce low side effects of tegafur (Fig. 3).

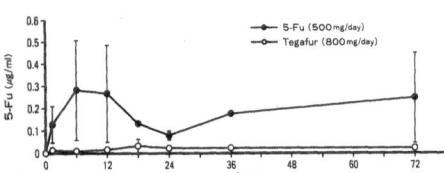

Fig. 2   Plasma concentration of 5-Fu

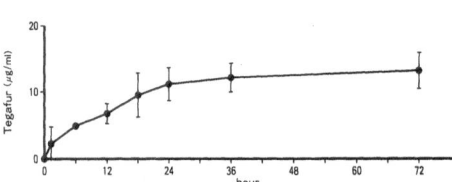

Fig. 3   Plasma concentration of Tegafur (Tegafur 800 mg/day)

Tissue concentration

1) The continuous intravenous infusions of 800 mg/body/day of tegafur and 500 mg/body/day of 5-fluorouracil were carried out for 3 days, and after 12 hours from the end of drug infusion, the operations, subtotal gastrectomy or total gastrectomy, were started. Tumor tissues, lymphnodes, and plasma were obtained, and stored at −80°C. The concentrations of 5-Fu or tegafur were measured as described above.

The durations from the end of the drug infusion to the excision of stomach were 15.0−17.0 hr (16.0 hr) in 5-Fu group and 15.6−17.0 hr (16.5 hr) in tegafur group. There was not significant difference between two groups.

2) The mean 5-Fu concentrations of gastric normal tissues, gastric cancer tissues, non-metastatic lymphnodes, metastatic lymphnodes, and plasma in 5-Fu infusion group were 27.7±14.0 ng/ml, 37.0±18.0 ng/ml, 23.0±10.2 ng/ml, 25.3±11.4 ng/ml, and 18.0±10.0 ng/ml respectively. (Fig. 4)

The mean 5-Fu concentration of gastric cancer tissue was 1.3 times higher than that of gastric normal tissue, and 2.1 times higher than that of plasma. The 5-Fu concentration of metastatic lymphnode was 1.1 times higher than that of non-metastatic lymphnode. The statistical differences among these groups were not present.

3) The mean tegafur concentrations of gastric normal tissues, gastric cancer tissues, non-metastatic lymphnodes, metastatic lymphnodes, and plasma in tegafur infusion group were 2.26±0.51 μg/ml, 2.46±0.34 μg/ml, 1.78±0.65 μg/ml, 1.99±0.37 μg/ml, 3.26±0.34 μg/ml respectively, and no significant difference was admitted (Fig. 5).

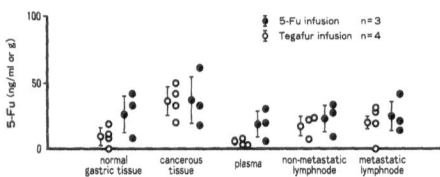

Fig. 4   Tissue concentration of 5-Fu

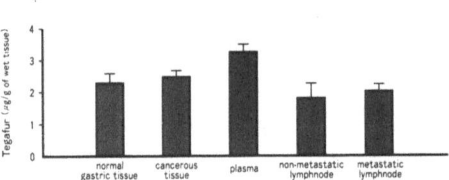

Fig. 5   Tissue concentration of Tegafur (800 mg/day)

The mean 5-Fu concentrations of gastric normal tissues, gastric cancer tissues, non-metastatic lymphnodes, metastatic lymphnodes, and plasma in tegafur infusion group were 9.5±6.81 ng/ml, 36.0±11.0 ng/ml, 17.0±7.7 ng/ml, 19.5±5.1 ng/ml, and 4.3±1.9 ng/ml respectively (Fig. 4).

The 5-Fu concentration of gastric cancer tissues was 3.8 times higher than that of gastric normal tissues, and 8.4 times higher than that of plasma. The difference among these three groups was statistically significant. The 5-Fu concentration of metastatic lymphnode was 1.1 times higher than that of non-metastatic lymphnode. There was not significant difference between these two groups.

DISCUSSION

The continuous intravenous infusions of 5-Fu or tegafur were applied to gastric cancer patients undergoing resectable gastrectomy in this pharmacological study.

Selective accumulation of 5-Fu was admitted after continuous intravenous infusion of tegafur. This result supported the reports that high activity of thymidine phosphorylase in cancer tissue facilitated the reaction of tegafur to 5-Fu.

These results indicated that continuous intravenous infusion of tegafur could introduce selective high concentration of 5-Fu in cancer tissues and was expected to bring an excellent therapeutic effect in patients with gastric cancer.

REFERENCE

1. T. Marunaka, Umeno, Y., Yoshida, K., Nagamachi, M., Minami, Y., Fujii, S., (1980), High-pressure liquid chromatographic determination of ftorafur [1-(tetrahydro-2furanyl)-5-fluorouracil] and GLC-mass spectrometric determination of 5-fluorouracil and uracil in biological materials after oral administration of uracil plus ftorafur. *Journal of Pharmaceutical Sciencses* 69:1296-1300.

Adhesive Tumor Cell Culture System (ATCCS) — Chemosensitivity Assay in Gastric Cancer with Emphasis on the Possibility of Preoperative Analysis by Data of Gastrobiopsy

V.A. Kouzmitchev, T. Suzuki, T. Ochiai, M. Nagata, Y. Gunji, T. Kouzu, and K. Isono

Department of Surgery (II), Chiba University School of Medicine, Chiba, 260 Japan

ABSTRACT

Adjuvant preoperative and postoperative chemotherapy is supposed to improve long term results of surgical treatment of gastric cancer. In order to optimise effect of chemotherapy determination of individual chemosensitivity seems reasonable. ATCCS-assay was chosen because of reported low amount of cells sufficient for completion of the test and inhibition of fibroblasts proliferation produced by properties of CAM-plates. Specimens of tumors were disintegrated, treated by anticancer drugs and cultured for 14 days. Four drugs-adriamycin (ADM), cisplatin (CDDP), 5-fluorouracil (5-FU) and mitomycin C (MMC) in 4 concentrations were tested. Assay was applied in 15 cases (gastrobiopsy — 5 cases, operation specimens — 10 cases). Results of the assay were expressed in terms of inhibition concentration of 90 % (IC90) and percentile (PCTL). In 4 cases we failed to complete test due to the lack of viable cells, there were no cases of contamination. By results of the test it was possible to select patients with high sensitivity (n = 3), complete resistance (n = 4) and intermidiate conditions (n = 4). Assesment of chemosensitivity by data of gastrobiopsy makes it possible to compare results of the test with clinical response in patients with preoperative chemotherapy.

KEY WORDS
adhesive tumor cell culture system, gastric cancer, chemosensitivity

INTRODUCTION

Chemotherapy for gastric cancer is often recommended in inoperable cases as well as in advanced cases after curative operations as an adjuvant treatment. Prediction of response can recommend drugs with high probability of patient benefit and avoid ineffective agents with unnecessary toxicity.

MATERIALS AND METHODS

ATCCS-assay of chemosensitivity (1) was performed in patients with gastric cancer treated in department of surgery (II) Chiba University School of Medicine from August 1992 untill February 1993. In all cases diagnosis was verified by histological examination of resected specimen and /or biopsy. Specimens of human tumors were obtained during operations (n = 10) or endoscopic examinations (n = 5) of gastric cancer patients. Tumors were minced with scalpels into 1 mm pieces and incubated in enzyme disaggregation medium for 16 hours with constant stirring. Cell suspension was diluted with methylcellulose attachment medium to 3000 cells/ml and was inoculated into 24-well plates (Life Trac, Irvine, CA) in duplicate for titration of 3000, 1500, 1000, 750, 500, 375 cells/well and 3000 cells in other wells. After 24 hours incubation the medium was changed to culture medium with drugs. We tested 4 different drugs, which proved to be most efficient in gastric cencer (2). The concentration of drugs in wells was determined according to the test of blood stem cells inhibition (table 1).

(Table 1) DRUGS AND DRUG CONCENTRATIONS

| | CONCENTRATION (mg/ml) | | | |
	L	M	H	VH
ADM	0.0025	0.005	0.01	0.015
CDDP	0.125	0.25	0.5	0.75
5-FU	0.08	0.16	0.32	0.48
MMC	0.015	0.03	0.06	0.09

After 5 days of incubation with drugs the medium was exchanged and cells were cultured till 13th day without drugs. Finally cultures were fixed in 70% ethanol and stained with 0.05% cristal violet. The survival of cells was determined quantitatively by image analysis using Nikon /Joyce-Loeble Magiscan-2 analysis system.

Results of the assay were expressed in terms of IC90 and PCTL, which shows degree of sensitivity comparing IC90 of tested specimen with cumulated data obtained previously and devided as high sensitive (PCTL < 15%), sensitive (15% < PCTL < 30%), low sensitive (30% < PCTL < 50%), resistant (50% < PCTL).

RESULTS

Amount of cells obtained after disaggregation varied from 4×10^4 to 38×10^4 according to the size of specimen, from biopsy specimens (5-6 pieces of tissue obtained by usual biopsy forcepses) that amount was about $4 \times 10^4 - 12 \times 10^4$ cells, depending on cellularity of tumor. Active growth was in 11 cases. In 4 cases although after disaggregation there was sufficient amount of tumor cells we failed in culturing. We could not find any relation between degree of differenciation and pattern of growth in culture. There was no case of contamination.
Results of sensitivity assay are presented in the table 2.

(Table 2) CHEMOSENSITIVITY OF EXAMINED SAMPLES

	ADR n (%)	CDDP n (%)	5-FU n (%)	MMC n (%)
high sensitivity (PCTL < 15%)	1 (9)	2 (18)	0 (0)	1 (9)
moderate sensitivity (15% < PCTL < 30%)	1 (9)	1 (9)	3 (27)	3 (27)
low sensitivity (30% < PCTL < 50%)	4 (36)	1 (9)	3 (27)	2 (18)
resistance (50% < PCTL)	5 (45)	5 (45%)	5 (45)	4 (36)

Tested tumors were sensitive for 3 drugs in 1 case, for 2 drugs in 4 cases, for 1 drug in 2 cases. Resistance for treatment was found in 4 cases.

DISCUSSION

Most of methods of in-vitro analysis of chemosensitivity needs a large amount of cells. ATCCS-assay has obvious advantage over other methods since this amount is not so large, so that analysis of sensitivity is possible from biopsy specimens.
Another advantage of this method is high rate of successful results (74% of completion by our data). Interpretation of results is not difficult, although accuracy of method should be confirmed in prospective clinical trials comparing results of chemosensitivity assays with real

response of gastric cancer for chemotherapy. Important improvement of assay can be reached if it becomes possible to evaluate polychemotherapy since treatment of gastric cancer is effective only in combined programs (2).

REFERENCES

1. Ajani JA, Baker FL, Spilzer G, Kelly A, Brock W, Tomasovic B, Singletary SE, McMurtrey M, Plager C (1987) Comparison between clinical response and in vitro drug sensitivity of primary human tumors in the adhesive tumor cell culture system. J Clin Oncol 5 : 1912 – 1921.
2. Saini A, Waxman J (1992) Chemotherapy for gastric cancer. Gut 33 : 1153 – 1154.

Effects of Surgical Adjuvant Chemotherapy and Combined Resection of Adjacent Organs on the Survival Rate of Gastric Cancer Patients

JIRO FUJIMOTO and TAKESADA MORI

Department of Surgery II, Faculty of Medicine, Osaka University, Suita, Osaka, 565 Japan

ABSTRACT

The effect of surgical adjuvant chemotherapy and combined resection of the spleen and pancreas on the survival rate in 505 patients who underwent total or proximal gastrectomy for gastric cancer was evaluated. Anticancer drugs administered perioperatively were mitomycin C, 5-fluorouracil, and other fluorinated pyrimidines, etc. Among 283 ps(+) cases who underwent combined resection for curatively or noncuratively resected tumors, chemotherapy improved the survival rate. However, among 64 ps(+) patients who did not undergo combined resection, chemotherapy did not improve the survival rate. Among 138 ps(-) patients, regardless of whether they underwent combined resection for curatively resected tumors, the 3-year survival rate was significantly higher in those who received chemotherapy.

KEY WORDS : stomach, cancer, surgery, chemotherapy, survival

INTRODUCTION

Surgical resection remains the only established curative technique for gastric cancer. Patients whose early gastric cancer was detected and treated properly usually have a good prognosis, but the prognosis of patients with serosal invasion is not always favorable. To improve the rate of cure for patients with serosal invasion, the optimal extent of surgical resection and the introduction of adjuvant chemotherapy should be considered. This study investigated whether adjuvant chemotherapy and combined resection of the spleen and pancreas improved the survival rate of patients with serosal invasion.

PATIENTS AND METHODS

The clinical background and treatment results in 505 patients who underwent total or proximal gastrectomy for gastric cancer at this institute between 1963 and 1987 were retrospectively analyzed. Prognostic factors, such as the extent of cancer spread, and the therapy modality are described using the terminology employed by the Japanese Research Society for Gastric Cancer [1]. Chemotherapy groups consisted of patients perioperatively and systemically receiving 30 mg or more mitomycin C per person, 1.0 g or more cyclophosphamide per person, 2.0 g or more 5-fluorouracil per person or other fluorinated pyrimidines (tegafur, carmofur, a combined preparation of tegafur and uracil, 5'-deoxy-5-fluorouridine) of equal potency to 2.0 g or more 5-fluorouracil. Cumulative survival rates of each treatment group were computed by acturial methods and tested for significant difference by normal approximation.

RESULTS

The 505 patients who underwent total or proximal gastrectomy for gastric cancer were divided into two groups by depth of invasion. There were 347 ps(+) cases (ssγ to sei) and 158 ps(-) cases [m to (ssγ)]. The 347 ps(+) cases consisted of 182 curatively resected cases and 165 noncuratively resected cases (Fig. 1). Among 160 ps(+) patients who underwent combined resection of adjacent organs, such as the spleen, pancreas and so on for curatively resected tumors, the 3-year survival rate was significantly higher in the 86 patients who received chemotherapy than in the 74 patients without chemotherapy (56.7% vs. 24.7%, p < 0.001). Among the 123 ps(+) patients who underwent combined resection for noncuratively resected tumors, the 1-year survival rate was significantly higher in the 55 patients who received chemotherapy than in the 68 patients without chemotherapy (48.6% vs. 25.0%, p <0.001). However, among 64 ps(+) patients who did not undergo combined resection for curatively (22 patients) or noncuratively (42 patients) resected tumors, chemotherapy did not improve the survival rate. In addition, among 182 curatively resected ps(+) patients, the

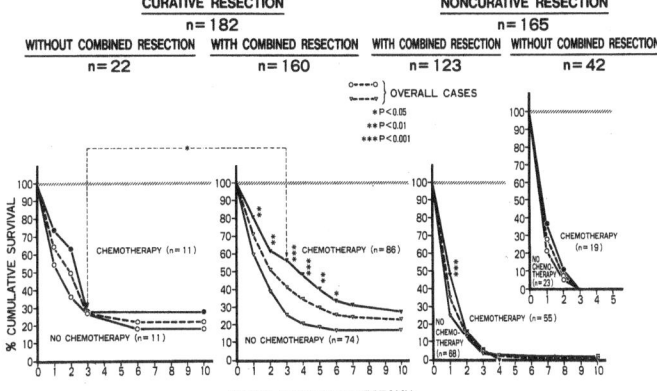

Fig.1 The effects of chemotherapy on survival of
patients undergoing surgery
for ps(+) gastric cancers
(stage II-IV)

3-year survival rate was significantly higher in 86 patients who underwent combined resection
and received chemotherapy than in 22 patients who did not undergo combined resection either
with or without chemotherapy (56.7% vs 27.3%, p < 0.05).

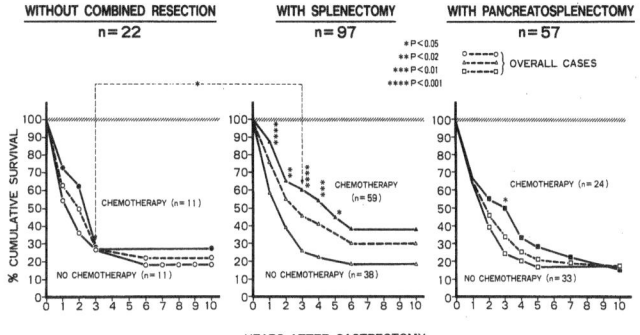

Fig.2 The effects of chemotherapy on survival of
patients undergoing curative
resection of ps(+) gastric
cancers (stage II-IV)

In Fig. 2, the combined resection group of curatively resected ps(+) cases were divided into
the splenectomy group (97 cases) and the pancreatosplenectomy group (57 cases), and compared
with those who did not receive combined resection (22 cases). In the splenectomy group, the
3-year survival rate was significantly higher in the 59 patients who received chemotherapy
than in the 38 patients without chemotherapy (60.6% vs. 25.1%, p < 0.001). The 3-year
survival rate of 59 patients receiving both splenectomy and chemotherapy was significantly
higher than that of 22 patients without combined resection irrespective of chemotherapy
(60.6% vs. 27.3%, p < 0.05). In the pancreatosplenectomy group, the 3-year survival rate
was significantly higher in 24 patients who received chemotherapy than in 33 patients without
chemotherapy (50.3% vs. 24.0%, p < 0.05).

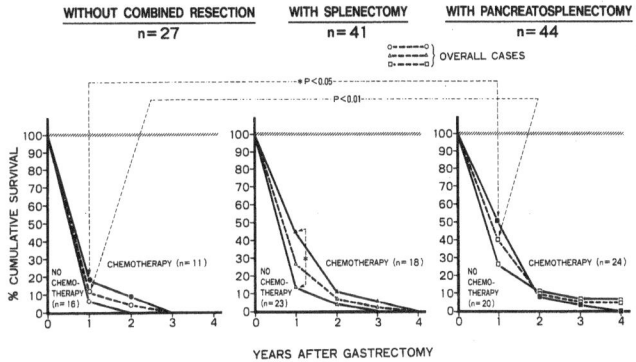

Fig.3 The effects of chemotherapy on survival of
patients undergoing noncurative resection of ps(+)
stage IV gastric cancers

In Fig. 3, the combined resection group of noncuratively resected ps(+) stage IV cases were
divided into the splenectomy group (41 cases) and the pancreatosplenectomy group (44 cases),

and compared with those who did not receive combined resection (27 cases). In the splenectomy group, the 1-year survival rate was significantly higher in 18 patients who received chemotherapy than in 23 patients without chemotherapy (44.4% vs. 13.0%, p <0.05). Both those who did not receive combined resection and in the pancreatosplenectomy group, chemotherapy showed a tendency to improve the 1-year survival rate. The 1-year survival rates of the chemotherapy group (24 cases) and 44 cases overall with pancreatosplenectomy were significantly higher than those of the chemotherapy group (11 cases) and 27 cases overall without combined resection, respectively (with chemotherapy : 50.0% vs. 18.2%, p < 0.05 ; overall : 40.4% vs. 11.2%, p < 0.01)

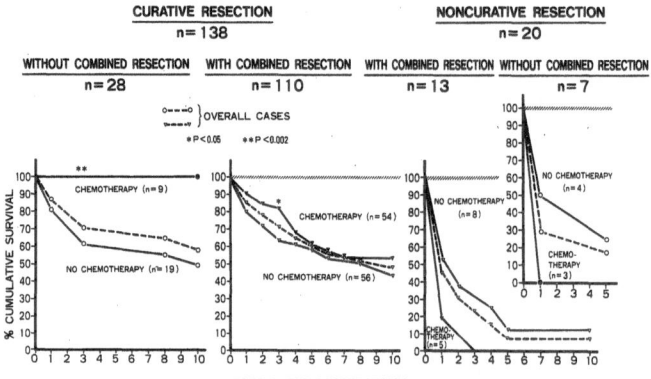

Fig.4 The effects of chemotherapy on survival of
patients undergoing surgery
for ps(-) gastric cancers
(stage I-IV)

Fig. 4 shows the 158 ps(-) cases consisting of 138 curatively resected cases and 20 non-curatively resected cases. Among both those who did and those who did not receive combined resection for curatively resected tumors, the 3-year survival rate was significantly higher in those who received chemotherapy. That is, the combined resection group : 81.9% for 54 patients with chemotherapy vs. 63.9% for 54 patients without chemotherapy, p < 0.05 ; those who did not receive combined resection : 100% for 9 patients who received chemotherapy vs. 60.8% for 21 patients without chemotherapy, p < 0.002. Among 20 patients undergoing noncurative resection who either received or did not receive combined resection, chemotherapy rather showed a tendency to decrease the survival rate.

DISCUSSION

This paper described the effect of surgical adjuvant chemotherapy and combined resection of adjacent organs, such as spleen, pancreas and so forth, on the survival rate of the patients who underwent total or proximal gastrectomy for gastric cancers with serosal invasion. Among both curatively (182 cases) and noncuratively (165 cases) resected ps(+) cases, the survival rate was slightly increased in the combined resection groups than in those who did not receive combined resection (Fig. 1, 2 and 3). There was a report demonstrating that with more advanced clinical stages, gastrectomy combined with resection of the adjacent organs produced a better prognosis than gastrectomy alone [2]. Among the combined resection groups of both curatively and noncuratively resected ps(+) cases, chemotherapy significantly improved the survival rate, but among those who did not receive combined resection, chemotherapy did not. Even among the noncuratively resected ps(+) cases, the survival rate increased in sequence relative to those who did not receive combined resection, those who received splenectomy and those who received pancreatosplenectomy (Fig. 3). Those findings suggest that minimal residual cancer after surgery could be potentially controlled by adjuvant chemotherapy.

Among both the combined resection group (110 cases) and those who did not receive combined resection (28 cases) of the curatively resected ps(-) cases, chemotherapy significantly improved the survival rate (Fig. 4). Thus, it was thought that combined resection was rarely required for the curatively resected ps(-) cases. In the 20 noncuratively resected ps(-) cases, it is possible that chemotherapy might decrease the survival rate.

REFERENCES

1. Japanese Research Society for Gastric Cancer (1981) The General Rules for the Gastric Cancer Study in Surgery and Pathology. Jpn J Surg 11:127-139
2. Nakajima T and Nishi M (1989) Surgery and adjuvant chemotherapy for gastric cancer. Hepato-gastroenterol 36:79-85

Evaluation of Combination Chemotherapy Using 5-FU, Leucovorin, and CDDP (FLP Therapy) Against Recurrent or Advanced Stomach Cancer

Tamotsu Okugawa, Yasushi Rino, Kenzo Okada, Osamu Kobayashi, Motonori Sairenji, and Hisahiko Motohashi

Department of Surgery, Kanagawa Cancer Center Hospital, Yokohama, 241 Japan

ABSTRACT

Between July 1991 and October 1992, we performed combination chemotherapy consisting of 5-FU, leucovorin, and CDDP (FLP therapy) against recurrent or advanced stomach cancer. The outcome was CR in 1, PR in 7, NC in 2, and PD in 11 of the 1 1evaluable patients, resulting in an overall response rate of 72.7%. Performance status was improved in all patients. All toxicities were grade 3 or below. Consequently, FLP therapy was, hereafter, expected to be safety and effective against recurrent and advanced stomach cancer, and to improve the QOL.

KEY WORDS : combination chemotherapy, 5-FU, leucovorin, CDDP, stomach cancer

INTRODUCTION

Recently, chemotherapy appling biochemical modulation has been offen carried out. We performed combination chemotherapy consisting of 5-FU, leucovorin, and CDDP (FLP therapy), appling biochemical modulation, against recurrent or advanced stomach cancer from July 1991. We reported the efficiency of FLP therapy against stomach cancer.

PATIENTS AND METHODS

Patients Selection

All patients had recurrent or advanced (unoperable and noncurative resected) stomach cancer. At entry, all patients were rquired to have adequate bone marrow reserve (leukocyte count $\geqq 3000/mm^3$; platelet count $\geqq 100,000/mm^3$), renal function (serum creatinine level $\leqq 2.0mg/dl$; creatinine clearance $\geqq 60ml/min$), and not to have inflammatory diseases and other malignancy. If patients had recieved any prior chemotherapy, they had to have completed those therapy more than 4 weeks before entry into FLP therapy. All patients or their families were given informed consent.

Therapeutic Regimen

In the inpatients, 5-FU, leucovorin, and CDDP were administered at $250mg/m^2$ (days 1-8) by continuous intravenous injection, 30mg/body (days 1-8) by intravenous bolus, and $60mg/m^2$ (days 1 and 8), respetively. 4 to 5 weeks defined one course of therapy in the inpatients. In the outpatients, they were administered at 500mg/body by 2 to 3-hour intravenous infusion, 30mg/body by intravenous bolus, and 20-30mg/body, respectively. 2 to 4 weeks defined one course of therapy in the outpatients. If toxicity more severe than grade 2 was encountered, the does of 5-FU and CDDP were reduced by 30%. During FLP therapy, peroral administration of fluoropyrimidines and biological response modifiers was left to the doctor in charge. This therapy was over when patients refused this therapy, grade 4 toxicity was encountered, the recurrent or metastatic lesions fell into PD, 4courses in the inpatients was recieved, or 10 times in the outpatients was recieved.

Administration of CDDP

We selected the route of administration of CDDP according to the sites of recurrence or metastasis for the purpose of reducing toxicities and increasing concentration of CDDP in the tumor. CDDP was administered by semi-selective intraaortic infusion (IA) for local recurrence, invasion of other intraperitoneal organs, intraperitoneal lymph node recurrence or matastasis (N_3 and N_4), and liver metastasis as a 3-hour infusion in the inpatients or a 2-hour infusion in the outpatients. IA was performed by advancing a catheter from the branch of lateral circumflex femoral artery into the aorta at the height of the lower margin of the 9th thoracic vertebra and subcutaneously implanting a reservoir. CDDP was administered by intraperitoneal infusion (IP) mixed with 1000ml of normal saline solution for peritoneal dissemination as a 2-hour infusion.

IP was performed by placing a catheter in Douglas' cul-de-sac and subcutaneously implanting a reservoir. CDDP was administered by intravenous injection (IV) for extraperitoneal metastasis, and the patients who were performed noncurative resections proving after the operation and not implanted a reservoir, as a 3-hour injecion in the inpatients or a 2-hour injecion in the outpatients.

Countermeasures for Toxicities

Administration of CDDP was performed with hydration at least 2000ml of physiological solution, and furosemide was administered at 10mg by intravenous injection on the day of CDDP injection for the renal toxicity. Moreover in the outpatients, furosemide (20mg/day) was taken once a day for 3 days Granisetron hydrochloride as antiemetics was administered at 3mg on the day of CDDP injection. If nausea and vomiting above grade 2 was encountered, granisetron hydrochloride was administered at 3mg/day for 2 more days. The solution of alloprinol as antistomatitis was gargled during 5-FU injection in the inpatients. If the leukocyte count was less than 1500/mm³, G-CSF was administered at 100 μg/day for 3 days by subcutaneous injection.

Evaluation

All patients who had recieved at least 1 course in the inpatients or at least 3 times in the outpatients were considered evaluable for response, toxicity, and performance status (PS). The histological findings, response criteria, and Grade of PS were determined using The General Rules for Gastric Cancer Study in Surgery and Pathology of the Japanese Research Society for Gastric Cancer. The therapeutic responses were evaluated by imaging techniques every 4-6 weeks. Only complete or partial responses were considered to be objective responses. PS before FLP therapy was reported just before this therapy, and after start in FLP therapy was reported minimum Grade kept for at least 4 weeks. The toxicities were evaluated twice a week in the inpatients, and every 2 weeks in the outpatients during this therapy. The toxicities were determined using WHO criteria for the most part.

RESULTS

Patients Characteristics

Between July 1991 and October 1992, FLP therapy had been carried out in 16 patients. 10 men and 6 women with a median age of 58.4 years (range, 44-72 years). All patients had been resected stomach. 11 patients had recurrent stomach cancer, 5 patients had advanced stomach cancer undergone noncurative resection. 11 of the 16 patients had the evaluable lesions. 11 of the 16 patients had been recieved this therapy also in the outpatients. CDDP was administered by IA in 6 patients, by IV in 5 patients, and by IP in 3 patients.

Responses

The outcome was CR in 1, PR in 7, NC in 2, and PD in 1 of the 11 evaluable patients, resulting in an overall response rate of 72.7%. In 4 patients with lymph node metastases, 1 CR and 3 PRs were achieved. In 2 patients with abdominal subcutis metastases, 2 PRs were achieved. In 1 patient with liver metastasis, and 1 with local recurrence, both PR were achieved. Of 6 patients with moderately differentiated adenocarcinoma, the outcome was CR in 1, PR in 3, and NC in 2. In 3 patients with poorly differentiated adenocarcinoma, 3 PRs were achieved. PR was achieved in 1 patient with signet ring cell carcinoma. But NC was resulted in 1 patient with mucinous adenocarcinoma.

Evaluation of Performance Status

PS was improved in all patients. PS was improved 3 grades in 1, 2 grades in 8, and 1 grade in 7 of the 16 patients.

Toxicity

All toxicities were grade 3 or below. The most frequent toxicities were nausea and vomiting, and appetite loss. They were observed in 87.5% of the 16 patients. The most frequent grade 3 toxicity was leukopenia which was encountered in 12.5% of the 16 patients. Toxicities in patients who were administered CDDP by IV were likely worse than those by IA.

DISCUSSION

The regimen of FLP therapy was made referring to FLEP therapy [1] against stomach cancer. We administered leucovorin at 30mg/body because there was the report on high response rate of combination chemotherapy using leucovorin at 20mg/m² and 5-FU[2]. For the purpose of reducing toxicities and increasing concentration of CDDP in tumor, CDDP was administered by one of three methods according to the sites of metastatic lesions. The toxicities by IA and IP of CDDP were likely more easy than those by IV of CDDP. FLP therapy was reported the efficasy against colon cancer of which the pathological classification was comparative well differentiated adenocarcinoma. In this study, FLP therapy was effective against stomach cancer which was composed of the comparative poor differentiated carcinoma such as poorly differentiated adenocarcinoma and signet ring cell carcinoma. The respnses by the sites of metastatic lesions suggested FLP therapy was especially effective against lymph nodes. An overall response rate was 72.7%, all patients were improved PS, and all toxicities were grade 3 or below. Consequently FLP therapy was, hereafter, expected to be safety and effective against stomach cancer, and to improve the QOL.

REFERENCES

1. Nakajima T, Ohta K, Ishihara S, Nishi M (1990) The operation and neoadjuvant chemotherapy (especially FLEP therapy) against advanced stomach cancer. Therapy 72 : 1607-1616
2. O'Connel, ML (1989) A phase III trial of 5-fluorouracil and leucovorin in the treatment of advanced colorectal cancer. Cancer 63 : 1026 − 1030

Local Immunotherapy for Gastric Cancer Using a Mixture of OK-432 and Fibrinogen

Taro Wakasugi, Tsutomu Takeda, Takushi Monden, Yoshihiro Katsumoto, Isao Sakita, Hirohito Nagaoka, Mutsumi Fukunaga, Takashi Shimano, Hitoshi Shiozaki, and Takesada Mori

Department of Surgery II, Osaka University Medical School , Osaka, 553 Japan

Introduction

OK-432 is an immunomodulatory agent prepared from a strain of Streptococcus pyogenes. We have previously reported that OK-432 displays considerably enhanced antitumor activity when injected intratumorally together with fibrinogen [1]. In the present study, we administered a mixture of OK-432 and fibrinogen (OK/fbg) into gastric carcinoma and examined the immune reactions induced in the tumors and in spleen.

Materials and Methods

OK/fbg was prepared by dissolving 0.5mg of OK-432 in 1ml of aprotinin and mixing this solution with 80mg of heat-treated human fibrinogen. Seven days before operation, a single intratumoral injection of OK/fbg was performed under endoscopy in 28 patients with gastric carcinoma. A control group of 10 patients with gastric cancer who received no therapy prior to operation were also included in this study. First, histopathologic examinations of tumor and spleen were carried out. Secondly, observations of immunohistochemical staining of spleen with anti-Su (specific for OK-432) and anti-CD68 (specific for macrophage) antibodies were made. Thirdly, functional analyses of spleen cells (flow cytometry for phenotypic analysis and fluorescein fluorochromasia cytotoxicity assay [2]) were performed. In addition, in order to determine the lymphokine-activated killer (LAK) activity, spleen cells were cultured with 700 JRU/ml recombinant IL-2 for 7 days.

Results

There were no differences in background characteristics between the two groups of patients studied. Histopathologic examinations disclosed the formation of fibrin fibers at the site of injection, marked infiltration of inflammatory cells, and destruction of cancerous tissue 7 days after the injection of OK/fbg. Immunohistochemical staining of spleens resected from patients pretreated with OK/fbg demonstrated large number of macrophages phagocytizing OK-432 in the splenic sinuses. Phenotypical analyses demonstrated that the CD4/CD8 ratio and expression of HLA-DR, CD25 and LeuM3 of spleen cells obtained from pretreated patients were significantly higher than those obtained from untreated patients. Cytotoxicity assays demonstrated that spleen cells from OK/fbg treated patients had significantly higher killing activity against K562 and Daudi cells than did those from control patients (Table). Furthermore, we were able to induce LAK cells from spleens of OK/fbg-pretreated patients by culture with IL-2 for a period of only seven days.

Table. Cytotoxicity of spleen cells from OK/fbg treated patients by 4h C-FDA assay
(E/T=10/1)

Target	OK/fbg treated	no treated
DAUDI	43.0±19.0 *	16.4±13.0 *
K562	48.0±17.8*	21.0±9.0 *

* p ‹ 0.01

Conclusion

1. Local immunotherapy for gastric cancer with OK/fbg augments the antitumor immunity of spleen cells.
2. Spleen cells from patients treated with OK/fbg may be a useful source of LAK cells.

References

1. Monden T, Morimoto H, Shimano T, Yagyu T, Murotani M, Nagaoka H, Kawasaki Y, Kobayashi T, Mori T (1992) Use of Fibrinogen to Enhance the Antitumor Effect of OK-432. Cancer 69 : 636-642
2. Nagaoka H, Monden T, Sakita I, Katsumoto Y, Wakasugi T, Kawasaki Y, Tomita N, Takeda T, Yagyu T, Morimoto H, Kobayashi T, Shimano T, Mori T (1992) Establishment of cytotoxic CD4+T cell clones from cancer patients treated by local immunotherapy. Biotherapy 5: 241-250

Intralymph Nodal Injection of the Mixture of OK-432 and Mitomycin C (MMC) Adsorbed onto Fine Activated Carbon Particles (CH$_{40}$) for the Treatment of Lymph Node Metastasis

S. Okano, K. Sawai, H. Minato, T. Fujioka, M. Yamaguchi, K. Kanemitsu, A. Hagiwara, and T. Takahashi

First Department of Surgery, Kyoto Prefectural University of Medicine, Kyoto, 602 Japan

ABSTRACT

Intralymph nodal injection of a mixture of an immunopotentiator (OK432) and an anticancer agent (Mitomycin C ; MMC) is an important locoregional immunotherapy. By combining these drugs into fine activated carbon particles (CH$_{40}$) the efficacy of the drugs in treating lymph node metastases should be increased as the nodes are selectively targeted and the local concentrations of chemotherapeutic agent and immunopotentiator will remain high for extended periods of time. When P388 murine leukemic cells ($5 \times 10^5/0.05$ ml of normal saline) were inoculated subcutaneously into the left hind footpad of BDF1 mice, they transferred to the left popliteal and the left lumbar lymph nodes within 8 days. At this time various combinations of MMC, OK432 and CH$_{40}$ were injected into the left popliteal lymph nodes, and three hours after drug administration the left popliteal lymph node and the left hind foot at the knee joint were surgically removed. Six days after excision, the left lumbar lymph node, a source of cancer cells, was transplanted intraperitoneally to a recipient mouse and the survival curves for the recipients were evaluated. The injection of a mixture of 80µg MMC, 0.2 KE OK432 and 0.004ml CH$_{40}$ into lymph nodes enhanced survival and is probably an effective treatment for distant lymph node metastases.

KEY WORDS : lymph node metastasis, intralymph nodal injection, OK432, Mitomycin C, CH$_{40}$.

INTRODUCTION

In solid cancer treatments, surgical resection of the tumor and regional lymph nodes is commonly carried out. Removal of regional lymph nodes, however, has certain drawbacks as they play important roles in establishing tumor immunity [1], and their resection is technically difficult. In addition, many of these patients cannot endure a great deal of stress, and they should experience minimal surgical interventions. Intralymph nodal injection therapy using anticancer agents and immunopotentiators can be used to remove metastasized lymph nodes and at the same time enhance the anti-tumor activity of regional lymph nodes. Intralymphatic infusion has been described as an effective means of delivering chemotherapeutic agents to regional lymph nodes [2]. In this study we examined the effect of intralymph nodal injection of a mixture of an anticancer agent and an immunopotentiator in mice.

MATERIALS AND METHODS

Animals, tumor cell line and agents
(1)Animals : Five-week-old male BDF1 mice, purchased from the Shizuoka Laboratory Animal Center (Hamamatsu, Japan), were used in this study. Five-week-old male DBA2 mice, purchased from the same center, were used to maintain the P388 tumor cells.
(2)Tumor cell line : P388 murine leukemic cells, syngeneic for BDF1 mice and DBA2 mice, were supplied by Nippon Kayaku Co. Ltd. (Tokyo, Japan). These cells, which were maintained by intraabdominal transplantation to DBA2 mice, were obtained aseptically from the peritoneal cavity to produce a suspension of 1×10^7 cells/ml normal saline. The tumor cell viability, determined by the Trypan-blue exclusion test, was higher than 95%.
(3)Immunopotentiator : OK432 (a streptococcal preparation) was donated by the Chugai Pharmaceutical Company (Tokyo, Japan).
(4)Anti-tumor agent : Mitomycin C (MMC), which was purchased from Kyowa Hakko Co. Ltd. (Tokyo, Japan), has anticancer activities against P388 cells.
(5)Fine Activated Carbon Particles (CH$_{40}$) (Mitsubishi Chemicals Co. Ltd., Tokyo, Japan) : Fine activated carbon

particles (21nm in diameter) , purchased from Mitsubishi Chemicals Co. Ltd., were used as an adsorbent for MMC. The particles, 50mg/ml, were combined with 20mg/ml of polyvinylpyrrolidone (Nakarai Chemicals Co. Ltd., Kyoto, Japan) in saline. Large amounts of anticancer agents can be adsorbed onto the numerous pores on the surface of the CH_{40} carbon particles. The agent is then released according to the concentration gradient around the particle.

All drug compositions (dose/mouse)
> (a)The MMC+OK+CH (1) group (n=16): 80 μg MMC and 0.2 KE OK432 in 0.096 ml of normal saline combined with 0.004ml CH_{40}.
> (b)The MMC+OK+CH (2) group (n=15): 25 μg MMC and 0.5 KE OK432 in 0.095 ml of normal saline combined with 0.005ml CH_{40}.
> (c)The MMC+OK group (n=14): 25 μg MMC and 0.5 KE OK432 in 0.1 ml of normal saline.
> (d)The OK+CH group (n=16): 0.5 KE OK432 in 0.095ml of normal saline combined with 0.005ml CH_{40}.
> (e)The MMC+CH group (n=15): 25 μg MMC in 0.095ml of normal saline combined with 0.005ml CH_{40}.
> (f)The control group (n=10): No intralymph nodal injections were made.

Injected site : All drugs were given into the left popliteal lymph nodes.

Induction of lymph node metastasis : A P388 cells suspension of 5×10^5 cells/0.05ml was inoculated into the hind footpad of 86 BDF1 mice with a 27 gauge needle (on day 0).

Intralymph nodal immunochemotherapy for lumbar lymph node metastasis : Tumor-bearing BDF1 mice were randomly divided into 6 groups. To treat the lumbar lymph node metastasis, OK432 and/or MMC mixed with or without CH_{40} (see above) was injected directly into the left popliteal lymph node on day 8 under intraperitoneal anesthesia with pentobarbital (40mg/kg). Three hours after the injection the popliteal lymph node and the tumor were excised. Mice in the control group underwent excision of the left popliteal lymph node and the tumor. On day 14 (6 days after drug treatment) the mice were sacrificed and the left lumbar lymph nodes were excised and weighed. Each node was minced with scissors in 0.5ml of normal saline and the node cells were transplanted intraperitoneally to another normal BDF1 mouse. Recipient mice were observed for 90 days. Survival curves were drawn after following the Kaplan-Meier method and differences in the survival curves were analyzed statistically by the generalized Wilcoxon test. The weight of the left lumbar lymph nodes was analyzed using the unpaired t-test.

RESULTS

Induction of lymph node metastasis in BDF1 mice : P388 tumor cells inoculated into the left footpad transferred to the left popliteal lymph node and the left lumbar lymph node by day 8 (Fig.1).

The weights of the left lumbar lymph node : The weights of the left lumbar lymph nodes were similar in both the MMC+OK+CH and MMC+OK groups. The weight of the nodes in the MMC+CH group, however, was statistically smaller than in the former three groups (P<0.05). (Fig.2)

Intralymphatic immunochemotherapy : If the MMC+OK and MMC+OK+CH(2) groups were not considered, the survival rate was higher for the MMC+OK+CH(1) group than for the control, OK+CH and MMC+CH groups (p<0.05-0.01). There were no significant differences between the MMC+OK+CH (1) group, the MMC+OK+CH (2) group and the MMC+OK group. (Fig.3)

DISCUSSION

Intralymphatic injection of anticancer agents has been applied in the treatment of lymph node metastases [2]. In our Department, we have found that anticancer agents adsorbed onto fine activated carbon particles (CH_{40}) offers many advantages for the treatment of lymph node metastases. First, this preparation flows immediately to the lymph nodes via lymphatic vessels and turns both tissues black in color. Second, anticancer agent remains at blackened sites at high concentrations[3,4]. In gastric cancer operations, the sites injected are chosen from N1 or N2 (UICC) lymph nodes, and these lymph nodes are usually removed with the primary tumor. In our animal model, the injected site (the primary lymph node) was removed and the efficacy of the treatment on the secondary lymph node metastases was evaluated. P388 cells inoculated into the left footpad transferred to the left popliteal lymph node and the left lumbar lymph node by day 8 [5]. Although it was reported previously that intralymph nodal injection of OK432 had a therapeutic effect on secondary lymph node metastases [6], we were unable to confirm this observation after coinjection of OK432 and CH_{40}. Since CH_{40} competitively inhibits the uptake of OK432 by macrophages, less OK432 is then available to activate the immune reactions necessary to kill the cancerous cells. Consequently, lower survival rates were observed. The improved survival for the MMC+OK group demonstrates a beneficial therapeutic effect of this drug combination on the left lumbar lymph node. Due to lack of statistical significance the best drug combination cannot be clearly defined and further studies may be needed to determine if MMC+OK+CH(1) is actually better than MMC+OK and MMC+OK+CH(2). The weight gain in the left lumbar lymph nodes has been attributed to lymphocyte infiltration, although we did not find any correlation between the weight of the nodes and the survival curves with the various drug treatments. Stimulation of local immune responses by OK432 along with the actions of a chemotherapeutic agent probably accounts for the enhanced survival without associated weight gain. In conclusion, the intralymph nodal injection of the mixture of MMC, OK432 and CH40 was effective in the treatment of lymph node metastases.

Fig.1 Induction of lymph node metastasis

On day 8 after inoculation of P388 cells into the left hind footpad the left popliteal and the left lumbar lymph nodes became swollen. This figure shows the left popliteal(➤) and the left lumbar($\lozenge$) lymph nodes, which were stained black by the intratumoral injection of CH_{40}.

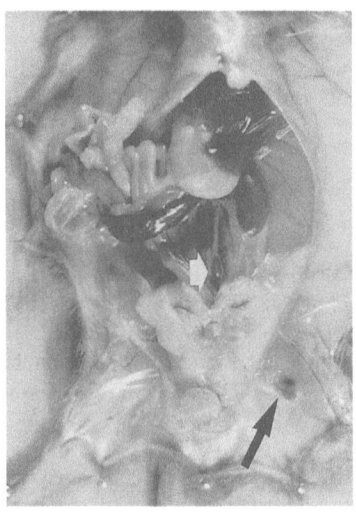

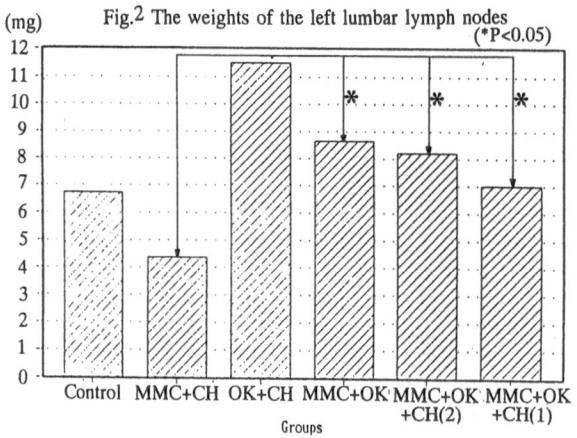

Fig.2 The weights of the left lumbar lymph nodes (*P<0.05)

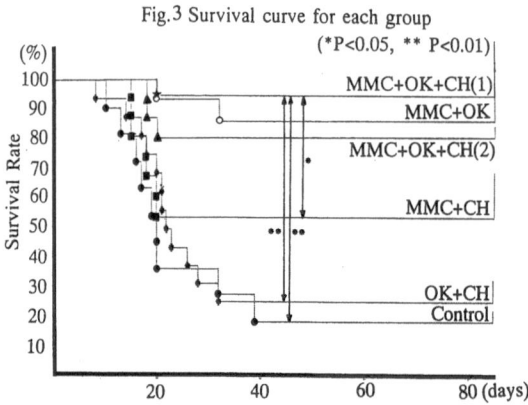

Fig.3 Survival curve for each group (*P<0.05, ** P<0.01)

References

[1] Fisher,B. and Fisher,E.R. : Studies concerning the regional lymph node in cancer. 1. Initiation of immunity. Cancer,27 : 1001–1004, 1971.

[2] Jackson,G.L., Wallace,S. and Weiss,A. : Chemotherapy by intralymphatic infusion. Cancer,15 : 955. 1962.

[3] Takahashi,T., Hagiwara,A., Sawai,K., et al : Targeting chemotherapy to lymph node and peritoneal metastases of gastric cancer using high–dose mitomycin C adsorbed on activated carbon particles. Mitomycin C in Cancer Chemotherapy Today, Excerpta Medica : 124–136, 1991.

[4] Hagiwara,A., Takahashi,T., Sawai,K., et al : Enhanced therapeutic efficacy of intralymph nodal etoposide on distal lymph node metastases using a new dosage format –activated carbon particles adsorbing etoposide. Anti–Cancer Drug Design 7 : 163–168,1992.

[5] Seiki,K., Takahashi,T., Okano,S., et al : A study on topical injection of small activated carbon particles suspension in ethanol into the metastatic lymph node in mice. Japanese Journal of Lymphology, Vol.13 No.2 : 31–38 1990 (in Japanese)

[6] Okano,S., Sawai,S., Fujioka,T., et al : Intra–lymph nodal injection of OK–432 for treatment of lymph node metastasis. Jpn J Cancer Chemotherapy 19(10) : 1598–1600, 1992.

Clinical and Immunological Effects of Locoregional Immunochemotherapy for Either Liver Metastases or Peritoneal Dissemination of Gastric Cancer

YASUYUKI SUGIYAMA and SHIGETOYO SAJI

Second Department of Surgery, Gifu University School of Medicine, Gifu, 500 Japan

ABSTRACT

Intermittent locoregional administration of BRM and chemotherapeutics for either liver metastases or peritoneal dissemination of gastric cancer was performed. For liver metastases, partial response was observed in 4 of 9 patients and administration of BRM brought about increase of IL-6 production and decrease of NK activity in the peripheral blood. For carcinomatous peritonitis, it resulted in disappearance of cancer cells from ascites followed by decrease of ascites. In the peritoneal cavity, neutrophils were predominant for a few days after the treatment and then lymphocytes increased. Furthermore, production of cytokines such as IL-6, interferon-γ and TNF-α was observed in the ascites.

KEY WORDS: locoregional immunochemotherapy, gastric cancer, liver metastases, carcinomatous peritonitis, cytokine production

INTRODUCTION

In order to augment the antitumor effect, intermittent locoregional administration of both biological response modifiers (BRM; OK-432, a streptococcal preparation and interleukin(IL) 2) and chemotherapeutics such as mitomycin C(MMC) and Adriamycin was performed for either the liver metastases or peritoneal dissemination of gastric cancer. In this study, clinical and immunological effects of this locoregional immunochemotherapy were examined.

MATERIALS AND METHOD

Liver metastases

Nine gastric cancer patients with simultaneous liver metastases were included in this study. Clinical profile of the patients and operative factors according to the general rules for the gastric cancer study in Japan[1] are listed in Table 1. The patients underwent the placement of catheter in the hepatic artery and thereafter intermittent transarterial administration of chemotherapeutics and BRM was performed. The schedule was as follows; MMC (10mg) was administered on day 0, OK-432(0.5~1.0KE) on day 1, IL-2(40×10⁴JRU)on day 4, 7 and 11. This regimen was repeated as many times as possible and occasionally modified depending on the physical condition of patients. All patients were assessed by computed tomographic examination and by measurement of serum concentration of several tumor markers. Performance status was also evaluated. In addition, the concentration of 3 kinds of cytokines suchas IL-6, interferon(IFN)-γ and tumor necrosis factor(TNF)-α in the peripheral blood sera was measured by ELISA immediately before and after the administration of agents. Natural killer (NK) activity of peripheral blood mononuclear cells(PBMC) was measured by 4 hours ^{51}-Cr release assay using K562 as a target.

Peritoneal dissemination

Ten of gastric cancer patients with microscopic peritoneal dissemination diagnosed by irrigation cytology were treated by intraoperative intraperitoneal administration of some anticancer agents and immunological response in the peritoneal cavity was investigated. Depending on the administered agents, patients were divided into 3 groups. Four patients were given both MMC(10mg) and OK-432(15KE), 3 patients were given cisplatinum(CDDP: 75~100 mg) and as a control group 3 patients underwent surgery alone. The exudate from peritoneal cavity was harvested every day from Day 1 through Day3 and subpopulation of immunocyte in it was examined by staining with May-Giemsa solution. Moreover, 3 kinds of cytokines (IL-6,

IFN-γ and TNF-α) in the exudate were quantified on Day 1,2 and 3 after operation by ELISA. Two patients with carcinomatous peritonitis originating from gastrc cancer were given intermittent intraperitoneal administration of MMC(5~10mg), OK-432(0.5~1.0KE)and IL-2(4×10⁴ JRU) in this sequence by use of implantable injection port and the investigation into immunological response in the peritoneal cavity was performed by measuring subpopulation of immunocytes and by quantifying cytokines (IL-6, IFN-γ and TNF-α) in the ascites at the indicated period of time after administration in the same way as described above.

RESULTS

Liver metastases

In terms of direct antitumor effect on liver metastases, partial response was observed in 4 of 9 cases, minor response 1, no change 3 and progressive disease 1, which indicated that the response rate was 44%. In addition, decline in serum tumor marker levels was observed in 7 of 9 patients(77%) and improvement of performance status was seen in 4 of 9 patients. Even though 8 of 9 patients died, 6 of them could survive more than 300 days after treatment (Table 1). Moreover, the patients who received locoregional immunochemotherapy had a significantly higher survival rate than the patients who received systemic immunochemotherapy in our department over the past 10 years(Fig.1).
As for cytokines in the peripheral blood sera, the concentration of IL-6 increased by BRM, whereas chemotherapeutics could not alter the level of it. Without respect to administered agents, TNF-α was not detectable at any time. Although IFN-γ was detectable, no particular pattern was observed. On the other hand, administration of BRM caused the decrease of NK activity of PBMC, whereas chemotherapeutics did not (Fig.2).

Table. 1 Clinical profile of the patients and antitumor effects of locoregional therapy for liver metastases of gastric cancer
(1989. 1~1992. 12 : 2nd Dep. of Surg. Gifu Univ. School of Medicine)

	Sex	Age	Operative Mode and degree of lymphnodes dissection	Macroscopic Operative Factors H	P	N	S	Histological Type	ADM (mg)	MMC (mg)	5-FU (mg)	OK-432 (KE)	IL2 (U)	Antitumor Effect	Tumor Markers	Change of Performance Status	Prognosis	Survival Days
1	M	55	Total gastrectomy R₀	2	2	3	3	tub₂	80			2.0	5000	NC	CEA (186→341)	No Change	Died	389
2	M	68	Subtotal gastrectomy R₁	3	0	2	1	por	270*	20		22.0	22000	PR	CEA (100→37)	Improved	Died	310
3	F	53	Subtotal gastrectomy R₁	3	0	3	2	pap	60*			3.0	7000	PR	CEA (31→4)	No Change	Died	488
4	M	57	Total gastrectomy R₁	3	3	4	2	pap	40*	90		24.0	60000	PR	CEA (1320→22)	Improved	Died	318
5	M	45	Exploratory laparotomy	3	1	2	3	por	90*			4.0	5000	NC	CEA (22→7)	Worsen	Died	364
6	M	56	Total gastrectomy R₁	3	0	4	1	tub₂		60		6.0	16000	PD	CEA (142→262)	Worsen	Died	126
7	M	59	Partial gastrectomy R₀	3	1	0	2	pap	200*	32	9250	7.5	20500	NC	AFP (2125→107)	Improved	Died	349
8	F	64	Partial gastrectomy R₂	1	0	4	2	muc	40**	16	200	4.0	9000	MR	CEA (34→8)	No Change	Died	174
9	F	52	Subtotal gastrectomy R₂	3	0	2	0	por	140**	26		14.4	16000	PR	AFP (89728→2751)	Improved	Alive	149

*: THP-ADM   **: Epi-ADM

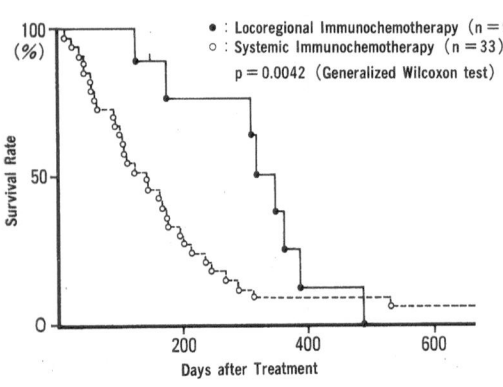

• : Locoregional Immunochemotherapy (n = 9)
○ : Systemic Immunochemotherapy (n = 33)
p = 0.0042 (Generalized Wilcoxon test)

Fig. 1 Survival curves of gastric cancer patients with liver metastases

a) IL-6 Production

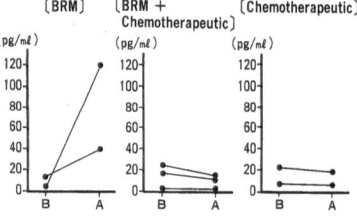

b) NK activity

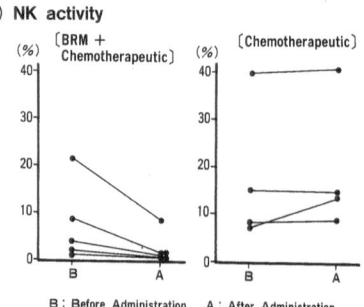

B : Before Administration   A : After Administration

Fig. 2 Effects of the administered agents on IL-6 production and on NK activity in peripheral blood

Peritoneal dissemination

When intraoperative intraperitoneal administration of either MMC in combination with OK-432 or CDDP, neutrophils were predominant and thereafter lymphocytes increased for the first 3 days, whereas no increase of the population of lymphocytes was observed in the control group. In terms of concentration of cytokines in exudate from peritoneal cavity, the pattern of fluctuation of IL-6 after operation was almost similar among those 3 groups, that is, the concentration of IL-6 was highest on Day 1 followed by gradual decrease. With regard to IFN-γ and TNF-α, however, a different pattern was observed dependingon the given agents. The administration of MMC in combination with OK-432 caused gradual increase of IFN-γ and that of CDDP caused gradual increase of TNF-α (Fig. 3).

Intermittent intraperitoneal administration of MMC, OK-432 and IL-2 was also applied to gastric cancer patients with carcinomatous peritonitis and resulted in disappearance of the cancer cells from ascites followed by decrease of ascites. The investigation into immunological response in the peritoneal cavity demonstrated that the neutrophils were predominant for the first several days and thereafter lymphocytes increased. Furthermore, production of cytokines such as IL6, IFN-γ and TNF-α was observed in the ascites and their quantity increased in proportion to the number of treatment courses (Fig. 4)

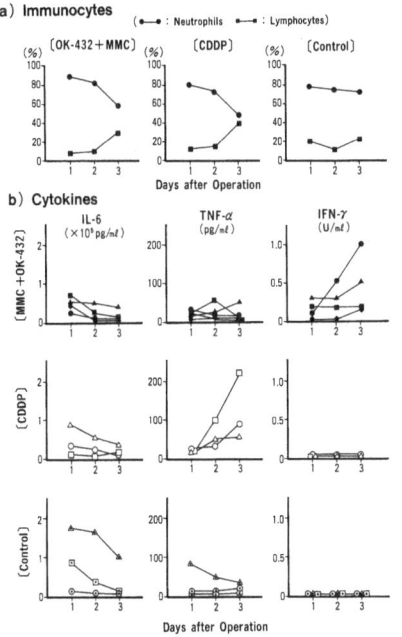

Fig. 3 Serial follow-up of immunocytes and cytokines in exudate from peritoneal cavity

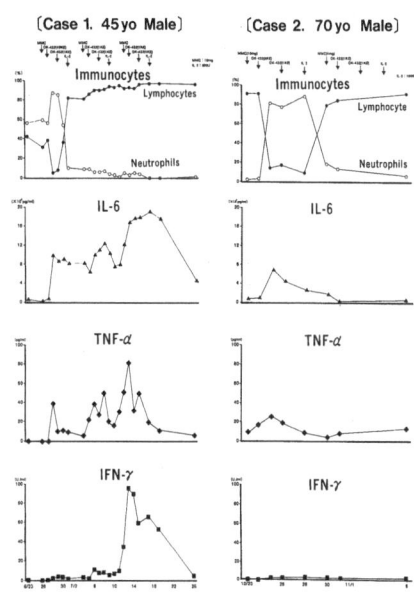

Fig. 4 Serial follow-up of immunocytes and cytokines in the ascites

DISCUSSION

We supposed that incomplete destruction of cancer cells by moderate ammount of anticancer drugs might result in the presentation of tumor associated antigen to the host and it could cause the augmentation of tumor specific immunity. Alternatively OK-432 is multi-cytokine inducer followed by augmentation of cellular immunity against cancer, where neutrophils, macrophages and T lymphocytes expressed IL-2 receptor on their surface could play important roles. Taking these efficacy into account, intermittent locoregional administration of anticancer drugs in combination with BRM(OK-432 and IL-2) for either liver metastases or peritoneal dissemination of gastric cancer was devised.Fortunately this therapy was effective to a considerable extent. In addition it was proved that both immunocytes and some cytokines were induced by administration of the agents. However, the degree of the production of cytokines was different among the patients and endogenously induced immunocytes were various and many. Therefore further examination is necessary, in which detailed mechanism of each agent must be made clear. Moreover, the important factors which influenced the response of tumor bearing host to the agents should be elucidated.

REFERENCES

1. The general rules for the gastric cancer study (The 11th Edition). Japanese Research Society for Gastric Cancer. 146p, 1985.

Suppression of Cytokines Production in Peripheral and Regional Lymph Node Lymphocytes from Patients with Gastric Cancer and the Augmentative Effect of BRM

MIKIHIRO KUSAMA, KOZABURO KIMURA, YASUHISA KOYANAGI, and KAZUNOBU SUZUKI

Department of Surgery, Tokyo Medical College, Shinjuku-ku, Tokyo, 160 Japan

ABSTRACTS

Lymphocytes of regional lymph nodes and peripheral blood were analyzed to determine the immunosuppressive state of gastric cancer patients. the γ-interferon (γ-INF) and interleukin-2 (IL-2) producing ability of lymphocytes of both regions were decreased in the advanced cases. As to the lymphocyte subset, remarkable suppression of helper T and NK cells was recognized.
Administration of lentinan (β-Glucan) as a BRM agent ameliorated the suppression of γ-INF and IL-2 producing ability and the population of immunopotent cells. It is suggested that the augmentative effect on γ-INF and IL-2 production with lentinan might play a role in the activation of immunopotent cells in gastric cancer patients.

KEY WORDS: γ-Interferon, Interleukin-2, Gastric cancer, Immunopotent cells, Lentinan (β-Glucan)

INTRODUCTION

It has long been known that immunosuppression occurs in the cancer bearing host. Recently, it has been reported that one of the factors in such immunosuppression is related to the functional insufficiency of helper T cells. We reported that the cytokines that were released from T cells in advanced cancer patients were significantly lower than in patients with other diseases [1]. In this study, we examined immunosuppression in relation to the stage of gastric cancer patients by measuring cytokine-producing ability. Also, by giving β-Glucan (lentinan) as a BRM before and after surgery, we studied the amelioration of lymphocyte function in regional lymph nodes and peripheral blood, and also measured the change of lymphocyte subset populations in the peripheral blood.

MATERIALS AND METHODS

Analysis was performed on 62 cases of gastric cancer patients who were given lentinan (stage I: 30 cases, stage II: 20 cases, stage III: 4 cases, stage IV: 3 cases) and on 20 cases of non-treated gastric cancer patients (stage I: 9 cases, stage II: 4 cases, stage III: 4 cases, stage IV: 3 cases). Stagings of gastric cancer was based on the classification of the Japanese Research Society for Gastric Cancer. Both groups had undergone absolutely curative operation at Tokyo Medical College. 25 cases of volunteers were used as non-cancer controls. In 22 cases in the pre-operative treatment group, 2 mg of lentinan was given about one week before operation. The lymph nodes located along the lesser or greater curvatures were collected under sterile conditions intraoperatively, and were evaluated. In the post-operative treatment group 40 cases received 4 mg of lentinan every two weeks. Blood samples were collected before treatment, after the first week and after the second week. Thereafter, the samples were collected once every two weeks.

METHODS:
1) Lymphocyte Separation of Lymph Nodes and Blood:
Lymph nodes were finely cut and floated in RPMI 1640 medium for lymphocyte separation. In Ficoll-Hypaque gradient centrifugation, mononuclear cells were collected from the heparinized peripheral blood and regional lymphnodes.
2) Lymphocyte Subset Analysis:
Single and two color subset analysis were conducted with flow cytometry using Leu 2a, Leu 3a, Leu 4, Leu 11, Leu HLA-DR, MOI and 4B4, and the rate of positive cells to all peripheral blood lymphocytes was evaluated.

3) γ-Interferon (γ-INF) Producing Ability:
The cells were adjusted to $2 \times 10^8/2$ ml with culture medium with 10% fetal bovine serum and 10 μg/ml of Concanavalin A was added. The mixture was cultured for 24 hours, and measured with the RIA method using the anti-γ-INF monoclonal antibody (Centcor Assay Kit).

4) Interleukin-2 (IL-2) Producing Ability:
Lymphocytes (5×10^5/ml) were stimulated with phytoheamgglutinin-P(PHA-P, 0.5 μ/ml) and cultured for 48 hours. Supernatant was then added to the culture medium for the IL-2 dependent cell line CTLL, cultured for 24 hours, and pulsed with 0.5 μCi $[^3H]$TdR to measure the uptake within 6 hours.

5) LAK cell activity measurement:
Lymphocytes cultured for three days with recombinant IL-2 10 U/ml were used as effector cells, and D audi cells were used as target cells. Four hours later, cell damaging capacity was measured by ^{51}Cr-release assay with an E/T ratio of 20/1.
The cytotoxity was calculated according to the following equation:

Cytotoxicity (%)= (experimental cpm - spontaneous cpm)/(total cpm - spontaneous cpm)x100

RESULTS

1) Lymphocyte Subset Analysis:
Using single color analysis, the proportion of CD3, CD4 positive cells and the CD4/8 ratio were increased in peripheral blood with lentinan treatment. CD8 positive cells slightly decreased and HLA-DR positive cells did not show any tendency. But no statistically significant difference by this treatment was found. In two-color analysis, pre-treatment CD4$^+$CD29$^+$ cells, which belong to helper T lymphocyte and CD57$^+$CD16$^+$ cells, which are NK cells were decreased in comparison with the control group. This decreasing was related to the tumor growth. Administration of lentinan ameliorated the decreasing of the proportion of these lymphocyte subsets. Especially, in stage IV gastric cancer patients, it was ameliorated with statistical significance. The fluctuation of CD8$^+$CD11$^-$ cytotoxic T cells was similar. However, the reduction with CD8$^+$CD11$^+$ suppressor T cells was quite the reverse, and no significant differences were found in these cell groups (Table 1).

2) Cytokine Producing Ability and LAK Cell Activity:
There was significant decreasing between the advanced gastric cancer patients and the control group in γ-INF and IL-2 production of peripheral blood lymphocytes ($p<0.01$)(Fig. 1, 2). Peripheral lymphocytes in gastric patients following lentinan administration significantly increased γ-INF and IL-2 production compared to what it was before treatment (Fig. 3, 4). However, analysis of patients who had undergone several administrations revealed that such production ability was not dependent on the total dose. Production of both cytokines increased significantly in the regional lymph nodes and peripheral lymphocytes following preoperative lentinan-administrated group. Also, LAK cell activity in lymphocytes of regional lymph nodes and peripheral blood increased significantly by preoperative treatment of lentinan ($p<0.01$) (Table 2).

Table 1. Peripheral lymphocyte subpopulation (Two-Color Analysis)

Table 2. Effect of lentinan on IL-2, γ-INF production and LAK cell activity in lymphocytes of regional lymph nodes and peripheral blood in patients with gastric cancer

| | MoAb Sub popu ation | pre-Lentinan Treatment | | | | | post-Lentinan Treatment | | | | |
| | | Control (n=25) | Gastric Caucer | | | | Control (n=25) | Gastric Caucer | | | |
			Stage I (n=30)	Stage II (n=20)	Stage III (n=11)	Stage IV (n=9)		Stage I (n=30)	Stage II (n=20)	Stage III (n=11)	Stage IV (n=9)
CD 4 "CD29"	Lymp34 4B4	10.6±3.4	12.3±7.3	11.8±6.1	12.6±4.9	10.9±5.0	11.4±6.0	12.8±7.2	11.8±9.0	13.8±5.9	11.9±4.2
CD 4 "CD29"	(Tsi)	33.9±8.9	32.4±5.3	32.3±1.9	32.9±5.1	30.8±4.7	33.4±7.6	32.8±1.9	33.0±2.2	34.0±4.1	30.7±4.9
CD 4 "CD29"	(Th)	10.7±6.2	10.4±8.2	10.8±8.3	9.8±6.9	7.3±3.8	11.8±9.2	13.3±9.4	13.2±7.8	13.0±4.1	12.6±3.0
CD11b"CD 8"	MO1 Leu2a	15.8±7.4	14.1±6.5	13.4±8.1	13.4±5.9	14.1±6.9	14.9±4.9	12.0±4.4	12.8±6.3	13.3±3.5	13.7±6.5
CD11b"CD 8"	(Tc)	12.8±6.0	13.0±8.0	11.9±2.3	10.2±5.4	10.2±6.3	13.0±4.2	15.0±6.9	13.2±4.7	12.6±5.9	11.8±4.7
CD11b"CD 8"	(Ts)	17.3±3.5	17.4±6.8	19.2±3.4	22.7±4.0	22.4±5.1	15.1±3.5	17.2±4.3	18.8±3.8	21.2±4.7	20.9±5.1
CD57 "CD16"	Lew11 INK1	11.0±7.9	9.8±3.7	10.3±4.9	8.8±6.0	9.5±4.2	12.2±6.3	12.4±6.3	11.9±2.8	12.2±7.1	13.8±3.9
CD57 "CD16"	(NK)	5.4±3.9	5.3±2.9	5.3±4.4	5.0±3.7	4.1±2.3	6.0±1.1	6.3±4.4	6.8±5.3	6.1±1.9	6.1±2.8
CD57 "CD16"	(NK)	10.1±6.3	11.8±7.6	12.3±4.8	9.5±4.0	8.5±2.8	10.8±5.6	13.6±8.2	13.5±4.9	13.3±3.9	13.5±3.5

* : p < 0.05
** : p < 0.05

| pre-operative treatment | No. of patient | IL-2 production (U/ml) | | γ-INF production (U/ml) | | LAK cell activity (% specific lysis) E/T:20 | |
		RLN	PB	RLN	PB	RLN	PB
non treated	10	17.3±20.9	4.3±3.2	1.8±0.7	1.4±1.3	6.3±6.0	53.7±23.9
treated stage(I·II)	14	63.8±32.3**	8.4±6.8**	3.1±1.6*	2.3±0.9**	16.3±14.9**	69.2±20.4**
stage(III·IV)	8	48.2±43.7**	6.8±8.0**	2.7±0.6**	1.8±1.4*	14.3±12.6**	63.4±18.3*

Patients were injected intravenously with 2mg of lentinan a week before operation.
Statistical significance of difference from non-treated group : * p· 0.1 and ** p· 0.05.
RLN : regional lymph nodes
PB : peripheral blood

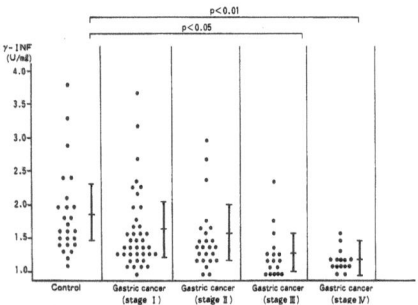

Fig. 1 γ-INF producing ability in lymphocytes of peripheral blood

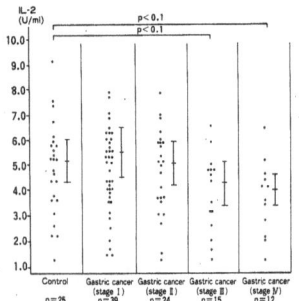

Fig. 2 IL-2 producing ability in lymphocytes of peripheral blood

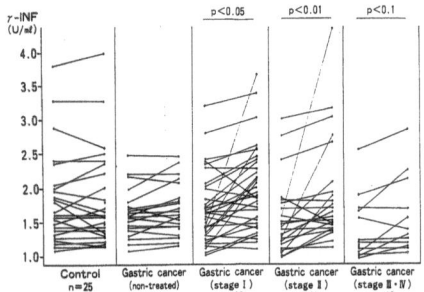

Fig. 3 Fluctuation of γ-INF producing ability in peripheral lymphocyte

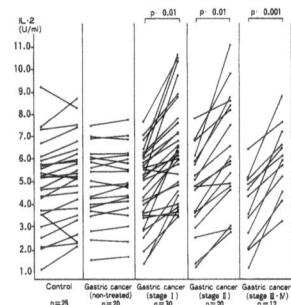

Fig. 4 Fluctuation of IL-2 producing ability in peripheral lymphocyte

DISCUSSION

Immunological responses to tumors are mainly related to T cell cellular immunity. It is generally thought that an anti-tumor immunoreaction appears in regional lymph nodes and plays a leading role in defending the host against tumors. However, the immunoreaction decreases with tumor growth, and then the tumor metastasizes to lymph nodes. General immunocompetence weakens gradually and the tumor grows. Also, in the lymphocyte subset in peripheral blood of stomach cancer patients. NK cells, helper T cells, and cytotoxic T cells decreased, and suppressor T cells increased. The cytokine secretion ability of lymphocytes in peripheral blood weakened with the progress of tumors. Lentinan, a purified polysaccharide of (1-3)-D-glucan isolated from Lentinus edodes, is one of the "host-mediated anti-cancer drug" which exert anti tumor activity through potentiation of host defense mechanisms [2]. Lentinan initially potentiates the PMN and macrophages (Mφ), followed by activating of helper T cells by cytokines produced by PMN and Mφ resulting in the production of IL-2. Then the produced IL-2 in turn activates NK and LAK cells [3]. Our experiment revealed that the IL-2 and γ-INF production ability of lymphocytes in peripheral blood and regional lymph nodes of stomach cancer patients who were given lentinan pre-operatively was significantly higher than in a group given no lentinan, the LAK cell activity of regional lymphocyte increased, and the lymphocyte subset in peripheral blood was activated to protect the host. These facts suggest that when lentinan is administered systemically, systemic immunocompetence is activated, and at the same time regional lymphocytes are activated. Lentinan promotes effector cell response to cytokines produced from helper T cells activated by the specific recognition of cancer cells. Two signals are thought to start the activation of these effector cells. We believe that polysaccharides, including lentinan and cytokines from helper T cells, contribute to the activation of these effector cells as a second signal.

REFERENCES

1. Kusama M, Kimura K, Koyanagi Y, Suzuki K, Tsuchida A, Tsurui S, Kawahara S, Kaise H (1992) Biotherapy 6:744-746
2. Chihara G, Maeda Y, Hamuro J (1969) Nature 222:687-688
3. Miyakoshi H, Aoki T, Mizukoshi M (1984) Int J Immunopharmac 6:373-379

Effect of Splenectomy on Prognosis in Immunochemotherapy After Total Gastrectomy for Gastric Cancer

TAKAYOSHI SEKIKAWA, TADAHIKO OGAWARA, KOHJI KOHNO, and
YOSHIRO MATSUMOTO

The First Department of Surgery, Yamanashi Medical College, Tamaho-cho, Yamanashi, 409-38 Japan

ABSTRACT

This retrospective study was undertaken to gain insight into the relationship between spleen and immunochemotherapy after total gastrectomy. The patients were stratified into two groups in stage II and III : a splenectomized group and a spleen preserved group. Furthermore the patients in each group were divided into immunotherapy and non-immunotherapy group. Survivals of splenectomized group was lower than spleen preserving group. The 5-year survival rate of spleen preserved group with immunotherapy in stage III was 41.7%. It was significantly higher level compared with 0% of splenectomized group with non-immunotherapy in stage III. These results suggest that the spleen is necessary for effective immunotherapy.

KEY WORDS : splenectomy, immunochemotherapy, gastric cancer

INTRODUCTION

Controversy continues over the appropriateness of splenectomy for complete systematic lymph node dissection compared to spleen preserving surgery for effective immunochemotherapy after gastric surgery [1]. The purpose of this study is to evaluate the splenic effectiveness in postoperative immunochemotherapy after total gastrectomy.

PATIENTS AND METHODS

From October 10, 1983, to September 30, 1991, 500 patients of gastric cancer had surgery at our hospital. One hundred sixty-seven patients underwent total gastrectomy for primary tumors mainly located in the upper or middle third of stomach. These patients were classified by histologic stage, as delineated by the General Rules of the Japanese Research Society for Gastric Cancer Study, as follows : stage I 25.7% (n = 43), stage II 15.0% (n = 25), stage III 22.8% (n = 38) and stage IV 36.5% (n = 61). These patients of each stage were subdivided into two groups those who underwent total gastrectomy with splenectomy (SP (+) group) and without splenectomy (SP (−) group). Furthermore, in the stage II and III group, patients were subdivided into two groups those who was received immunotherapy with the streptcoccal pyogenes preparation, OK-432, intramuscularly (OK-432 (+) group) and was not received by the request of patients individually for the side effects (OK-432 (−) group).

All patients with advanced gastric cancer were given mitomycin-C (10 to 20mg) and tegafur (400 to 600mg/day) after surgery. Post operative immunotherapy was started from the 2nd or 3rd postoperative day with OK - 432 and was continued for 1 to 2 years.

Survival rates were compared either with SP (+) group and SP (−) group or OK-432 (+) group and OK-432 (−) group in each stage. Survival rates were calculated on an acturial basis with the Kaplan-Meier method. These curves were compared with the use of the logrank test and the generalized Wilcoxon test. For calculation of intercurrent death-corrected survival, patients who died causes unrelated to carcinoma were withdrawn from the study at the moment of death. Chi-square test was used to compare patients background factors of the four groups in stage II and III.

Table 1 Background Factors

	Stage II				Stage III			
	SP (+)		SP (−)		SP (+)		SP (−)	
	OK(+)	OK(−)	OK(+)	OK(−)	OK(+)	OK(−)	OK(+)	OK(−)
Sex								
M	3	8	0	4	11	3	6	5
F	2	3	3	2	7	3	2	1
Depth of invasion								
m, sm	0	1	2	0	0	0	1	0
pm, ss	5	10	1	6	3	1	2	1
se	0	0	0	0	15	5	4	5
Nodal involvement								
(−)	4	10	1	3	6	2	3	0
n1	1	1	2	3	7	2	1	3
n2	0	0	0	0	5	2	4	3
n3	0	0	0	0	0	0	0	0
Histologic findings								
Well to moderately differentiated	3	8	0	5	12	3	3	5
Poorly differentiated	2	3	3	0	4	2	4	1
Other	0	0	0	1	2	1	1	1
Curability								
Curative	5	11	3	6	17	6	5	3
Palliative	0	0	0	0	1	0	3	3
Total	5	11	3	6	18	6	8	6

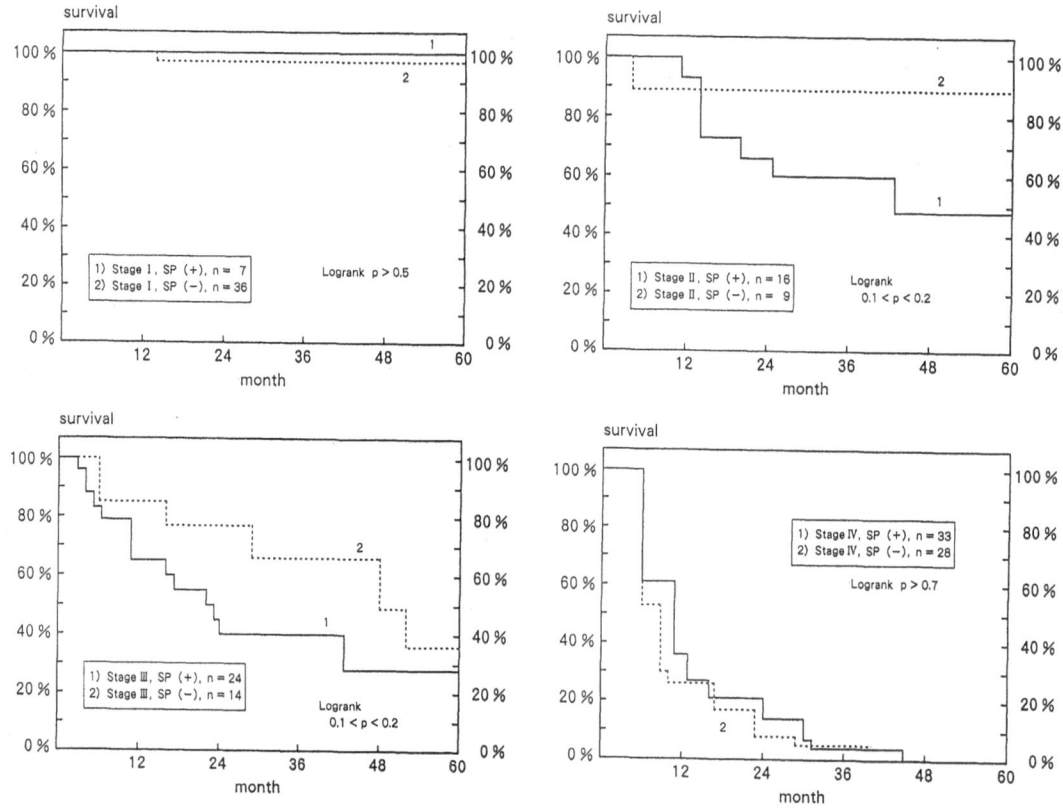

Fig.1. Survival after Total Gastrectomy with Splenectomy or without Splenectomy according to Stage.
SP (+) : Splenectomy, SP (−) : Spleen Preserving Operation,
St : Stage delineated by the General Rules of the Japanese Reserch Society for Gastric Cancer Study.

RESULTS

There was no significant difference in background factors between SP (+) and SP (−) group in each stage (Table 1). Although the 5-year survival rates of SP (−) group were almost same as SP (+) group in stage I and IV, those of SP (−) group in stage II and III were higher than SP (+) group (Fig. 1). Furthermore, to evaluate the postoperative immunotherapy in SP (+) group and SP (−) group, we compared the survival between OK-432 (+) group and OK-432 (−) group. These results were shown in Fig. 2 and 3. The number of patients with palliative resection in the SP (−) group was higher in the SP (+) group (Table 1). However, as shown in Fig. 3, the survival of SP (−) OK-432 (+) group was significantly higher than SP (+) OK-432 (−) group (p < 0.05 Logrank test and generalized Wilcoxon test).

DISCUSSION

Total gastrectomy with splenectomy for the lymph node dissection of the splenic hilum is performed for the effective radical curative resection with the complete systematic lymph node dissection in the advanced gastric cancer patients for primary tumors chiefly located in the upper or middle third of stomach. However, in case of no metastasis of splenic hilum lymph node, there is still debate whether or not splenectomy is the best treatment from the point of postoperative immunochemotherapy. In experimental study, a previous report by Yamagishi demonstrated that the spleen had a biphasic role on the tumor growth in mice [2]. In stage II and III, the survival of the SP (−) group was higher than the SP (+) group. The benefits of immunotherapies are shown when they are used as an ajuvant therapy after surgery or in conjunction with chemotherapy [3]. This current study demonstrates that OK-432 immunotherapy significantly improved the survival of stage III gastric cancer patients who underwent gastrectomy without splenectomy. This effect was not seen in patients who were received gastrectomy with splenectomy, however. These results suggest that the spleen is necessary for effective immunochemotherapy with OK-432.

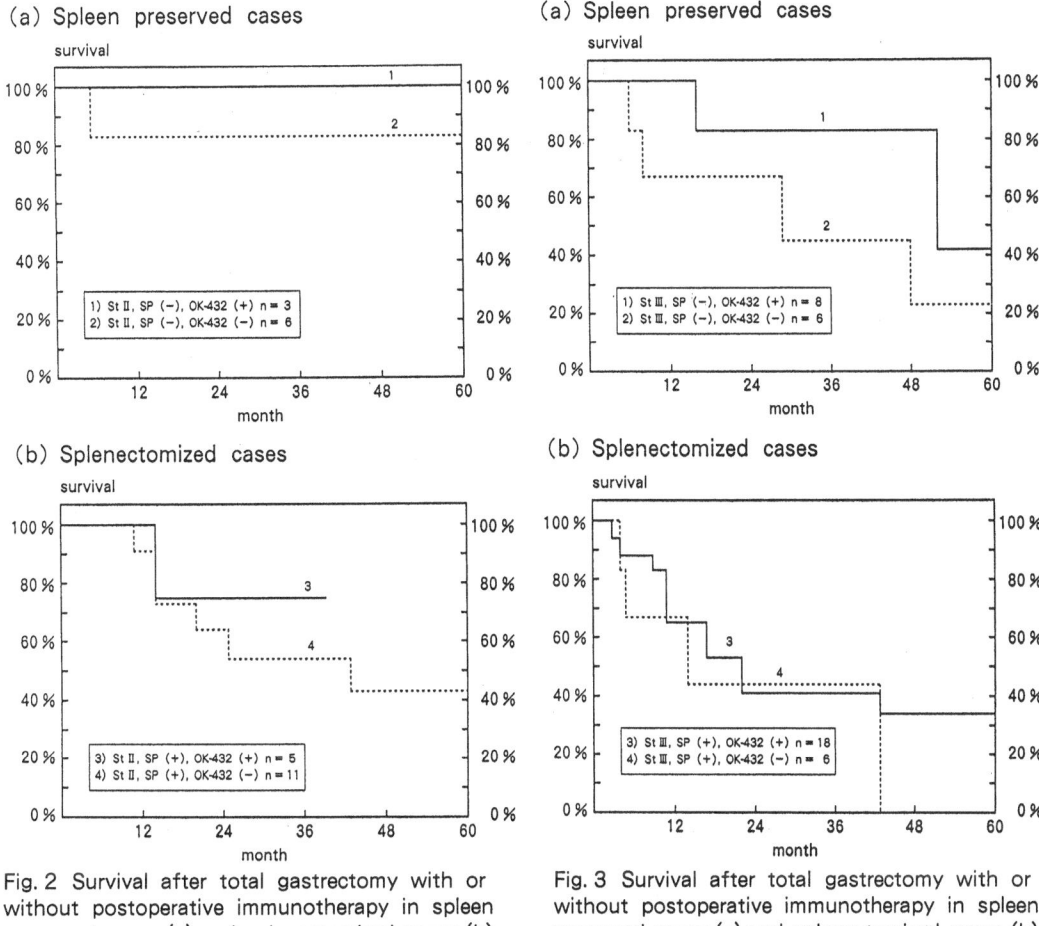

Fig. 2 Survival after total gastrectomy with or without postoperative immunotherapy in spleen preserved cases (a) and splenectomized cases (b)
1 vs 2, 3 vs 4 ; Logrank 0.4 < p < 0.5
1 vs 4 ; Logrank 0.1 < p < 0.2

Fig. 3 Survival after total gastrectomy with or without postoperative immunotherapy in spleen preserved cases (a) and splenectomized cases (b)
1 vs 2 ; Logrank 0.1 < p < 0.2, 3 vs 4 ; Logrank p > 0.5
1 vs 4 ; Logrank p < 0.05, generalized wilcoxon p < 0.05

CONCLUSION

It is suggested that the spleen is necessary for effective immunochemotherapy with OK-432. Because the survival rate of the OK-432 (+) group was significantly improved in patients whose spleen was preserved when compared with OK-432 (−) group in splenectomied patients.

REFERENCES

1. Saji S, Nalazato H, Koike A, Ohashi Y, Tanemura H, Katou K, Sakamoto J and Teramukai S (1992) Advantages and disadvantages of splenectomy and significance of preoperative serum IAP level for adjuvant immunochemotherapy in gastric cancer patients. BIOTHERAPY 6 : 175 − 182
2. Yamagishi H, Pellis NR, and Kahan, BD (1980) Effect of splenectomy upon tumor growth ; characterization of splenic tumor-enhancing cells in vivo. Surgery 87 : 655 − 661
3. Kim JP, Kwon OJ, Oh ST and Yang HK (1992) Results of surgery on 6589 gastric cancer patients and immunochemosurgery as the best treatment of advanced gastric cancer. Ann Surg 216 : 269 − 279

Immunosuppressive Acidic Protein and Postoperative Immunotherapy in Gastric Cancer

Kyoji Ogoshi, Kenji Nakamura, Masao Miyaji, Kunihiro Iwata, Yasumasa Kondoh, Tomoo Tajima, and Toshio Mitomi

Department of Surgery, School of Medicine, Tokai University, Isehara, Kanagawa, 259-11 Japan

ABSTRACT

One hundred ninety-five gastric cancer patients who underwent total gastrectomy were examined for serum immunosuppressive acidic protein (IAP). Multivariate analysis utilizing Cox's model was performed with seven variables including as age, sex, pTNM stage, postoperative adjuvant therapy, preoperative serum levels of IAP and histopathological grading. Postoperative chemotherapy with or without PSK was a significant prognostic factor in patients with abnormal levels of IAP. These results indicate that if patients with abnormal levels of IAP who had immunosuppressive status, they showed good results with postoperative immunotherapy, probably in combination with splenectomy.

KEY WORDS; immunosuppressive acidic protein, PSK, gastric cancer, splenectomy, total gastrectomy

INTRODUCTION

The received wisdom is that the spleen plays an important role immunologically in the tumor-bearing host. On the other hand, prophylactic excision of lymph nodes with splenectomy during total gastrectomy for gastric cancer has been shown to improve the survival rate and it has become a standard therapy for gastric cancer in Japan. However, Japanese retrospective studies on curative patients reported that non-splenectomy patients showed better results than those with splenectomy[1,2].

The aim of this study was to evaluate the clinical usefulness of preoperative serum levels of IAP in gastric cancer patients receiving total or proximal gastrectomy in predicting the indication of splenectomy and the response to postoperative adjuvant therapy.

MATERIALS AND METHODS

Preoperative serum levels of immunosuppressive acidic protein (IAP) were examined in 195 gastric cancer patients who underwent total gastrectomy and had histologically confirmed primary adenocarcinoma. Tables 1 shows the characteristics of patients with or without splenectomy and the two therapies among patients with normal or abnormal levels of IAP. All resected specimens were subjected to a detailed pathological examination, and the patients were then staged according to the 1987 Unio Internationalis Contra Cancrum(UICC) on pTNM staging. Postoperative adjuvant chemotherapy which consisted of intravenous administration of mitomycin C(MMC)(Kyowa Hakko Kogyo Co., Ltd., Tokyo, Japan) (20 mg intraoperatively and 10 mg on postoperative day(POD) 1). This was followed on POD 14 with the oral administration of fluoropyrimidines, such as N1-(2'-tetrahydrofuryl)-5-fluorouracil(Futraful)(Taiho Pharmaceutical Co., Ltd., Tokyo, Japan) (600 mg/day) or 5-fluorouracil(5-FU)(Kyowa Hakko Kogyo Co., Ltd, Tokyo, Japan) (150 mg/day). PSK(Kureha Chemical Industry Co., Ltd., Tokyo, Japan) (3.0 g/day), started on POD 14 after gastrectomy as a postoperative adjuvant immunochemotherapy. Patients received oral administration of fluoropyrimidines or PSK over a period of 3 months.

Survival was assessed from the day of surgery until death or the most recent update. Follow-up information for all patients was obtained by direct patient contact or by telephone contact with the patients or their families. The percentages of patients who have been followed up until death or for over

400

5 years and 3 years were 51% and 73%, respectively.
Multivariate analysis utilizing Cox's model was performed with seven
variables including as age, sex, pTNM stage, postoperative adjuvant therapy,
preoperative serum levels of IAP and histopathological grading.
The IAP level was determined by the single radial immunodiffusion method(IP
plate;Sanko Junyaku Co. Ltd., Tokyo, Japan). The mean and standard deviation
of IAP values for 61 healthy subjects were 356.6±100.5 μg/ml(180-610 μg/ml).
In this study the upper limit of normal IAP was defined as 558 μg/ml[3].

Table 1. Characteristics of patients with or without splenectomy and two
therapies among patients with normal levels of IAP.

		IAP(-)		IAP(+)	
		CH	CH+PSK	CH	CH+PSK
No. case		72	59	35	29
median age(range)		57(36-82)	56(25-83)	64(26-79)	65(39-82)
sex male:female		48:24	42:17	32:3	22:7
pTNM	IA	2	12	1	1
	IB	6	10	2	1
	II	13	7	4	3
	IIIA	13	10	4	4
	IIIB	12	9	1	1
	IV	23	8	22	19
Histology					
	well	25	28	14	11
	poor	47	31	21	18

CH:Gastrectomy+chemotherapy
CH+PSK:gastrectomy+chemotherapy+PSK
well:papillary, well or moderately differentiated adenocarcinoma, and
mucinous cancer.
poor:poorly differentiated adenocarcinoma and signet ring cell
carcinoma

RESULTS

(1)Splenectomy, sex and pTNM stage were significantly related to survival in
patients with normal IAP levels. Postoperative adjuvant therapy and pTNM stage
were significantly related to survival in patients with abnormal IAP
levels(Table 2).
(2)In patients who had abnormal levels of IAP with splenectomy was related to
survival(p<0.1).

Table 2. Results of multivariate analysis of factors related to the
survival of patients according to the IAP levels.

	IAP(-)		IAP(+)	
	χ^2	p value	χ^2	p value
Age	1.681	NS	0.603	NS
Sex	9.513	0.002	0.293	NS
pTNM stage	27.295	<0.0001	10.983	0.0009
IAP	1.728	NS	10.697	0.0010
Therapy	0.010	NS	3.888	0.0485
Splenectomy	4.577	0.032	2.581	NS
Histology	2.206	NS	2.494	NS

DISCUSSION

It is unclear whether the immunological function of the spleen in cancer bearing hosts is defensive or offensive with respect to the cancer and whether postoperative adjuvant therapy is effective in prolonging survival of the patients. Therefore markers by which the results of splenectomy and postoperative adjuvant therapy in cancer patients can be predicted should be investigated. We reported an association between the serum levels of sialic acid and the effectiveness of immunotherapy. Pretreatment sialic acid levels are a good marker for treatment with PSK in gastric cancer[4]. Immunosuppressive acidic protein(IAP) is a glycoprotein containing 31.5% carbohydrates with a molecular weight of 50,000 and a single acidic isoelectric point of 3.0. It has been described a new subfraction of the acute phase reactant alpha1-acid glycoprotein and suppresses both phytohemagglutinin induced lymphoblast formation and mixed lymphocyte reaction in vitro. Preoperative IAP values showed a significant negative correlation with CD4 and the CD4/CD8 ratio and significant positive correlation with CD8. PSK (Krestin) is a protein-bound polysaccharide prepared from Coriolus vesicolor(Fr.) Quel, a member of the Basidiomycetes. It has a molecular weight of approximately 100,000. PSK has been shown to exert a beneficial therapeutic effect on gastric and colon cancer[5,6] and on experimental models. The possibility of biological modulation was raised by the findings that PSK potentiates the activity of interferon, interleukin-2 and natural killer cells and PSK is considered to be a potent inducer of gene expression for some interleukins(interleukin-1α, $-\beta$, -6, -8), tumor necrosis factor-α and monocyte chemotactic and activating factor. The antitumor activity of this nonspecific immunopotentiator is considered to be based on its regulation of host immunity and its ability to normalize the immunosuppressed condition of cancer patients. The present investigation also suggested that the indication of splenectomy depends on both the preoperative IAP value and postoperative adjuvant therapy in gastric cancer patients undergoing total gastrectomy. Using tumor transplantation system in mice, Fujii reported that splenectomy in combination with PSK administration is more effective for survival at an early period than at a late period after transplantation[7]. These reports indicate that cancer patients who have become immunosuppressed following tumor progression show high serum IAP levels probably derived from liver cells stimulated by cytokines associated with immunosuppressive factors of spleen cells. Therefore, we assume that if patients who show high IAP levels undergo splenectomy and are given PSK, beneficial results are achieved.

REFERENCES

1.Yoshino K, Haruyama K, Nakamura S, Matumoto S, Yamada K, Isobe K, Kubota T, Kumai K, Ishibiki K, Abe O (1979) Evaluation of splenectomy for gastric carcinoma. Jpn J Gastroenterol Surg 12:944-949(Japanese)
2.Sugimachi K, Kodama Y, Inokuchi K, Kumashiro R, Kanematu T, Fukuda S, Noda S (1980) Appraisal of prophylactic splenectomy in patients with gastric cancer. J J S S 81:731-735(Japanese)
3.Ogoshi K, Kondoh Y, Nakasaki H, Tajima T, Mitomi T (1983) Immunosuppressive acidic glycoprotein(IAP) and immunosuppressive substance. Jap J Cancer Clin 29:987-990(Japanese)
4.Ogoshi K, Kondoh Y, Tajima T, Mitomi T(1992) Glycosidically bound sialic acid levels as a predictive marker of postoperative adjuvant therapy in gastric cancer. Cancer Immunol Immunother 35:175-180
5.Torisu M, Hayashi Y, Ishimitsu T, Fujimura T, Iwasaki K, Katano M, Yamamoto H, Kimura Y, Takesue M, Kondo M, Nomoto K (1990) Significant prolongation of disease-free period gained by oral polysaccharide K(PSK) administration after curative surgical operation of colorectal cancer. Cancer Immunol Immunother 31:261-268
6.Mitomi T, Tsuchiya S, Iijima N, Aso K, Suzuki K, Nishiyama K, Amano T, Takahashi T, Murayama N, Oka H, Oya K, Noto T, Ogawa N (1992) Randomized, controlled study on adjuvant immunochemotherapy with PSK in curatively resected colorectal cancer. Dis Colon Rectum 35:123-130
7.Fujii M, Fujii T, Saito K, Kobayashi Y, Takahashi N, Yoshikumi C, Taguchi T (1987) Effect of PSK on the serum level of immunosuppressive substance in splenectomized rats. In Vivo 1:151-156

Prevention of Growth of a Human Gastric Cancer Xenograft in Nude Mice with Anti-EGF Receptor Antibody

Akira Tokunaga[1], Masahiko Onda[1], Takeshi Okuda[1], Tadashi Teramoto[1], Tsuyoshi Oguri[1], Itsuo Fujita[1], Takashi Mizutani[1], Yasuhito Shimizu[1], Toshiro Yoshiyuki[1], Teruo Kiyama[1], Norio Matsukura[1], Kiyohiko Yamashita[1], and Goro Asano[2]

[1]First Department of Surgery, [2]Department of Pathology, Nippon Medical School, Bunkyo-ku, Tokyo, 113 Japan

ABSTRACT

Previously, we established seven human gastric cancer xenografts with different concentrations of EGF receptor in nude mice. A close correlation was seen between the concentration of ^{125}I-EGF binding activity and the doubling time of these tumors. The present study was therefore designed to clarify whether anti-EGF receptor antibody would prevent the growth of the xenografts. Twenty micrograms of anti-EGF receptor monoclonal antibody (MoAb528) in an Alzet mini-osmotic pump, which releases its contents over 2 weeks, was given to each animal bearing a xenograft (NMS12) containing 1,000 fmol/mg protein EGF receptor. The treatment inhibited tumor growth completely when it was started on the day after tumor cell inoculation, whereas tumors in control animals grew to 0.8 to 1.0 g in 3 weeks. No toxic effects on the liver, kidney or spleen were evident either macro- or microscopically. The growth of an EGF receptor-hyperproducing xenograft derived from human gastric cancer in nude mice was thus shown to be inhibited by MoAb528. Therefore, MoAb528 is suggested to be an effective antitumor agent against gastric cancer showing overexpression of EGF receptor.

KEY WORDS: EGF recptor, anti-EGF receptor antibody, human gastric cancer xenograft

INTRODUCTION

Epidermal growth factor (EGF) is a polypeptide which, via its receptor (EGF receptor), stimulates the growth of epithelial and stromal cells. EGF may play a role in regulating the growth of some cancer cells in vivo because it produces mitogenic effects on them in vitro. In studies of gastric cancer, EGF-positive cells detected immunohistochemically showed a greater degree of gastric wall invasion and lymph node metastasis, and patients with EGF-positive tumors had a much worse prognosis[1,2]. Furthermore, EGF-positive cancer cells were shown to have higher transplantability in nude mice[3]. Subsequently, seven human gastric cancer xenografts with different concentrations of EGF receptor were established in nude mice. EGF receptor was found mainly in squamous cell or epidermoid carcinoma and was thought to regulate the growth of these cancer cells. Recent studies on surgically resected gastric cancer tissues, considered to have a low concentration of EGF receptor, have revealed the presence of EGF receptor immunohistochemically and shown that cases positive for EGF receptor have a poor prognosis[4]. In studies with nude mice, the expression of EGF receptor has been shown to be associated with the growth of human gastric cancer xenografts. A close correlation between the concentration of ^{125}I-EGF binding activity and the doublimg time of these tumors in nude mice has been demonstrated[5]. Therefore, we rationalized that anti-EGF receptor MoAb might prevent the growth of these tumors, since increased levels of EGF receptor would confer a growth advantage in response to physiological levels of EGF.

MATERIALS AND METHODS

Human gastric cancer xenografts in nude mice

One (NMS 12) of the 7 human gastric cancer xenografts in nude mice, originally obtained from patients with gastric cancer, was used for this study. Relative tumor volume (mm^3) was calculated as $1/2ab^2$ (a: long diameter, b: short diameter). The data for exponentially growing tumors were analyzed by linear regression, and the doubling time was calculated as described previously [5,6].

Identification of EGF receptor in human gastric cancer xenografts

EGF receptor was detected by Western blotting, ^{125}I-EGF ligand binding assay and immunohistochemisry.

Effect of anti-EGF receptor MoAb528 on the growth of a human gastric cancer xenograft

Pieces of tumor 2 mm in diameter were implanted by trocar into the flank of each animal. On the following day, an Alzet mini-osmotic pump containing 20 ug of MoAb528 or 200 ul of PBS was implanted into the back of the animal. The pump released its contents over 2 weeks. The animals were inspected daily, and tumor size was determined with a caliper along two dimensions. On day 21 after pump implantation, the animals were sacrificed and the tumors and viscera were removed for histological examination. Student's t test was used for statistical analysis. Significance was set at the 5% level .

RESULTS

Identification of EGF receptor in human gastric cancer xenogafts in nude mice

EGF receptor in the xenografts was detected as doublet bands at 150 kDa and 170 kDa by Western blotting. The specific binding to EGF was calculated by Scatchard analysis and the binding concentration was found to show a broad range with a mean of 1400 fmol/mg protein. The EGF binding of NMS 12 was 1000 fmol/mg protein. Five of 7 xenografts were positive for EGF receptor by immunohistochemical staining. EGF receptor was positive predominantly on the apical border of the gland, the cell membrane and in the cytoplasm of the cancer cells. Details of the expression of EGF receptor in the xenografts are summarized in Table 1.

Table 1. Expression of EGF receptor in human gastric cancer xenografts in nude mice

	Histologic type	EGF receptor			Doubling time (days[*])
		Western	EGF binding (fmol/mg protein)	IHS	
NMS 2	tub	+	9,000	+	12.5+5.2
6	tub	+	36	+/-	26.2+4.4
10	tub	+	117	+	14.1+1.6
11	sig	+	49	+	17.6+2.8
12	por	+	1,000	+	8.6+1.8
13	por	+	537	+	10.6+0.7
24	tub	+	60	+/-	30.6+5.2

Western; Western blotting, IHS; Immunohistochemical staining, NMS; Serial number of transplantation of human gastric cancer in our laboratory, tub; tubular adenocarcinoma, sig; signet-ring cell carcinoma, por; poorly differentiated adenocarcinoma, +; positive, -; negative, +/-; Left of the bar predominates, * mean+SD

Effect of anti-EGF receptor MoAb528 on the growth of a human gastic cancer xenograft in nude mice

The treatment with MoAb528 inhibited the growth of NMS 12 completly when it was started on the day after tumor inoculation, whereas tumors in control animals grew to 0.8 to 1.0 g in 3 weeks. No toxic effects on the liver, kidney or spleen were observed either macro- or microscopically.

DISCUSSION

The growth of an EGF receptor-hyperproducing xenograft derived from human gastric cancer in nude mice was shown in this study to be inhibited by MoAb528. Inhibitory effects of anti-EGF receptor MoAb on the growth of human cancer xenograts in nude mice have been reported by Mendelsohn and Masui[7]. They have shown that most tumor cells were necrotic by day 7, and that most of the tumor tissue had been replaced with connective tissue by 14-21 days after the antibody treatment[8] . In the present study, marked fibrosis and lack of tumor cells were observed on hematoxylin- and eosin stained sections on day 21 of the treatment. There was no evidence of small round cell infiltration. As antibody-mediated treatments for human cancer xenografts, blockade of the type I insulin-like growth factor[9] receptor in breast cancer and interference with the c-erbB-2 receptor[10] in gastric cancer have been shown to be effective. Selective blockade or interference with the receptors for growth factors, which stimulate the proliferation of cancer cells, by antibody therapy may thus provide a new treatment strategy.

REFERENCES

1. Tokunaga A, Onda M, Shimizi Y, Yoshiyuki T, Nishi K, Matsukura N, Tanaka N (1987) Estrogen, estradiol and epidermal growth factor in gastric cancer as biological markers of proliferation and progression. Jpn J Surg Soc 88:1113-1116
2. Onda M, Tokunaga A, Nishi K, Yoshiyuki T, Shimizu Y, Kiyama T, Mizutani T, Matsukura N, Tanaka N, Yamashita K, Asano G (1990) The correlation of epidermal growth factor with invasion and metastasis in human gastric cancer. Jpn J Surg 20:269-274
3. Yoshiyuki T, Shimizu Y, Onda M, Tokunaga A, Kiyama T, Nishi K, Mizutani T, Matsukura N, Tanaka N, Akimoto M, Asano G (1990) Immunohistochemical demonstration of epidermal growth factor in human gastric cancer xenografts of nude mice. Cancer 69:953-957
4. Yasui W, Hata J, Yokozaki H, Nakatani H, Ochiai A, Tahara E (1988) Inter-action between epidermal growth factor and its receptor in progression of human gastric carcinoma. Int J Cancer 41:211-217
5. Kiyama T, Onda M, Tokunaga A, Fujita I, Okuda T, Mizutani, Yoshiyuki T, Shimizu Y, Nishi K, Matsukura N, Tanaka N, Todome Y, Ohkuni H, Asano G (1992) Correlation between epidermal growth factor receptor concentration and the growth of human gastric cancer xenografts in nude mice. Gastroent Jpn 27:459-465
6. Tokunaga A, Onda M, Kiyama T, Nishi K, Mizutani T, Yoshiyuki T, Shimizu Y, Matsukura N, Tanaka N, Asano G (1989) Contrasting actions of estradiol on the growth of human gastric cancer xenografts in nude mice. Jpn J Cancer Res 80:1153-1155
7. Masui H, Kawamoto T, Sato D, Wolf B, Sato G, Mendelsohn (1984) Growth inhibition of human tumor cells in athymic mice by anti-epidermal growth factor receptor monoclonal antibodies. Cancer Res 44:1002-1007
8. Tachikawa T, Boman B, Mendelsohn J, Matsui H (1992) Tumor cytotoxity mediated by anti-epidermal growth factor receptor (EGFR) monoclonal antibody (MAb). Proc AACR 33:345
9. Arteaga CL, Kitten LJ, Coronado EB, Jacobs S, Kull Jr FC, Allred DC, Osborne CK (1989) Blockade of type I somatomedin receptor inhibits growth of human breast cancer cells in athymic mice. J Clin Invest 84:1418-1423
10. Kasprzyk PC, Uk Song S, Di Fiore PP, King CR (1992) Therapy of an animal model of human gastric cancer using a combination of anti-erbB-2 monoclonal antibodies. Cancer Res 52:2771-2776

Intraperitoneal Administration of Recombinant Interleukin-2 (rIL-2) Against Peritoneal Dissemination of Gastric Cancer

Kenichi Shiiba, Yoshihiro Saito, Ryoichi Anzai, Takahiko Ogoshi, Hiroaki Koseki, Yukimasa Suzuki, Taku Asanuma, Ko Miura, Masayuki Sato, and Seiki Matsuno

The First Department of Surgery, Tohoku University School of Medicine, Sendai, 980 Japan

ABSTRACT

Postoperative intraperitoneal (i.p.) daily administration of recombinant interleukin 2 (rIL-2) was performed in gastric cancer patients with or without peritoneal metastasis. A remarkable increase in NK activity as well as LAK activity in peritoneal exudate cells (PEC) was observed during the treatment, and cytological examinations revealed a disappearance of malignant cells in peritoneal effusions or intraperitoneal washings in either patient examined. Preventive effects against peritoneal metastasis were achieved in 2 out of 4 patients receiving i.p. rIL-2. However, this treatment could not lead to a clinical efficacy in patients with peritonitis carcinomatosa.

KEY WORDS: recombinant interleukin 2, intraperitoneal administration, peritoneal metastasis, gastric cancer, LAK cells

INTRODUCTION

Peritoneal dissemination is a type of metastasis most frequently encountered in gastric cancer at recurrence after a curative operation [1]. As the prognosis of the patients with peritoneal metastasis is unfavorable, it is important to establish preventive and therapeutic modalities against peritoneal dissemination. Interleukin-2 (IL-2) is a 15,000 dalton glycoprotein that serves as the second signal in lymphocyte mitogenesis [2] and also stimulates directly to the generation of LAK cells that lyse fresh human tumor cells [3]. Systemic administration of IL-2 to a variety of cancer patients were conducted to elicit LAK cells endogeneously, but had limited efficacy in a restricted number of tumor types with significant toxicity [4,5]. In the process of peritoneal metastasis, peritoneal exudate cells (PEC) were supposed to play an important role as the immunologically competent cells against cancer cells in the peritoneal cavity. Intraperitoneal administration (i.p.) of IL-2 would allow direct interaction of IL-2 activated PEC with tumor cells, therefore this approach is expected to improve the response rates of the treatment for peritoneal metastasis and decrease toxic effects. In this study, postoperative daily i.p. administration of recombinant IL-2 was performed in 21 cancer patients including 19 gastric cancer, and the clinical efficacy in the treatment and the prevetion for peritoneal dissemination was evaluated with consideration to its immunological effects.

PATIENTS AND METHODS

Patients : Eleven patients with peritoneal disseminated tumors due to primary gastric cancer or cancers of other origins (Table1) were treated by i.p. administration of rIL-2 immeadiately after the exploratory laparotomy. Ten patients with gastric cancer whose lesions invaded serosal layer macroscopically but free of peritoneal metastasis (Table2) were also received i.p. administration of rIL-2 after gastrectomy to prevent peritoneal disseminations.

Administration of rIL-2 : Atom tubes (8Fr) were inserted at the time of laparotomy and the catheter tips were placed in the left subhepatic space and the Douglas pouch. All patients receivd rIL-2 (Shionogi Pharmaceutical Company) intraperitoneally as a bolus dose, $35 \times 10^4 - 140 \times 10^4$ JRU (Japan Reference Unit) in warmed saline solution of 50-100ml through the catheter every day.

Sample Collection : Peritoneal effusions or peritoneal washings were serially obtained through the catheters, and the cells (PEC) were obtained by centrifugation and suspended in 10% FCS/RPMI 1640 medium. When a separation of tumor cells from mononuclear cells was required, Ficoll-Isopaque (FI) gradient centrifugation was employed as mentioned before [6]. Peripheral blood mononuclear cells (PBMC) were separated from a heparinized blood by centrifugation through a FI gradient.

Flow Cytometry and Cytotoxicity assays : Analysis of cell surface markers with monoclonal antibodies was carried out by a method described before with modification [7]. A four-hour ^{51}Cr release assay was used to asssay the cytotoxicity of PEC or PBMC against K-562 cells (NK activity), Raji cells (LAK activity) and fresh tumor cells as described befofe [6].

Clinical assessments : An extent of peritoneal effusion was assesed by a combination of physical examination and US,CT examinations. Performance Status (PS) was estimated according to the ECOG criteria [8].

RESULTS

Clinical effects of i.p. administration of rIL-2 were summarized in Table 1 & 2. Peritoneal effusion was observed in 9 patients (Patient 3-11) at the time of operation and it disappeared in 2 patients (22.2%) after starting the i.p. treatment (Table 1). Cytological examinations revealed malignant cells in peritoneal effusions or intraperitoneal washings in 9 patients (Patient 1,5,7,10,11,14,19-21), and those cancer cells disappeared during the treatment without exception. Performance status of the patients estimated by ECOG criteria was not affected in the course of the treatment. All of the 11 patients with peritoneal disseminated tumors (Patient 1-11) died within one year, which indicated prolongation of survival time was not achieved by i.p. administration of rIL-2 (Table 1). In contrast, two out of 4 patients (Patient 14,19,20,21) without macroscopic peritoneal metastasis but microscopically identified for cancer cells in their intraperitoneal washings were alive for 66 mo (Patient 14) and 93 mo (Patient 20) respectively without any evidence of cancer recurrence (Table2).

Table 1　Effects of i.p. rIL-2 in gastric cancer with peritoneal disseminations

Patient	Total dose ($\times 10^4$ JRU)	Disappearance of peritoneal effusion	Disappearance of cancer cell	Prognosis
1	805	(−)a	Yes	8M died
2	2,520	(−)	N.D.b	10M died
3	210	Yes	N.D.	9M died
4	1,120	No	N.D.	3M died
5	700	No	Yes	1M died
6	2,100	Yes	N.D.	8M died
7	2,345	No	Yes	2M died
8	980	No	N.D.	9M died
9	1,400	No	N.D.	7M died
10	1,540	No	Yes	5M died
11	875	No	Yes	8M died

a (−) Patient 1,2 had no peritoneal effusion before treatment.
b cytological examination was not done.

Table 2　Effects of i.p. rIL-2 for prevention of peritoneal disseminations in gastric cancer

Patient	Resectiona of the primary tumor	Total dose ($\times 10^4$ JRU)	Disappearance of cancer cells	Prognosis
12	AC	1,960	(−)b	1y9M died
13	AC	105	(−)	2y9M died
14	AC	210	Yes	5y6M alive
15	AC	525	(−)	5y6M alive
16	AC	350	(−)	1y died
17	RC	2,100	(−)	4y2M died
18	RC	980	(−)	9M died
19	NC	1,750	Yes	2y3M died
20	NC	1,400	Yes	7y9M alive
21	NC	1,540	Yes	8M died

a AC; absolute curative, RC; relative curative, NC; non-curative
b (−) cancer cells were not identified in the peritoneal washings before and after treatment.

Fig.1 shows the cytotoxic activity of PEC recovered from peritoneal effusion (patient 7) and peritoneal washing (patient 19). NK and LAK activities of PEC were extremely low before therapy but significant increases of those activities were observed after the initiation of i.p. rIL-2 administration. Disappearance of malignant cells in the peritoneal effusions or washings occurred when significant LAK activity was induced in either case. These activated PEC manifested a strong cytotoxicity against autologous cancer cells derived from peritoneal effusions as shown in table 3.

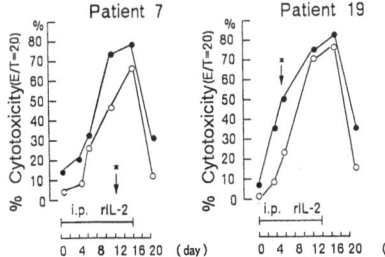

Fig.1　Cytotoxic activity of PEC in the course of i.p. administration of rIL-2
(—●—NK—○—LAK, ＊Disappearance of cancer cells)

Table 3　Cytotoxic activity of PEC derived from Patient 7

Target (E/T = 20)	Days on treatment	
	Day 0	Day 12
K-562	15.0	75.2
Raji	5.5	45.0
Kato-3	0.2	21.6
Cancer cell in ascites		
┌ Auto	1.0	75.9
└ Allo.	−1.0	40.2

a % cytotoxicity

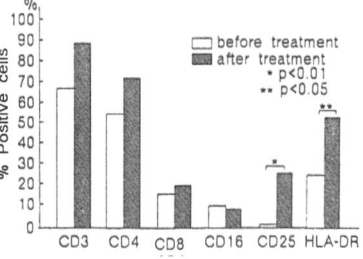

Fig.2　Phenotype of PEC before and after i.p. administration of rIL-2 (N=5)

Fig.2 indicates serial changes of cell markers of PEC with i.p. administration of rIL-2. The large majority of the mononuclear cells from peritoneal effusions possesed CD3 antigen and i.p. administration of rIL-2 induced significant increase of CD25 and/or HLA-DR positive cells, that indicated these activated PEC must be of T cell lineage. NK activity but not LAK activity was significantly augmented in PBMC of patients receiving i.p. rIL-2 and concomitant increase of CD25 positive cells was observed (Data not shown). Main side effects of i.p. administration of rIL-2 were fever (61.9%), eosinophilia (28.6%) and a transient increase of peritoneal effusion (38.1%), but no serious side effect was observed during the treatment.

DISCUSSION

IL-2, discovered as a T cell growth factor in 1976 by Morgan et al. [2], can produce LAK cells that lyse fresh human tumors [3]. Rosenberg et al. applied IL-2 and LAK cells for anticancer treatment, but limited efficacy in a restricted number of tumor types were obtained [4,5]. In these studies, severe toxic effects, rapid clearance of IL-2 from circulating blood, and poor homing of transfered LAK cells at the tumor sites were pointed out as disadvantages of the systemic administrations. In the present study we employed i.p. administration of rIL-2 to overcome those disadvantages expecting a direct potentiation of the effector mechanism against peritoneal metastasis. As a result i.p. administration of rIL-2 leads to a remarkable increase in NK activity and a generation of LAK activity in the peritoneal exudate cells, which is maintained as long as rIL-2 injection continues, and cytological examinations revealed disappearance of cancer cells from peritoneal effusions and/or intraperitoneal washings. Continuing activation of effector cells at the site of disease is induced probably due to slow peritoneal clearance of macromolecules like rIL-2 shown in the pharmacokinetic study by Urba et al [9]. As rIL-2 activated PEC manifested strong cytotoxicity against autologous cancer cells isolated from peritoneal effusions, they must be responsible for the disappearance of cancer cells. Yasumoto et al. reported pleural effusions and cancer cells in the effusions disappeared in 9 out of 11 patients with malignant pleurisy by intrapleural instillation of rIL-2 accompanied by LAK cell induction, and indicated the induction of LAK cells may result in the disappearance of cancer cells and pleural effusions [10]. In the present study only 2 out of 9 patients manifested the disappearance of peritoneal effusions though the disappearance of cancer cells from peritoneal effusions and the generation of LAK activity were obseved in all cases examined. The discrepancy between the findings of Yasumoto et al. and ours might be attributed to a difference of the anatomical sites and the type of the tumors or the dose of rIL-2. Patients without macroscopic peritoneal metastasis but microscopically identified for cancer cells in their intraperitoneal washings recurred in a short time even if radical operations were performed in gastric cancer [11]. The observations of malignant cells in the intraperitoneal washings disappeared during the therapy in 4 patients without macroscopic peritoneal metastasis, in which two patients were alive for 66 Mo and 93 Mo without any evidence of peritoneal recurrence, should give a rationale for a preventive i.p. administration of rIL-2 against peritoneal metastasis. We conclude that this approach has various advantages such as to allow direct and continuing activation of the effector cells at the site of the tumor with decreased systemic side effects, and is justified as a modality for prevention of peritoneal metastasis through LAK cell-mediated cytotoxicity against intraperitoneal cancer cells, but needs to be refined in treating the patients who have already developed peritonitis carcinomatosa.

REFERENCES

1. Kano T, Kumasiro R, Masuda H, Okamura T, Inokuchi K (1983) Jpn J Surg 13: 106-111
2. Morgan DA, Rusetti FW, Gallo RC (1976) Science 193: 1007-1009
3. Grimm EA, Mazumder A, Zhang HZ, Rosenberg SA (1982) J Exp Med 155: 1828-1840
4. Rosenberg SA, Lotze ML, Muul LA, Chang AE, Avis FP, Leitman S, Linehan WM, Robertson CN, Lee RE, Rubin JT, Seip CA, Simpson CG, White DE (1987) N Eng J Med 316: 889-897
5. Rosenberg SA, Lotze M, Yang J, Linehan M, Seipp C, White D (1989) Ann Surg 210: 474-485
6. Shiiba K, Suzuki R, Kawakami K, Ouchi A, Kumagai K (1986) Cancer Immunol Immunother 21: 119-128
7. Shiiba K, Stohl W, Gray JD, and Horwitz DA (1990) Cell Immunol 127: 458-469
8. Oken MM, Creech R, Tormey DC, Horten J, Davis TE, McFadden ET, Carbone PP (1982) Am J Clin Oncol 5: 649-655
9. Urba WJ, Clark JW, Steis RG, Bookman MA, Smith II JW, Bckner S, Maluish AE, Rossio JL, Rager H, Ortaldo JR, Longo DL (1989) J Natl Cancer Inst 81: 602-611
10. Yasumoto K, Miyazaki K, Nagashima A, Ishida T, Kuda T, Yano T, Sugimachi K, Nomoto K (1987) Cancer Res 47: 2184-2187
11. Rai Y, Kanamori H, Tohgi K, Yaita A, Nakamura T, Nagaoka S, Koike M (1985) Jpn J Gastroenterol Surg 18: 2000-2005 (In Japanese)

The Prognostic Effect of the Immuno-Chemotherapy to Gastric Cancer with Peritoneal Metastasis

Yoshio Moriguchi, Norimichi Kan, Seiji Yamasaki, Takehisa Harada, You Ichinose, Li Li, Tomoharu Sugie, Kazuhisa Ohgaki, Kazutomo Inoue, and Masayuki Imamura

The First Department of Surgery, Kyoto University, Kyoto, 606 Japan

ABSTRACT

We evaluated the prognostic factors of gastric cancer patients with peritoneal metastasis who received various treatment including OK-432 combined adoptive immunotherapy (AIT). The univariate analysis revealed that age, resection of the primary lesion, extent of the peritoneal metastasis, chemotherapy and AIT were significant prognostic factors. The multivariate analysis revealed that the resection of the primary lesion, chemotherapy and AIT were the most significant prognostic factors (p=0.0174, 0.01724 and 0.02292, respectively). This study demonstrated that the intensive therapy including chemotherapy and AIT improved the prognosis of the gastric cancer with peritoneal metastasis.

KEY WORDS: adoptive immunotherapy, OK-432, interleukin-2, peritoneal metastasis, gastric cancer

INTRODUCTION

The control of disseminated peritoneal metastasis, which is a major determinant of morbidity and mortality in gastric cancer, is still difficult. No standard therapeutic protocol has been established yet against peritoneal metastasis from gastric cancer. In our previous study on adoptive immunotherapy (AIT) in a murine malignant ascites model, we found that local preadministration of OK-432, a streptococcal preparation, augmented the therapeutic efficacy of AIT (1). Moreover, a consecutive therapy with OK-432, mild chemotherapy, and AIT was most effective (2). Since 1986, we have used OK-432-combined AIT for peritoneal metastasis from gastric cancer. In present study, we retrospectively analyzed the effect of this therapy and several prognostic factors on patient survival.

PATIENTS AND METHODS

Patients

Between 1979 and 1991, 61 patients with advanced peritoneal metastasis (P2 or P3) from gastric cancer, and with no liver metastasis, underwent laparotomy and postoperative therapy at the First Department of Surgery, Kyoto University Hospital. Thirty-two of the patients were male and 29 were female; the median age was 60 years old (range, 29 to 88). Various treatment including chemotherapy in 35 patients, OK-432 (Chugai Pharmaceutical CO., Japan) in 28 and OK-432-combined AIT in 23 patients. In some patients, these treatments were performed in combination. Grading of the extent of peritoneal metastasis (P factor) was based on the General Rules for Gastric Cancer Study in Surgery and Pathology in Japan (3).

Schedule for OK-432-combined Adoptive Immunotherapy

Ten KE (Klinische Einheit: 1KE contains 0.1 mg constituent of killed streptococcus pyogenes A3) of OK-432 was injected intraperitoneally at laparotomy and a catheter was placed in the peritoneal cavity. One, 2 and 5 KE were injected via the catheter on days 4, 6 and 8, respectively, after laparotomy. Lymphocytes isolated from heparinized peripheral blood, regional lymphnodes, mesenteric lymphnodes or peritoneal effusion were cultured with T cell growth factor (TCGF: a supernatant of PHA-P-stimulated human spleen cells) (4) and sonicated tumor extract (5) for 13 days, as previously described. Cultured lymphocytes were transferred intraperitoneally via the same catheter on days 14 to 17 after laparotomy.

Prognostic Factors and Statistical Analysis

In this study, we evaluated the influence of several factors on the prognosis of the patients with peritoneal metastasis (Table 1, 2). Preoperative factors were age, sex, serum hemoglobin, serum albumin and serum carcinoembryonic antigen (CEA). Intraoperative findings were resectability of the primary lesion, Borrman's classification of cancer type, grade of P factor, serosal invasion (S factor) and grade of lymphnode metastasis (N factor). Postoperative therapeutic factors were chemotherapy, hyperthermia, OK-432 and OK-432-combined AIT. Survival distribution of various prognostic factors was estimated by Kaplan-Meier method. Differences in this distribution were compared by the generalized Wilcoxon test. To assess the relative prognostic importance of factors, Cox's proportional hazard model was employed. A p value less than 0.05 was considered significant.

RESULTS AND DISCUSSION

Among the 5 preoperative factors, age alone influenced the survival. The survival of the patients under 60 years old was significantly longer than that of patients over 60 (p=0.00726), as shown in Table 1. With regard to the intraoperative findings, resection of the primary lesion and the grade of the P and S factors influenced survival (p=0.00342, 0.03571, and 0.03110, respectively) as shown in Table 1. Cancer type and grade of N factor did not influence the prognosis. As for treatment factors, chemotherapy, OK-432, and OK-432-combined AIT prolonged the survival significantly (p=0.00845, 0.04451, and 0.02672, respectively), as shown in Table 2. The 6-month, 1-, and 2- year survival rates of the patients treated with OK-432-combined AIT were 69%, 31% and 13%, respectively. MST of treated patients was 7.5 month which was longer (p=0.02672) than those who did not receive AIT (MST=4.3 months) as shown in Table 2. In unresectable cases with poor prognosis, the survival of 11 patients given OK-432-combined AIT was significantly (p=0.02068) longer than that of the 18 patients not given OK-432-combined AIT.

Moreover, the multivariate analysis showed that chemotherapy (p=0.01724), resection of the primary lesion (p=0.01740) and OK-432-combined AIT (p=0.02292) were significant factors.

Based on our previous studies (1), we developed OK-432-combined AIT as a new approach against peritoneal metastases from gastric cancer (6). Our culture and therapy system are different from those of LAK (Lymphokine Activated Killer) therapy (7) in the following points: (a) addition of TCGF and sonicated tumor extract to augment the killer-activity, (b) local administration of OK-432 before the lymphocytes transfer to induce host's effector cells (8). Our present study demonstrated that age, resection of primary lesion, grade of P and S factors, chemotherapy, OK-432 and OK-432-combined AIT were significant prognostic factors by univariate analysis. Moreover, the multivariate analysis showed that chemotherapy, OK-432-combined AIT and resection of primary lesion are deeply involved in the prognosis of those patients. In conclusion, intensive therapy including OK-432-combined AIT may be useful to control peritoneal metastasis from gastric cancer.

Table 1. Prognostic effect of the pre-and-intraoperative factors

Characteristics	Number		MST*	P value
1. Age	<60	30	7.0	0.00726
	>60	31	2.9	
2. Gastric resection	(+)	32	7.7	0.02672
	(−)	29	3.2	
3. P factor	P2	25	8.2	0.03571
	P3	39	3.9	
4. S factor	S1, 2	23	7.2	0.03110
	S3	38	4.3	

*median survival time (month)

Table 2. Prognostic effect of the therapeutic factors

Characteristics	Number		MST*	P value
1. Chemotherapy	(+)	35	7.2	0.00845
	(−)	26	3.7	
2. OK-432	(+)	28	7.0	0.04451
	(−)	33	4.2	
3. OK-432-combined AIT	(+)	23	7.5	0.02672
	(−)	38	4.3	

*median survival time (month)

1. Kan N, Ohgaki K, Inamoto T, Kodama H (1984) Antitumor and therapeutic effects of spleen cells from tumor-bearing mice cultured with T cell growth factor and soluble tumor extract. Cancer Immunol Immunother 18: 215-222

2. Kan N, Okino K, Nakanishi M, Satoh K, Mise K, Yamasaki S, Teramura Y, Ohgaki K, Tobe T (1989) Therapeutic efficacy of sequential therapy with OK-432, cyclophosphamide, IL2-cultured lymphocytes and in vivo IL-2 against advanced murine plasmacytoma. Biotherapy 1: 197-206

3. Japanese Research Society for Gastric Cancer (1981) The general rules for the gastric cancer study in surgery and pathology. Part 1: Clinical classification. Jpn J Srug 11: 127-139

4. Nakanishi M, Kan N, Okino T, Mise K, Teramura Y, Yamasaki S, Ohgaki K, Tobe T (1990) Comparison between crude interleukin-2 and recombinant interleukin-2 in maintaining killing activity of cultured lymphocytes. Biotherapy 2: 21-32

5. Kan N, Okino T, Kodama H, Ohgaki K, Tobe T, Inamoto T (1987) Breast cancer-specific immunity evaluated by a new in vitro method: IL-2 enhanced MLTR (in Japanese with English abst.). Nippon Geka Gakkai Zasshi (J Jpn Surg Soc) 88: 1624-1631

6. Okino T, Kan N, Mise K, Nakanishi M, Satoh K, Yamasaki S, Teramura Y, Hori T, Inoue K, Ohgaki K, Tobe T (1990) Adoptive immunotherapy against peritoneal metastases from stomach cancer: Application of regional lymph node lymphocytes (in Japanese with English Abst.). Nippon Gan Chiryo Gakkai Shi (J Jpn Soc Cancer Ther) 25: 613-620

7. Grimm EA, Mazumder A, Zhang HZ, Rosenberg SA (1982) Lymphokine-activated killer cell phenomenon: Lysis of natural killer-resistant fresh solid tumor cells by interleukin 2-activated autologous human peripheral blood lymphocytes. J Exp Med 155: 1834-1841

8. Yamasaki S, Kan N, Mise K, Harada T, Ichinose Y, Moriguchi Y, Kodama H, Satoh K, Ohgaki K, Tobe T. : Cellular interaction against autologous tumor cells between IL-2-cultured lymphocytes and fresh peripheral blood lymphocytes in patients with breast cancer given immuno-chemotherapy. Biotherapy: in press

Continuous Hyperthermic and Normothermic Peritoneal Perfusion for the Prevention of Peritoneal Recurrence of Gastric Cancer — A Randomized Control Study

T. Fujimura, Y. Yonemura, K. Muraoka, H. Takamura, Y. Hirono,
H. Sahara, I. Ninomiya, H. Matsumoto, K. Tsugawa, G. Nishimura,
K. Sugiyama, K. Miwa, and I. Miyazaki

The Second Department of Surgery, School of Medicine, Kanazawa University, Kanazawa, 920 Japan

ABSTRACT

We had reported advantage of continuous hyperthermic peritoneal perfusion (CHPP) for the prevention of peritoneal recurrence after surgery for gastric cancer in a historical control study. We performed CHPP (CHPP group, n=22) or continuous normothermic peritoneal perfusion (CNPP group, n=18) combined with cisplatin and mitomycin C for the prevention of peritoneal recurrence. The survival curve of the CHPP group was significantly better than of the CNPP group in log-rank test (p<0.01). This fact showed that not only intraperitoneal perfusion combined with chemotherapy (CNPP) but also intraperitoneal hyperthermia(CHPP) are effective procedures for prevention of peritoneal recurrence.

KEY WORDS: continuous hyperthermic peritoneal perfusion, peritoneal recurrence, gastric cancer

INTRODUCTION

Advanced gastric cancer with serosal invasion is associated with a high risk of peritoneal recurrence predicting a poor prognosis. It is very important to prevent peritoneal recurrence but there is no means of prophylaxis. Koga et al [1] introduced continuous hyperthermic peritoneal perfusion (CHPP) combined with mitomycin C (MMC) as a prophylactic treatment for peritoneal recurrence after surgery in gastric cancer. The CHPP is perfusion with massive saline heated to 42 ℃ containing anticancer drugs having synergestic effects between hyperthermia. We performed CHPP with cisplatin (CDDP) and MMC to prevent peritoneal recurrence and reported better results in the CHPP group as compared with the control group with respect to survival time after operation [2]. It is uncertain that perfusion with saline heated to body temperature(37-38 ℃) with chemotherapy has the same effect as CHPP. Since March 1988 we have performed CHPP and continuous normothermic peritoneal perfusion (CNPP) with CDDP and MMC in a randomized control study to determine which modality of the treatment took the preventive effect, perfusion, chemotherapy, hyperthermia, or some combination.

MATERIALS AND METHODS

Forty patients received intraperitoneal perfusion with CDDP and MMC for 60 minutes at the Second Department of Surgery, Kanazawa University, between March 1988 and March 1992(Table 1). Twenty-two of 40 patients were operated for gastric cancer with macroscopic curative resection, and before the closure of the abdominal wound they were treated with perfusion by about 10-liters of saline heated to 41-42℃ (CHPP group) at the peritoneal cavity; 18 patients were treated in a similar manner by saline heated to 37-38℃ (CNPP group) at the peritoneal cavity; and 18 patients underwent only gastric surgery without the perfusion(control group) in a randomized control study. The preheated perfusate containing 300mg of CDDP(Nihon Kayaku Co.Ltd. Japan) and 30mg of MMC(Kyouwa Hakkou Co.Ltd. Japan) was infused into the peritoneal cavity through a peritoneal cavity expander (PCE, Nihon Kayaku Co.Ltd. Japan)(Fig. 1). The peritoneal cavity was expanded by a PCE large enough to allow the small intestine to float in the perfusate, and the perfusate infused to the peritoneal cavity was sufficiently circulated by manual stirring. Refer to the previous paper [3] about detailed procedures. The intraperitoneal temperatures, which were simultaneously and cotinuously monitored with Copper-Constantan thermocouples(Type IT-18 Sensortek Co.Ltd.USA), were measured on Douglas' pouch and bilateral subphrenic cavities.

The pharmacokinetics of CDDP and MMC were analyzed under CHPP. The concentrations of perfusate and plasma of total and free CDDP and MMC were measured before perfusion, every 10 minutes from the start to the finish of perfusion, and 20, 40, 60, 120 minutes, 6, 12, and 24 hours thereafter. Survival curves were obtained by means of the method of Kaplan-Meier. For the comparison of different survival curves the p value from the log-rank test was used.

Table 1   Treatments

	Temperature	Anticancer Drugs
CHPP(n=22)	41-42 ℃	CDDP 300mg, MMC 30mg
CNPP(n=18)	37-38 ℃	CDDP 300mg, MMC 30mg
Control(n=18)		no peritoneal perfusion

Table 2   Background of the patients

	P		N					S		
	0	1	0	1	2	3	4	1	2	3
CHPP(n=22)	21	1	3	11	3	2	3	2	18	2
CNPP(n=18)	17	1	3	6	7	0	2	5	11	2
Control(n=18)	15	3	2	7	4	1	4	3	8	7

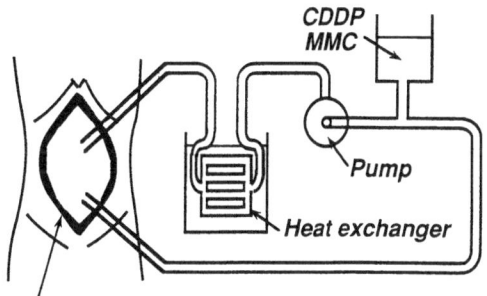

PCE ; Peritoneal Cavity Expander

Fig.1 Schema of Peritoneal Perfusion

RESULTS

The patients with peritoneal dissemination of P_0 and P_1 were 21 and one in the CHPP group; 17 and one in the CNPP group; and 15 and three in the control group(Table 2). The nodal and serosal status were also summarized in Table 2. There were no significant differences in the background features of the patients in the CHPP, CNPP, and control groups. Twenty-two patients died of the recurrent disease after surgery. Deaths due to recurrences numbered five(23%) in the CHPP group, six(33%) in the CNPP group, and 11(61%) in the control group(Table 3). Recurrent sites included peritoneum, in 10 patients; liver, in five; lymph node, in four; local site, in one; and others, in two. Deaths due to peritoneal recurrences numbered two(9%) in the CHPP group, four(22%) in the CNPP group, and four(22%) in the control group. The one-, two-, and three-year-survival rates were 95, 89, 68%, in the CHPP group; 81, 75, 51%, in the CNPP group; and 43, 23, 23%, in the control group, respectively. There was a significant difference between the three survival curves in log-rank test (p<0.01)(Fig. 2).

Table 3   Deaths due to recurrence after surgery

Recurrent site	CHPP(n=22)	CNPP(n=18)	Control(n=18)
Peritoneum	2(9%)	4(22%)	4(22%)
Liver	1	1	3
Lymph node	1	1	2
Local site	1		
Others			2
Total	5(23%)	6(33%)	11(61%)

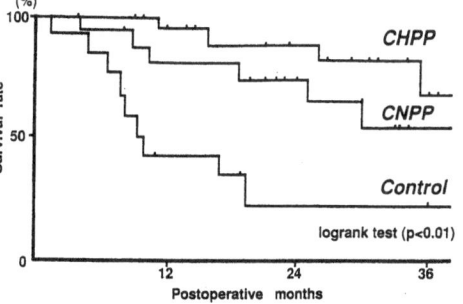

Fig.2 Survival Curves in All Groups

The maximal concentrations in the perfusate of total and free CDDP under 300mg administration were 12.2 and 10.1 μg/ml at the finish of the perfusion. The maximal plasma concentrations of total and free CDDP under 300mg administration were 2.1 and 1.0 μg/ml at the finish of perfusion. While this concentration in the perfusate of total CDDP is much higher than the peak plasma concentation (PPC) of CDDP, 2.5 μg/ml, the plasma concentration of this drug was lower than the PPC. The maximal concentration in the perfusate of MMC under 30mg administration was 1.00 μg/ml at 50 minutes from the start of the perfusion. The maximal plasma concentrations of MMC under 30mg administration was 0.05 μg/ml at the finish of perfusion. The concentration of MMC in the perfusate was lower than the PPC of MMC, 1.5 μ

g/ml, and plasma concentration was much lower than the PPC.

DISCUSSION

Free viable cancer cells in the peritoneal cavity are frequently demonstrated by Douglas' pouch washing cytology in gastric cancer with serosal invasion [4] . Intraperitoneally free cancer cells which can migrate and adhere to the peritoneum may develop peritoneal seedings. Extended peritoneal dissemination, which is never resectable, results in intestinal obstruction, ascites, and malnutrition followed by death. Nakajima et al [5] reported that the 5 year survival rate was 86% for patients with intact serosa and negative cytology in peritoneal washing, whereas none of patients with involved serosa and positive cytology survived more than 5 years.
The purpose of CHPP is to wash away free cancer cells in the peritoneal cavity by irrigation with massive perfusate and to kill cancer cells by anticancer drugs combined with hyperthermia. Koga et al [1] first introduced CHPP combined with MMC for prophylaxis of peritoneal recurrence in gastric cancer. According to their randomized control study the survival rate(83%) of patients in the CHPP group(n=26) was higher than that(67.3%) of those in the control group(n=21) confirming the superiority of CHPP in their previous historical control study. We have also tried CHPP with CDDP and MMC since 1983 in a historical control study and already reported that the 2-year survival rate of the CHPP group was 90% significantly higher than 63% in the control group [2] . It is not evident, however, which modality of the treatments contributes to the prevention of peritoneal recurrence, perfusion, chemotherapy, hyperthermia, or some combination. Since March 1988 we performed CHPP and continuous normothermic peritoneal perfusion (CNPP) with CDDP and MMC in a randomized control study to determine the effect of hyperthermia. This study indicated that not only intraperitoneal perfusion combined with chemotherapy (CNPP) but also intra-peritoneal hyperthermia (CHPP) are effective procedures for prevention of peritoneal recurrence.
The independent effect of hyperthermia against cancer cells strongly increases over 42.5-43.0 ℃ but the injury to normal tissues also increases. Because complete selective heating of only tumor tissue is very difficult today, treatment strategy with a synergestic effect between hyperthermia and chemotherapy is available for the clinical use. The cytotoxicity of CDDP is enhanced by hyperthermia. Fisher et al [6] proposed three possibili-ties about the mechanism of the synergism: 1) A heat-induced increase in membrane permeability to CDDP; 2) a thermodynamic effect of increasing the reaction rate of drug with the target molecule; 3) a thermal inhibition of cellular repair processes capable of eliminating drug induced lesions. Los et al [7] demonstrated increased penetration of CDDP into a peritoneal rat tumor when intraperitoneal administration was combined with abdominal hyperthermia.

REFERENCES

1. Koga S, Hamazoe R, Maeta M, Shimizu N, Murakami A, Wakatsuki T(1988) Prophylactic therapy for peritoneal recurrence of gastric cancer by continuous hyperthermic peritoneal perfusion. Cancer 61: 232-237
2. Fujimura T, Yonemura Y, Urade M et al(1989) Continuous hyperthermic peritoneal perfusion with cisplatin and mitomycin C for peritoneal dissemination in gastric cancer. J Jpn Soc Cancer Ther 24: 1415-1424(In Japanese)
3. Fujimura T, Yonemura Y, Fushida S et al(1990) Continuous hyperthermic peritoneal perfusion for the treatment of peritoneal dissemination in gastric cancers and subsequent second-look operation. Cancer 65:65-71
4. Iitsuka Y, Kaneshima S, Tanida O, Takeuchi T, Koga S(1979) Intraperitoneal free cancer cells and their viability in gastric cancer. Cancer 44:1476-1480
5. Nakajima T, Harashima S, Hirata M, Kajitani T(1978) Prognostic and therapeutic values of peritoneal cytology in gastric cancer. Acta cytologica 22:225-229
6. Fisher GA, Hahn GM: Enhancement of cis-platinum(Ⅱ) diamminedichloride cytotoxicity by hyperthermia. National Cancer Institute Monograph 61:255-257,1982.
7. Los G, Sminia P, Wondergem J, et al: Optimization of intraperitoneal chemotherapy with regional hyperthermia. Eur J Cancer 27:706-713,1991.

Peritoneum

Establishment of Human Gastric Cancer Cell Line (SGC-7901) Intraperitoneally Transplantable in Nude Mice

WANG LONG-BAO[1], QIAN BO-WEN[2], and XIA YAN-XING[2]

[1]Second Department of Surgery, Toyama Medical and Pharmaceutical University, Toyama, 930-01 Japan
[2]Shanghai College of Traditional Chinese Medicine, Shanghai, 200031, China

ABSTRACT

A gastric cancer cell line (SGC-7901) was established in our laboratory from the surgically resected metastatic lymphnode of a female patient. SGC-7901 cells induced tumors in the flanks of nude mice after inoculation. The tumor was minced mechanically, and cancer cell suspensions (8×10^6 cells/ml) were inoculated intraperitoneally into nude mice. After about 2 0 days, marked abdominal distentions were recognized and cancer cells were collected. The cancer cells were transplantable and were maintained continuously by intraperitoneal inject- ion of the ascites into other nude mice with 100% transplantability.

INTRODUCTION

Of all malignant tumors, gastric cancer is the most prevalent. To further study the mechan- ism of the therapeutic effects of Chinese traditional medicine on gastric cancer, a gastric cancer cell line (SGC-7901) was transplanted in nude mice subcutaneously and intraperitonea- lly. After 6 months' experimental observation and examination of pathological sections, chromosomes, histochemical staining and transmission electron microscopic ultrastructure, the cancer cells growing in the nude mice were proven to maintain the structure of human cancer cells. The establishment of this model has great practical value in screening effec- tive anti-cancer medicines in vivo.

MATERIALS AND METHODS

Cell line:

Human gastric cancer cell line (SGC-7901) was established in cooperation with Shanghai No.6 People's Hospital and other institutions in China. The gastric cancer was staged 4 as S(+) N(+) H_0 P_3, with remarkable peritoneal invasion. The shape was Borrmann $3 \sim 4$. Cell line was maintained in RPMI-1640 supplemented with 10% fetal calf serum, 100u/ml penicillin.

Method of transplantation:

Twelve flasks of cells (8×10^6) were digested and cultured with pancreatin in a sterile envi- ronment. After being centrifuged at 1000g $\times$10 min., the precipitated cells were mixed with sterile physiological saline (up to 0.2ml) to produce cell suspension which was then inocu- lated subcutaneously in the right flank of nude mice. The recultured cells of the original generation of transplanted tumor were used for intraperitoneal inoculation. 0.4ml of physio- logical saline was added and the solution was inoculated into the nude mice intraperitoneal- ly (8×10^6 cells each).

Pathological sections:

After the transplanted tumor was minced and suspended in Canoy's solution, cellular morpho- logical observation was made with paraffin section H-E staining. As histochemical study, AB/P AS staining was used to differentiate between neutral and acid mucopolysaccharides.

Examination of chromosomes:

The transplanted cancer cells were serially cultured for three generations. When the transplanted cancer cells had been cultured for 44 hours, 0.8μg/ml colchicine was added. Then, they were cultured in a 37℃ incubator for 10 hours, before hypotonic suspension and Gimsa staining.

Transmission electron microscopic examination:

The tumor tissue was suspended in glutaraldehyde solution made with 2% sodium dimethylarsenate buffer. After being refrigerated at 4℃ for 2 hours and washed with buffer, the tissue was suspended for one hour with 1% osmic acid, dehydrated with graded alcohol series, embedded in 618 resin, and sectioned with a Swedish LKB ultramicrotone. The ultrathin sections were doubly stained with aldehydic acid uranium and citric acid lead, observed and photographed with Model H-600-4 Hitachi electron microscope.

EXPERIMENTAL RESULTS

Observation of shape:

SGC-7901 cancer cell line suspension saline (8X10⁶/0.2ml) was inoculated subcutaneously into the right front flank of nude mice. Protuberances as big as mung beans were recognized under the skin immediately after inoculation. No reduction was observed for 7 days. On the 8th day , the protuberances increased and by the 10th day, they were as big as red beans, while on the 16th day, as big as soy beans. Twenty days after inoculation, the tumor developed rapidly, and had a diameter of about 15mm. On the 21st day, small nodes as big as mung beans appeared around the tumor. These nodes became as big as soy beans on the 24th day, with the diameter of the main tumorincreasing to about 20mm. Ascites occured 10days after intraabdominal inoculation and phlebectasio was observed on the abdomen (Fig.1).

Collection of ascites:

0.3ml bloody ascites was collected on the 12th day after intraperitoneal inoculation in the first generation nude mice. By microscopic observation, most of the cells were red blood cells. 0.15ml of the bloody ascites was cultured in a culture flask for 24 hours. The floating red blood cells were drained after the cancer cells adhered to the flask wall. These cells grew vigorously on the next day.

Pathological examination:

Conglobation or divergent arrangement of cells was recognized in the sections, while glandular lumen structure was not observed. Cells were of different sizes and deeply stained. The karyons were big and the karyosomes were clear. There were multi-karyon tumor giant cells and typical or atypical diversion phase. The ratio of the karyoplasm was high. Histochemical staining, abundunt red neutral mucopolysaccharide was mostly seen in the cytoplasm. By electron microscopic examination, the cells were either oval or irregular with a few microvilli spreading unevenly over the cell surface. The karyons were big and irregular in shape. Nuclear membranes were depressed locally. The karyosomes were clear. Mitochondria, free ribosomes and endoplasmic reticulum were seen in the cytoplasm. Mucous vesicles also existed (Fig.2).

Examination of chromosomes:

With the nude mice transplanted tumor as stained preparation, the characteristics of human tumor cell chromosomes were shown. The chromosomes usually numbered 44-67. Most of them were noneuploid, with the number and the form of chromosomes homogenous to the established SGC cell line as reported. Aberrant dikinetochore chromosomes and giant chromosomes could be seen on the slide glass. The chromosome showed the apical kinetochore in the blood vessels and other mouse tissues extending into the tumor.

DISCUSSIONS

According to the present study on histogenesis, gastric cancers could be divided into two types; the undifferentiated type (similar to intrinsic gastric mucosa) and the differentiated type (similar to intestinal metaplastic mucosa). The transplanted tumor human gastric cancer cell line (SGC-7901) was homologous with undifferentiated type. After AB/PAS staining it was found that reactions in the cell reaction neutral mucous adhering to the wall of the coverglass was mostly PAS. Only a few eres Alsian blue. This result supports the idea that the cancer cell line originated from the epithelium of intrinsic gastric mucosa. A few micro villi were observed by electron-microscope, and mucous vesicles were found. In this case of SGC-7901, gastric cancer had a serosal invasion and marked peritoneal dissemination. Nevertherless, liver metastasis was absent. All these characteristics showed that the cancer categorically undifferentiated type.

According to Miyagi, ascites occurred 4-6 weeks after inoculation. We experimented with inoculating 6×10^6 cells into the peritoneal cavity of nude mouse. Ascites occurred on the 19th day. Abdominal distension was recognized and the skin became brighter. The success of the transplantation of human gastric cancer in nude mice was marked by the following: (1) Growth of the transplanted tumor (2) Pathological verification (3) serial transplantation to other nude mice for at least one other generation. In this experiment, the recultured cells of the transplanted tumor not only had a 100% survival rate in transplantation, but also remain ed unchanged morphologically in serial growth. Histochemical, ultra-microstructural and chromosomal examinations all showed that the recultured cells maitained the structure and function of human cancer cells. A cancer model serially transplantable in nude mice will greatly help research on biological characteristics and experimental therapy for human tumors.

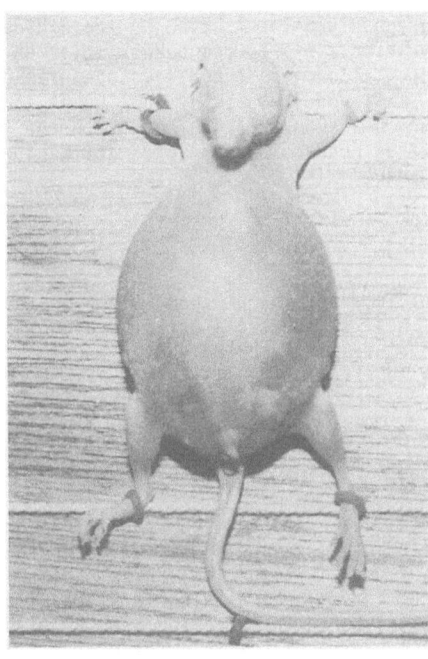 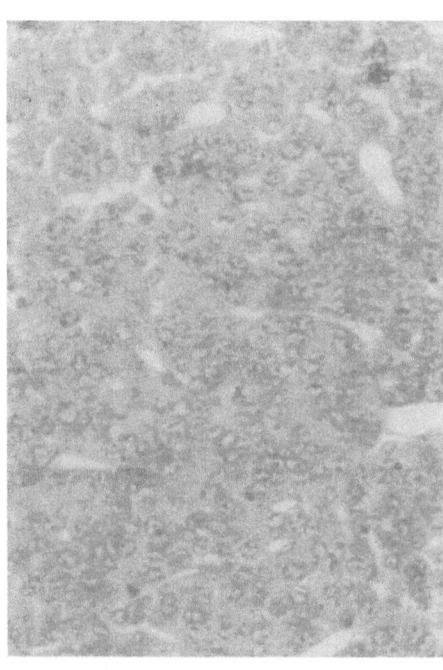

Fig.1 Bloody ascites were observed, 10 days after intraperitoneal inoculation of SGC-7901 cells.

Fig.2 Glandular lumen structure was not observed. The karyons were big and karyosomes were clear.

REFERENCES

1. Kajitani T, et al (1976) Surgical treatment for gastric cancer, Their contribution to improvement in the five-year survival rate. Asian Med. J. 19:915-939
2. Nakamura K, et al (1977) Carcinoma of the stomach in incipient phase; Its histogenesis and histological appearance. Gann 59:251-258
3. Lauren P (1965) The two histological main types of gastric carcinoma. Acta Patholo Microbio Scand 64:31-49
4. (1981) "Application of the Theory and Method of Pathological Tissue Staining", People's Health Publisher, p.72,
5. Yang Jin-long, et al.(1982) Acta Scientia 27:12

Effect of Laminin Receptor Ligands on Peritoneal Metastasis

Akira Yamamoto, Masaki Fujimura, Masamitu Hirano, Masashi Suwo, and Atsumi Mori

The Second Department of Surgery, Shiga University of Medical Science, Otsu, 520-21 Japan

ABSTRACT

Laminin receptor ligand (laminin or YIGSR:synthetic laminin pentapeptide) was injected intraperitoneally into Ehrlich ascites tumor-bearing mice. The group receiving laminin only showed a shorter survival time than the group receiving tumor cells only. The injection of laminin with mitomycin C resulted in a longer survival time than mitomycin C inoculation alone. In the scanning electron-microscopic study, the mice injected with a single dose of laminin were observed to have many implanted cells. On the other hand, the laminin with mitomycin C group showed fewer implanted cells. YIGSR had no effect.

KEY WORDS: peritoneal metastasis, laminin receptor, receptor ligand, YIGSR, anti-adhesion therapy

INTRODUCTION

It is known that the basement membrane acts to prevent cancer metastasis. In this process, laminin in the basement membrane has an important role. The tumor cell binds to laminin of the basement membrane via the laminin receptor and secretes hydrolytic enzyme which chemically dissolve the basement membrane [1]. We have reported on the degradation process of peritoneal basement membrane by metastasizing tumor cells in a immunoelectron-microscopic study[2]. Our study and others have suggested that the blocking of tumor cell-attachment to the basement membrane inhibits peritoneal implantation. As a result, the blocking activities of anti-laminin receptor antibody, TIMP (tissue inhibitor of mettalloproteinases) and others have been investigated[3, 4]. The purpose of this study was to examine the effect of laminin receptor ligand (laminin or YIGSR:synthetic laminin pentapeptide) on the implantation of tumor cells into the peritoneal basement membrane.

MATERIALS AND METHODS

1, An Ehrlich ascites tumor specimen was incubated with laminin for 2 hours, and fixed by a fixative containing 4% paraformaldehyde. The specimen was incubated with anti-laminin antibody for 2hr, following with the avidin-biotin-peroxidase complex, and nickel ammmonium sulfate-DAB. The specimen was observed by microscopy.

2, Ehrlich ascites tumor cells (2×10^6), suspended in 0.2ml saline, were injected into the peritoneal cavity of DDY mice. Each group was consisted of ten mice. The control group received tumor cell injection only. In one injection series (3 groups), 10 μg laminin(LN) (E-Y LABO.), 10 μg mitomycin C (MMC) (Kyowa Hakko Ltd. Japan) or 10 μg LN+10 μg MMC was injected intraperitoneally (ip) on the 1st day after inoculation. In a three injection series (3 groups), 10 μg LN, 10 μg MMC, or 10 μg LN+10 μg MMC was injected ip on the 1st, 3rd and 5th day after inoculation (MMC was injected 2 hours after LN injection). In another one injection series, 500 μg and 1mg YIGSR (Peninsula Labo.Ins.) were used instead of LN according to the same schedule . The survival time was determined in each group of comparison for purpose.

3, In the one injection series (10 μg LN only, 10 μg LN+10 μg MMC, 100 μg LN only, 100 μg LN+10 μg MMC, MMC10 μg only), the peritoneal specimens were obtained on the 3rd, 5th and 7th day after inoculation. These specimens were treated conventionally in order to carry out scanning electron-microscopic examinations. The number of implanted cells were counted.

RESULTS

1, Laminin was detected on the surface of many tumor cell, but the immunoreactivity was not distributed uniformly. No immunoreactivity was detected on several cells.(Fig.1).

2, The group injected with LN only showed a shorter survival time than the control group (15.1±1.9 days versus 18.1±1.9 days, MN± SD). There were no significant differences in the survival times of the groups in the one injection series (LN+MMC:23.3±5.3 versus MMC:22.0±4.3). In the three injection series, administration of LN+MMC resulted in longer survival times than MMC injection alone (29.8±5.1 versus 23.8 ± 6.2). The group injected with YIGSR only did not result a shorter survival time than the control group.

One injection series had no effect (YIGSR 500 μg+ MMC:20.0±2.5, YIGSR 1mg+MMC:24.1±2.3).

3, In the scanning electron-microscopic study, the mice injected with a single dose of 100 μg LN only were observed to have many more implanted cells than the control mice as early as the 5th day after injection. On the other hand, the receiving 100 μg LN and 10 μg MMC showed fewer implanted cells than the group administered MMC only even on the 7th day after injection(Fig.2). The 10 μg LN group did not show any significant difference.

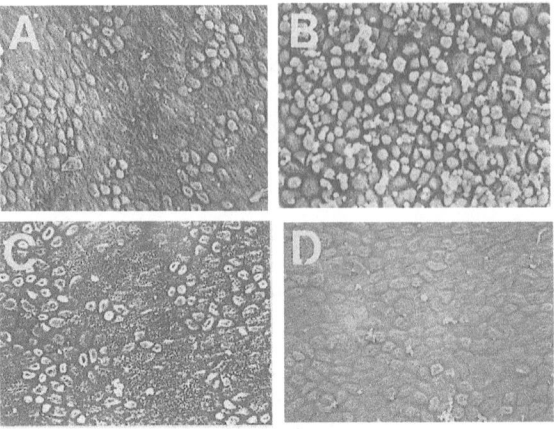

Fig 2 : Scanning electronmicroscopic study.

A : Control group at 5th day after inoculation. Several cells were observed.

B : LN100 μ g injection at 5th day. Many more implanted cells were observed.

C : MMC10 μ g injection at 7th day. A few implanted tumo cells were observed.

D : LN100 μ g with MMC10 μ g injection group at 7th day. Fewer implanted cell were observed.

DISCUSSION

Peritoneal metastasis is the most uncontrolable type of metastasis from the viewpoints of prevention and treatment. At present, anti-cancer agent or immuno-potentiator (OK432 etc.) are usually administered into the intraperitoneal cavity. These treatments have shown good results. Recently, it was elucidated that the extracellularmatrix (fibronectin, laminin etc.)is related to tumor cell metastasis. Laminin promote the haptotactic migration of tumor cells [5] and laminin receptor

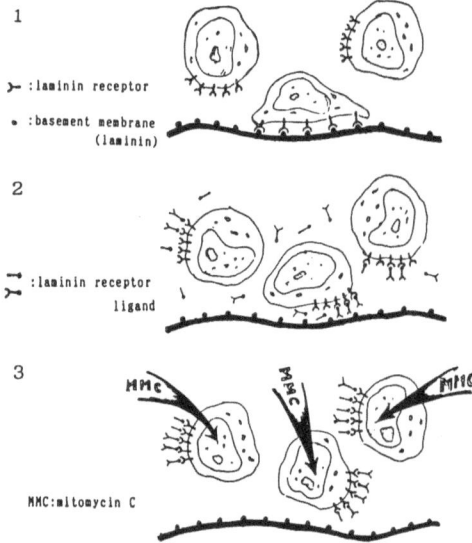

Fig 3 : Block of metastasis with receptor ligands and anticancer agents.

1 : Tumor cells adhere to basement membrane by laminin receptor.

2 : Laminin receptor ligands bind to laminin receptor, and tumor cells can not adhere to the basement membrane and remain suspended in the peritoneal cavity.

3 : Anticancer agents can work more effectively on suspended cancer cells.

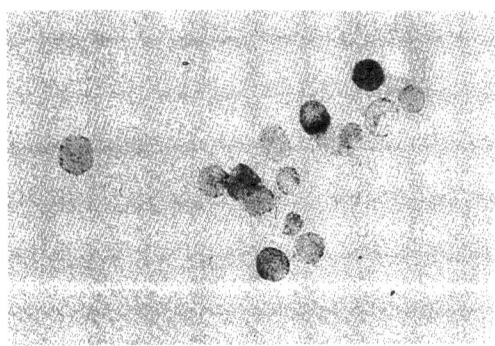

Fig 1: Immunoreactivity of laminin.

Immunoreactivity was not destributed uniformly and did not detected on several cells.

expression was augmented in highly malignant tumor cells [6]. In addition, after exposure to laminin the tumor cells were more likely to invade the basement membrane and they produced more lung colonies [7]. Our previous study indicated that the basement membrane is the major physical barrier blocking the passage of cells across the peritoneum (tumor cells proliferate in the submesothelial space). The inhibition of adhesion to the besement membrane prevents it's degradation and block tumor cell-implantation. Furthermore, we proposed the following sequence which explains the usefulness of laminin receptor ligands in the treatment of peritoneal metastasis (Fig.3). 1) The injected laminin receptor ligand binds to the laminin receptor of tumor cells. 2) The tumor cells cannot adhere to the basement membrane and remain suspended in the peritoneal cavity. 3) Since the anti-cancer agent can work more effectively on suspended cancer cells than on implanted or invaded cancer cells, treatment efficacy is enhanced. Laminin itself was used as a laminin receptor ligand in the present study. Laminin bound to the tumor cell, was detected on the tumor cell surface. The immunoreactivity was not distributed uniformly and the differences may be due to the heterogeneity of tumor cells or to their different stages of development in the cell cycle. Laminin was also useful for anti-adhesion therapy, but laminin only injection promoted the attachment and implantation of tumor cells, resulting in a shorter survival time than observed for the controls. Therefore, laminin should not be used practically. YIGSR is a synthetic laminin pentapeptide whose amino acid sequence was identified in laminin mediating cell attachment and receptor binding [8]. YIGSR was found to reduce the formation of lung colonies in mice injected with melanoma cell [9]. In our study YIGSR had no effect. This result indicates that Ehrlich ascites tumor cells have no YIGSR receptor binding site.

This study was supported in part by a Grant-in-Aid for Scientific Research from the Japanese Ministry of Education, Science and Culture(No. 03670617).

REFERENCES

[1]Liotta LA, Rao CN, Wewer UN, (1986) Biochemical interactions of tumor cells with the basement membrane. Ann Rev Biochem 55:1037-1057

[2]Yamamoto A, Fujimura M (1991) Degradation of peritoneal basement membrane by metastasizing tumor cells-An immunoelectronmicroscopic study-. Acta Histochem Cytochem 24:285-294

[3]Rahman A, Panneerselvam M, Guirguis R, Castronova V, Sobel ME, Abraham K, Daddona PE, Liotta LA (1989) Anti-laminin receptor antibody targeting of liposomes with encapsulated doxorubicin to human breat cancer cells in vitro. J Natl Cancer Inst 81:1794-1800

[4]Albini A, Melchiori M, Santi L, Liotta LA, Brown PD, Stetler-stevenson WG (1991) Tumor cell invasion inhibited by TIMP-2. J Natl Cancer Inst 83:775-779

[5]McCarthy JB, Furcht LT (1984) Laminin and fibronectin promote the haptotactic migration of B16 mouse melanoma cells in vitro. J CELL Biol 98:1474-1480

[6]Wewer UN, Taraboletti G, Sobel ME, Albrechtsen R, Liotta LA (1987) Role of laminin receptor in tumor cell migration. Cancer Res 47:5691-5698

[7]Terranova VP, Williams JE, Liotta LA, Martin GR (1984) Modulation of the metastatic activity of melanoma cells by laminin an fibronectin. Science 226:982-985

[8]Graf J, Iwamoto Y, Sasaki M, Martin GR, Kleinman HK, Robey FA, Yamada Y (1987) Identificaion of an amino acid sequence in laminin mediating cell attachment, chemotaxis, and receptor binding. Cell 48:989-996

[9]Iwamoto Y, Robey FA, Graf J, Sasaki M, Kleinman HK, Yamada Y, Martin GR (1987) YIGSR, a synthetic laminin pentapeptide, inhibits experimental metastasis formation. Science 238:1132-1134

Adjuvant Intraperitoneal High-Dose Chemotherpay with Mitomycin C in Patients with Primary Advanced Gastric Cancer

MASAHIRO HIRATSUKA, HIROSHI FURUKAWA, TAKESHI IWANAGA, SHOJI NAKAMORI, MASAO KAMEYAMA, YO SASAKI, TOSHIYUKI KABUTO, OSAMU ISHIKAWA, HIROKI KOYAMA, and SHINGI IMAOKA

Department of Surgery, The Center for Adult Diseases, Osaka, 537 Japan

ABSTRACT

Gastric cancer patients (n=53) with peritoneal dissemination defined macroscopically or microscopically underwent resection of the stomach (n=29) or resection plus intraperitoneal chemotherapy using mitomycin C (MMC) (n=24). Forty mg MMC dissolved in 1000 ml saline was intraperitoneally administered and withdrawn 60 min later. This treatment schedule was found to be relevant in terms of attaining an intraperitoneal MMC concentration over IC_{50}, 7.6 μg/ml for 60 min, which was determined from the *in vitro* colony formation assay using human gastric cancer cells. Two year overall survival of the patients treated with intraperitoneal chemotherapy (25 %) was significantly (p=0.03) higher than that of those without it (14 %). These results suggest that intraperitoneal chemotherapy is a useful adjuvant treatment for gastric cancer patients with peritoneal dissemination.

KEY WORDS: gastric cancer, intraperitoneal chemotherapy, pharmacokinetics, mitomycin C

INTRODUCTION

Carcinomatous peritonitis accounts for more than 50 % of recurrence in gastric cancer patients. Lower intraperitoneal lavage cytology is positive in as high as 17 % of patients with macroscopic cancerous involvement of the gastric serosa. For these patients, some treatment should be given in order to prevent the subsequent development of intraperitoneal tumor dissemination. Intraperitoneal chemotherapy seems to be a treatment of choice for the prevention of peritoneal dissemination since a high intraperitoneal concentration of anticancer drug is attainable with less systemic toxicity. Mitomycin C (MMC) has been used for intraperitoneal chemotherapy due to its high activity to gastric cancer cells. Conventional i.p. chemotherapy, however, was shown to be ineffective in the prevention of peritoneal dissemination probably because intraperitoneal MMC concentration over IC_{50}, 7.6 μg/ml for 60 min [1], was hard to be attained by the conventional method and contact time must be insufficient. In the present study, we have developed a new modality of intraperitoneal chemotherapy in order to overcome the drawbacks of the conventional method.

MATERIALS AND METHODS

Patients and Intraperitoneal MMC Chemotherapy

Fifty-three gastric cancer patients with macroscopic- or microscopic-intraperitoneal tumor dissemination who underwent resection of the stomach from January 1985 to December 1989 were entered in this study. Patients over 80 years old or those with hepatic metastasis were excluded. Immediately after the surgery, 40 mg MMC dissolved in 1000 ml saline was intraperitoneally administered through a drainage catheter of which tip was placed in the Douglas' cul-de-sac, and it was withdrawn 60 min later. Of 53 patients, 24 were treated with the intraperitoneal MMC chemotherapy (i.p. (+) group) and other 29 were not (i.p. (−) group).

Statistics
Difference in the distribution of background factors were evaluated by a chi-square test. Overall survival rate was calculated according to the method of Kaplan-Meier and difference in survival was evaluated by a generalized Wilcoxon's test.

RESULTS

Table.1 shows background factors of patients enrolled in this study. There was no significant difference in background factors except for age between the i.p. (+) (n=24) and i.p. (−) (n=29) groups.

Table.1 Background factors of patients with macroscopically or microscopically positive peritoneal dissemination who underwent gastric resection

Variable	No. of patients		p value
	i.p.(−) (n=29)	i.p.(+) (n=24)	
Sex 　male / female	16 / 13	12 / 12	NS
Age (mean ± SD)	61 ± 11	54 ± 12	p<0.05
Tumor Type# 　IIc advanced / Borr.3 / Borr. 4	1 / 14 / 14	1 / 8 / 15	NS
Lymph node metastasis# 　n(−) / n_1 / n_{2-4}	3 / 9 / 17	3 / 7 / 14	NS
Depth of tumor Invasion# 　ssγ / se / si	3 / 20 / 6	7 / 14 / 3	NS
Mode of Peritoneal Dissemination# 　P_0 / P_1 / P_2 / P_3	9 / 5 / 15 / 0	10 / 3 / 8 / 3	NS
Tumor Stage# 　stage III / stage IV	6 / 23	7 / 17	NS
Intraperitoneal Lavage Cytology 　negative / positive	11 / 18	7 / 17	NS

NS: not significant (p≥0.05).
#: According to the criteria of the Japanese Research Society for Gastric Cancer

Two year survival of patients in the i.p. (+) group (25 %) was significantly (p=0.03) higher than that in the i.p. (−) group (14 %) (**Fig. 1**).

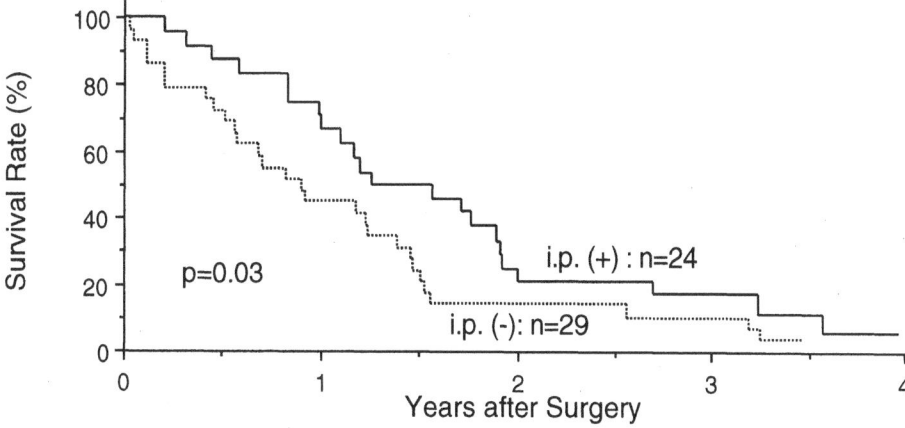

Fig. 1 Survival rate of patients with macro- or microscopic-peritoneal dissemination
　who underwent gastric resection

In 15 patients who had no evident macroscopic intraperitoneal dissemination but were disclosed to be positive after lower intraperitoneal lavage cytology, there was no significant difference in any background factors between the i.p. (+) (n=8) and i.p. (−) (n=7) groups. Two year survival of patients in the i.p. (+) group (63 %) was higher than that in the i.p. (-) group (29 %) but statistical significance was not attained (**Fig. 2**). In 20 patients who had evident macroscopic intraperitoneal dissemination and underwent palliative resection, no statistically significant difference was found in the distribution of background factors between the i.p. (+)(n=10) and i.p. (–)(n=10) groups though three P3 patients were included only in the i.p. (+) group. One year survival of patients in the i.p. (+) group (60 %) was significantly (p=0.004) higher than that in the i.p. (–) group (10 %) (**Fig. 3**).

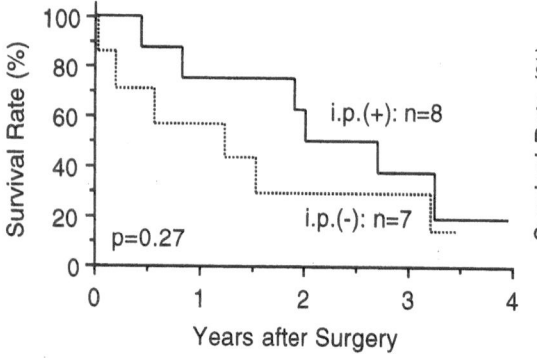

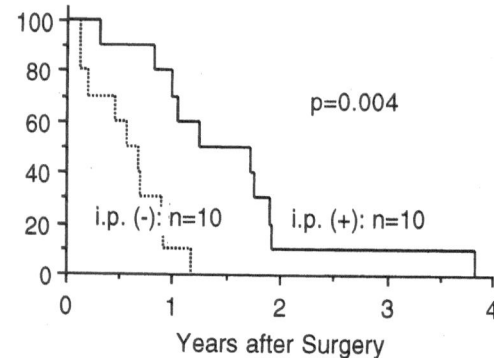

Fig.2 Survival rate of curative-resected patients with positive peritoneal cytology

Fig. 3 Survival rate of non-curative-resected patients with peritoneal dissemination

DISCUSSION

We have previously shown that intraperitoneal MMC concentration over IC_{50} can be attained by administrating 40 mg MMC dissolved in 1000 ml saline for 60 min [2,3]. In the present study, clinical effect of this method was evaluated by comparing the survival of patients treated with or without the intraperitoneal chemotherapy. Reichman *et al.* reported intraperitoneal chemotherapy with 5FU [4] and Sugarbaker *et al.* reported intraperitoneal chemotherapy with MMC at a dose, 12mg/m², which is less than our dose performed in this study [5]. They did not evaluate the contribution of their i.p. therapy to patients' survival. We could demonstrate a significant efficacy of this treatment in patients who had macroscopic peritoneal dissemination. Tendency, though not significant, toward a better survival in the i.p. (+) group over the i.p. (–) group was observed in patients who had no macroscopic peritoneal dissemination but were disclosed to be positive after lower intraperitoneal lavage cytology. Systemic and local side effects of the intraperitoneal chemotherapy was acceptable and no serious complication was encountered in any patients. These results suggest that the intraperitoneal MMC chemotherapy at a dose of 40 mg in 1000 ml saline is a useful adjuvant therapy for gastric cancer patients who have intraperitoneal dissemination.

REFERENCES

1. Kurihara H (1986) Experimental study on clonogenic assay– *in vitro* and *in vivo* chemosensitivity tests of human tumor xenografts serially transplanted into nude mice–. *Keio igaku* 63:387-397.
2. Hiratsuka M, Ogawa A, Ohigashi H, Kameyama M, Sasaki Y, Ishikawa O, Kabuto T, Fukuda I, Furukawa H, Imaoka S, Koyama H, Iwanaga T (1988) Dosage and its safety on intraperitoneal high dose mitomycin C administration as postoperative adjuvant therapy for gastric ancer. *J Jpn Soc Cancer Ther* 23:1574-1579.
3. Hiratsuka M, Furukawa H, Iwanaga T, Nagano H, Yasuda T, Masutani S, Ohigashi H, Kameyama M , Sasaki Y, Kabuto T, Ishikawa O, Fukuda I, Imaoka S, Koyama H (1990) Pharmacokinetics and prophylactic effect of intraperitoneal administration of mitomycin C resulting in IC_{50} of gastric cancer. *Jpn J Cancer Chemother* 17:1541-1545.
4. Reichman B, Markman M, Hakes T, Kemeny N, Kelsen D, Hoskins W, Rubin S, Lewis L Jr (1988) Phase I trial of concurrent intraperitoneal and continuous intravenous infusion of fluorouracil in patients with refractory cancer. *J Clin Oncol* 6:158-162.
5. Sugarbaker PH, Graves T, DeBruijin EA, Cunliffe WJ, Mullins RE, Hull WE, Oliff L, Schlag P (1990) Early postoperative intraperitoneal chemotherapy as an adjuvant therapy to surgery for peritoneal carcinomatosis from gastrointestinal cancer. *Cancer Res* 50:5790-5794

The Effects of Intraperitoneal Administration with High-Dose MMC and OK-432 Against Far Advanced Gastric Cancer

Toshihiro Fujimoto, Masayoshi Mai, Huang Chengdong, Hidehiro Nomura, Nakaba Fujioka, Yasushi Deguchi, Tohru Itoh, and Yutaka Takahashi

Department of Surgery, Cancer Research Institute, Kanazawa University, Kanazawa, 921 Japan

ABSTRACT

As a new therapeutic approach, we have attempted a high-dose intraperitoneal administration of MMC (40mg) and OK-432 (50KE) to control and prevent peritoneal dissemination in patients with gastric cancer. In the cases with peritoneal dissemination and even in the high risk group of peritoneal dissemination, significantly good survival rates were found in the high-dose MMC+OK-432 group as compared with that of the high-dose MMC group and the historical control group. It was of great therapeutic interest that MMC might exert a direct cytocidal effect and OK-432 might enhance the immune system against cancer cells in the peritoneal cavity.

KEY WORDS: gastric cancer, peritoneal dissemination, intraperitoneal immunochemotherapy, OK-432

INTRODUCTION

Carcinomatous peritonitis is a most common metastatic pattern in far advanced gastric cancer. The median survival of gastric cancer patients with peritoneal dissemination upon surgery is about 7 months after surgery, with extremely poor prognosis. Therefore, to control cancer cells in the peritoneal cavity, we have administered several kinds of anti-cancer drugs into peritoneal cavity in these 16 years. Since 1986, we have attempted a high-dose intraperitoneal administration of Mitomycin-C (MMC) and OK-432 (Streptococcal preparation, one of the biological response modifiers).

MATERIALS AND METHODS

Subjects

The subjects of this historical control study include 1) 11 cases with peritoneal dissemination and 2) 13 cases who were clearly supposed to be at high risk of peritoneal dissemination upon surgery. As shown in Table 1, high risk group of peritoneal dissemination was determined here according to the histopathological characteristics.

Table 1. Histopathological characteristics of high risk group of peritoneal dissemination

1. Gross appearance	: Infiltrative type
2. Histological type	: Poorly differentiated adenocarcinoma
	Signet ring cell carcinoma
	Moderately differentiated tubular adenocarcinoma
	Mucinous adenocarcinoma
3. Cancer stroma	: Scirrhous pattern
4. Cytologically positive for cancer cells by saline lavage at surgery	

* Mucinous adenocarcinoma is a high risk for peritoneal dissemination, unrelated to gross appearance and its stroma.

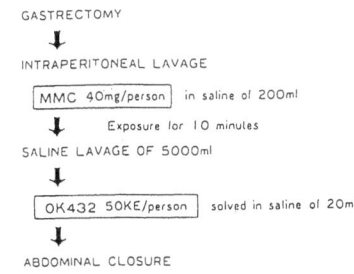

Fig. 1 Method of intraperitoneal administration, emlpoying high-dose of MMC and OK-432

Method of intraperitoneal administration

A high-dose of MMC (40mg/person) and OK-432 (50KE/person) was administered into the peritoneal cavity after the gastrectomy, according to the method shown in Figure 1.

Data analysis

The postoperative survival rate was determined by the Kaplan-Meier method. The significance of differences was analized by the generalized Wilcoxon method. The patients' characteristics such as age, severity of histological lymphnode metastasis and depth of cancer invasion, were compared among the groups by U- test.

RESULTS

Postoperative survival rate

In gastric cancer patients with peritoneal dissemination upon surgery, as shown in Figure 2, excellent survival rates were found in the high-dose MMC+ OK-432 group, which showed significant good survival as compared with that of the high-dose MMC group (9 to 16 months) and the control group (4 to 15 months). In the high risk group of peritoneal dissemination, as shown in Figure 3, excellent survival rates were found in the high-dose MMC+OK-432 group, which showed significant good survival as compared with that of the high-dose MMC group (8 to 14 months) and the control group (5 to 14 months, 22 to 34 months). There was a case of 73 years old male, who was one of the high risk group of peritoneal dissemination, that is, cancer cells were positive by cytological findings in the peritoneal cavity at surgery. He was undergone intraperitoneal immunochemotherapy with high-dose of MMC and OK-432 after gastrectomy. Then he has been alive for more than 5 years, which is supposed to be an effective case of our therapy.

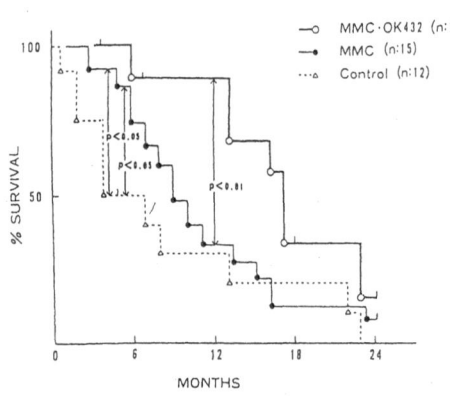

Fig.2 Postoperative survival of gastric cancer patients with peritoneal dissemination upon surgery

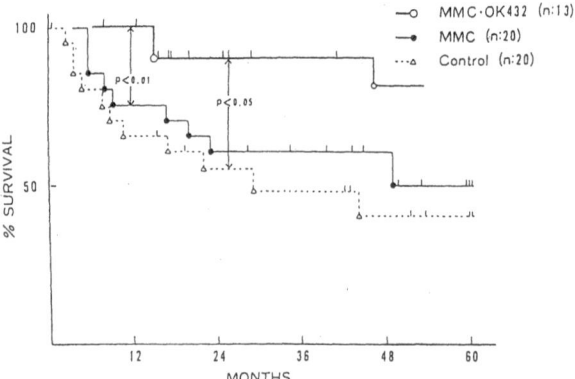

Fig.3 Postoperative survival of gastric cancer patients without peritoneal dissemination upon surgery but in the high risk group of peritoneal dissemination

Side effects

Several side effects of intraperitoneal administration of MMC and OK-432 were observed as follows, that is, fever for more than 5 days in 4 cases, delayed evacuation for more than 5 days in 2 cases, leukocytopenia in a case, thrombocytopenia in 2 cases and anastomotic leakage in a case.

DISCUSSION

In gastric cancer, peritoneal dissemination is the highest incidental metastatic and relapsing pattern and is difficult to treat with. Out of 240 dead cases of gastric cancer reviewed in our department, 120 cases (50%) were died of carcinomatous peritonitis. This fact suggest that an urgent need for the establishment of an effective therapeutic method for peritoneal dissemination. On the other hand, cancer spreading and metastatic patterns presented a good correlation with histopathological type of primary gastric lesion[1], so the high risk group of peritoneal dissemination was designed as shown in Table 1 . The present method was established with the intention of obtaining the greater anti-cancer effects by combining high-dose i.p. lavage of MMC (according to Sasaki et al.' method[2]) and massive OK-432 spray. In this therapy, we administer MMC to obtain a direct cytocidal effect on residual cancer cells in the peritoneal cavity. Subsequently, the effector cells in the peritoneal cavity were activated, and then OK-432 was administered to enhance the anti-cancer effect. In other words, as proposed by Sasaki et al.[2], MMC administered intraperitoneally is expected to exert a cytocidal effect on residual cancer cells by its contact with the cells in 10 minutes, and in addition, about 12 mg of the drug is considered to be transported into the circulation via the portal vein. Our previous study of changes in blood MMC concentration also revealed similar results. Then by the i.p. administration of OK-432, as shown in Figure 4, neutrophils, macrophages and lymphocytes are induced in the peritoneal cavity, and those effectors exert anti-cancer effects via Interleukin-2 (IL-2), Interferon (IFN) and Tumor necrosis factor (TNF) etc[3,4]. As a result of our trial, in patients with peritoneal dissemination and even in the high risk group of peritoneal dissemination, excellent survival rates were found in the high-dose MMC+OK-432 group, which showed significantly better results than those in the high-dose MMC group and the control group. These results suggest the usefulness of the present therapeutic approach. In addition, the advantage of our therapy is that it can be performed easily everywhere, and there is almost no side effect except for fever. But on the other hand, the possibility of destroying effector cells in the peritoneal cavity by massive administration of MMC is also likely that optimal doses of MMC and OK-432 and suitable protocol for administration should be further considered in the future.

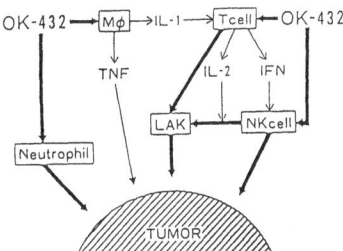

Fig 4. Effects of OK-432 in the peritoneal cavity

REFERENCES

1. Mai M, Takahashi Y, Ueno M (1987) Multimodal therapy for gastric cancer based on biological variability. Oncologia 20:66-76
2. Sasaki M, Ogita M (1980) Mass washing-off therapy of Mitomycin-C in the peritoneal cavity in the surgery of gastric cancer. Jpn J Cancer Chemother 7:1421-1431
3. Fujimoto T, Mai M, Omote K, Ueda H, Takahashi Y, Ogino T (1989) Intra-operative immunochemotherapy against peritoneal dissemination of gastric cancer with high-dose administration of intraperitoneal Mitomycin-C and OK-432. Biotherapy 4:95-100
4. Toge T, Yamada H, Hattori T (1985) Effects of intraperitoneal administration of OK-432 for patients with advanced cancer. Jpn J Surg 15:260-265

Intraperitoneal Administration of Cisplatin for Patients with Gastric Cancer and Peritoneal Dissemination

SHUNICHI TSUJITANI[1], AKIHIRO WATANABE[2], YOSHISHIGE ABE[2], and NOBUAKI KAIBARA[1]

[1]The First Department of Surgery, School of Medicine, Tottori University, Yonago, Tottori, 683 Japan
[2]The Department of Surgery, Saga Prefectural Hospital, Saga, 840 Japan

ABSTRACT

We investigated the efficacy of intraperitoneal administration (IP) of cisplatin in 82 patients with gastric cancer having peritoneal seeding but no liver metastases. Cisplatin IP was given to 45 patients immediately after gastrectomy while 37 controls were treated with intravenous mitomycin C on the day of their gastrectomy and daily oral tegafur (N1-(2'-tetrahydrofuryl)-5-fluorouracil) postoperatively. The dose of cisplatin was 25 to 200 mg (89.4 mg in average). Side effects and postoperative complications after cisplatin IP were limited as much as mitomycin C and tegafur. Patients given cisplatin survived longer than the controls (P<0.05). The 3-year survival rate was 14.2% in those given cisplatin, but only 3.2% in the control group. Significant difference in survival was seen particularly in those with the undifferentiated type gastric cancer which often spread to the peritoneum. Cisplatin IP was effective in patients with severe peritoneal dissemination. These results demonstrate that intraperitoneal cisplatin after gastrectomy is safe and suitable for the treatment of patients with gastric cancer and peritoneal dissemination.

KEY WORDS: gastric cancer, intraperitoneal chemotherapy, cisplatin

INTRODUCTION

Peritoneal dissemination of gastric cancer is one of the most common cause of surgical incurability. Patients with severe peritoneal dissemination are likely to die within 1 year. Although cytoreductive surgery results in relapse of the disease, patients treated with gastrectomy survive longer than those undergoing laparotomy alone. There has been no effective therapy with intravenous or oral administration of antitumor drugs for gastric cancer with peritoneal dissemination. In our laboratory, the feasibility of continuous hyperthermic peritoneal perfusion (CHPP) with a solution that contains anti-cancer drugs for peritoneal cancer was studied experimentally [1]. CHPP with mitomycin C is a safe, effective and clinically available therapy for peritoneal dissemination of gastric cancer [2]. When combined with gastrectomy, however, CHPP is complicated in setting the instrument and takes an additional or 2 hours for treatment. Recently, intraperitoneal administration (IP) of the immunological response modifier OK-432 [3], or mitomycin C adsorbed onto activated charcoal [4] have been tried in Japan on attempt to control the disease. Many investigators reported that cisplatin is one of the most effective agents in gastric carcinoma [5]. We have administered intraperitoneal cisplatin during gastric resection for treating peritoneal dissemination. We report here on the therapeutic effects and side effects of cisplatin IP on patients with gastric cancer and peritoneal dissemination.

MATERIALS AND METHODS

From 1978 to 1990, cisplatin IP was given during surgery to 45 gastric cancer patients with peritoneal seeding and no liver metastasis, at the Department of Surgery, Saga Prefectural Hospital. No patient had undergone preoperative chemotherapy. Immediately after gastrectomy, cisplatin was injected into the peritoneal cavity before the closing of the abdominal wall. Twenty-five to 200 mg of cisplatin was administered without dilution to each patient. An additional 1500 ml of saline and 300 ml of 20% D-mannitol were given intravenously to prevent postoperative renal failure. One patient died from cerebral infarction within a month after surgery. The control group in this study consisted of 37 gastric cancer patients with peritoneal seeding and no liver metastasis who underwent gastrectomy. In these patients, 20 mg of mitomycin C was given on the day of operation, and 600 mg of daily oral tegafur (N1-(2'-tetrahydrofuryl)-5-fluorouracil) was started 2 weeks after the operation. One patient died from cerebral infarction within a month after surgery. The patients were not randomized into each group although cisplatin IP was given to patients without selection. There was no significant difference between those given cisplatin IP and the controls in a number of clinicopathologic features including patient's age, sex and histologic type of tumor. All patients were scrutinized according to the criteria described in the general rules from the Japanese Research Society for Gastric Cancer [6]. The findings of peritoneal dissemination were classified as follows: P1; disseminating metastasis to the adjacent peritoneum (above the transverse colon and including the greater omentum), P2; a few scattered metastases to the distant peritoneum (applicable to cases in which there is only ovarian metastasis), P3; numerous metastases to the distant peritoneum. Lymph node metastases were observed in all patients, however, the extent of lymph node metastasis could not be confirmed histologically because of lack of radical lymph node dissection.

RESULTS

Complications

The complications experienced in the cisplatin and control groups were respectively as follows; 3 (7%) and 2 (5%) in nausea or vomiting, 4 (9%) and 7 (19%) in pleural effusion, 2 (4%) and 2 (5%) in ileus, 2 (4%) and 1 (3%) in anastomotic leakage, 1 (2%) and 1 (3%) in subphrenic abscess, 1 (2%) and none in renal dysfunction (creatinine>1.5 mg/100ml), 5 (11%) and 1 (3%) in liver dysfunction (GOT>100 unit/L), 3 (7%) and 2 (5%) in leukopenia (<3,000) and 3 (7%) and none in thrombocytopenia (<100,000). No patient required vigorous antiemetic therapy and only three experienced nausea and vomiting in the cisplatin IP group. The incidence of these symptoms was nearly the same in the two groups. No patient developed signs or symptoms of peripheral neuropathy. Serum creatinine levels were elevated in one patient but no one suffered severe renal toxicity. There were no drug-related deaths in the current study.

Survival

The postoperative survival for the patients studied was compared (Table 1). The 3-year survival rate of those given cisplatin IP was 14.2%, whereas that of the controls was only 3.2%. A log-rank test revealed that those given cisplatin IP survived longer than the controls (P<0.05). According to the criteria for gastric cancer, the extent of peritoneal dissemination was classified into the P1, P2 and P3 groups. There was no significant difference in survival between those given cisplatin IP and the controls in the limited peritoneal dissemination (P1 and P2 groups). However, patients with severe peritoneal dissemination (P3 group) given cisplatin IP survived longer (P<0.05) and had a better 1-year survival rate (47%) than the controls (0%). Survival was also compared between the groups with special reference to the histologic type of cancer. There was no significant difference between the groups in those with differentiated adenocarcinoma. In patients with undifferentiated adenocarcinoma, however, those given cisplatin IP survived longer than the controls (P<0.01). The 3-year survival rate of patients with cisplatin IP was 20.1%, whereas that of the controls was 0% .

Table 1. Survival of patients with gastric cancer and peritoneal dissemination

Extent of Peritoneal Dissemination	Chemotherapy	No. of Patient	Survival Rate		
			1-year	2-year	3-year
Limited (P1, P2)	Cisplatin IP	27	52.3%	39.2%	29.4%
	Control	31	46.5%	11.6%	3.8%
Severe (P3)	Cisplatin IP	18	47.1%	17.7%	5.8%
	Control	6	0.0%		
All cases	Cisplatin IP	45	50.2%	18.9%	14.2%
	Control	37	38.0%	9.5%	3.2%

DISCUSSION

The prognosis of gastrointestinal cancer patients with peritoneal effusions is poor. The 50% survival rate for patients with malignant effusions was 2 months when the primary focus was resected, irrespective of any intraperitoneal or intravenous administration of antitumor drugs [7]. Bleomycin IP showed no efficacy on peritoneal dissemination of gastric cancer [8,9]. Since anti-tumor drugs given intraperitoneally can transfer through the large surface of the peritoneum into the blood, it is difficult to maintain a high intraperitoneal drug level to achieve maximal cytocidal effects [10]. Hagiwara et al. [4] reported IP of mitomycin C adsorbed onto activated charcoal (2.0 to 2.4 mg/kg of mitomycin C) to effect a slow, steady release of the drug. This approach may maintain a certain level of intraperitoneal mitomycin C. Biological response modifier OK-432, a compound composed of penicillin-treated, attenuated Streptococcus pyogenes of human origin, was given intraperitoneally to patients with peritoneal effusion and showed a favorable response [3]. It may be an excellent strategy for peritoneal dissemination to use immunological defense mechanisms against cancer, if its cytocidal potential can be activated continuously.

In the current study, we investigated the effects of intraoperative cisplatin IP in combination with gastrectomy in patients with gastric cancer and peritoneal dissemination but no liver metastasis. Intravenous mitomycin C and oral tegafur in the control group is one of the most popular regimens of postoperative chemotherapy for gastric cancer in Japan [11]. Survival in the cisplatin IP treated group was significantly superior to those given mitomycin C and tegafur. Direct tumor penetration from free-surface diffusion is quite limited with intraperitoneal cisplatin. The highest cisplatin concentrations were in the outermost 1 to 3 mm of the tumor from the peritoneal surface [12]. Following cisplatin IP, drug is also delivered to tumor by capillary flow as a result of significant uptake into the systemic circulation. In cisplatin IP, both of direct and systemic routes of drug delivery may be important to overcome the resistance of peritoneal metastases to antitumor drugs.

The toxic effects of cisplatin are bone marrow suppression, impaired renal function, nausea and vomiting, and hearing loss. The clinical use, however, is mainly limited by nephrotoxicity and nausea. Clinical nephrotoxicity is manifested by elevations of blood urea nitrogen and serum creatinine. In the current study, renal functional impairment was not more frequent in the cisplatin IP group than in the control group. Furthermore, nausea and vomiting with cisplatin IP were rare, and vigorous antiemetic therapy was not required. This is probably attributable to the lingering effect of anesthesia and the slow elevation of the plasma cisplatin concentration. IP chemotherapy results in a high concentration of drug in the peritoneal cavity, while its plasma concentration and systemic toxicity remain low [13]. Therefore, cisplatin IP is not only tolerable but also reasonable route of administration.

The dose of cisplatin IP ranged from 25 to 200 mg, with an average of 89.4 mg to each patient. It ranged from 16.8 to 138.9 mg/m^2 with an average of 63.5 mg/m^2. In the current study, toxicity did not correlate with the dose of cisplatin. However, in the past one patient with gastric cancer having both peritoneal and liver metastases was given 200 mg (150 mg/m^2) of cisplatin IP after gastrectomy and died due to a leakage of the anastomosis. We therefore recommend a cisplatin IP dose of 60 to 130 mg/m^2. Although previous studies have suggested a dose-dependent response to cisplatin for the treatment of ovarian cancer [14], our study revealed no correlation between the dose of cisplatin and patients' survival times.

Tumor heterogeneity between the primary and metastatic lesions has long been discussed. The relationship between the metastatic potential and the properties of tumor cells such as growth rate, adhesive character, biochemical change on the cell surface, have been studied. However, little is known about the heterogeneity of drug sensitivity. With some chemosensitivity tests for antitumor drugs, there has been poor correlation between the primary and metastatic lesions and the results have been attributed to heterogeneity [15,16]. Undifferentiated adenocarcinoma of the stomach often spreads to the peritoneum, and the difference in survival was observed in patients with undifferentiated carcinoma. Therefore, cisplatin would be expected to be more effective for patients with peritoneal dissemination than the other agents.

Although this is not a randomized study, its results are important and likely to be confirmed by randomized studies because there was no intentional selection of less ill patients for the cisplatin IP arm. These promising results indicate that a randomized, controlled study of cisplatin IP for the treatment of peritoneal seeding of gastric cancer is required.

REFERENCES

1. Koga S, Hamazoe R, Maeta M, Shimizu N, Kanayama H, Osaki Y (1984) Treatment of implanted peritoneal cancer in rats by continuous hyperthermic peritoneal perfusion in combination with an anticancer drug. Cancer Res 44:1840-1842
2. Koga S, Hamazoe R, Maeta M, Shimizu N, Murakami A, Wakatsuki T (1988) Prophylactic therapy for peritoneal recurrence of gastric cancer by continuous hyperthermic peritoneal perfusion with mitomycin C. Cancer 61:232-237
3. Torisu M, Katano M, Kimura Y, Ito H, Takesue M (1983) New approach to management of malignant ascites with a streptococcal preparation, OK-432: Improvement of host immunity and prolongation of survival. Surgery 93:357-364
4. Hagiwara A, Takahashi T, Lee R, Ueda T, Takeda M, Ito T (1987) Chemotherapy for carcinomatous peritonitis and pleuritis with MMC-CH, mitomycin C adsorbed on activated carbon particles. Cancer 59:43-49
5. Elliott TE, Moertel CG, Wieand HS, Hahn RG, Gerstner JB, Tschetter LK, Mailliard JA (1990) A phase II study of etoposide and cisplatin in the therapy of advanced gastric cancer. Cancer 65:1491-1494
6. Japanese Research Society for Gastric Cancer (1981) The general rules for gastric cancer study in surgery and pathology. Jpn J Surg 11:291-296
7. Yamada S, Takeda T, Matsumoto K (1983) Prognostic analysis of malignant pleural and peritoneal effusion. Cancer 51:136-140
8. Pladine W, Cunningham TJ, Sponzo R, Donavan M, Olson K, Horton J (1976) Intracavitary bleomycin in the management of malignant effusions. Cancer 38:1903-1908
9. Ostrowski MJ (1986) An assessment of the long-term results of controlling the reaccumulation of malignant effusions using intracavitary bleomycin. Cancer 57:721-727
10. Dedrick RL, Meyers CE, Bungay PM, Devita VT (1978) Pharmacokinetic rationale for peritoneal drug administration in the treatment of ovarian cancer. Cancer Treat Rep 62:1-11
11. Inokuchi K, Hattori T, Taguchi T, Abe O, Ogawa N (1984) Postoperative adjuvant chemotherapy for gastric carcinoma: Analysis of data on 1805 patients followed for 5 years. Cancer 53:1393-1397
12. McVie JG, Dikhoff T, van der Heide J, et al. (1985) Tissue concentration of platinum after intraperitoneal cisplatin administration in patients (pts). Pros Am Assoc Cancer Res 26:112 (abstr)
13. Casper ES, Kelsen DP, Alcock NW, Lewis Jr JL (1983) Ip cisplatin in patients with malignant ascites: Pharmacokinetic evaluation and comparison with the iv route. Cancer Treat Rep 67:235-238
14. Ozols RF (1985) Pharmacologic reversal of drug resistance in ovarian cancer. Semin Oncol 12:7-11 (supple 4)
15. Schlag P, Schreml W (1982) Heterogeneity in growth pattern and drug sensitivity of primary tumour and metastases in the human tumour colony-forming assay. Cancer Res 42:4086-4089
16. von Hoff DD, Clark GM, Forseth BJ (1986) Simultaneous in vitro drug sensitivity testing tumors from different sites in the same patient. Cancer 58:1007-1013

Intraperitoneal Cisplatin Microspheres for the Management of Malignant Ascites*

AKEO HAGIWARA[1], TOSHIO TAKAHASHI[1], KIYOSHI SAWAI[1], HIROKI TANIGUCHI[1], MASATAKA SHIMOTSUMA[1], CHOUHEI SAKAKURA[1], SHOZO MURANISHI[2], YOSHIHITO IKADA[3], and SUONG HYU-HYON[3]

[1]First Department of Surgery, Kyoto Prefectural University of Medicine, Kyoto, Japan
[2]Department of Biopharmaceutics, Kyoto College of Pharmacy, Kyoto, Japan
[3]Research Center for Medical Polymers and Biomedical Engineering, Kyoto University, Kyoto, Japan

ABSTRACT

A new formulation (CDDP-MS), comprising lactic acid oligomer microspheres incorporating cisplatin was, administered intraperitoneally, at a cisplatin dose of 100 mg to 14 patients and at 200 mg to one patient, for the treatment of malignant ascites. The ascites disappeared completely in 8 of the 15 patients, and partially in 5 patients, for an overall response rate of 87 %. The side effects were mild, temporary and tolerable for the patients. Intraperitoneal CDDP-MS was determined to have good efficacy with minimal side effects, when used for the treatment of malignant ascites.

KEY WORDS: cisplatin microsphere, intraperitoneal chemotherapy, drug delivery system, peritoneal carcinomatosis, malignant ascites.

INTRODUCTION

A new formulation (CDDP-MS), composed of lactic acid oligomer microspheres incorporating cisplatin, has been developed for the treatment of malignant ascites. CDDP-MS is designed to be retained in the peritoneal cavity for long periods, releasing an active form of cisplatin slowly and over a long time. Animal experiments [1], have shown that, compared with the administration of aqueous cisplatin solution, intraperitoneally injected CDDP-MS maintains the cisplatin concentration in the peritoneal cavity at a higher level and for a longer period, while exposing the rest of the body tissues to a lower concentration of cisplatin, Furthermore, CDDP-MS shows decreased systemic toxicity and increased local therapeutic effects. This paper describes clinical trials involving the administration of intraperitoneal CDDP-MS for the treatment of malignant ascites induced by cancers or pseudomyxoma peritonei of the digestive organs.

METHODS AND PATIENTS

Drug Preparation

Ten mg/ml of cisplatin, (donated from Nippon Kayaku Co., Ltd., Tokyo), and 90 mg/ml of poly d,l-lactide were dissolved in dimethylformamide. The resulting solution and 10 volumes of castor oil were mixed and emulsified by agitation at 250 rpm. The dimethylformamide was evaporated by stirring at 45°C for 24h so that the remaining poly d,l-lactide formed microspheres incorporating cisplatin. After drying under vacuum for 2 days to completely remove the dimethylformamide, these microspheres were sieved and those with a diameter of 50 to 150 micro-meter were used [1] for the clinical trials.

Pharmacologic Effects of CDDP-MS in Animal

CDDP-MS was tested to determine tissue distribution of cisplatin in rats, acute toxicity in mice, and therapeutic effects on peritoneal carcinomatosis induced by M5076 in mice, when administered intraperitoneally. The experiment revealed that CDDP-MS resulted in a higher cisplatin concentration in tissues adjacent to the

---

* This work was supported, in part, by a Grant-in-Aid for Cancer Research from the Ministry of Health and Welfare, and from the Ministry of Education, Science and Culture, Japan.

peritoneum for a longer period, and that the concentration in the rest of the body was lower than that delivered by the cisplatin aqueous solution. These experiments also showed that the 50% lethal dose value, determined by Litchfield–Wilcoxon method, was 23.8 mg/kg body weight in CDDP–MS in terms of cisplatin, whereas in cisplatin aqueous solution it was 13.5 mg/kg body weight, and that CDDP–MS enhanced therapeutic effects when compared with the same toxicity doses of cisplatin aqueous solution.

Patients and Drug Administration

Eight male and 7 female patients, who were diagnosed to have malignant ascites due to histologically proven cancers or due to pseudomyxoma peritonei, received CDDP–MS therapy. The primary lesions in the 15 patients comprised 9 gastric cancers, 2 colon cancers, 2 pseudomyxoma peritonei, one adenocarcinoma of the pancreas and one adenocarcinoma of unknown origin (probably pancreatic cancer). None of the patients had received anticancer drugs prior to the initiation of CDDP–MS therapy. After the removal of 0.5 to 1.5 L of ascites fluid, through laparotomy in 2 patients with pseudomyxoma peritonei or through paracentesis in the other 13 patients, each patient received a bolus intraperitoneal injection of a 0.5 to 1.5 L saline suspension of CDDP–MS. The drug was administered at a dose of either 100 mg of cisplatin (14 patients) or 200 mg of cisplatin (one patient). The patients were asked to change their position and respire abdominally for one hour in order to distribute the CDDP–MS particles throughout the peritoneal cavity. The patients received hydration using an intravenous drip–infusion of electrolyte solutions for 3 days after CDDP–MS administration, so that the urine volume exceeded 1.5 L/day. Neither supplimentary anticancer drugs nor diuretics were given from 2 weeks before, to 6 weeks after, the initiation of CDDP–MS therapy. Responses to the treatment were classfied into 3 categories: (1) a complete response (CR) defined as the complete disappearance of ascites for more than 4 weeks with negative cytological findings in the ascites taken within 10 days before the disappearance of the fluid, (2) a partial response (PR) defined as a definite improvement (more than 50% reduction) in ascites, with negative cytological findings for more than 4 weeks, and (3) a failure (F) defined as any response less than a CR or a PR. In patients with pseudomyxoma peritonei, the response was evaluated for 3 months.

The blood was checked for biochemical and hematological changes once and twice a week, respectively. Urine was also moniored biochemical, twice a week. Nausea and vomiting caused by the CDDP–MS therapy were evaluated by the criteria of WHO [2]: in grade 1 (nausea), grade 2 (transient vomiting), grade 3 (vomiting requiring therapy) and grade 4 (intractable vomiting).

RESULTS

Of the 15 patients given CDDP–MS therapy, 8 (53%) demonstrated a complete response, and 5 (33%) demonstrated a partial response, while 2 (13%) did not respond, for an overall response rate of 87% (Table 1). Of the 9 patients with ascites induced by gastric cancer, 8 (CR=6, PR=2) responded to the CDDP–MS treatment. Of the 2 patients with pseudomyxoma peritonei, one responded completely and the other did not. The two colon cancer patients responded completely. A partial response was seen in one patient with ascites caused by pancreatic cancer and in one patient with ascites due to a cancer of unknown origin (probably pancreatic cancer). The response durations for the 13 CR and PR individuals ranged from 1.5 to 12 months. All 13 responders demonstrated clinical improvements in the symptoms of peritoneal

Table 1. Therapeutic effects of CDDP–MS

Primary cancers	Response			Total
	CR	PR	F	
Gastric cancer	6	2	1	9
Pseudomyxoma peritonei	1	0	1	2
Colon cancer	2	0	0	2
Pancreas cancer	0	1	0	1
Cancer of unknown origin (probably pancreas)	0	1	0	1
Total	9	4	2	15

No of responders: 13

Response rate : 13/15 = 87 %

CR: complete response; PR: partial response; F: failure

carcinomatosis such as ileus, abdominal fullness and dyspnea. Seven of these 13 responders were discharged from the hospital.

The side effects of CDDP-MS treatment were mild (Table 2). A fever higher than 38°C was seen in 8 patients (53%), and nausea and/or vomiting which lasted for one to 3 days was noted in 8 (54%) patients. An elevation of blood urea nitrogen was noted in one patient (7%). In 4 patients (27%) an increase of less than two times normal serum levels of glutamic oxaloacetic transaminase and/or glutamic pyruvate transaminase was noted. No abnormalities in serum creatinine, lactic dehydrogenase or alkaline phosphatase were reported. Anemia, leukopenia and thrombocytopenia were not observed. In 3 patients (23%), proteinuria of only less than 50 mg/dl was seen, which disappeared within one month.

Table 2. Side Effects in Clinical Trials

Side Effect		No. of Patients	Percentage
Fever(>38°C)		8	53%
Nausea and/or vomiting		8	53%
Grade 1	3		
Grade 2	4		
Grade 3	1		
Grade 4	0		
Elevation of BUN		1	7%
Elevation of GOT and/or GPT		4	27%
Proteinuria(< 50 mg/dL)		3	23%

BUN: blood urea nitrogen. GOT, GPT: glutamic oxaloacetic transaminase, glutamic pyruvate transaminase.

DISCUSSION

Since the anticancer activity of cisplatin depends both on the concentration of the drug and on the contact time [3], enough concentration of cisplatin in an active form should be delivered selectively to the peritoneal cavity for the desired length of time. When administered intraperitoneally in a solution form, however, cisplatin quickly binds to proteins in the ascites [4], and thus loses its anticancer activity [5]. Furthermore, small molecules, like active form of cisplatin, are rapidly absorbed the through blood-capillary wall into the circulatory blood [6]. Therefore, it is difficult for an intraperitoneal solution of cisplatin to maintain its anticancer activity at a high enough level for a long time to effectively control ascites induced by peritoneal carcinomatosis. In animal experiments [1], however, CDDP-MS has been shown to selectively deliver an active form of cisplatin to the peritoneal cavity for a prolonged period. Furthermore, this cisplatin formulation has been shown to exhibit superior therapeutic effects in the treatment of peritoneal carcinomatosis, with less systemic toxicity. Yamada et al [7] reported that an aqueous solution of intraperitoneal cisplatin demonstrated therapeutic effects in the treatment of malignant ascites induced by gastroenteral cancers. However, this therapy induced relatively strong systemic side effects. In our clinical study, intraperitoneal CDDP-MS brought about very torelable side effects with good therapeutic benefits.

We concluded that intraperitoneal CDDP-MS was very useful in the control of malignant ascites.

REFERENCES

1. Hagiwara A, Takahashi T, Kojima O, Yamaguchi T, Sasabe T, Masaki Lee et al.(1993) Cancer 71: 844-850.
2. WHO handbook for reporting results of cancer treatment (1979) World Health Organization. Geneva.
3. Drewinko B, Brown WB, Gottlieb AJ (1973) Cancer Res 33: 3091-3095.
4. Oku M, Moda T, Kiyozuka Y, Ninomiya Y, Hino K, Okamura Y et al(1988) J Jpn Society for Cancer Therapy 23: 657-664 (in Japanese).
5. Takahashi K, Seki T, Nishikawa K, Minamide S, Iwabuchi M, Ono M et al (1985) Jpn J Cancer Res 76: 68-74.
6. Pretorius GR, Petrilli ES, Kean C, Ford CL, Hoeschele DJ, Lagasse DL. (1981) Cancer Treat Rep 65: 1055-1062.
7. Yamada T, Ohira M, Hikishima H, Hashizume Y, Yamashita R, Kawaura Y et al (1986) Jpn J Cancer Chemother 13: 1004-1009.

Endoscope

Role of Dye Endoscopy with Lugol in the Diagnosis of Esophageal Carcinoma

Necati Ormeci, Ilker Okten, Adem Gungor, Isinsu Kuzu, Hadi Akay, Ali Resit Beyler, Ozden Uzunalimoglu, and Serdar Yol

Departments of Gastroenterology, Thoracic Surgery and Pathology, Ankara University School of Medicine, Ankara, Turkey

ABSTRACT

Ninetynine patients, 67 male and 32 female, who applied to endoscopy laboratory of gastroenterology department of the Ankara University School of Medicine were diagnosed to esophageal carcinoma between the years 1986 and 1993. Lugol was routinely used in selective cases. Four out of 99 cases were in early stages. Two cases had submucosal invasion without lymph node metastasis. One case showed flat undyed area with lugol and she was proved to have squamous cell carcinoma but she refused the operation. One case showed severe dysplasia and she had liver metastasis after three years of operation.
Lugol which is used in selective cases during endoscopy is not only useful for early diagnosis but also provides the proximal margin of the lesion.

KEY WORDS: Lugol, Esophageal Carcinoma

INTRODUCTION

Esophageal carcinoma is seen as an endemic disease in some countries such as Transkei area of the Capp province, Kasakstan, Puerto Rico and North China. It has been encountered as the second common disease in especially eastern Turkey.
Esophageal cancer in which infiltration is limited to the submucosa without metastasis to lymph nodes is defined as "early" cancer of the esophagus by the guideline established by the Japanese Study Group for Esophageal Disease.[1] If there is a metastasis in cases with superficial cancer, the results are the same as in the advanced one.[2]
There are several tools such as X-ray, brush cytology, endoscopic ultrasonography, computed tomograpy, nuclear magnetic resonance and endoscopy. Of these methods, endoscopy plays extremely important role in the diagnosis of early stage esophageal carcinoma.
We will present our experiences with esophageal carcinoma in this article.

MATERIALS AND METHODS

Ninetynine patients, 67 male and 32 female, who applied to our endoscopy laboratory were diagnosed to have esophageal carcinoma between the years 1986 and 1993. Average age was 58.2 years (range 22-80).
When any abnormality of the mucosa was detected, Lugol solution, 3 % was sprayed to the mucosa and if there appeared any undyed area, at least four biopsies were taken. When there was esophageal carcinoma, Lugol solution was also used to evaluate the oral margine of lesion.

RESULTS

Localization of the lesions were 2 % at upper one-third, 11 % at middle
one-third of the esophagus, 54 % at lower one-third, 2 % at upper and
middle one-third, 31 % at middle and lower one-third.
Four out of 99 cases were in early stages. One case showed severe
dysplasia by biopsy and she had distal esophagectomy.Carcinoma could not
be proved but she had liver metastasis after three years of operation.
Two cases were diagnosed as early esophageal carcinoma possessing
submucosal invasion without lymph node metastasis (Figs. 1,2). One case
showed flat undyed areas with lugol and she was proved to have squamous
cell carcinoma but refused the operation.

DISCUSSION

Staining endoscopy was first used by Schiller in 1933 for the early
diagnosis of cervix cancer.[3] Voegali applied this technique to the
gastrointestinal system for defining the boundary between the esophagus
and the stomach. Nothman used the same technique for diagnosis of
esophagitis.[4] In recent years staining endoscopy has been succesfully
used not only for the selective diagnosis of esophageal disease but also
for the stomach, duodenum and colon diseases in many endoscopy centers.
[5,6,7] Normal esophageal mucosa contains significant amounts of
glycogene. Iodine in lugol and glycogene give a chemical reaction
forming iodite. Iodite is responsible for the blackish color change in
the mucosa. When normal mucosa loses its features, the amount of
glycogene decreases and staining does not occur. This is the major
indication to recognize the pathological mucosa.[4] Staining endoscopy
facilitates detection of the tumour at the mucosal level and clearly
defines its boundaries. This is particularly important for biopsy and
determination of the resection line.
We have found multifocal tumour in some of our cases.
In conclusion, staining endoscopy should be widely used as a highly
sensitive screening method for the early diagnosis and determination
of the boundaries of the esophageal lesions.

REFERENCES

1. Japanese Society for Esophageal Disease (1976), Guidelines for the
   clinical and pathological studies on carcinoma of the esophagus.
   Jpn.J.Surg.6:69.
2. Endo M.,Takeshita K.,Yoshida M.,(1986) How can we diagnose the early
   stage of esophageal cancer?Endoscopic diagnosis. Endoscopy 18:11-18.
3. Richart M.R.(1963), A clinical staining test for the in vivo
   delineation of dysplasia and carcinoma in situ. American Journal of
   Obstetrics and Gynaecology, 86(6):703-712
4. Nothmann J.B.,Wright R.J.,Schuster M.M.(1972), In vivo vital staining
   as an aid to identification of esophagogastric mucosal junction in man,
   Digestive Diseases, 17(10): 912-924.
5. Kawai K.,Takemoto T.,Suzuki T.,Ida K.,(1979), Proposed nomenclature
   and classification of dye-spraying techniques in endoscopy. Endoscopy
   1:23-25.
6. Suzuki S.,Groitl H.I.,Suzuki H.,Endo M.,Takemoto T.,Nakayama K. (1974)
   Differential diagnosis endoscopically dyed lesions by gastroscopic
   close-up appearences.Endoscopy 6:99-104.
7. Tada M.,Katoh S.,Kohli Y.,Kawai K. (1976) On the dye spraying method
   in colonofiberscopy. Endoscopy 8:7-74.

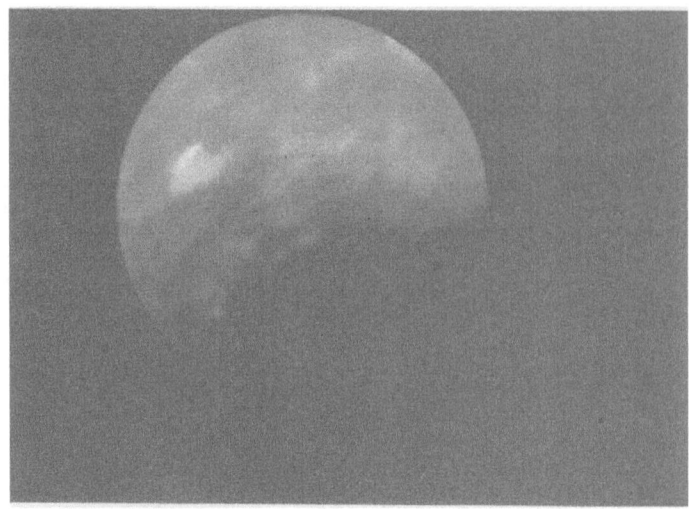

Fig. 1   Undyed areas after lugol staining caused by the ulceration
          with irregular margin and the granular base.

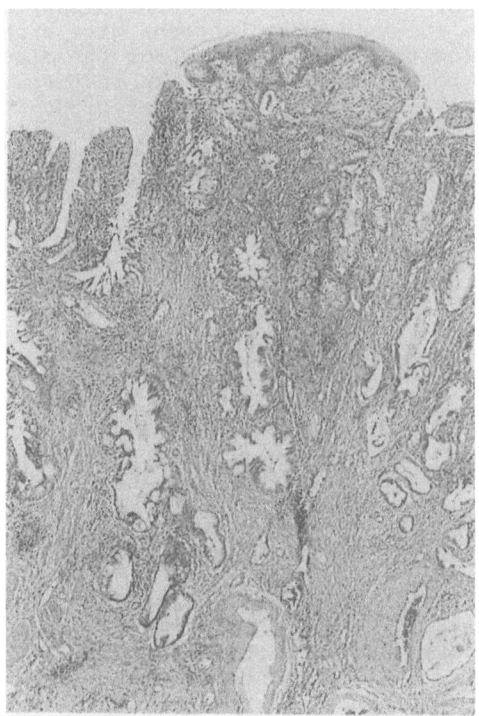

Fig. 2   The surface epithelium is lacking at the ulcerated areas
          and the submucosa is infiltrated by the tumour, which is
          characterized by the malignant adenoid formations [x40,H.E.].

Endoscopic Examination for the Early Esophageal Cancer in Patients with Head and Neck Cancers

Hitoshi Shiozaki, Kenji Kobayashi, Masatoshi Inoue, Shigeyuki Tamura, Hiroshi Oka, Yuuichiro Doki, Keisuke Iihara, Takatoshi Kadowaki, and Takesada Mori

Department of Surgery II, Osaka University Medical School, Osaka, 553 Japan

ABSTRACT

Endoscopic screening of the esophagus with Lugol-dye staining was performed on 304 patients with head and neck cancers at the Department of Surgery II, Osaka University Medical School between June 1987 and August 1992. We found 19 patients with esophageal cancer (6.3%) and 21 patients with esophageal dysplasia (6.9%). Fifteen (78%) of 19 esophageal cancer patients were early stages (within submucosal invasion) with no lymph node metastases. Twelve (63%) of 19 esophageal cancer patients coexisted with multiple areas of dysplasia and/or cancer. The esophageal epithelium in patients with head and neck cancers may have tendency of field cancerization and multicentric potency for carcinogenesis.

KEY WORDS: esophageal cancer, head and neck cancer, endoscopicscreening, second primary cancer, Lugol-dye staining

INTRODUCTION

Esophageal cancer has a poor prognosis despite radical surgical treatment combined with radiotherapy and/or chemotherapy because of its aggressive character. However, cases with no lymph node metastases have a good prognosis after simple resection[1]. The normal esophageal epithelum is stained by a modified Lugol's solution, but dysplastic and cancerous mucosa of the esophagus is not. Endoscopic examinaton with Lugol-dye method is widely used to find dysplastic and cancerous lesions of the esophagus[2,3]. In order to detect early esophageal cancer, we performed endoscopic screening of the esophagus with Lugol-dye method for patients with head and neck cancer regarded as being high risk for synchronous or metachronous esophageal cancer.

PATIENTS AND METHODS

PATIENTS

Three hundred four patients with head and neck cancers who were treated at the Osaka University Hospital and who had no symptoms related to the esophagus were enrolled in this study from June 1987 to August 1992. They consisted of 146 cases of tongue cancer, 56 of mouthfloor cancer, 12 of nasopharyngeal cancer, 18 of oropharyngeal cancer, 23 of hypopharyngeal cancer, 33 of laryngeal cancer and 16 of other sites(Table 1). The primary tumors were successfully treated by radiation therapy with or without chemotherapy or surgical resection in all of cases. The ages of the patients ranged from 25 to 80 years (mean age, 59.2 years). There were 233 male and 71 female patients. The mean time interval from the first diagonsis of head and neck cancer to the endoscopic examination was approximately 50 months.

ENDOSCOPIC EXAMINATION

In the Department of Surgery II, Osaka University Medical School, both esophagoscopy and gastroscopy were performed with an electronic endoscope(V-10, Olympus, Tokyo, Japan) or an optical panendoscope (P-10, Olympus, Tokyo, Japan) to find second primary cancers in the esophagus and the stomach. The entire surface of the esophageal mucosa was sprayed with Lugol's solution with the aid of esophagoscopy, and unstained lesions were biopsied for histological examination. The terminlogy used in this report was derived from theJapanese Research Siciety for Esophageal Disease Classification[4].

440

RESULTS

ENDOSCOPIC EXAMINATION

The endoscopic findings for the screened head and neck cancer patients are shown in Table 1. In 77 cases (25.3%) of 304 screened cases, unstained lesions by Lugol's
solution were detected and biopsied endoscopically. By histologic examination of these 77 biopsy specimens, 19 cases of squamous cell carcinoma, 6 cases of severe dysplasia and 15 cases of moderate dysplasia were shown respectively(Table 1). Within these unstained lesions by Lugol's solution only 9 cancerous lesions could be detected by barium studies and ordinary endoscopic studies without the Lugol-dye method.

CLINICOPATHOLOGIC FINDINGS OF THE ESOPHAGEAL CANCER PATIENTS

Endoscopic examination found a total of 26 second primary cancers (19 esophageal and 7 gastric cancers), indicating a second cancer incidence of 8.5%. The 19 second esophageal cancers were accompanied by head and neck cancers of the tongue and hypopharynx in each 5 cases, of mouthfloor in 4 cases, of oropharynx and others in 2 cases and larynx in only one case. The incidence of second cancer was 21.7% in hypopharyngeal cancer cases, 11.1% in oropharyngeal cancer cases, 7.1% in mouthfloor cancer cases, 3.4% in tongue cancer cases and 3.0% in laryngeal cancer cases (Table 1). Thus, the incidence of second cancer in hypopharyngeal cancer cases was highest. Table 2 details the clinical and pathologic findings of the esophageal cancer cases. The esophageal cancers in 9 cases were synchronous and those in 10 cases were metachronous to head and neck cancers. Sixteen of the detected 19 cases were treated surgically withor without radiation therapy. Two cases with severe circulatory dysfunction were treated by exposure toa laser beam and radiation therapy. Only one case with small unstained lesions was treated by the endoscopic mucosal resection.There were multiple lesions scattered widely througout the esophagus in six of nine synchronous and one of ten metachronous esophageal cancer patients. Of the 26 cancerous lesions in these 19 cases, only 8 lesions(30.8%) could be detected by barium studies and 9 lesions (34.6%) by ordinary endoscopic studies because they were slightly depressed or elevated. The other 17 lesions(65.4%)could not be detected by these two methods because they were completely flat. Of the 19 esophageal cancer cases in 14 cases tumors did not invade deeper than the submucosal layer and accompany without lymph node metastases. All of the esophageal cancers have been succcessfully controlled by the therapies without recurrence at the end of 1992.

DISCUSSION

Twenty six cases of the 304 head and neck cancer cases screened in present study were accompanied by second primary cancers of upper gastro-intestinal tract (19 esophageal and 7gastric cancers). The incidence of the esophageal cancer(6.3%) as second cancer was a significantly higher ratio than the expected number of esophageal cancer patients calculated from the Osaka Cancer Registration[5]. Fourteen patients (73.7%) of 19 esophageal cancers had early stage disease with no clinically accurate lymph node

metastases. Clinicopathological evaluations of the patients with esphageal cancer showed that most of the lesions (17 of 26 lesions) were not detectable by balium studies and ordinary endoscopic studies. The prognosis after surgical resection of the esophageal cancer patients who had not invasion deeper than the submucosal layer and no lymph node metastases is exellent[1].
The esophageal cancer with head and neck cancer had multiple cancerous and dysplastic lesions. Especially in 6 cases of 9 synchronous cancers multiple cancerous lesions were detected. The hypothesis of field carcinogenesis can offer a plausible explanation of why head and neck cancer and esophageal cancer frequently develop in the same indivisual. Since the oral cavity, pharynx and esophagus are covered with seriel squamous epithelium, these area are subject to the simultaneous development of dysplasia and cancer in chronic exposure to mutagens contained in tobacco and alcohol. Specifically, tobacco and alcohol are known to play a crucial role in the development of multiregional and multicentric cancer in head and neck cancer patients[6,7].
We conclude that it is necessary to examine throughly the upper gastro-intestinal tract of head and neck cancer patients. For the detection of small and superficial esophageal cancer with head and neck cancer, the endoscopic examination and biopsy of the esophagus after application of a modified Lugol's solution to the esophageal epithelium might be very useful.

Table 1 Histological findings of unstained lesions by Lugol's solution (June 1987-Aug. 1992)

primary ca.	unstained lesins	dysplasia		cancer
		moderate	severe	
tongue (146)	21	2	3	5 (3.4%)
mouth floor (56)	14	3	1	4 (7.1%)
nasopharynx (12)	1			
oropharynx (18)	8	3	1	2 (11.1%)
hypopharynx (23)	11	5	1	5 (21.7%)
larynx (33)	13	2		1 (3.0%)
others (16)	9	1		2 (12.5%)
total (304)	77 (25.3%)	16	6	19 (6.3%)

Table 2 Clinical and pathological findings of the cases with esophageal cancer

No.	age	sex	primary cancer	timing[1]	lode unstained lesion	location	gross[2] type	size(cm)	depth[3]	management
1.	49	F	hypopharynx	syn	multiple	middle	0-IIb	0.8x0.5	mm	blunt dissection+
						lower	0-IIb	0.6x0.4	ep	laryngectomy
2.	49	M	hypopharynx	syn	multiple	middle	0-IIc	1.0x0.6	pm	irradiation+
									ep	esophagectomy
3.	72	M	neck	syn	multiple	middle	0-IIa+IIb	2.0x3.0	sm	blunt dissection
4.	61	M	hypopharynx	syn	multiple	lower	0-IIa+IIb	-	ep	irradiation+blunt.
5.	72	M	oropharynx	meta	multiple	everywhere	0-IIb	-	ep susp	Laser therapy
6.	54	M	mouth floor	meta	multiple	lower	0-IIb	3.0x3.5	mm	blunt dissction
							0-IIb	-	ep	blunt dissction
7.	61	M	mouth floor	meta	single	lower	0-IIc	1.0x1.0	ep	blunt dissction
8.	75	M	mouth floor	meta	single	upper	0-IIc+IIb	1.5x2.0	mm	blunt dissction
9.	62	M	larynx	meta	multiple	middle	0-IIb	1.5x1.0	ep	blunt dissction
10.	64	M	tongue	meta	single	middle	type 2	5.8x2.3	pm	esophagectomy
11.	52	M	tongue	meta	single	middle	type 2	-	pm	esophagectomy
12.	56	F	mouth floor	meta	single	middle	type 2	8.0x4.0	a2	esophagectomy
13.	56	M	tongue	syn	multiple	middle	0-IIa+IIb	1.5x1.5	mm	endoscopic mucosal
							0-IIb	1.5x1.5	ep	resection
14.	35	M	hypopharynx	syn	multiple	middle	0-IIc+IIa	3.5x1.5	mm	blunt dissection+
							0-IIb	1.0x0.7	mm	laryngectomy
15.	67	M	oropharynx	meta	single	lower	0-IIb	2.5x2.5	mm	lower esophagect.
16.	53	F	tongue	meta	single	lower	type 2	4.5x2.6	pm	esophagectomy
17.	54	M	tongue	syn	multiple	middle	0-IIc	1.0x1.0	mm susp	irradiation
						lower	0-IIb	1.0x1.0	ep susp	
18.	55	M	hypopharynx	syn	multiple	cervical	0-IIa+IIc	2.2x1.8	mm	blunt dissection+
						lower	0-IIc	3.6x3.3	mm	laryngectomy
19.	60	M	hypopharynx	syn	multiple	middle	0-IIa+IIb	2.0x2.0	mm	blunt dissection

*1 timing--- syn:synchronous, meta:metachronous

*2 gross type--- 0-IIa:slightly elevated , 0-IIb: flat, 0-IIc: slightlydepressed, type 2: ulcerative and localized

*3 depht of invasion--- ep:limited the epithelium, mm:muscularis mucosa, sm:submucosa, pm:muscularis propria

REFERENCES

1. Isono K, Sato H, Nakayama K. (1991) Results of a nationwide study on the three-field lymph node dissection of esophageal cancer. Oncology, 48:411-420.

2. Sugimachi K, Ohno S, Matsuda H, Mori M, Kuwano H. (1988) Lugol combined endoscopic detection of minute malignant lesions of the thoracic esophagus. Ann Surg, 208:179-183.

3. Goodner JT, Watson WL, (1956) Cancer of the esophagus : Its association with other primary cancers. Cancer, 9:1248-1252.

4. Japanese Society for Esophageal Disease. Guidelines for the Clinical and Pathologic Studies on Carcinoma of the Esophagus, ed. 7. (1989)Tokyo: Kanehara

5. Shiozaki H, Tahara H, Kobayashi K, Yano H, Tamura S, Imamoto H, Yano T, Oku K, Miyata M, Nishiyama K, Kubo K, Mori T. (1990) Cancer 66:2068-2071.

6. McGuirt WF, (1982) Panendoscopy as a screening examination for simultaneous primary tumors in head and neck cancer: prospective sequential study and review of literature. Laryngoscope 92:569-576.

7. Okumura T, Aruga H, Inohara H, Matsunaga T, Shiozaki H, Kobayashi K, Kubo K, Yoshida J. (1993) Endoscopic examination of the upper gastrointestinal tract for the presence of second primary cancers in head and neck cancer patients. Acta Otolaryngol 501:103-106.

Effect of Routine Endoscopy on Critical Assessment in Diagnosis of Intestinal Metaplasia at Mexico General Hospital

Rafael Barreto Z.[1], Isaias Garduño[1], Fernando Bernal S.[1], Jose Jessurum[2], Rosario Valdes L.[1], Daniel Murguia D.[1], and Jorge Huerta T.[1]

Department of [1]Gastroenterology and [2]Pathology, General Hospital, Mexico City, Mexico

ABSTRACT

Had been described low frequency of intestinal metaplasia (I.M.) in gastric biopsies from Mexican patients as comparision with other ethnic groups. The cause responsible remains unclear.But,there is the possibility that other endoscopist recognize more easily gastric areas with I.M. for tissue sampling than Mexican endoscopist. In order to clarify that, we reviewing 1807 consecutive upper gastrointestinal endoscopies at General Hospital in Mexico during January to November 1991, with endoscopic and pathological diagnosis of chronic gastritis with or without I.M. The interobserver reliability of endoscopic diagnosis was analyzed compared with histological diagnosis. Of total of 1807 endoscopies, 270 (15%) had I.M. their positive predictive value were found in 61% of the patients with positive endoscopic test result had pathological diagnosis, and 72% of sensitivity. The study indicates that I.M. primarily represents and histological diagnosis with relatively good correlation (61%) with endoscopic defined macroscopic findings. In conclusion the low frequency of I.M. should be another factor then interobserver reliability of endoscopic diagnosis.

KEY WORDS: intestinal metaplasia, endoscopy, diagnosis.

INTRODUCTION.

Although there has been a decline in the incidence of gastric adenocarcinoma in Mexico, there are still new cases every year, and more than 90% of these are diagnosed at well advanced stage with predominant diffuse type[1]. The low proportion of intestinal type adenocarcinoma contrasts with a much higher frequency in other populations. Thus, the low frequency of this tumor variant in Mexican appears to correlate well with a low frequency of I.M. [4,6] Previous investigations have demonstrated the low frequency of I.M. in gastric biopsies from Mexican patients a comparison with Japanese and Swedish patients [5]. It is know that environmental factors decide the geographic differences of I.M. However, the accuracy of diagnosis of I.M. has not been determined, In order to clarify that, the purpose of this study was to determine the accuracy of the endoscopic method for estimating the gastric mucosal changes of I.M. in Mexican population .

MATERIALS AND METHODS

We reviewing 1807 consecutive upper gastrointestinal endoscopies at General Hospital in Mexico during January to November 1991, with endoscopic and pathological diagnosis of chronic gastritis with or without I.M. .Several endoscopist was participate in the study. After overnight fasting the patients undergoing gastroscopy using endoscope Olympus K10 and video Pentax 3000 intestinal metaplasia (I.M.) in this paper refer to gray-white patches with a villus and slightly opalescent appearance (7) and unevenness mucosa or slight dye-spraying technique with indigo carmin solution 0.5%. Four gastric mucosal biopsy specimen were then taken from the gastric mucosa . Additional specimens were taken from any pathological lesions seen. All sections will examine by the same pathologist without knowledge of other patient data. Data was reported as likelihood ratio and the critical assessment of diagnostic endoscopic test in comparision with pathology "gold standard" diagnosis.

RESULTS

Table 1 shows the sensitivity, specificity, and predictive values of endoscopic test in Intestinal Metaplasia among Mexico General Hospital patients. The patients value had positive (72%) and negative (92%) endoscopic diagnosis for intestinal metaplasia, with the proportion of diseased patients among all tested group (14.9%). Another hand, the index " likelihood ratio" contrasts the proportions of patients with (9.15) and without (0.30) intestinal metaplasia. That means that endoscopy result for a sort are 9.5 times is likely to come from patients with I.M. and less than one (0.30) as likely to come from patients with I.M.

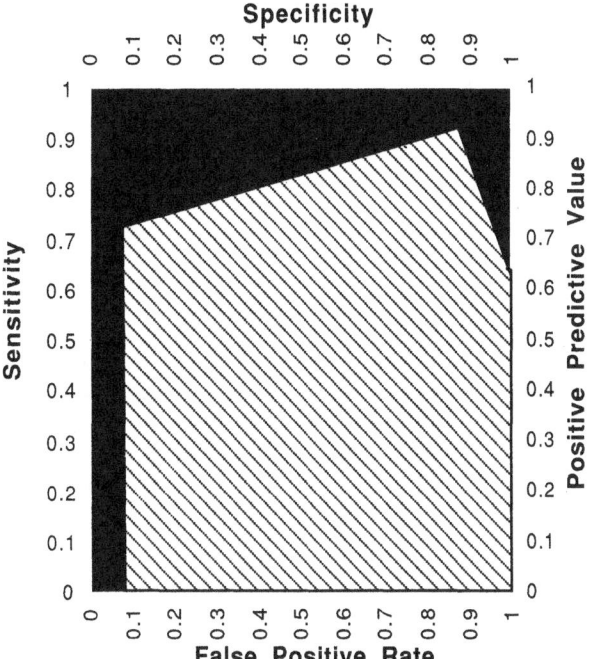

This figure provides tha a picture of implications for using different cutoffs and such ROC curve have some interesting properties: The upper left corner denotes a relatively good test diagnosis a sensitivity of .72, patients with I.M. was detected and the probability is 1.60: 1

DISCUSSION

Previous investigators suggested that low incidence of Mexican population is due to environmental component [4,5]. However, the accuracy of diagnosis of I.M. has not been determined, The question addressed by the present study was whether the discriminating ability of diagnosis by Mexican endoscopist of I. M. is a one factor to explain the low incidence in our population. The imprecision we detected in this study could have arisen from limitations of the method. One limitation is that not blind study. Another limitation of our method is exist several endoscopist. Despite these limitations, our method of data analysis has disvantages. This study, which incorporates and confirms the observations of previous investigators [2,4,5] includes new observations that provide a more complete understanding of the I.M. in Mexico General Hospital. This study in Mexican population demonstrates that in the accuracy of endoscopic method to evaluate I.M. not is the factor to explain the low incidence in Mexican population.

REFERENCES

1. De la Torre B. A., Torres R. M., (1988)Carcinoma gástrico incipiente, Rev Gastroenterol Méx,53 (1):27-31
2. Garduño I. H., Bernal S. F., Barreto Z. R., Valdes L. R., Espino C. H., Huerta T. J., Bardales I., (1991) Metaplasia Intestinal: Correlacion endoscopico-patologica. (Reporte preliminar). Endoscopia (Mexico), II, 3:118-119
3. Llanos, O., S. Guzman and I. Duarte, Accuracy of the first endoscopic procedure in the differential diagnosis of gastric lesions. Ann. Surg 195:224,1982.
4. Rubio C. A.,Jessurum J.,Alonso De Ruiz P., (1991) Geographic variations in the Histologic Characteristics of the Gastric Mucosa, Am J Clin Pathol. 96:330-333
5. Rubio, C. A., Kato Y., Sugano H., and Kitagawa T., (1987) Intestinal metaplasia of the stomach in Swedish and Japanese patient without ulcers or carcinoma. Jpn. J. Cancer Res., 78, 467-472
6. Pedroza-Herrera, G. E. and Jessurum, J. (1990) Carcinoma gastrico intestinal y difuso en la poblacion del Hospital General de Mexico. Estudio comparativo. Patologia (Madrid), 28, 5-17

Management of Early Colorectal Carcinoma Defined by Endoscopic Findings

K. Ikeuchi, N. Ohno, S. Toyota, T. Yoon, M. Ohtsuka, Y. Takao,
R. Katayama, S. Anazawa, and K. Sakurai

The First Department of Surgery, The Jikei University School of Medicine, Tokyo, 105 Japan

ABSTRACT

Two hundred seventy-one cases (330 lesions) of early colorectal carcinoma were analyzed to assess the primary treatment modality by endoscopic findings. All cases were classified into two groups, namely intramucosal polypoid growth-type (PG-ca; 287 lesions), and nonpolypoid growth-type (NPG-ca; 41 lesions), according to histological findings. Two hundred forty-one lesions of PG-ca were intramucosal carcinomas (m-ca) and 46 were submucosal carcinomas (sm-ca). All 43 lesions of NPG-ca were sm-ca. The incidence of massive invasion to submucosa was greater in NPG-ca (53.8%) than in PG-ca (8.9%). Lymph node metastasis was detected in 5 lesions, (11.6%) of NPG-ca and in 4, (1.4%) of PG-ca. In contrast, over 80% of nodular tumors with depressions defined by colonoscopic findings were NPG-ca and all of the lobular type were PG-ca.

Conclusions : Nodular tumors with depressions observed by endoscopy should be resected by a surgical procedure including lymphadenectomy as they tend to be NPG-ca with a high risk of lymph node metastasis. Lobular tumors should be removed by endoscopy when possible; then, the necessity for additional surgical procedures should be decided.

KEY WORDS : early colorectal carcinoma, growth type, endoscopic findings

INTRODUCTION

Since the technical advance of flexible endoscopy, the number of patients diagnosed with early colorectal carcinoma has increased and colonic polyps can now be resected safely by endoscopy . Several authors have described the histological criteria for polypectomy, distinguishing cases for endoscopic polypectomy should be sufficient and those for which additional colectomy might be necessary after polypectomy. However, it also important to determine whether colectomy should be performed or not when early carcinoma is observed by endoscopy. We retrospectively reviewed 273 cases of early carcinoma to assess the primary treatment modality by endoscopic findings.

MATERIALS AND METHODS

Between 1977 and 1992, 273 patients who had early colorectal carcinomas (330 lesions)were treated in our department. In this study, all patients who had familial polyposis, Gardner syndrome, or early colorectal carcinoma associated with advanced colorectal carcinoma were excluded. Of the 273 patients (330 lesions) included in this study, 185 had intramucosal carcinomas (m-ca; 241 lesions) and 86 submucosal carcinomas (sm-ca; 89 lesions).

The depth of invasion of the carcinomas to submucosa was divided into three levels. In level 1, the carcinoma invaded to the upper third of the submucosa (sm+; minimum invasion). In level 2, the carcinoma invaded to the middle third of the submucosa (sm++). Level 3 involved massive invasion to the lower third of the submucosa but above the muscularis propria (sm+++).

The growth type of early colorectal carcinomas was divided into two groups, namely polypoid-growth carcinoma (PG-ca) from intramucosal proliferation of adenoma or carcinoma, and nonpolypoid-growth carcinoma (NPG-ca) without intramucosal protuberant growth (fig.1).

Other histologic findings were included the histologic grade of the carcinoma (well moderately or poorly differentiated), the presence of lymphatic or blood vessel invasion and the status of the surgical margins of the specimens. In resected cases, the polypectomy site was checked for residual carcinoma and lymph nodes were examined for metastasis.

The shape of the tumor was defined by colonoscopy as nodular type, lobular type or irregular type with or without a depression.

RESULTS

Two hundred seventy-three patients (330 lesions) were analyzed in this study; 241 lesions were of m-ca and 89 lesions of sm-ca type. The patients included 139 men and 46 women in the m-ca group, and 57 men and 31 women in the sm-ca group. The mean age of the patients was 61.8 years. Two hundred and five lesions (m-ca 195, sm-ca 10) were treated by endoscopic resection alone. Forty-eight lesions (m-ca 7, sm-ca 41) were removed by endoscopy followed by surgical resection. A total of 77 lesions (m-ca 39, sm-ca 38) were surgical resected.

In 7 lesions of m-ca, the additional resection was performed because of positive margins of polypectomy specimens; the other 2 lesions of this type had residual carcinoma of the surgical margin. Surgical resection was performed because the tumor had a broad base and endoscopic resection would have been difficult. In the sm-ca group, 9 of 41 lesions for which additional resection were performed after polypectomy had positive status at the surgical margin and residual carcinoma was detected at the polypectomy site of the surgical specimen in 3 lesions (33 %). Three (7%) of the 41 lesions were associated with lymph node metastasis. These had sm+++ invaded carcinoma and positive lymphatic and blood vessel invasion. One of these patients died of lymph node metastasis despite surgical resection with lymphadenectomy.

Among 38 lesions of sm-ca type which underwent surgical resection, lymph node metastasis was seen in 6 (15.8%). Two of these had sm+ and positive lymphatic and blood vessel invasion. One had sm++ and negative vessel invasion. One had sm+++ and positive vessel invasion, and 2 lesions had sm+++ and negative vessel invasion. With respect to the histological grade of the carcinoma, 9 lesions of sm-ca were moderately differentiated adenocarcinoma with sm+++. Lymph node metastasis was seen in 2 lesions.

All lesions were classified into two groups: intramucosal polypoid growth-type lesions (PG-ca; 287), and nonpolypoid growth-type lesions (NPG-ca; 43). Two hundred forty-one (84.0 %) of the PG-ca lesions were of the m-ca type and 46 (16.0 %) were sm-ca. All 43 lesions of NPG-ca were sm-ca. In the sm-ca group, 53.8% of NPG-ca lesions had sm+++ while 8.9% of PG-ca lesions had this type of invasion (fig.2). Tumor size was 10mm or smaller in 25.6%, 11~20 mm in 56.4% and larger than 20mm in 18% of the patients who had NPG-ca. Tumors were 10 mm or smaller in 11.4%, 11~20 mm in 63.6% and larger than 20 mm in 25.5% of PG-ca cases. Lymph node metastasis was observed in 5 patients (11.6%) with NPG-ca and 4 (1.4%) with PG-ca.

We analyzed whether NPG-ca or PG-ca could be defined by endoscopic findings. All tumors were classified into three types, nodular, lobular, and irregular by endoscopic findings. Also, the presence of a central depression was recorded. All lesions of the lobular type were PG-ca with sm-ca. NPG-ca was seen in 85.7% of the nodular type, and PG-ca was observed in 14.3%. NPG-ca was observed in 87.2% of the lesions with a central depression and 4.5% of those without a depression, while PG-ca was seen in 12.8% and 95.5% of the two types, respectively (fig. 3).

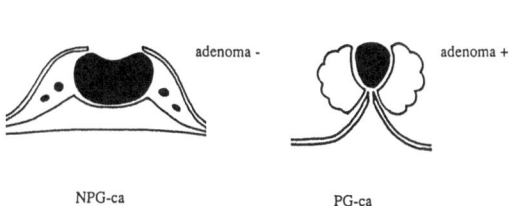

Fig.1 Growth type of early colorectal carcinoma polypoid growth-type (PG-ca) from intramucosal proliferation of adenoma or carcinoma and nonpolypoid growth type (NPG-ca) without intramucosal protuberant growth.

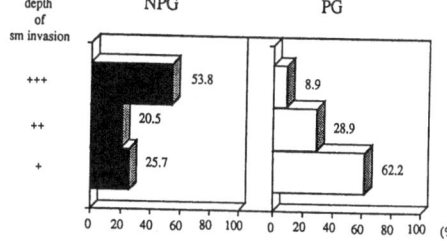

Fig.2 The relation between the depth of sm invasion and the growth type.

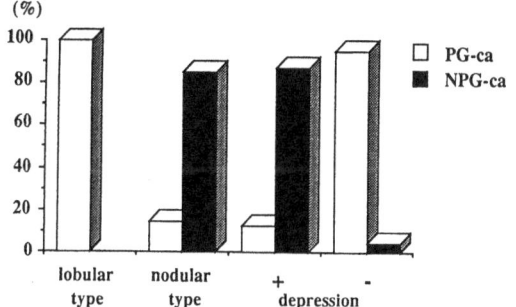

Fig.3 The incidence of PG-ca and NPG-ca in the lesions of lobular or nodular type with or without depression defined by endoscopic findings.

DISCUSSION

The management of patients with colorectal polyps or early carcinomas remains controversial. Several authors have reported that endoscopic polypectomy should be sufficient if it completely removes the lesion, the margins are negative with no lymphatic or blood vessel invasion, and if the lesion is not poorly differentiated adenocarcinoma. Others have suggested that endoscopic resection alone might not be adequate for treatment. Kyzer et al. reported that in the absence of vascular and lymphatic invasion or poorly differentiated adenocarcinoma, only level 4 lesion according to Haggitt's classification should be resected. Our classification using the depth of invasive carcinoma to the submucosa suggests a different approach. Our sm+ is similar to Haggitt's level 1, sm++ compares with level 2 or 3, and sm+++ is similar to level 4, with a high risk of lymph node metastasis or vessel invasion. Sm+++ lesions should be resected. In addition, sm++ lesions should be resected because they are associated with a high risk of lymph node metastasis. Even in the sm+ group, lymph node metastasis was observed if there was lymphatic or blood vessel invasion. However, sm+ lesions without lymphatic or blood vessel invasion had no lymph node metastasis. Thus, all sm-ca lesions except sm+ without lymphatic or blood vessel invasion should be resected. In m-ca lesions, no lymph node metastasis was seen, so if the margin of the polypectomy specimen is negative, endoscopic polypectomy should be sufficient

We analyzed whether or not additional surgical resection was necessary after polypectomy. However, it is important to stress that polypectomy may be sufficient or in some cases, surgical resection should be done when the lesion is observed by endoscopy. Therefore, all lesions were classified into two groups, PG-ca and NPG-ca, and analyzed. All m-ca lesions (241) were classified in the PG-ca group. Forty-six lesions in the PG-ca group were sm-ca, while all of those in the NPG-ca group were sm-ca. Although the incidence of sm+++ in NPG-ca lesions was higher than that in the PG-ca group, NPG-ca tended to be smaller than PG-ca. Lymph node metastasis was detected in 13% of NPG-ca lesions, and in 1.4% of PG-ca lesions. NPG-ca had a high risk of massive invasion to the submucosa and lymph node metastasis. Thus, NPG-ca lesions should be resected surgically rather than endoscopically. On the other hand, NPG-ca or PG-ca could be defined by endoscopic findings. All of the lobular type were PG-ca, while 85.7% of the nodular type were NPG-ca. Furthermore, in 87.2% of the lesions with a depression, NPG-ca was observed.

In summary, we believe that nodular tumors with a depression observed by endoscopy should be resected by surgical procedures with lymphadenectomy, as they tend to be NPG-ca lesions with a high risk of massive invasion to submucosa and lymph node metastasis. Lobular tumors should be removed by endoscopy when possible. Endoscopic resection should be sufficient in cases of m-ca with negative margins, and sm+ lesions of well differentiated adenocarcinoma with negative margins, and no vessel invasion. Otherwise, additional surgical procedures should be performed.

REFERENCES
1. Kyzer S, Begin LR, Gordon PH, Mitmaker B (1992) Cancer 70: 2044-2050
2. Shimoda T, Ikegami M, Fujisaki J, Matsui T, Aizawa S, Ishikawa E (1989) Cancer 64: 1138-1146
3. Ikegami M (1987) Acta Pathol Jpn 37: 21-37
4. Ishida S, Ohno N, Toyota S, Yoon T, Ikeuchi K, Otsuka M, Katayama R, Anazawa S, Sakurai K (1992) Jpn J Gastroenterol Surg 25: 1975-1983

Intraportal Endovascular Ultrasonography for Pancreatobiliary Carcinoma

Tetsuya Kaneko, Akimasa Nakao, and Hiroshi Takagi

Department of Surgery II, Nagoya University School of Medicine, Nagoya, Japan

ABSTRACT

Intraportal endovascular ultrasonography (IPEUS) was performed to diagnose the portal vein invasion of pancreatobiliary carcinoma. The study group consisted of 15 patients, six men and nine women, with a mean age of 65.5 years who underwent IPEUS between Feb 1992 to Dec 1992. Basically, the wall of portal vein was visualized as echogenic band with a thickness 0.5mm to 1.0mm. When this echogenic band was seen, portal invasion was diagnosed as negative. When this band was destroyed, portal invasion was diagnosed as positive. In 14 out of 15 patients, portal invasion of the tumor was diagnosed correctly. In one case of bile duct cancer of hepatic hilum, tumor invasion of right hepatic artery could also be diagnosed. This finding could not be detected by conventional imaging technology such as CT, angiography. IPEUS was considered to give important information about pancreatobiliary carcinoma.

INTRODUCTION

Pancreatobiliary carcinoma is liable to invade the major vessels, particularly the portal vein and hepatic artery. In recent years, aggressive surgery for these carcinoma including combined resection of portal vein and hepatic artery has been reported[1-4]. Information about portal vein invasion is important in deciding the operative strategy for radical resection of pancreatobiliary carcinoma. Recently, intravascular ultrasonography (IVUS) has been applied in the vascular field to evaluate vascular lesions and the results of angioplasty[5]. IVUS has also been used to localize intravascular tumors. IVUS was used preoperatively to determine the vena caval extension of recurrent renal cell carcinoma and to help plan a successful resection[6] We perfomed IPEUS for pancreatobiliary carcinoma to diagnose the portal invasion of tumor. This is a preliminary report of our results.

MATERIAL AND METHODS

The study group consisted of 15 patients, six men and nine women, with a mean age of 65.5 years (range, 53 to 78 years) who underwent intraportal endovascular ultrasonography (IPEUS) between Feb 1992 and Dec 1992. A breakdown of individual cases shows 9 pancreatic cancers, 5 bile duct cancers and 1 gallbladder cancer. Extened pancreaticoduodenectomy with portal vein resection was performed in 5 patients. Extended distal pancreatectomy with portal vein resection was performed in 1, extended total pancreatectomy with portal vein and celiac arterial resection in 1 left hepatic lobectomy with caudate lobe and right hepatic arterial resection in 1, right hepatic posterior segmentectomy in 1, proximal bile duct resection with caudate lobe in 1, proximal bile duct resection in 1, by-pass operation in 3 and exploratory laparotomy in 1. After all, resected cases were 10 in which histological comparison was done with the results of IPEUS. In all patients contrast enhancement CT, arterial portography and ultrasonography were performed in all patients.

Technique: IVUS catheter used in this study was comprized of a 20 MHz transducer mounted on the tip of 8-French catheter (CVIS, Sunnyvale, Ca). The ultrasound beam is reflected onto a rotating mirror revolving at 900 rpm, creating a 360° real-time image perpendicular to the catheter. The 20 MHz frequency of provided axial resolution of 0.12mm, lateral resolution of 0.3mm and maximum penetration of 20 mm. This catheter was used intraoperatively. 20 MHz transducer on the tip of 6-French catheter (Aloka, Tokyo, Japan) was used preoperatively.

Inraoperative procedure; Following laparotomy, a branch of the superior mesenteric vein was exposed and 8.5-French introducer was inserted. The IVUS catheter was inserted into the portal vein through this introducer. The catheter was advanced carefully into the intrahepatic portal vein. The catheter was then gradually withdrawn as the cross-sectional images of the area under investigation were recorded on a thermal paper printer and super VHS videotape. After examination, Anthron by-pass catheter (Toray Industries, Inc. Tokyo, Japan) was inserted from the cut-down portion of the superior mesenteric vein in the cases of combined resection of the portal vein. Under portosystemic shunt by this catheter, portal vein resection and anastomosis was performed safely[1]. This procedure was performed in 12 patients.

Preoperative procedure; This procedure was performed by percutaneous transhepatic approach. Following placing 7-French introducer into the intrahepatic portal vein, IVUS catheter was insreted into the superior mesenteric vein. From this point, IVUS catheter was gradually withdrawn with recording as the intraoperative procedure.

RESULTS

The wall of the portal vein was visualized as echogenic band with a thickness of 0.5mm to 1.0 mm. When the echogenic ring of the portal vein was preserved, the portal vein invasion of the tumor was diagnosed as negative. The destruction of the echogenic band of the portal vein wall with distortion of the lumen of the portal vein by the tumor was considered diagnostic of portal vein wall invasion. Basically, normal pancreatic tissue was visualized as echogenic speckled pattern. Pancreatic cancer was visualized as a hypoechoic speckled pattern. 14 out of 15 patients, portal invasion of the tumor was diagnosed correctly. In 7 patients who underwent extended resection of the pancreas, tumor was in contact with the wall of the portal vein and portal invasion of the tumor was diagnosed as negative. The average distance between the advanced portion of tumor and the adventitia of the portal vein was 0.66 mm (range, 0.42 mm to 0.9 mm). This distance was considered to reflect the fibrosis associated with the advanced portion of the tumor. In one patients in whom the diagnosis could not be made correctly, the associated pancreatitis was severe. In this case, the margin between tumor and pancreatitis was unclear.

Another important information obtained by IPEUS was hepatic arteial iavasion. In case of proximal bile duct cancer, left branch of the portal vein and right hepatic arterial invasion was diagnosed. Right hepatic arterial invasion could be diagnosed only by IPEUS. In another case of pancreatic cancer, common hepatic arterial invasion was diagnosed by angiography. In this case, right hepatic artery originated from superior mesenteric artery. Right hepatic arterial invasion could also be diagnosed only by IPEUS. In both cases, the finding of IPEUS was confirmed by operation and resected specimen.

Lymph nodes along the potal vein was clearly visualized and the possibility of visualization of intrapancreatic lymph nodes could be suggested.

DISCUSSION

Recently, aggressive radial operation for pancreatobiliary carcinoma including portal vein resection has been reported. In spite of progress of imaging diagnosis, detection of areas of subtle cancer invaion into portal vein wall as difficult. Arterial portography provides the luminal profile and CT scan provides the cross-sectional shape of the portal vein. These modalities can therefore only reveal tumor invasion when it is at an advanced stage. IPEUS could visualize the wall of the portal vein and decide between compression and invasion of the tumor. Right hepatic artery commonly runs between proximal bile duct and portal vein. So, this artery is liable to be invaded by the carcinoma of hepatic hilum. IPEUS could diagnose this arterial invasion which could not be detected by conventional imaging technology.

Lymph nodes along the portal vein and intrapancreatic lymph nodes were clearly visualized. But judgement of metastasis was difficult in our experience.

IPEUS was considered to give important information about pancreatobiliary sugery.

REFERENCES

1. Nakao A, Nonami T, Harada A, et al (1990) Portal vein resection with a new antithrombogenic catheter. Surgery 108:913-918
2. Tashiro S, Uchino R, Hiraoka T, et al (1991) Surgical indication and significance of portal vein resection in biliary and pancreatic cancer. Surgery 109:481-487
3. Mimura H, Takakura N, Kim H, et al (1991) Block resection of the hepatoduodenal ligament for carcinoma of the bile duct and gallbladder: surgical technique and a report of 11 cases. Hepatogastroenterology 38:561-567
4. Nimura Y, Hayakawa N, Kamiya J, et al (1991) Hepatopancreatoduodenectomy for advanced carcinoma of the biliary tract. Hepatogastroenterology 38:170-175
5. Tobis JM, Mallery J, Mahon D, et al (1991) Intravascular ultrasound imaging of human coronary arteries in vivo. Circulation 83:913-926
6. Barone GW, Kahn MB, Cook JM, et al (1991) Recurrent intracaval renal cell carcinoma: The role of intravascular ultrasonography. J Vasc Surg. 13:506-509

New Endoscopic Mucosectomy Technique for Early Cancer of Esophagus, Stomach, and Colon

Haruhiro Inoue[1], Kimiya Takeshita[2], Satoshi Okabe[2], Tatsuyuki Kawano[2], Kunihide Yoshino[2], and Mitsuo Endo[2]

[1]Department of Surgery, Kasukabe-Syuwa Hospital, Saitama, 344 Japan
[2]First Department of Surgery, Tokyo Medical and Dental University, Bunkyo-ku, Tokyo, 113 Japan

ABSTRACT

A new, simplified technique for endoscopic mucosal resection using a transparent plastic cap (EMRC) was introduced. A total of fifty-four cases of mucosectomy of the esophagus, stomach and colon were successfully performed using this procedure causing no severe complications such as mass bleeding and perforation. During the short-term follow-up period, no recurrence of tumor was evident. We believe that because of its technical simpleness and safety this EMRC procedure will become accepted by many digestive endoscopists.

KEY WORDS: Endoscopic mucosal resection, Mucosectomy, EMRC

INTRODUCTION

Endoscopic mucosectomy has become accepted in many institutes in Japan as a strategy for mucosal cancerous lesions of the esophagus, stomach and colon (1-3). Full-thickness mucosal reseciton poses the definite advantage of contributing to accurate histopathological analysis. We developed a considerably simplified technique of mucosectomy using a cap-fitted panendoscope (EMRC) for early esophageal, gastric and colonic cancer (4). This EMRC procedure is also useful not only as a therapeutic measure for the mucosal cancer lesion but also as a diagnostic approach even for the polypoid mucosal lesion.

PATIENTS AND METHODS

Fifty-four consecutive cases underwent this novel jumbo biopsy or polypectomy technique for the resection of esophageal, gastric or colonic mucosal lesion. Specifically, these cases included six esophageal cancer patients, ten early gastric cancer lesions, and four colon malignant polyps.

The tip of the endoscope (XV-100, XQ-200, Q-200, 200-I, 2T200 Olympus Optical Co.) used in the procedure is covered with a specially designed transparent endoscope cap (12-mm in outer diameter, 10.5-mm in inner diameter and 10-mm depth for upper gastrointestinal tract mucosectomy, or a 16 mm in outer diameter cap for colonoscope; Olympus Optical Co.) (4). We also designed a novel pre-looped plastic cap (5). A small-size snare (SD-7P, Olympus Optical Co.) is inserted through the biopsy channel of the endoscope, and opens inside the cap fitted at the tip of the scope. We selected a fine snare so that a shallow free space is maintained inside the biopsy channel to facilitate development of sufficient endoscopic suction.

More than 10 ml of normal saline mixed with low-volume epinephrine is injected into the submucosal layer around the target mucosal lesion sufficient to lift up the entire mucosal lesion (Fig. 1a). A loop of snare wire is formed inside the cap prior to resection (5) or during the procedure (4). Under full endoscopic suction, the lesion-involved mucosa becomes tightly packed inside the cap of the endoscope and is then snared tightly (Fig. 1b). After reconfirming the size and shape of the snared mucosa to ensure procedural safety, resection is performed by high-frequency waves (Fig. 1c).

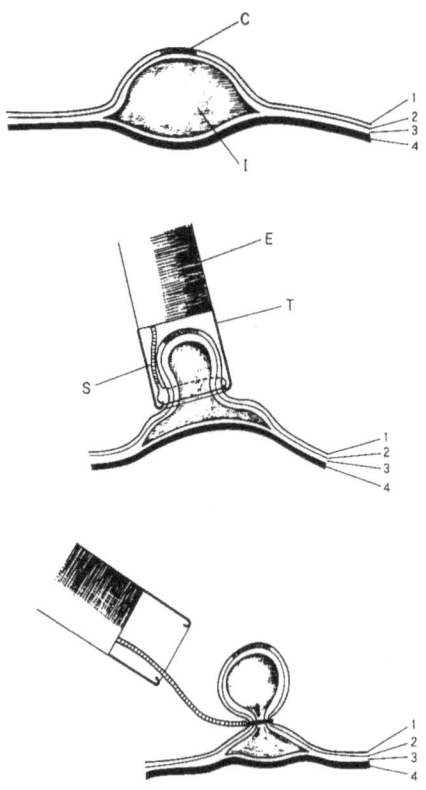

Fig. 1 Outline of EMRC procedure.

a. Epinephrine-added saline is injected into the submucoal layer underlining the mucosal cancerous lesion.

b. Cancer-bearing mucosa is captured inside the cap attached to the endoscope tip under full suction.

c. Mucosal lesion is snared tightly using the snare device passed through the biopsy channel of the panendoscope.

C, cancer lesion
I, injected saline
E, endoscope
T, transparent plastic cap
S, snare
1,2,3,4, number of echoic layer.

$$\frac{a}{\dfrac{b}{c}}$$

RESULTS

Fifty-four patients received this EMRC procedure under topical anesthesia. During upper gastrointestinal endoscopy the endoscope bearing the cap relatively easily passed through the pharynx with only slight resistance. In addition, insertion of the specially designed cap-fitted colonoscope was also smoothly achieved.

In every case mucosal resection was easily and safely performed causing no severe complications. Resected specimens were within about 2 cm in diameter, and repeated mucosectomy could also be safely performed. Regarding the esophagus, the uncolored portion that underwent lugol staining was resected in each of the nine patients. About one-fourth of circumferential mucosal resection was possible constantly in each cauterization. Half of the circumferential resections could be performed only by two-times cauterization. Thirty-eight polypoid lesions of the colon were also resected using this EMRC procedure. Fouyr of the resected polyps was clarified to be adenocarcinoma, and its surgical margin was confirmed to be free of cancer.

Actually lesions positioned in any direction could be easily captured inside the cap under full endoscopic suction without causing laceration of the target mucosa. Resected specimens were also easily transported outside the body by capturing them inside the cap under the continued endoscopic suction.

DISCUSSION

Mucosal cancers of the esophagus, stomach and colon usually have neither lymph node invovement nor vscular invasion (2,6,7). Therefore, they are good candidates for local treatment. The establishment of a considerably simplified technique which also prevents the complications of perforation and bleeding is particularly desirable.

Preoperative diagnosis of mucosal cancer can be achieved mainly by actual
endoscopic findings. Either a slightly depressed or elevated superficial
lesion of less than 2 cm in size presents the possibility of being a mucosal
cancer. Usually a amall lesion of less than 1 cm in size is a appropriate
candidate for this local resection (2,6,7).

Concerning the esophagus we have already introduced an endoscopic mucosal
resection technique employing a transparent overtube for treating early-stage
esophageal cancer (EMRT) (3). EMRT has been proven to be a safe and effective procedure (8), but demands a certain degree of skillfulness on the part of
the endoscope operator. Based on the clinical experience of this EMRT-proce-
dure, we developed a considerably more simplified mucosectomy technique using
a cap-fitted panendoscope (EMRC) for early esophageal cancer (4), and extended
its application to gastric and colonic mucosal lesions. Using this technique
enables any part of the esophageal, gastric and colonic mucosa to be resected easily and safely under topical anesthesia without leading to major
complications such as perforation and bleeding.

Furthermore, the resected specimen sizes of about 2 cm are sufficient for
promoting accurate histopathological evaluation including invasion depth and
vascular permeability. If histopathological assessment reveals that the
cancer invasion penetrates through the lamina muscularis mucosae into the
submucosal layer and demonstrates some possibility of lymph node involvement, performance of concomitant surgical resection should be considered
(2,6,7).

We believe that cecause of its technical simpleness and safety this EMRC
procedure will become accepted by many endoscopists, and, as a diagnostic
measure, indication for the procedure will become extended to the entire
digestive tract.

REFERENCES

1. Tada M, Karita M, Yanai H, Takemoto T (1987) Treatment of early gastric
cancer using a strip biopsy, a new technique for jumbo biopsy, In; Takemoto
T, Kawai K, eds. Recent topics of digestive endoscopy. Tokyo: Excerpta Medica
:137-142
2. Morson BC, Bussey HJR, Samoorian S (1977) Policy of local excision for
early cancer of the colorectum. Gut 18:1045-1050
3. Inoue H, Endo M (1990) Endoscopic esophageal mucosal resection using a
transparent tube. Surg Endosc 4:198-201
4. Inoue H, Takeshita K, Hori H, Muraoka Y, Yoneshima H, Endo M (1993) Endoscopic mucosal resection with a cap-fitted panednoscope for esophagus, stomach and colon mucosal lesions. Gastrointest Endosc 39:58-62
5. Inoue H, Noguchi O, Saito N, Takeshita K, Endo M. Easy, safe procedure
for endoscopic mucosectomy for early cancer of entire gastrointestinal tract
using a pre-looped plastic cap (letter) Gastrointestinal Endosc, contributed.
6. Endo M, Takeshita K Yoshida M (1989) How can we diagnose the early-stage
of esophageal cancer? Endoscopic diagnosis. Endoscopy 18:11-18
7. Takemoto T, Tada M, Yanai H (1989) Significance of strip biopsy, with
particular reference to endoscopic "Mucosectomy". Digestive Endosc 1:4-9
8. Inoue H, Endo M, Takeshita K, Kawano T, Yoshino K (1991) Endoscopic
resection of early-stage esophageal cancer. Surg Endosc 5:59-63

Endoscopic Mucosal Resection of Early-Stage Esophageal Cancer

Masatoshi Inoue, Hitoshi Shiozaki, Shigeyuki Tamura, Kenji Kobayashi, Hiroshi Oka, Keisuke Iihara, Yuichiro Doki, Takatoshi Kadowaki, Shigeo Matsui, and Takesada Mori

Second Department of Surgery, Osaka University Medical School, Osaka 553 Japan

ABSTRACT

Endoscopic mucosal resection (EMR) was performed for the treatment of 8 early stage esophageal cancers. All of the resected specimens were available for histological examinations, and were found out that no cancer cells remained at any margin. As for depth of invasion, five lesions were limited to the epithelium and three to the muscularis mucosae. Large ulcers by endoscopic mucosal resection disappeared without any stenotic change within four weeks. No signs of recurrence were observed during the follow up period (mean = 9.3 months). We found no severe postprocedural complications except one with a perforation which demanded surgical repair. Thus, EMR is a useful technique for the treatment of early-stage esophageal cancer.

KEY WORDS: early-stage esophageal cancer, endoscopic mucosal resection

INTRODUCTION

Surgical procedures such as transthoratic esophagectomy and blunt dissection have been popular to treat early-stage esophageal cancer. In some institutes, laser therapy [1] and radiation therapy [2] are chosen for this disease. Recently, a newmethod of endoscopic mucosal resection for this disease has been developed with the advance of the endoscopic equipment [3]. Futhermore, using a new type of over-tube for EMR, which was designed by Makuuchi, esophageal mucosal lesions can be resected easily and certainly. We resected eight early-stage esophageal cancerous lesions endoscopically using this over-tube.

PATIENTS AND METHODS

Patients

Six patients with eight early-stage esophageal cancerous lesions were treated by EMR between June, 1991 and December, 1992. The lesions were detected radiologically and endoscopically using iodine staining. In the endoscopical observasions, eight lesions were classified into three superficial types; elevated, flat and depressed type [4]. Computed tomography was preformed preprocedurally, and warranted no metastasis to the distant organs or to the legional lymphnodes. All patients were informed of the risks due to EMR and consented to undergo the therapy.

Procedure of EMR and Fllow-up

The patients received lidocaine liquid local anesthic and intramuscular injection of mild sedatives. EMR was carried out with the patient in supine position for the over-tube, which remained in the esophagus throughout the procedure. All procedures were performed using a fiber-optic gastroscope (GIF V-10, Olympus), a snare(SD6L,Olympus), over-tube, and an electrosurgical unit(PSD-2) (figure 1). To follow the repair of ulcer and to detect any recurrence in situ, endoscopic examinations has been performed routinely at 1 week, 4 weeks, 3 months of after EMR and every 6 months.

Histopathological Evaluation

All resected lesions were spread on rubber plates, fixed in neutral buffered formalin and enbedded in paraffin. The specimens were cut into 5 μm sections, stained with hematoxylin/eosin and examined nicroscopically.

RESULT

Preprocedural characteristics of patients and cancerous lesions

The mean age of the patient was 65.6 years (range 55 to 78 years). Men outnumbered women by 6 to 1. The reasons for the selection of this procedure in six patients were the high surgical risks to their general conditions in 4 cases and the disapproval to undergo surgery in 2 cases. All the lesions, located in intrathoratic esophagus, could be visualized by spraying of iodine dye solution, and classified into three superficial types; two, slightly elevated type; five, flat type; and one was both elevated and depressed type (Table 1). All of the lesions were perprocedurally diagnosed that the depth of them were limitted to the muscularis mucosae with no distant metastasis.

Histopathological features and follow-up

The size of the resected mucosa was about 4x4cm in one procedure. Two cases demanded additional EMR since cancerous lesions could not be resected completely in one procedure. All of the specimens were found out to be squamous cell carcinoma, resected at the submucosal layer. The diameter of the lesions ranged from 0,7 to 2.5cm (mean = 1.8cm). Histological examination of all the resected specimens revealed that no cancer cell remained at any margin, five lesions were limited to the epithelium and three to the muscularis mucoal (table 2). Just after EMR, the resected area formed a large artificial ulcer, in which the muscle layer proper could be seen (Fig. 2). We found no severe postprocedural complications except one with a minor perforation which was repaired surgically. In the follow-up period, all ulcers were re-epithelialized within 4 weeks, and no stenotic changes could not be seen (Fig. 2). No signs of recurrence were observed during the follow-up period (mean = 9.3 months).

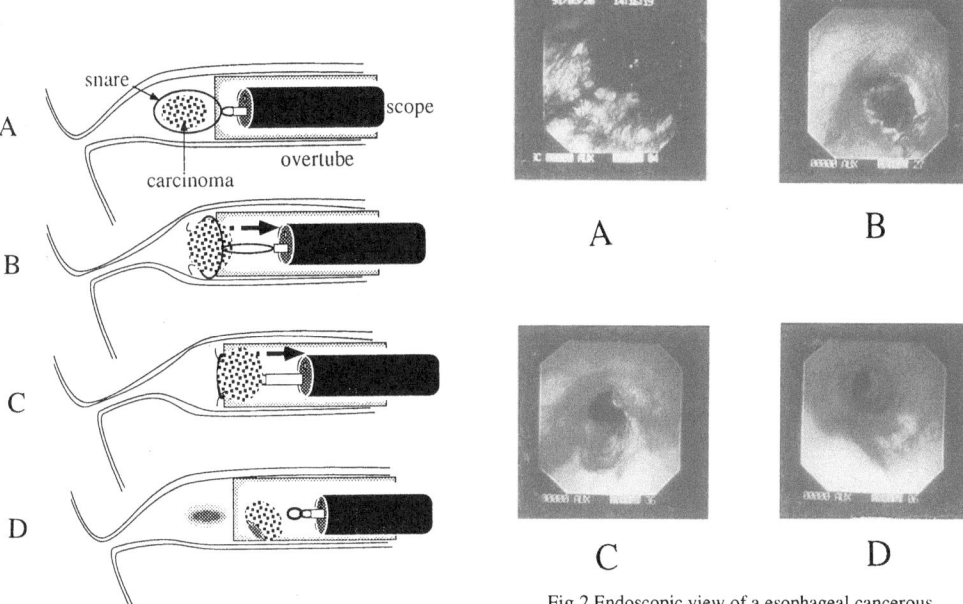

Fig.1 Method of endoscopic mucosal resection using over-tube which was desined by Makuuchi. A; Over-tube is aimed at the lesion and the snare is opened. B; The lesion is absorbed into the tube. C,D; The snare is closed and the lesion is cut.

Fig.2 Endoscopic view of a esophageal cancerous lesion and resected area. A; The cancerous lesion shows white color by spraying iodine dye solusion. B; Just after EMR, the muscle layer proper can be seen. C; At 7 days after EMR, the large artificial induced ulcer can be seen. D; At the 4weeks after resection, the large ulcer has completely disappeared.

DISCUSSION

Since early stage cancer limited to epithelium or musclaris mucosae has no lymph node involvement nor distant metastasis[5], local treatment may be effective in the treatment of early stage esophageal cancer. Moreover, endoscopic examination using iodine dyeing has detected

454

Table 1. Chalacteristics of patients and evaluation of early-stage esophageal cancerous lesions at the endoscopic observations

Patient No.	Age	Sex	Location	Endoscopic classification	Risk factor
1	55	M	Iu	IIb	-
2	71	M	Im Ei	IIa IIb	Liver cirrhosis
3	53	M	Im Ei	IIa IIb	Tongue cancer
4	76	M	Ei	IIc+IIa	Colon cancer
5	78	M	Ei	IIb	Gastric cancer
6	61	F	Im	IIb	-

Abbrevations: M=male; F=female; Iu=upper intrathoratic; Im=middle intrathoratic; Ei=lower intrathoratic;IIa=superficial and elevated; IIb=superficial and flat; IIc=superficial and deppressed

Table 2. Histopathological findings of specimens resected by EMR

Lesion No.	Size (cm)	Histological classification	Depth
1	0.7X0.7	SCC	ep
2	2.0X2.0	SCC	mm
3	2.0X1.3	SCC	ep
4	1.5X1.5	SCC	mm
5	2.0X1.0	SCC	ep
6	2.5X2.5	SCC	mm
7	2.0X0.5	SCC	ep
8	2.0X1.5	SCC	ep

Abbrevations: SCC=squamous cell carcinoma; ep=intraepithelium; mm=limited to the lamina muscularis mucosae.

esophageal cancer in early stage frequently[6]. Although radiation and/or laser therapy are selected for non surgical treatment of this disease, they can not offer any samples for the histopathological evaluation. On the other hand, EMR, newly developed technique to resect esophageal mucosa[3], can provide specimens available to histopathological assessment.

In our institute, eight early-stage esophageal cancerous lesions were resected using EMR. they resected completely without any complication except one with a minor perforation, where the lesion seemed too large for EMR retrospectively.

REFERENCE

1. Tai ME, Qui SL, Ji Q (1985) Preliminary result of hematoporphyrin derivative-laser treatment for 13 cases of early esophageal carcinoma. Adv Exp Med Biol 193:21-25
2. Hishikawa Y, Tanaka S, Miura T (1985) Early esophageal carcinoma treated with intracavitary irradiation. Radiology 156:519-522
3. Inoue H, Yoshino H (1991) Endoscopic resection of early-stage esophageal cancer. Surg Endosc 5:59-62
4. Japanese Society for Esophageal Disease. Guidelines for the Clinical and Pathologic Studies on Carcinoma of the Esophagus, ed. 8. (1992) Tokyo:Kanehara
5. Isono K, Sato H, Nakayama K. (1991) Results of a nationwide study on the three-field lymph node dissection of esophageal cancer. Oncology 48:411-4205.
6. Shiozaki H, et.al (1990) Endoscopic screening of early esophageal cancer with lugol-dye method in patient with head and neck cancer Cancer 66:2068-2071

The Elevated Type Early Gastric Cancer as the Subject of the Endoscopic Resection or the Conservative Surgical Operation

Hiroshi Furukawa, Masahiro Hiratsuka, Takeshi Iwanaga, and Shingi Imaoka

Department of Surgery, The Center for Adult Diseases, Osaka, 537 Japan

ABSTRACT

We tried to decide on a new rule which would allow endoscopic resection or the conservative small surgery from a total of 1667 early gastric cancers which underwent common surgery with R2 lymph node dissection. In the elevated type cancer (I or IIa) invading within the mucosal layer (E-EGC-m) we experienced only two cases of E-EGC-m with lymph node metastasis (1.1%) whose sizes were 3.0 and 3.2 cm in diameter. The indication of endoscopic resection for E-EGC-ms is a tumor smaller than 2.0 cm and for E-EGC-ms larger than 3.0 cm, a preserving surgery with limited lymph node dissection is recommended.

KEY WORDS: early gastric cancer, lymph node metastasis, conservative surgery, endoscopic resection

INTRODUCTION

Since early cancer can be detected frequently in clinics the ratio of early cancer was increased to over 50% in our hospital. A total of 1800 patients with early gastric cancer have undergone common resection and R2 lymph node dissection (1) during the last 30 years. Recently, endoscopic surgery (ES)(2) and conservative small surgery (CS) (3) have been performed for a good QOL. Now the new indicator for ES or CS should be decided on for early gastric cancer, and it is necessary to establish a new rational method of CS.

PATIENT AND METHODS

A total of 1667 early gastric cancers were evaluated in their lymph node metastases. Macroscopic findings, size, and the depth of invasion in the node positives were compared with tumors without node metastasis. The frequecyof correct preoperative diagnosis of the depth of invasion is estimated by comparison with the results of the resected specimen. A case of early IIa gastric cancer involved within mucosal layer and having a metastatic node is presented on its macroscopic and microscopic findings. Finally, a trial of conservative small surgery, which is performed for early gastric cancer in our hospital, is proposed for a surgery with good QOL.

RESULTS

Lymph Node Metastasis in Early Gastric Cancer

Lymph node metastasis was noted in 5% of intramucosal carcinomas and in 20% of cancers invading to the submucosal layer. In the intramucosal cancer the node metastasis was observed in 5.7% of depressed type with ulceration, 0.6% of depressed type without ulceration, and 1.1% of elevated type.

Preoperative Diagnosis of The Depth of Invasion

It is difficult to diagnose the depth of invasion in early gastric cancer before operation. Recently, we tried to diagnose the depth of invasion before operation by endoscopy and x-ray examination. **Table 1** shows the results of preoperative diagnosis (PD) and final diagnosis (FD). For protruded type (I and IIa) PD was correct in a high percentage of the tumor (90%), but for depressed type (IIc) it was insufficient(70%).

Table 1. Final diagnosis (FD) of tumors invading within mucosal layer diagnosed before operation

Macroscopic Classification	Depth of invasion (FD)	
	m (%)	sm ≤ (%)
elevated	27 (90)	3 (10)
depressed with ulcer	51 (71)	21 (29)
depressed without ulcer	30 (70)	13 (30)

A Case Report of an Elevated Type Early Gastric Cancer Invading Within Mucosal Layer With Lymph Node Metastasis

A 62 year old female was diagnosed with early gastric cancer at a clinic. In x-ray examination, the IIa lesion was located at the greater curvature in the antrum (Fig. 1). The size of the tumor was 3.2 cm in diameter and the depth of invasion was diagnosed M (within mucosal layer). In the endoscopy the diagnosis was almost the same as x-ray examination. A subtotal gastrectomy with R2 lymph node dissection was performed, and a IIa tumor whose size was 3.2 cm in diameter accompanied with a lymph node metastasis along the lesser curvature was found. Microscopically, primary tumor involved within the mucosal layer was a tubular adenocarcinoma, and the metastatic node showed the the same appearance as the primary one.

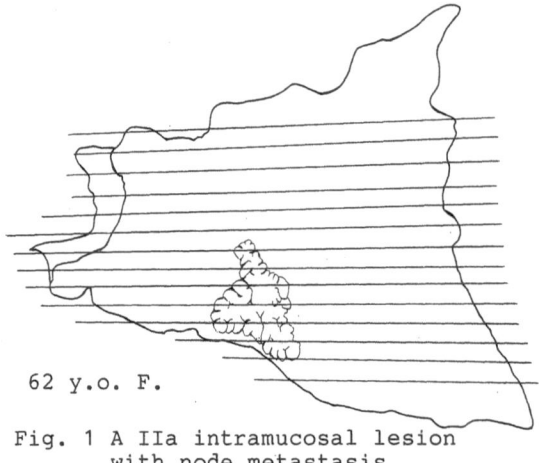

62 y.o. F.

Fig. 1 A IIa intramucosal lesion
with node metastasis

A Review of Early Gastric Cancer Characterized Elevated, m and n(+)

Some authors (4)(5)(6) reported a total of 6 patients with early gastric cancer (IIa or I) involved within mucosal layer and having a metastatic node. Their sizes were between 3.2 cm and 11.6 cm in the 4 cases.The location of the metastatic node was not written in any reports.

A Trial of Conservative Surgery for Early Gastric Cancer

We are trying a small resection and limited lymph node dissection for early gastric cancers which are diagnosed as being without lymph node metastasis. The indicator for this operation are as follows; I or IIa intramucosal cancer or IIc smaller than 2.0 cm in diameter. The surgical methods are proximal resection for cancers in the upper stomach, segmental resection for those in the middle stomach and distal resection for those in the antrum. Vagal nerve was preserved at the liver branch and the celiac branch. Over 50 patients underwent conservative surgery during the last 3 years and a lymph node metastasis was found in only one patient. The intraoperative diagnosis (frozen section) on the node was negative but the metastatic focus was found on a specimen fixed by formalin after operation.

DISCUSSION

The endoscopic resection (ER) or conservative small surgery (CS) is proposed for early gastric cancer without lymph node metastasis. The criteria for ER is the I or IIa intramucosal cancer less than 2.0 cm in diameter. It is important to diagnose whether the margin of the lesion is well defined and whether or not there is node metastasis. In these series we experienced only two cases of early cancer which involved within the mucosal layer, was of IIa type, and had node metastases. The ratio of node positives in these cases (IIa, m) is still very low (1.1%) but the number of node positives will increase with cases of early gastric cancer. The oppotunities to performing ER and CS will increase, but for safety the CS is better than the ER when the size or the depth of invasion is unclear before operation.

REFERENCES

1. Iwanaga T, Furukawa H, Hiratsuka M (1991) Treatment of early gastric carcinoma. *Jpn J Digest Organs* 2:361-370.
2. Mimura S, Ichii M, Imanishi K, Tatsuta M, Otani T, Okuda S (1990) Evaluation of photodynamic therapy for gastric cancer. Dig2. Mimura S, Ichii M, Imanishi K, Tatsuta M, Otani T, Okuda S (1990) Evaluation of photodynamic therapy for gastric cancer. *Dig Endosc* 2:265-274.
3. Sowa M, Kato Y, Nishimura M, Kubo T, Maekawa H, Umeyama K (1989) Surgical approach to early gastric cancer with lymph node metastasis. *World J Surg* 13:630-636.
4. Ota H, Takagi K, Ohashi I, Tamura S, Kuno K, Kajitani T (1981) Studies of the 1000 cases of early gastric cancer —with special reference to macroscopic classification—. *Jpn J Gastroenterol Surg* 14:1399-1408.
5. Kuriyama Y, Higashi H, Miyamoto T, Maeura G, Kozaki G (1982) Studies on lymphatic invasion in early gastric cancer. *Jpn J Gastroenterol Surg* 15:1314-1317.
6. Korenaga D, Kamekawa T, Okamura K, Kumashiro R, Inokuchi K, Furusawa G, Era S, Noda S, Matsusaka T (1984) Studies on intramucosal carcinoma of the stomach with lymph node metastasis. *Jpn J Gastroenterol Surg* 17:1501-1506.

Endoscopic Surgery for Early Gastric Cancer and the Points Which Demand Special Attention

ATSUSHI NASHIMOTO[1], JUEI SASAKI[1], MASAYUKI NIWA[2], and KAZUEI OGOSHI[2]

[1]The Department of Surgery, [2]The Department of Internal Medicine, Niigata Cancer Center Hospital, Niigata, 951 Japan

ABSTRACT

Endoscopic therapy for early gastric cancer has recently progressed. Our methods are endoscopic resection, and our criteria for endoscopic resection are as follows: ①well defined mucosal cancer of the elevated or flat type less than 2cm in size, ②well defined mucosal cancer of the depressed type less than 1cm in size and histologically differentiated adenocarcinoma, and with no peptic ulcer within the lesion. Eighty-five cases and 94 lesions were treated by endoscopy. Seven patients later died: six died of other diseases but one died of cancer itself after laser therapy. Seventeen patients were subsequently treated by surgical procedures after endoscopic therapy. Two patient died, namely, one died of myeloma and the other of suicide. The points which demand special attention are as follows: ①observance of strict indication, ②combination with superficial spreading of flat cancer ③multiple lesions of cancer, ④ill-defined minimal cancer, and ⑤other malignancies which occur during post-treatment after endoscopic therapy. It is important to select and perform the most appropriate endoscopic therapy according to strict criteria. However, endoscopic therapy must be undertaken even if the criteria does not so warrant. We emphasize that the surgical treatment should be selected on the incomplete endoscopic resection or recurrence, because the margin of the cancer lesion will have become ill-defined after endoscopic therapy.

KEY WORDS: early gastric cancer, endoscopic therapy, endoscopic resection

INTRODUCTION

Progress of diagnostic endoscopy has resulted in the detection of an increasing number of minute or small lesions in early cancer. Early cancer has been found in the aged more and more as society is faced with an increasing percentage of elderly. Endoscopic treatment for early gastric cancer has recently progressed (1,2,3). Therefore endoscopic therapy for early gastric cancer is going to become more necessary. Radical endoscopic therapy is applicable for early gastric cancer without lymph node metastasis. We have already reported the applications for endoscopic treatment based on the results of histopathological studies of many cases of early gastric cancer surgically resected, and the usefulness of endoscopic resection as a means of practical treatment (4,5). The features of early gastric cancer without lymph-node metastasis, which are indicated for endoscopic resection, are as follows: ①Well-defined mucosal cancer of the elevated or flat type less than 2cm in size, ②Well-defined mucosal cancer of the depressed type less than 1cm in size and histologically differentiated adenocarcinoma, and with no peptic ulcer within the lesion. We studied the patients who underwent endoscopic resection, and also referred those who were treated by surgical resection after endoscopic therapy. Now we would like to describe the points which demanded special attention for endoscopic resection.

PATIENTS AND METHODS

Eighty-five cases and 94 lesions were treated at Niigata Cancer Center Hospital from 1966 to 1991, and continued follow-up examinations (Table 1). They were mainly treated by 3 endoscopic procedures; strip biopsy, polypectomy, and laser therapy. As a rule, we have selected the method of high frequency electric current, but when it was not possible, we preferred laser therapy.

RESULTS

Early gastric cancer patients treated by endoscopic therapy

Eighty-five cases and 94 lesions were treated and seven patients later died: six died of other diseases but one died of cancer itself after laser therapy. Table 2 shows characteristics of the patients and lesions treated by endoscopic therapy. Tumor size was: 5-9mm in 37 cases, 10-19mm in 33, more than 20mm in 9, and 15 are unknown. Gross type was 79 for type II a, and 15 for type II c. Concerning the depth of invasion, 79 lesions were limited to the mucosa, but 2 were invaded to the submucosa, 1 was proper muscular layer, and 12 were unknown.

Table 1

ENDOSCOPIC THERAPY FOR EARLY GASTRIC CANCER

Endoscopic therapy	No.of cases (No.of lesions)	Operation	Death
strip biopsy	35(38)	11	4
polypectomy	38(44)	4	1
laser therapy	12(12)	2	2(1)
total	85(94)	17	7

( )cancer death

Table 2

ENDOSCOPIC THERAPY FOR EARLY GASTRIC CANCER
— 85 cases, 94 lesions —

sex	age		tumor size (mm)		gross type		depth of invasion	
male 48	<50	5	5-9	37	II a	79	m	79
female 37	≥50	8	10-19	33	II c	15	sm	2
	≥60	40	≥20	9			pm	1
	≥70	24	unknown	15			unknown	12
	≥80	8						

The correct rate of preoperative diagnosis for the depth of early gastric cancer

We investigated 454 consecutive cases diagnosed as early cancer in preoperative examination (Table 3). The correct rate of preoperative diagnosis for mucosal cancer was 87.1% and for submucosal cancer was 54.5%. The rate of correct preoperative diagnosis for the depth of invasion of total early gastric cancer was 72.9% (331/454). This data revealed that the correct preoperative rate for mucosal cancer was almost satisfactory, but that for submucosal cancer was difficult. The correct rate of preoperative diagnosis for several gross types of mucosal cancer was almost equal. Even in some cases of mucosal cancer, it was difficult to determine the correct depth of invasion.

Table 3

THE CORRECT RATE OF PREOPERATIVE DIAGNOSIS FOR DEPTH OF INVASION OF EARLY GASTRIC CANCER

Preoperative diagnosis	Histological diagnosis m	sm	pm—	total
m	223(87.1%)	33(12.9%)		256 cases
sm	77(38.9%)	108(54.5%)	13(6.6%)	198 cases

*The rate of preoperative correct diagnosis for the depth of invasion of whole early gastric cancer was 72.9%(331/454)

Surgical resection cases after endoscopic therapy

Table 4 shows 17 patients who were subsequently treated by surgery after endoscopic therapy. Four cases were treated after polypectomy, 2 cases after laser therapy, and 12 cases after strip biopsy. All cases were negative in lymph node metastasis. Concerning the depth of invasion, the 14 lesions were limited to the mucosa, but two were invaded to the submucosa and one to the proper muscular layer. The histological type of all cases were differentiated tubular adenocarcinoma. Resected tumor size ranged from 5 to 40mm. The stump of 13 resected specimens were positive, 2 were negative, and 2 were unknown because of laser therapy. Four cases were accompanied with superficial spreading of flat cancer. Four resected specimens revealed double lesions which were overlooked before the operation. Two lesions were minute cancers but the margins were ill-defined. Case number 17 was demonstrated malignant lymphoma of the stomach by follow-up endoscopy 50 months after the endoscopic resection, and had a total gastrectomy and splenectomy with lymph node dissection. The surgical procedures were total gastrectomy for 4 cases and subtotal gastrectomy for 11 cases. Surgical local resection was also indicated for 2 cases with residual cancer after endoscopic resection. Two cases died from other causes, and the other cases remained alive and healthy. There were no deaths caused by gastric cancer.

Table 4   SURGICAL RESECTION CASES AFTER ENDOSCOPIC THERAPY

NO.	Age	Sex	Depth	n	Hist.	Gross	Size	Stump	Therapy	Ope**	Prognosis	Notes
1.	60	F	pm	0	tub2	I,IIc	40mm	+	polypectomy	T	46m dead	double ca., IgM(k)myeloma
2.	59	F	m	0	tub	IIa+IIb	23	+	polypectomy	B1	73m alive	IIb(+)
3.	68	M	m	0	tub1	I,IIa	10	+	polypectomy	B1	11m alive	double ca.
4.	73	M	m	0	tub1	IIa	10	/	laser	B1	62m alive	
5.	70	F	m	0	tub1	IIa	10	/	laser	SLR	14m alive	colon ca with liver meta.
6.	60	M	m	0	tub1	IIc,IIc	22	+	strip biopsy	T	8m alive	double ca.
7.	75	M	m	0	tub1	IIa	24	+	SB*+laser	B1	2m dead	suicide
8.	78	M	sm	0	tub2	IIa+IIb	15	+	strip biopsy	T	42m alive	IIb(+)
9.	83	F	m	0	tub1	IIa	25	−	strip biopsy	B1	40m alive	near pylorus ring
10.	61	M	m	0	tub1	IIa	15	+	strip biopsy	B1	30m alive	
11.	82	F	m	0	tub1	IIc	5	+	strip biopsy	B1	18m alive	minute ca.
12.	77	F	m	0	tub2	IIa+IIb	11	+	strip biopsy	B1	16m alive	IIb(+)
13.	74	M	m	0	tub1	IIa	8	−	strip biopsy	B1	21m alive	
14.	75	M	m	0	tub1	IIa+IIb	15	+	strip biopsy	SLR	18m alive	IIb(+)
15.	69	F	m	0	tub1	IIa	5	+	strip biopsy	B1	17m alive	minute ca.
16.	70	M	sm	0	tub1	IIa,IIc	20	+	strip biopsy	B1	13m alive	double ca.
17.	79	M	m	0	tub1	IIa	20	+	strip biopsy	T	8m alive	lung ca. postope., malig. lymphoma

* SB   strip biopsy
** Ope   ⌈ B1   subtotal gastrectomy
           ⌊ T   total gastrectomy
           SLR surgical local resection

DISCUSSION

The technique of endoscopic therapy has improved and the correct rate of pretreatment diagnosis for depth of intramucosal cancer has increased up to about 80%. Therefore, endoscopic radical resection has been performed frequently and positively. But we must discuss the remnant rate, recurrent rate, surgical rate after treatment, second malignancies and multiple lesions. Oizumi et al (6) reported that endoscopic resection was undertaken for 256 lesions of early gastric cancer, and the rate of residual lesions was 9.7% and the recurrence rate was 12.9%. New lesions of cancer were found in 11 cases in follow-up endoscopy, and surgical resection was performed in 35 cases. We must also treat the cases whose lesions do not warrant for endoscopic resection. We have experienced 17 cases (20%) who underwent surgical resection after endoscopic therapy. Four cases were accompanied with superficial spreading flat cancer. Four resected specimens revealed double lesions which were overlooked before the operation. Two lesions were minute cancers in which the margins were ill-defined and difficult to detected. The frequency of multiple cancers in surgically treated early gastric cancer was high (more than 10%) including minute cancer. After endoscopic resection, careful follow-up is necessary so as not to overlook local recurrence and residual foci of cancer. Conclusively these are points which demand special attention: ①Observance of strict criteria ②Combination with superficial spreading of flat lesion, ③Multiple lesions of cancer, ④Ill-defined minimal cancer, ⑤Other malignancies which occur during post-treatment after endoscopic therapy. Endoscopic therapy can be repeated on the same lesion and can be done with combination methods. Additional endoscopic therapy may be enough for some primary cancer lesions, even if the margins of the resected specimens positive. But the surgical treatment should be selected on the incomplete endoscopic resection or recurrence, because the margins of the cancer lesions will have become ill-defined after endoscopic therapy.
If this advice is not heeded, additional endoscopic therapy may fail again.

REFERENCES

1. Hirano M, Masuda K, Asanuma T, Naka H, Noda K, Matsuura K, Yamaguchi O, Ueda N (1988) Endoscopic resection of early gastric cancer and other tumors with local injection of hypertonic saline-epinephrine. Gastrointest Endosc 34: 264-269.

2. Tada M, Shimada M, Yanai H (1984) New technique of gastric biopsy. Stomach Intestine 19: 1107-1116 (in Japanease)

3. Oguro Y (1990) Recent advances in endoscopic treatment. Gann Monograph on Cancer Research 37: 89-99

4. Nashimoto A, Maeda T, Sasaki K, Muto T (1988) The significance of endoscopic treatment for early gastric cancer. J Jpn Surg Soc 89: 655-663 (in Japanease)

5. Nashimoto A, Tanaka S, Miyashita K, Sasaki K, Muto T, Soga J (1988) Clinicopathological study for early gastric cancer. -Indication of conservative surgery and radical endoscopic treatment for early gastric cancer- J Jpn Surg Soc 89: 1780-1788 (in Japanease)

6. Oizumi H, Matsuda T, Fukase K, Furusawa A, Mito S, Takahashi E (1991) Endoscopic resection for early gastric cancer. Stomach Intestine 226: 289-300

Endoscopic Treatment of Early Gastric Cancer and Evaluation of Submucosography in the Diagnosis of the Depth of Cancer Invasion

SHIGERU ASAKI, AKIRA SATO, SHUICHI OHARA, JIN SEKINE, YO HATOYAMA, and YUICHI NAKAYAMA

The Third Department of Internal Medicine, Tohoku University School of Medicine, Sendai, 980 Japan

ABSTRACT

More than ten years have passed since we introduced laser coagulation therapy
for gastric cancer. 149 cases and 164 lesions were performed endoscopic
therapy. Of the 149 cases, cancer did not disappear in 8 cases(5.4%), and
cancer became positive again during postoperative course in 10 cases(6.7%).
Three patients died from gastric cancer. All these three cases were surgically
inoperable and also were histologically poorly differentiated type adenocarcinoma with massive cancer invasion into submucosal layers. From these
results, to facilitate the selection of cases indicated for endoscopic therapy
, a suitable means of evaluating the depth of cancer invasion is needed. We
have developed a technique for submucosography(SMG) utlizing water-soluble
contrast medium and have used it for the diagnosis of cancer invasion since
1984. SMG accurately diagnosed the depth of cancer invasion in 89% of mucosal
cancers and 88% of submucosal cancers. SMG was evaluated to be an accurate
method for small lesions which are often indicated for endoscopic treatments.

KEY WORDS: early gastric cancer, endoscopic treatment, submucosography(SMG)

INTRODUCTION

With the advancement in treatment employing endoscopy, endoscopic therapy
has become prevalent among cases with high surgical risk due to complications
and cases in which patients themselves refuse operation due to advanced age.
In 1974, we started performing endoscopic therapy on a small number of cases
of early gastric cancer as a part of polypectomy, excision by snare using
high-frequency current. Full-fledged treatment began after July 1981 with the
introduction of YAG laser irradiation equipment made by MBB Co. in Germany
into our department. Since then untill December 1991, endoscopic therapy was
conducted on 149 cases(164 lesions) of early gastric cancer. To accomplish the
objective of endoscopic therapy, it is important to determine prior to the
operation whether the lesions can be sufficiently treated by endoscopy. The
following tests are performed as preoperative tests to determine suitability
of the lesions. Evaluation of gastric cancer's depth of invasion has also been
performed through normal X-ray and endoscopic examination. With these methods,
early gastric cancer and advanced gastric cancer can be distinguished to a
certain extent. However, the distinction between m and sm types and the extent
of infiltration into the submucosal layer are difficult to estimate. Therefore
, special methods to evaluate the depth of invasion became necessary. Two
highly accurate and objective methods of diagnosing depth of invasion are
employed: one is endoscopic ultrasonography, and the other is submucosography
developed by our department.

MATERIALS AND METHODS

Endoscopic Therapy

Clinical profiles of the 149 cases(164 lesions) were as follows. Patients
consisted of 96 males and 52 females, slightly more males than females. Ages
ranged from 39 to 89 years, with a mean age of 72 years and 33 subjects over
80 years of age, comprising 22% of the total. Macroscopic configuration of the
lesions displayed 100 protruded types(67%), followed by 42 depressed types
(28%), 6 flat types(4%), and 16 combined types(11%). As for location,50
lesions(31%) were found in the pyloric antrum, 79 lesions(48%) in the gastric
angle, and 35 lesions(21%) in the gastric body. Histopathological examination

461

revealed 3 lesions(2%) of papillary adenocarcinoma, 149 lesions(91%) of tublar adenocarcinoma, and 12 lesions(7%) of poorly differentiated adenocarcinoma.

Submucosography

Among this period, SMG was performed for 62 lesions(55 early cancers, 7 advanced cancers) in 59 cases of gastric cancer as well as in one case of esophageal cancer. Thirty-eight cases were males and 22 cases were females. Patients' mean age was 68 years. Fifty-five lesions were early gastric cancers . Twenty-six lesions were elevated type, 10 lesions mixed type and 19 lesions depressed type. The cancer was classified as m for 38 lesions and sm for 17 lesions, with advanced cancer of pm or more accounting for 8 lesions. As to histlogic type, 3 lesions were classified as papillary adenocarcinoma, 44 lesions as tubular adenocarcinoma and 15 lesions as poorly differetiated adenocarcinoma.

METHODS

Endoscopic Therapy

With high-frequency resection, a snare is used to remove the main part of the lesion, enabling histological examination of the collected specimen. The laser method excels in reaching into depths and completing treatment in a short period of time. Thus, we decided to adopt a combined therapy of high-frequency resection and laser coagulation. As the heat coagulation methods have limitation in obtaining sufficient deep effects without causing perforation, the pure ethanol method is used to complement this major weak point. As pure ethanol has strong dehydration and fixation actions, it can safely destroy cancer cells by diffusing between the muscle fasciculus of the tunica muscularis propria, in which the cancer has deeply infiltrated. Thus, in cases where submucosal infiltration was suspected, pure ethanol was locally injected into the depth of laser coagulation sites and ulcerated floor high-frequency resection sites.

Submucosography

In SMG, depth of cancer invasion is evaluated by injecting a water-soluble contrast medium into the submucosal layer surrounding the focus, and estimating the depth of invasion from X-ray pictures. We prepared 330γ/ml Mytomycin chacoal(MMC-CH) containing water-soluble contrast medium by mixing 2 mg of MMC ,2 ml of 5% activated carbon containing physiological saline and 4 ml of 80% iodamine sodium meglmine solution. Under endoscopic observasion, 1 to 2 ml each of the contrast medium was injected into the submucosal space in both the oral and the anal side of the tumor using a topical injection needle and immediately after the injection the frontal and lateral X-ray pictures were taken. A solution of MMC-CH having excellent retention properties and lymphotaxis developed by Takahashi and Hagiwara et al., Kyoto Prefectural University of Medicine. Film findings obtained by injecting our contrast medium could be classified into four patterns. Diffuse pattern without any hindrance in diffusion in either the frontal or the lateral view was defined as Type I. Relative diffuse pattern with slight hindrance in diffusion in the frontal view and small defect in the upper area in the lateral view was defined as Type II. Relative defect pattern with hindrance in diffusion in the frontal view and irregular defect in the lateral view desingnated as Type III. Defect pattern showing clear-cut defect was defined as Type IV. Then, we examined the relation between submucosographic findings and pathohistologic depth. Many of m cases gave diffuse Type I pattern. Among sm cases Type II and Type III pattern were prevailing. All cases of progressive cancer with pm or more, submucosographic findings were classified as Type IV.

RESULTS

Endoscopic Therapy

Results of endoscopic therapy performed on 149 cases and 164 lesions of early gastric cancer are described below. Of the 116 protruded and combined type lesions, 9 lesions(7.8%) could not be treated with high-frequency resection. Of the 48 flat and depressed type lesions, high-frequency resection was performed on 18 lesions(38%). Of the 149 cases, cancer did not disappear in 8 cases(5.4%), and cancer became positive again during postoperative course in 10 cases(6.7%). Three patients died from gastric cancer. All these three cases were surgically inoperable and also were histologically poorly differentiated type adenocarcinoma with cancer invasion into submucosal layers. The survival rate for early gastric cancer was 96% for 5 years and 94% for 8 years.

Submucosography

As shown in the Table 1 ; SMG accurately diagnosed the depth of cancer invasion in 89% of mucosal cancer and 88% of submucosal cancers, and in 96% of ele-

Table 1. Judgement of cancer invasion by submucosography

SMG pattern / Ca. depth	I	II	III	IV	Total
m	34(89%) 97%	3(8%) 30%	1(3%) 11%		38(100%)
sm	1(6%) 3%	7(41%) 70%	8(47%) 89%	1(6%) 11%	17(100%)
More than pm				8(100%) 89%	8(100%)
Total	35 100%	10 100%	9 100%	9 100%	63

vated type early cancers and 74% of depressed type early gastric cancers. By endoscopy the corresponding values were 74% and 65% in mucosal and submucosal carcinomas, respectively.

DISCUSSION

There is no doubt that surgery is the optimal treatment for early gastric cancer. However, with the increase in discovery of early gastric cancer among the aged and the prevalence of complications of basic diseases, which pose higher risk to surgery for the aged, there are many patients not wishing to undergo surgery. For this reason, there has been a demand for the development of therapies with less invasion to take the place of surgery. Amid such circumstances, endoscopic mucosal resection using a snare employing high-frequency current was developed. Early gastric cancer can become advanced cancer with the passage of time, treating early gastric cancer by less invasive endoscopic therapy is considered extremely significant. In any report of endoscopic therapy for early gastric cancer, with initial treatment alone, there are 10 to 20% residual cancer and recurrence. The results of endoscopic therapy are poor in cases of massive invasion into the submucosal layer and poorly differentiated adenocarcinoma. SMG excels in picking up microscopic findings, especially when evaluating the depth of slight invasion of gastric cancer into the mucosal and submucosal layers, which are the target of endoscopic therapy, it is far more superior than endoscopic ultrasonography. SMG was evaluated to be an accurate method for assessing the depth of cancer invasion, especially for small lesions which are often indicated for endoscopic treatment.

REFERENCES

1.Asaki S,Nishimura T,Ohara S,et al:Diagnosis of the depth of cancer invasion by submucosography.Tohoku J Exp Med 147: 427-428,1984
2.Asaki S,Nakayama Y,Ohara M,et al:Comparison of the efficacy of endoscopic ul trasonography and submucosography in diagnosing the depth of gastric cancer invasion.Tohoku J Exp Med 159: 227-235,1989
3.Hagiwara A,Takahashi T, Okamoto M, et al:The preparation and properties of anticancer agents absorbed to activated carbon. Akita J Med 9: 439-444,1983 (Japanese)
4.Asaki S,Sato A,Kinpara T,et al:Endoscopic treatment of early gastric cancer and its long-term prognosis.Endoscopia Digestiva 2: 1537-1544,1990(Japasese)

Endoscopic Treatment for the Cancer and Submucosal Tumor of the Upper Gastrointestinal Tract

Mamoru Hiraishi, Toshiro Konishi, Ken-Ichi Mafune, Takeshi Miyama, Tooru Hirata, Kiyoshi Mori, Haruhiro Nishina, and Yasuo Idezuki

Second Department of Surgery, University of Tokyo, Bunkyo-ku, Tokyo, 113 Japan

SUMMARY

Endoscopic treatment was performed for 38 patients of gastric cancer and 6 patients of esophageal cancer and 3 patients of submucosal tumor of the upper gastrointestinal tract. Thirty-four patients of gastric cancer were treated by laser irradiation. In these patients, 26 were considered as early cancer, and 8 were considered as advanced cancer. Four patients of gastric cancer and one patient of esophageal cancer were treated by strip biopsy. All these patients were considered as intolerable for surgical operation or refused for operation. In the laser therapy, Nd:YAG laser irradiation of 40-90 watts with 1-0.5 second duration was repeated for the lesions. The prognosis of early gastric cancer was good in case of protruded type or small ulcerative type which was less than 2cm in diameter. Three patients of submucosal tumor of the upper GI tract were treated by laser and electro-surgery. The lesion was in the esophagus, stomach and duodenum. KTP laser with bare quartz fiber of 0.3 mm in diameter was used. The surface of mucosal layer was cut with laser at the base of the tumor. Then the tumor was grasped by forceps and resected by electro-surgery. The resected specimens revealed myoma of the esophagus, fibrosis with calcified tissue of the stomach, and lipoma of the duodenum.
Endoscopic treatment for gastric cancer was effective for early cancer of protruded type and small cancer of ulcerative type less than 2 cm in diameter. Endoscopic treatment with KTP laser for the submucosal tumor was useful to remove the tumor.

KEY WORDS : endoscopic treatment, laser, strip biopsy, gastric cancer

INTRODUCTION

Endoscopic treatment for the bleeding or malignant disease of the gastro-intestinal tract has been performed using laser and electrosurgery (1). Nd:YAG laser irradiation therapy was a relatively easy method, and the photo-coagulation effect was strong enough to kill the cancer cells. For the small superficial type cancer, laser irradiation therapy was effective. On the other hand, after laser therapy, we could not take a resected specimen, it was difficult to confirm the therapeutic effect. So in the recent cases, we tried endoscopic resection such as strip biopsy for the superficial type cancer (2). In this study, we evaluated the therapeutic effect and indication of laser irradiation therapy for the cancer and submucosal tumor of the upper gastro-intestinal tract.

MATERIALS AND METHODS

Endoscopic treatment was performed for 38 patients of gastric cancer and 6 patients of esophageal cancer and 3 patients of submucosal tumor of the upper gastrointestinal tract. Thirty-four patients of gastric cancer were treated by laser irradiation. In these patients, 26 were considered as early cancer, which meant the cancer invaded within the submucoasa of the stomach, and 8 were considered as advanced cancer, which meant the cancer invaded deeper than the muscular layer of the stomach. Four patients of gastric cancer and one patient of esophageal cancer were treated by strip biopsy.

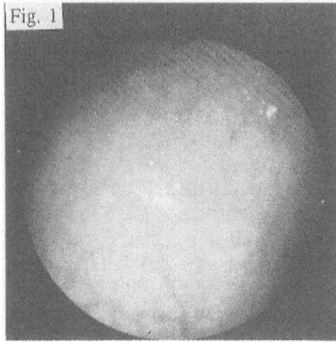 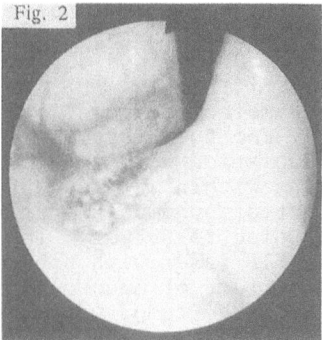 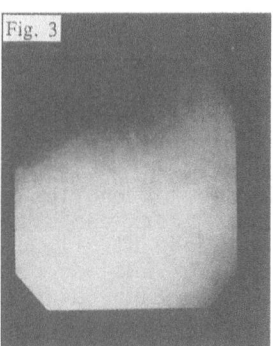

Fig. 1 shows the small gastric cancer in diameter of about 1 cm before laser treatment. Nd:YAG laser irradiation with a shot of 50 watts with 1 second duration was repeated. The total dosage was about 5000 joules for the lesion.

Fig. 2 shows the same lesion during the Nd:YAG laser irradiation.

Fig. 3 shows the same lesion 1 year after the laser irradiation. The ulceration was dissapeared and no malignant cell were seen by biopsy specimen.

DISCUSSION

For the treatment of malignancies in the gastro-intestinal tract using endoscopy, Nd:YAG laser irradiation with photocoagulaticn is one of the strong and minimum invasive procedue. As other treatments using laser, there are photodynamic therapy and laserthermia. But after these treatments, the therapeutic effect was sometimes unstable. In the laser therapy, it is very difficult to confirm the therapeutic effect, because of the absence of resected specimens. In this point of view, endoscopic resection is excellent to obtain the lesion. For the complete healing by the endoscopic treatment, we can only treat the lesion which has no metastatic lymph nodes. In case of gastric cancer, it is the suitable lesion for the endoscopic laser treatment that the size was within 2 cm in diameter and the depth of invasion is limiting within the mucous layer. In patients of the advanced gastric cancer, we have no case which was completely healed by the endoscopic treatment. To mention about the indication of the endoscopic treatment for malignancies in the upper gastro-intestinal tract, we consider the indication that the lesion is limiting within the submucosa, and the size is less than 2 cm in diameter. In the recent cases, we try a strip biopsy to remove the lesion at first, unfortunately the cancer has not been removed completely, a local resection of the lesion by surgical operation, or the laser irradiation therapy is performed. Nd:YAG laser irradiation therapy has been also performed for the palliation of the tumor. For the wide spread shallow ulcerative lesion and stenosis by the cancer, laser irradiation is sometimes very effective in palliation. For the treatment of submucosal tumor, KTP laser was effective to cut the surface of the tumor. We reported about the cutting ability of KTP laser in the gastric mucosa of rat (3).

REFERENCES

1) Fruhmorgen P., Bodem F., Reidenbach H.D., et al.(1976) Endoscopic laser coagulation of bleeding gastrointestinal lesions with report of the first therapeutic application in man. Gstrointestinal endoscopy 23 : 73-75
2) Tada M., Shimada M., Takemoto T., et al. (1984) New technique of gastric biopsy. Stomach and Intestine 19 : 1107-1116
3) Hiraishi M., Konishi T., Idezuki Y., et al. (1992) A new treatment of endoscopic surgery using KTP/YAG laser. Laser applications in medicine and surgery. ed. by Galletti G., Bolognani L. and Ussia G. : 327-332, Monduzzi Editore.

All the patients were considered as intolerable for surgical operation or refused for operation. In laser therapy, Nd:YAG laser irradiation of 40-90 watts with one second or 0.5 second duration time was repeated for the lesions.

The equipments were Molectron model 6000 (Molectron Co.) and KTP/YAG laser (Laserscope Co.). For the treatment of gastric cancer, we usually performed a laser irradiation with non-contact method. The therapeutic dosage for one lesion was within the range from 296 to 29282 joules at one time. For the treatment of subumcosal tumor of the upper GI tract, we utilized KTP laser and electro-surgery. The lesion was in the esophagus, stomach and duodenum. KTP laser with a bare quartz fiber of 0.3 mm in diameter was used. The surface of mucosal layer was cut with KTP laser at the base of the tumor. Then the tumor was grasped and pulled to the luminal site by forceps, then resected by electro-surgery at the root of the tumor.

Table 1) THERAPEUTIC EFFECT OF LASER IRRADIATION FOR THE PROTRUDED TYPE EARLY GASTRIC CANCER

| size of the lesion | number | 6 month after laser therapy | | |
		cancer(-)	cancer (+)	not evaluable (died within 6 month)
less than 1 cm	5	5 (100%)	0	0
1 - 2 cm	8	6 (75%)	0	2 (1)
more than 2cm	3	2 (67%)	0	1 (1)
total	16	13 (81.2%)	0	3 (2)

Table 2) THERAPEUTIC EFFECT OF LASER IRRADIATION FOR THE ULCERATIVE TYPE EARLY GASTRIC CANCER

| size of the lesion | number | 6 month after laser therapy | | |
		cancer(-)	cancer (+)	not evaluable (died within 6 month)
less than 1 cm	5	5 (100%)	0	0
1 - 2 cm	6	4 (66.7%)	0	2 (2)
more than 2cm	8	1 (12.5%)	4	3 (2)
total	19	10 (52.6%)	4	5 (4)

RESULTS

Endoscopic laser therapy was effective for the early cancer of protruded type and a small cancer of ulcerative type. Table 1 and 2 showes the results of laser irradiation therapy for the gastric cancer. We calculated the required shots of laser irradiation from the surface areas of the lesion. We usually took 100 shots for one square cm area of the lesion. The power of the Nd:YAG laser was set to coagulate the surface and submucosa of the lesion, which we considered about 40-60 watts power with the duration time of 1-0.5 second. After laser irradiation in these power and duration time, the color of the lesion changed to white or brown . After laser therapy, the prognosis of small early gastric cancer was very good both in case of protruded type and ulcerative type which was less than 1 cm in diameter. The prognosis of the large cancer more than 2 cm in diameter was not good, especially in the ulcerative type. In patients of advanced gastric cancer, or the wide spread type cancer, it was very difficult to coagulate the tumor ccmpletely. In patients of submucosal tumor, KTP laser was very effective to cut the mucosal tissue. The resected specimens revealed myoma of the esophagus, fibrosis with calcified tissue of the stomach, and lipoma of the duodenum.

Colon and Rectum

Characteristics of Cancer of the Large Bowel and Implication of Intestinal Flora and Bile Acids as Causal Factors

KYOTARO KANAZAWA[1], TOMOTARI MITSUOKA[2], and YUKIYOSHI ESAKI[3]

[1]Department of Gastroenterological and General Surgery, Jichi Medical School, Minamikawachi-cho, Kawachi-gun, Tochigi, 329-04 Japan
[2]Department of Veterinary Medicine, University of Tokyo, Bunkyo-ku, Tokyo, 113 Japan
[3]Department of Pathology, Tokyo Metropolitan Geriatric Hospital, Itabashi-ku, Tokyo, 173 Japan

ABSTRACT

The "Adenoma-Carcinoma Sequence" is a real phenomenon, but, the incidence of "cancer in adenoma" is too high compared with the incidence of lethal cancer of the large bowel, most of which develop as de novo cancer. These lesions are usually flat or excavated in shape, and tend to develop in the female right-half of the colon. Fecal bile acid levels are not parallel with the development of colorectal cancer. No strong correlation between particular intestinal microfloral group and the development of colorectal cancer can be seen, although some possible implications of Veillonellae, Lecithinase-negative clastridia and Enterobacteriaceae in the colorectal carcionogenesis among the female have been alluded.

KEY WORDS : Adenoma-Carcinoma Sequence, de novo cancer, fecal bile acid, intestinal microflora.

INTRODUCTION

The "Adenoma-Carcinoma Sequence" theory of Dr.Morson [1] has been well-established, but, those lesions compatible with this category are seen mainly among large adenomas, bigger than 10mm, and more definitely those large than 20mm in size. Having been able to collect tiny cancerous lesions without any sign of residual adenomatous component, we should like to close-up so-called de novo cancer of the large bowel.
Analysis of background factors, such as fecal bile acid level and intestinal microflora, were also analyzed to examine their implication in the development of colorectal cancer.

MATERIALS AND METHODS

The large bowels of 5,100 individuals, who have been consecutively autopsied at the Tokyo Metropolitan Geriatric Hospital, were scrutinized for the existence of cancerous foci.
The fecal bile acid levels were analyzed by the modified method of Grundy et al.. [2] [3] Samples were obtained from patients with cancer of the right and left-half of the colon as well as rectum. Patients with cataracta were selected as the control.

RESULTS

Incidence of colorectal cancer

Figure 1 shows the incidence of colorectal adenoma. More than 50% of individuals older the 60 years old in Tokyo had colorectal adenoma. The incidence is quite similar to the data reported by Chapman from the U.S.A.[4]

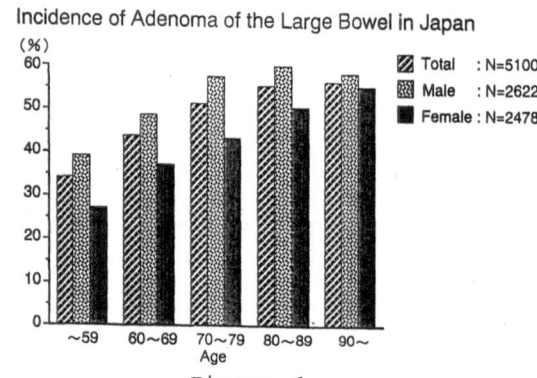

Incidence of Adenoma of the Large Bowel in Japan

Figure 1

Cancerization rate of colorectal adenoma

Cancer in adenoma was common among adenomas bigger than 10mm in size, especially larger than 20mm in size. Papillotubular adenoma had much more higher cancerization rate than the ordinary tubular adenoma Table 1.

Distribution of colorectal cancer

In total 312 clinically definite cancer of the large bowel were observed among the individuals of this series. The incidence was quite similar to the data reported by Berg from the U.S.A..[5] Caecoascending cancer found to be more popular among the aged, especially among the female.(Fig.2)

Age versus Size and Cancerization of Adenoma

Size (cm) Age	≦5	5<≦10	10<≦20	20<	
~59	0/70 (0/0)	0/21 (0/6)	1/3 (1/3)	0/3 (0/3)	1/97 (1/12)
60~69	1/475 (0/15)	3/176 (1/30)	3/38 (1/17)	1/6 (1/6)	8/695 (3/68)
70~79	5/1933 (0/58)	6/605 (1/122)	18/24 (13/68)	9/24 (8/19)	38/2686 (22/262)
80~89	5/2068 (0/63)	14/753 (7/161)	19/193 (10/99)	8/27 (7/22)	46/3041 (24/345)
90~	1/620 (1/17)	2/206 (0/34)	5/54 (5/32)	5/9 (3/6)	13/889 (9/89)
	12/5166 (1/148)	25/1761 (9/353)	46/412 (30/219)	23/69 (19/56)	106/7408 (59/776)

Adenoma with Focal Cancer / Adenoma
(Papillotubular Adenoma with Focal Cancer / Papillotubular Adenoma)

Table 2

Age-Related Distribution of Cancer in Each Segment

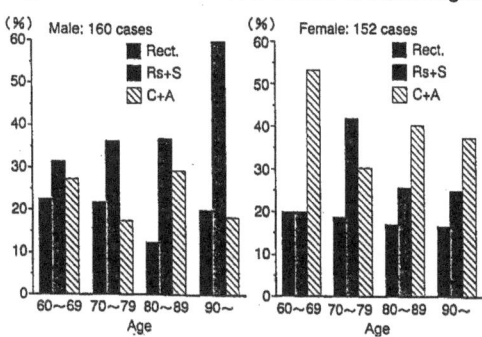

Figure 2

Lesions which may be called as de novo cancer

Collecting all cancerous foci confined either to the mucosa or submucosa, one can see there are flat or excavated foci without any remnant of adenomatous component. These lesions tend to penetrate through the Lamina muscularis mucosae into the submucosa before they get to the size of 10 mm, and regional lymph node metastasis can be seen among the lesions beyond 10mm in size. Typical features of these lesions are shown in Figure 3a 3b.[6]

Figure 3a

Colorectal Cancer
less than 10mm in Size

	Male	Female
P+Rb+Ra	8	2 / 5 / 8
Rs+S	3 / 5 / 6 / 10 / 10 / 6 / 8	1 / 5 / 6 / 8 / 8 / 3 / 7
A+C	5	1.5 / 3 / 7 / 8 / 8 / 3 / 5 / 7

3b

Fecal bile acid levels.

No definite correlationship between fecal bile acid profiles and colorectal cancer. The control group showed very high fecal bile acid levels.(Fig.4)

Intestinal microflora

Considerable difference in number of each group of flora was encountered. veillonellae and Lecithinasw-negative clostridia were increased among the colorectal cancer group, but, other floral group showed no definite tendencies, except for slight increase in Enterobacteriaceae and slight decrease in Bifidobacteria among the female with cancer of the colon.(Fig.5)

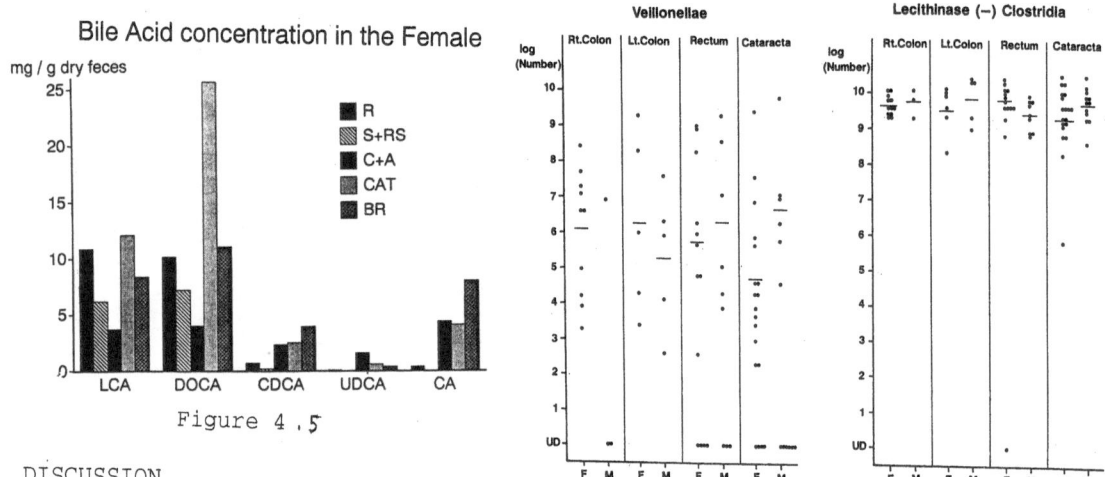

Figure 4 , 5

DISCUSSION

Colorectal adenoma is quite a popular lesion in Japan. The incidence of colorectal cancer calculated by the adenoma incidence and its cancerization rate, is too high compared to the incidence of real clinical or lethal cancer. The incidence of so-called de novo cancer does correspond to the incidence of lethal cancer. These lesions are flat or excavated in shape, and show a definite tendency to penetrate through the Lamina muscularis mucosa into the submucosa. These are the lesions, which and surely kill the patient; lethal cancer. The incidence of de novo cancer is markedly different among both genders, they are more common in the caecoascending part among the female. Thus different cancerization factors may be responsible for cancer of each different colorectal regions and different gender. Bile acids seems not so strongly involved in carcinogenesis of all colorectal segments. Microflora analyzed in the order of "Group" seems not so definitely involved in colorectal carcinogenesis as had been debated before. More detailed studies in the level of each species are necessary.

REFERENCES

[1]. Morson BC (1968) Precancerous and early malignant lesions of the large intestine. Br. J. Surg. 55:725-731.
[2]. Grundy SM, Ahrens EH Jr., Miettinen TA (1965) Quantitative isolation and gas-liquid chromatographic analysis of total fecal bile acids. J. Lipid Res. 6:397-410.
[3]. Imai K, Tamura Z, Mashige E, Osuga T (1976) Gas Chromatography of bile acids as their hexafluoisopropyl ester-trifluoroacetyl derivatives. J. Chromatography 120:181-186
[4]. Chapman I (1963) Adenomatous polypi of large intestine: incidence and distribution. Am. Surg. 157:223-226
[5]. Berg JW, Downing A, Lukes RJ (1970) Prevalence of undiagnosed cancer of the large bowel found at autopsy in different races. Cancer 25:1076-1080.
[6]. Kanazawa K, Konishi F, Saito Y, et al. (1991) Histgenesis of colorectal carcinoma. Proc Jpn Res Soc Gastroenteral Carcinog 3:169-173.

Effect of Apple Pectin on Azoxymethane-Induced Colon Carcinogenesis — Fecal Enzyme Activities and Prostaglandin E2 Level in Colonic Mucosa

KENJI TAZAWA[1], HIDEO OOKAMI[1], IWAO YAMASHITA[1], TETSURO SHIMIZU[1], MASAO FUJIMAKI[1], KENJI MURAI[2], KYOICHI KOBASHI[2], and TAKASHI HONDA[3]

[1]Second Department of Surgery, [2]Faculty of Pharmaceutical Sciences, [3]Department of Radiological Sciences, Toyama Medical and Pharmaceutical University, Toyama, 930-01 Japan

ABSTRACT

The diet including 10 or 20% apple pectin decreased dependently the multiplicity and occupied area of colon tumors. Furthermore, prostaglandin (PG) E2 level in distal colonic mucosa in 20% pectin-fed rats were significantly lower than those in basal diet group. In a separate experiment, apple and citrus pectin induced a 2-fold increase in fecal β-glucuronidase activity after dosing Azoxymethan(AOM) treatment. Fecal β-gluco-sidase and azoreductase activity, however, decresed in only apple pectin-fed rats. These results thus indicate that the effect of pectin on the colon carcinogenesis may depend on the type of pectin and be related to fecal enzyme activities, especially β-glucosidase and azoreductase.

KEY WORDS : colon cancer, pectin, prostaglandin E2, fecal enzyme activity

INTRODUCTION

Epidemiological data strongly suggest the importance of dietary factors in the etiology of colon cancer. A protective effect of dietary fiber has been suggested [1]. In chemically induced experimental colon cancer in animals, however, the kind of dietary fiber influences the number of colon tumors. As to pectin, there are various reports that pectin has been effective in experimental colon carcinogenesis or not [2-3]. We used low methoxyl apple pectin and investigated the tumor incidence and PGE2 level in colonic mucosa induced by AOM in rats. Furthermore, we investigated fecal enzyme activities.

MATERIALS AND METHODS

Experiment-1

6-week- old male Donryu rats were given subcutaneous injections of 7.4 mg AOM (Sigma chemical company, St Louis, USA) per kg body weight once weekly for 11 weeks. We placed 20 rats in each of 3 groups that received: 1) a basal diet 2) the basal diet with 10% apple pectin (OM type Herbstreith & Fox), and 3) the basal diet with 20% apple pectin. The rats were weighed weekly, and most were killed 30 weeks after the first injection. Grossly visible colonic tumors were recorded and tabulated. All tissues were fixed in formalin and processed for histology. The colonic mucosa was scraped off, immediately frozen and stored at −80°C until extraction for the measurement of PGE2. The amount of PGE2 in extract of homoginized colonic mucosa was measured by a radioimmunoassay method at Minase Research Institute, Ono Pharmaceutical Co., Ltd.

Experiment-2

3 groups of 20 rats were fed the following diets under the same conditions as in the experiment-1: 1) a basal diet 2) the basal diet with 20% apple pectin and 3) the basal diet with 20% citrus pectin (GENU pectin 150 grade USA-SAG type DD slow set, COPENHAGEN PECTIN A/S). Feces were collected 3 times from 5 rats in each group, that is, 1).before AOM injection 2) 12 weeks after the first injection and 3) 19 weeks after the first injection. Fecal sumples were then processed and analyzed for fecal

enzyme activities as described by Rowland et al [4-5] .

RESULTS

Experiment-1

The rats fed the pectin diet gained weight significantly less than rats fed the basal diet. Colon tumor incidence in control group was 100% (20/ 20), but that in 20% pectin group was 45% (9/20)(p<0.001). The difference in number of colon tumors per rat in control group (3.2±0.6) and pectin (10%:1.4±0.3, 20%:0.9±0.3) group was statistically significant (p<0.01, p<0.005). Occupied tumor area per rat in 20% pectin group (10.5±2.2 mm³) was significantly smaller than those in other group (Table 1).

Table 1. Colon tumor incidence and occupied tumor area induced by Azoxymethane (AOM) in rats fed diets containing pectin

Diet	Animals with colon tumors		No. of tumors			No. of tumors per rat (Mean±SE)	Occupied tumor area per rat[a] (Mean±SE)
	No.	Percent	Dist.	Prox.	Total		
Control (N=19)	19	100	41	20	61	3.2±0.6	79.7±39.5
10% Pectin (N=20)	14	70[b]	24	3	27	1.4±0.3[c]	60.0±23.0
20% Pectin (N=20)	9	45[e]	15	2	17	0.9±0.3[d]	10.5±2.2[b]

a) $xy^2/2$ (x > y) (mm³), x : long diameter, y : short diameter
b) p<0.05, c) p<0.01, d) p<0.005, e) p<0.001 compared with control group

PGE2 level in colonic mucosa are in Fig.1. There was significant difference on PGE2 level in distal colonic mucosa between control group and 20% pectin group, but no significant difference in proximal colonic mucosa existed.

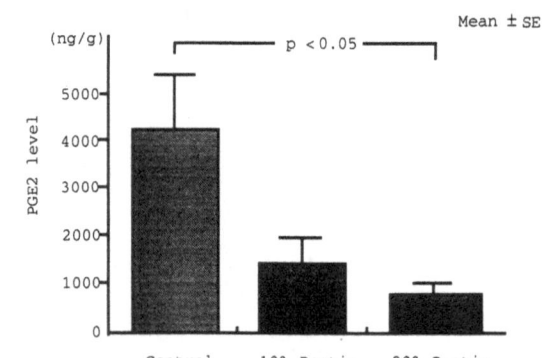

Fig.1 Prostaglandin E2 levels in distal colonic mucosa induced by AOM in rats fed diets containing pectin (rats killed at 30th weeks)

Experiment-2

Table 2 shows the fecal enzyme activities. Apple and citrus pectin induced a 2-fold increase in fecal β-glucuronidase activity after finishing AOM treatment. Fecal β-glucosidase and azoreductase activity, however, decreased in only apple pectin-fed rats.

Table 2. Effect of pectin on fecal enzyme activities

1) β-glucuronidase (μmol / min·g)

	before AOM injection (after 2weeks' diets)	12 Weeks	19 Weeks
Control	2.47 ± 0.94	1.58 ± 0.28	1.21 ± 0.20
Citrus pectin	1.10 ± 0.22	3.11 ± 0.27**	3.72 ± 0.66*
Apple pectin	0.23 ± 0.03*	4.06 ± 0.33***	2.56 ± 0.41*

2) β-glucosidase (μmol / min·g)

	before AOM injection (after 2weeks' diets)	12 Weeks	19 Weeks
Control	2.50 ± 0.46	1.88 ± 0.22	0.92 ± 0.16
Citrus pectin	1.40 ± 1.10	1.34 ± 0.05	1.31 ± 0.27
Apple pectin	0.73 ± 0.06*	1.02 ± 0.10**	1.02 ± 0.06

3) Azoreductase (nmol / min·g)

		12 Weeks	19 Weeks
Control		7.35	15.67
Citrus pectin		7.35	17.63
Apple pectin		5.88	6.86

DISCUSSION

*p<0.05, **p<0.01, ***p<0.005 compared with control group

Pectin is a partially methoxylated polymer of galacturonic acid obtained from fruits. Among pectin, apple pectin exerts a bacteriostatic action on Staphylococcus aureus, Streptococcus faecalis, Pseudomonas aeruginosa and Escherichia coli compared with citrus pectin [6]. So, it is thought that apple pectin may change the composition of the intestinal flora. There are various reports that pectin has been effective in experimental colon carcinogenesis or not [2-3]. In this study, we used water-soluble methoxylated pectin from apple. The rats fed 20% apple pectin especially decreasesd multiplicity and occupied area of colon tumors. Many of tumors were observed in distal colon and interestingly, PGE2 level in distal colonic mucosa in 20% pectin fed rats were lower than those in basal diet fed rats. It has been known that PGE2 leads to regulation of the immune response directly or indirectly [7], and activation of ornithine decarboxylase (ODC) which is necessary for the proliferation of tumors [8]. These results thus indicate that the effect of apple pectin on the colon carcinogenesis may partially depend on the decrease of PGE2 concentration in colonic mucosa.

Bacterial β-glucuronidase has been considered a key enzyme for the final activation of Dimethylhydrazine metabolites to carcinogens in the colonic lumen [9]. In our present study, fecal β-glucuronidase activities in the pectin-fed group were significantly higher than those in control group. Thus, it is thought that β-glucuronidase activity in the pectin group was not associated with a lower tumor incidence. In the case of apple pectin, the concentrations of β-glucosidase and azoreductase were decreased compared with control and citrus pectin. Apple pectin has a bacteriostatic action, which suggest that the composition of the colonic microflora changes and the alternations in the concentrations of fecal bacterial enzyme activities occures. In conclusion, the effect of pectin on the colon carcinogenesis may depend on the type of pectin and be related to fecal enzyme activities, especially β-glucosidase and azoreductase.

REFERENCES

1. Buritt DP (1971) Epidemiology of cancer of the colon and rectum. Cancer (Phila.), 28:3-13
2. Watanabe K, Reddy BS, Weisburger JH, and Kritchersky D. (1979) Effect of dietary alfalfa, pectin, and wheat bran on azoxymethane or methylnitrosourea-induced colon carcinogenesis in F344 rats. J. Natl. Cancer Inst. 63: 141-145
3. Bauer HG, Asp NG, Dahlqvist A, Fredlund PE, Nyman M, and Oste R. (1981) Effects of two kinds of pectin and guer gum on 1,2-dimethylhydrazine initiation of colon tumors and fecal β-glucuronidase activity in the rat. Cancer Res., 41:2518-2523
4. Rowland IR, A Wise, and AK Mallet (1983) Metabolic profile of caecal microorganisms from rats fed indigestible plant cell wall components. Food Chem. Toxicol. 21:25-29
5. Wise A, AK Malleett, and IR Rowland. (1982) Dietary fibre, bacterial metabolism and toxicity of nitrate in the rat. Xenobiotica 12:111-118
6. Tazawa K (1988) Bacteriostatical properties of skin barriers. Proceedings of the 7th biennial congress of the world council of enterostomal therapists 37-41
7. Goodwin JS, Ceuppens J (1983) Regulation of the immune response by prostaglandins. J. Clin. Immunoi. 3:295-315
8. Narisawa T, Hosaka S, Niwa M (1985) prostaglandin E2 counteracts the inhibition by ornithine decarboxylase induction by deoxycholic acid. Jpn. J. Cancer Res. (Gann) 76:338-344
9. Reddy BS, Mangat S, Weisburger JH, and Wynder EL (1977) Effect of high risk diets for colon carcinogenesis on intestinal mucosal and bacterial β-glucuronidase activity in F344 rats. Cancer Res. 37:3533-3536

Inhibitory Effect of Green Tea Extract Against Azoxymethane-Induced Colon Carcinogenesis in Rat

MASAO INAGAKE, TETSURO YAMANE, YOSHITAKA KITAO, KATSUYA KUWATA, KAZUHIKO OYA, AKIRA OKUYAMA, and TOSHIO TAKAHASHI

First Department of Surgery, Kyoto Prefectural University of Medicine, Kyoto, 602 Japan

ABSTRACT

We investigated the effect of green tea polyphenol (GTP) on azoxymethane(AOM)-induced colon carcinogenesis in male Fisher rats. AOM was given (7.4mg/kg body weight) s.c. once a week for ten weeks. A week after the treatment, they were divided into three groups. AOM-GTP1 and AOM-GTP2 groups received 0.01 and 0.1% GTP in drinking water respectively from weeks 11 to 26. The AOM-control group received tap water. The tumor incidence in the AOM-GTP1 and AOM-GTP2 groups was significantly lower than that of the AOM-control group. We concluded that GTP supprssed AOM-induced colon carcinogenesis.

KEYWORDS: colon carcinogenesis, green tea extract, Azoxymethane, polyphenols

INTRODUCTION

We reported that (-)-epigallocatechin gallate (EGCg) inhibited the promotion stage of duodenal carcinogenesis induced by N-ethyl-N'-nitro-N-nitrosoguanidine[1], and suggested that polyphenols such as EGCg may have a chemopreventive effect on carcinogenesis in the alimentary tract. The evidence prompted us to study the influence of polyphenol-enriched extract of green tea(GTP) on colon carcinogenesis. We examined the inhibitory effect of GTP on colon carcinogenesis induced by AOM in rats.

MATERIALS AND METHODS

Eight-week-old male Fisher rats were purchased from Japan SLC Inc., Shizuoka, Japan, and they were allowed free access to drinking water and standard laboratory chow MF (Oriental Yeast Co., Tokyo,

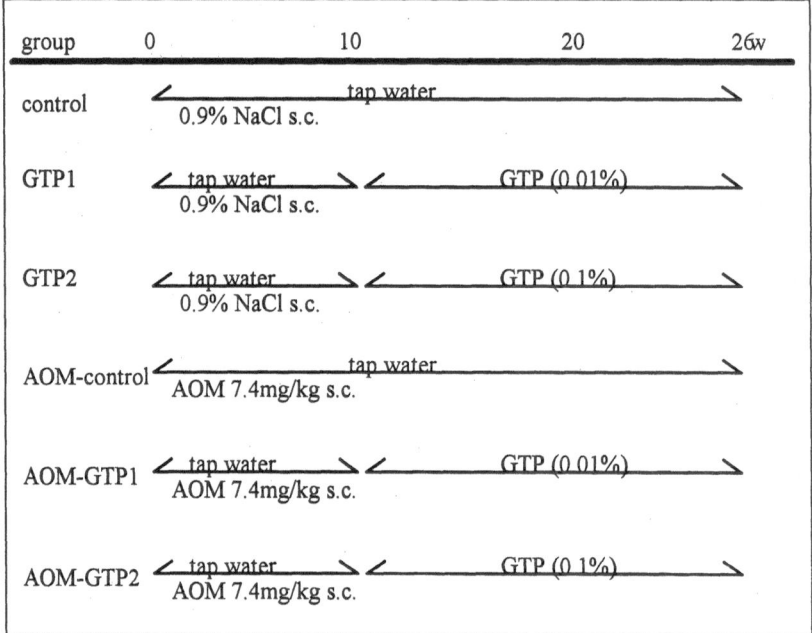

Fig.1 Experimental schedule

474

Japan). Throughout the experiment, the rats were maintained on a 12-h light-and-dark cycle in a 25°C. AOM (Sigma Chemical Co., St. Louis, MO, U.S.A.), kept at -80°C before use, was dissolved in 0.9% NaCl solution, and injected s.c. at a dosage of 7.4 mg/kg body weight once a week for the first 10 weeks. One week after the last AOM treatment, the treated rats were divided randomly into three groups: AOM-control (35 rats), AOM-GTP1 (34 rats) and AOM-GTP2 (21 rats). The AOM-control group received tap water throughout the experiment. The AOM-GTP1 and AOM-GTP2 groups respectively received 0.01 and 0.1% GTP dissolved in tap water as drinking water from week 11 to 26. GTP used in this study was Sunphenon®, a product of Taiyo Kagaku Co., Ltd.(Yokkaichi, Japan). It is composed mainly of polyphenolic compounds: (+)-catechin (3.5%), (-)-epicatechin (7.0%), (+)-gallocatechin (14.8%), (-)-epigallocatechin (15.0%), (-)-epicatechin gallate (4.6%), (-)-gallocatechin gallate (11.6%) and EGCg (18.0%).

Table 1. Inhibitory effects of green tea polyphenol fraction on colon carcinogenesis induced by AOM

Treatment groups[a]	Tumor incidence ratio[b]	Total number of tumors	Average numbers of tumors per rat[c]	Diameter of tumors (mm)[d]
AOM-control	24/35 (68.6)	42	1.45 ± 0.22	5.6 ± 3.4
AOM-GTP1	13/34[e] (38.2)	21	0.62 ± 0.20[g]	5.4 ± 2.8
AOM-GTP2	10/21[f] (47.6)	12	0.67 ± 0.17[g]	6.4 ± 3.0

[a] See the material and methods
[b] Numbers in parentheses are percent of tumor-bearing rats.
[c] Mean $\pm$ S.E.
[d] Mean $\pm$ S.D.
[e,f,g] Significantly different from the AOM-control group at $p<0.005$, $p<0.05$ and $p<0.01$, respectively

The residue of GTP includes caffeine, sugars, amino acids and moisture. In addition, three groups without the AOM treatment, *i.e.*, control, GTP1 and GTP2 alone(each 10 rats), were prepared as the counterparts of the above AOM-treated groups. The rats in these groups were also injected s. c. for the first 10 weeks, but with 0.9% NaCl solution containing no AOM. All rats were killed on week 26. Their esophagus, stomach, small intestine and large intestine were removed, and dissected longitudinally. The location, shape, size and number of tumors were recorded. At week 25, the rats feces was examined and at the time of death, the blood was also taken. In the blood we examined the total and free cholesterol, neutral fat, ß-lipo protein. From feces, bile acids were examined by gas-chromatography. Fig.1 shows the experimental protocol. The significance of difference in tumor incidence was analyzed using Chi-square test, and the remaining data were analyzed using Student's t-test.

Table 2 Blood lipid level

Group	AOM-control	AOM-GTP1
Total Cholesterol (mg/dl)	74.9 ± 10.1	67.1 ± 8.7
Free Cholesterol (mg/dl)	10.0 ± 6.8	7.8 ± 2.7
Triglyceride (mg/dl)	164.8 ± 51.4	145.3 ± 54.1
β-lipo protein (mg/dl)	6.7 ± 4.0	7.5 ± 3.1

N.S.

Results are expressed by Mean $\pm$ S.D

Table 3 Bile acid in feces

Group	AOM-control	AOM-GTP2
LCA (mg/g of dried feces)	0.117 ± 0.066	0.160 ± 0.046
DCA	0.524 ± 0.142	0.495 ± 0.083
CDCA	0.054 ± 0.019	0.047 ± 0.009
HDCA	1.222 ± 0.404	1.083 ± 0.194
HCA	0.151 ± 0.062	0.139 ± 0.069
Total Bile Acid	2.553 ± 0.847	2.356 ± 0.358

N.S.

Results are expresssed by Mean $\pm$ S.D.
LCA:Lithocholic acid
HDCA:Hyodeoxycholic acid
DCA:Deoxycholic acid
HCA:Hyocholic acid
CDCA:Chenodeoxycholic acid

RESULTS

Autopsy on week 26 showed that the body weight was not significantly different among the six groups. Table 1 shows the inhibitory effect of GTP. The percentage of tumor-bearing rats in the AOM-control group was 68.6%, whereas those in the AOM-GTP1 and AOM-GTP2 groups were 38.2% ($p<0.005$) and 47.6%($p<0.05$), respectively. Two groups, AOM-GTP1 and AOM-GTP2, did not show any significant difference in dose response. GTP may have an optimum dose to inhibit the colon carcinogenesis. Rats without the AOM treatment (*i.e.*, control,

GTP1 and GTP2) had no colon tumors. The average number of tumors per rat in the AOM-control group was 1.45, whereas those in the AOM-GTP1 and AOM-GTP2 groups were 0.62 ($p<0.01$) and 0.67 ($p<0.01$), respectively. The mean tumor diameter was not significantly different among the three AOM-treated groups. Table 2 shows the biochemical laboratory data of lipids. There were no significant differences in total cholesterol, free cholesterol, neutral fat, and ß-lipo protein between the groups. Table 3 shows the excretion of the bile acids in rat feces. There was no definite tendency between the listed groups. The proportion of primary and secondary bile acids was also showed no difference among them.

DISCUSSION

EGCg was shown to be an anti-tumor promoter in two-step carcinogenesis experiment on mouse skin[2] and in N-ethyl-N'-nitro-N-nitrosoguanidine-induced mouse duodenal carcinogenesis experiment[1]. In the present study, green tea polyphenols were administered to the AOM-treated rats one week after the last AOM treatment. Therefore, they might have inhibited the promotion stage of the AOM-induced colon carcinogenesis. The reduction of tumor incidence and average numbers of tumors per rat in this experiment was consistent with those found in the above experiments. GTP contained 74.5% of polyphenolic compounds including EGCg. These polyphenols are closely similar in their structure and biological activity. Although the inhibition of AOM-induced colon carcinogenesis could be due to components other than the polyphenols, from circumstantial evidence[1,2], it is safe to conclude that the polyphenols exerted their anti- tumor promoting activity against colon carcinogenesis. The relationship between lipid metabolism and colon carcinogenesis has been suggested. Elevated lipid consumption is said to increase the risk of colon cancer. However, in this experiment, the group without green tea polyphenols showed lower levels of cholesterol. Polyphenols may elevate the blood cholesterol level directly, or they may help lipid digestion. There was no significant difference in body weight between control and GTP treated groups. This suggests that polyphenols do not contribute to the lipid digestion. Bile acids have been suggested to promote colon carcinogenesis. The lack of any difference in the bile acid level in the feces between the AOM-control, AOM-GTP1 and AOM-GTP2 groups in this experiment indicate that the polyphenols do not change the fecal bile acid level. There would be another way to suppress the colon carcinogenesis. GTP was administered to rats in the drinking water at concentrations of 0.01 and 0.1%. In terms of mg/kg body weight, the daily GTP intake by these rats was comparable to that by average Japanese people. A recent epidemiological study showed a lower risk of gastric cancer among individuals with a high consumption of green tea (10 or more cups per day)[3]. These findings suggest that green tea polyphenols are useful in preventing carcinogenesis in the alimentary tract. However, the mechanism of their suppressive effect against tumorigenesis remains to be determined in future studies.

REFERENCES

1.   Fujita Y, Yamane T, Tanaka M, Kuwata K, Okuzumi J, Takahashi T, Fujiki H, Okuda T (1989) Inhibitory effect of (-)-epigallocatechin gallate on carcinogenesis with N-ethyl-N'-nitro-N-nitrosoguanidine in mouse duodenum. Jpn. J. Cancer Res. 80: 503-505

2.   Yoshizawa S. Horiuchi T, Fujiki H, Yoshida T, Okuda T, Sugimura T(1987) Antitumor promoting activity of (-)-epigallocatechin gallate, the main constituent of "tannin" in green tea. Phytother. Res. 1:   44-47

3.   Kono S, Ikeda M, Tokudome S, Kuratsune M (1988) A case-control study of gastric cancer and diet in northern Kyusyu, Japan. Jpn. J. Cancer Res.79: 1067-1074

Significance of Fecal Bile Acid Ratio in Colorectal Cancer Patients

TOSHIKI KAMANO[1], KEI NAKAMURA[1], YOUSHI MIKAMI[1], NOBURU SAKAKIBARA[1], MOTONARI KANO[2], and MASARU MATSUMOTO[3]

[1]The First Department of Surgery, Juntendo University School of Medicine, Bunkyo-ku, Tokyo, 113 Japan
[2]Daito College of Medical Technology, [3]Tokyo Health Service Association

ABSTRACT

Fecal bile acid values in 10 colorectal cancer patients have been demonstrated to have diagnostic significance. Deoxycholic acid (DCA) and cholic acid (CA) were measured by Emzyme Linked Immunosorbent Assay (ELISA) method and their composition ratio (DCA/CA) was used for the pre and post operative comparison. The post operative ratio was found to be lower than the pre operative ratio in every patient. The result can be anticipated the clinical utility in the diagnosis of colorectal cancer patients.

KEY WORDS: fecal bile acid, deoxycholic acid (DCA), cholic acid (CA), DCA/CA ratio, colorectal cancer patients

INTRODUCTION

Recently, the incidence of colorectal cancer is increasing in Japan. Westernization of dietary habits of Japanese people which take high fat[1] and low fiber foods has been pointed out as a likely cause of the increase. Fecal bile acid has been confirmed to be a diagnostically significat factor in the epidemiological analysis[2,3] of the incidence of colorectal cancer in Japan, but no results have been obtained from clinical application of the measurement of fecal bile acids in assessing the diagnosis of colorectal cancer patients. In this report we have investigated the diagnostic significance in measuring fecal bile acids in colorectal cancer patients.

MATERIALS AND METHODS

Subjects of this study were 10 patients who were diagnosed as colorectal cancer and undernent curative operation. There was no particular tendency in characteristics of the patients including age, site and stage of cancer. The composition ratio of fecal bile acids one week before resection with that 2 weeks after resection were compared. Deoxycholic acid (DCA), the secondary bile acid, and cholic acid (CA), the primary bile acid, were measured by Enzyme Linked Immunosorbent Assay (ELISA) method and their composition ratio (DCA/CA) was used for the pre and post operative comparison. The DCA/CA ratio was also calculated in 10 normal individuals for reference.

RESULTS AND DISCUSSION

The pre and post operative DCA, CA levels and DCA/CA ratio in colorectal cancer patients are shown in Table 1 and in normal individuals in Table 2. The postoperative DCA concentrations were found to be lower than preoperative concentrations in all the patients except for 2 patients who showed slight increase of DCA after resection. On the contrary the post operative CA concentrations tended to be higher than pre operative in all the patients with the exception of 1 patient with unchanged and 2 with decreased concentrations after resetion. The postrative ratio (DCA/CA) was found to be lower than the preoperative ratio in every patient which was similar to the ratio in normal individuals (Fig.1).

477

Fecal Bile Acid Composition and Ratio in Colorectal Cancer Patients

	Sex	Age	Site of Cancer	Dukes classificasion	DCA nmol/ml before R.	DCA nmol/ml after R.	CA nmol/ml before R.	CA nmol/ml after R.	DCA/CA before R.	DCA/CA after R.
No.1	♀	54	S	A	365.7	70.4	149.0	844.6	2.454	0.083
2	♂	62	A	B	85.9	99.7	99.5	1310.1	0.863	0.076
3	♂	56	R	C	555.0	46.1	152.9	42.3	3.630	1.096
4	♂	58	S	C	768.4	173.8	213.1	136.3	3.606	1.275
5	♂	52	R	C	183.9	70.6	139.7	134.6	1.316	0.525
6	♂	54	R	C	59.6	70.4	53.0	1916.2	1.125	0.036
7	♂	62	T	A	653.8	170.2	341.2	754.4	3.841	0.452
8	♀	62	S	A	895.8	433.1	131.8	5453.6	6.797	0.079
9	♂	56	R	B	866.8	90.9	416.4	1133.2	2.082	0.080
10	♂	45	T	B	230.9	81.5	221.1	594.5	1.044	0.137

Site of Cancer :　A : ascending colon　　T : transverse colon　　S : sigmoid colon　　R : rectum

DCA : deoxycholic acid　　CA : cholic acid　　R. : resection

Fecal Bile Acid Composition and Ratio in Normal Individuals

	Sex	Age	DCA nmol/ml	CA nmol/ml	DCA/CA
No.1	♂	59	310.4	213.1	1.45
2	♂	45	232.2	612.7	0.37
3	♂	55	108.5	266.0	0.40
4	♂	46	289.8	268.9	1.07
5	♂	59	23.7	132.5	0.17
6	♀	44	504.7	759.2	0.66
7	♀	41	56.2	154.6	0.36
8	♀	53	29.0	120.0	0.24
9	♀	49	91.5	101.1	0.90
10	♀	54	153.0	255.0	0.60

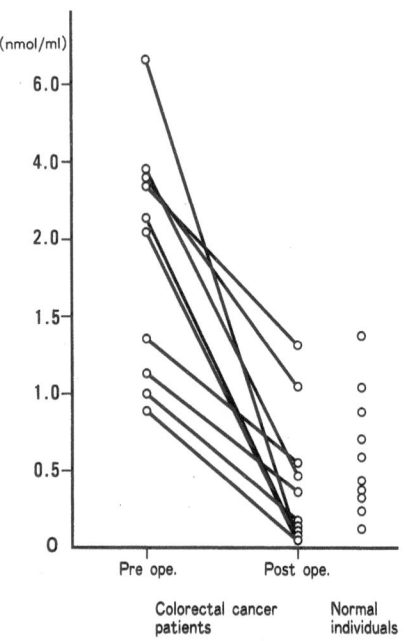

DCA/CA RATIO

Table.1	Fig.1
Table.2	

The observation in our study that curative operation in colorectal cancer patients brought about reduction in the composition ratio of fecal bile acids to the level in normal individuals can be anticipated high clinical utility in the diagnosis of colorectal cancer patients. In addition it may be appliciable to normal individuals in screening for high risk factors for colorectal cancer and in dietary counselling to prevent it. We are currently engaged in comparison of the fecal bile acid composition ratio in normal individuals with that in colorectal cancer patients and in investigation of its day to day fluctuation in advanced colorectal cancer patients.

REFERENCES

1. Wynder EL, Reddy BS (1977) Diet and cancer of the colon. Curr Concepts Nutr 6:55-71
2. Kaibara N, Sasaki T, Koga S, Ikawa S (1983) Fecal bile acids and neutral sterols in Japanese with large bowel carcinoma. Oncology 40:255-258
3. Hikasa Y, Tanida N, Ohno T, Shimoyama T (1984) Fecal bile acid profiles in patients with large bowel cancer in Japan. Gut 25:833-838

Effect of Short Chain Fatty Acids on Histopathological Type of Colon Cancer Induced by 1,2-Dimethylhydrazine in Rat

Kazuhito Masaki[1], Hiroshi Tanimura[1], Kiwao Ishimoto[1], Hirohumi Yukawa[1], Kohichi Murakami[1], Yoshiya Umemoto[1], and Shigeaki Matsuura[2]

[1]Department of Gastroenterological Surgery, [2]Second Department of Pathology, Wakayama Medical College, Wakayama, Japan

ABSTRACT

Short chain fatty acids (SCFAs) in cecal contents and feces were assessed in relation to the histological type of colon cancer induced by 1,2-dimethyl-hydrazine. When the amounts of SCFAs were changed by the ingestion of different types of dietary fibers, colon cancers showed differences in the distribution and differentiation. The incidence of the well differentiated type in large intestine containing a large amount of SCFAs and that of poorly differentiated type in large intestine containing a small amount of SCFAs were particularly high. SCFAs, butyric acid in particular, are considered to be closely involved in the histological type of colon cancer.

KEY WORDS: 1,2-dimethylhydrazine, short chain fatty acid, colon cancer

INTRODUCTION

Short chain fatty acids, such as acetic acid, propionic acid and butyric acid, which are formed by fermentation of dietary fibers by the large bowel flora, are known to absorb water and Na$^+$ in the large intestine, to stimulate the contraction of the colon and to accelerate the proliferation of the colon epithelium[1]. However, whether short chain fatty acids related with the carcinogenesis of colon cancer remains unknown. We determined the amounts of short chain fatty acids in the feces and cecal contents of rats with colon cancer induced by 1,2-dimethylhydrazine(DMH), to which different types of dietary fiber were administered, and investigated the relationship between short chain fatty acids and the colon carcinogenesis.

MATERIALS AND METHODS

Five-week-old SD male rats (n=88) were divided into 4 groups. The basal diet group was given only a basal diet deficient in cellulose (group FF). The other three groups were given a basal diet to which three types of dietary fiber, cellulose, pectin, and fructo-oligosaccharides, were added at weight ratios of 15% each (groups C15, P15 and F15). DMH, a carcinogenic agent, was subcutaneously injected into the dorsal region at a dose of 20 mg/kg once a week, 20 times in total. Fecal samples were collected 16 weeks after the start of experiment, and cecal content samples were collected 26 weeks after the start of the experiment when animal were sacrificed. The amount of short chain fatty acids in the individual samples was determined by gas-liquid chromatography (Fig. 1).

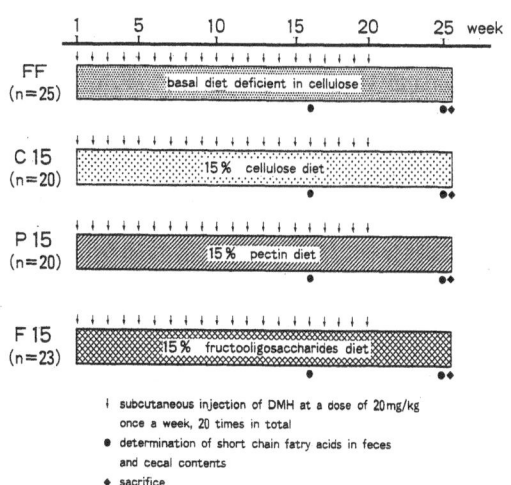

Fig. 1 Materials and methods

479

RESULTS

The total amount of short chain fatty acids in 1g wet weight of feces was 1,775±1,083 µg in group FF, 890±154 µg in group C15, 3,735±1,516 µg in group P15 and 5,000±1,229 µg in group F15. The total amount of short chain fatty acids in cecal contents was 2,814±657 µg in group FF, 2,293±443 µg in group C15, 4,425±1,350 µg in group P15 and 4,656±675 µg in group F15. The amounts in group C15 were thus less than those in group FF, and those in groups P15 and F15 were significantly greater than those in group FF ($p<0.01$) (Fig. 2). Although there was no difference in the site of occurrence of adenoma or carcinoma between the proximal and distal colon in group FF or C15, the incidence of tumor in the distal colon was twice as high as that in the proximal colon in groups P15 and F15 (Table 1). The number of adenomas or carcinomas per animal was 1.6 in group FF, 0.8 in group C15, 2.0 in group P15 and 2.0 in group F15, showing a significant decrease in group C15 ($p<0.05$) (Table 2). The proportion of well differentiated adenocarcinoma was 0%. In group FF, 15% in group C15, 35% in group P15 and 56% in group F15 (Table 3). The proportion of poorly differentiated adenocarcinoma was 36% in group FF, 39% in group C15, 6% in group P15 and 9% in group F15 (Table 4). The incidence of the well differentiated type was significantly higher in the distal colon than in proximal colon in groups P15 and F15, in which the amount of short chain fatty acids was large, while the incidence of poorly differentiated type was significantly higher in the proximal colon in groups FF and C15, in which the amount was small ($p<0.01$).

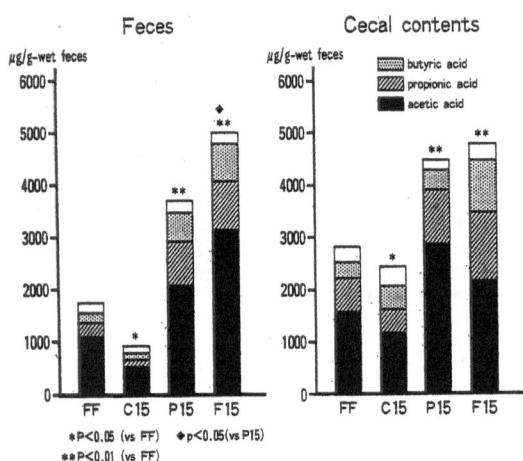

Fig. 2   Amount of short chain fatty acid in four diet groups.

Table 1   Number and distribution of DMH-induced colon tumors in four diet groups.

	proximal colon		distal colon	
	adenoma	carcinoma	adenoma	carcinoma
FF (n=23)	1	16	6	12
C15 (n=18)	0	7	2	6
P15 (n=14)	0	9	10	8
F15 (n=17)	0	12	11	10

Table 2   Effects on DMH-induced colon tumors in four diet groups.

	ratio of carcinoma bearing rat	adenoma and/or carcinoma	Tumor volume (mm³)
		one rat	Tumor bearing rat
FF (n=23)	87%	1.6	46.3±14.2
C15 (n=18)	50%*	0.8*	40.9± 9.1
P15 (n=14)	79%	2.0	129 ±38.1+
F15 (n=17)	88%	2.0	137 ±50.0+

* P <0.05 (vs FF),   + P <0.1 (vs FF),   Mean±SE

Table 3   Proportion and distribution of well differentiated adenocarcinoma in four diet groups.

(%)

	proximal colon	distal colon	total
FF (n=23)	0 (0/16)	0 (0/12)	0 (0/28)
C15 (n=18)	0 (0/7)	33 (2/6)	15 (2/13)
P15 (n=14)	0 (0/9)	75 (6/8)	35 (6/17)
F15 (n=17)	42 (5/12)	70 (7/10)	56 (12/22)

Table 4   Proportion and distribution of poorly differentiated adenocarcinoma in four diet groups.

(%)

	proximal colon	distal colon	total
FF (n=23)	38 (6/16)	33 (4/12)	36 (10/28)
C15 (n=18)	57 (4/7)	17 (1/6)	39 (5/13)
P15 (n=14)	11 (1/9)	0 (0/8)	6 (1/17)
F15 (n=17)	8 (1/12)	10 (1/10)	9 (2/22)

DISCUSSION

With regard to the relationship between the occurrence of colon cancer and histological type, most cases of colon cancer are of the well differentiated type, with the incidence of the poorly differentlated type being about 5% in Japan[2]. In Western countries, by contrast, the incidence of the poorly differentiated type is about 17.5%[3]. As the Japanese life style becomes more westernized, poorly differentiated type of colon cancer with poor prognosis may increase. Measures to counter this possibility are waited.

Of the dietary fibers used in this experiment, cellulose is insoluble in water, whereas pectin and fructooligosaccharides are highly soluble in water. Fructooligosaccharides have been found to be nondigestible by humans but selectively utilized by bifidobacteria in the large intestine[4].

The total amounts of short chain fatty acids in feces and cecal contents were small in group FF and C15, and large in groups P15 and F15. The proportion of butyric acid was higher in group F15, in which the incidence of the well differentiated type was high, than in the other three groups. Butyric acid is involved in cell differentiation, and is believed to protect the colon epithelium from dysplastic change[5]. It is considered to be closely related to the histological type of DMH-induced colon cancer. This finding suggests an explanation for the epidemiological fact that many cases of poorly differentiated colon cancer that develop in patients with ulcerative colitis, in whom the amounts of short chain fatty acids in feces less than in healthy persons, are of the poorly differentiated type[6][7].

However, the inhibitory effect of cellulose on the development of DMH-induced colon cancer was greater than that of a basal diet deficient in dietary fibers, while such an effect was not observed in group P15 or F15. This suggests that short chain fatty acids accelerate epithelial cell proliferation the colon as a co-initiater of DMH-induced colon cancer. However, the action of short chain fatty acids in actual human cases of colon cancer should be further assessed in the future.

REFERENCES

1) Yajima T., Sakata T.: Influence of Short Chain Fatty Acids on the Digestive Organs. Bifidobact Microflora. 6: 7-14, 1987.

2) Okuzumi J., Hagiwara A., Seiki K., Takahashi T.: Clinicopathological study on colonic poorly differentiated carcinoma and undifferentiated carcinoma. Jpn. J. Gastroenterological Surgery 22: 2404-2407, 1989.

3) Chung C.K., Zaino R. J., Stryker J.A., et al: Colorectal carcinoma: Evaluation of histologic grade and factors influencing prognosis. J Surg Oncol 21: 143-148, 1982.

4) Hidaka H., Eida T., Takizawa T.: Effects of fructooligosaccharides on intestinal flora and human health. Bifidobact Microflora. 5: 37-50, 1986.

5) Cumming J.H., Bingham S.A.: Dietary fibre, Fermentation and large bowel cancer. Cancer Surveys 6: 601-621, 1987.

6) Morson, B.C., Dawson, I.M.P.: Gastrointestinal Pathology, Blackwell Sci, Pub., 2nd ed Oxford pp.534-542, 1979.

7) Fukushima T., Kawamoto M., Kubo A., et al.: Fecal bacteria and short chain fatty acid in patients with ulcerative colitis. Saishin Igaku 38: 1501-1504, 1983.

Relationship Between Gastrin Receptor Values in Colorectal Cancer Tissues and Clinical Stage

Masao Kameyama[1], Ichiro Fukuda[1], Shoji Nakamori[1], Shinzaburo Noguchi[1], Shingi Imaoka[1], Takeshi Iwanaga[1], Kazushige Mori[2], Yu Miura[2], and Masanori Miwa[2]

[1]The First Department of Surgery, The Center for Adult Diseases, Osaka, 537 Japan
[2]The Department of Oncology, Nippon Roche Research Center

ABSTRACT

We have measured gastrin receptor (GR) in cancer tissue and adjacent normal mucosa of the colon and rectum from 12 patients. GR was detectable in all cancer tissues, and in 11 of 12 normal mucosa. GR levels were higher in the colorectal cancer tissues (mean±SD; 7.7±7.7) than in colorectal mucosa (mean±SD; 3.6±3.3) ($p < 0.05$). Negative relationship was implicated by the observation that the mean GR content in cancer tissue in Dukes' stage C (6.8±3.0) was significantly ($p < 0.05$) higher than that in stage D (2.4±0.8). However, no other significant correlation was found between GR content and other clinicopathologic factors (age, sex, serum levels of gastrin and carcinoembryonic antigen (CEA), macroscopic appearance, histologic differentiation, and serosal invasion in primary cancer lesions).

KEY WORDS: gastrin receptor, colorectal cancer

INTRODUCTION

We have reported that serum gastrin levels serve as a significant predictor of liver metastasis [1]. It has been shown that gastrin stimulates colorectal cancer growth and its effect is inhibited by a gastrin receptor antagonist in animal experiment (under submission). Since gastrin exerts its effect through GR, it is of interest to study the GR levels in human colorectal cancer. In this study, we investigated GR content in cancer tissue and normal mucosa and attempts were also made to elucidate the relationship between GR levels and clinical stage.

PATIENTS AND METHODS

Patients

Colorectal cancer tissues and adjacent normal mucosa were obtained from twelve patients with colorectal cancer who underwent surgery from January to June 1992. Mean age was 59 years (33 - 72), and there were 7 males and 5 females. We examined preoperative fasting serum gastrin and CEA levels, macroscopic appearance, histologic differentiation, serosal invasion and clinical Dukes' staging of primary lesions.

Methods

We measured gastrin receptor levels in the plasma membrane by the ligand-binding assay according to Singh's method [2]. In brief, frozen specimens were minced. The pellet was suspended in 10 volume of buffer (10 mM Tris: HCl, pH 7.4, 137 mM NaCl, 5 mM KCl, 2 mM $CaCl_2$, 2.5 mM $MgCl_2$, 250 mM sucrose, 1 mg/ml BSA, 10μg/ml APMSF, 0.2 mg/ml Bacitracin, 0.2 mg/ml sodium azide) and then homogenized with a glass homogenizer. The homogenate was filtered through nylon mesh and centrifuged at 1,500g at 4°C for 10 min. The supernatant was centrifuged at 30,000g at 4°C for 45 min. The pellet was resuspended in 2 ml PBS and homogenized again with a glass homogenizer. The homogenate thus collected was stored at -70°C until assay. Plasma membrane fractions were incubated with 200pM ^{125}I-gastrin (Amersham), either in the presence (for non-specific binding) or in the absence (for total binding) of a 3μM of unlabeled gastrin (Sigma) at room temperature for 120 min. Specific binding sites were estimated by subtraction non-specific binding from total binding.

RESULTS

1) In all colorectal cancer, GR was detectable in all cancer tissues and 11 of 12 normal mucosa. The GR levels (mean±SD) in the primary lesions 7.7±7.7 (1.6 - 29.1) were significantly ($p<0.05$) higher than that in colorectal mucosa 3.6±3.3 (0-11.5) (Fig. 1).

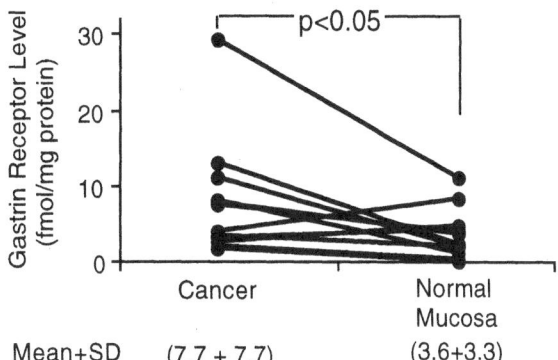

Fig.1. Gastrin receptor levels of cancer and normal mucosa   Mean±SD   (7.7 ± 7.7)   (3.6±3.3)

2) GR levels were significantly ($p<0.05$) lower in tumors larger than 6 cm in diameter (2.3±0.7) than those less than 6 cm in diameter (9.5±8.2).

3) GR levels were 14.7±13.6 in Dukes' A and B patients (n=3), 6.8±3.0 in Dukes' C patients (n=6) and 2.4±0.8 in Dukes' D patients (n=3). These results indicated the negative relationship between GR and clinical stage (Table 1).

Table 1. Relationship between gastrin receptor and clinical stage in colorectal cancer

	Clinical Stage		
	Dukes'A & Dukes'B (n=3)	Dukes'C (n=6)	Dukes'D (n=3)
Gastrin Receptor(mean±SD) (fmol/mg protein)	14.7±13.6	6.8±3.0	2.4±0.8[#]

#: $p<0.05$ versus Dukes' C

4) No significant association was found between GR and macroscopic appearance, histologic differentiation, serosal invasion, preoperative fasting serum gastrin or CEA levels.

DISCUSSION

In this study, we have shown that every colorectal cancer has detectable GR. This result suggests a possible involvement of gastrin in the growth and metastasis of colorectal cancer.

REFERENCES

1. Kameyama M, Fukuda I, Imaoka S, Nakamori S, Iwanaga T (1993) Level of serum gastrin as a predictor of liver metastasis from colorectal cancer. *Dis Colon Rectum* in press
2. Singh P, Le S, Beauchamp RD, Townsend CMJr, Thompson JC (1987) Inhibition of pentagstrin-stimulated up-regulation of gastrin receptors and growth of mouse colon tumor in vivo by proglumide, a gastrin receptor antagonist. *Cancer Res* 47:5000-5004

DNA Index and p53 Immunoreaction in Colorectal Cancer and Its Relationship to Prognosis

Akio Yamaguchi, Takanori Goi, Masanori Maehara, Kazuo Hirose, Yoshiaki Isobe, and Gizou Nakagawara

The First Department of Surgery, Fukui Medical School, Matsuoka-cho, Yoshida-gun, Fukui, 910-11 Japan

ABSTRACT

The DNA ploidy pattern and p53 immunoreactivity was studied in colorectal cancers and the results correlate with prognosis. There was no significant correlation between the DNA ploidy pattern and clinicopathological findings. However, patients with aneuploid tumor ran significantly poorer than diploid ones. The 5- and 10-year survival rates were 60.4% and 53.4% for those with diploid tumor. On the other hand, p53 immunoreactivity was found 57.1% of 203 colorectal cancers. The 5-year survival rate was 62.8% of patients with p53-positive tumors, and 74.2% for ones with p53-negative tumors: there was a significant differece between these two groups. We suggest therefore that DNA ploidy pattern and p53 immunoreactivity may possible be a useful prognostic marker of colorectal cancers.

KEY WARDS: DNA ploidy pattern, DNA index, p53 immunoreactivity, colorectal cancer

INTRODUCTION

Many reports discussed the relation between the nuclear DNA content of colorectal cancers determined by flow cytometry and prognosis in the patients; many authors found that aneuploid tumors had generally a poorer prognosis than diploid tumors(1,2). On the other hand, the inactivation of suppressor gene p53 through point mutation or deletion plays an important role in carcinogenesis. Also, p53 over-expression has been reported in a number of human tumors, including those of the breast, lung, and colorectum. Several authors have shown the relationship between p53 over-expression and prognosis in breast cancer(3,4). In this study, we analyzed for the DNA ploidy pattern and p53 expression in colorectal cancer and studied the correlation between prognosis and DNA ploidy pattern or p53 immunoreactivity.

MATERIAL AND METHODS

Flow-cytometric analysis of nuclear DNA content was performed on 323 colorectal cancers. Each tissue sample was deparaffinized with xylen, and then progressively dehydrated in decreasing concentration of alcohol. After the specimen was washed with distilled water, it was incubated in a 0.5% pepsin solution. The specimen was then filtered through a 40-μm filter and centrifuged. The remaining pellet was washed with saline solution and incubated in Hanks' solution containing 0.2% EDTA and 0.01% RNase at 37°C for 30 min. Propidium iodide solution (Sigma Chemical) in RPMI, at a final concentration of 100mg/l, was added to the single-cell preparation as a DNA stain. Cell analysis was performed with EPICS PROFILE (Coulter, USA). Tumors were judged DNA diploid when the DNA profile showed one G0/1 population, and diploid samples were assigned a DNA index of 1.00. The findings of an additional G1 peak indicated the presence of aneuploidy.

p53 protein expression was detected by immunohistochemical methods. Tissue specimens taken by endoscopic biopsy from 203 patients with colorectal cancers. The sections were stained with a monoclonal antibody against p53 (Ab1801, Novocastra Labo.). The sections were dewaxed, and the endogenous peroxidase activity was blocked by incubation of the sections in 1% hydrogen peroxidase in methanol for 30 min. The sections were covered with normal goat serum for 15 min and incubated with a 1:20 dilution of primary antibody at 4°C overnight After being washed with TBS, the slides were incubated with a 1:30 dilution of biotinylated goat anti-mouse IgG at room temperature for 30min and finally covered with a 1:100 dilution of streptoavidin-biotin-peroxidase complex (DAKO Patts) at room temperature for 30 min. The antibody was located with 3,3'-diamino-benzene tetrahydrochloride. Negative control studies were carried out in the abscence of the primary antibody to p53.

Statistical Processing

Statistical analysis was performed by the $\chi 2$ test. Differences were taken as significant when p was less than 0.05. The outcomes from different groups of patients were compared by generalized Wilcoxon test. By the proportional hazards model of Cox, multivariate analysis was done of the factors said to affect the prognosis in patients with colorectal cancer.

RESULTS

The DNA ploidy patterns of the 323 primary colorectal cancers were diploid in 131 tumors
(40.6%) and aneuploid in 192 tumors (59.4%). DNA ploidy patterns did not correlate with any
background factors such as histologic type, depth of invasion, lymphatic invasion, venous
invasion, lymph node metastasis, liver metastasis, and peritoneal metastasis.
However, patients with aneuploid tumor ran significantly poorer than diploid ones. The 5-
and 10-year survival rates were 60.4% and 53.4% for the patients with aneuploid tumor, 77.4%
and 69.0% for those with diploid tumor (Fig 1). Figure 2 shows the survival curves of
patients with colorectal cancers subdivided according to DNA index. Patients with increasing
DNA index had an increasingly worse prognosis, especially those with DNA index of above 2.0
had a most unfavorable prognosis.

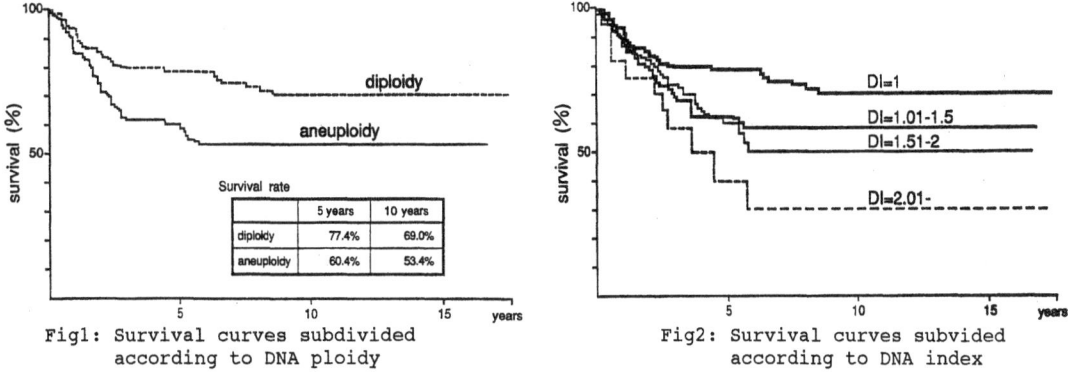

Fig1: Survival curves subdivided
according to DNA ploidy

Fig2: Survival curves subvided
according to DNA index

We found p53-immunoreactive cells in 117(57.6%) of the 203 endoscopic biopsy specimens from
patients with colorectal cancers. The pattern of p53 immunoreactivity was detected mainly in
the nuclei of almost all cancers. There was no correlation between the p53 immunoreactivity
and histologic type, depth of invasion, lymphatic invasion, venous invasion, lymph node
metastasis, liver metastasis, or peritoneal metastasis. However, the patients with p53-positive
tumors had a greater relative risk of death compared with those with p53-negative tumors.
Figure 3 shows the Kaplan-Meier survival curves for these two groups of all patients.

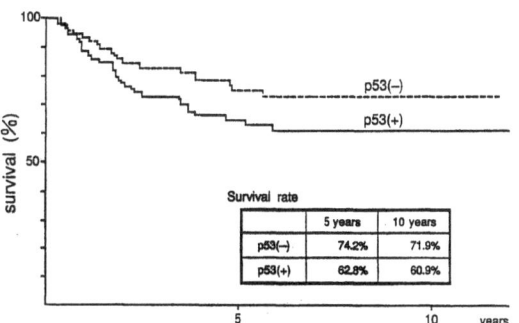

Fig 3: Survival curves subvided according
to p53 immunoreactivity

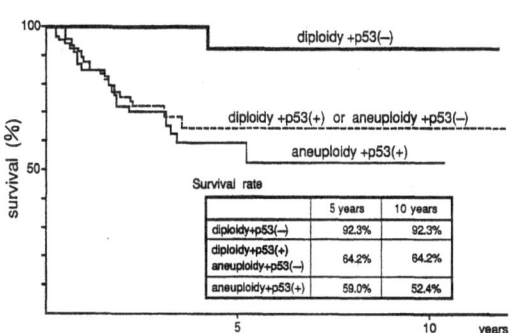

Fig 4: Survival curves subdivided according
to DNA ploidy and p53 immunoreactivity

The 5- and 10-year survival rate were 62.8% and
60.9% of patients with p53-positive tumors,
and 74.2% and 71.9% for ones with p53-negative
tumors. In the cases of Dukes' stage C, especially,
p53-positive tumors were related to poor prognosis,
whereas p53-negative tumors were associated with
a favorable prognosis. By combining DNA ploidy
pattern and p53 immunoreactivity, DNA diploids
together with p53 negative were associated with a
favorable prognosis, whereas DNA aneuploids with
p53-positive were related to the poorest prognosis
with significantly higher relative risk of death
than DNA diploids with p53-negative (Fig 4).
In addition, the prognostic factors in patients
with colorectal cancer were examined according to
the proportional hazard model of Cox. The results
showed that p53 immunoreactivity, DNA ploidy
pattern, and DNA index were judged to bean
independent prognostic factor(Table 1).

Prognostic variable	F value	P value
Histologic type	6.947	0.0094
Depth of invasion	4.012	0.0473
Lymphatic invasion	0.128	0.7210
Venous invasion	4.332	0.0394
Lymph node metastasis	8.146	0.0050
Liver metastasis	24.905	0.0000
Peritoneal metastasis	7.236	0.0081
DNA ploidy pattern	5.320	0.0227
DNA Index	4.695	0.0321
P53 immunoreactivity	8.722	0.0038

Table 1: Variable of independent
prognostic importance

DISCUSSION

It has been thought that the prognosis of patients with colorectal cancers is largely dependent on the stage of disease, grade of malignancy and host immunity. The grade of malignancy is determined by proliferative activity, DNA ploidy, and expression of protooncogenes. The DNA ploidy pattern has been shown to be correlated with the prognosis in patients with colorectal cancers(1,2). In this study, there was no correlation with DNA ploidy pattern and clinicopathplogical findings. The prognoses in patients of colorectal cancer, however, were such that aneuploid tumor patients had poor prognoses compared with diploid tumor patients. In addition, DNA index was strongly associated with prognosis of colorectal cancer. Patients with increasing DI values had an increasingly worse prognosis. It is possible to analyse preoperatively the DNA index in several biopsy specimens by flow cytometry. In the other hand, several report demonstrated that intratumoral DI heterogeneity has been found at rate of about 30%(5). However, Kosaka et al(6) reported that there is a good correlation between DI of biopsy specimens and those of resected specimens from patients with colorectal cancers. Regarding heterogeneity of DNA index, it may be possible to avoid overlooking small clones of cancer cells in several biopsy specimens.

Overexpression of p53 has been reported immunohistochemically in colon cancers. The cellular concentration of wild-type p53 is low, with short half-life, therefore those p53 is undetectable by immunohistochemically(7). Whereas mutant p53 in tumors with an extended half-life may be recognized immunohistochemically. Several investigator demonstrated that immunohistochemical detection for p53 correlates with mutations of p53 genes(8). We analyzed immunohistochemically the p53 expression in formalin-fixed paraffin-embedded biopsy specimens. In our study, 117(57.6%) of the 203 colorectal cancers were positively stained for p53 product by using a PAb1801. We, therefore, thought that analysis of p53 by use of PAb1801 enables to preoperatively in biopsy specimens. There are recent reports that over-expression of p53 provides a reliable prognostic indicator of malignant tumor, including those of the breast, colorectum, lung, and bladder. In addition, Kern et al.(9) reported that the deletion of 17p and 18q were associated with the increase predilection for distant metastasis and cancer-related death. In this study, there was no significant correlation between p53 immunoreactivity and clinicopathological findings. However, the 5- and 10-year survival rate were 72.4% and 71.9% for patients with p53-negative tumors, but it was as low as 62.8% and 53.4% for those with p53-positive tumors. The results of multivariate analysis indicated that the DNA ploidy pattern, DNA index, and p53 immunoreactivity were an independent prognostic indicator of colorectal cancer. We previously reported that poor survival of patients with p53-positive tumors may be associated with a high cell proliferation. By combining DNA ploidy and p53 immunoreactivity, in addition, DNA diploids together with p53-positive were related to the poorest prognosis. In conclusion, our findings suggested that analysis of DNA ploidy and immunohistochmical determination of p53 might be useful indicator in projecting the prognosis of colorectal cancers and that it would be possible to analyze them preoperatively in biopsy specimens.

REFERENCES

1. Armitage NC, Robins RA, Evans DF, Turner DR, Baldwin RW, Hardcastle JD (1985) The influence of tumor cell DNA abnormalities on survival in colorectal cancer. Br J Surg 72:828-830
2. Schutte B, Reynders MM, Wigger T, Arends JW, Volovics L, Bosman FT, Blijam GH (1987) Retrospective analysis of the prognostic significance of DNA content and proliferative activity in large bowel carcinoma. Cancer Res 47:5494-5496.
3. Cattoretti G, Rilke F, Andreola S, D, Amant L, Delia D (1988) p53 expression in breast cancer. Int J Cancer 41:178-183.
4. Iwaya K, Tsuda H, Hiraide H, Tamaki K, Tamakuma S, Fukutomi T, Mukai K, Hirohashi S (1991) Nuclear p53 Immunoreaction associated with poor prognosis of breast cancer. Jpn. J Cancer Res 82:835-840.
5. Hiddemann W, Von Bassewitz DB, Kleinemeier H-J (1986) DNA stemline heterogeneity in colorecal cancer. Cancer 58:258-263.
6. Kosaka T, Ii T, Matsumoto H, Ishida T, Takegawa S, Ohyama S, Kamata T, Kanno M, Yamaguchi A, Yonemura Y, Miwa K, Miyazaki I (1990) Flowcytometric measurement of DNA index and BrdUrd labeling index in endscopic biopsy specimens of colorectal carcinoma. Dig Endosc 3:317-322.
7. Rodrigues NR, Rowan A, Smith MEF, Kerr IB, Bodmer WF, Cannon JV, Lane DP (1990) p53 mutations in colorectal cancer. Proc Nat Acad Sci 87:7555-7559.
8. Thompson AM, Anderson TJ, Condie A, Prosser J, Chetty U, Carter C, Evans HJ, Steel CM (1992) p53 allele losses, mutations and expression in breast cancer and their relationship to clinico-pathological parameters. Int J Cancer 50:528-532.
9. Kern SE, Fearon ER, Tersmette KWF, Enterline JP, Leppert M, Nakamura U (1989) Allelic loss in colorectal carcinoma. JAMA 261:3099-3103.
10. Yamaguchi A, Kurosaka Y, Fushida S, Kanno M, Yonemura Y, Miwa K, Miyazaki I (1992) Expression of p53 protein in colorectal cancer and it's relationship to short-term prognosis. Cancer 70:2778-2784.

Relationship Between Fecal Mutant p53 Protein and Colorectal Cancers

Ryo Fukuda, Tomoyuki Hashimoto, Kazuya Hirakawa, Noriyuki Arima, Kyoichi Adachi, Nobuo Ashizawa, Satoru Ikeda, Makoto Watanabe, and Shiro Fukumoto

Second Department of Internal Medicine, Shimane Medical University, Izumo, Shimane, 693 Japan

ABSTRACT

Mutant p53 protein was investigated by ELISA using the stool of 132 patients with various colorectal diseases. Mutant p53 protein was detected in 41 cases (31.1%). The positive rates of fecal mutant p53 protein were 68.2% of colorectal cancer, 29.4% of colon polyps, 21.2% of colon diverticulosis, 0% of inflammatory bowel diseases and 27.7% of the patients with normal findings. The frequency of fecal mutant p53 protein in patients with colorectal cancers was significantly high compared with those without cancers (P<0.01, X^2 test).

KEY WORDS   mutant p53 , colorectal cancer

INTRODUCTION

Although the colorectal cancer is a poor prognostic disease, they are removable by surgically or endoscopically if found in early stage. For this purpose, early detection of colorectal cancer is very important. Screening tests for colorectal cancer, therefore, must be selective and specific. However, until now, there has been no specific and effective screening test for these diseases.   Recently, molecular biological studies revealed that many genetic changes have great roles on the carcinogenesis of colorectal cancers including deletion of FAP gene[1], DCC gene [2], mutation in ras gene[3], p53 gene[4]. Some of these genetic changes may be a good marker for detection of colorectal tumors. Practically, identification of K ras gene mutation in the stool was reported to correlate to the existence of colorectal tumors [5]. Since the mutation of p53 gene has been reported to have close association with the final step in the colorectal carcinogenesis and p53 protein has been detected in cancer cell but not in normal cells immunohistochemically [6], detection of mutant p53 in the stool may be a good marker for colorectal cancer.   In the present work, we tried to detect mutant p53 protein by ELISA assay from the stool of 132 patients of various colorectal diseases to investigate the relationship between mutant p53 protien in the stool and colorectal diseases, particularly colorectal cancer.

MATERIALS AND METHODS

Patients

Stools were collected from 132 patients who came to the 2nd Department of Internal Medicine of University hospital of Shimane Medical University from August to October in 1992 with complaints related to colon diseases such as changes of bowel movement, anal bleeding, lower abdominal discomfort. All these patients received both X ray examination of the colon and colonoscopy to investigate the colonic lesions.

Methods

A small amount of stool was stacked by fine sticks several times and dissolved in 1ml of OC-HEMODIA'Eiken'(an immunological detection Kit for fecal heamoglobin, EIKEN CHEMICAL. CO.,LTD). All these samples were stored

487

in 4°C until detection of mutant p53 protein. A 100 µl of the solution was applied to Mutant p53 Selective Quantity ELISA Assay (Oncogene Science. INC.).

RESULTS

Diagnoses of these 132 patients on X ray and endoscopic examinations of the colon were complising from 22 colorectal cancers, 34 colon polyps, 15 inflammatory bowel diseases(13 ulcerative colitis, one Crohn's disease, one Behcet disease), 14 colon diverticulosis and 47 normal cases. Of these 132 patients, 41 patients (31.1%) showed mutant p53 protein in the stool. The potitive and negative rate of fecal mutant p53 protein in each disease were shown in Table.1. Concerning colorectal cancers, mutant p53 protein in the stool was positive in 68.2% and 31.8% was negative. Although about one thirds (29.4%) of colon polyp showed positive fecal mutant p53 protein, the majority of this disease was fecal mutant p53 protein negative. Inflammatory bowel diseases were all fecal mutant p53 protein negative. In colon diverticulosis, 21.2% of cases showed positive fecal mutant p53 protein. About 28% of normal cases also showed fecal mutant p53 positive. The frequencies of each colorectal disease in patients with positive fecal mutant p53 protein were 36.6% of colorectal cancers, 24.3% of colon polyps, 0% of inflammatory bowel diseases, 7.3% of colon diverticuloses and 31.8% of normal cases. Statistical analysis between colorectal disease and positive fecal mutant p53 in the stool showed a siginificance only in colorectal cancers($P < 0.01$, $X2$ test).

Table.1 Relationship between fecal mutant p53 protein and colorectal diseases.

Disease	Fecal mutant p53 protein	
	positive	negative
Cancer	68.2% (15/22)	31.8% (7/22)
Polyp	29.0% (10/34)	71.0% (24/34)
IBD	0.0% (0/15)	100.0% (15/15)
Diverticulosis	21.2% (3/14)	78.8% (11/14)
Normal	28.0% (13/45)	72.0% (32/45)

IBD:Inflammatory bowel disease, (positive case/ examined case)

DISCUSSION

Until now, screening tests for colorectal cancer including measurement of serum CEA, CA19-9 and detection of occult blood in the stool have been used. In the present work, The frequency of colorectal cancer was 36.6% in cases with positive mutant p53 in the stool. This frequency was high compared with tose in other usual screening tests. As a method of detection of tumor-associated substance from the stool, Sidransky reported the identification of the mutation of K ras gene from the stool(6). However, their method was very expensive because of the applications of advanced molecular biological techniques. In addition, K ras gene mutation has been reported in about 50% of colorectal tumors at most. On the contrary, mutations in p53 gene have been reported about in 80% of colorectal cancers. Accordingly, detection of mutant p53 protein or mutation of this gene seem more specific to colorectal cancers than those of K ras gene.
The reason why mutant p53 protein was detected in the stool was probably that tumor cells containing p53 protein were comming off from the tumor by erosion or ulceration on the tumor surface. This seems the same reason why

we can detect mutations of K ras gene from the stool. Or alternatively, this protein might be excreted from these colorectal tumors.

Concerning the cases showing mutant p53 in the stool without colorectal cancer, other gastrointestinal tumors including one esophagial cancer[7] and three gastric cancers were found. Since the mutations in p53 gene had been reported in all these diseases, fecal mutant p53 protein may associate with any gastrointestinal cancer. However, we can not deny the possibility of both fales positive and cases despite the high frequency of colorectal cancers in fecal p53 protein positive cases ,since this ELISA system detect the mutation at an epitope of aminoacide accoding to the instraction. Therefore, the colorectal cancers with mutations in other epitopes of p53 protein seem undetectable. Further studies are necessary including the preparation of anti-mutant p53 protein antibody used in ELISA system, investigation of the stability of mutant p53 protein during the passage of the stool for the application of this system to detection of colorectal cancers.

RERERENCES

1. Nishisho I, Makamura Y, Miyoshi Y (1991) Mutation of chromosome 5q21 gene in FAP patients and colorectal cancer patients. Science 253:665-669
2. Fearon FR, Cho KR, Nigro JM (1990) Identification of a chromosome 18q gene that is altered in colorectal cancer. Science 247:4956
3. Vogelstein B, Fearon ER, Stanley R(1991) Genomic alteration during colorectal tumor developement. N.Engl.J. Med 319: 525-532
4. Baker SJ, Fearon ER, Nigro JM (1989) Chromosome 17 deletion and p53 gene mutation in colorectal carcinomas. Science 244:217-221
5. Sidransky D, Tokino T, Hamilton SR(1992) Identification of ras oncogene mutations inthe stool of patients with curable colorectal tumors. Science 256:102-105.
6. Gannon JV, Greaves R, Iggo R and Lane DP(1990) Activation mutations in p53 produce a common conformational effects. A monoclonal antibody specific for the mutant form. The EMBO J 9:1595-1602.
7. Hollstein M, Metcalf RA, Welsh J, Montesano R, Hrris Al(1990) Frequent mutation of the p53 gene in human esophageal cancer. Proc.Natl.Acad.Sci.U.S.A 87:9958.

Proliferating Cell Nuclear Antigen Expression in Colorectal Cancer According to the Depth of Invasion

Nariyuki Shibano, Mitsuo Namba, Munenori Azuma, and Shigemitsu Shida

Department of Surgery, Dokkyo University School of Medicine, Mibu-cho, Shimotsuga-gun, Tochigi, 321-02 Japan

ABSTRACT

Fifty eight cases of colorectal cancer treated in our department were classified into 4 groups according to the depth of invasion of tumor. In each group, proliferating cell nuclear antigen(PCNA) expression were compared between the superficial and deep part of the tumor. These results showed that the differences in the positive rates between the superficial and deep portions tended to be greater in the more advanced cases, although those of the deep part were almost the same in all groups. It was suggested that proliferative activity of the superficial part of the tumor became to be decreased with the progression of the disease.

KEY WORDS: colorectal cancer, monoclonal antibody, Proliferating cell nuclear antigen(PCNA), the depth of invasion

INTRODUCTION

Proliferating Cell Nuclear Antigen (PCNA) [1] is present in the cell nucleus during the late presynthetic(G1) and early synthetic(S) phase . Its expression is considered to reflect proliferative activity of cells [2]. Immunohistochemistry for the expression of PCNA was performed on the colorectal carcinomas resected in our Department and the PCNA expression and clinico-pathological findings were compared with the depth of invasion of tumor to clarify the relation between tumor progression and proliferative activity.

MATERIALS AND METHODS

Fifty eight cases of colorectal cancer resected in our department were classified into 4 groups according to the depth of invasion of tumor ; Group 1: sm, pm Group 2: ss, a_1 Group 3: s, a_2 and Group 4 : si, ai and these cases were examined PCNA expression both the superficial and the deep part in the cancer lesion. And then, 32 cases were performed to stain in the deep part only. These tissue samples were used regular paraffin-embedded blocks, and 3-μm sections were sliced on poly-L-lysine coating slides. The first antibody was used anti-PCNA antibody(PC-10, DAKO), and the method for immunohistochemical study was performed on Labelled Streptavidin Biotin(LSAB)Kit with Alkaline Phosphatase method(DAKO). Specific immunostaining was identified by a colored product using New Fuchsin with alkaline-phosphatase, then the tissue was counterstained with Methyl Green. The positive rate was determined by calculating the number of positive nucleus in 1000 cells, and it was expressed by percentage. Five years survival results were examined 292 cases of colorectal cancer in our department, these cases certified clinico-pathological findings. The comparisons of PCNA expression were analyzed by paired or unpaired Student's t test, and five years survival results were analyzed by log rank test. Furthermore, all terms was used according to Japan Research Society for Cancer of Colon and Rectum: General Rules for Clinical and Pathological Studies on Cancer for Colon, Rectum and Anus, The 4th edition. July 1985.

RESULTS

Table 1 showed the PCNA positive rate of the superficial part and deep part that were no significant correlation with the deep part of each groups. In the superficial part of the tumor, the PCNA positive rate became to be decreased with the progressive disease. On the whole, the positive rates of PCNA had significant correlation between the superficial and the deep part. ($p < 0.01$)
Due to the difference of PCNA positive rate with the depth of invasion in the superficial part, the expression of PCNA was investigated in the deep part of 90 cases and clinico-pathological findings were compared with depth of invasion of tumor.

Table 2 showed the PCNA expression and these were classified into three groups according to histological defferentiation. Same histological differentiation group was not correlated with depth of invasion. There was a tendency that its expression of moderately ,poorly differentiated and mucinous adenocarcinoma were more higher expression than well differenti- ated adenocarcinoma. As for Table 3, a significant correlation was recognized between PCNA expression and v factor in Group 4 only. The correlation between PCNA expression and ly, n factor were not recognized.
Table 4 shows that these survival results were mostly influenced by the progressive n factor.

Table 1 Comparison of PCNA expression between superficial part and
deep part and five years survival results according to depth of invasion

	PCNA positive rate (%)		5 years survival
	superficial part	deep part	results (%)
Group 1	57.5 ± 4.9	67.2 ± 2.6	95.1 (n= 42)
Group 2	56.7 ± 3.5	65.5 ± 3.4	63.3 (n= 65)
Group 3	53.2 ± 2.6	61.1 ± 2.2^a	51.0 (n=154)
Group 4	47.8 ± 5.0	60.4 ± 3.1	11.3 (n= 31)
Total	53.7 ± 1.8	62.7 ± 1.5^b	55.1 (n=292)

Note. Results are expressed as mean ± SE. ^{a}p<0.05, ^{b}p<0.01 compared
with superficial part of same group. There were significant defference
in survival results between each groups (p<0.01)

Table 2 Relation between PCNA expression and histological differentiation

Histological	PCNA positive rate (%)		
type	well diff.	mode. diff.	poor.& muci.
Group 1	58.7 ± 4.5	65.4 ± 4.2	no cases
Group 2	58.1 ± 3.8	68.8 ± 6.4	64.3 ± 6.3
Group 3	56.4 ± 1.9	60.5 ± 2.6	60.4 ± 5.7
Group 4	57.6 ± 2.4	62.0 ± 2.2	58.0 ± 8.7
Total	57.1 ± 1.5	63.1 ± 2.1	60.4 ± 4.2

Note. Results are expressed as mean ± SE.

Table 3 Relation between PCNA expression and clinico-pathological findings (such as ly,v,n factor)

Factor	PCNA positive rate (%)					
	ly		v		n	
	(+)	(−)	(+)	(−)	(+)	(−)
Group 1	56.3 ± 6.1	63.9 ± 3.6	63.2 ± 3.6	57.6 ± 6.4	63.9	60.9 ± 3.7
Group 2	57.1 ± 3.1	77.9 ± 2.6	59.8 ± 4.7	64.4 ± 4.1	57.9 ± 1.6	63.9 ± 4.4
Group 3	58.4 ± 1.9	56.2 ± 2.5	58.4 ± 2.0	57.4 ± 2.1	58.6 ± 2.2	56.5 ± 2.1
Group 4	58.6 ± 3.5	60.7 ± 2.8	62.3 ± 2.6	50.9 ± 3.8^a	60.6 ± 4.5	57.8 ± 1.9
Total	58.0 ± 1.4	61.5 ± 2.1	60.1 ± 1.6	58.2 ± 1.8	59.0 ± 1.8	59.3 ± 1.7

Note. Results are expressed as mean ± SE. ^{a}p<0.10 compared with same group.

Table 4 Relation between 5 years survival result and clinico-pathological findings(such as ly,v,n factor)

Factor	5 years survival result (%)					
	ly		v		n	
	(+)	(−)	(+)	(−)	(+)	(−)
Group 1	83.1 (n= 13)	100.0 (n= 28)	90.9 (n= 11)	96.8 (n= 37)	62.5 (n= 6)	100.0 (n= 38)^a
Group 2	70.1 (n= 40)	60.3 (n= 36)	73.7 (n= 31)	59.1 (n= 34)	43.9 (n= 17)	71.5 (n= 47)^a
Group 3	48.7 (n= 95)	54.8 (n= 71)	37.0 (n= 45)	56.8 (n=109)^b	43.4 (n= 66)	59.3 (n= 85)^a
Group 4	16.3 (n= 23)	0 (n= 9)	9.4 (n= 16)	13.3 (n= 15)	5.6 (n= 18)	22.2 (n= 9)
Total	48.9 (n=171)	62.2 (n=144)^c	45.1 (n=103)	61.0 (n=195)^b	36.6 (n=107)	68.6 (n=179)

Note. ^{a}p<0.10; ^{b}p<0.05; ^{c}p<0.01 compared with same group

Now, 62 cases with histological curative resection were classified into two groups according to each mean value of PCNA positive rate in ly, v, n factors, and then two groups were com- pared with 5 years survival rate. (Table 5)

Those results were no significant correlation with survival results in each factor.

Table 5 Relation between ly,v,n factor - and 5 years survival result

factor		mean value (%)	5 years survival result (%)	
			PCNA ≦ M	PCNA > M
ly	+	58.0	75.4 (n=20)	70.6 (n=17)
	−	63.0	67.0 (n=14)	80.0 (n=10)
v	+	60.0	70.3 (n=13)	84.6 (n=13)
	−	60.0	63.6 (n=17)	72.2 (n=18)
n	+	59.0	68.5 (n=12)	53.0 (n=11)
	−	61.0	69.0 (n=18)	85.0 (n=20)
Total		60.0	64.7 (n=30)	77.2 (n=31)

CONCLUSION

1. In colorectal cancer, PCNA positive rate had a significant correlation between the superficial and the deep part. ($p < 0.01$) The decreasing proliferative activity in the superficial portion of tumor might be related to ulcer formation on the luminal side.
2. The correlations between PCNA expression and ly, v, n factors were not recognized except for v factor in Group 4.
3. The presence of vascular permeation and regional or distant metastases had greater prognostic significance than cellular proliferative activity.

DISCUSSION

PCNA was regarded as an auxiliary protein for DNA polymerase-δ [3], and its expression was indicated of proliferative activity of the cell. Many papers [4-6] have shown that PCNA expression was valuable and easy technic for the study of cancer, and agreed to other analysis such as a use of Bro-modeoxyurdine (BrdU), [^{3}H]thymidine, and flow cytometry. But in another report [7], PCNA expression was decreased by condition of formalin fixation.
Our study showed that PCNA was valuable investigation for retrospective study, although some tissue samples were not stained. In the deep part, proliferative activity of colorectal cancer cells showed difinite value that were no correlation with the depth of invasion. In superficial part, it was thought that proliferative activity became decreased according to the depth of invasion, on account of digested foods, digestive fluid and feeding artery of the tumor, that may also related to ulcer formation.
Therefore it implied that the progress of tumor could not defined by preoperative biopsy, and tumor of massive type was inferred the process of cancer invasion. As no correlation between PCNA expression and clinico-pathological findings, survival rate, PCNA expression do not consist of its malignant degree. It was suggested that as for indication of malignancy metastatic ability was more important factor than proliferative ability.

REFERENCES

1. Miyachi K, Fritzler MJ, Tan EM (1978) Autoantibody to a nuclear in proliferating cells. J Immunol 121:2228-2234
2. Robbins BA, de la Vega D, Ogata K, Tan EM, Nakamura RM (1987) Immunohistochemical detection of proliferating cell nuclear antigen in solid human malignancies. Arch Pathol Lab Med 11:841-845
3. Bravo R, Frank R, Blundell PA, MacDonald-Bravo H (1987) Cyclin/PCNA is the auxiliary protein of DNA polymerase-δ. Nature 326:515-517
4. Celis JE, Celis A (1985) Cell cycle-dependent variations in the distribution of the nuclear protein cyclin proliferating cell nuclear antigen in cultured cell:Subdivision of S phase. Proc Natl Acad Sci USA 82:3262-3266
5. Dierendonck JH, Wijsman JH, Keijzer R, Cornelis JH, van de Velde Cornelisse CJ (1991) Cell-cycle-related staining patterns of anti-proliferating cell nuclear antigen monoclonal antibodies. Am J Pathol 138:1165-1172
6. Yamada K, Yoshida K, Sato M, Ahnen DJ (1992) Proreferating cell nuclear antigen expression in normal, preneoplastic, and neoplastic colonic epithelium of the rat. Gastroenterlogy 103:160-167
7. Hall PA, Levison DA, Woods AL, Yu CC-W, Kellock DB, Watkins JA, Barnes DM, Gillett CE, Camplejohn R, Dover R, Waseem NH, Lane DP (1990) Proliferating cell nuclear antigen(PCNA) immunolocalization in paraffin sections:an index of cell proliferation with evidence of deregulated expression in some neoplasms. J Pathol 162:285-294

The Expression of Neural Cell Adhesion Molecule in Advanced Rectal Cancer

Teruo Sasatomi, Akira Okita, Yoshito Akagi, Yasumi Araki,
Yutaka Ogata, Tatsuhisa Morodomi, Kazuo Shirouzu,
Hiroharu Isomoto, and Teruo Kakegawa

The First Department of Surgery, Kurume University School of Medicine, Kurume, Fukuoka, 830 Japan

ABSTRACT

The expression of neural cell adhesion molecule (NCAM) was studied immunohistochemicaly in 164 cases of advanced rectal cancer (Stage II and Stage III). Fourteen cases (8.5%) were positive for NCAM, and NCAM positive cases had a high incidence of perineural invasion of cancer and poor prognosis compared with NCAM negative cases. These results suggest that NCAM plays an important role in perinural invasion of tumor and survival rates for rectal cancer.

KEY WORDS: neural cell adhesion molecule (NCAM), rectal cancer, survival rate

INTRODUCTION

The neural cell adhesion molecule (NCAM) was the first intercellular adhesion molecule to be isolated, characterized and cloned. Although, NCAM was originally identified in neural tissues, it is now known to be broadly expressed in embryonic development, and probably plays an important role in cell-cell interactions in many different tissues such as malignant tumors.

PATIENTS

164 patients with advanced rectal cancer who had undergone curative resection from 1982 to 1986 at Kurume University Hospital.

METHODS

Histopathological Diagnosis

Surgical specimens were fixed in 10 % formalin, and the whole tumor was cut into longitudinal sections 5 mm thick. After all sections were cut 5-micro meters thick and stained with hematoxylin-eosin and elastica van Gieson, histopathological examination was made. Pathological stageing was defined according to UICC TNM Classification.

Immunohistochemical Dignosis

Using the deepest resion of cancer, thin sections were stained with anti-NCAM monoclonal antibody (CHEMICON) by ABC method. NCAM positive ceses were defined over 80 % stained with antibody on each sections.

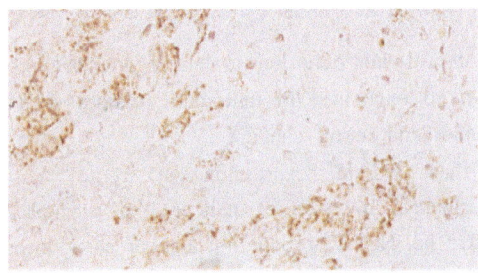

Fig.1 ABC Staining with Anti-NCAM Antibody

Statstical Analysis

The chi-square test was used to determined the statistical significance, and the Kaplan-Meier and Logrank test was used for survival rates.

RESULTS

The incidence rate of NCAM expression was 8.5% (14/164).

Table 1 shows the incidence of NCAM expression acccording to perineural invasion (PNI) of rectal cancer. The incidence of rectal cancer with PNI was significantly high rate of 30.6% compared with the cases without PNI.

Table 1. Incidence of NCAM expression according to perineural invasion (%)

	PNI (-)	PNI (+)
NCAM (-)	97.7 (125/128)	69.4 (25/36)
NCAM (+)	2.3 (3/128)	30.6 (11/36)
		$P<0.01$ ($\chi^2=6.63$)

Fig. 2 shows in the case of UICC Stage Ⅱ ten-year survival rate of NCAM positive was 71.4% and that of NCAM negative was 79.2%. No significant differnces were found between the positive and negative NCAM expression. On the other hand, as shown in Fig. 3 of the case of UICC Stage Ⅲ, a significant differences of ten-years suvival rates were observed between the positive and negative NCAM expression.

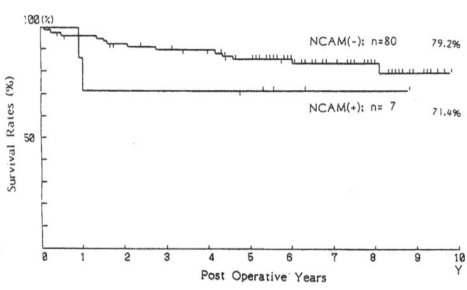

Fig. 2 Relation between NCAM expression and survival rates for UICC Stage Ⅱ

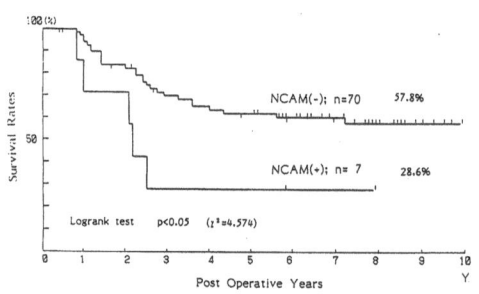

Fig. 3 Relation between NCAM expression and survival rates for UICC Stage Ⅲ

DISCUSSION

NCAM is one of the intercellular adhesion molecule and belongs to super immunogloblin family, NCAM is known to expressed in malignant tumors such as malignant melanoma, lung cancer, pancreas cancer and rectal cancer.

Our results indicate that NCAM expression of rectal cancer has a significant relationship with the perineural invasion of cancer and prognosis in the UICC Stage 3, and it is considered that the NCAM producing cancer gets into and skips to perineural space from the main tumors of rectum easier compared with nagative expression of the NCAM.

This study shows that NCAM plays an important role in perineural invasion of the tumor and prognosis of rectal cancer.

REFERENCE

Cunningham B, Hemperly J, Murray B, Predinger E, Brankenbury R, Edelman G (1987) Neural Cell Adhesion Molecule: Structure,Immunogloblin-Like Domains,Cell Surface Modulation,and Alternative RNA Splicing. SCIENCE 236:799-806

Sialyl Lewis-X Antigen Expression in Human Colorectal Carcinomas: Relationship Between Expression Level and Prognosis

Shoji Nakamori[1], Masao Kameyama[1], Shingi Imaoka[1], Hiroshi Furukawa[1], Yo Sasaki[1], Toshiyuki Kabuto[1], Osamu Ishikawa[1], Takeshi Iwanaga[1], and Tatsuro Irimura[2]

[1]Department of Surgery, The Center for Adult Diseases, Osaka, 537 Japan
[2]Division of Chemical Toxicology and Immunohistochemistry, Faculty of Pharmaceutical Science, The University of Tokyo, Bunkyo-ku, Tokyo, 113 Japan

ABSTRACT

Levels of sialyl Lewis-X antigen (SLX) in 132 human colorectal carcinomas were immuno-histochemically examined. The positive SLX staining for the primary tumors was significantly correlated with the depth of tumor invasion ($p < 0.05$), the presence of lymphatic invasion ($p < 0.005$) and lymph node metastasis ($p < 0.001$), and tumor stage($p < 0.001$). Patients with colorectal carcinoma showing positive SLX staining had higher relapse rate ($p < 0.001$) and poorer survival rate ($p < 0.001$) after surgery. Multivariate analysis suggested that SLX expression was an independent prognostic factor in the patients with colorectal carcinomas. Careful follow-up and intensive postoperative therapy are required for the patients with an SLX-positive colorectal carcinoma.

KEY WORDS: sialyl Lewis-X antigen, colorectal cancer, prognostic factor, carbohydrate antigen, adhesion molecule

INTRODUCTION

Altered expression of cell surface glyco-conjugate molecules is most frequently found to be associated with tumor progression and metastatic phenotype [1,2]. These influence specific phenotypes of tumor aggressiveness such as metastasis. Our recent studies demonstrated that changes in the expression of SLX play an important role in the acquisition of metastatic phenotype of colorectal carcinoma cells [3-6]. In this study, to investigate the prognostic value of the SLX expression in patients with colorectal carcinoma, we immunohistochemically examined the expression levels of SLX in 132 patients of colorectal carcinomas undergoing surgery.

PATIENTS AND METHODS

The 132 patients who underwent resection of the primary colorectal carcinoma at Department of Surgery, The Center for Adult Diseases, Osaka, were used for this study. All tumors were macroscopically and microscopically examined and classified according to pTNM staging system [7]. All patients received standardized follow-up examinations until death or until the end of the observation period (December 31, 1992). Immunohistochemical staining was performed as follows; Sections from paraffin blocks of 132 primary colorectal carcinomas and adjacent normal colonic mucosa were dewaxed and stained with anti-SLX monoclonal antibody FH6 [8] under the avidin-biotin system using 3,3'-diaminobenzide tetrahydrochloride as chromogen. The percentage of positively stained tumor cells was calculated and graded as follows: SLX negative: 0 to 5% of tumor cells stained, SLX positive; more than 6% of tumor cells stained, as previously described [3]. Statistical comparisons between SLX negative and positive groups were performed using the chi-square test or Student's t test. Statistical analysis of the difference between the relapse or survival curve of each group was made by the Log-rank test. Factors related to survival were analyzed by the Cox's proportional hazards regression model. The difference was considered to be significant when $p < 0.05$.

RESULTS

Of 132 primary colorectal carcinomas, 51 (39%) were classified into SLX positive, and 81 (61%) were SLX negative. Significant difference was found between the SLX expression and the depth of invasion ($p < 0.05$), lymphatic invasion ($p < 0.005$), the presence of lymph node metastasis ($p < 0.001$), and tumor stage ($p < 0.001$). No statistically significant differences in age, sex, location of primary tumor, tumor size, histological type, or the presence of venous invasion were found between the groups.

To investigate prognostic value of SLX, we compared the overall survival rates between the patients with SLX positive or negative staining tumor. Poorer overall survival rate was found in the patients with SLX positive staining tumor than in the patients with SLX negative staining tumor (p<0.001; Fig.1.). To avoid influence of non-curative resection on the patients' survival, survival rates were calculated from the data on 114 patients undergoing curative resections. The difference of survival rates between the SLX negative and positive groups was significant (p<0.001). As for recurrence of the disease, relapse rate in SLX positive group was significantly higher than in SLX negative group (p<0.001; Fig. 2.). Incidence of primary relapse at distant organs (liver, lung, bone) in the patients with SLX positive staining tumors was more frequent than with SLX negative staining tumors (9 of 40 vs. 6 of 74; p<0.05).

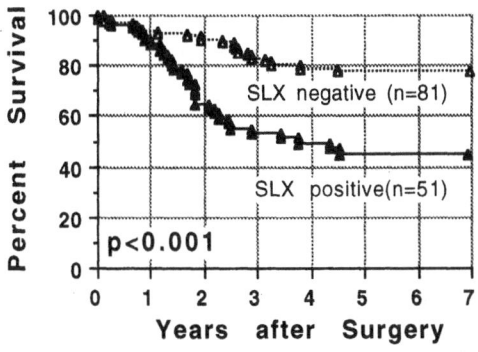

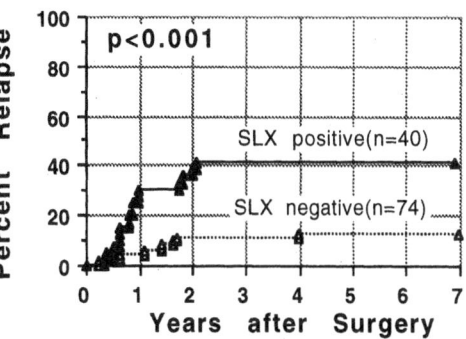

Fig. 1. Overall survival for all patients according to SLX staining status in tumor

Fig.2. Percent relapse for 114 patients with curative resections according to SLX staining status in tumor

Cox's proportional-hazards model showed that SLX expression was judged to be an independent prognostic factor for the 114 patients undergoing curative resection, although univariate analysis showed the significant correlation of several clinicopathologic factors, including SLX staining, with poorer survival (Table 1).

Table 1 *Clinicopathologic Features and SLX Expression as Prognostic Factors for 114 Patients with Colorectal Carcinoma: According to Univariate and Multivariate Analysis*

Variables	Univariate Analysis		Multivariate Analysis	
	chi-square	p Value	F value	p Value
Age				
< 60 vs. ≥ 60	0.10	0.76	0.48	0.49
Sex				
male vs. female	0.06	0.81	0.07	0.40
Tumor location [a]				
Rt. vs. Lt. vs. Rectum	0.09	0.96	1.10	0.29
Histologic type [b]				
well vs. mod. vs. poor/muc	7.94	0.047	0.056	0.81
Depth of invasion [c]				
m, sm vs. pm, ss, vs. se, si	24.2	<0.0001	11.2	0.001
Lymphatic invasion				
negative vs. positive	4.92	0.027	0.72	0.40
Venous invasion				
negative vs. positive	2.71	0.100	1.95	0.17
Tumor size (cm)				
< 4.8 vs. ≥ 4.8	1.51	0.22	1.55	0.22
Lymph node metastasis				
negative vs. positive	6.60	0.010	0.03	0.86
SLX staining				
negative vs. positive	14.0	0.002	8.24	0.005

[a] Rt.; right side colon (Caecum, Ascending, Transverse colon), Lt.; left side colon (Descending, Sigmoid colon), Rec.; Rectum.

[b] well; well differentiated, mod.; moderately differentiated, por.; poorly differentiated, muc; mucinous

[c] m; mucosa, sm; submucosa, pm; musclaris propria, ss; cancer cells extend to subserosa, se; cancer cells present on the serosa surface, si; cancer cells infiltrating neighboring tissue.

498

DISCUSSION

Altered expression of carbohydrate molecules during malignant transformation and tumor progression of cells is well known, and utilized for diagnosis or follow-up of cancer patients as a tumor associated antigen. SLX is one of such carbohydrate antigens, and expression of SLX was commonly found on the cell surfaces of a variety of adenocarcioma such as lung cancer, gastric cancer, and colorectal cancer. Recently, it has been proposed that one function of this antigen is to serve as a ligand of endothelial adhesion molecule, ELAM-1 [9-11]. Possible role of this antigen expression in metastasis formation is focused on. We have recently reported that human colon carcinoma variant cells expressing higher levels of SLX are more metastatic than those expressing lower levels of SLX in metastatic model system in vivo and in vitro [3-6]. In this study, we found this is the case in patients with colorectal carcinoma. We demonstrated that high SLX expression level in the tumors of human colorectal carcinoma was correlated with the extent of local invasiveness, such as depth of tumor invasion, lymphatic invasion, and lymph node metastasis. SLX expression was also correlated with poor prognosis of patients. The patients with SLX positive tumors exhibited a poor survival (44.9%: 5-year survival rate after surgery), whereas patients with SLX negative tumors had a rate of 77.4%. Furthermore, relapse rate of the disease after curative resection was significantly higher in the patients with SLX positive tumors than in those with SLX negative tumors. Incidence of disease relapse at the distant organs was higher in the SLX positive patients than that in the SLX negative patients.These results suggest that altered expression of SLX in human colorectal carcinoma cells might be associated with changes of phenotypes of tumors from less malignant to more malignant. Multivariate analysis for patients' survival revealed that SLX staining status was one of the independent prognostic factors which affect patients survival. Therefore, the SLX expression appears to be a useful independent prognostic marker for colorectal carcinoma patients. Examining SLX expression will be useful for clinicians to obtain further information on the prognosis. Careful follow-up and intensive postoperative therapy will be required for the patients with an SLX positive colorectal carcinoma.

ACKNOWLEDGMENT

This work was supported in part by Grant from Osaka Association for Cancer Research to S.N..

REFERENCES

1. Irimura T, Reading CL (1987) Surface properties of metastatic tumor cells. Cancer Bull 39: 132-141
2. Hakomori S (1989) Aberrant glycosilation in tumors and tumor-associated carbohydrate antigens. Adv Cancer Res 52: 257-331
3. Matsushita Y, Cleary KR, Ota DM, Hoff SD, Irimura T (1990) Siaryl-dimeric Lewis-X antigen expressed on mucin-like glycoproteins in colorectal cancer metastasis. Lab Invest 63: 780-791
4. Irimura T, Matsushita Y, Hoff SD, Yamori T, Nakamori S, Frazier M.L, Giacco GG, Cleary KR, Ota DM (1991) Ectopic expression of mucins in colorectal cancer metastasis. Semin Cancer Biol 2: 129-139
5. Matsushita Y, Nakamori S, Seftor EA, Hendrix MJC, Irimura T (1991) Human colon carcinoma cells with increased invasive capacity obtained by selection for sialyl-dimeric Le^X antigen. Exp Cell Res 196: 20-25
6. Nakamori S, Matsushita Y, Seftor EA, Hendrix MJC, Dohi DF, Ota DM, Frazier ML, Cleary KR, Irimura T (1991) Characterization of colon carcinoma cell variants selected for their different expression of sialyi-dimeric Lewis-X antigen. Proc. Am. Assoc Cancer Res 32: 61
7. Harmanek P, Sobin LH. (1987) Colon and Rectum. TNM classification of Malignant Tumors 4th ed: 47-49, Berlin: Springer-Verlag
8. Fukushi Y, Nudelman E, Leavery SB, Hakomori S (1984) Novel fucolipids accumulating in human adenocarcinoma: A hybridoma antibody (FH6) defining a human cancer-associated difucoganglioside (VI^{3}NeuAcV^{3}III^{3}Fu$_2$NLc$_6$). J Biol Chem 259: 10511-10517
9. Lowe JB, Stollman LM, Nair RP, Larsen RD, Berhend TL, Marks RM (1990) ELAM-1-dependent cell adhesion to vascular endothelium determined by a transfected human fucosyltransferase cDNA. Cell 63: 475-484
10. Phillips ML, Nudelman E, Gaeta FCA Perez M, Singhal AK, Hakomori S, Paulson, JC (1990) ELAM-1 mediates cell adheshion by recognition of a carbohydrate ligand, sialyl-Le^X. Science. 250: 1130-1132
11. Walz G, Aruffo A, Kolanus W, Bevilacqua M, Seed B (1990) Recognition by ELAM-1 of the sialyl-Le^X determinant on myeloid and tumor cells. Science 250: 1132-1135

A Scanning Electron Microscope Study of the Fibrous Stroma Adjacent to the Tumor Acini of Invasive Colonic Cancers

Hisayasu Aoki[1], Seiji Miura[1], Susumu Kodaira[1], Ichiro Takahashi[2], and Yuri Amakawa[2]

[1]Department of Surgery I, [2]Central Laboratory for Electron Microscopy, Teikyo University School of Medicine, Itabashi-ku, Tokyo, 173 Japan

ABSTRACT

To examine how colonic cancer foci affect on the fibrous stroma, the stroma adjacent to the infiltrating tumor acini was investigated by scanning electron microscopy. In the lower part of normal colonic glands the percentage of the area occupied by collagen fibrils appeared larger, and the fibrils ran more parallel to the gland. In cancer stroma the percentage of fibrils was larger and angles(direction)were more widely distributed, and in the invasive portion fibril diameter was increased, implying that the collagen fibers in the stroma are more randomly generated and that tumor glands are poorly supported by them.

KEY WORDS: collagen, stroma, interstitium, colon cancer, scanning electron microscopy

INTRODUCTION

Far advanced or recurrent colonic cancers are often unmanageable, i.e., they respond poorly to chemotherapy, and surgical resection tends to be unsuccessful in cases of invasion of the bony pelvis. These facts may be attributable to desmoplastic fibrous stroma forming a hard and sclerotic tumor mass, however, its fine structure has not been fully elucidated. To examine how colonic cancer foci affect or are dependent on fibrous stroma, the stroma adjacent to infiltrating tumor acini was investigated by scanning electron microscopy[SEM].

MATERIALS AND METHODS

Surgically resected colonic segments, including advanced adenocarcinomas of well-differentiated type cancer together with the normal colon, were perfused with 1/15M phosphate buffer, pH 7.4 at 37°C, and then with 1% paraformaldehyde for 30 min. Cutout samples, after rinsing with buffer solution, were successively immersed in 25 and 50% dimethyl sulfoxide for 30 min each. Samples were frozen in liquid nitrogen, cut into pieces with a razor blade, rinsed in the buffer solution, and then transferred into 0.5% glutaraldehyde and allowed to stand for 20 min. After rinsing with the buffer solition, samples were treated with 2% tannic acid for 2 hr and 1% osmium tetroxide for 2 hr. Following dehydration in graded ethanol, the pieces were replaced into isoamyl acetate, dried in a critical-point dryer, coated with Pt in an ion coater, and examined with a scanning electron microscope(S-800, Hitachi Co. Ltd.,Tokyo) at 10 kV. Cancer acini were divided into an upper part(upper portion facing the mucosal side) and an invasive part(middle and lower portion on the serosal side)for the sake of description. Normal colonic glands(crypts)were divided into upper(mucosal side), middle and lower(serosal side)parts, and observations were made focusing on the surface of the gland and on the interstitium between glands(observing the interstitium of the lamina propria in both). Collagen bundles and fibrils appearing on photographs taken at 30,000 magnification were measured with respect to the percentage of area occupied by them, the in numbers, (per approximately $10.5\mu m^2$), angle(the direction of fibrils running parallel to the longitudinal axis of the gland is defined as 90° and those at right angles to it as 0°)and their diameter (width), using a Nexus Qube image processing system(Nexus Co., Tokyo). To test for statistical significance the unpaired t test was used.

499

RESULTS

SEM Examination of the Cut Surface of Normal Colonic Interstitium Surrounding Glands

In the glandular surface(Fig.1)fibroblasts were arranged in longitudinal rows in close
proximity to and surrounding the crypt. Collagen fibrils ran longitudinally(parallel to the
longitudinal axis of the gland), obliquely or horizontally, occasionally exhibiting branching.
Collagen bundles and fibrils seemed broader and more densely distributed closer to the bottom
of the gland. In the interglandular interstitium thick bundles were prominent, and ran
parallel to and several micrometers to the side of the gland. Fine fibrils connected the thick
bundles and basement membrane side of the gland, and their distribution seemed to become dense
as the bottom of the gland was approched.

SEM Observation of the Cut Surface of the Stroma Adjacent to Infiltrating Tumor Acini(Fig.2)

Collagen distribution seemed more dense, but there appeared to be fewer fibrils connecting
the bundles and basement membrance side of the tumor acini(tumor glands)than in normal
interstitium. In the invasive part, the bundles were greater in diameter and fewer in number
than in the upper part, and mainly ran parallel to the outer margin of the acini.
The percentage of the area occupied by collagen fibrils and the angle of the fibrils were
larger in cancers than in normal colon(Fig.3).

The percentage occupied seemed larger in the lower part of normal glands(Fig.4). The number
of fibrils seemed greater in the lower part of normal glands, and smaller in the invasive
part of cancerous glands than in the upper part. The angle was smaller in the invasive part
of the cancers. Fibril diameter was larger in the lower part of the glandular surface and in
the invasive part of the cancer. The variance of the angle data was in creasingly larger in
the following order:glandular surface, interglandular interstitium and cancer stroma.

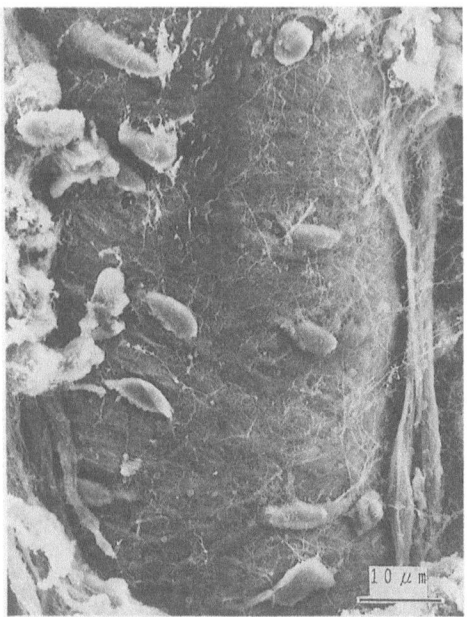

Fig.1 Surface of a normal colonic gland.

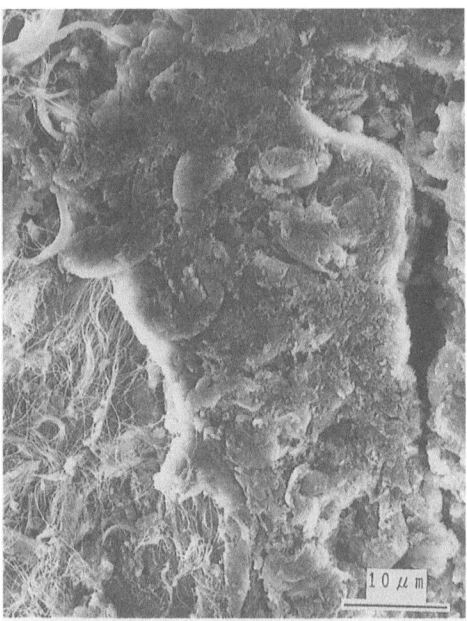

Fig.2 Tumor acinus and collagenous stroma of
advanced colon cancer.

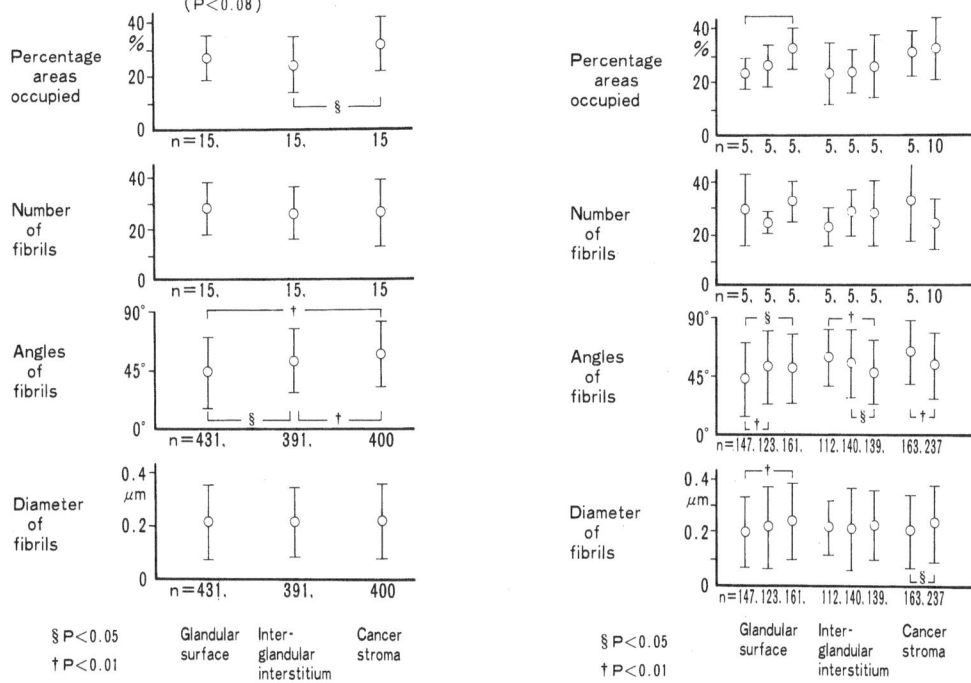

Fig.3 Morphometric data in normal vs. cancerous colonic glands.

Fig.4 Morphometric data comparing different parts of the gland.

DISCUSSION

Not much attention has been paid to the stromal elements in cancer research, however, vigorous desmoplastic reactions are only induced after carcinoma cells have invaded beyond the muscularis mucosae[1,2]. Kaye et al., in their transmission electron microscopic study on pericryptal fibroblast sheaths, reported that pericryptal collagen deposition was maximal at the mouth of the crypt, but minimal around the deeper portions of the crypt[3]. In our study, however, in the lower part of the gland the percentage of the area occupied seemed larger, at the glandular surface, which may be the result of tissue organization aimed at supporting functioning colonic glands. In the cancer stroma, percentage of the area occupied was larger than in normal interstitium and the angle of the fibrils showed greater variance, and in the invasive part, fibril diameter was increased. Fewer connections between thick collagenous bundle and the glandular surface were recognized than in normal interstitium. All these findings may imply that collagen fibers in the stroma were generated more randomly and that tumor glands were not as well supported by them as in normal interstitial structures.

REFERENCES

1. Ohtani H, Sasano N(1983)Stromal cell changes in human colorectal adenomas and carcinomas. Virchows Arch A 401:209-222
2. Miura S, Kodaira S, Hosoda Y(1993)Immunohistologic analysis of the extracellular matrix components of the fibrous stroma of human colon cancer. J Surg Oncol 53(in press)
3. Kaye GI, Lane N, Pascal RR(1968)Colonic pericryptal fibroblast sheath: Replication, migration, and cytodifferentiation of a mesenchymal cell system in adult tissue. Gastroenterology 54:852-865

Diagnostic Significance of Serum CEA and CA19-9 Levels in Colorectal Cancers

Kiwao Ishimoto, Hiroshi Tanimura, Kazuto Masaki, Kouichi Murakami, Kazuhisa Uchiyama, and Minoru Ochiai

Department of Gastroenterological Surgery, Wakayama Medical College, Wakayama, 640 Japan

ABSTRACT

We investigated the clinical significance of measuring serum CEA and CA19-9 levels for the early diagnosis of colorectal cancer in 157 cases. In the present study, the preoperative positive rate of serum CEA and CA19-9 levels in patients with curatively resected primary cancer was only 14.5% (11/76), 12.1% (4/33) of Dukes A, B, and 22.0% (11/50), 27.6% (8/29) of Dukes C, respectively, however, we found that serum CEA or CA19-9 levels were positive in 82.4% (14 cases) of 17 recurrent colorectal cancers after curative resection and that the elevation of these tumor markers was the first diagnostic method of recurrence in 38.1% of 21 cases. Thus, we conclude that the measurement of serum CEA and CA19-9 levels is not useful for the diagnosis of primary colorectal cancers, but is very useful for the early detection of recurrent colorectal cancers.

KEY WORDS: colorectal cancer, recurrence, serum CEA and CA19-9 levels

INTRODUCTION

If colorectal cancers are diagnosed earlier and resected curatively, postoperative prognosis is relatively well. Primary colorectal cancers are diagnosed by secal occult blood test, barium enema, colonoscopy or serum tumor marker levels, and recurrent colorectal cancers by ultrasonography, CT scanning, chest X-ray film, barium enema, colonoscopy, or serum tumor marker levels. We investigated the clinical significance of measuring serum CEA and CA19-9 levels for the early diagnosis of primary and recurrent colorectal cancers.

MATERIALS AND METHODS

Serum CEA levels were measured in 157 cases of primary colorectal cancer, which were divided into three groups according to the histopathological stage-grouping (group I; 76 cases of Dukes A+B, group II; 50 cases of Dukes C, group III; 31 cases of noncurative resection with a distant metastasis or carcinomatous peritonitis). Serum CA19-9 levels were combined with 80 of 157 cases (group I; 33, group II; 29, group III; 18 cases). CEA was measured with EIA method (normal range <5ng/ml), and CA19-9 with RIA method (<37U/ml) (Table 1).

Table 1. Serum CEA and CA19-9 levels in colorectal cancers

Group	staging	CEA	CA19-9
I	Dukes A Dukes B (early cancer	76 (cases) 9	33 (cases) 4)
II	Dukes C	50	29
III	Distant metastasis Peritonitis carcinomatosa	31	18
		157 (cases)	80 (cases)

CEA : EIA method (normal range < 5ng/ml)
CA19-9 : RIA method (normal range < 37U/ml)

In 21 cases which developed recurrence after curative resection, we investigated the clinical significance of measuring serum tumor markers as a diagnostic method for recurrence from the correlation between the elevation of serum CEA, CA19-9 levels and the recurrence pattern.

RESULTS

The positive rate of serum CEA was only 14.5% in group I, 22.0% in group II, but jumped sharply to 77.4% in group III. Preoperatively, serum CEA level was positive in 11 cases of group I and II (126 cases), of which only 2 cases resulted in recurrence of cancer after curative resection (Fig.1).
The positive rate of serum CA19-9 level was only 12.1% in group I, 27.6% in group II, but elevated to 66.7% in group III (Fig.2).
These two tumor markers showed almost the same sensitivity.

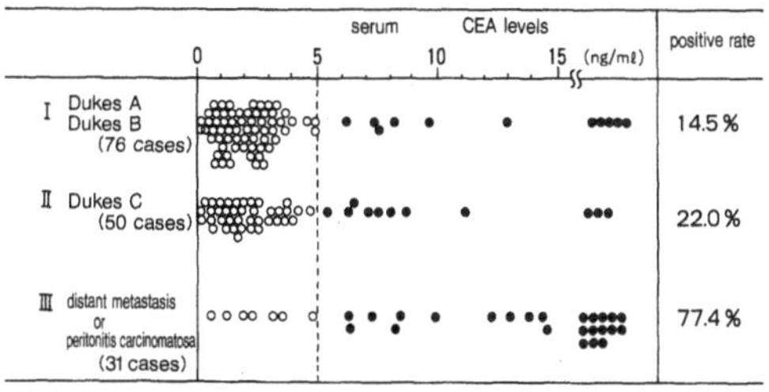

Fig.1 Serum CEA levels of colorectal cancer according to Dukes

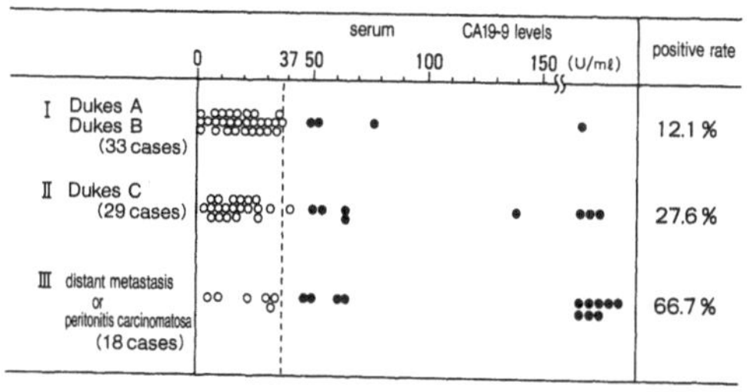

Fig.2 Serum CA19-9 levels of colorectal cancer according to Dukes

Recurrence has developed in 21 among 126 cases who were resected curatively. Of 21 cases, 8 (38.1%) were diagnosed firstly with the elevation of serum CEA or CA19-9 level, 4 (19.0%) with CT scanning, 4 (19.0%) with ultrasonography, 3 (14.5%) with chest X-ray film (Table 2). In 17 cases in which we investigated the correlation between the elevation of serum CEA, CA19-9 levels and the recurrence pattern, these tumor markers were positive in 14 cases (82.4%). In 77.8% of 9 cases with liver metastasis, both markers remarkably elevated. In 75.0% of 4 cases with local recurrence, both markers elevated. Three, including 2 cases with lung metastasis, showed normal level of tumor markers (Fig.3).

Table 2. First diagnostic method of recurrent colorectal cancers

1) tumor markers (CEA, CA19-9)	38.1 % (8 cases)
2) CT scanning	19.0 (4)
3) ultrasonography	19.0 (4)
4) chest X-ray film	14.5 (3)
5) colonoscopy	4.8 (1)
6) DIP	4.8 (1)

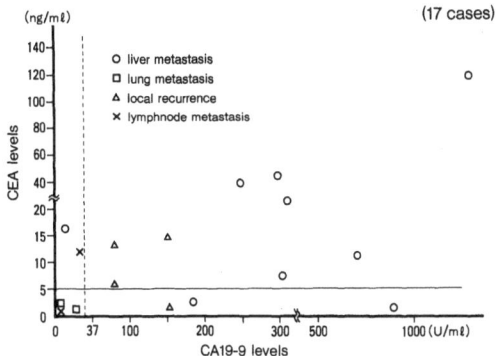

Fig.3 Correlation between serum CEA, CA19-9 levels and recurrence of colorectal cancer

The patient is 60-year-old male, who had sigmoid resection with R_2 lymphnode dissection for sigmoid colon cancer on June, 1990. Postoperative histopathological stage was Dukes C. After 6 months passed postoperatively, serum CEA and CA19-9 levels elevated from 4.9 to 58 ng/ml, from 35 to 298 U/ml, respectively. CT scanning demonstrated liver metastasis at left lateral segment and posterior segment. On January 1991, left lateral segmentectomy with partial resections of posterior segment was performed. His postoperative course has been uneventful, and serum CEA and CA19-9 levels has declined within normal range. He is well without recurrence as of March, 1993 (Fig.4).

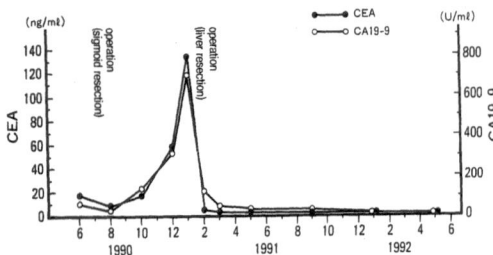

Fig.4 Postoperative course and the change of serum CEA and CA19-9 levels

DISCUSSION

The diagnosis of colorectal cancers by serum tumor markers is simple comparing with barium enema or colonoscopic examination. But the question is whether or not they have enough sensitivity for the diagnosis of colorectal cancers. In the present study, we revealed that serum CEA and CA19-9 had low sensitivity for primary colorectal cancers which can be resected curatively by operation, and particularly had no sensitivity for early colorectal cancers.
We follow up the postoperative course of patients after curative resection of colorectal cancer with tumor markers (every 3 months), ultrasonography or CT scanning (every 6 months), chest X-ray film (once a year), and barium enema or colonoscopy (every 1∿2 years). The elevation of secum CEA and/or CA19-9 levels led to the first diagnosis of recurrence in 8 (38.1%) of 21 patients, and had the most useful diagnostic ability for the recurrence of colorectal cancer. If liver metastasis, lung metastasis, or local recurrence is detected earlier, metastatic lesion will be able to be resected again and the postoperative long-term survival of patients with colorectal cancer will be remarkably improved.

Evaluation of Preoperative Serum CEA and IAP Levels in the Patients with Colorectal Cancer

Takao Umemoto, Yasuyuki Sugiyama, and Shigetoyo Saji

The Second Department of Surgery, Gifu University School of Medicine, Gifu 500, Japan

ABSTRUCT

The usefulness of the preoerative measurement of serum CEA and IAP level as prognostic factors in colorectal cancer patients was investigated. The cases were divided into negative or positive groups acording to cut off points of CEA of 5ng/ml ,IAP of 500µg/ml orIAP of 580µg/ml respectivly. In comparison of survival rates in colon cancer , the groups of CEA negative, IAP500 negative or IAP580 negative were all significantly better than those of positive ones respectivly. But in rectal cancer , only the rate of IAP580 negative one was significantly better than that of positive one. To further investigation of above results , according to the general rules for clinical and pathological studies on cancer of colon ,rectum and anus in Japan , distributions of cases by histological backgrounds and by these cut off points were analized. Results were those both in colon and rectal cancer , CEA correlated almost all bacgrounds except histological type and lymphnode metastasis. But IAP500 correlated only operative curability in rectal cancer ,and also IAP580 corelated only operative culability in both colon and rectal cancer and lymphnode metastasis in colon cancer.

KEY WORDS: serum CEA level,serum IAP level, colo-rectal cancer,survival rate

INTRODUCTION

Carcinoembryonic antigen (CEA) was a well-known tumor marker and was believed as useful for the evaluation of surgical resectability and for early diagnosis of recurrence in colo-rectal cancer. Immunosuppresive acidic protein (IAP) was observed as one of serum immunosuppresive proteins in patients with various carcinomas. Recently it was used as a tumor marker for evaluating the humoral immunity of cancer patients. However serum IAP level has been considered to be not so useful for early diagnosis of colo-rectal cancer. In present study , the clinical usefulness of preoperative plasma CEA and IAP levels for a diagnostic or prognostic significance in patients with colo-rectal cancer was examined and re-evaluated.

MATERIALS AND METHODS

Preoperative plasma CEA or IAP values were measured in 276 patients with colo-rectal cancer (149:colon and 127:rectum) during the period from 1981 to 1991. In terms of cut off points, 5ng/ml of CEA and 500 or 580µg/ml of IAP were emploid . 580µg/ml of IAP was derived from SIP[1](Study of Immunochemotherapy with PSK) for gastric cancer and was considered as more useful prognostic factor than conventional cut off value of 500µg/ml. Acording to above cut off values, the differences of survival curves were investigated for prognostic factor, and its statistical significance was tested by Generalized Wilcoxon method. Thereafter the distribution of the number of patients by general rules for clinical and pathological studies on cancer of cohlon ,rectum and anus in Japan, and cut off values were evaluated for diagnostic and histologic factors by CHI-square test.

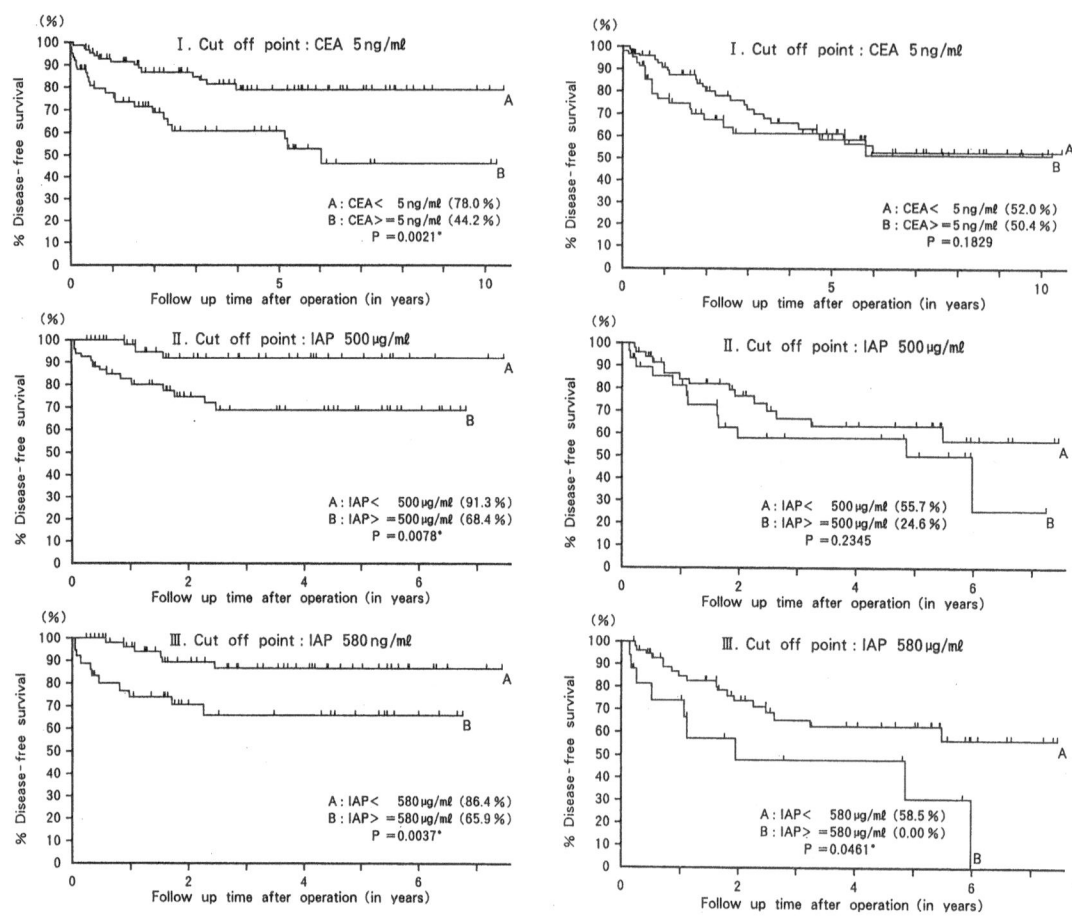

Fig-1, Survival Curves of Colon Cancer Patients   Fig-2, Survival Curves of Rectal Cancer Patients

Table1, Summary of CHI-square tests of distributions by histological backgrounds

	CEA		IAP500		IAP580	
	Colon	Rectum	Colon	Rectum	Colon	Rectum
Historogical typing	n.s	n.s	n.s	n.s	n.s	n.s
Depth of invasion	p=0.01*	p=0.001*	n.s	n.s	n.s	n.s
Lympphnode metastasia	n.s	n.s	n.s	n.s	p=0.035*	n.s
Imvasion of lymphvessels	p=0.018*	p=0.003*	n.s	n.s	n.s	n.s
Invasion of vessels	p=0.007*	n.s	n.s	n.s	n.s	n.s
Operative curability	p=0.01*	p=0.02*	n.s	p=0.02*	p=0.038*	p=0.001*
Gross findings of primary lesions	p=0.019*	p=0.012*	n.s	n.s	n.s	n.s
Tumor size (4cm)	n.s	p=0.002*	n.s	n.s	n.s	p=0.002*
Hepatic metastasis	p=0.042*	n.s	n.s	n.s	n.s	p=0.015*
Peritoneal dssemination	n.s	n.s	n.s	n.s	n.s	n.s

RESULTS

As shown in Fig 1-I,1-II and 1-III ,in colon cancer, suvival rates of negative CEA , negative IAP500 or negative IAP580 were significantly better than
those of positive ones respectivly. So there might be some correlation between
preoperative serum CEA or IAP levels and the prognosis of colon cancer patients . Howener in rectal cancr , significant differences were noted only between the rates of negative IAP580 and positive IAP580 (Fig 2-III). While in
terms of cut off point of serum CEA of 5ng/ml or that of serum IAP of
500ug/ml, there were no significant differences (Fig 2-I,2-II).

Table1 shows the summary of the CHI-square test among the distribution of
histological backgrounds and above cut off points. The cut off points of CEA
of 5ng/ml was able to detect the significant differences of almost all backgrounds except histological typing, lymphnode metastasis , peritoneal dissemination etc. However the cut off point of IAP of 500ug/ml correlated hardly
any backgrounds excpt operative curability. While the cut off point of IAP of
580ug/ml corelated somemore factors, those were lymphnode metastasis, operative curability, tumor size , hepatic metastasis etc.

DISCUSSION

Serum CEA value was a well-known tumor marker for colo-rectal cancer[2] and
serum IAP value was used as a tumor marker for detection of immunosupresive
state of cancer patients[3] In the present study preoperative serum CEA or IAP
value in colorectal cancer were re-evaluated for a prognostic factor. In colon
cancer, the cut off points of CEA or IAP were well able to detect the difference of survival rates , but not in rectal cancer except the IAP of 580ug/ml.
The result of analysis of the frequency distributions of histological backgrounds showed that there was the well correlation of CEA for histological
factors and hardly any of IAP in contrast , and that in comparison between
IAP500 and IAP580, IAP580 is considerd more sensitive than IAP500. In this
study only histological factors were analized, sothat CEA was only able to
show the well corelation. It might be because that CEA was produced by carcinoma cells and strongly affected by the amounts of tumor cell and its sor-
roundings. Among the histological factors, IAP was affected by operative curability ,lymphnode metastasis, tumor size or hepatic metastasis. It was suggested that IAP was affected mainly by the factos far from the tumor. And
also it was suggested that in colon cancer, measurments of both serum IAP or
CEA levels were useful to evaluate its survival rates, but in recteal cancer,
only serum IAP level was thought as useful. However to explain why preoerative serum CEA or IAP value were able to show the differences in suvival
curves , the further statistical analysis about the another humoral factors
shouhd be necessary.

REFFERENCES

1.Sakamoto J, Kato K, Tanemura H, Watanabe T, Nagata I, Kishikawa H, Itou y,
   Teramukai S, Oohashi Y, Ogawa T, Nakasato H (1989) Serum immunosuppresive
   acidic protein in patients with gastric cancer - statistical resaerch for
   the cut-off level and evaluation of the effect of biological response modifier PSK -. The 9th Reports of Japan Tumor Makar Association 9:217-220
2.Gold P, Freedman SO (1965) Demonstration of tumor specific antigen in human
   colonoc carcinoma by immunological tolerance and absorption teqniques.
   J.Exp.Med. 121:439-462
3.Currie GA, Basham C (1972) Serum mediated inhibition of the immunological
   reactions of the patient to his own tumour: A possible role for circulating
   antigen. Br. J. Cancer 26:427-438

The Meanings of CEA in Gallbladder Bile in Colorectal Cancer

KATSUKI ITO, KOUZOU KIRIYAMA, TAKAYUKI UMEDA, KAZUHIKO NAKATA,
CHUN-LIN YE, KEN KONDOU, SEIJI AKIYAMA, and HIROSHI TAKAGI

Department of Surgery II, School of Medicine, Nagoya University, Nagoya, 466 Japan

ABSTRACT

To clarify the meaning of the CEA level in bile, the measurements of CEA level
in the serum and in the bile were done, by the method of enzyme immunoassay
after Takita and Yamamura, in 18 cases (group 1) of cholelithiasis without
cancer, 12 cases (group 2) of colorectal cancer without hepatic metastasis, 8
cases (group 3) of colorectal cancer with hepatic metastasis. The mean of
serum CEA of group 1, 2 and 3 were 1.4 ± 1.1 (n=18) ng/ml, 8.5 ± 9.8 (n=12) and
329 ± 665.3 (n=8), respectively and the mean of bile CEA level of group 1, 2 and
3 were 22.0 ± 37 (n=18), 42.6 ± 74.2 (n=12) and 1485 ± 2215.8 (n=8), respectively.
And the higher level of bile CEA of the colorectal cancer groups than those of
non-cancerous groups was statistically different, $p<0.01$, as serum CEA. The
CEA of bile in hepatic metastatic group was also higher statistically than
those of non-metastatic group. Therefore the high value of bile CEA can be a
predictive indicator of hepatic metastasis in colorectal cancer, but in 3 of
18 non-cancerous cases they were more than 100 ng/ml and were not able to
neglect the presence of false positive cases.

KEY WORDS : CEA in bile, predictive indicator of hepatic metastasis

INTRODUCTION

The early detection of liver metastasis of colorectal cancer is great concern
among the surgeons who had curative operation to the patients, because the
early developed liver metastasis can be treated surgically to obtain the
complete cure or to obtain the benefit from effective chemotherapy. It is
said that bile CEA level correlates significantly well the size of metastatic
tumor mass, as serum CEA. In this investigation by the measurement of CEA
level in bile to compare to serum CEA, it is aimed to know if the prediction
of hepatic metastasis of colorectal cancer is possible and to know if the data
can be the indicator of the therapy or recurrence.

MATERIAL AND METHODS

Patients : Eighteen cases (group 1) of benign cholecystolithiasis or/and
choledocholithiasis, 12 cases (group 2) of colo-rectal cancer without hepatic
metastasis, 8 cases (group 3) of colorectal cancer with hepatic metastasis.
The bile was obtained by a puncture of gall bladder during or after operation.
The bile was mixed with same volume of 0.5M buffer (pH 5) solution for 15
minutes in 70 °C, then was spined for 10 minutes in 3000 rpm and was measured
the CEA level by Enzyme-immunoassay method after Takita and Yamamura, using

508

CEA-RIABEAD kit of Dinabot co.

RESULTS

The mean of serum CEA of group 1.2 and 3 were 1.4±1.1(n=18) ng/ml,
8.5±9.8(n=12) and 329±665.3(n=8), respectively and the mean of bile CEA of
group 1.2 and 3 were 22.0±37(n=18), 42.6±74.2(n=12) and 1485±2215.8(n=8),
respectively (Fig.1). The levels of bile CEA of the colorectal cancer group
were higher statistically, p<0.01, than those of non-cancer group as serum
CEA, and in the hepatic metastatic group those CEA were also higher
statistically, p<0.01, than those in non-metastatic group (Fig.2). And as for
the degree of hepatic metastasis concern, it is suggested that it has some
correlation between the value of bile CEA (Fig.3). In 3 of 18 non-cancerous
cases the level of bile CEA were more than 100 ng/ml and extensive surveys
were done to detect the cancerous lesions but failed to find out.

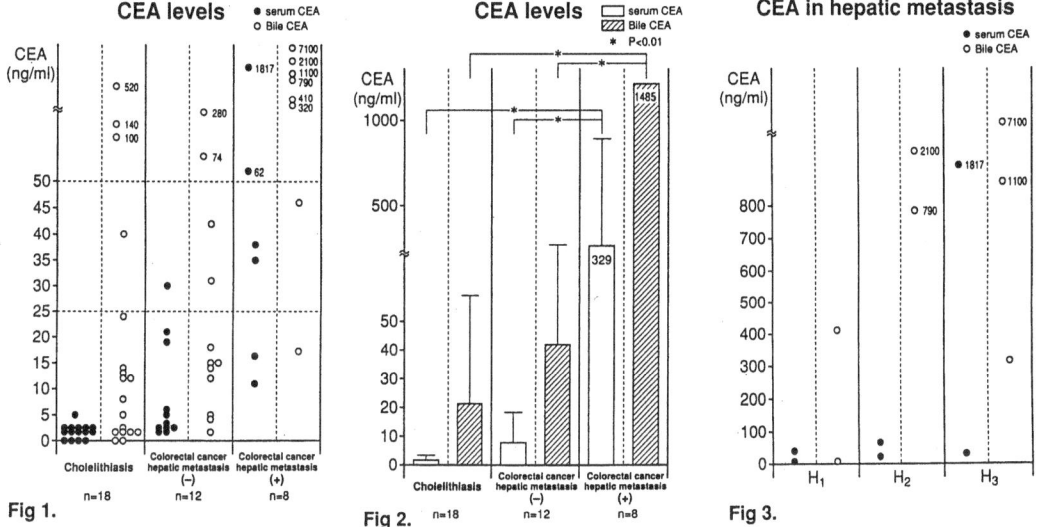

Fig 1. Fig 2. Fig 3.

DISCUSSION

From this investigation it was concluded that the high value of bile CEA could
be a good predictive indicator of hepatic metastasis, and there was some
correlation between the value of bile CEA and degree of metastasis. The cut-
off value concern, it was still in the process to find out and more
accumulation of cases should solve that by itself. Other problem of this
study was the presence of false positive and in 3 cases of 18 non-cancerous
cases the values of bile CEA were more than 100 ng/ml and extensive diagnostic
surveys failed to find out cancer lesions and in all those 18 cases of
cholelithiasis serum CEA level were normal.

References

1) Yeatman T.J., Bland K.I., Copeland E.M., et al.; Relationship between

colorectal liver metastases and CEA levels in gallbladder bile. Ann. Surg. 210:505-512 1989

2) Yeatman T.J., Kimura A.K., Copeland E.M.: Rapid analysis of carcinoembryonic antigen levels in gallbladder bile. Ann.Surg.213:113-117 1991

3) Yano Y.:Biliary carcinoembryonic antigen, non-specific cross-reacting antigen and biliary glycoprotein-lts analysis and clinical aspect-.Jap. J. Surg. 87:1432-1442 1990

The Relationship Between Metastatic Potential and the Expression of Sialyl Lewis A (CA 19-9) and Sialyl Lewis X Antigens in Colorectal Cancer

Masanori Maehara, Akio Yamaguchi, Takanori Goi, Kazuo Hirose, Yoshiaki Isobe, and Gizo Nakagawara

The First Department of Surgery, Fukui Medical School, Matsuoka-cho, Yoshida-gun, Fukui, 910-11 Japan

ABSTRACT

The relationship between metastatic potential and the expression of sialyl Le^a or sialyl Le^x antigens was studied in 128 advanced colorectal cancer. Hematogenous metastasis was observed more often in the Grade II-III group of sialyl Le^a or sialyl Le^x staining than in Grade 0-I. The recurrence rates in the Grade II-III group of sialyl Le^x staining was significantly higher than those in the Grade 0-I, and the prognosis in the Grade II-III group of sialyl Le^x staining was significantly poorer than that in the Grade 0-I. These results suggested that sialyl Le^a and sialyl Le^x antigens in colorectal cancer might be involved in the hematogenous metastasis.

KEY WARDS: sialyl Le^a, sialyl Le^x, hematogenous metastasis, colorectal cancer

INTRODUCTION

The adhesion of tumor cells to endothelial cells of the target organ is one of the most important steps of hematogenous metastasis [1.2]. Endothelial leukocyte adhesion molecule-1 (ELAM-1) is reported to be expressed on endothelial cells and interacts with carbohydrate sialyl Le^a or sialyl Le^x [3-5]. Therefore, it is of particular interest to consider that these antigens might be involved in hematogenous metastasis as the ligand for ELAM-1. This study was undertaken to determine whether the expression of these antigens have some relation to the hematogenous metastatic properties in colorectal cancer

MATERIALS AND METHOD

For this study, the tissues of primary advanced colorectal cancer were obtained from 128 patients undergoing surgical resection at the First Department of Surgery, Fukui Medical School. Seventy-two were colon cancer and fifty-six were rectal cancer. The tissue samples from primary colorectal cancer were studied by immunohistochemical examination using monoclonal antibodies against sialyl Le^a (KM-231 MAb) and sialyl Le^x (CSLEX-1 MAb). KM-231 [anti-sialyl Le^a MAb (mouse IgG)] was kindly provided by Kyowa (Tokyo). CSLEX-1 [anti-sialyl Le^x MAb (mouse IgM)] was kindly provided by Dr. P. Terasaki (UCLA Tissue Typing Laboratory, Los Angeles, CA). All tissue samples were fixed in 10% formalin for 24 h and embedded in paraffin. Serial 4- μm sections were cut and the expression of these antigens were detected immunohistochemically by the labelled streptavidin-biotin methods (DAKO LSAB KIT). Staining results were scored from "Grade 0" to "Grade III": Grade 0, negative; Grade I, apical type or cytoplasmic type (polarity (+)); Grade II, cytoplasmic type (polarity (-)); Grade III, stromal type. This classification corresponds with that of Ichihara. Statistical significance was assayed using the chi-square test. Curves for survival were drawn according to the Kaplan-Meier method. Differences were taken as significant when p was less than 0.05.

RESULTS

Synchronous or recurrent metastasis in liver, lung or bone was counted as hematogenous metastasis. The positive rates of sialyl Le^a and sialyl Le^x in all tissues of primary advanced colorectal cancer were 77.3% and 71.9% respectively. As shown in Fig. 1, the incidence of hematogenous metastasis in the Grade II-III groups of sialyl Le^a and sialyl Le^x staining were 43.7% (21/48) and 67.5% (21/48) respectively, whereas those in the Grade 0-I groups were 17.5% (14/80) and 11.3% (10/88). There was a significant difference between two groups ($p < 0.01$). These results suggested that these antigens might be involved in the metastatic properties of colorectal cancer. Therefore, we investigated the relationship between recurrence pattern in patients after curative resection and the expression of these antigens. Distribution of 99 patients who underwent curative resection is presented in Table 1. There was no statically significant difference between the pathologic features and the Grade of sialyl Le^a or sialyl Le^x staining. However, the incidence of recurrent hematogenous metastasis in the Grade II, III group of sialyl Le^x staining was significantly higher than that in the Grade 0, I group (Table 2).

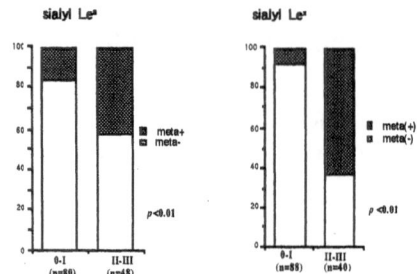

Fig. 1 The relationship between hematogenous metastasis and the expression of sialyl Le^a or sialyl Le^x antigen.

Table 1. Pathologic features and staining results

Variables	sialyl Le^a Grade 0-I	Grade II-III	P value	sialyl Le^x Grade 0-I	Grade II-III	P value
Histological type			NS(not significant)			NS
well	46 (66.7%)	21 (70.0%)		53 (68.8%)	14 (63.6%)	
mode	18 (26.1%)	8 (27.7%)		20 (26.0%)	7 (31.8%)	
por	4 (5.8%)	1 (3.3%)		3 (3.9%)	1 (4.5%)	
muc	1 (1.4%)	0		1 (1.3%)	0	
Depth of invasion			NS			NS
pm	15 (21.7%)	4 (13.3%)		15 (19.5%)	4 (18.2%)	
ss	33 (47.8%)	15 (50.0%)		40 (52.0%)	8 (36.4%)	
s	17 (24.6%)	11 (36.7%)		19 (24.7%)	9 (40.9%)	
si,ai	4 (5.8%)	0		3 (3.9%)	1 (4.5%)	
Lymphnode metastasis			NS			NS
n0	44 (63.8%)	12 (40.0%)		45 (58.4%)	11 (50.0%	
n1	16 (23.2%)	11 (36.7%)		20 (26.0%)	7 (31.8%)	
n2	7 (10.1%)	6 (20.0%)		10 (13.0%)	3 (13.6%)	
n3	2 (2.9%)	1 (3.3%)		2 (2.6%)	1 (4.5%)	

Table 2. Staining results and recurrent pattern

	Sialyl Le^a	Sialyl Le^x	
	Recurrence rate		
Grade 0-I	12/69(17.4%)	10/77(13.0%)	
hematogenous	9	7	$p<0.01$
local	2	2	
peritoneum	1	1	
Grade II-III	8/30 (27.7%)	10/22(45.4%)	
hematogenous	8	10	
local	0	0	
peritoneum	0	0	

Fig. 2 shows the relationship between prognosis and sialyl Le^a or sialyl Le^x immunoreactivity. The correlation between the survival after curative resection and expression of sialyl Le^a was no statistically significant. However, the 5-year survival rate was 87.5% of patients with Grade 0-I tumors of sialyl Le^x, and 57.5% for ones with Grade II-III tumors; there was a significant difference between these two groups.

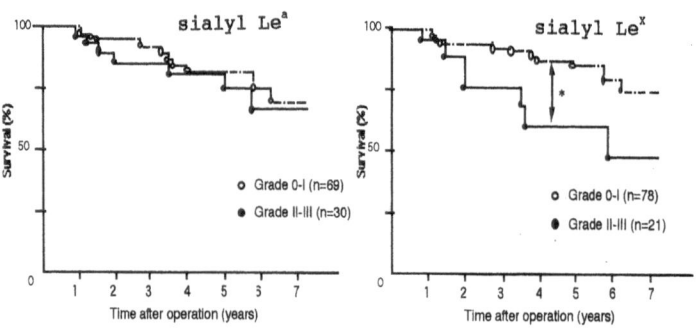

Fig. 2 The relationship between prognosis and sialyl Le^a or sialyl Le^x immunoreactivity.

DISCUSSION

Sialyl Le^a and sialyl Le^x, generally accepted as serum markers for diagnosis of cancer, are expressed on the surface of malignant cells [6,7]. ELAM-1 is reported to recognize this carbohydrate structure of sialyl Le^x [3,4] or sialyl Le^a [5]. Therefore, these authors suggested that the interaction of these antigens with ELAM-1 is involved in the cell-adhesive step of hematogenous metastasis of cancer cells. In this study, we demonstrated that the expression of sialyl Le^a or sialyl Le^x in advanced colorectal cancer was correlated with synchronous or recurrent hematogenous metastasis. Our results stressed that sialyl Le^a and sialyl Le^x are not only tumor-associated antigens but also important carbohydrate structures determining the metastatic properties of colorectal cancer.

The combined use of two monoclonal antibodies against sialyl Le^a and sialyl Le^x antigens has been reported to detect a wider range of sera from patients with cancer than the use of a single monoclonal antibody alone [8]. In our present study the sialyl Le^x-positive patients with liver metastasis who were negative with sialyl Le^a was shown, and some patients showed the opposite reaction.

The correlation between the survival after curative resection and expression of sialyl Le^a was not statistically significant. However, the survival in the Grade II, III group of sialyl Le^x staining was significantly poorer than that in the Grade 0, I group. The patients who are Le($^{a-b-}$) can not synthesize the sialyl Le^a antigen [9]. However, the expression of sialyl Le^x was not restricted by Lewis blood type. Although further studies are evidently necessary, this might be one of the reasons for the higher specificity of sialyl Le^x compared with sialyl Le^a.

In conclusion, the expression of sialyl Le^a and sialyl Le^x antigens in primary colorectal cancer might be correlated with their hematogenous metastatic potential and that the immunohistochemical analysis for these antigens might be useful in determining prognosis or the need for further treatment or closer follow-up of patients at high risk for the development of metastasis.

REFERENCES

1. Irimura T, Reading CL (1987) Surface properties of metastatic tumor cells. Cancer Bull. 39: 132-141

2. Dennis JW, LAFERTE S (1987) Tumor cell surface carbohydrate and the metastatic phenotype. Cancer Metastasis Rev. 5: 185-204

3. Phillips ML, Nudelman E, Gaeta FCA, Peretz M, Singhal AK, Hakomori S, Paulson JC (1990) ELAM-1 mediates cell adhesion by recognition of a carbohydrate ligand, sialyl-LeX. Science 250: 1130-1132

4. Walz G, Aruffo A, Kolanus W, Bevilacqua M, Seed B (1990) Recognition by ELAM-1 of the sialyl-LeX determinant on myeloid and tumor cells (1985) Science 250: 1132-1135

5. Berg EL, Robinson MK, Mansson O, Butcher EC, Magnani JL (1991) A carbohydrate domain common to both sialyl Le^a and sialyl Le^x is recognized by the endothelial cell leukocyte adhesion molecule ELAM-1. J. biol. Chem. 266: 14869-14872

6. Fukushima K, Hirota M, Terasaki PI, Wakisaka A, Togashi H, Chia D, Suyama N, Fukushi Y, Nudelman E, Hakomori S (1984) Characterization of sialosylated Lewis X as a new tumor-associated antigen. Cancer Res. 44: 5279-5285

7. Magnani JL, Nilsson B, Brockhaus M, Zopf D, Steplewski Z, Koprowski H, Ginsburg V (1982) A monoclonal antibody-defined antigen associated with gastrointestinal cancer is a ganglioside containing sialylated lacto-N-fucopentaose II J. biol. Chem. 257: 14365-14369

8. Chia D, Terasaki PI, Suyama N, Galton J, Hirota, M, Katz D. Use of monoclonal antibodies to sialylated Lewis^x and sialylated Lewis^a for serological tests of cancer (1985) Cancer Res. 45: 435-437 .

9. Koprowski H, Blaszcyk M, Steplewski Z, Brockhaus M, Magnani JL, Ginsburg V (1982) Lewis blood type may affect the incidence of gastrointestinal cancer. Lancet i: 1332-1333

Laminin Levels and Stage of Vascular Invasion as Predictive Factors of Liver Metastasis in Colon Cancer

Toshio Imada[1], Toshitaka Takehana[1], Makoto Takahashi[1],
Kuniyasu Fukuzawa[1], Yasushi Rino[1], Yuji Yamamoto[1], Akihiko Matsumoto[1],
Kenzo Okada[2], Takashi Suda[2], and Hiroshi Takemura[2]

[1]The First Department of Surgery, Yokohama City University School of Medicine, Yokohama, 232 Japan
[2]Department of Surgery, Saiseikai Yokohamashi Nambu Hospital, Yokohama, Japan

ABSTRACT

The glycoprotein laminin mediates the adhesion of tumor cells to the basement membrane prior to invasion. In this study, we determined the laminin levels of the peripheral and returned venous blood in 46 colon cancer patients without detectable liver metastasis. The laminin levels of both peripheral and returned blood were significantly higher in the cases with vascular invasion compared to the group without it. However, no correlation was observed between the stage of vascular invasion and laminin levels.
These data show the possibility that the laminin levels can serve as a predictive factor of liver metastasis from colon cancer.

KEY WORDS:laminin, vascular invasion, colon cancer

INTRODUCTION

The glycoprotein laminin mediates the adhesion of tumor cells to the basement membrane prior to invasion[1]. In patients with colon cancer, the liver is the primary site of hematogenous metastases followed by the lung[2]. Colon cancer can present with or without vascular invasion. Liver metastases are three times as frequent in patients with vascular invasion as in patients without it[3]. In the present study, we determined the laminin levels of the peripheral and returned venous blood and their relationship to vascular invasion in colon cancer patients without detectable liver metastasis.

MATERIALS AND METHODS

Peripheral and venous blood were collected from the tumor site of 46 colon cancer cases without liver metastasis.
Laminin levels were determined by RIA method (LamininP1 Kit,Hoechst).
Values between 0.85 to 1.41 U/ml are considered to be within the normal range.
Stage of vascular invasion was evaluated according to the general rules for clinical and pathological studies on cancer of colon,rectum and anus[4].
Staining with hematoxylin eosin (HE) and victoria blue was performed to classify the stage of invasion in V_1, V_2 and V_3 indicating increasing invasion.

RESULTS

Twenty of the total 46 cases (43.5%) showed evidence of vascular invasion. Ten cases were classified as V1, two cases as V2, and eight cases as V3 (Table.1). The average laminin levels of the peripheral and returned blood of the cases with evidence of vascular invasion were 1.52+/−0.50 U/ml and 1.52+/−0.48 U/ml, respectively. In the cases with no vascular invasion the corresponding values were 1.16+/−0.26 U/ml and 1.17+/−0.22 U/ml. The laminin levels of both peripheral and returned blood were significantly higher in the cases with vascular invasion compared to the group without it ($p < 0.05$, $p < 0.001$) (Table.2). The difference between the laminin level of the peripheral blood and that of the returned blood was minimal in the individual cases with a correlation coefficient of 0.96 (Fig.1).

No correlation was observed between the stage of vascular invasion and laminin levels.

Table.1 The stage of vascular invasion

Vascular invasion	Number of cases	
V0	26(56.5%)	
V1	10(21.7%)	⌐
V2	2(4.4%)	20(43.5%)
V3	8(17.4%)	⌐
	46(100 %)	

Table.2 The relati onship between laminin levels and vascular invasion

	Positive invasion	Negative invasion
Peripheral blood	1.52+/−0.48(U/ml)*	1.16+/−0.26(U/ml)*
Returned blood	1.52+/−0.50(U/ml)**	1.17+/−0.22(U/ml)**
	*P‹0.05	**P‹0.01

Laminin level of
peripheral blood

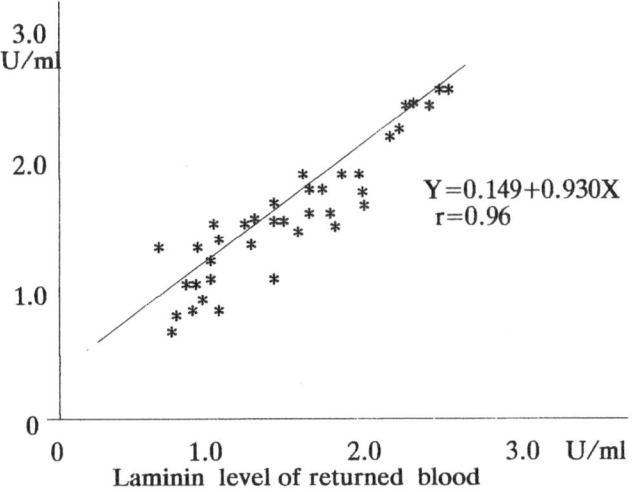

$Y=0.149+0.930X$
$r=0.96$

Fig.1 Correlation between laminin level of peripheral blood and that of returned blood

DISCUSSION

One of the decisive factors of the treatment outcome of colon cancer is liver metastasis. Vascular invasion shows a close relation to liver matastasis, and the incidence of liver metastasis in colon cancer cases with vascular invasion is reported to be significantly higher than that in those without[5]. The stage of vascular invasion is often difficult to determine accurately by usual HE staining alone. By also employing victoria blue staining we obtained more accurate results for the classification of stage.

Cell surface receptors for the basement membrane glycoprotein laminin participate in the metastasis of cancer. Laminin mediates the adhesion of tumor cells to the basement membrane before invasion. Cancer cells invade blood vessels and destroy the basement membrane of the sites, showing an increase in laminin which is a predictive factor of liver metastasis[6] Serum laminin levels were reported to be higher in colon cancer cases with liver metastasis. It is likely that, in cases without evident liver metastasis, blood laminin concentration increases with vascular invasion. Comparing the laminin level of peripheral blood and that of venous blood returning from the tumor site did not show any difference.

We have shown that a relationship between the laminin levels and vacular invasion exist, indicating the possibility that the laminin levels of peripheral or returned blood can serve as a predictive factor of liver metastasis from colon cancer. Further studies should bring this observation into clinical use.

REFERENCE

1. Rao C.N.,Margulies M.,Tralka S.et.al. (1982) Isolation of a subunit of laminin and its role in molecular structure and tumor cell attachment. J Biol Chem 257: 9740

2. Weiss L.,Grundmann E.,Torhorst J.et.al. (1986) Haematogenous metastatic patterns in colonic carcinoma: An analysis of 1541 necroscopies. J Pathol 150: 195–203

3. Knudsen J.B.,Nilsson T.,Sprechler M.,et.al. (1983) Venous and nerve invasion as prognostic factors in postoperative survival of patients with resectable cancer of the rectum.Dis Colon Rectum 26:613–617

4. Japanese Research Society for Cancer of Colon and Rectum (1985) The general rules for clinical and pathological studies on cancer of colon, rectum and anus. 4th ed. Tokyo :Kanehara Shuppan

5. Yamaguchi A.,Kurosaka N.,Oota N.,et.al. (1990) Examination of hematogenous metastasis cases after operation of colon cancer. J.Jpn Soc Clin Surg. 51:256–260

6. Izumi K. (1992) A study on relationship between liver metastasis of colon cancer and serum laminin level. Jpn J Gastroentrol Surg. 25:1234–1242

Elevated Serum Levels of Soluble Tumor Necrosis Factor Receptors in Patients with Colorectal Cancer

KATSUHIKO KIMURA, YASUHITO ABE, ATSUSHI HORIUCHI, and SHIGERU KIMURA

The Second Department of Surgery, Ehime University School of Medicine, Shigenobu-cho, Onsen-gun, Ehime, 791-02 Japan

ABSTRACT

To evaluate the clinical significance of serum levels of soluble tumor necrosis factor receptors (sTNF-Rs), we investigated the relationship between serum levels of sTNF-Rs (sTNF-R-p55 and sTNF-R-p75) and clinical parameters in 8 patients with colo-rectal cancer. Serum levels of sTNF-R-p55 were correlated with their stages. Serum levels of both sTNF-Rs were correlated with the extent of microscopic invasion of cancer cells into lymph vessels in the wall of colon or rectum and with the serum levels of carcinoembryonic antigen (CEA). Thus, serum levels of sTNF-Rs are indicated to be new tumor markers of colo-rectal cancer.

KEY WORDS: soluble tumor necrosis factor receptors, colo-rectal cancer, tumor marker

INTRODUCTION

TNF and lymphotoxin bind to the same cell surface receptors (TNF-Rs) and mediate numerous biological functions, such as hemorrhagic necrosis of transplanted tumors and cytotoxicity against cancer cells [1-5]. Soluble forms of TNF-Rs are the extracellular domains of the TNF-Rs shed from cell surfaces [1,2,4,6,7]. It was reported that serum levels of both sTNF-Rs are elevated in patients with malignancy [8]. In this retrospective study, to evaluate the clinical significance of serum levels of sTNF-Rs, we investigated the relationship between serum levels of sTNF-Rs and clinical parameters, including their stages, histopathological findings and tumor markers, in 8 patients with colo-rectal cancer.

PATIENTS AND METHODS

Patients

We studied 8 patients with colo-rectal cancer, who were hospitalized from June 1988 to December 1992 and underwent operations. These patients were not under treatment with immuno-chemotherapeutic agent and did not have apparent inflammatory diseases. Their renal function tests showed normal values. Their mean age was 61.2 ± 9.6 (SD) years. The 55 control samples were kindly provided by Ehime Red Cross Blood Center and their laboratory data, including liver functions tests, renal functions tests and serological tests for syphilis, hepatitis type B and hepatitis type C, were either within normal limits or negative.

Methods

Blood obtained by venipuncture was allowed to clot at room temperature for 1 hr. Serum samples were stored at −80°C until used. Stages and the extent of lymph node involvement (pN) in colo-rectal cancer were determined according to the UICC TNM Classification [9]. The extent of microscopic invasion of cancer cells into both lymph vessels (Ly) and veins (Ve) in the wall of the colon or rectum was clarified according to the General Rules for Clinical and Pathological Studies on Cancer of Colon, Rectum and Anus [10].

The serum levels of sTNF-Rs were measured using enzyme-linked immunosorbent assay (ELISA). ELISA plates (Corning, USA) were coated with rabbit polyclonal antibodies to either sTNF-R-p55 or sTNF-R-p75 at a concentration of 5μg/ml in 0.1M sodium carbonate and incubated overnight at 4°C. After washed with phosphate-buffered saline (PBS) containing 0.05% Tween 20 (washing solution), the plates were incubated with PBS containing 1% bovine serum albumin and 0.05% Tween 20 for 1 hr at 37°C to block the remaining sites for protein binding. 50μl of samples and 50μl of PBS containing 0.05% Tween 20 were added to the plates and incubated for 3hr at 37°C. After

517

washed with washing solution, peroxidase-conjugated rabbit polyclonal antibodies to either sTNF-R-p55 or sTNF-R-p75 was added to each well. The plates were incubated for 1hr at 37°C followed by washes with washing solution. Tetramethyl benzidine (Wako Pure Chemical Industries, Japan) was added to each well and incubated for 30 min. at room temperature. The absorbance was measured at 450nm in an automatic plate reader. Recombinant sTNF-Rs were used as standards. Serum levels of CEA were measured using an immuno-radiometric assay. The differences between groups were analyzed by t-test and correlation coefficients were calculated using the Stat View II, Macintosh.

RESULT

In healthy controls, serum levels of sTNF-R-p55 and sTNF-R-p75 (mean ± SE) were 0.14 ± 0.03 and 0.18 ± 0.02 ng/ml, respectively. Each level was not correlated with age and sex. In patients with colo-rectal cancer, serum levels of sTNF-R-p55 and sTNF-R-p75 were 0.18 ± 0.12 and 0.23 ± 0.13 ng/ml, respectively. There were no significant differences of sTNF-Rs levels between in controls and in patients with colo-rectal cancer (Fig.1). The serum levels of sTNF-R-p55, but not sTNF-R-p75, were correlated with stages of colo-rectal cancer (p55; r=0.71, p<0.05 p75; r=0.65, NS) (Fig.2).

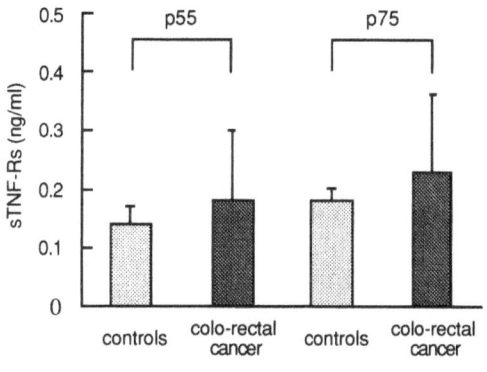

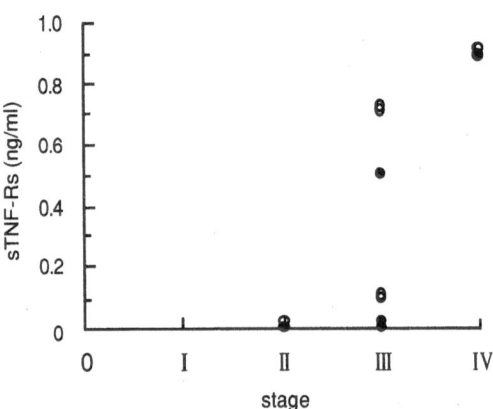

Fig. 1 Serum levels (mean ± SE) of sTNF-Rs in healthy controls and patients with colo-rectal cancer

Fig. 2 Correlation between stages of colo-rectal cancer and serum levels of sTNF-R-p55 (○; r=0.71, p<0.05) or sTNF-R-p75 (●; r=0.65, NS)

The serum levels of both sTNF-Rs in patients with colo-rectal cancer were correlated with the extent of Ly (Fig.3). However, they were correlated with neither the extent of pN nor the extent of Ve (data not shown).

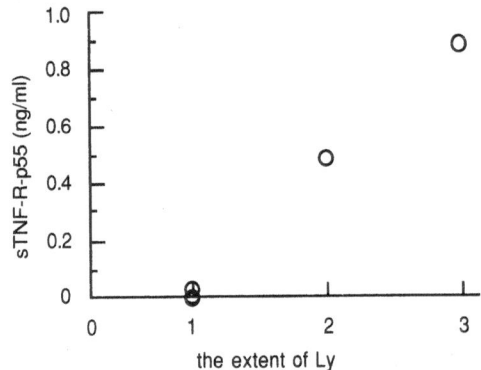

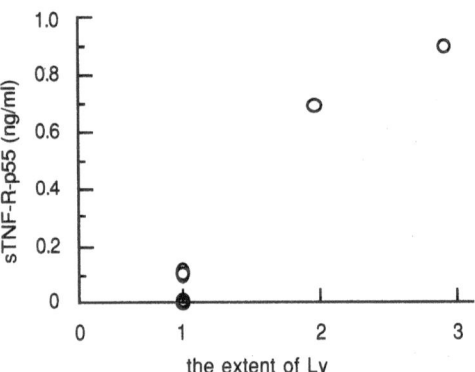

Fig. 3 Correlation between the extent of Ly and serum levels of sTNF-R-p55 or sTNF-R-p75 (p55; r=1.00, p<0.01 p75; r=0.97, p<0.01) The numbers of the extent of Ly indicate as follows: 0; No evidence of invasion, 1; Evidence of minimal invasion, 2; Evidence of moderate invasion, 3; Evidence of maximal invasion.

Serum levels of sTNF-Rs were also correlated with serum levels of carcinoembryonic antigen (CEA) (p55; r=0.98, p<0.01 p75; r=0.93, p<0.01) (Fig.4). However, they were correlated with neither α-fetoprotein (AFP) nor carbohydrate antigen 19-9 (CA 19-9) (data not shown).

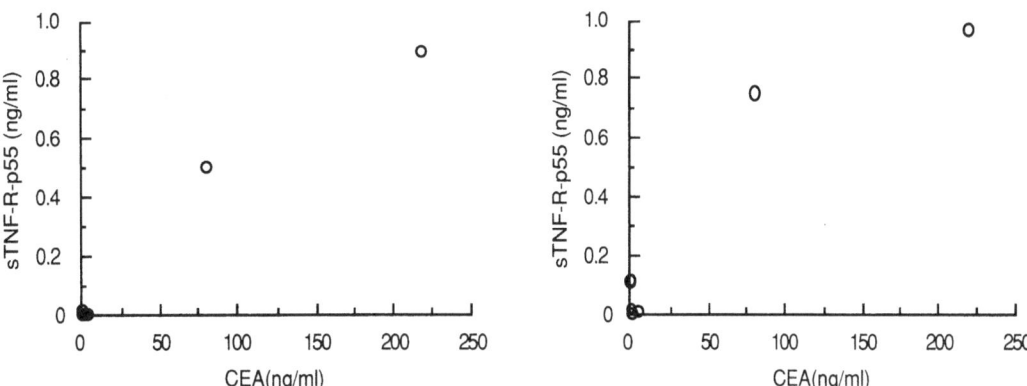

Fig. 4 Correlation between serum levels of CEA and serum levels of sTNF-R-p55 or sTNF-R-p75 (p55; r=0.98, p< 0.01 p75; r=0.93, p<0.01)

DISCUSSION

Our results show that serum levels of sTNF-R-p55 in patients with colo-rectal cancer are correlated with their stages. Also showed by our results are the fact that serum levels of both sTNF-Rs are correlated with the extent of Ly and the serum levels of CEA. In our data, serum levels of sTNF-Rs in patients at stage II–III were slightly, but not significantly, elevated. It was previously reported that serum levels of sTNF-Rs increased in more than one-half of the patients at stages I–III [8]. If further investigations on the relationship between serum levels of sTNF-Rs and stages of the colo-rectal cancer were carried out, the difference between controls and patients may become more obvious. In addition, serum levels of sTNF-Rs were found to be correlated with the extent of Ly. This results may suggest that the elevation of serum levels of sTNF-Rs is caused by shedding from cancer cells in the lymph vessels. However, these levels were correlated with neither the extent of pN nor the extent of Ve. Therefore, serum levels of sTNF-Rs can be markers of the extent of Ly in colo-rectal cancer. Furthermore, we found that serum levels of CEA were correlated with serum levels of sTNF-Rs and that they were not correlated with serum levels of AFP or CA 19-9. It was reported that the incidence of elevation of sTNF-Rs was higher than that of CEA at stages I-III colon cancer and a correlation was fairly observed between sTNF-Rs and CEA [8]. In conclusion, serum levels of sTNF-Rs are indicated to be new tumor markers of colo-rectal cancer. Further investigations should be carried out.

REFERENCE

1. Schall TJ, Lewis M, Koller KJ, Lee A, Rice GC, Wong GHW, Gatanaga T, Granger GA, Lentz R, Raab H, Kohr WJ, Goeddel DV (1990) Cell 61: 361-370
2. Loetscher H, Pan Y, Lahm H, Gentz R, Brockhaus M, Tabuchi H, Lesslauer W (1990) Cell 61: 351-359
3. Smith CA, Davis T, Anderson D, Solam L, Beckmann MP, Jerzy R, Dower SK, Cosman D, Goodwin RG (1990) Science 248: 1019-1023
4. Engelmann H, Novick D, Wallach D (1990) J Biol Chem 265: 1531-1536
5. Tartaglia LA, Goeddel DV (1992) Immunology Today 13: 151-153
6. Kohno T, Brewer MT, Baker SL, Schwartz PE, King MW, Hale KK, Squires CH, Thompson RC, Vannice JL (1990) Proc Natl Acad Sci USA 87: 8331-8335
7. Gray PW, Barrett K, Chantry D, Turner M, Feldmann M (1990) Proc Natl Acad Sci USA 87: 7380-7384
8. Aderka D, Engelmann H, Hornik V, Skornick Y, Levo Y, Wallach D, Kushtai G (1991) Cancer Res 51: 5602-5607
9. Hermanek P, Sobin LH (1990) TNM Classification of Malignant Tumours. Kanehara & Co., Ltd. Tokyo, pp 47-49
10. Japanese Research Society for Cancer of Colon and Rectum (1985) General Rules for Clinical and Pathological Studies on Cancer of Colon, Rectum and Anus. Kanehara & Co., Ltd. Tokyo,

Prognosis of Colorectal Cancer
Related to Histopathological Type and Stage

K. TOHYAMA, N. MIYAJIMA, M. MARUTA, J. KUROMIZU, and T. UTSUMI

Department of Surgery, Fujita Health University School of Medicine, Kutsukake-cho, Toyoake, Aichi, 470-11 Japan

ABSTRACT

770 cases of colorectal cancer; 240 cases of colonic cancer and 530 cases of rectal cancer were experienced. These cases were histologically divided into 4 types; well differentiated adenocarcinoma(well), moderately differentiated adenocarcinoma(mod), pooly differentiated adenocarcinoma(por) and mucinous carcinoma(muc). 5-year survival rate was calculated accoding to the stage. Furthermore, reccurent cases were studied on each histopathological type according to the stage. As a result, in colonic cancer the survival rate in well was low compared with other histopathological type, for it was caused of frequent hematogenous metastasis after curative resection. In rectal cancer at stage III, IV the survaival rate was poor, not related to histopathological type, because the frequency of local recurrence or lymphatic metastasis rate was high due to an anatomical characteristics and/or surgical difficulty.

KEY WORDS: 5-year survival rate, histopathological type, colorectal cancer

INTRODUCTION

In recent years, the incidence of colorectal cancer is increasing in Japan. Prognosis of colorectal cancer is relatively good. It is thought that one of the factors to determine the prognosis is histopathological type. We divided our cases of colorectal cancer that had been surgically treated into well differentiated adenocarcinoma, moderately differentiated adenocarcinoma, pooly differentiated adenocarcinoma and mucinous carcinoma, and calculated 5-year survival rate according to stage. We studied their correlation with the prognosis.

MATERIALS AND METHODS

During 18 years from 1974 to 1990, 770 cases of colorectal cancer underwent surgery at our department, including 240 cases of colonic cancer and 530 cases of rectal cancer. These cases were histologically divided into 4 types; well differentiated adenocarcinoma(well), moderately differentiated adenocarcinoma(mod), pooly differentiated adenocarcinoma(por) and mucinous carcinoma(muc). 5-year survival rate was caluculated according to the stage. Cases who died of other diseases were excluded. Furthermore, recurrent cases were studied on each histopathological type according to the stage. Moreover the histopathological type and the stage were decided by the Japanese Research Society for Cancer of Colon and Rectum, and the Kaplan-Meier method was used to caluculate 5-year survival rate.

RESULTS

I Age, sex, classification of histopathological type

In cases of rectal cancer the ratio of the male was slightly high. On each histopathological type the ratio of por in colonic cancer was slightly high compared with in cases of rectal cancer(Table 1). Curative resection rate was 68.3%(164 cases) in cases of colonic cancer and 82.5%(437 cases) in cases of rectal cancer.

Table 1 Ratio of each hitopathological
type in colonic and rectal cancer

	colonic cancer(n=240)	rectal cancer(n=530)
average age	62.0	59.1
male:female ratio	1.4:1	1.8:1
well	175 (72.9%)	382 (72.1%)
mod	32 (13.3%)	93 (17.5%)
por	9 (3.8%)	9 (1.7%)
muc	10 (4.2%)	22 (4.2%)
other	14 (5.8%)	24 (4.5%)

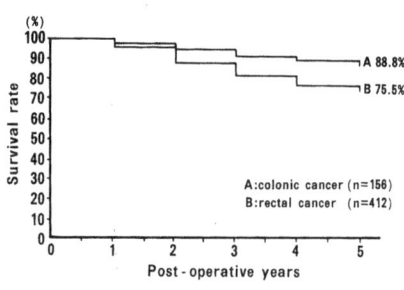

Fig.1 Survival rate in cases of colonic
and rectal cancer after curative resection

II Survival rate in cases of colorectal cancer after curative resection

The overall 5-year survival rate was relatively good(Figure 1). In cases of colonic cancer after curative resection the survival rate had high tendency in mod and por than in well(Figure 2). On the other hand, in cases of rectal cancer that was low except for well(Figure 3).

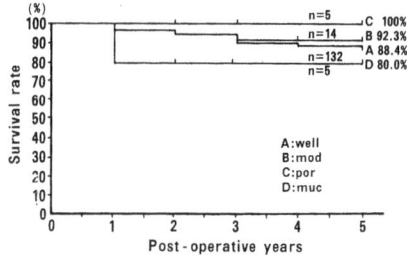

Fig.2 Survival rate on each histopathological type in cases of colonic cancer

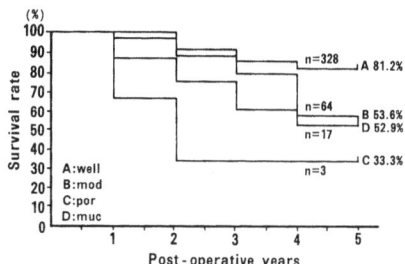

Fig. 3 Survival rate on each histopathological type in cases of rectal cancer

In cases of colonic cancer except stage V, 5-year survival rate was relatively good, not related to histopathological type. However in well with progress of the stage decreased 5-year survival rate was seen compared with other histopathological type. In mod and por except stage V all patients were alive, though there were a few cases(Table 2). On the other hand, in cases of rectal cancer at stage III and stage IV, 5-year survival rate was low, not related to histopathological type(Table 3).

Table 2 Survival rate on each stage in cases of colonic cancer

Stage	Histopathological type	n	Survival rate				
			1Y	2Y	3Y	4Y	5Y
I	well	28	100	91.4	91.4	91.4	91.4
	mod	1	100	100	100	100	100
	por	0	—	—	—	—	—
	muc	1	100	100	100	100	100
II	well	54	96.2	92.3	88.1	88.1	85.0
	mod	6	100	100	100	100	100
	por	3	100	100	100	100	100
	muc	1	100	100	100	100	100
III	well	33	97.0	97.0	89.2	84.8	84.8
	mod	2	100	100	100	100	100
	por	0	—	—	—	—	—
	muc	2	100	100	100	100	100
IV	well	17	80.0	80.0	80.0	80.0	80.0
	mod	4	100	100	100	100	100
	por	2	100	100	100	100	100
	muc	2	0	0	0	0	0
V	well	34	51.6	41.9	38.1	33.9	24.2
	mod	12	41.7	33.3	33.3	0	0
	por	4	50.0	50.0	50.0	50.0	50.0
	muc	2	50.0	50.0	50.0	50.0	50.0

Table 3 Survival rate on each stage in cases of rectal cancer

Stage	Histopathological type	n	Survival rate				
			1Y	2Y	3Y	4Y	5Y
I	well	77	98.7	98.7	97.3	95.9	94.2
	mod	10	100	100	87.5	87.5	87.5
	por	0	—	—	—	—	—
	muc	1	100	100	100	100	100
II	well	122	99.2	99.2	96.2	95.0	95.0
	mod	15	92.9	92.9	85.1	85.1	85.1
	por	0	—	—	—	—	—
	muc	5	100	100	100	100	100
III	well	72	94.3	80.0	72.6	66.3	66.3
	mod	20	85.0	60.0	43.6	38.2	31.8
	por	2	100	50.0	50.0	50.0	50.0
	muc	5	100	100	75.0	75.0	75.0
IV	well	57	91.2	77.2	65.3	61.0	53.6
	mod	21	76.2	61.9	43.3	43.3	34.7
	por	2	0	0	0	0	0
	muc	8	100	75.0	50.0	0	0
V	well	33	59.4	37.5	29.2	25.0	15.0
	mod	18	33.3	22.2	11.1	5.6	5.6
	por	1	100	0	0	0	0
	muc	2	0	0	0	0	0

III Recurrent pattern in cases of colorectal cancer after curative resection

In well with colonic cancer hematogenous metastasis frequentely appeared after curative resection with progress of the stage(Table 4). On the other hand, in cases of rectal cancer at stage III and stage IV the frequency of local recurrence or lymphatic metastsis was high, not related to histopathological type(Table 5).

Table 4 Recurrent pattern in cases of colonic cancer

Stage	Histopathological type	Hematogenous metastasis	Lymphatic metastasis	Local recurrence	Peritoneal dissemination
I	well	1			
	mod				
	por				
	muc				
II	well	6			
	mod				
	por				
	muc				
III	well	3			1
	mod				
	por				
	muc				
IV	well	6			
	mod				
	por				
	muc				

Table 5 Recurrent pattern in cases of rectal cancer

Stage	Histopathological type	Hematogenous metastasis	Lymphatic metastasis	Local recurrence	Peritoneal dissemination
I	well	1			
	mod	2			
	por				
	muc				
II	well	1	1	1	
	mod	2		1	
	por				
	muc				
III	well	18	1	2	
	mod	13		2	
	por				
	muc	2			
IV	well	21	1	7	
	mod	3	2	1	1
	por				2
	muc	2	1	2	

DISCUSSION

In cases of colonic cancer, not related to histopathological type the cases to be done curative resectoin had a good survival rate. However in well with progress of the stage the survival rate decreased compared with other histopathological type, for it was caused of frequent hematogenous metastasis after curative resection. In rectal cancer, on the other hand, the cases with stage III and stage IV had a low survival rate, not related to histopathological type, because the frequency of local recurrence or lymphatic metastasis was high, which was probably attributed to the factor of an anatomical characteristics and/or surgical difficulty.

A Clinicopathological Study
of Surgically Treated Colorectal Cancer

Kouichi Murakami, Hiroshi Tanimura, Kiwao Ishimoto, Yosirou Maniwa, Kazuhisa Uchiyama, Minoru Ochiai, and Tadashi Kontani

Department of Gastroenterological Surgery, Wakayama Medical College, Wakayama, 640 Japan

ABSTRACT

One hundred ninety three patients with colorectal cancer surgically treated at our department were reviewed from 1987 to 1992. The age of patients receiving surgical treatment ranged 33 to 86 years, with an average of 61.6 years. Location of colorectal cancers was as the following, rectum; 76 (39.4%), sigmoid colon; 56 (29.0%), descending colon; 10 (5.2%), transverse colon; 12 (6.2%), ascending colon; 23 (11.9%), cecum; 16 (8.3%). Curative operations were performed for 152 cases (78.8%). Thirty two cases (16.6%) were done with non-curative operations. Non-curative operations were performed more frequently for right-sided colon cancers than for left-sided colon and rectal cancers. Patients of Dukes' A, B and C were 77 (39.9%), 24 (12.4%) and 92 (47.7%) cases. Furthermore, lesions of Dukes' A and B cancers were found more frequently in left-sided colon and rectal than in right-sided colon. Thus, it is important for the total colonoscopy to be done for not only symptomatic but also asymptomatic patients because of the discovery of early or curative colorectal cancers, especially right-sided colon cancers.

KEY WORDS: colorectal cancer, total colonoscopy

INTRODUCTION

Recently, the mortality of colorectal cancer is increasing in Japan, despite improvement of diagnostic technique, adjuvant chemotherapy, radiotherapy and immunotherapy. Colonoscopically, we have been able to find a lot of small colorectal lesions, but still frequently encounter more advanced colorectal cancers. We retrospectively reviewed the chart of all patients surgically treated for colorectal cancer at our hospital for the purpose of revealing the present state of colorectal cancer.

MATERIALS AND METHODS

One hundred ninety three patients with colorectal cancer surgically treated in the Department of Surgery, Wakayama Medical College from 1987 to 1992. Age distribution, sex, location of cancers, histological classification, stage (Dukes' classification) of cancers and curativity of cancers were investigated.

RESULTS

There were one hundred ninety three patients found to be eligible for the study. There were 110 males and 83 females with sex ratio of 1.3:1.0. The age of patients receiving surgical treatment ranged 33 to 86 years with an average of 61.6 years. The age of patients at the peak was 60~69 years (Fig. 1).

Location of colorectal cancers was as the following, rectum; 76 (39.4%), sigmoid colon; 56 (29.0%), descending colon; 10 (5.2%), transverse colon; 12 (6.2%), ascending colon; 23 (11.9%), cecum; 16 (8.3%) (Table 1). Seventy three point six percent of all colorectal cancers existed in left-sided colon and rectum.

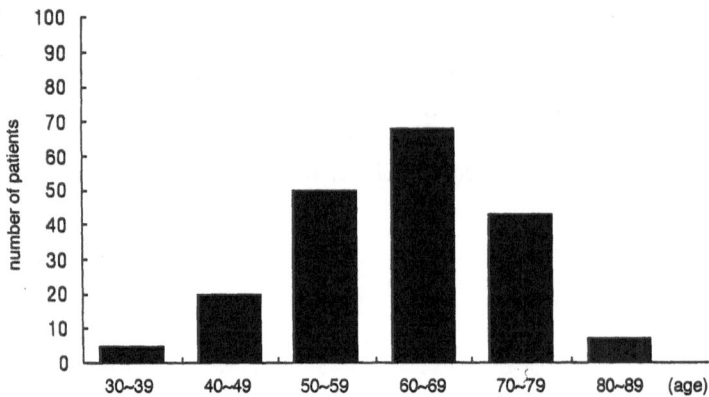

Fig.1 Distribution of age

Table 1. Location of colorectal cancer

location	n	%
Rectum	76	39.4
Sigmoid colon	56	29.0
Descending colon	10	5.2
Transverse colon	12	6.2
Ascending colon	23	11.9
Cecum	16	8.3
total	193	100

Twenty one (10.9%) cases among patients of colorectal cancers were intramucosal (m) and submucosal (sm) cancers as an early cancers and these cases were found in the rectum (12; 57.1%) and sigmoid colon (9;42.9%).
Colonoscopically excised early colorectal cancers were 42 cases from 1987 to 1992. Most of early colorectal cancers existed in rectosigmoid colon.
Pathological classification of colorectal cancers was as the following, well differentiated adenocarcinoma; 132 (73.7%), moderatery one; 19 (16.2%), poorly one; 11 (6.2%), mucinous carcinoma; 5 (2.8%), signet ring cell carcinoma; 2 (1.1%).
Curative operations were performed for 152 cases (78.8%). Thirty two cases (16.6%) were done with non-curative operations. Non-curative operations were performed more frequently for right-sided colon cancers than for left-sided colon and rectal cancers (Table 2).

Table 2. Curativity of colorectal cancer

location	curative	relative curative	non-curative	total
Rectum	63 (82.9%)	2 (2.6%)	11 (14.5%)	76
Sigmoid colon	46 (82.1%)	3 (5.4%)	7 (12.5%)	56
Descending colon	9 (90.0%)	0	1 (10.0%)	10
Transverse colon	7 (58.3%)	2 (16.7%)	3 (25.0%)	12
Ascending colon	17 (73.9%)	1 (4.4%)	5 (21.7%)	23
Cecum	10 (62.5%)	1 (6.2%)	5 (31.3%)	16
total	152 (78.7%)	9 (4.7%)	32 (16.6%)	193

Patients of Dukes' A, B and C were 77 (39.9%), 24 (12.4%) and 92 (47.7%) cases. Furthermore, lesions of Dukes' A and B cancers were found more frequently in left-sided colon and
rectum than in right-sided colon (Fig. 2).

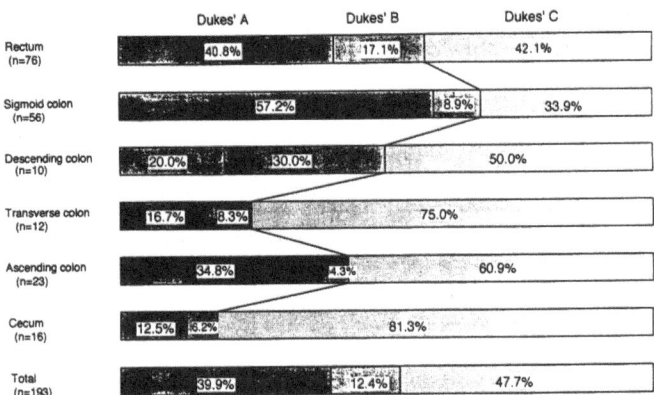

Fig.2 Stage of colorectal cancer by Dukes' classification

DISCUSSION

Most of colorectal cancers existed in left-sided colon and rectum (73.6%), and all early
colorectal cancers were found in rectosigmoid colon. On the other hand advanced cancers
were found more frequently in right-sided colon cancers.
Walter et al [1] reported that occult blood testing failed to detect a substantial number of
proximal colon cancers. And Wexner et al [2] reported that occult blood test was negative
in 44% of 100 patients with colorectal cancers. Besides Walter et al [1] reported that the
aggressive colonoscopy increases the detection rate of early colorectal cancers (Dukes' A).
Thus, it is important for the total colonoscopy to be done for not only symptomatic but also
asymptomatic patients because of the discovery of early or curative colorectal cancers,
especially right-sided colon.

REFERENCES

1. Walter E. L., Garth H. B. and Irvin M. M. Colonoscopic Detection of Early Colorectal
   Cancers. Ann. Surg. 207:174-178, 1988.
2. Wexner S. D., Gregory W. B. and Wichern W. A. Sensitivity of Hemoccult testing in
   patients with colorectal carcinoma Dis. Colon & Rectum 27:775-776, 1984.

Prognostic Features of Colorectal Cancer in the Young Adult

Fangxin Wang, Masaaki Oka, Tetsuji Uchiyama, Akira Inaba,
Hiroshi Morichika, and Takashi Suzuki

Department of Surgery II, Yamaguchi University School of Medicine, Ube, Yamaguchi, 755 Japan

ABSTRACT

Several prior studies have shown that the prognosis of young adult patients
with colorectal cancer is poor. A comparative clinical study was performed in
10 patients diagnosed in the third decade (group A) and 15 patients diagnosed
in the fourth decade (group B). The cumulative 5-year survival rate of
patients in group A was 32%, with a median survival of 83.7 months. Patients
in group B had a 5-year survival rate of 64%, with a median survival of 152.1
months. Moreover, colorectal polyposis was observed in 4 patients (40%) in
group A, but in none of the patients in group B. These data suggest that the
clinical characteristics of patients diagnosed with colorectal cancer in the
third decade were quite different from the characteristics of patients
diagnosed in the fourth decade.

KEY WORDS: colorectal cancer, young adult, clinico-pathologic findings,
colorectal polyposis

INTRODUCTION

The definition of what age group constitutes "young adult" remains
controversial. Many reports have selected patients younger than 40 years of
age, and some reports have selected only patients younger than 30. Thus, the
aim of this study was to determine if there are clinico-pathologic difference
between patients presenting with colorectal cancer in the third decade
compared to patients presenting in the fourth decade.

PATIENTS AND METHODS

Between 1970 and 1990, 511 patients with colorectal cancer underwent surgery
in our clinic. In this population, 10 patients were less than 30 years old
(group A) and 15 patients were between 30 and 39 years old (group B). None of
these patients had received any treatment prior to surgery. All the patients
received postoperative chemotherapy with 5-fluorouracil or tegaful.
The patients were evaluated for: cancer stage (Japanese Research Society for
Cancer of the Colon and Rectum <1> and Dukes classification), incidence of
associated colon polyp(s) or polyposis and prognosis.

Statistics

Fisher's exact probability test was used to compare differences in
distribution; $p < 0.05$ was considered statistically significant. The survival
of each patient was studied by the Kaplan-Meier method, and statistical
analysis was done with the generalized Wilcoxon test.

Patients result characteristics

Cancer stage (Table 1)

In group A, 7 of 10 patients had stage IV or V, whereas 4 0f 15 in group B
had stage IV or V. The difference approaches statistical significance,
p<0.10.

Table 1. CANCER STAGE

stage	<30 years 10 patients	30-39 years 15 patients	Dukes	<30 years 10 patients	30-39 years 15 patients
I	3	3	A	3	6
II	0	4	B	1	2
III	0	4	C	6	7
IV	1	2	* Dukes classification		
V	6	2			

* Japanese classification

The incidence of associated colon polyp(s) or polyposis (Table 2)

One patient in group A had colon polyp(s), and 3 patients in group B. had
colon polyp(s). In contrast, 4 patients in group A had colon polyposis, but
none of the patients in group B had colon polyposis (p<0.02).

Table 2. THE INCIDENCE OF ASSOCIATED COLON POLYP(S) OR POLYPOSIS

	<30 years 10 patients	30-39years 15 patients
Polyp(-)	4	12
Polyp(+)	1	3
Polyposis	4	0
Unknown	1	0

Prognosis

The cumulative survival rate of all patients in group A was 32% at 5 years,
with a median survival of 83.7 months. In group B, the overall 5-year
survival rate was 64%, with a median survival of 152.1 months. Patients in
group B had a higher survival rate than patients in group A, but this
difference was not significant (p=0.17702). In patients having tumor
resection, the 5-year survival rates in group a and B were 42% and 64%,
respectively, and following a curative resection, the 5-year survival rates
were 60% and 80%, respectively (see Figure 1).

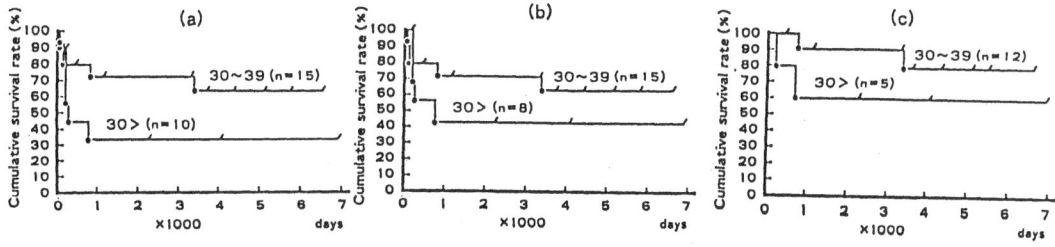

Figure 1. a: the overall cumulative survival rate in young adults with
colorectal. b: The cumulative survival rate in patients undergoing resection.
c: The cumulative survival rate in patients having curative resections.

DISCUSSION

The definition of age in young patients with colorectal cancer remains controversial. Many reports have selected patients younger than 40 years of age, but some reports have limited selection younger than 30. Katho et al. found that the survival rates among patients less than 40 years old were similar(2), and that compared to older patients, patients younger than 40 years of age tended to have a poorer prognosis, more advanced stage, and a high incidence of peritoneal dissemination or lymph node metastases (3). In our study, the 55-year survival rate in group B (80%) was slightly better than that in group A (60%). Thus, our result suggests the prognostic difference between two groups. Okumoto et al. found that patients younger than 30 years of age had a high incidence of poorly differentiated adenocarcinoma (4) and colon polyposis, which may suggest that hereditary factors play a stronger etiologic role in this age group (5). Mayo et al. (6) reported that 42 of 126 patients diagnosed with colorectal cancer at an age less than 30 had colon polyposis. This strongly suggests that hereditary factors play an etiologic role in patients diagnosed in the third decade. We observed 4 patients with colon polyposis in group A, but none in group B. Finally, although our numbers were small. there were differences in the cancer stage , prognosis, and incidence of colon polyposis between patients diagnosed with colorectal cancer in the third and fourth decades. Thus, "less than 30 years of age" may be the appropriate definition of "young adult" in patients with colorectal cancer.

REFERENCES

1. Japanese Research Society for Cancer of the Colon and Rectum: General rules for clinical and pathological studies on cancer of the colon, rectum and anus. Jpn. J. Surg., 13:557-573, 1983.
2. Katho, T., Morimoto, T., Watanabe, A. et al. Rectal cancer in the young adult. Geka, 40:802-807, 1978 (in Japanese).
3. Kanai, M., Takahashi, T., Katou, T. et al.: A study of rectal cancer by age-Primarily rectal cancer in young patients- Nippon Syoukakigeka Gakkaisi (Jpn. J. Gastroenterol. Surg.), 18:799-808, 1985(in Japanese).
4. Okumoto, S., Horita, Y., Kato, M. et al.: Colorectal cancer in patients less than 30 years of age. Nippon Syoukakigeka Gakkaisi (Jpn. J. Gastroenterol. Surg.), 24:831-839, 1991(in Japanese).
5. Ochi, A., Asai, T., Okamura, S., Yamaguchi, H., Ohashi, N., Mitake, M.: Clinicopathological studies in young patients with colon cancer including Cancer Family Syndrome. Gan no Rinsyou, 33:386-391, 1987 (in Japanese).
6. Mayo, C.W., Pagyalunan, R.J.G.: Malignancy of the colon and rectum in patients under 30 years of age. Surgery, 53:711-718, 1963.

Surgical Treatment for Juvenile Colorectal Carcinoma (Below the Age of 40)

Hitoshi Mizutani, Kunio Okajima, Taiichiro Kanagawa, Masao Toyoda, Osamu Marukawa, Katsumi Amioka, Kyowon Lee, and Hiroshi Nishino

The Department of Surgery, Osaka Medical College, Osaka, 569 Japan

ABSTRACT

The characteristics of juvenile colorectal carcinoma were determined in a comparative study of various clinical and pathological findings for 31 patients below the age of 40 and a control group of 569 patients aged 40 or older. Juvenile colorectal carcinoma was most common in the transverse colon (22.6%, P<0.01) and had significantly high incidence of peritoneal dissemination (22.6%, P<0.01). There were no significant differences between the two groups with regard to sex distribution, macroscopic type of tumor, tumor size, histological depth of invasion, tumor differentiation, hepatic metastasis or rate of lymph node metastasis. The long-term survival rate for the juvenile group following curative resection was close to that for the control group. These findings indicate the importance of radical lymphadenectomy and progressive treatment of peritoneal dissemination for improvement of the prognosis of patients with juvenile colorectal cancer.

KEY WORDS: colorectal cancer, juvenile cancer, surgical treatment

OBJECTIVES

The prognoses of all malignant tumors are generally reported to be very poor in young patients. In the present study, we considered people younger than 40 years of age as "juvenile" and attempted to determine what differences exist in various clinicopathological variables between the juvenile group and patients aged 40 or older who underwent surgical treatment for colorectal cancer. We discussed possible methods for the improvement of treatment of juvenile colorectal cancer.

SUBJECTS AND METHODS

In the past twelve years, 636 patients were surgically treated for colorectal cancer in our department. A total of 31 of these patients (4.9%) were included in the juvenile group, while the other 569 patients aged 40 or older made up the control group. Patients with mucosal carcinoma (36 cases) were excluded from this study. Statistical analysis was performed using the chi-square test and Student's t-test, with differences considered significant if p< 0.05.

RESULTS

The juvenile colorectal cancer group tended to have a higher proportion of women among its members than did the control group (Fig. 1). Colorectal cancer in juvenile patients tended to occur in the right colon, and had a higher rate of incidence in the . transverse colon (22.6%) in the juvenile group than in the control group (7.2%) (p<0.01) (Fig. 2). There were no significant differences between the juvenile and the control groups in macroscopic

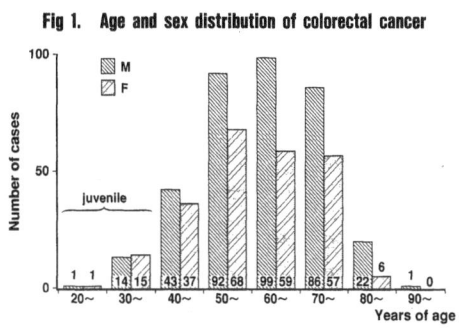

Fig 1. Age and sex distribution of colorectal cancer

type of tumor. There was no significant difference between the mean value of the maximum diameter of tumor for the juvenile group (5.4±2.0cm) and that for the control group (5.5±2.3 cm). No significant difference was observed in frequency of transmural invasion (s, a2) between the juvenile group (18 patients, 58%) and the control group (38%). Moderately differentiated adenocarcinoma was observed in 17 patients (54.8%) of the the juvenile group and 235 patients (41.3%) of the control group. This difference was not significant (Table 1). The rate of lymph node metastasis was 45.2% in the juvenile group and 40.8% in the control group. Para-aortic lymph node metastasis was observed in 4 patients (12.9%) of the juvenile group. This frequency was higher than that observed for the control group (5.3%), but not significantly so (Fig. 3). Hepatic metastasis was observed in 5 patients (16.1%) of the juvenile group and 75 patients (13%) of the control group, this difference was not significant. Peritoneal dissemination was observed in 7 patients (22.6%) of the juvenile group; this frequency was significantly higher than that in the control group (5.6%) (p<0.01) (Fig. 4). Curative resection of colorectal cancers was performed for 64.5% of the juvenile group. This frequency was slightly lower than that (78%) for the control group. There was no significant difference between the two groups in distribution of staging by Dukes' classification (Fig. 5). The overall 5-year and 10-year survival rates were 44.7% and 39.7% for the juvenile group, and 57.2% and 51.3% for the control group (Fig. 6). The 5-year and 10-year survival rates following curative resection were 66.7% and 59.3% for the juvenile group, and were not significantly worse than the corresponding rates of 69.1% and 64.3% for the control group (Fig. 6).

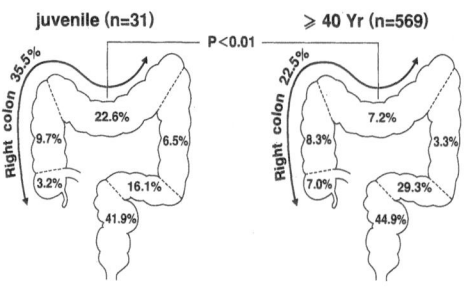

Fig 2. Site distribution of colorectal cancer

juvenile (n=31) P<0.01 ≥ 40 Yr (n=569)

Table 1 Pathologic findings

Characteristic	Age (Years)	
	<40	≥40
Macroscopic classification of tumor		
Superficial type	3.2%	3.7%
Protuberant type	12.9%	10.4%
Localized ulcer type	67.8%	76.4%
Infiltrative ulcer type	9.7%	8.3%
Diffuse infiltrating type	3.2%	0.5%
Unclassified	3.2%	0.7%
Tumor size (maximum diameter)		
0~19mm	0%	4.6%
20~39mm	19.4%	19.1%
40~59mm	45.1%	37.1%
60~79mm	19.4%	26.2%
80~99mm	16.1%	8.3%
100~	0%	4.7%
Histological depth of tumor invasion		
Submucosal (sm)	6.5%	6.3%
Intermediate (pm)	6.5%	9.3%
Subserosal (ss, a1)	29.0%	38.5%
Transmural (s, a2)	58.0%	38.0%
To neighboring organs (si, ai)	0%	7.9%
Histological type of tumor		
Well differentiated	32.2%	49.3%
Moderately differentiated	54.8%	41.3%
Poorly differentiated	6.5%	3.5%
Mucinous	6.5%	4.7%
Others	0%	1.2%

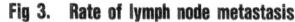
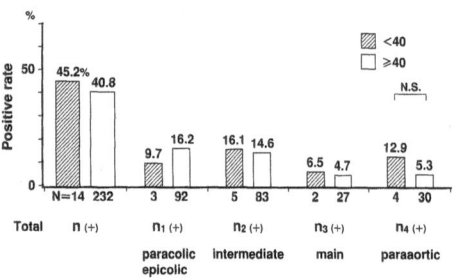

Fig 3. Rate of lymph node metastasis

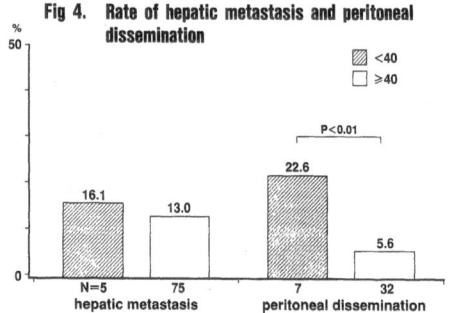

Fig 4. Rate of hepatic metastasis and peritoneal dissemination

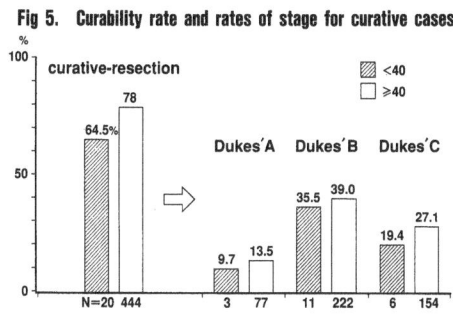

Fig 5. Curability rate and rates of stage for curative cases

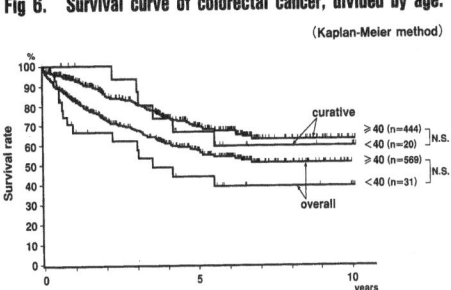

Fig 6. Survival curve of colorectal cancer, divided by age.

(Kaplan-Meier method)

DISCUSSION

Colorectal cancer in the young patient under the age of forty is reported to have an especially poor prognosis [1]. The reasons for this are thought to the higher percentage of poorly differentiated mucinous lesions in young patients [2]. In our series, however there was no difference in the pattern of histological grading between the juvenile and the control groups. Pratt et al.[3] reported in 1977 the frequent finding of disease which had advanced beyond the scope of surgical resection at the time of diagnosis. In this study, juvenile colorectal cancer was found to have a higher incidence of peritoneal dissemination (22.6% p<0.01) than did the control group. We found, in addition, a predominance of right-sided colonic lesions (22.6% p<0.01) in our this series of patients [4, 5]. In some recent studies survival rate in younger patients has been found to be as good as or better than that for older patients [6]. While in others younger patients have been found to have a poorer prognosis [7]. However, in our retrospective study the long-term survival rate for the juvenile group following curative resection was close to that for the older control group. The improved prognosis for younger patients may be due to earlier diagnosis and the use of better surgical techniques.

REFERENCE

1. Mills,S.E. & Allen,M.S. (1979) Colorectal carcinoma in the first three decades of life. American Journal of Surgical Pathology 3 : 443-448.
2. Recalde,M., Holyoke,E.D. & Elias,E.G. (1974) Carcinoma of the colon, rectum & anal canal in young patients. Surgery, Gynecology and Obstetrics 139 : 909-913.
3. Pratt,C.B., Rivera,G. Shanks,E. et al. (1977) .LM11
    Colorectal cancer in adolescents. Implications regarding etiology. Cancer 40 : 2464-2472.
4. Howard,E.W., Cavallo,C. Hovey,L.M. et al. (1975) Colon and rectal cancer in the young adult. American Surgery 41 : 260
5. Simstein,N.L., Kovalcik,P.J. & Cross,G.H. (1978) Colorectal carcinoma in patients less than 40 years old. Dis. Colon & Rectum 21 : 169-171
6. Martin,E.W., Joyce,S. Lucus,J. et al. (1981) Colorectal carcinoma in patients less than 40 years of age. Pathology and prognosis. Dis. Colon & Rectum 24 : 25-28
7. Enker,W.E., Paloyan,E., Kirsner,J.B. (1977) Carcinoma of the colon in the adolescent : a report of survival analysis of the literature. American Surgery of Surgery 133 : 737-741

Early Invasive Colorectal Carcinoma — A Retrospective Study About Risk Factors of Nodal Metastasis

CHENG-DONG HUANG[1], TOSHINARI MINAMOTO[2], TOHRU ITOH[2],
TOSHIHIRO FUJIMOTO[2], YASUSHI DEGUCHI[2], NAKABA FUJIOKA[2], HIDEHIRO NOMURA[2],
AKISHI OOI[2], YUTAKA TAKAHASHI[2], and MASAYOSHI MAI[2]

[1]Visiting Research Fellow from Second Medical University of Shanghai, Holder of Scholarship from Komatsu Green Found
[2]Department of Surgery, Cancer Research Institute Hospital, Kanazawa University, Kanazawa, 921 Japan

ABSTRACT

To decide adequate indication of endoscopic polypectomy, 46 cases of colorectal submucosal carcinoma including 6 cases with nodal metastasis were reviewed clinicopathologically. The six cases had at least one of the previously reported risk factors for lymph node metastas such as moderately-differentiated histologic characteristics, relatively high degree of submucosal invasion and lymphatic invasion. The most interesting finding of the present study was that all the 6 cases with nodal metastasis showed nonpolypoid growth feature and furthermore 5 of the cases had no coexistent adenomatous tissue. Therefore, nonpolypoid growth pattern and absence of adenomatous component were concluded to be significant risk factors predictive of nodal metastasis in the patients with colorectal submucosal carcinoma.

KEY WORDS: colorectal submucosal carcinoma, nonpolypoid growth pattern, degree of lymph node metastasis.

INTRODUCTION

Early colorectal carcinoma has been defined as primary adenocarcinoma with invasion confined to the mucosa or submucosa[1]. Because mucosal carcinomas almost never possess metastatic potential, their treatment is completed by endoscopic removal or limited surgery for the primary tumor. On the contrary, carcinomas invading the submucosa are capable of metastasizing to the lymph node or to other distant organs and their management is still controversial. Recently we experienced a patient with minute early invasive carcinoma of the rectum metastatic to the pararectal lymph node[2] (included in the present study). The primary tumor of this case showed nonpolypoid growth and was 5mm in size which, to our best knowledge of the literatures, is the smallest colorectal carcinoma with lymph node metastasis. This unique experience encouraged us to make a precise review of the clinicopathologic features of 46 cases of colorectal submucosal carcinoma including 6 cases with metastasis to lymph node treated in our institute.

PATIENTS AND METHODS

From 1980 to 1992, 124 tumors (122 cases) of early colorectal carcinoma were resected consecutively in our hospital. Forty six cases of colorectal submucosal carcinoma without any previous or concurrent advanced carcinoma were treated by endoscopic resection or surgery. Six of them were found to have metastasis to regional lymph nodes   and were investigated clinicopathologically in this study (Table 1). The investigated risk factors for lymph node metastasis were gross appearance, size, histology, co-existent adenomatous tissue, degree of submucosal invasion and lymphatic invasion. Gross appearance, endoscopic findings and pathologic types of each primary tumor and status of regional lymph nodes were classified according to the General Rules for Clinical and Pathological Studies on Cancer of the Colon, Rectum and Anus published in Japan[1]. Degrees of submucosal invasion were estimated as corresponding to sm_1, sm_2 and sm_3, described by Kudoh et al[5]. Paraffing-embedded tumors were sectioned with 2-3mm thickness and examined after hamatoxylin and eosing, and elastica van Gieson stainings. Gross appearances were divided into polypoid growth (PG)-type and nonpolypoid growth (NPG)-type according to the description of Shimoda T et al[6].

RESULTS

The clinicopathologic features of 6 cases of colorectal submucolsal carcinoma metastatic to lymph node are summarized in Table 1.

Table 1. Clinicopathologic findings of 6 cases of colorectal submucosal carcinoma with metastasis to the lymph node.

Case No.	Age/ Sex	Location	Gross Appearance	Size (mm)	Histologic Type	Degree of Invasion	Adenoma	Ly	V	Group of lymph Node	Treatment Procedure	Postoperative Outcome
1.	54/M	R	NPG(IIa)	5	M/D	sm_3	(-)	(+)	(-)	N_1	ER and OP	Alive; 46 Month
2.	39/F	S	NPG(IIa)	7	W/D	sm_3	(-)	(+)	(-)	N_2	ER and OP	Alive; 16 Month
3.	75/F	A	NPG(IIa)	10	M/D	sm_1	(-)	(+)	(-)	N_1	OP	Alive; 28 Month
4.	74/M	S	NPG(Is)	11	W/D	sm_3	(+)	(+)	(-)	N_1	ER and OP	Alive; 106Month
5.	69/F	S	NPG(Is)	17	M/D	sm_2	(-)	(-)	(-)	N_1	ER and OP	Alive; 13 Month
6.	75/M	R	NPG(IIa+IIc)	18	M/D	sm_3	(-)	(-)	(+)	N_1	OP	Dead ; 49 Month

Abbreviation: W/D and M/D: well and moderately differentiated adenocarcinoma; NPG:nonpolypoid growth; sm_1, cancer invasion to upper 1/3 of submucosal layer; sm_2, cancer invasion to middle 1/3 of submucosa layer; sm_3, cancer invasion to lower 1/3 of submucosallayer; ly, lymphatic permeation; v, venous invasion.

The tumor size in all cases with lymph node metastasis shows less than 20mm in diameter and 3 cases of them less than 10mm in diameter (Table 1). By gross observation, all the 6 cases with lymph node metastasis were categorized as NPG- type although 40 cases without nodal metastasis have no correlation to gross appearance (Table 2).
Histologically 2 cases were well differentiated adenocarcinoma and 4 were moderately differentiated adenocarcinoma. Most of the tumors showed massive invasion of the submucosal layer frequently accompanied by lymphatic and/or venous permeation of carcinoma cells (Figure 1).

Table. 2 Gross appearance of sm cancer with or without lymph node metastasis

	Polypoid	Nonpolypoid			
	Ip+Isp	Is	IIa	IIa+IIc	IIc
LN(+)	0	2	3	1	0
LN(-)	15	15	5	4	1

LN(+): Positive Metastasis.

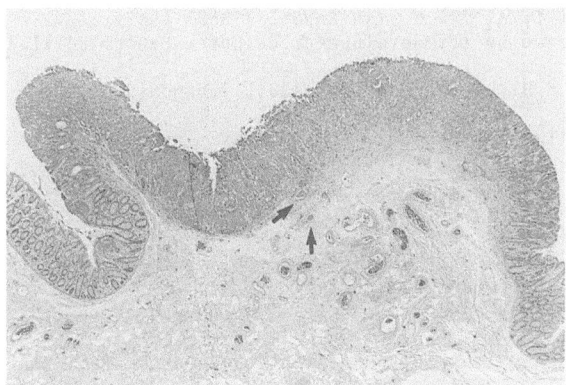

Figure 1. The cross section of the No.3 case showed adenocarcinoma proliferating in NPG (IIa) pattern. Remarkably lymphatic permeation of carcinoma cells was noticed (arrows).

The tumor without adenoma showed higher frequency of lymph node metastasis (20.8 %) than the cases with adenoma (4.5%) (Table 3). Cases with submucosal massive invasion showed higher frequency of lymph node metastasis (sm_2:12.5%, sm_3: 26.7%) thanthe cases of non massive invasion. (Table 4) As shown in Table 5 significant correlation was found between lymphatic permeation and nodal metastasis (p<0.01).
In 5cases metastatic carcinoma was limited to the paracolic or pararectal lymph nodes(N1), and Case 2 showed metastasis to a N_2 lymph node along the sigmoid colonic artery. No cases had operative complication and all patients left the hospital in good health. Five out of 6 patients are alive at present without recurrence. However the patient of Case 6 died of multiple hepatic metastasis about 4 years after surgery (Table 1).

DISCUSSION

Although the incidence of nodal metastasis from early invasive colorectal carcinoma has been controversial ranging from 0 to 31%[4,8], our incidence of 13% seems to be comparable with the mean value of 9% calculated from a nationwide questionnaire in Japan[9].
Based on a series of morphological studies of primary tumors for early invasive carcinomas with nodal metastasis[5,8,9], various histopathologic correlating to the risk of lymph node metastasis have been proposed. The accepted risk factors

Table. 3 Correlation between with or without
adenoma and lymph node metastasis of sm cancer

	N(+)	N(-)	Total
with adenoma	1(4.5%)	21(95.5%)	22(100%)
without adenoma	5(20.8%)	19(19.2%)	24(100%)

Table.4 Correlation between degree of submucosal
invasion and lymph node metastasis

	N(+)	N(-)	Total
sm_1	1(4.3%)	22(95.7%)	23(100%)
sm_2	1(12.5%)	7 (87.5%)	8 (100%)
sm_3	4(26.7%)	11(73.3%)	15(100%)

Table. 5 Correlation between lymphatic invasion
and lymph node metastasis of sm cancer

	N(+)	N(-)	Total
Ly(+)	4(66.6%)	2(33.3%)	6 (100%)
Ly(-)	2(5%)	38(95%)	40(100%)

(p<0.01).

are not necessarily acquittal for metastasis.

are as follows (1) moderately or poorly differentiated histological characteristics; (2) lymphatic invasion of tumor cells; (3) considerable degree of submucosal invasion described by Muto et al.,[9]. In the present study, NPG and absence of adenoma were found to be important risk factors in addition to the three accepted factors. It is intriguing that NPG and absence of adenomatous component are corresponding to characteristics of "de novo"carcinoma [11,12]. On the contrary PG and existence of concurrent adenoma are those of cancer developed through "carcinoma adenoma sequence"[13]. Therefore it is possible that the two different type of carcinoma divided based on histogenesis might have a different biological behavior such as early nodal metastasis. Reportedly in most cases with lymph node metastasis, the sizes of the primary tumor exceeded 1 cm, with a predominant population larger than 2cm in diameter. Thus the larger tumor sizes seems to relate, to some extent, to increasing rate of lymph node metastasis[5,8]. In our cases, however, all tumors were smaller than 2 cm and 3 of them were less than 10 mm. Although the number of our cases is small, we could suggest that tumors less than 1 cm in diameter

REFERENCES

1. Japanese Research Society for Cancer of the Colon and rectum(1983).General rules for clinical and pathological studies on cancer of the colon, rectum and anus. Part I.Clinical classification and Part II Pathological classification. Jpn J Surg. 13: 557-598.
2. Waye JD ,Haggitt RC (1990) When is colonoscopic resection of an adenomatous polyp containing a "malignancy " sufficient? Am J Gastroenterol 85:1564-1568.
3. Ohta T, Mai M, Ogino T, Kida Y, Minamoto T, Takahashi Y, Sawaguchi K, Jinkawa S, Yasuda Y(1991). Minute rectal cancer associated with nodular involvement. A case study. Dig Endosc. 90-94.
4. Sugihara K, Muto T, Morioka Y (1989) Management of patients with invasive carcinoma removed by colonoscopic polypectomy.Dis Colon Rectum 32:829-834.
5. Kutoh S, Kusaka H, Kimata H, Fujii T (1992) The diagnosis and treatment of colorectal sm cancer. Stomach and Intestine. 26: 764-775(in Japanese).
6. Shimoda T, Ikegami M, Fujisaki J, Matsui T, Aizawa S, Ishikawa E (1989) Early colorectal carcinoma with special reference to its development de novo. Cancer 64:1138-1146.
7. Cohen AM, Tremiterra S, Candela F, Thaler HT, Shigurdson ER (1991) Prognosis of node positive colon cancer. Cancer 67:1859-1861.
8. Colacchio TA, Forde KA, Scantlebury VP (1981) Endoscopic polypectomy. Inadequate treatment for invasive colorectal carcinoma. Ann Surg 194:704-707.
9. Muto T, Nishizawa M, Kodaira S, Shimoda T, Tada M (1991) Risk factors of lymph node metastasis of colorectal submucosal carcinoma: A quantitative analysis of 857 cases. Stomach and Intestine 26:911-918 (in Japanese).
10. Brodsky JT, Richard GK, Cohen AM, Minsky BD (1992) Variables correlated with the risk of lymph node metastasis in early rectal cancer. Cancer 69:322-326.
11. Spratt JS, Ackerman LV. (1962) Small primary adenocarcinomas of colon and rectum. JAMA 179:337-346.
12. Castleman B, Krickstein HI. (1962) Do adenomatous polyps of the colon become malignant? N Engl J Med 267:469-475.
13. Morson BC (1966) Factors influencing the prognosis of early cancer of the rectum. Proc Roy Coll Med 59:607

Perioperative Blood Transfusion Adversely Affects Prognosis of Colorectal Cancer Patients

Hisashi Onodera, Yoshihiro Yamazoe, Tae Bun Park, Masato Hasegawa, Tadahiro Sakamoto, Hiroshi Inoue, Yoshiki Takeuchi, Daisuke Ikeuchi, Masayuki Imamura, and Shunzou Maetani

First Department of Surgery, Faculty of Medicine, Kyoto University, Kyoto, 606 Japan

Abstract

In order to evaluate the effect of blood transfusion on prognosis of colorectal cancer, data of 905 patients having been operated on in our department were analyzed by the multivariate analysis. The predictor valuables were age, tumour location, Turnbull's modification of Dukes stage, preoperative hemoglobin (HB), anesthetic time (AT), intraoperative blood loss (BL) and perioperative blood transfusion (BT). Not only the Cox model but also the logistic analysis confirmed that blood transfusion is an important prognostic factor of colorectal cancer unrelated to other valuables. Its adverse effect of survival is of higher significance than BL and HB.

Key Words: blood transfusion, colorectal cancer, multivariate analysis, prognostic factor

Introduction

Since kidney graft survival was found to be improved in transfused patients, blood transfusion has been incriminated as a potential immunosuppressive agent, thus leading to a number of retrospective studies to evaluate adverse effect of blood transfusion in cancer patients [1]. However, their results have yet to be convincing because of background biases and insufficient number of patients [2-4]. The purpose of our study is to statistically evaluate the effect of transfusion by controlling background factors in our large series of colorectal cancer patients.

Patients and Methods

We reviewed 905 patients who had been operated on in our department with diagnoses of colorectal cancer during 1965-1989. From the patients' medical records information was obtained on age (yr), location of tumour (colon=1, rectum=2), Turnbull's modification of Dukes stage (A=1, B=2, C=3, D=4), preoperative hemoglobin values (g/dl), anesthetic time (min), operative blood loss (g) and blood transfusion (ml) administered during hospitalization. The Cox proportional hazards model was used to evaluate multiple factors in relation to survival [5]. The logistic regression model was also applied to analyze not only short term survival but also long term survival [6]. Cumulative 5 year survival was calculated by the Kaplan-Meier method. Significance of the observed differences was evaluated by the Mantel-Haenszel test in which stratum-to-stratum comparisons were made.

Results

Analysis of the association of blood transfusion with other valuables was presented tables 1 and 2. Factors that might be related to the need for blood transfusion included intraoperative blood loss, anesthetic time, tumour location (colon or rectum) and preoperative hemoglobin values. But no relation was noted between blood transfusion and age or Dukes stage.

The Cox regression analysis was presented in table 3. Blood transfusion was the second significant prognostic factor ($\chi 2$=16.55), following to Dukes Stage ($\chi 2$=34.25). Although tumour location and anesthetic time were significant factors, preoperative hemoglobin values and intraoperative blood loss did not reach the statistical significance. The same result was obtained by the logistic regression model in which prognostic valuables were appraised not only for short term survival but also for long term prognosis (table 4 and 5).

Table 1. Comparison between Transfusion and Non-transfusion Groups

Variable	Non-transfusion	Transfusion	χ^2	t
Age	61.41±12.83	60.40±12.51		0.24(NS)
Tumor site				
Colon	223	110	65.24	
Rectum	192	308	(P<0.00001)	
Dukes stage				
A	92	78		
B	115	113		
C	105	130	4.90	
D	83	94		
Hemoglobin	12.6±2.1	11.9±2.5	(NS)	3.98 (<0.001)
Blood loss	350.2±23.7	1146.7±88.7		404.4 (<0.00001)
Anesthetic time	238.0±69.2	328.0±107.2		14.27 (<0.00001)

Table 2. Correlation between Transfusion and Other Variables

Variable	Correlation coefficient
Age	$\gamma = 0.068$
Tumor site	$\tau = 0.3244$ ***
Dukes stage	$\tau = 0.0243$
Hemoglobin	$\gamma = 0.0986$ *
Blood loss	$\gamma = 0.8467$ ***
Anesthetic time	$\gamma = 0.5536$ ***

γ : Peason's correlation coefficient
τ : Kendall's correlation codfficient
*** P < 0.005 * 0.01 < P < 0.05

Table 3. Cox Regression Analysis

Variable	Coefficient	S. E.	χ^2
Anesthetic time	- 0.2194	0.0827	7.03
Transfusion	0.2215	0.0545	16.55
Hemoglobin	0.0932	0.0488	3.65
Tumor site	0.6507	0.2372	7.53
Blood loss	- 0.0697	0.0703	0.98
Dukes stage	0.7087	0.1211	34.25

Table 4. Logistical Regression Analysis (cut-off point = 1 year survival)

Variable	Coefficient	S. E.	χ^2
Anesthetic time	0.2645	0.288	1.834
Transfusion	- 0.4634	0.162	5.724
Hemoglobin	- 0.0646	0.158	0.818
Tumor site	- 0.4779	0.801	1.192
Blood loss	0.2159	0.218	1.982
Dukes stage	- 1.3673	0.522	5.242

Cumulative 5 year survival curves with the Kaplan-Meier method stratified by both Dukes stage and intraoperative blood loss were shown in Fig 1. A decreased survival was seen in transfused patients in both Dukes B stage and Dukes C stage (Mantel-Haenszel test, χ2=18.81, p<0.001).

Table 5. Logistical Regression Analysis (cut-off point = 5 year survival)

Variable	Coefficient	S. E.	χ^2
Anesthetic time	0.3198	0.124	5.146
Transfusion	- 0.2760	0.082	6.710
Hemoglobin	- 0.0680	0.073	1.870
Tumor site	- 0.7751	0.342	4.532
Blood loss	0.0350	0.106	0.662
Dukes stage	- 1.3340	0.195	13.650

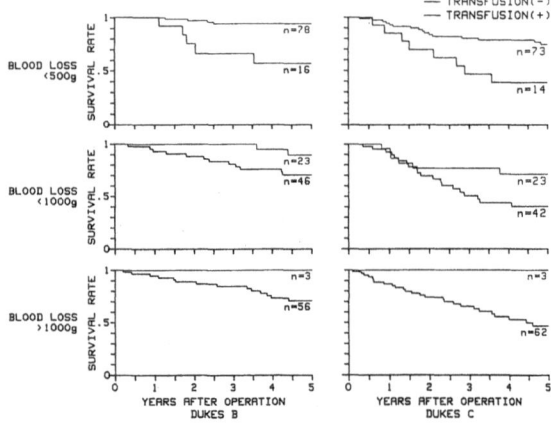

Fig. 1 SURVIVAL OF COLORECTAL CANCER PATIENTS WITH AND WITHOUT BLOOD TRANSFUSION   MANTEL-HAENSZEL TEST: CHI SQR=18.8, p<0.001

Discussion

In this report we have studied the treatment outcome of 905 patients with colorectal cancer to determine whether perioperative blood transfusion influenced the prognosis. Although quite a number of studies have been reported so far to evaluate the effect of blood transfusion on prognosis of cancer patient, some of them are insuffcient because of the background biases and small number of patients. Our method with the multivariate analysis recruiting large number of colorectal cancer patients is aimed to yeild some definitive results for this issue. Prognostic values we used are age, tumour site, Turnbull's modification of Dukes stage, preoperative hemoglobin value, anesthetic time, intraoperative blood loss and perioperative blood transfusion administered during the hospitalization. Both the Cox regression model and the logistic analysis revealed that blood transfusion is an important prognostic factor of colorectal cancer patients unrelated to other variables. Moreover its adverse effect on survival is of higher significance than blood loss and preoperative anemia. This indicates that the observation can not be attributed to differences in operative difficulties, as suggested in some reports.

In considering the mechanism of this adverse effect, a number of observations have pointed out the nonspecific immune suppression caused by blood transfusion [7]. Although deteriorations of immune parameters have been observed in some patient shortly before recurrent malignancy became clinically apparent, it is still unclear whether such changes are of major importance of not [8]. Whatever the mechanism of this effect may be, our current study appears to highlight the need for careful secrutiny of the indication for transfusions in cancer patients untill the issue is clarified by further study [9].

References

1. Opelz G, Senger DP, Mickey MR, et al. (1973) Effect of blood transfusion on subsequent kidney transplants. Transplant. Proc. 5: 253-259
2. Blumberg N, Agarwal MM and Chuang C. (1985) Relation between recurrence of cancer of the colon and transfusion. Brit. Med. J. 290: 1037-1039
3. Foster RS Jr, Costanza MC, Foster JC et al. (1985) Adverse relationship between blood transfusion and survival after colectomy for colon cancer. Cancer 55: 1195-1201
4. Franscis DMA and Judson RT. (1987) Blood transfusion and recurrence of cancer of the colon and rectum. Br. J. Surg. 74: 26-30
5. Cox DR. (1972) Regression model and life tables. J. Roy. Stat. Soc. 34: 187-220
6. Ranson JH and Pasternack BS. (1977) Statistical methods for quantifying the severity of clinical acute pancreatitis. J. Surg. Res. 22: 79-91
7. Waymack JP, Gallon L, Barcelli U, et al. (1987) Effect of transfusions on immune function. III alterations in macrophage arachidonic acid metabolism. Arch. Surg. 122: 56-60
8. Younes RN, Rogatko A and Brennan MF. (1991) The influence of intraoperative hypotension and perioperative blood transfusion of desease-free survival in patients with complete resection of colorectal liver metastases. Ann. Surg. 214: 107-113
9. Maetani S, Nishikawa T, Hirakawa A et al. (1986) Role of blood transfusion in organ system failure following major abdominal surgery. Ann. Surg. 203: 275-281

Laparoscopic-Assisted Partial Colectomy for Early Colon Carcinoma

Y. Kawachi, S. Kawai, T. Inoue, T. Iwama, and Y. Mishima

The Second Department of Surgery, Tokyo Medical and Dental University, Bunkyo-ku, Tokyo, Japan

ABSTRACTS

Laparoscopic technique to assist in the performance of partial colectomy is presented. A 55-year-old male had 1/5 circumference flat elevated lesion with central depression at the middle transverse colon. The colonoscopic diagnosis was early colon carcinoma and unable to resect endoscopically. Instead of performing a laparotomy with its potential morbidity, the lesion was resected by laparoscopic assisted partial transverse colectomy. Post operative course was uneventful, and patient was discharged on 13th post operative day. This technique can be applied to selected patients with early colon carcinoma.

KEY WORDS: Laproscopy, Laparoscopic colectomy, Early colon carcinoma

INTRODUCTION

In recent years, laparoscopic cholecystectomy has become widely available in the treatment of gallstone disease. The extension of surgical laparoscopy beyond the biliary tract has been done. In this work, we present a technique of laparoscopic assisted transverse colectomy.

PATIENT AND METHODS

A 55-year-old male, who had undergone endoscopic polypectomy, had follow up examination. Colonoscopy revealed a 1/5 circumferece oval flat elevated lesion with central depression at the middle transverse colon. Barium enema study showed a flat elevated lesion with irregular central depression. Endoscopic ultrasound sonography (20 MHz Sonoprobe system; Fuji Photo Optical Co.,LTD.) showed the tumor invasion limited to the submucosal layer. Because of the size of the tumor, endoscopic resection was not indicated. Instead of performing a laparotomy with its potential morbidity, the lesion was resected by laparoscopic assisted colectomy. The day before operation, CH40 was injected in the submucosa of the transverse colon 5cm apart from the tumor by colonoscopically.

Patient was placed in the supine position with his legs open. Under small abdominal incision, 11mm trocar was placed in the lower middle portion for insertion of the flexible videolaparoscope. The abdomen was distended with carbon dioxide and 4 trocars were inserted for instruments (Fig.1). The patient was then placed in a 20-degree reversed Trendelenburg's position.

Before mobilization, general visual exploration of the peritoneal cavity was undertaken. It was possible to visualize the operating field in many directions by using the flexible videolaparoscop (Fuji Photo Optical Co.,LTD.).

The stomach was detached from the transverse colon (Fig.2). The vessels located near the hepatic flexure were ligated with endoscopic surgical clips. The intestine was grasped with specifically designed non crushing intestinal clamps. The detached transverse colon was held upward so that its mesocolon

538

could be inspected (Fig.3). The middle colic vessels were ligated with Endo-Clip for three times at near their origins and divided (Fig 4). The transverse mesocolon was incised in an inverted V up to the bowel edge at the site selected for resection that was marked by CH40. At this point, the colon was movable. A 3cm skin incision was made at upper middle of the umbilicus. The bowel was delivered through this incision, and end-to-end anastomosis was performed by hand sewing on the outside. After the largest incision was closed, carbon dioxide was again insufflated into the peritoneal cavity. Hemostasis was checked, and the trocars were then removed under direct vision.

Operative duration was 250 minutes. Post operative course was uneventful, and patient was able to take oral fluids on 3rd post operative day. He was discharged on 13th postoperative day.

Histologic examination revealed that carcinoma invaded the submucosal layer of the colon without lymph node meatstasis (Fig 5).

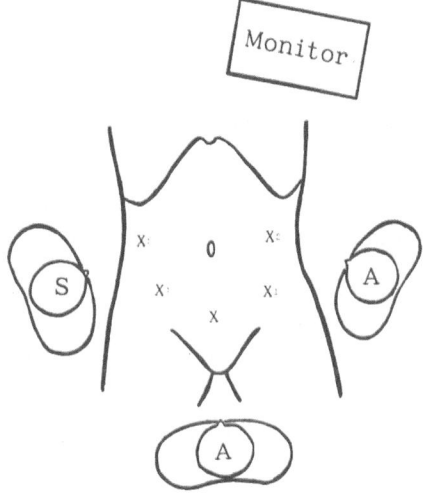

Figure 1. Illustrated is the patient, port, personnel, and monitor placement for a laparoscopic transverse colectomy. (X; Camera port, X1; 10mm port, X2; 5mm port)

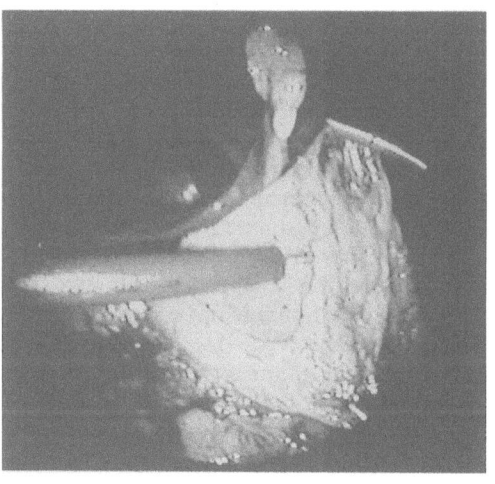

Figure 2. The stomach was detached from the transverse colon

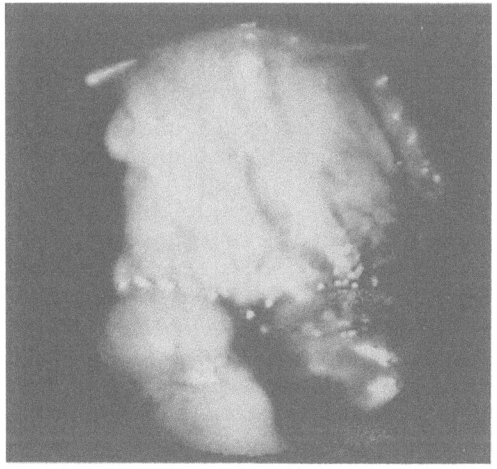

Figure 3. The transverse mesocolon could be inspected

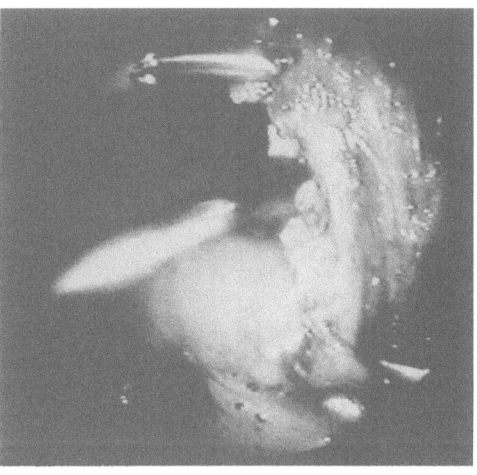

Figure 4. The middle colic vessels were ligated with Endo-Clip at near their origins and divided

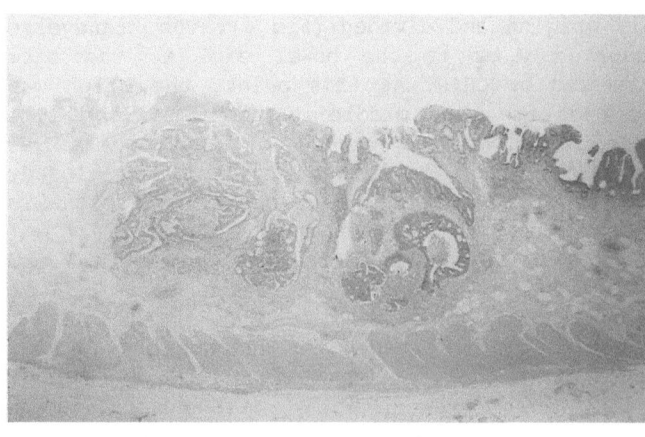

Figure 5. Carcinoma invaded the submucosal layer of the colon

DISCUSSION

Some reports concerning the use of laparoscopy in colorectal surgery were presented from 1991[1-4]. The indications for the laparoscopic approach to colon surgery are broad, from inflammatory to malignant disease.

Cancer operation should be performed just as in "open" cases. In this case, the lymph node dissection was performed at pericolic and intermediate nodes. The main nodes of the middle colic artery were considered unnecessary to be dissected. In general the dissection of main nodes along the middle colic artery was complex operations. Therefore, the extent of lymph node dissection is dependent on the skill of the operators. Concerning the technique of the anastomosis, laparoscopic technique for intracorporeal anastomosis could allow this procedure to be performed completely within the abdominal cavity. Intracorporeal anastomosis is complex operation, and the specimen should be removed intact with making small incision. In this case, extracorporeal anastomosis was done with a 3cm skin incision. The most limiting aspect of laparoscopic intestinal surgery is the lack of appropriate instruments. Current indications for laparoscopic colectomy for malignant disease should be limited for early carcinoma.

The most useful result of this technique was the decrease in postoperative pain, ileus and post operative stay.

CONCLUSION

We report laparoscopic assisted partial transverse colectomy for early transverse colon carcinoma. The procedure appears to be safe, and available for early colon carcinoma.

The true mobidity, mortality and long term results of this technique remain unknown. Further studies are being performed to determine the long term results of this technique.

REFERENCES

1.Jacobs M, Verdeja JC, Goldstein HS (1991) Minimally invasive colon resection (laparoscopic colectomy), Surgical Laparosc Endosc 1: 144-150
2.Richard T.S., (1991) Laparoscopic-assisted right hemicolectomy, Dis Colon Rectum 34: 1030-1031
3.Edward H.P., Morris F., Brendan J.C., Moses J.F., Raul Ramos, Daniel Rosenthal, (1992) Laparoscopic Colectomy, Ann. Surg. 216:
703-707
4. Steven D.W., Olaf B.J., Juan J.N., David G.J. (1992)
Laparoscopic total abdominal colectomy, Dis Colon Rectum 35: 651-655

Local Recurrence After Local Excision of Early Rectal Cancer

YASUHISA YAMAMOTO, TSUTOMU MURE, SUEHARU IWAMOTO, and KAISO SANO

Department of Surgery, Kawasaki Medical School, Kurashiki, Okayama, 701-01 Japan

ABSTRACT

The advantage of local excision for early rectal cancer, excluding fiberscopic polypectomy, is that it allows preservation of the anal function of the sphincter. We treated 75 patients with early rectal cancer and carried out local excision in 29 of these cases during the period from 1974 to 1992. Three of these 29 patients were reoperated upon immediately because of massive invasion to the submucosa at the margin of the removed specimen. Two other cases experienced local recurrences and required additional surgery.

KEY WORDS: early rectal cancer, local excision, local recurrence

INTRODUCTION

It is highly desirable to preserve the anal function of the sphincter when surgery for rectal cancer is performed. Local excision for early cancer of the lower rectum can usually achieve this goal without sacrificing cure of the cancer. However, we have experienced two cases of local recurrences after local excision for early rectal cancer.

MATERIALS AND METHOD

We treated 75 patients with early rectal cancer (Rs: 10 cases, Ra :32 cases, Rb: 31 cases, P: 2 cases according to the General Rules of the Japanese Research Society for Cancer of the Colon and Rectum) during the period from 1974 to 1992. Local excisions were carried out in 29 of these 75 patients (transanal: 23 cases, transabdominal: 5 cases, transsacral: 1 case). Three of these 29 patients were treated immediately with additional reresection because pathological findings revealed massive invasions to the submucosa at the margin of the removed specimen. Two other cases experienced local recurrences and required additional surgery (Table 1).

Table 1   Number of patients with rectal cancer

Sites	No.	Early* Cancer	Local Excision	Immediate Additional Surgery	Recurrence after Local Excision
Rs	72	10	2		
Ra	207	32	6		1
Rb	198	31	21	3	1
P	12	2	0		
Total	489	75	29	3	2

(1974–1992)
*Mucosal or submucosal invasion

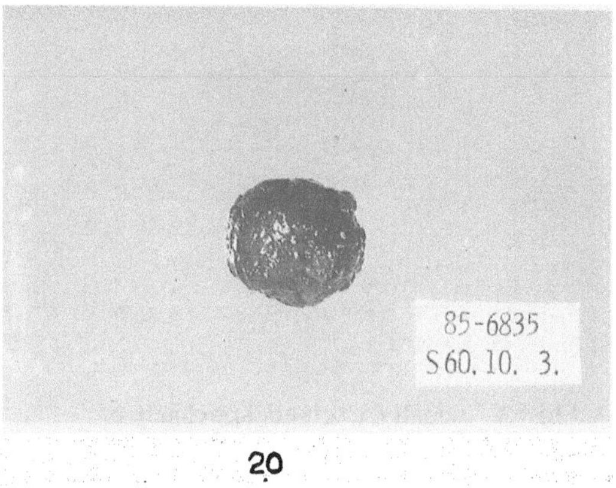

20

Fig. 1 Macroscopic findings after local excision of Case 1.

RESULTS

Case 1. This patient was a 56-year-old male with cancer of the middle rectum (Ra) who had been treated transabdominally with local excision in 1985 and had experienced a local recurrence (Fig. 1). It was diagnosed by elevation of the CEA levels and colonofiberscopy two months before he was admitted to the hospital in 1992 for an expected additional operation. The pathological findings after anterior resection of the rectum revealed a local recurrence with a huge submucosal tumor (11 x 8 cm) invading to the mesenteric side and involving the lymph nodes (n_2)(Fig 2). Five months after the second operation, reelevated CEA levels suggested liver metastases (Fig. 3).

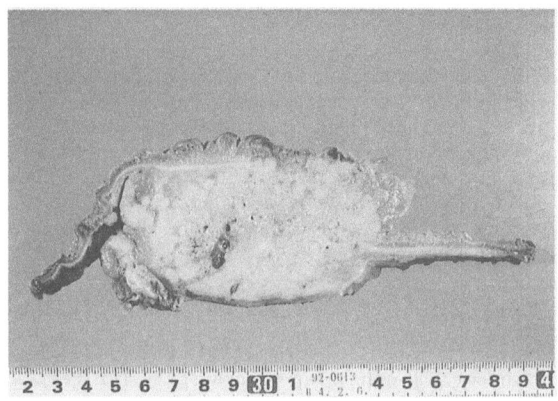

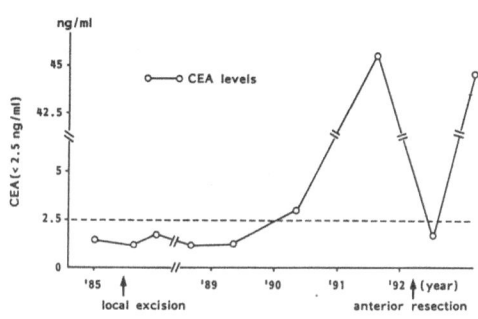

Fig. 2   Cross section of Case 1 showed a huge submucosal tumor.

Fig. 3   Clinical course of Case 1.

Case 2. This patient was a 51-year-old female with cancer of the lower rectum (Rb) who had been treated transanally with local excision in September 1991 and had experienced a local recurrence in November 1992 (Fig. 4). The pathological findings after Miles' operation revealed an invasion to the rectal adventitia (a_2) without lymph node involvement or intravessel spread (Fig. 5).

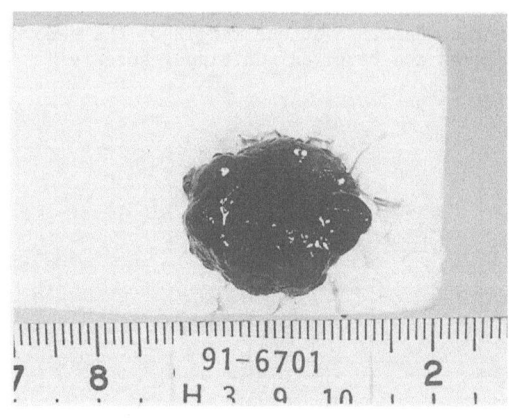
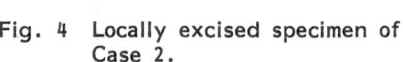

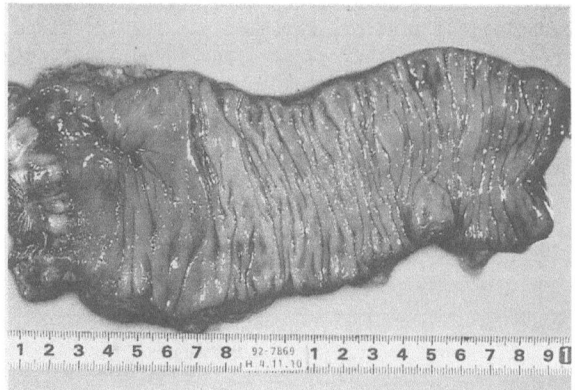

Fig. 4   Locally excised specimen of Case 2.

Fig. 5   Macroscopic findings after Miles' operation of Case 2 revealed a local recurrence.

Among our patients, three (14.3%) of 21 patients with mucosal invasion were found histologically to have moderately differentiated adenocarcinomas. The remainder had well differentiated adenocarcinomas. Four (50.0%) of eight patients with submucosal invasion were found to have moderately differentiated adenocarcinomas and the other four had well differentiated adenocarcinomas (Table 2). There were 16 cases (76.2%) with tumors 0.5-2 cm in diameter with mucosal invasion and four cases (50.0%) with tumors 2-3 cm in diameter with submucosal involvement (Tble 3). With regard to shape, there were 13 patients (44.8%) with a tumor of the sessile type (Is), 15 patients (51.7%) with a tumor of the semipedunculated type (Isp) and 1 patient (3.5%) with a tumor of the pedunculated type (Ip). The local recurrences

543

after local excision were detected in two cases of the Isp type. Twenty (95.2%) of the 21 patients with mucosal invasion and all of the cases with submucosal involvement had tumors of the Is or Isp type (Table 4).

DISCUSSION

Determination of whether or not the local excision for early cancer of the rectum was adequate is based on pathological examination of serial sections of the excised specimen. Further surgery after local excision should be recommended when the pathological findings reveal incomplete excision, poorly differentiated adenocarcinomas and/or intravessel spread.

Table 2   Diameter and depth of lesions after local excision

Location*	Mucosa				Submucosa			
	~1	~2	~3	~4 (cm)	~1	~2	~3	~4 (cm)
Rs		1	1					
Ra	1	3[1]				1	1	
Rb	6(1)	5	1	3	1	2[1]	3(2)	
Total	7(1)	9[1]	2	3	1	3[1]	4(2)	

□: Recurrence
( ): Additional surgery
*Japanese Classification

Table 3   Shape of lesion and diameter after local excision

Type	Mucosa				Submucosa			
	~1	~2	~3	~4 (cm)	~1	~2	~3	~4 (cm)
Is	2	3	1	2	1	1	3(1)	
Isp	4(1)	6[1]	1	1		2[1]	1(1)	
Ip	1							
Total	7(1)	9[1]	2	3	1	3[1]	4(2)	

Is: Sessile type, Isp: Semipedunculated type,
Ip: Pedunculated type, □: Recurrence,
( ): Additional surgery

Table 4   Shape of lesion and depth after local excision

Location*	Mucosa			Submucosa		
	Is	Isp	Ip	Is	Isp	Ip
Rs		2			1	
Ra	1	2[1]	1	1		
Rb	7	8(1)		4(1)	2[1](1)	
Total	8	12[1](1)	1	5(1)	3[1](1)	

Is: Sessile type, Isp: Semipedunculated type
Ip: Pedunculated type, □: Recurrence,
( ): Additional surgery, *Japanese Classification

Table 5   Summary of two cases

	Case 1 (56 y. Male)	Case 2 (51 y. Female)
Local excision	6 y. ago transabdominal	1 y. ago transanal
Location*	Ra	Rb
Clinico-pathological findings	2 × 1.5 cm Ips m well ly(-) v(-)	1.7 × 1.7 cm Ips sm mod. ly(-) v(-)
Additional surgery	anterior resection	Miles' operation
Outcome	1 y. alive liver metastases	0.5 y. alive

*Japanese Classification

As indicated in our summary of two recurring cases (Table 5) after local excision, the histological grade and shape of the tumor are important risk factors for local recurrence. Retrospectively, the CEA levels in the clinical course of case 1 revealed malignant development at five years after local excision. The exact reason why local recurrence after local excision occurred in these two cases could not be determined.

REFERENCES

1. Morson B C, Bussey H J R, Samoorian S (1977) Policy of local excision for early cancer of the colorectum. Gut 18: 1045-1050
2. Killingback M J (1985) Indications for local excision of rectal cancer. BR J Surg 72: S54-S56
3. Muto T, Sawada T, Sugihara K (1991) Treatment of carcinoma in adenomas. World J Surg 15: 35-40

Management of Colorectal Cancer

G.R. Verma[1], S.M. Bose[1], R.N. Kataria[1], B.D. Gupta[2], and S.K. Khanna[1]

The Departments of [1]Surgery and [2]Radiotherapy, Postgraduate Institute of Medical Education and Research, Chandigarh 160 012, India

ABSTRACT

The study describes our experience of management of 212 patients of colorectal cancer. Frequency of occurrence of these tumours at an younger age was high compared to western countries. Majority of patients (72.5%) had advanced locoregional spread or distant metastasis. 17.4% of patients presented to emergency with intestinal obstruction. The resectability rate was 51.4%. All the patients with advanced disease (Duke's C and D stage) had received chemotherapy and/or radiotherapy. The overall incidence of metastasis following definitive treatment was 37.5%. Duke's C tumours, obstructing and mucin secreting carcinoma had high incidence of recurrence.

KEYWORDS: Coloretal cancer, Carcinoma rectum, Obstructing colorectal tumours, Large bowel malignancy.

INTRODUCTION

Colorectal cancer is not a common malignancy in India. Bhansali [1] and Paymaster [2] have reported the incidence of colon cancer as 3-10% of all gastrointestinal malignancies in Bombay. In contrast, the incidence of colorectal carcinoma in western countries is second only to carcinoma to lung in frequency [3]. The diagnosis is invariably made late when the tumour is far too advance. Treatment is essentially surgical and despite the efficacy of adjuvant treatment, the incidence of recurrence is 40%. [4]. The present study describes our experience of management of colorectal cancer at Nehru Hospital attached to Postgraduate Institute of Medical Education and Research, Chandigarh.

MATERIAL AND METHODS

Nine years (1983-91) record of 212 patients of colorectal cancer was analysed. The tumours were classified according to site. Lesions of caecum, ascending colon and hepatic flexure were classified as right sided lesions and tumours of splenic flexure, descending colon, sigmoid colon and rectosigmoid junctions were classified as left sided lesions. The extent of the tumour spread was assessed by Duke's classification. Patients deemed to have had definitive treatment were those in whom the tumour was either resected only or followed by chemoradiotherapy or was subjected to curative radiotherapy. In palliative treatment group, the tumour was left insitu.

RESULTS

Of the 212 patients, 144 (68%) were over the age of 40 years and had significantly high incidence of diseas (Table 1) compared to younger patients (P < 0.01). Tumours were classified accordingly to Duke's classification. Ninetyfive patients (72.5%) had advanced locoregional spread or distant metastasis (Table 1). One hundred and forty three patients (67.4%) had ulceroproliferative type of tumour and it was the commonest variety of macroscopic lesion. Treatment modalities are shown in Table 2. Overall resectability rate was 51.4% (109/212). Sixtytwo patients were offered only palliative treatment.

Eighty patients who received definitive treatment were followed up from 1-72 months with a mean of 17.6 months. The tumour recurred in 30 patients (37.5%). Incidence of recurrence in relation to site, nature, stage and histopathology of tumour has been shown in Table III. Obstructing tumours, stage C and mucin secreting tumours had higher incidence of recurrences in their respective groups. Thirty patients in palliative treatment group were followed up to a mean of 6.2 months. Nine of them died due to disseminated malignancy.

Table 1. Age of the patients, Duke's staging and type of tumours

	No of patients	Percentage
AGE		
< 40 years	68	32.1 (P < 0.01)
> 40 years	144	67.9
DUKE'S STAGE		
A	10	7.7
B	26	19.8
C	70	53.4
D	25	19.1
TYPE OF TUMOUR		
Ulceroproliferative	143	67.4
Ulcerative	13	6.1
Stricturus	21	9.9
Infiltrative	12	5.7
Not known	23	10.8

Table 2. Treatment modalities

A. DEFINITIVE (121 patients)	
Curative resection alone	37
Resection and radiotherapy	39
Resection, chemotherapy ± radiotherapy	33
Curative radiotherapy	12
B. PALLIATIVE (62 patients)	
Diversion colostomy ± chemoradiotherapy	46
Palliative radiotherapy	11
Laparotomy, biopsy and chemotherapy	5

Table 3. Relationship of recurrence with site, nature and staging and H/P of tumours

	No of patients	No recurrences (%age)
SITE		
Anorectum	49	18 (36.7)
Colon	31	12 (38.7)
NATURE OF TUMOUR		
Nonobstructing	62	21 (33.8)
Obstructing	18	9 (50.0)
DUKE'S STAGING		
A	8	1 (12.5)
B	19	8 (42.1)
C	39	18 (46.1)
HISTOPATHOLOGY		
Nonmucin secreting adenocarcinoma	52	21 (40.3)
Mucin secreting adenocarcinoma	14	7 (50.0)
Squamous cell carcinoma	8	0 -
Others	6	2 (33.3)

DISCUSSION

Colorectal cancers in younger patients are found to be more common (32.1%) in this study compared to 3% in western population [5]. Due to late presentation and advanced disease in our patients, the resectable rate was low, 51.4% compared to close to 90% reported in one series [6]. The cause of high incidence of recurrence (37.5%) in the present series was due to the fact that 60% of them had Duke'C stage of the disease. Obstructing lesions and mucin secreting tumours have also shown higher tendency to recurrence. Difference in the pattern of the recurrences in colorectal cancer has been reported [7]. However, we did not find the difference between local and distant metastasis following definitive surgery in colon or rectal carcinomas.

REFERENCES

1. Bhansali SK,(1968). Geographical distribution of gastrointestinal cancer in India. Ind Jour Surg 30:33-35

2. Paymaster JC, Sarighari LD, Gangadharan P (1968). Cancer of gastrointestinal tract in western India. Cancer 21:279-82

3. Cancer (1990). Survival statistics 1990 CA,40:10-19

4. Moertal, CG, Fleming TR, Mac Donald, JS (1990). Levamisole and fluorouracil for adjuvant therapy of resected colon carcinoma. N Eng J Med 322:352-358

5. Mc Ardle CS, Hole D, Hansell D, Blumgart LH and Wood CB (1990). Prospective study of colorectal cancer in western Scotland : 10-year follow up. Br Jr Surg 77:280-282

6. Cohen JR, Theile DE, Evans EB, Quinn RL and Davis NC (1983). Colorectal cancer at the Princess Alexandra Hospital : a prospective study of 729 cases. Aus NZ J Surg 53:113-9

7. Wirth A, Green M, Zalcberg JR (1991). Adjuvant therapy of colorectal cancer : An overview. Aus NZ J Surg 61:13-22

Surgical Trial for Rectal Cancer Using a Tissue Expander in Association with Pelvic Partition to Prevent Radiation-Induced Bladder Dysfunction

A.F.M. Matin, Shozo Baba, and Hiroyuki Ogiwara

Second Department of Surgery, Hamamatsu University School of Medicine, Hamamatsu, Shizuoka, Japan

ABSTRACT

Postoperative pelvic radiation therapy after surgery for rectal cancer leads to serious voiding dysfunction in patients. To reduce the postoperative radiation injury, the tissue expander (TE) of 320 ml was inserted into the pelvic cavity after abdominoperineal resection of rectum, and polyglycolic acid mesh was placed at the upper region of the pelvic cavity to prevent invasion of small intestine into pelvis. Tissue expander was removed under local anesthesia 3 to 8 weeks after surgery. Comparative urodynamic study shows, residual urine volume was 70 ml or less in 10 patients treated with TE. On the other hand urinary volume in 18 patients without TE was average 215 ml (p< 0.001). Animal experiment was carried out to observe the role of free radicals after radiation therapy in urinary bladder. Free radicals was directly detected using electron spine resonance. In radiation group free radical generation increased 7 folds (p<0.01) in compare to control. In conclusion TE minimize the side effect of radiation to bladder and preserve good bladder function, further more, free radicals are generates after radiation which may play a vital role for bladder injury.

INTRODUCTION

After surgery for rectal cancer, symptom of voiding dysfunction, which are serious for the patients, usually occur due to the interruption of the pelvic autonomic nerve plexuses in the course of radical dissection (1), exacerbation of pre-existing outlet obstruction (2), and posterior displacement of the bladder (3). We have found that new technique (mesh partition, tissue expander) can reduce bladder complications after post operative pelvic radiation therapy. The purpose of this study to compare urodynamic studies in patients so treated with a recent group of patients who had a conventional abdominoperineal resection. The role of free radicals in bladder injury was also evaluated.

MATERIALS METHODS

Clinical Study

The subjects were 28 patients (17 male and 11 female, 35 to 75 years old) underwent abdominoperineal resection of rectum for rectal cancer. Among them 10 patients under went insertion of a tissue expander 320 ml to 400 ml of tissue expander was inserted into the pelvic cavity after abdominoperineal resection of rectum, polyglycol acid mesh was placed at the upper region of the pelvic cavity to prevent small intestine invasion of pelvic cavity Tissue expander was removed under local anesthesia 3 to 8 weeks after surgery. Tissue expander group patients received radiation therapy (4600 to 6660 cGy). Residual urinary volume and rate flow per unit time was measured after removing catheter.

Animal Study

In rat butyl-phenyl-nitrone (50mg/kg, I.V) was administered 10 mi before radiation of lower abdomen. Urinary bladder lipid was extracted using chloroform : methanol. Free radicals of tissue lipid extract was measured using electron spine resonance.

RESULT

One patient died of heart failure 3 months after surgery. One patient had hepatic metastasis and had curative liver resection. The other 8 patients are living well with out any evidence of recurrence.

Table 1 shows the residual urinary volume after removal of catheter. The residual urinary volume was 70 ml or less with an average of 35 ml in tissue expander treated group. On the other hand, conventional group volume range from 100 to 400 ml with an average of 215 ml. The MRI study showed tissue expander prevent backward displacement of the bladder whereas in conventional group bladder remained at recession.

	n	Range(ml)	Average(ml)	
Tissue Expander Miles	10	0 – 78	33.3	p<0.001
Conventional Miles	18	40 –400	215	

Table 1 Residual Urinary Output after Abdominoperineal Resection

Animal experiment

In sham operation group no free radicals were detected. In radiation treated group free radicals increased 7 folds (p< 0.01).

CONCLUSION

Our surgical procedure has a possibility to minimize the side effect of radiation to small intestine and urinary bladder, and cancer killing dose of radiation to micrometastasis can be given.

Free radical generation was observed in urinary bladder after radiation in rat model, which may play a vital role for bladder injury.

REFERENCES

1. Fowler J.W, Bermner D.N and Moffat L.E.F. The incidence and consequences of damage to the parasympathetic nerve supply to the bladder after abdominoperineal resection of rectum for cancer. Br.J.Surg., 1978, 50: 95-99

2. Eickenberg H.U, Amin M, Klompus W. Urologic complications following abdominoperineal resection. J. Urol., 1976, 115: 180-182.

3.. Neal D.E, Bouge R.P, Williams R.E. Histological appearances of the bladder in patients with denervation of the bladder after excision of rectum. Br.J.Urol., 1982, 54: 658-662

A Novel Method for Restoration of Postoperative Defecation Function in the Patients with the Lower Rectal Cancer

Nobuhiko Tanigawa, Tetsuya Horiuchi, Takumi Shimomatsuya,
Masaru Uchinami, Yasuhiko Masuda, and Ryusuke Muraoka

The Second Department of Surgery, Fukui Medical University, Matsuoka-cho, Yoshida-gun, Fukui,
910-11 Japan

ABSTRACT

A new attempt with purpose of preserving the anal canal as much as possible was conducted
in the patients with distal rectal cancer in which the anal canal would be resected
when a usual sphincter sparing operation is applied. The novel point about this technique
is that the everted anal canal in the perineum at the time of the invaginated technique
of the Maunsell-Weir method is resected diagonally to permit the preservation of the
maximum length of the anal canal. Indications for this procedure included the low
region at a distance less than 4 cm from the dentate line, less than T2 for mural stage,
and less than 1/3 the circumference for size. Four patients on which this technique
was sequentially performed since 3 years ago were favarably reviewed from the various
aspects such as tumor size, site, mural stage, lymph node metastasis, postoperative
urination/defecation function, and stool soilage. We believe that this method should
be the operation of choice in selected patients with low rectal cancer.

KEY WORDS: lower rectal cancer, anal sphincter-preserving operation, invagination method

INTRODUCTION

The choice of operative procedures for rectal carcinoma has in recent years undergone
a marked revolution. Recently surgery preserving anal sphincter muscle function has
been variously applied (1). This is because anastomosis in the pelvic cavity can be
performed with safety and certainty with the introduction of stapled anastomosis.
Another relevant factor is that the study on the mode of cancer progression has made
clear that wide resection for carcinoma at a relatively early stage is not necessary
(2-5). Most of the anal sphincter function preservation operations performed today
are anterior resections. From the aspect of postoperative defecation function the
anterior resection is most favorable, and is the main reason for its frequent use.
  However, in some cases with lower rectal cancer it is impossible to preserve a sufficient
length of the anal canal because the region occupied is too low. There are those who
leave a several centimeter rectal mucosal segment proximal to the anoderm in ileal
pouch-anal anastomosis in order to preserve involuntary continence (6-8). Therefore,
we have made a new attempt with the purpose of preserving mucosa just above the dentate
line as much as possible in cases in which the anal canal must be partially resected.

MATERIALS AND METHODS

Indication for surgery

Cases in which it is impossible to preserve a sufficient length of the anal canal by
anterior resections are the subjects of our procedure. Since the length of the anal
canal is normally about 2 cm from the dentate line, if the cancer safety margin of
at least 2 cm is included, then the lower border of the carcinoma must be at a distance
of more than 4 cm from the dentate line when an anterior resection is applied. The
cases of a tumor closer than this to the dentate line, therefore, are indicated for
our procedure. In addition, since the anal canal is diagonally resected during this
technique, cases exhibiting continuous extension of the carcinoma into the adjacent
wall must be excluded. Since extension of the carcinoma into the adjacent wall is
almost not observed at a mural stage of T2 (invasion into muscularis propria but not
beyond) or less, such cases of mural stage are indicated for our technique. Depth

of invasion through the bowel wall by the primary tumor is assessed with endorectal ultrasound in each case preoperatively. Since the anal canal mucous membrane on the opposite side from the tumor region must be preserved as much as possible, there is a limit to the size of tumors for this procedure. For these reasons, indications for grade and size included less than T2, and less than 1/3 the circumference.

Surgical Technique (figure 1)

(1) Abdominal procedures: At a point 1-2 cm from the juncture it is doubly ligated, **and the inferior mesenteric lymph nodes are dissected** en bloc (upper dissection).

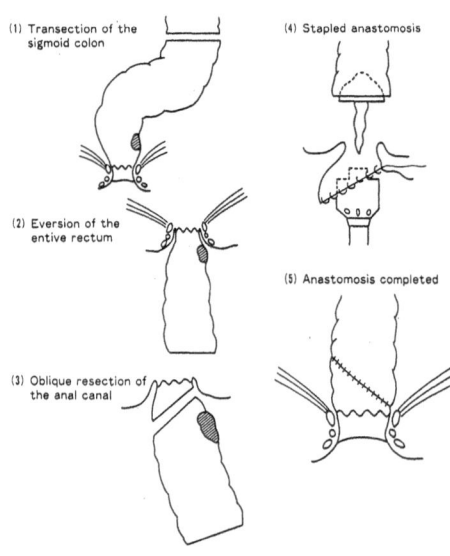

Fig.1 Operative procedures

The sigmoid colon is transected by applying a purse string suture. The mesosigmoid is dissected toward the cul-de-sac up to the peritoneal reflexion. The hypogastric nerve trunk and pelvic nerve plexus are exposed along the anterior surface of the sacral bone. In all 4 cases, we took care to preserve one side of the pelvic nerve plexus and the vesicorectal ligament, in which its branches run through, for saving defecation/unination functions. Lateral dissection proceeds from the juncture of the internal iliac artery toward the periphery. The internal iliac artery and its external fatty tissue is dissected using CUSA (Cavitron Ultrasonic Surgical Aspirator System Ns-100, Cavitron Co. Ltd., USA). The obturator nerve in its depth is easily observed, and the fatty tissue on its peiphery are dissected with the lymph nodes. Amputation of the middle rectal artery on the side where the pelvic nerve plexus is preserved is done more toward the rectal wall side away from the nerve plexus. The rectum can be elevated several centimeters by dividing the right and left lateral ligaments, so that the levator ani muscle can come into view.

(2) Perineal procedures: The forcep is inserted into the rectum, and after grasping the sigmoid stump at the tip of the forcep, it is slowly pulled, so that the rectum everts its mucosal membranes toward the outside and is pulled outside the anus. By pulling the rectal wall toward the operator, the distance between the lower margin of the tumor and the dentate line can be confirmed. The anal canal is resected circumferentially at 2-3 cm apart from the tumor border, leaving the anal canal on the side opposite the tumor as long as possible. By this procedure, the anal canal on the tumor side is shortened, and by resecting diagonally the anal canal on the opposite side remains long. After performing stapled anastomosis with the oral colon, the procedure is concluded.

RESULTS

The breakdown of the 4 cases on which this technique was performed since about 3 years ago is shown in Table 1. In all cases we conducted surgery so as to preserve unilateral autonomous nerves, mainly the pelvic nerve plexus, on the right side in case no. 1 and 2 and on the left in case no. 3 and 4. Transient urinary retention occurred in only case no. 1 at 1 month after surgery and thereafter he perceived no problem with urination. The frequency of defecation was 5-7 times per day at 6 months and at 1 year postoperatively it stabilized at a 2-3 defection frequency in each case. No anastomotic strictures occurred and none of patients experienced frank incontinence during walking hours. Nocturnal soilage occured in case 4 at 3 months after surgery, but by 6 months no patients experienced nocturnal soilage. During the postoperative course at 24 - 38 months respectively no signs of relapse including local recurrence have been observed.

Table 1. Details of 4 patients

Case	Age	Gender	Tumor site (from dentate line)	Tumor size (mm)	Mural stage	Lymph node metastasis	Pelvic plexus saving	n. at 1 year defecation frequency	at 3 months stool soilage
1	49	male	3.5	25	subserosa	(-) (0/27)	right	2	(-)
2	37	female	2.5	30	muscularis propria	(-) (1/59)	right	3	(-)
3	47	female	4.0	27	muscularis propria	(-) (0/36)	left	2	(-)
4	70	female	2.5	35	muscularis propria	(-) (0/24)	left	2	(-)

DISCUSSION

The novel point about this operative technique is that the everted anal canal in the perineum at the time of the invaginated technique of the Maunsell-Weir method (9,10) is resected diagonally to permit the preservation of maximum length of the anal canal.
This technique differs from the anterior resection in which procedures are carried out in the deep and narrow pelvic base. While measuring the distance from the tumor border under direct vision rectal resection can be performed.
There has been a great debate about what level the rectal mucosal dissection should be extended to (8). Martin LW has pointed out that the trasitional epithelium covering the anorectal column provides the sensation above the sphincter mechanism and is the necessary afferent limb of the reflex arc of involuntary continence (11). Rectal carcinomas at the early or intermediate stage, which are the subjects of our technique, have already been demonstrated to exhibit an extremely low frequency of continous extension into the adjacent rectal wall (12). Therefore, this is a good reason for preserving as much as possible the rectal wall/mucous membrane on the side opposite the tumor site. Postoperative defection pattern of each patient in the current study can be compared favorably with sphincter sparing procedures, such as low anterior resection, colo-anal anastomosis or ileo-anal pull-through (8).

REFERENCES

1. Goligher J (1984) Surgery of the Anus, Rectum and Colon. 5th ed, London, Bailliere Tindall, chap 19, pp 590-789
2. Grinnel RS (1954) Distal intramural spread of carcinoma of the rectum and rectosigmoid. Surg Gynecol Obstet 99:421-430
3. Waugh JM, Block MA, Gage RP (1955) Three and five year survival following combined abdominoperineal resection, abdominoperineal resection with sphincter preservation and anterior resection for carcinoma of the rectum and lower part of the sigmoid colon. Ann Surg 142:752-757
4. Lock MR, Cairns DW, Ritchie JK, Lockhart-Mummery HF (1978) The treatment of early colorectal cancer by local excision. Br J Surg 65:346-349
5. Williams NS, Johnston D (1984) Survival and recurrence after sphincter saving resection and abdominoperineal resection for carcinoma of the middle third of the rectum. Br J Surg 71:278-282
6. Johnston D, Holdsworth DJ, Nasymth DG (1987) Preservation of the entire anal canal in conservative proctocolectomy for ulcerative colitis: a pilot study comparing end-to-end ileo-anal anastomosis without mucosal resection with mucosal proctectomy and endoanal anastomosis. Br J Surg 74:940-944
7. Sagar PM, Holdsworth DJ, Johnston D (1991) Correlation between laboratory findings and clinical outcome after restorative proctocolectomy: serial studies in 20 patients with end-to-end pouch-anal anastomosis. Br J Surg 78:67-70
8. Becker JM, Raymond JL (1986) Ileal pouch-anal anastomosis. A single surgeon's experience with 100 consecutive cases. Ann Surg 204:375-383
9. Maunsell HW (1892) A new method of excising the two upper portions of the rectum and the lower segment of the sigmoid flexure of the colon. Lancet 2:473-476
10. Weir FR (1901) An improved method of treating high seated cancers of the rectum. J Am Med Ass 37:801-803
11. Martin LW, Fischer JE (1982) Preservation of anorectal continence following total colectomy. Ann Surg 196:700-704
12. Yasutomi M, Maruyama, J (1988) Standard surgical procedures of sphincter preservation for the rectal cancer. Gastroentetrol Surg (Japanese) 11:1225-1234

Patterns of Recurrence in Rectal Carcinoma Following Curative Resection: What Did the Post-Operative Radiotherapy Do?

Kwang Wook Suh, Choong Bai Kim, and Jin Sik Min

Department of Surgery, Yonsei University College of Medicine, Seoul, Korea

ABSTRACT

To elucidate the precise roles of postoperative radiotherapy, 200 high-risk rectal cancer patients were reviewed. Patients were divided into two groups: 83 patients in group I had undergone curative resection alone and 117 in group II, curative resection followed by radiotherapy. Two groups were compared according to overall rate of recurrence, patterns of recurrence, location of recurrence and the types of treatment of recurrent lesions. Rate of recurrence was 42.2% in group I and 38.5% in group II ($p > 0.1$) but it was significantly lower in group II at stage C2 (85.0% vs 44.8%, $p < 0.05$). Local-regional recurrence was the dominant pattern of recurrence in group I and it was significantly lower in group II(32.5% vs 16.2%, $p < 0.05$) but distant metastasis was significantly higher in group II(7.2% vs 15.4%, $p < 0.05$). Pelvic soft tissue and liver were the ususal locations of localrecurrence and distant metastasis. Minor locations were similar in both groups but anastomotic recurrence was more prominent in group I. Time interval to diagnosis of initial recurrence was significantly delayed in group II($p < 0.001$). Surgical treatment for recurrent lesion was possible in 13 patients(12 of group I, 1 of groupII). The result of this study reassure a logical background of chmoradiation protocols as adjuvant treatment for high risk rectal cancer but revealed that radiotherapy could interfere the surgical plan for the recurrent lesions.

KEY WORDS: patterns of recurrence, rectal cancer, radiotherapy

INTRODUCTION

For past 3 decades, numerous informations about the patterns of recurrence of rectal carcinoma have been reported (1-4). Recent protocol of adjuvant treatment for high risk rectal cancer (5) is largely indebted to those studies. Adjuvant radiotherapy, preceded or followed by curative resection, has been shown to improve the recurrence. But roughly 20% of patients will be destined to recurrence in spite of adjuvant treatment (6). Thus, treatment strategy for recurrent rectal cancer should be considered and the present study was undertaken to elucidate how the postoperative radiotherapy changed the patterns of recurrence of rectal cancer and to discuss their clinical implications.

MATERIALS AND METHODS

Between 1971 to 1987, at the Yonsei University Hospital, 484 patients underwent curative resections for rectal cancer. Among them, 200 patients staisfied the prerequisites for study; 1)adenocarcinoma of rectum, 2)complete removal of tumor and regional lymph nodes, 3)higher risk group for recurrence,i.e., Dukes' B2,C1 and C2., 4)followed more than 60 months, 5) alive more than 30 days after operation. Age ranged from 26 to 82(median, 52), 115 were male and 85 were female. 118 underwent abdominoperineal resection and 82 underwent anterior resection. The distribution of patients by staging is in Table 1. Patients were divided into 2 groups; I included 83 who underwent curative resection alone and II included 117 who underwent curative resection plus radiotherapy(external beam irradiation of 5040 rads). Median follow up time was 9.5 years. Recurrence was confirmed histologically in 25 out of 80 cases. Other recurrences were diagnosed by combination of physical examination, X rays and serum level of CEA. Imaging studies(abdominal CT scan, ultrasonography, bone scan) were performed every 6 months within first year of operation and yearly thereafter.

Table 1. Comparison of 2 groups by stage according to modified Dukes' classification

Stage	Group I(N=83)	Group II(N=117)
B2	53	38
C1	10	12
C2	20	67

RESULTS

A diagnosis of recurrent or metastatic carcinoma was made in 80 patients(40.0%). Recurrence rate was 42.2% in group I and 38.5% in group II and difference didn't reach the statistical significance. But comparing by individual stage, recurrence rate was lower in group II at C2. Table 2 lists the pattern of recurrence found in 80 patients. Locoregional recurrence(LR) was

Table 2. Comparison of 2 groups by patterns of recurrence

	Group I(N=83, %)	Group II(N=117, %)	p value
Local recur.	32.5	16.2	<0.05
Distant met.	7.2	15.4	<0.05
Concomitant	2.4	6.8	NS

the dominant pattern of recurrence in group I and distant metastasis(DM) was significantly higher in group II. Table 3 shows the locations of recurrence. The pelvic soft tissue was the major site of recurrence of LR in both groups and liver was counterpart of DM. Distribution of minor site of recurrence was similar in both groups except the anastomotic recurrence.

Table 3. Comparison of 2 groups by location of recurrence

	Group I	Group II
Local recurrence		
Pelvic soft tissue	16(14)	10(5)
Anastomosis	6(6)	2(2)
Vagina	3(3)	2(2)
others	6(4)	6(2)
Undetermined	0	8(8)
Distant metastasis		
Liver	5(4)	12(8)
Paraaortic node	1(1)	2(0)
others	2(1)	6(4)

( ) means being the solitary recurrence

Time interval from the operation to the initial recurrence is shown in Fig. 1. Half of the recurrence had been diagnosed at 7.2 months in group I and 16.6 months in group II($p<0.001$).

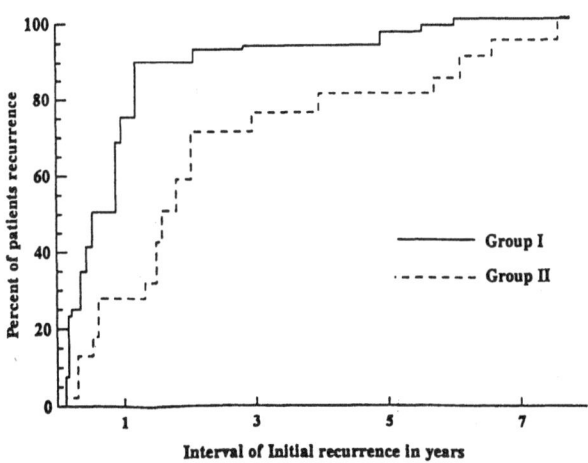

Fig. 1 Cumulative per cent of patients showing interval to recurrence

In group I, surgical resection was possible in 12 patients for their recurrent lesions but in group II, only 1 patient underwent operation. 12 patients of group I included 6 anastomotic lesions ,3 pelvic recurrences, 2 vaginal recurrences and 2 perineal recurrences. Most of recurrent lesion in group II, even the LR lesions, should be treated by palliative chemo-

DISCUSSION

Although there is considerable disparity in the literature regarding incidences of recurrence after surgery for rectal cancer (1-4), an almost unanimous acceptance is taken regarding the risk factors and patterns of recurrence (5); first, local-regional recurrence is the dominant pattern of recurrence and second, depth of primary lesion and regional lymph node metastases are the most important risk factor for recurrence. The present study based upon an accumula- tion of clinical experiences of adjuvant radiotherapy; many patients who had undergone the radiotherapy showed firm and fibrotic pelvis mimicked the local recurrence and indiscernible findings on imagings even in the computed tomography. Moreover, even in the lucky situations in which the histological diagnosis of early local recurrence was made, surgical resection of curative intent could be possible onle in a small proportion of patients. Obviously, it is likely that adjuvant radiotherapy improved the local recurrence and delayed the initial recur- rence as observed by others (5,7). But in our series, radiotherapy improved overall recurrence rate only in Dukes' C2 patients. It meant substantial proportion of our series did not take advantage from radiotherapy. This could be explained by increased proportion of distant meta- stasis in the irradiated group. Our results reassure the conclusion of the North Central Can- cer Treatment Group (8), i.e., the combined chemoradiation played significant role in reducing distant metastsis. But we inquire; Can we exclude the possiblility that a true recurrent le- sion hides in the fibrotic pelvis ? and Whether the outcomes changed if surgery was eliminate the locoregional recurrence after radiotherapy ?. It is anecdotal to recall the Minnesota se- ries of second look operations for high risk patients (9) but their efforts should not be un- derestimated. Only 6.2% of salvage rate had been reported (10) and their works had been cha- llenged by many authors, but their pioneer works should be remined. It seemed to be very di- fficult to attempt to resect the recurrent lesions but outcomes after resection would be hopeful. In this view point, the radiotherapy absolutely interfere the surgical plan for recurrent lesions. We could resect the recurrent lesion in 12 patients and 10 out of them with curative intent. The patients who underwent resections for their recurrent lesions are still alive 25 to 60 months from the diagnosis. This was beyond the expectations. In summary, it was found that the radiotherapy improved tha rate of locoregional recurrence, delayed the initial recurrence but could improve the overall rate of recurrence only in Dukes' C2 patient. It was also found that the radiotherapy was enough to change the patterns of recurrence. If the surgical treatment is planned for the recurrent lesions, radiotherapy obviously interfere it. Beneficial as well as negative effects, rather than a complication, of radiotherapy should be regarded and an adequate selection of high risk patients who are going to undergo radio- therapy will be a problem.

REFERENCES

1. Gunderson LL, Sosin H (1974) Areas of failure found at reoperation(second or symptomatic look) following "curative surgery" for adenocarcinoma of the rectum. Cancer 34:1278-1292
2. Cass AW, Million RR, Pfaff WW (1976) Patterns of recurrence following surgery alone for adenocarcinoma of the colon and rectum. Cancer 37:2861-2865
3. Rich T, Gunderson LL, Lew R (1983) Patterns of recurrence of rectal cancer after potentia- lly curative surgery. Cancer 52:1317-1329
4. Galadiuk S, Wieand HS, Moertel CG (1992) Patterns of recurrence after curative resection of the colon and rectum. Surg Gynecol Obstet 174:27-32
5. Krook JE, Moertel CG, Gunderson LL (1991) Effective surgical adjuvant therapy for high- risk rectal carcinoma. N Engl J Med 324:709-715
6. Gastrointestinal Tumor Study Group (1985) Prolongation of the disease-free interval in surgically treated rectal carcinoma. N Engl J Med 312:1465-1472
7. Gastrointestinal Tumor Study Group (1986) Survival after postoperative combination treat- ment of rectal cancer. N Engl J Med 315:1294
8. NIH Consensus Conference (1990) Adjuvant therapy for patients with colon and rectal cancer. JAMA 264:1444-1450
9. Wangensteen OH, Lewis FJ, Arhelger SW (1954) An intrim report upon the 'second-look' pro- cedure for cancer of the stomach, colon and rectum for 'limited intraperitoneal carcino- sis'. Surg Gynecol Obstet 99:257-267
10. Griffen WO Jr, Humphrey L, Sosin H (1969) The prognosis and management of recurrent abdo- minal malignancies. Curr Probl Surg 6:2-43

The Role of Lateral Lymphnode Dissection in the Prevention of Recurrence for Rectal Cancer

NELSON TSUNO, TOSHIO SAWADA, YOSHIRO KUBOTA, KOKI SUNOUCHI,
MASATOSHI OHYA, KIMITAKA SUZUKI, TOSHIAKI WATANABE, SHIN'ICHI SAMESHIMA,
MASARU SHINOZAKI, MASAYUKI UCHIYAMA, MASATAKA SAKAGUCHI,
YOSHIKI HIGUCHI, and TETSUICHIRO MUTO

The First Department of Surgery, University of Tokyo, Bunkyo-ku, Tokyo, 113 Japan

ABSTRACT

In an attempt to clarify the role of lateral node dissection in preventing the local recurrence of rectal cancer, 203 patients undergoing surgery for advanced lower rectal cancer in our surgical department from 1963 to 1991 were studied retrospectively. The incidence of lateral lymphnode metastases was higher in patients with tumors invading beyond the subserosa and a higher recurrence rate was observed in patients with lymphnode metastasis diagnosed at or before operation. Lymphnode metastases were found in 18.2% of the patients undergoing lateral node dissection, and surgery was succeeded in 66.7% of these patients, although 50% of the cases had tumors invading beyond the subserosal layer. The recurrence rate was 33.3%. We concluded that the lateral node dissection plays an important role in preventing local recurrence of rectal cancer, and should be indicated for all patients with either lymphnode metastases or tumors invading beyond the subserosal layer.

KEY WORDS: rectal cancer, lymphnode, metastasis, prevention

INTRODUCTION

The incidence of local recurrences after surgery for rectal cancer varies between 3 and 40% in the literature [1,2,3], and a significant proportion of these recurrences should be attributed to inadequate surgical clearance [1]. Most of the recurrences are thought to be extramural than intramural. Healed et al. [4] found a neoplastic involvement of the cellulolymphatic tissue of the mesorectum, even in the absence of a distal spread along the wall of the rectum and concluded that most of pelvic recurrences after curative operation for rectal cancer do not arise from the bowel wall, but from the regional cellulolymphatic structures. Cohen et al. [5] reported that from 25-50% of patients with pelvic disease relapses die in the absence of distant metastases. In resectable rectal surgery, the extent of the dissection to the extraregional nodes (lumboaortic, pelvic, or others) has been the object of numerous retrospective studies. Moriya et al. [6] reported an excellent survival rate of 49 percent of patients with lateral node metastasis by the lateral node dissection. They described three techniques of systematic lymphadenectomy: the upward, the lateral, and the downward dissection. Although the results of lateral and lumbo-aortic lymphadenectomy are satisfying, the postoperative genitourinary morbidity is undoubtedly worsened by the extraregional extension of the lymphadenectomy and this good results may also be obtained with radical surgery and adjuvant pelvic radiotherapy, without pelvic lymphadenectomy [2]. Having these conflicting opinions, we proposed to evaluate the importance of lateral dissection in preventing local recurrence.

PATIENTS

Two-hundred and three patients undergoing surgery for advanced low rectal cancer (lower edge < 7.0 cm from the anal verge) at the First Department of Surgery, University of Tokyo, from 1963 to 1991, were studied retrospectively. The metastatic lymphnode spreading was classified as upward when the pararectal, superior rectal, or inferior mesenteric lymphnodes were involved, and as lateral when the middle rectal, obturator, or internal iliac groups of lymphnodes were involved. Indication for lateral node dissection were either the tumors infiltrating beyond the subserosa, or the presence of lymphnode metastasis. Radical lateral node dissection without nerve preservation is routinely indicated for the tumors infiltrating beyond the subserosa, associated with lymphnode metastasis. When the tumor is confined to the subserosal layer, but lymphnode metastasis is positive, or lymphnode metastasis is negative, but the tumor is infiltrating beyond the subserosa, we indicate partial nerve preservation, i.e., partial or complete preservation of the hypogastric nerve, and of the pelvic plexus.

RESULTS

From the 203 cases studied, lymphnode metastasis was found in 65 (32.0%). The recurrence rate was 21.5% (14/65) in these patients. In comparison, the patients without lymphnode metastasis had a recurrence rate of 10.9% (15/138). Among the patients with lymphnode metastasis, 47 had only upward spreading, 6 (3.0%) had lateral spreading only, and 12 (5.9%) had both upward and lateral spreading, giving an incidence of lateral spreading of 8.9% (18/203). Lateral lymphnode dissection was performed in 99 (48.7%) cases, and among them 18 (18.2%) had lymphnode metastases. Recurrence was found in 33.3% (6/18) of these patients with lymphnode metastases, whilst in the group without lymphnode metastasis receiving lateral dissection, the recurrence rate was 11.1% (9/81), giving a total recurrence rate of 15.2% (15/99) for the patients who received lateral dissection. The local recurrence rate was 13.5% (14/104) for the patients without lateral dissection. (See Figure 1 for details). According to the depth of tumor invasion, 145 cases were of tumors limited to the subserosa, and 58 beyond the subserosa. In the first group, 5 (3.4%) had lateral spreading, and 17 (11.0%) had local recurrence. In the second group, 13 (22.3%) had lateral spreading, and 6 (10.0%) had local recurrence. Analyzing the 18 cases with lateral spreading, 10 had metastases localized in only one space, the middle rectal lymphnodes being predominant. The other 8 cases had metastases in various spaces, including the middle rectal, obturator, and internal iliac. In the first group, the incidence of recurrence was 40% (4/10), compared with 25% (2/8) in the second group.

LATERAL LN DISSECTION		UPWARD LN META	LOCAL RECURRENCE	CASES	% TOTAL
Not performed (104 cases)		Negative (73 cases)	negative	64	31.5
			positive	9	4.4 (12.3)
		Positive (31 cases)	negative	26	12.8
			positive	5	2.5 (16.1)
Performed (99 cases)	Metastasis (-) (81 cases)	Negative (65 cases)	negative	59	29.1
			positive	6	3.0 (9.2)
		Positive (16 cases)	negative	13	6.4
			positive	3	1.5 (18.8)
	Metastasis (+) (99 cases)	Negative (6 cases)	negative	3	1.5
			positive	3	1.5 (50.0)
		Positive (12 cases)	negative	9	4.4
			positive	3	1.5 (25.0)

Fig 1. Incidence of local recurrence, according to lymphnode metastases.

DISCUSSION

Besides depth of penetration, the presence or absence of lymphnode metastases is one of the two most important factors determining the decision for local therapy [7]. Cavaliere et al. [2] in a retrospective study, found the locoregional relapse of 5.3-20.0% in the literature. Hojo et al. [3] found local recurrence rates, including iliopelvic recurrences following surgery for rectal cancer patients, of 20 to 30% in the literature. Di Matteo [1] found it in 3 to 40%. In our series, the total recurrence rate was 14.3 (29/203). The patients with lymphnode metastasis had a higher incidence of recurrence than those without metastasis (21.5% vs. 10.9%). The incidence of lateral spreading was higher in the group with tumors invading beyond the subserosa than in that with tumors limited to the subserosal layer. In the 90 cases without indication for lateral dissection, tumor invasion was confined to the subserosal layer in 78 (86.7%). Lateral lymphnode dissection was indicated for 99 patients, and lymphnode metastasis was found in 18.2%. A high recurrence rate of 33.3% (6/18) was observed in these patients, whilst in those without lymphnode metastasis it was 11.1%. From the 18 patients with lateral spreading, lateral dissection was succeeded in 12 (66.7%), and 9 of them had tumors invading beyond the subserosa. From the 6 recurrent patients, thought to have incomplete lateral dissection, the tumor was invading beyond the subserosa in 4 (66.7%). Recurrence was found in 13.5% of patients without lateral lymphnode dissection, but all these cases were operated before 1982, when the concept of lymphnode dissection was not completely established. We concluded that lateral lymphnode spreading and the depth of tumor invasion are important prognostic factors, and that lateral node dissection plays an important role in preventing the local recurrence of rectal cancer. We believe that although the increase in the risk of genitourinary and sexual disfunctions [3,8] due to this procedure, it should be indicated for all patients with either lymphnode metastasis or tumors invading beyond the subserosa. Recently, nerve preserving operations are being performed [3,8] that can give better results in respect to the postoperative quality of life.

REFERENCES

1. Di Matteo G, Mascagni D, Tarroni D (1991) J Surg Oncol Suppl 2:32-35
2. Cavaliere R, Tedesco M, Giannarelli D, Aloe L, Perri P, Di Filippo F, Crecco M, Gabrielli F, Cosimelli M, Stipa S (1991) J Surg Oncol Suppl 2:24-31
3. Hojo K, Sawada T, Moriya Y (1989) Dis Colon Rectum 32:128-133
4. Healed RI, Husband EM, Ryall RDM (1982) Br J Surg 69:613-616
5. Cohen AM, Minsky BD (1990) Dis Colon Rectum 33(5):432-438
6. Moriya Y, Hojo K, Sawada T, Koyama Y (1989) Dis Colon Rectum 32:307-315
7. Hildebrandt U (1991) Int J Colorect Dis 6:74-76
8. Hojo K, Kernava AM, Sugihara K, Katumata K (1991) Dis Colon Rectum 34:532-539

Indications of Operative Modalities and Analysis of Local Recurrence After Curative Surgery for Rectal Cancer

Kenichi Shiiba, Takashi Migita, Ko Miura, Yoshihiro Saito, and Seiki Matsuno

The First Department of Surgery, Tohoku University School of Medicine, Sendai, 980 Japan

ABSTRACT

Two hundred and eight patients who underwent curative resection for rectal cancer were reviewed in order to identify the factors which influence local recurrence. The incidence of recurrence depended on Dukes' stage (C > B,A), depth of tumor invasion (a_1,ss ~ ai,si > m ~ pm), lymph node involvement (n+ > n-), lymphatic invasion (ly+ > ly-), and histological type (poorly, moderately > well differentiated adenocarcinoma). When the maximum diameter of the tumor was greater than 5 cm, an increased rate of local recurrence was observed in the low anterior resection (LAR) group compared to the abdominoperineal resection (APR) group. LAR or other function preserving operations should be carefully employed in case these factors were identified in the patient pre- or intraoperatively.

KEY WORDS: rectal cancer, local recurrence, abdominoperineal resection, low anterior resection

INTRODUCTION

Local recurrence is a major clinical problem after the surgical treatment for rectal carcinoma. The introduction of stapling instruments has led to an increasing tendency to treat rectal cancer by sphincter-saving operation, i.e. low anterior resection (LAR), in order to warrant the increased quality of life for patients who avoid permanent colostomy. In addition, pelvic autonomic nerve preservation technique has been developed to decrease the urinary and sexual morbidity which follows radical pelvic lymphadenectomy. Although radical treatment should remain the ultimate goal, these procedures reduce the perirectal clearance leading to an increased risk of local recurrence. Indeed a higher rate of local recurrenc after LAR compared to APR has been reported by several investigators [1,2]. Various clinicopathological factors have been also attributed to predicting a higher rate of local recurrence [3-6] but there is still no definite criteria in selecting sphincter-saving surgery. In the present study 208 patients with rectal cancer who had curative operation were reviewed in order to identify the factors which influence local recurrence and reveal the clinical parameters on which to base in selecting operative modalities.

PATIENTS AND METHODS

Two hundred and eight patients who underwent curative surgery for cancer of the rectum between January 1979 and December 1991 were evaluated. The operation was considered curative if the resection satisfies the following criteria: there are no distant metastases, no involvement of the resected margins by tumor, and the extent of regional lymph node resection exceeds or equal to the extent of lymph nodes metastases. The selection of APR or LAR was based on the distance of tumor from the anal verge evaluated prior to surgery. The histories of the 208 patients were reviewed to determine local recurrence rate and the influence on local recurrence of the following parameters: patient's age, stage of disease, tumor differentiation, surgical procedure and length of the distal cuff. The location of the tumor was presented by the site where the lesion predominantly occupied: i.e. Rb; below the peritoneal reflection, Ra; above peritoneal reflection to the level of the lower margin of the 2nd sacral bone, Rs; below promontry. Tumor stage was classified according to Dukes' classification. Histological classification was done using the criteria by the Japanese Research Society for Cancer of the Colon and Rectum (JRSCCR) The depth of invasion of the tumor was described as follows: m or sm -cancer limited in mucosa or submucosa, pm -limited to propria muscle layer, a1 or ss -reaching on adventitia or serosa, a2 or s -fully exposed on adventitia or serosa, and ai or si -invading into other organs after penetrating adventitia or serosa. In those patients who underwent sphincter-saving resection, the length of distal cuff was measured when the operation sample was obtained. Most patients underwent determination of blood CEA level, physical examination every two months, liver ultrasound every six months, and chest x-ray, barium enema and CT scan every year. Further investigations, i.e. intrarectal ultrasound, pelvic MRI and total colonofiber were carried out when local recurrence was suspected. Final diagnosis of local recurrnce was obtained by biopsy or reoperation. Statistical analysis was performed using chi square and unpaired Student t tests.

RESULTS

Two hundred and eight patients underwent curative surgery for rectal cancer at our department between January 1979 and December 1991. The group of patients comprised of 100 females and 108 males with median age of 58 years (range 26-82 years) (Table 1). One hundred and twenty-three patients underwent APR and 85 patients had LAR. Local recurrence occurred in 21 patients (10.1%); 10 (8.1%) in the APR group and 11 (12.9%) in the LAR group. The average time between initial operation and diagnosis of local recurrence was 17.1 months (2-51months); 24.3 months in the APR group and 12.9 months in the LAR group. Survival time after recurrence was 10.7 months (2-27 months); 13.2 months in the LAR goup and 8.9 months in the APR group. Time to recurrence as well as survival after recurrence were shorter for patients who had undergone LAR but the differences were not statistically significant.

Table 1. Clinical data on 208 patients undergoing curative resection for rectal cancer

	APR	LAR	Total
No. Patients	123	85	208
Age,Mean(years)	57.8	58.3	58.0
No. Local recurrence	10	11	21
% Local recurrence	8.1	12.9	10.1
Time to recurrence			
Mean (months)	24.3	12.9	17.1
median(months)	21	8	16
Survival after recurrence			
Mean (months)	13.2	8.9	10.7
median(months)	10	6	10

Table 2. Local recurrence in relation to one pathologic variable

Dukes' stage		Depth of invasion	
A	1.5%	m-pm	4.9%
B	6.3%	a_1-ai	13.2%*
C	18.1%*		
		Lymph node metastasis	
Histologic type		n(-)	2.7%
well	3.4%	n(+)	17.5%*
moderately	23.1%*		
poorly	50.0%*	Lymphatic invasion	
signet	100.0%	ly(-)	3.8%
undiff.	100.0%	ly(+)	16.7%*

* statistically significant

Neither patient age, sex, site of tumor, size of tumor, surgical procedure; APR or LAR nor vascular invasion appears to influence overall local recurrence rate. As shown in Table 2, recurrence was significantly increased in Dukes C tumors compared to Dukes A ($p<0.005$) or B ($p<0.05$), and moderately ($p<0.005$) or poorly differentiated ($p<0.05$) tumors recurred more frequently than well differentiated tumors. Moreover a significant increase in recurrence was observed when the tumors invaded beyond pm layer ($p<0.05$), or accompanied by lymph node involvement ($p<0.005$) or lymphatic invasion ($p<0.005$).

Next, local recurrence rates after APR and LAR were compared according to each pathologic variable (Table 3). In patients with maximum tumor diameter of greater than 5 cm, the LAR group manifested significantly higher rate of recurrence than the APR group (29.4%vs7.4%, p=0.05). Tumor staging, histologic type and site, depth of invasion, lymph node involvement, lymphatic invasion and vascular invasion did not statistically discriminate the recurrence rate between the two groups, however the recurrence rate in the LAR group was two-fold higher than that in the APR group in either the case with moderately differentiated tumors, a2 ~ ai in the depth, lymphatic invasion, or lymph node involement which was restricted to epi- or paracolic and anorectal nodes (data not showna). In the LAR group, a moderate increase in recurrence was observed when the distal cuff was ≤ 2 cm in length, paticularly in Dukes C patients, though the difference was not statistically significant (Table 4).

Table 3. Comparison of local recurrence after APR and LAR

	APR	LAR	p		APR	LAR	p
Site				Histologic type			
Rb	8.5%	11.4%		well	3.5%	3.3%	
Ra	6.7%	17.1%	NS	moderately	14.3%	33.3%	NS
Rs	0 %	6.7%		poorly	33.3%	100 %	
				signet	100 %		
Dukes' stage				undiff.	100 %		
A	0 %	3.2%					
B	3.4%	10.5%	NS	Tumor size			
C	15.3%	22.9%		≤ 5 cm	10.0%	7.5%	
				> 5 cm	7.4%*	29.4%*	p=0.05

Table 4. Local recurrence according to length of distal cuff

Distal cuff	DukesA	DukesB	DukesC	Total	Distal cuff	DukesA	DukesB	DukesC	Total
≤ 2.0 cm	9.1%	0 %	20.0%	13.6%	≤ 3.0 cm	4.8%	9.1%	16.7%	10.7%
> 2.0 cm	0 %	6.3%	14.8%	8.5%	> 3.0 cm	0 %	0 %	15.4%	8.0%

DISCUSSION

The local recurrence rate of 10.1% observed in this series of 208 patients who had undergone curative surgery for rectal cancer was compatible with the previous reports in which the rates varied between 5% and 35% [7-9]. The location of the tumor in the rectum may influence local recurrence [3,10] particularly in those who had LAR. Secco et al reported that extraperitoneal primary lesions were associated with a greater incidence of local relapse compared to intraperitoneal tumors [3]. In our study location of the tumor had no prognostic significance regarding local recurrence in either case with APR or LAR, which might give a rationale of selecting LAR for extraperitoneal (Rb) lesions. Some investigators showed tumor stage, histologic differentiation had no prognostic significance in local recurrence [6,11], while others reported patients with advanced Dukes' stage tumors as well as poor histological grade had markedly higher rates of local recurrence [4]. Our results were consistant with the latter findings. Moreover it was proven that lymph node involvement was an important risk factor of local recurrence corresponding to the higher rates of recurrence in Dukes C. Another findings that the incidence of local recurrence depended on the depth of invasion suggested the importance of local invasion. In that respect Russell et al showed locally invasive tumors (Stage B2,C2) are more predictive of local recurrence than regional node involvement (Stage C1) [12]. The findings that a histologic evidence of lymphatic invasion in the primary tumor had increased the risk of recurrence must be related to the invasion around perirectal tissues through lymphatic vessels as well as lymph node involvement. These findings concerning local invasion claim a precise and wide resection of the perirectal tissues including the numerous lymphatic connections. A higher rate of local recurrence after LAR in comparison to APR has been documented in various reports [1,2], but other investigators have shown no such differences [1,2,4,5,7]. In this study, there was no significant difference in the local recurrence rate between APR and LAR, but patients with maximum tumor diameter of greater than 5 cm had significantly higher incidence of recurrence in the LAR group than the APR group (p=0.05). Although tumor size was closely related to other pathological factors, the other factors did not discriminate the recurrence rate between the two groups. Among those factors either moderately differentiated tumors, a2 and ai in the depth, invasion of lymphatic vessels, or lymph node involvement, which were recognized as significant prognostic factors for local recurrence in our study, gave a two-fold increase of local recurrence in LAR group compared to APR group. If the preoperative or intraoperative examinations revealed the patients with a higher risk of local recurrence, surgeons should employ suitable operations like wider pelvic dissection and minimize the morbidity of recurrence. In the case of LAR, the distal margin of resection necessary to limit local recurrence has been controversial even though pathologic observations have established that distal spread of rectal carcinoma beyond 2 cm is a rare event [13]. In this study no significant difference in recurrence with margins less than or equal to 2 cm and greater than 2 cm was observed, but in Dukes C patients a 5% increase in local recurrence rate was observed when the distal cuff was inferior to 2 cm in length. In conclusion, local recurrence of rectal cancer are highly related to lymph node involvement, invasion of lymphatic vessels, depth of tumor invasion and histologic type. In selecting operative modalities, LAR are preferably employed when tumor size is less than 5 cm and at least 2 cm of distal margin is sequred. Autonomic nerve preservation operation is not recommended for patients with Dukes C, Dukes B with a2, s2 or and ly(+) as well as moderately/poorly differentiated adenocarcinoma because extensive and complete removal of regional lymph nodes with sufficient external surgical margin is required to reduce local recurrence.

REFERENCES

1. Phillips RS, Hittinger R, Bleovsky L, Fry JS, Fielding P (1984) Br J Surg 71: 12-16
2. Reid JD, Robins RD, Atkinson KG (1984) Am J Surg 147: 629-632
3. Secco GB, Fardelli R, Campora E, Rovida S, Bertoglio S (1989) Oncology 46: 10-13
4. Vlasak JW, Wagner D, Passaro E (1989) J Surg Oncol 41: 236-239
5. Amato A, Pescatori M, Butti A (1991) Dis Colon Rectum 34: 317-322
6. Fuhrman G, Davidson BS, Larach SW, Williamson PR (1992) Southern Medical Journal 85: 502-505
7. Lasson ALL, Ekelund GR, Lindstrom CG (1984) Acta Chir Scand [Suppl] 150: 85-89
8. Pheils MT, Chapuis PH, Newland RC, Colquhoun K (1983) Dis Colon Retum 26: 98-102
9. Williams N, Johnston D (1984) Br J Surg 71: 278-282
10. Warneke J, Petrelli NJ, Herrera L (1989) Am J Surg 158: 3-5
11. Habib NA, Daeson PM, Peck MA (1988) Br J Clin Prac 42: 225-227
12. Russel AH, Pelton J, Reheis CE, Wisbeck WM, Tong DY, Dawson LE (1985) Cancer 56: 1446-1451
13. Polett WG, Nicholls RJ (1983) Ann Surg 198: 159-163

Cryosurgical Treatment for Local Recurrence of Rectal Cancer

Yasuhisa Yamamoto, Sueharu Iwamoto, Tsutomu Mure, and Kaiso Sano

Department of Surgery, Kawasaki Medical School, Kurashiki, Okayama, 701-01 Japan

ABSTRACT

During the last 19 years we have used cryosurgery as part of a multidisciplinary therapy to treat 12 patients with local recurrence of rectal cancer. This treatment was chosen to provide these patients with the palliative benefits of minimal bleeding and to reduce tumor bulk. The survival time following resection therapy in 30 cases after relapse was significantly greater than that for the 12 cases receiving cryosurgical treatment. However, local destruction of the recurring cancer by cryosurgery resulted in effective control of the tumor.

KEY WORDS: rectal cancer, local recurrence, cryosurgical treatment

INTRODUCTION

The goal of treatment for tumor recurrence after the resection of rectal cancer is effective control of the tumor. Not all patients with relapses involving local spread of the tumor expect further curative surgery when some symptoms are subjectively noticed. Inveterate complaints, such as intractable bleeding or pain, require multidisciplinary therapy in some cases. The purpose of this study was to demonstrate that cryosurgical treatment for local recurrence of rectal cancer could offer the palliative benefits of minimal bleeding as well as reduce tumor bulk as part of a multidisciplinary therapy.

MATERIALS AND METHOD

The Japanese Research Society for Cancer of the Colon and Rectum set up the General Rules for Clinical and Pathological Studies on Cancer of Colon, Rectum and Anus in 1977 (Fig. 1). We have treated 489 patients (Rs: 72, Ra: 207, Rb: 198, P: 12) with rectal cancer according to these rules between 1974 and 1992 (Table 1).

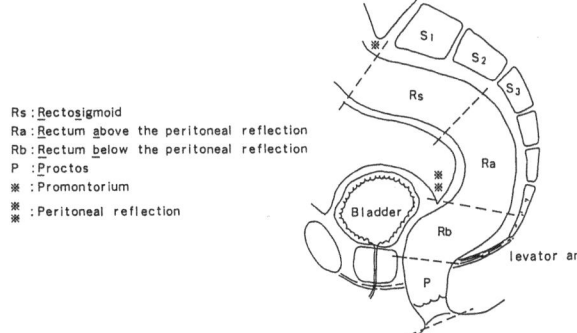

Rs : Rectosigmoid
Ra : Rectum above the peritoneal reflection
Rb : Rectum below the peritoneal reflection
P : Proctos
※ : Promontorium
※ : Peritoneal reflection

Fig. 1 Division of the Rectum

Table 1 Patients with Rectal Cancer

| Site | Stages of Japanese Classification | | | | | Total |
	I (A)*	II (B)*	III (C1)*	IV (C2)*	V (D)*	
Rs	13(10)	27	9	4	19	72(10)
Ra	44(30)	53	46(2)	24	40	207(32)
Rb	66(31)	44	35	17	36	198(31)
P	3(2)	1	1	3	4	12(2)
Total	126(73)	125	91(2)	48	99	489(75)

*Dukes' classification
( ): Early cancer
1974-1992

Local recurrences including intrapelvic relapse and inguinal lymph node metastases were found in 55 patients (11.2%) (Table 2). Among these 55 patients, 45 underwent surgery; traditional surgery in 33 cases and additional cryosurgery in 12 cases. The other 10 patients were treated conservatively without resection (Table 3).

Table 2　　　　　　　　　　　　　Recurrences after Surgery

Recurrence Site	Local Recurrences	Liver Metastases	Lung Metastases	Lymph Nodes Metastases	Dissemination	Brain Metastases	Total
Rs	5(1)	6(1)	1(1)	1	1		14(3)
Ra	23(2)	12(3)	8(3)	5(3)	2(1)		50(12)
Rb	25(3)	11(3)	12(7)	4(1)		2(2)	54(16)
P				2			2
Total	53(6)	29(7)	21(11)	12(4)	3(1)	2(2)	120(31)

( ): Overlapping cases

RESULTS

Among 489 patients with rectal cancer we have had 75 cases of early cancer involving the mucosa or submucosa. Two of these 75 patients had regional lymph node metastases (n_1) and were classified into stage III (Table 1).

The frequency of relapse was highest for local recurrences (53 cases), followed by liver metastases (29 cases) and lung metastases (21 cases). The rates of recurrence with regard to each tumor location were as follows; local recurrences (Rs: 6.9%, Ra: 11.1%, Rb: 12.6%), liver metastases (Rs: 8.3%, Ra: 5.8%, Rb: 5.6%) and lung metastases (Rs: 1.4%, Ra: 3.9%, Rb: 6.1%) (Table 2).

Six of 12 patients who underwent cryosurgery for local recurrences received it as part of a multidisciplinary therapy that also included palliative resection and administration of anticancer agents. The remainder received cryosurgical treatment for perineal relapses along with generalized chemotherapy (Table 3).

The tumor stages at the time of the first operation and following treatment after local recurrence are shown in Table 4. The parenthesized numbers indicate the number of patients receiving cryosurgery and/or chemotherapy.

The survival period for resection therapy of local relapses was significantly greater than that following cryosurgical treatment (Fig. 2). Comparison of the survival period following cryosurgery and that following conservative therapy showed no significant difference (Fig. 3).

Table 3　Following Treatment for Local Recurrence

Site	Cryosurgery	Resection	Conservative	Colostomy
Rs	1	2	1	1
Ra	7	10	4	2
Rb	4	16	5	
P		2*		
Total	12	30	10	3

*Inguinal Lymph Node Metastases

Table 4　Stages at First Operation and Following Treatment for Local Recurrence

Stage(Dukes)		Cryosurgery	Resection	Conservative	Colostomy
I	(A)		6		
II	(B)	3	8		
III	(C1)	5(3)	10	2	
IV	(C2)		4	7	3
V	(D)	4(3)	2	1	
Total		12(6)	30	10	3

( ): Cryosurgery and/or chemotherapy

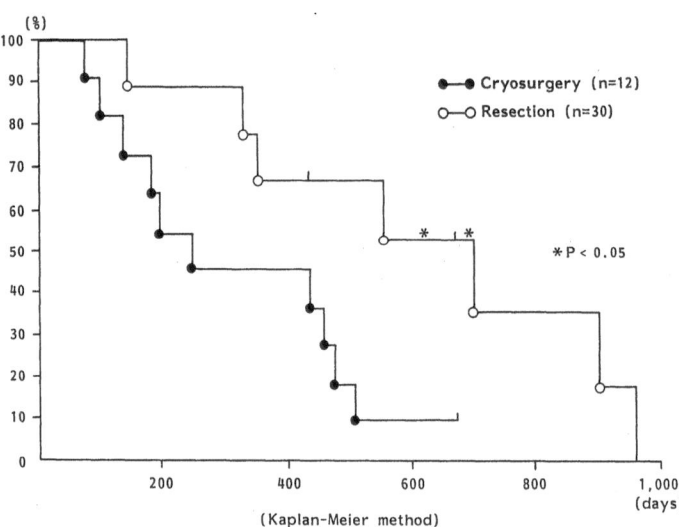

Fig. 2　Survival Period after Recurrences of Rectal Cancer (Comparison between Cryosurgery and Resection)

DISCUSSION

The Japanese General Rules for Clinical and Pathological Studies of Colorectal Cancer divide the location for such cancer into four sites in the rectum from the promontorium to the anal verge (Fig. 1). The n_1 lymph node of the rule corresponds to the regional lymph node, and the n_2 or n_3 lymph node has metastases equal to the high metastases of Dukes' classification (Fig. 4). Small differences between the Japanese stages and Dukes' classification were roughly noted in stages I and II (Table 5).

The first choice of treatment for local recurrence is thought to be resection by traditional surgery if possible. The significant difference in the survival time between resection therapy for local relapse of rectal cancer and cryosurgical treatment was due to the disparity between the two groups, that is, most patients undergoing cryosurgery were at the end stage. A multidisciplinary therapy should be applied when a patient has had some symptoms due to local recurrence of rectal cancer.

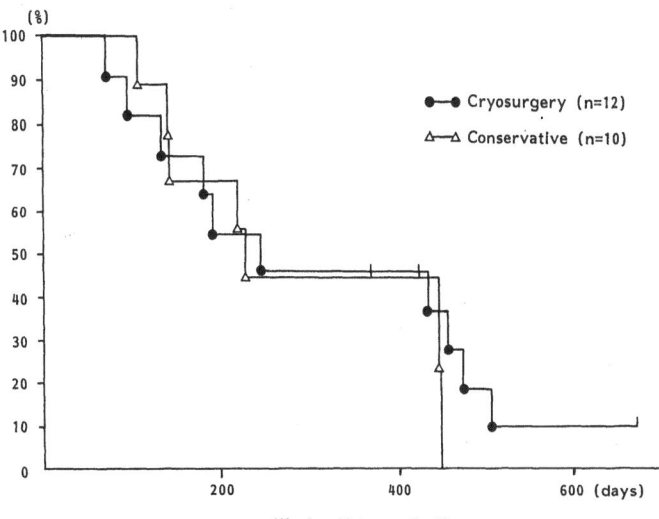

(Kaplan-Meier method)

Fig.3   Survival Period after Recurrences of Rectal Cancer
(Comparison between Cryosurgery and Conservative Therapy)

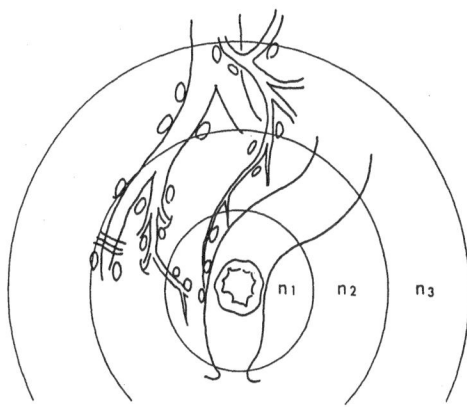

Fig. 4 Lymph Node Metastases
n_1: regional
n_2, n_3: high

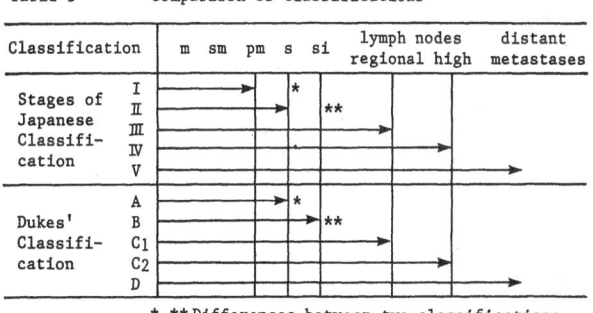

Table 5   Comparison of Classifications

Classification		m	sm	pm	s	si	lymph nodes regional	high	distant metastases
Stages of Japanese Classification	I II III IV V				*	**			
Dukes' Classification	A B C1 C2 D				*	**			

*,** Differences between two classifications
m: mucosa, sm: submucosa, pm: proper muscle
s: serosa, si: extracolonic invasion

Although there was no significant difference in the survival time between cryosurgical treatment for local relapse and that for conservative therapy, cryosurgery was judged to provide significant palliation. Local destruction of the recurring cancer by cryosurgery provides effective control of the tumor. Bleeding was controlled, pain was lessened or relieved, and the tumor bulk was reduced in size. These results encourage further study and clinical application of cryosurgery for the treatment of local recurrences of rectal cancer as part of a multidisciplinary therapy.

REFERENCES

1. Yamamoto Y, Sano K, Kimoto M (1989) Cryosurgical treatment for anorectal cancer--A method of palliative or adjunctive management--. Am Surg 55: 252-256
2. Asbun H J, Hughes K S (1993) Management of recurrent and metastatic colorectal carcinoma. Surg Clin North Am 73: 145-166

An Application of 201Tl-SPECT for Evaluating in Carcinoma of Digestive Diseases (Thallium-Technetium Subtraction SPECT of Hepatobiliary Carcinoma)

S. Yamada[1], I. Honda[1], T. Togawa[2], N. Yui[2], M. Yanagisawa[2], F. Kinoshita[2], K. Watanabe[1], H. Yamamoto[1], W. Takayama[1], S. Watanabe[1], Y. Fujita[1], and M. Ryu[3]

[1]Division of Gastrointestinal Surgery, [2]Division of Nuclear Medicine, Chiba Cancer Center, Chiba 260
[3]Division of Surgery, National Cancer Center East Hospital, Kashiwa, Chiba, 277 Japan

ABSTRACT

We evaluated 10 patients with hepatobiliary carcinoma, using thallium(Tl)-technetium(Tc) subtraction SPECT to assess its usefulness in the diagnosis of this condition. All ten patients (100%) had positive findings on Tl-Tc subtraction SPECT. Three of them underwent Tl-Tc subtraction SPECT after radiotherapy and chemotherapy. A significant decrease in Tl uptake was observed in all patients. Tl-Tc subtraction SPECT appears to be a sensitive method for detecting hepatobiliary carcinomas and measuring the effect after radiotherapy and chemotherapy.

KEY WORDS:Thallium-Technetium subtraction SPECT, Hepatobiliary Carcinoma, Radiotherapy

INTRODUCTION

Technologic advances in SPECT have resulted in continued improvement in spatial resolution. Recently 201Tl-SPECT(single photon emission computed tomography) has been used for tumor imaging in some neoplasms, including thyroid cancer and lung cancer[1,2]. But there are few reports on the diagnosis of hepatobiliary carcinomas using 201Tl-SPECT, because thallium is also taken up by the liver. Thallium-technetium subtraction scintigraphy has been used as a method to visualized enlarged parathyroid glands[3]. Applying this method,we have used a subtraction technique which removes a 99mTc liver image, leaving the hepatobiliary tumor as a "hot" area.

MATERIALS AND METHODS

Ten patients (seven male, 3 female) admitted to the Chiba Cancer Center Hospital between July 1992 and February 1993 were enrolled in the study. The mean age was 61 years (range: 50-87). Eight patients had bile duct cancer, two gallbladder carcinomas and one hepatocellular carcinoma. Cytologic or histologic proof of the malignant character of the tumor was obtained (either by percutaneous or endoscopic route or by laparotomy) in all but nine patients.
SPECT imaging

Double tracer image technique was described by Togawa et al(1993)[4]. The patients were simultaneous given an i.v. injections of 185MBq technetium phytate and 111MBq thallium chloride. Data acquisition was started 5 min. after the injection, by means of a three-headed rotating gamma camera (Toshiba GCA 9300A). After the rotation of each gamma camera with 6° step angle, one step in 60 seconds, and with acquisition matrix of 128×128, projection data from 60 steps were acquired in 20 minutes. Transaxial images with a 3.4mm slice were reconstructed by means of Butterworth and Ramp filters for preprocessing and back-projection, respectively.

Table.1 Summary of 10 patients of hepatobilliary carcinoma

Case	Age	Sex	Diagnosis	Histology*	Tl-Tc subtraction**
1	74	M	Bile duct carcinoma	adenocarcinoma	Positive
2	55	F	Bile duct carcinoma	adenocarcinoma	Positive
3	50	M	Bile duct carcinoma	Well	Positive
4	59	M	Bile duct carcinoma	Poor	Positive
5	65	F	Bile duct carcinoma	Pap	Positive
6	45	F	Bile duct carcinoma	Well	Positive
7	87	M	Bile duct carcinoma		Positive
8	48	M	Gallbladder carcinoma	Poor	Positive
9	52	F	Gallbladder carcinoma	Mod	Positive
10	74	M	Hepatocellular carcinoma		Positive

*Pap:papillary adenocarcinoma, Well: well differentiated tubular adenocarcinoma, Mod: moderately differentiated tubular adenocarcinoma, Poor: poorly differentiated tubular adenocarcinoma
**Overall positive rate of Tl-Tc scan in hepatobiliary carcinoma was 10/10(100%).

Standardized gradual computer subtraction was thereafter performed, removing the liver image and leaving an image of abnormal tissue. The technetium image, representing the normal liver tissue, was subtracted from the thallium image. The final image showed areas of increasing thallium uptake.

RESULTS

As shown in Table 1, in all of 10 patients with hepatobiliary carcinomas, 'hot spots' corresponding to the lesions were shown by the Tl-Tc subtraction technique. In patient 4, a tumor of the polypoid type, measuring 2.2 × 1.5cm, was located in the common hepatic duct. The Tl-Tc subtraction SPECT was able to detect such a small tumor, so our findings demonstrated an extremely high sensitivity for detecting hepatobiliary carcinomas. Three patients who received Tl-Tc subtraction SPECT before treatment had positive results with Tl-201, and Tl-uptake disappeared following the completion of irradiation and transcatheter arterial embolization(TAE). Therefore, Tl-Tc subtraction SPECT was thought to be useful for assessing the tumor response after irradiation and TAE.

An example of a patient with bile duct carcinoma prior and after radiotherapy is shown in Figure 1. Cholangiography showed obstruction at the junction of the right and left hepatic duct (Fig.1A), and a computed tomography scan of the abdomen showed dilated biliary ducts (Fig1B). The Tl-Tc subtraction SPECT (Fig.1C) demonstrates porta hepatis mass with an intense Tl accumulation. The patient was treated with intraluminal irradiation using a remote after loading system. The radiation dose was set at 5Gy at a depth of 1.5cm from energy source, and 30Gy totally. There was a significant decrease in Tl accumulation (Fig1D). The patient showed recurrence 5 months after radiotherapy. At the time of recurrence, there was again an increase in Tl accumulation (Fig.1E).

In another patient with hepatocellular carcinoma, a CT scan showed the main tumor mass in the right lobe (Fig.2A)

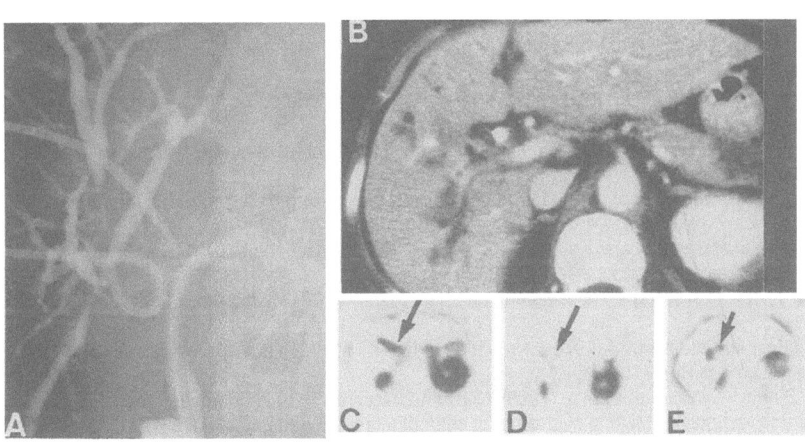

Fig.1 Patient with bile
duct carcinoma
(A)cholangiography
(B)Dynamic CT
(C,D,E)Tl-Tc subtraction
SPECT

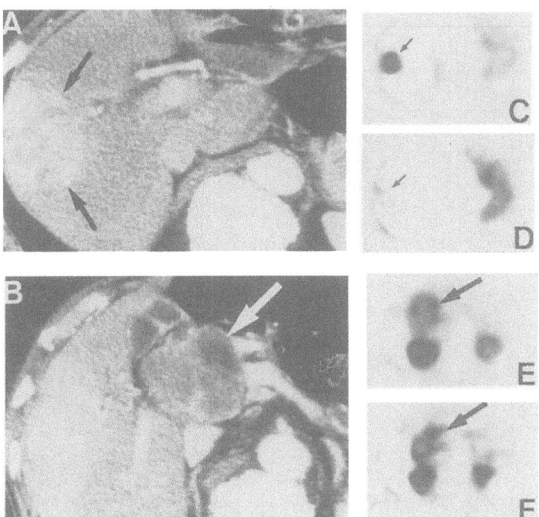

Fig2.Patient with hepatocellular carcinoma
(A,B) Dynamic CT (C,D,E,F) Tl-Tc subtraction
SPECT

and a swelling lymph node in the hepatoduodenal ligament (Fig.2B). Both tumor lesions were shown as 'hot spots' on the Tl-Tc subtraction SPECT image (Fig .2C and 2E).The patient was treated with TAE from the right hepatic artery. There was decreased Tl uptake in the right lobe mass(Fig.2D), but no changes in the hepatoduodenal lymph node mass(Fig.2F).

DISCUSSION

Our results demonstrate that thallium accumulates well in hepatobiliary carcinomas by SPECT, using the Tl-Tc subtraction technique. The mechanism for thallium accumulation in the tumor cells is not fully understood. Part of the thallium uptake is mediated by Na-K-ATPase where the uptake of potassium is replaced by thallium[5]. Levels of Na-K-ATPase in malignant cells were correlated with growth[6].Therefore, thallium is thought to accumulate in malignant tumors. Thallium uptake in several tumors has been shown to be related to viability[7]. Recently thallium has been shown to be an effective radiopharmaceutical in the detection of many types of malignancies[8].
It is difficult to evaluate hepatobiliary tumors radiologically. Tl SPECT was expected to be an effective means of detecting malignancy in hepatobiliary lesion. However, thallium is also taken up by the liver. We have used a subtraction technique which removes a 99mTc liver image, leaving the hepatobiliary tumor as a "hot" area. The results of our study showed that the sensitivity of Tl-Tc subtraction SPECT in detecting hepatobiliary carcinoma was 100%. The CT scan could not differentiate acute reaction lesion by irradiation from a viable tumor, even if a contrast enhanced medium was used. There was a significant decrease in Tl accumulation after radiotherapy and chemotherapy. Tl uptake is a sensitive parameter for the follow-up of recurrences.
In conclusion, we can state that SPECT using the Tl-Tc subtraction technique is a sensitive method for detection of hepatobiliary carcinomas, and for measuring effect after radiotherapy and chemotherapy.

REFERENCES

1. Tonami N, Shuke N, Yokoyama K,Seki H, et al (1989) Thallium-201 single photon computed tomography in the evaluation of suspected lung cancer. J Nucl Med. 30:997-1004
2. Senga O, Miyakawa M, Shirota H, Makiuchi M, et al (1982) Comparison of Tl-201 chloride and Ga-67 citrate scintigraphy in the diagnosis of thyroid tumor. J Nucl Med. 23:225-228
3. Ferlin G, Borsato N, Camerani M, Conte N, et al (1983) New perspectives in localizing enlarged parathyroids by technetium-thalliun subtraction scan. J Nucl Med 24:438-441
4. Togawa T, Yui N, Kinoshita F, Yanagisawa M and Kuniyasu Y (1993) Clinical application of 201Tl SPECT to pancreatobiliary tumors. J.Biliary Tract and Pancreas14:243-254
5. Ito Y, Muranaka A, Harada T, et al (1979) Experimental study on tumor affinity of 201Tl-chloride. Eur J Nucl Med 3:81-86
6. Elligsen JD, Thompson JE, Frey HE and Kruuv J (1974) Correlation of (Na-K)-ATP ase activity with growth of normal and transformed cells. Exp Cell Res 87:233-240
7. Ramanna L, Waxman AD, Binney G, Waxman S, et al (1990) Thallium-201scintigraphy in bone sarcoma: comparison with gallium-67 and technetium-MDP in evaluation of chemotherapeutic response. J Nucl Med 31:567-572
8. Togawa T, Yui N, Kinoshita F, Koakutu M, et al (1991) Diagnosis of pancreatic cancer using 201Tl-chloride and three-head roating gamma camera SPECT system. Jpn J Nucl Med 28:1475-1481

Radioimmunoimaging of Local Recurrence of Rectal Cancer by Radiolabeled Mouse Monoclonal Antibody A7

Toshiharu Yamaguchi[1], Takuya Miyagaki[1], Kazuya Kitamura[1], Eigo Otsuji[1], Nobuki Yamaoka[1], Tatsuya Kotani[1], Makoto Kato[1], Katsunori Taniguchi[1], Hiroki Taniguchi[1], Kiyoshi Sawai[1], Toshio Takahashi[1], Masato Yamashita[2], and Tomoho Maeda[2]

[1]The First Department of Surgery, [2]Department of Radiology, Kyoto Prefectural University of Medicine, Kyoto, Japan

ABSTRACT

Though the definite diagnosis of local recurrence of rectal carcinoma is still difficult, recent rapid development of new diagnostic tools such as ultrasonography, X-ray CT and MRI brought us many information of mass lesion in the body.   One of the most promising approaches to clarify the nature of mass lesion is radioimmunoimaging by radiolabeled tumor specific monoclonal antibody. We had developed mouse monoclonal antibody A7 that is reacted with human adenocarcinoma including colorectal cancer. A7 reacted with glycoprotein that is expressed on the cell surface of cancer. The molecular weight of glycoprotein is 42kD and is proved to be different from CEA and CA19-9. Selective accumulation of 131I-labeled A7 to human cancer tissue was observed in nude mouse model. And 131I-labeled A7 is applied for patients who had mass lesion which suspected to be local recurrence of colorectal carcinoma. Five Mci of radiolabeled A7 diluted in saline was administered intravenously for five patients. One, 2, 3 and 7 days after injection the planner or/and SPECT images of the lesion were obtained by digital gamma camera.

In four out of five patients, the accumulation of radiolabeled A7 could be detected by digital gamma camera. No serious side effects were observed in this series. Though the image was not satisfactory in the case of small lesion, these results suggested that such new approach may be useful in early diagnosis of recurrence of colorectal carcinomas in the future.

Key Words: Radioimmunoimaging, Colorectal carcinoma, Monoclonal antibody

INTRODUCTION

Though the definite diagnosis of local recurrence of rectal carcinoma is still difficult, one of the most promising approaches to clarify the nature of mass lesion is radioimmunoimaging by radiolabeled tumor specific monoclonal antibody. We had developed mouse monoclonal antibody A7 that is reacted with human adenocarcinoma including colorectal cancer. Radiolabeled A7 had been proved to accumulate selectively in primary colon cancer tissue. So we applied radiolabeled A7 for radioimmunoimaging of recurrent colorectal cancer.

MATERIALS AND METHOD

Characters of Monoclonal Antibody A7 : Characters of monoclonal antibody A7 is summarized in Table 1. Immunogen of A7 is human colon cancer serially transplanted in the back of nude mice. A7 belongs to IgG1 class of mouse immunoglobulin and reacts with human colorectal carcinoma, breast cancer, pancreatic cancer, stomach cancer and lung cancer. The epitope detected by A7 was supposed to be protein part of glycoprotein molecular weight around 42kD. The epitope detected by A7 is different from CEA(carcinoembryonic antigen) or CA19-9. Only a trace amount of antigen reacted with A7 could be detected in culture medium of cancer cell lines that had been proved to express epitopes of A7 on cell surface. And clinical study had proved that only a trace amount of antigen was detected by A7 in sera of colon cancer patients. This non-shedding character of epitope of A7 is favorable to apply A7 to radioimmunoimaging of cancer lesion or immunotargeting chemotherapy with antibody-drug conjugate.

(Table 1)Character of Monoclonal Antibody A7

(1)Immunogen:Human colon cancer
(2)IgG1 class mouse monoclonal antibody
(3)Epitope:42kD of glycoprotein on cell membrane, different from CEA and CA19-9.
(4)Reacted with human colon cancer, stomach cancer, pancreas cancer and breast cancer.
(5)Selective accumulation of ^{131}I-labeled A7 to human cancer tissue was observed in nude mouse model.

Preparation of F(ab')2 : A7 was digested with pepsin and the optimal conditions employed were an enzyme-antibody ratio of 1:50. F(ab')2 fraction was separated by gel-filtration on Sephacryl S-200 column.

Clinical Trial : A7 was labeled with ^{131}I by chrolamin T and was administered intravenously to 5 patients who had mass lesion which suspected to be local recurrence of colorectal carcinoma. Three to 6 mCi of radiolabeled A7 or F(ab')2 fragment of A7 diluted in 100ml of saline that contained human albumin was administered intravenously. One, 2, 3 and 7 days after injection the planner or/and SPECT images of the lesion were obtained by digital gamma camera. Total of five patients with metastatic lesion after operation for colorectal carcinoma were entered in this clinical trial.

RESULTS

Monoclonal A7 was successfully digested with pepsin and the purity of F(ag')2 fragments of A7 was confirmed by SDS-PAGE. In four out of five patients, the accumulation of radiolabeled A7 could be detected by digital gamma camera(Table 2). No serious side effects were observed in this series. The image was not satisfactory in the case of small lesion.

Clinical Cases(Table 2)

Pt No.		Dose of ^{131}I-A7	Type of MoAb	Imaging
IM-1	RK	6mCi/1mg	whole A7	positive
IM-2	CK	3mCi/0.5mg	whole A7	positive
IM-3	CK	3mCi/0.5mg	whole A7	negative
IM-4	RK	3mCi/0.5mg	whole A7	positive
IM-4	RK	5mCi/1mg	F(ab')2	positive

(Fig.1)X-ray CT and SPECT Image of Case IM-1
(A) (B)

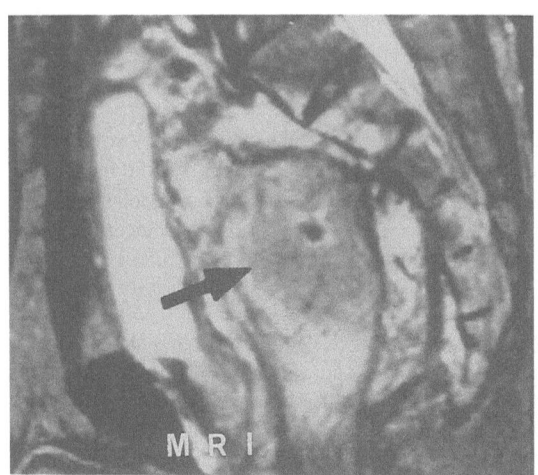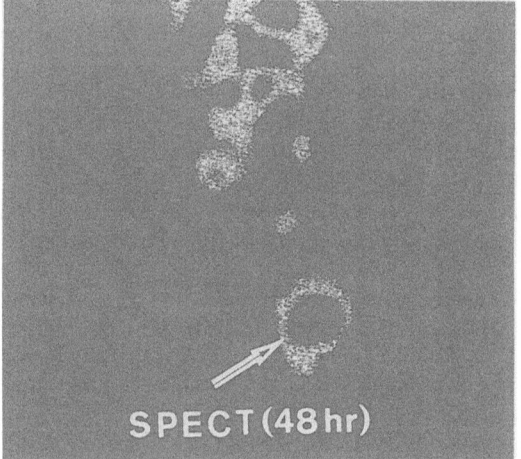

Tumor mass, that was suspected to be recurrence of rectal cancer, was found presacral region of the patient(A). SPECT image clearly showed hot area at the same location(B).

DISCUSSION

Development of new biotechnology had made it possible to apply large amount of high specific monoclonal antibody for diagnosis and treatment of cancer patients. A7 was developed by immunization with human colon cancer cell and it reacts with many kinds of human adenocarcinoma cell lines. We have already applied A7 for immunotargeting chemotherapy of colorectal carcinoma(1). And the possibility of immunoimaging of colorectal cancer using A7 or its fragments were studied extensively(2). Clinical trial of radioimmunoimaging of colorectal cancer had started from 1992(3). In this paper the results of clinical trial of radioimmunoimaging of colorectal cancer with radiolabeled A7 or its fragments. The results was satisfactory for large size lesions though small lesion was difficult to identify. Another kinds of radionuclide such as 111-In or 99m-Tc were reported to be superior to

131-I. We should try to use such radionuclides after confirming the localization in nude mice models before clinical use. We believe that the development of more sensitive machine and application of protein engineering technology will show us more clear image of small caner lesions in the near future.

SUMMARY AND CONCLUSION :

Radioimmunoimaging of recurrent colorectal cancer was tried in 5 patients using ^{131}I-labeled anti-human colorectal carcinoma monoclonal antibody A7. In 4 cases accumulation of radiolabeled A7 could be confirmed, though the image was not clear in cases of small mass lesion. These results suggested that more refined device is necessary for successful imaging of early staged recurrence of colorectal cancers using A7.

This work was supported in part by a Grant-in-Aid for Cancer Research from the Ministry of Education,Science and Culture,Japan and a grant form the Ministry of Health and Welfare,Japan.

REFERENCES

1.Takahashi,T.,Yamaguchi,T.,Kitamura,K.,Suzuyama,H.,Honda,M,Yokota,T.,Kotanagi,H.,Takahashi,M., Hashimoto,Y. Clinical application of monoclonal antibody-drug conjugates for immunotargeting chemotherapy of colorectal carcinoma(1988) Cancer 61:881-888

2.Kitamura,K.,Takahashi,T.,Yamaguchi,T.,Kitai,S.,Amagai,T.,Imanishi,J.MonoclonalantibodyA7tumor localization enhancement by its F(ab')2 fragments to colon carcinoma xenografts in nude mice(1990) Jpn.J.Clin.Oncol.20:139-144

3.Miyagaki,T.,Yamaguchi,T.,Kotani,T.,Yamaoka,N.,Tsurumi,H.,Otsuji,E.,Kitamura,K.,Taniguchi,H.,Sawai,K., Takahashi,T.,Yamashita;M. Radioimmunoimaging of local recurrence of colorectal cancer using 131I-labeled murine monoclonal antibody A7(1992) Jpn.J.Gastrointestinal Surg. 25:2878

Investigation of Thymidylate Synthase Induction in Colorectal Carcinoma Tissues After Administration of Anticancer Drug, Fluorinated Pyrimidine Fluoride Derivatives

KITARO FUTAMI and SUMITAKA ARIMA

Department of Surgery, Chikushi Hospital, Fukuoka University, Chikushino, Fukuoka, 818 Japan

ABSTRACT

Patients with colorectal carcinoma were treated with UFT or Tegafur for 7 days repeated (600mg per day), and 5-FU concentration and inhibition rate of Thymidylate Synthase (TS) in tissues were compared. As a control, total amount of TS was determined in tissues from patients who did not receive any drug. Total amount of TS was compared between UFT or Tegafur group and control group. Both 5-FU concentration and inhibition rate of TS in tumor tissues were significantly higher in UFT group than Tegafur group. Total amounts of TS in tumor tissue, normal mucous membrane, and lymph node were significantly higher in patients treated with drugs than patients who did not receive any drug. Paticularly, high level of TS was induced in patients treated with UFT. Relationship between total amount of TS and inhibition rate of TS in tumor tissues were then studied. Inhibition rate of TS remained 50 to 55 % regardless of total amount of TS.

Key words; TS induction, TS inhibition rate, Colorectal cancer, UFT

INTRODUCTION

It is generally bilieved that 5-FU manifests antitumor activity primarily by inhibiting DNA replication by inhibiting Thymidylate Synthase (TS) by way of its active metabolite, 5-fluorodeoxyuridinemonophosphate (FdUMP). UFT is a masked compound of 5-FU and one of the most widely used antitumor drugs for gastrointestinal carcinoma today. It has been reported that high levels of 5-FU concentration in tumor tissues were achieved after the administration of UFT and that TS was greatly inhibited from basic and clinical studies. Higher levels of TS were detected in tumor tissues than normal mucous membranes, and it has been pointed out that TS was induced in tissues after the administration of pyrimidine fluoride derivatives from basic study. We investigated 5-FU concentration and inhibition rate of TS in tissues after the repeated administration of UFT or Tegafur in patients with colorectal carcinoma and monitored TS activity as compared with cases who did not receive any drug as a control.

MATERIALS AND METHODS

Forty-eight resection cases with colorectal carcinoma were studied. Thirty seven cases were treated with drugs, UFT or Tegafur was administered repeatedly and orally for 7 days, 600 mg daily, 200 mg per administration, 3 times a day before surgery. Tumor tissue, mucous membrane in normal area, and regional lymph node were collected at the timeof surgery. 5-FU concentration, total amount of TS and inhibition rate of TS in various tissues were measured. Twenty cases received UFT, 17 cases received Tegafur, and these two groups were compared. Eleven cases did not receive any drug. various tissues were collected from these 11 patients as well at the time of surgery, and total amount of TS was measured. Total amount of TS was compared between dose group and control group. 5-FU concentrations in tissues were measured by Gas Chromatogfaphic Mass Fragmentgraphic Method. TS was measured according to a modified method by Spears, total amount of TS and

570

free TS were measured, and inhibition rate of TS was calculated by [(1-TS free/TS total) × 100%].

RESULTS

1. Comparison of 5-FU concentration among Dose groups (Fig. 1); 5FU concentration in tumor tissues was 0.208 ± 0.143 μg/g among UFT group, and 0.077 ± 0.027 μg/g among Tegafur group. UFT group showed significantly higher ($p<0.05$). In metastasized lymph node, UFT group showed higher 5-FU concentration, but no statical significance was detected. No difference was seen in normal mucous membrane and non-metastasized lymph node between two groups.

2. Comparison of Inhibition Rate of TS among Dose Groups (Fig. 2); Inhibition rates of TS in Tumor tissue was 56.12 % among UFT group and 45 % among Tegafur group. UFT group showed a significantly higher inhibition rate. In normal mucous membrane, It was 39 % among UFT group and 38 % among Tegafur group.

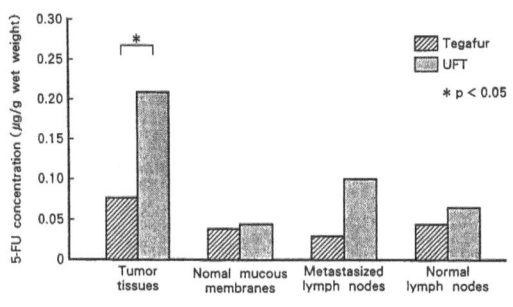

Figure 1. 5-FU concentrations after UFT or Tegafur administration

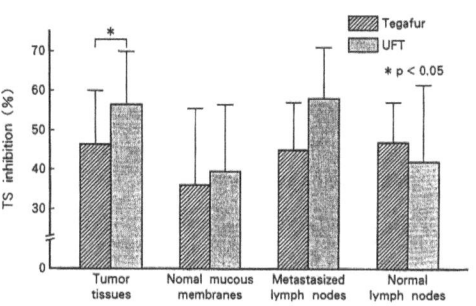

Figure 2. Inhibition rate of TS after UFT or Tegafur administration

3. Comparison of TS total in Normal Mucous Membrane and Lymph Node (Table.1); In normal mucous membrane and lymph node, both UFT and Tegafur group showed stastically higher total TS than control group.

Table. 1

TS total	mucous membrane	lymph node
UFT group	4,80±3.05 p mol/g	13.6 ±11.0 p mol/g
Tegafur group	3.52± 1.63	6.43± 3.86
control group	1.52± 1.35	2.43± 3.70

4. Comparison of Total TS in Tumor Tissues (Fig. 3); Total TS in tumor tissue were 16.35 ± 13.15 p mol/g among UFT group, 11.90 ± 9.84 p mol/g among TS group, and 4.95 ± 5.96 p mol/g among control group. Both UFT group and Tegafur group showed stastically higher total TS than control group.

5. Relationship between Total TS and Inhibition Rate of TS in Tumor Tissues (Fig. 4); Inhibition rate of TS was 50 to 55 % regardless of total TS.

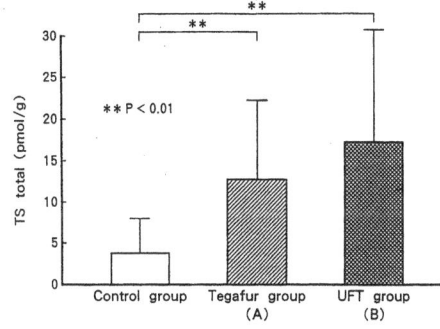

Figure 3. Total amounts of TS in tumor tissues

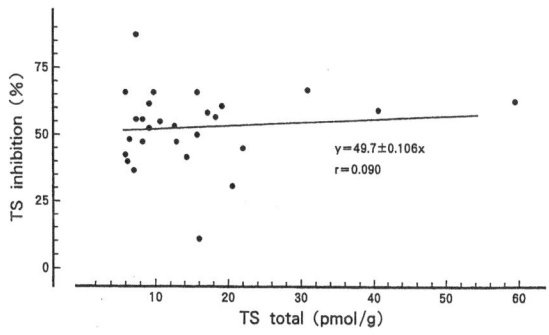

Figure 4. Relationship between total amounts of TS and inhibition rate of TS in tumor tissues

DISCUSSION

We investigated 5-FU concentration and inhibition rate of TS in tissues after administration of UFT or Tegafur. Both 5-FU concentration and inhibition rate of TS in tumor tissue after administration of UFT were higher than Tegafur. Consequently, UFT may have a component which is responsible for more potent antitumor activity against colorectal carcinoma than Tegafur. The mechanism of antitumor activity of 5-FU is at clinical dose as follows. 5-FU is taken up in tumor tissues, 5-FU is converted to FdUMP in tumor cells, FdUMP-TS-methylene hydrofolate binds, and then the ternary complex is formed.TS activity will be inhibited by the ternary complex, DNA replication will be inhibited, and eventually antitumor effect will be manifested. Our clinical study showed that TS was induced in various tissues, especially tumor tissue, after administration of pyrimidine fluoride (UFT and Tegafur), but inhibition rate of TS remained 50 to 55 % regardless of total TS. This level of inhibition rate of TS may be the limitation by administration of clinical dose of UFT alone. It could be due to depletion of methylene hydroforate, but in order to prove this theory, determination of methylene hydroforate as well as TS in tumor tissue may be required.

REFERENCE

1)Cohen, S.S., Flaks, J.G., Barner, M.D., et al.: The mode of action of 5-fluorouracil and its derivatives. Proc. Natl. Acad. Sci. USA, 44: 1004-1012, 1958.
2)Fujii, S, Ikenaka, K., Shirasaka, T., et al.: Effect of Uracil and its derivatives on antitumor activity of 5-fluorouracil and 1-(2-tetrahydrofuryl)-5-fluorouracil. Gann, 69 ; 763-772, 1978.
3)Nakamura, H., Wang Y.Q., Miyauchi, S., et al.: Studies on the mechanism of antitumor activity of 5-FU and its derivatives-Relationship between the inhibition of tumor growth and the inhibition of thymidylate synthase in vivo. Jp. J. Cancer Chemother, 11: 1049-1056, 1984.
4)Walberg, W.H. and Moris, J.: Thymidylate synthase activity and fluorouracil sensitivity of human colonic cancer and normal mucosal tissues preparations. Cancer, 47: 1313-1317, 1981.
5)Takeda, S., Uchida, J., Yamada, Y., et al.: The significance of measuring inhibition of thymidylate synthase activity as a parameter for antitumor activity of 5-fluorouracil derivatives. Jpn. J. Cancer Chemother, 15: 2125-2130, 1988.
6)Oie, S., Okabe, H., Takeda, S., et al.: Analysis of the mechanism of increased antitumor activity of UFT after combined treatment with CDDP. Jpn. J. Cancer Chemother, 17: 132-1326, 1990.
7)Shirasaka, T., Shimamoto, Y., Kinoshita, H., et al.: Mechanism for synergistic antitumor effect in the combination of 5-fluorouracil with cisplatin in vivo tumor models: from the view of biochemical moduration of 5-fluorouracil. Jpn. J. Cancer Chemother, 18: 403-409, 1991.
8)Spears, C.P., Gustarsson, B.G., Berne, M., et al.: Mechanism of innate resistance to thymidylate synthase inhibition after 5-fluorouracil. Cancer Res., 48: 5894-5900, 1988.

Effect and Action Mechanism of Prostaglandin E2 on Proliferation of Human Colon Cancer Cells in Culture

Michio Kato[1], Satoru Okumoto[2], Yoichi Saitoh[2], Yuichi Hori[1],
Daisuke Kuroda[1], Hideaki Nomura[1], Shinichi Nishimatsu[1],
and Harumasa Ohyanagi[1]

[1]Department of Surgery II, Kinki University School of Medicine, Osaka-Sayama, Osaka, 589 Japan
[2]Department of Surgery I, Kobe University School of Medicine, Kobe, 650 Japan

ABSTRACT

The effect of prostaglandin E2(PGE2) on the growth of human colon cancer cell line HT-29 was investigated. PGE2 significantly inhibited the growth of HT-29 cells without increasing cyclicAMP production. Furthermore, the proliferation of HT-29 cell was not suppressed by the administration of vasoactive intestinal peptide or dibutyryl cyclicAMP. The metabolism of PGE2 in the culture medium showed that a considerable amount of PGA2 was produced from PGE2. These observations suggest that PGE2 inhibits the cell growth of HT-29 without stimulation of cAMP production, and that this inhibitory effect was due to the metabolic change of PGE2 to PGA2.

KEY WORDS: prostaglandin E2, colon cancer, cyclic AMP

INTRODUCTION

Inflammatory cell infiltration is often observed in colon tumor tissues, and these inflammatory cells are considered to include prostaglandin-producing cells. Some tumor cells are also reported to produce prostaglandins. We studied the effects of PGE2 on the proliferation of colon tumor cells.

MARERIALS AND METHODS

Chemicals

Prostaglandin E2(PGE2) provided by Ono Pharmaceutical Co. Ltd., vasoactive intestinal peptide(VIP) and 3-isobutyl-1-methylxanethine(IBMX) of Sigma, and dibutyryl cyclic AMP(dbcAMP) of Yamasa Shoyu were used.

Cell culture and growth experiments

HT-29 cells established from well differentiated human colon adenocarcinoma were used. The culture medium was Dulbecco's modified Eagle's medium supplemented with 5% fetal calf serum. Penicillin G and streptomycin were added to the medium. The cells were cultured at 37℃ in 5% CO2 and the medium was changed every other day.

Tumor cells were suspended at 4.0×10^4 cells/ml in the medium, and 0.5ml of the cell suspension was placed in each well of a 24-well plate. PGE2 was added to this culture medium every other day at a final concentration of 1, 3, 5, or 10 μ g/ml. The cells were counted on Days 4 and 6 of culture.

Stimulation of cyclic AMP(cAMP) production in HT-29 cells by PGE2 and VIP.

Tumor cells were suspended at 1.0×10^6 cells/ml with the culture medium, and 1 ml of the cell suspension was placed in each well of a 6-well plate. The cells were cultured for 24 hours and were washed with PBS. Next, at a BSA concentration of 1 mg/ml, 0.8 ml of 10^{-5} M IBMX was added to HEPES-buffered Krebs Ringer bicarbonate buffer containing 2.5 mM glucose(HKRBG), and the plate was incubated at 37℃ for 15 minutes. Next, various concentration of PGE2 and VIP were added to the wells, and the plate was incubated at 37℃ for 15minutes. One milliliter of cooled 12% TCA solution was added to the wells, and the plate was cooled with ice for 20 minutes. The suspension of detached cells was centrifuged at 3000rpm for 5 minutes , and the supernatant was washed 3 times with the same volume of diethyl ether. cAMP was measured by radioimmunoassay.

Effects of VIP and dbcAMP on cell proliferation

Similarly to the experiment using PGE2, 0.5ml of a cell suspension(2.0x10^4 cells/well) was placed in each well of a 24-well plate. VIP was added at a final concentration of 10^{-7}, 10^{-8}, 10^{-9},10^{-10}, 10^{-11}M, dbcAMP was added at a final concentration of 10^{-3}, 10^{-4}, 10^{-5}M, and the cells were cultured at 37℃ in 5% CO2 for 4 days. The medium was changed every day, and viable cells were counted on Day 4.

Metabolism of PGE2 to prostaglandin A2(PGA2) in the medium

To measure the amount of PGA2 resulting from progressive metabolism of PGE2 in the medium, the ratio between PGE2 and PGA2 in the culture medium was determined by high-performance liquid chromatography, and the percentage of PGE2 metabolized to PGA2 was evaluated.

RESULTS

Addition of PGE2 significantly inhibited the growth of HT-29 cells on Day 4 and on Day 6 after the biginning of culture(Figure 1a). The percentage of the cell count after culture with 1, 3, 5, and 10 μ g/ml PGE2 relative to the control value showed dose-dependent inhibitory effect of PGE2 both on Day 4(Fig. 1b) and on Day 6(Fig. 1c) of culture.
The intracellular cAMP concentration in the cells stimulated with 1, 5, and 10 μ g/ml PGE2 did not increase significantly as compared with the control group(Fig.2a). When the cells were stimulated with 10^{-11} to 10^{-7} M VIP, the intracellular cAMP concentration was increased by additioning of VIP at a concentration of more than10^{-10}M(Fig.2b).
The percentage of the cell count after culture with 10^{-11} to 10^{-7}M VIP relative to the control value on Day 4 showed growth stimulatory effect of VIP at the concentration of 10^{-10} and 10^{-9}M (Fig.3a). The cell count of the cells cultured with 10^{-5} to 10^{-3}M dbcAMP was not decreased, and the increase in the exogenous cAMP concentration had no inhibitory effect on cell proliferation(Fig.3b).
The ratio between PGA2 and PGE2(PGA2/PGE2 ratio) in the medium was expressed as the mean of 5 samples. The PGA2/PGE2 ratio was 35.8±10.2% after 24 hours and by 83.8±6.3% after 48 hours of incubation.

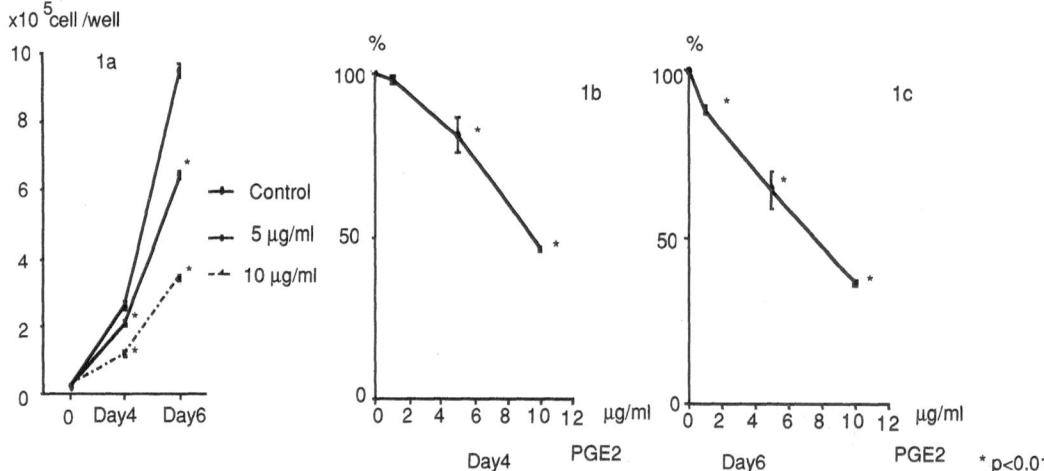

Fig. 1 Cell counts of HT-29 cells, cultured with 5 μ g/ml and 10 μ g/ml PGE2, on Day 4 and Day 6 after the beginning of culture were significantly smaller than in the control group(1a). The percentage of the cell counts after culture with PGE2 relative to the control value on Day 4 (1b) and on Day 6(1c) of culture showed dose-response inhibition of cell growth.

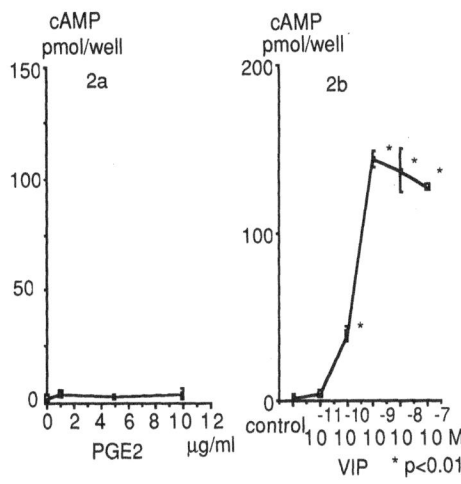

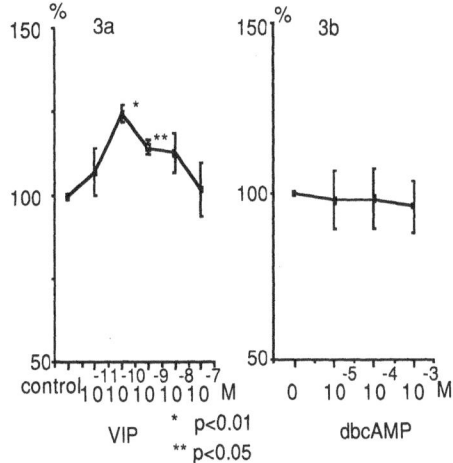

Fig. 2 Effects of PGE2 on cAMP production showed
no significant difference with the control group(2a).
Effects of VIP on cAMP production showed significant

increase of the intracelullar cAMP concentration (2b).

Fig. 3 The percentage of the cell count after culture with
VIP relative to the control value on Day 4 of culture
showed a growth stimulatory effect of VIP at the

concentration of 10^{-10} and 10^{-9}M (3a). Effects of
dbcAMP on the growth of HT-29 cells showed no
significant change(3b).

DISCUSSION

PGE2 has been reported to promote or inhibit tumor cell proliferation, and the findings vary with the cell type and other
factors. In this study, it inhibited proliferation of HT-29 colon cancer cells. Since the PGE2 concentration was reported to
exceed 1 μ g/g in some human colon cancer tissues, marked inflammatory cell infiltration in the tumor tissue may have an
inhibitory effect on tumor cell proliferation.
PGE2 has been reported to inhibit cell proliferation by increasing cAMP production by acting on the cell membrane(1), and
attempts to treat cancer with cAMP have been made. However, PGE2 inhibited the proliferation of HT-29 cells without
increasing the cAMP production. Also, proliferation of HT-29 cells was not inhibited even when the cAMP concentration in
tumor cells was exogenously or endogenously increased by the addition of VIP or dbcAMP. Therefore, the inhibition of
proliferation of HT-29 cells by PGE2 is not considered to be dependent on an increase in cAMP production.
In some reports, PGA2, a metabolite of PGE2, was considered to be responsible for the inhibition of cell proliferation(2). Also,
PGA2 is considered to act without affecting adenylate cyclase on the cell membrane(3). In this study, a considerable amount
of PGA2 was produced from PGE2 within 48hours from the beginning of culture. Tumor cell proliferation, therefore, may have
been inhibited by PGA2 generated by metabolism of PGE2.

REFERENCES

1. Nakamura A, Chiba T, Yamatani T, Yamaguchi A, Inui T, Morishita T, Kadowaki S, Fujita T(1989) Prostaglandin E2 and F2 α
inhibit growth of human gastric carcinoma cell line KATO Ⅲ with simultaneous stimulation of cyclic AMP production. Life Sci.
44:75-80
2. Ohno K, Fujiwara M, Fukushima M, Narumiya S(1986) Metabolic dehydration of prostaglandin E2 and cellular uptake of
the dehydration product: Correlation with prostaglandin E2 induced growth inhibition. Biochem. Biophys. Res. Commun.
139:808-815
3. Marumiya S, Fukushima M(1986) Site and mechanism of growth inhibition by prostaglandins. Ⅰ.Active transport and
intracellular accumulation of cyclopentenone prostaglandins, a reaction leading to growth inhibition. J. Pharmacol. Exp. Ther.
239:500-505

Combination Therapy with CPT-11 and Interferon-α Against Human Colon Carcinoma in Nude Mice

Isao Kobayashi[1], Susumu Ohwada[1], Yukio Miyamoto[1], Yasuo Morishita[1], Tetsuo Taguchi[2], and Masahide Fujita[2]

[1]The Second Department of Surgery, Gunma University, Maebashi, 371 Japan
[2]The Department of Surgery, Research Institute for Microbial Diseases, Osaka University, Suita, Osaka, Japan

ABSTRACT

We studied the antitumor effect of INF-α and CPT-11 against human colon carcinoma in nude mice. CPT-11 and INF-α were administered intraperitoneally every 4 days and subcutaneously every day, respectively. The results were as follows: 1) the INF-α (1×10^5 I.U./body) alone achieved no antitumor effects. 2) the CPT-11 alone significantly ($p<0.02$) achieved antitumor effects with the dose dependence. 3) The combination of CPT-11 and INF-α achieved better synergistic antitumor effects than the single dose of CPT-11 ($p<0.02$). The mechanism of synergistic antitumor effects of CPT-11 and INF-α remains unclear, but one of these mechanisms may be the cell cycle progression.

KEY WORDS: Interferon-alfa, CPT-11, Human Colon Carcinoma,
           Nude Mice, Cell Cycle Progression

INTRODUCTION

CPT-11 is a semisynthesized derivative of camptothecin that has the potent antitumor activity of inhibiting DNA topoisomerase I. CPT-11 is an effective agent for colorectal cancer in experimental models and clinical trials. The combination of interferons and fluorouracil or alkaloid has synergistic cytotoxic activity against human cancers. The aim of this study was to examine the antitumor effect of interferon-alfa (INF-α) and CPT-11 against human colon carcinoma in nude mice and the mechanism of combination effects on the cell cycle progression of tumor cells.

MATERIALS AND METHODS

Animals. Athymic BALB/c nude mice (6 to 8 weeks of age) were obtained from the Research Institute for Laboratory Animal Science of Gunma University. The mice were housed in laminar flow cabinets under specific pathogen-free conditions.

Human tumor cell lines-in vivo growth. The human colon carcinoma line, H-110, was a generous gift from Dr. T. Taguchi (The Department of Surgery, Research Institute for Microbial Diseases, Osaka University, Suita, Japan). Transplantation of tumor cells and evaluation of antitumor effects. H-110 was transplanted subcutaneously on the back of each mouse with a 14 Gage trocal needle. The diameter of growing tumors was measured with calipers every week. The tumor weight was calculated from the length (a) and the width (b) of tumors measured with calipers in milimeters according to the Battelle Columbus Laboratories Protocol. The calculation was done as follows:

$$\text{Tumor weight (mg)} = \frac{a \times b^2}{2}$$

The data were expressed as the relative weight using the following formula.

$$\text{Relative tumor weight} = \frac{\text{mean tumor weight at a given time}}{\text{initial mean tumor weight}}$$

Drug treatment. The tumor was allowed to grow for 4 weeks, then drug injection was started. The mice were randomly allocated into 4 groups with at least 5 mice in each group. Drugs were injected into mice of all groups for 41 days as follows; a) saline (0.1ml), subcutaneously (s.c.) every day and intraperitoneally (i.p.) every 4 days, (control group); b) INF-α (1 × 10^5 I.U./body), s.c. every day (INF-α group); c) CPT-11 (10, 25 or 50 mg/kg/body), i.p. every 4 days (CPT-11 group); d) INF-α (1 × 10^5 I.U./body), s.c. every day and CPT-11 (10 , 25 or 50 mg/kg/body) i.p. every 4 days (combination group). Then, the mice were sacrificed for the analysis of tumor cells.

Analysis of cell cycle progression. Mice were sacrificed 1 hour after the intravenous injection of BrdU (20mg/kg). The phase of the cell cycle was analyzed by flow cytometry.

Statistical analysis. The statistical significance of differences was examined by using Student's t test. A p value of less than 0.05 was considered significant.

RESULTS

Antitumor effect. No significant antitumor effect on H-110 was seen in the INF-α group (Fig. A). The single dose of CPT-11 showed antitumor effects at dosages of 10, 25 and 50 mg/kg each compared with the control group. Its effect was increased significantly ($p<0.02$) with the dose dependance three weeks after the treatment. The combination group achieved significantly better antitumor effects than the single dose of 10 or 25mg/kg of CPT-11 from three weeks after the treatment ($p<0.02$), and than the single dose of 50mg/kg of CPT-11 at six weeks after the treatment ($p<0.02$).

Cell cycle progression. The ratio of the cells in the G0/G1 phase vs the whole cells increased significantly in the INF-α group as opposed to those in the control group ($p<0.02$). The ratio of the cells in the G2/M phase vs the whole cells increased significantly in the combination group as opposed to those in the CPT-11 group ($p<0.02$) (Table 1).

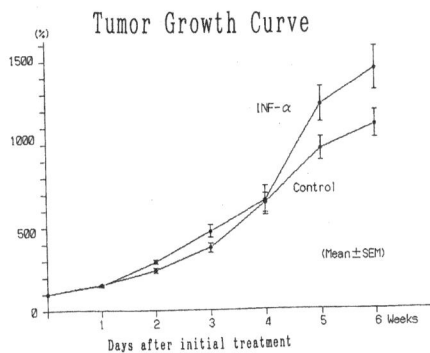

Fig. A No significant antitumor effect on H-110 was seen in the INF-α group compared with the control group.

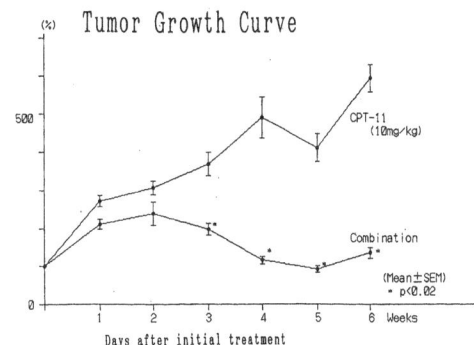

Fig. B The combination group achieved better antitumor effects than the single dose of CPT-11 (10mg/kg) from 3 weeks after the treatment (p<0.02).

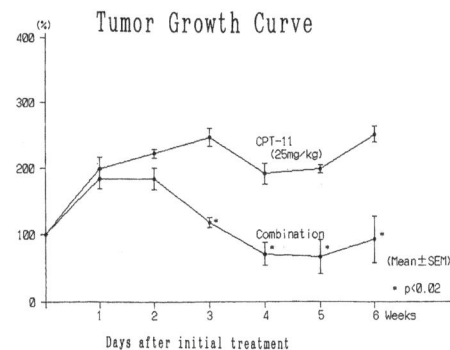

Fig. C The combination group achieved better antitumor effects than the single dose of CPT-11 (25mg/kg) from 3 weeks after the treatment (p<0.02).

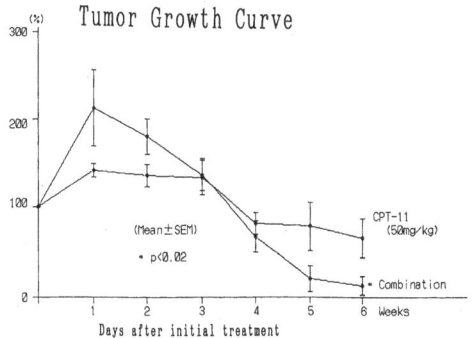

Fig. D The combination group achieved better antitumor effects than the single dose of CPT-11 (50mg/kg) at 6 weeks after the treatment (p<0.02).

Table 1. Cell Cycle Progression of H-110

	G_0/G_1	S			G_2/M
		early	middle	late	
control	75.0	4.0	2.0	2.3	16.7
INF-α	80.9*	8.1	2.0	1.8	7.2
CPT-11	69.1	12.3	3.6	3.9	11.3
combination	57.9	9.7	4.9	5.7	21.8*

Cell Cycle Phase (%)

* P< 0.02 vs control
Values = Mean

The ratio of cells in the G0/G1 phase vs the whole cells increased
significantly in the INF-α group as opposed to those in the control
group (p<0.02). The ratio of the cells in the G2/M phase vs the whole
cells increased significantly in the combination group as opposed to
those in the control group (p<0.02).

DISCUSSION

The administration of CPT-11 alone achieved significant dose dependent
antitumor effects on human colon carcinoma in nude mice. The combination
therapy of CPT-11 and INF-α achieved synergistic antitumor effects compared
with the CPT-11 alone. The mechanism of synergistic effects of CPT-11 and INF-
α remains unclear. CPT-11 inhibited DNA synthesis in the S phase and caused
a G2 accumulation[1]. In our study, CPT-11 caused an early S phase
accumulation. Some investigators have shown that INF-α delayed cell
transition of the G0/G1 phase to the S phase[2], whereas, others observed that
INF-α caused an S phase accumulation[3]. The present study showed INF-α
alone caused a G0/G1 phase accumulation. The combination therapy of INF-α
and CPT-11 caused a G2/M phase accumulation. An interaction of INF-α and
CPT-11 caused tumor cell cycle progression and achieved synergistic antitumor
effects.

REFERENCES

1) Gallo RC, Whang-Peng J, Adamson RH (1971) Studies on the antitumor
activity, mechanism of action, and cell cycle effects of camptothecin.
J Nat Cancer Inst 46: 789-795

2) Creasey AA, Bartholomew JC, Merigan TC (1980) Role of G0/G1 arrest in the
inhibition of tumor cell growth by interferon. Proc Natl Acad Sci 77:
1471-1475

3) Muro M, Naomoto Y, Orita K (1991) Mechanism of the combined antitumor
effect of natural human tumor necrosis factor-α and natural human
interferon-α on cell cycle progression. Jpn J Cancer Res 82: 118-126

Expressions of HLA and Adhesion Molecules in Colorectal Cancer and the Effects of Local Administration of Interferon (IFN) Gamma and OK-432

MASAHIKO SHIBATA, KATSUYUKI ANDO, HIDEHIRO TAKIZAWA, HIROSHI MIYAKE, SADAO AMANO, and YASUHIKO KUROSU

The First Department of Surgery, Nihon University School of Medicine, Itabashi-ku, Tokyo, 173 Japan

ABSTRACT

For a local control of the tumor, it is important for T lymphocytes to recognize tumor cells. For these, the expressions of HLA and adhesion molecules such as ICAM-I and LFA-3 on tumor cells are essential. The expressions of HLA-DR, ICAM-I and LFA-3 on tumor cells were highest in patients with Dukes A and decreased as the disease advanced to Dukes B and C. The populations of CD3(+), CD4(+) and CD8(+) cells in TIL were significantly higher in the cases in which HLA Class I or HLA-DR was highly expressed on tumor cells. IFN gamma and OK432 elevated expressions of these molecules on tumor cells as well as the percentage of certain subsets of T lymphocytes in TIL.

Key Words: Colorectal Cancer, Interferon gamma, OK-432, HLA, Adhesion Molecules

INTRODUCTION

The products of major histocompatibility complex and adhesion molecules play a major role in T lymphocytes' recognition of tumor cells(1). Thus, the interactions of these molecules on tumor cells and T lymphocytes may be very important in a local control of malignancy. Interferon gamma has been reported to enhance the expressions of HLA and ICAM-I in vitro and in vivo(2,3). OK-432 is reported to be one of the most effective biological responce modifiers(BRM) which is clinically applicable(4). To evaluate the expressions of these molecules on tumor cells of colorectal cancer, surgically obtained specimens were examined immunohistochemically for these molecules. IFN gamma and OK-432 were locally administered before surgery. Expressions of HLA Class I and DR and adhesion molecules on tumor cells were analysed according to clinicopathological findings of the cancer in non-treated group and the results obtained in IFN gamma and OK-432 groups were compared with those of control group in this study.

MATERIALS AND METHODS

Sixty five cases of colorectal cancers consisting 45 for control group, 7 for IFN gamma-treated group and 4 for OK-432-treated group were entered. For these BRM-injection groups, 10^6 units of IFN gamma(Shionogi pharmaceuticals) or 5KE of OK-432(Chugai pharmaceuticals) were locally injected on 7 days before surgery. The specimens were taken from surgery and sent to our laboratory. These were stained with Hematoxylin-Eosine and immunohistochemistry by ordinary ABC manner. Monoclonal antibodies used for immunohistochemistry were for HLA Class I and HLA-DR(Dako Inc.), ICAM-I and LFA-3(CD54 and 58, Cosmo Bio Inc.) for tumor cells and CD3, CD4, CD8, CD16(Beckton Dickinson Inc.), CD2 and CD11a(Dako Inc.) for tumor infiltrating lymphocytes(TIL). Expressions of HLA, adhesion molecules and subsets of TIL by immunohistochemistry were classified as (+) and (-), and infiltration of TIL were classified into the groups of (-), (+),(+) and (++).

RESULTS

Immunohistochemical staining with anti-HLA, ICAM-I and LFA-3 showed that
normal colorectal epithelium did not express HLA-DR, ICAM-I and LFA-3 antigens.
However cancer tissues expressed HLA-DR and LFA-3. Expressions of HLA Class I,
HLA-DR, ICAM-I and LFA-3 were analysed according to some clinicopathological
findins of the cancer. There were no statistically significant differences
in the expressions according to the types of histology or invasion(expansive
or infiltrative). Expressions of these molecules were higher in the cases
without metastases to liver or lymphnode or serosal invasion. As shown in
Figure 1, expressions of HLA-DR, ICAM-I and LFA-3 were highest in in patients
with Dukes A and these decreased as the disease advanced to Dukes B to C.
In the expressions of HLA ClassI, same tendency was observed. TIL subsets
were analysed according to the expressions of HLA Class I and HLA-DR on
tumor cells. Percentages of the patients with high infiltration of TIL(+,++)
were increased by administration of IFN gamma or OK-432(Figure 2), but these
changes were not statistically significant. Next, effects on expressions of
HLA Class I, HLA-DR, ICAM-I and LFA-3 were investigated. As shown in Figure 3,
HLA-DR, ICAM-I and LFA-3 were expressed more in OK-432-treated group and
HLA Class I and LFA-3, in IFN gamma-treated group, both compared with expressions in the control group. Subsets of TIL were also analysed. IFN gamma
increased percentages of CD3(+), CD8(+), CD2(+) and CD18(+) cells and OK-432
did that of CD2(+) cells. But the percentage of CD16(+) cells was not increased by the administration of these BRMs.

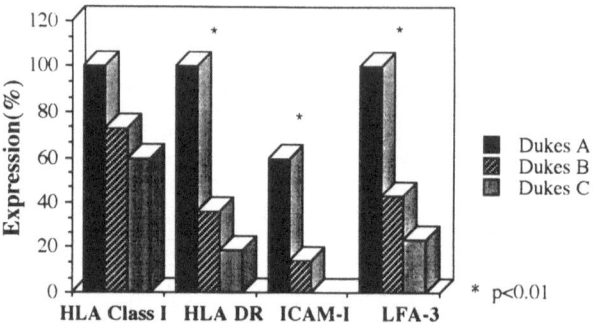

Figure 1. Expressions of HLA and Adhesion Molecules
on Colorectal Cancer Cells according to Dukes classification

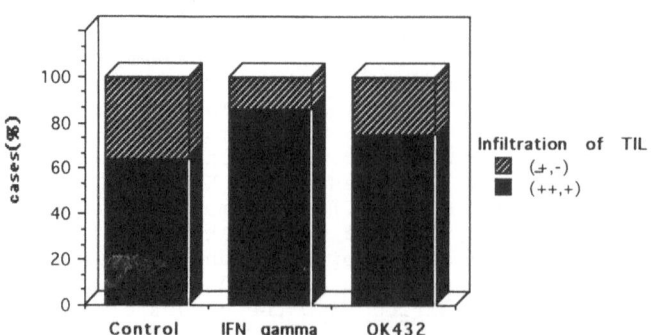

Figure 2. Effects of BRMs on Infiltration of Tumor
Infiltrating Lymphocytes in Colorectal Cancer

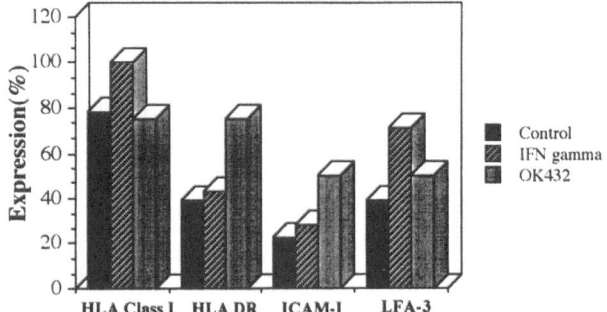

Figure 3. Effects of BRMs on the Expressions of HLA and Adhesion Molecules on Tumor Cells

DISCUSSION

It is very important for the tumor cells to be recognized by T lymphocytes. For these, local expressions of HLA and adhesion molecules such as ICAM-I and LFA-3 on the tumor cells are essential. In this study, not only the natural expression status of these molecules in colorectal cancers according to the clinicopathological findings but also the effects of local administrations of IFN gamma and OK-432 were reported in this study. In the control group, the expressions of these molecules were highest in the cases in which the disease was locally limited and decreased as the disease advanced. Since expressions of these molecules are necessary for localcontrol of malignant tumors, it is required to find an agent which can increase the levels of these expressions. We tested 2 BRMs in this study. IFN gamma and OK-432 both showed effectiveness in an enhancement of TIL infiltration, especially in T lymphocytes, and local expressions of HLA and adhesion molecules. It seemed to be useful to administer BRMs such as IFN gamma and OK-432 locally for the patients whose colon cancer does not express HLA and adhesion molecules such as patients with advanced colorectal carcinoma from our observations in this study. Further evaluation has to be done.

REFERENCES

1. Roitt IM, Brostoff J, Male DK (1985) Immunosurveillance. Immunology 18: 11-13
2. Marley GM, Doyle LA, Ordonez JV (1989) Potentiation of interferon induction of class 1 major histocompatibility complex antigen expression by human tumor necrosis factor in small cell lung cancer cell lines. Cancer Res 49:6232-6236
3. Rosa Mf, Fellous M (1988) Regulation of HLA-DR gene by IFN-gamma. Transcriptional and post-transcriptional control. J Immunol 140: 1660-1664
4. Kurosu Y, Matsumoto S, Nakanishi H, Morita K (1985) Adjuvant immunotherapy of gastric and colorectal cancers using streptococcal preparation OK-432. Recent advances in Chemotherapy, Univ of Tokyo Press:721-722

A New Chemotherapy to Reduce the Local Recurrence of Rectal Cancer

Kazuya Kitamura, Toshio Takahashi, Katsunori Taniguchi, Makoto Katoh, Tatsuya Kotani, Nobuki Yamaoka, Eigo Otsuji, and Toshiharu Yamaguchi

First Department of Surgery, Kyoto Prefectural University of Medicine, Kyoto, 602 Japan

ABSTRACT

This report investigates the application of monoclonal antibody A7 and its drug conjugate ininhibiting the local recurrence of rectal cancer. The experimental protocol consisted of local retension, lymphatic delivery andinhibitory effect of tumor development. These studies revealed that the locally injected immunoconjugate showed a high tumor localization, lymphatic delivery and highly inhibitory effect on tumor development. This finding indicates that local injection of immunoconjugate is a promising new field for inhibiting local recurrence of rectal cancer.

KEY WORDS : monoclonal antibody, colorectal cancer, local recurrence

INTRODUCTION

In spite of radical operations, a large number of patient have died of local recurrence without distant metastasis at rates of 19 to 42 percent[1]. Preventing local recurrence is vital to colorectal cancer treatment and consequently a new type of cancer therapy is required. For the most part, local recurrence of colorectal cancer is thought to result from a regrowth of remnant cancer cells surrounding the rectum. A new therapeutic mode of cancer chemotherapy, therefore, should be directed at eliminating residual cancer cells with target specificity and with fewer adverse side effects. Monoclonal antibody–drug conjugate may specifically target cancer cells and efficiently eliminate the cancer cells, especially with local administration. In this study, we focused on the application of Mab A7 and A7–NCS, which selectively react to human colorectal cancer, for the local control of colorectal cancer. This is the report describing the application of monoclonal antibody–drug conjugate in preventing local recurrence of colorectal cancer.

MATERIALS AND METHODS

Peri-tumoral injection of [125I]–Mab A7.

A solution containing human colon cancer cell line–SW1116 was injected into the posterior thigh of athymic nude mice (Balb/c, nu/u). The mice developed palpable tmor on their thigh 14 days after inoculation, which ranged from 0.2 g to 0.4 g in weight. [125I]–Mab A7[2–5] and non–specific IgG were administered locally to the thigh muscle at the distal portion of the tumor. The mice were sacrificed 6, 12, 18 and 24 h after injection. The tumor were resected and weighed, and the radioactivity was measured in a gamma counter. For comparison, [125]–Mab A7 was injected IV into the athymic nude mice. The following procedure was the same as described above.

Lymph node accumulation.

Ten μl of saline solution containing [125I]–Mab A7 was injected into the pelvis or foot pad of Balb/c mice via the anal mucosa. The mice were sacrificed 2 h after injection. The ipsilateral– and contralateral popliteal, para–aortic, and pericolic lymph node were removed and the radioactivity was measured in a gamma counter.

Local injection of A7-NCS into mice bearing cancer cells but no palpable tumor.
Initially, solution containing SW1116 cells was injected into the thighs of athymic nude mice. Three days after the injection, single local injections of 50 μl solution of A7-NCS equivalent to 5 U of NCS, 5 U of NCS in 50 μl of saline and saline alone were administered locally to the area near the cell-inoculated site. For comparison, an A7-NCS solution equivalent to 5 U of NCS and an A7-NCS solution mixed with 100-fold the amount of free Mab A7 were administered IV and locally to athymic nude mice 3 days after the cell injection, respectively. Tumor development in the thigh was followed 7, 14 and 21 days after the treatment. The mice, divided into five groups, were compared using the ratio of palpable tumor development after the treatment. In a separate experiment, a solution containing KB cells was injected into the thigh of athymic nude mice. Three days after the cell injection, single local injections of 50 μl solution of A7-NCS equivalent to 5 U of NCS , 5 U of NCS in 50 μl of saline and saline alone were administered locally to the area near the cell-inoculated site. The ratio of tumor development was followed as described above.

RESULTS

Local retension property.

[125I]-Mab A7 accumulation in the tumor was greater in the peritumoral injection than in the intravenous injection. Peritumoral injection of [125I]-non-specific IgG showed a lower accumulation in the tumor than that of [125I]-Mab A7 (Fig.1).

Lymph node accumulation.

In the pelvic injections, a significantly higher accumulation of [125I]-Mab A7 was observed in the para-aortic and pericoloic lymph nodes, compared to the popliteal nodes. In the foot pad injections, the ipsilateral popliteal and the para-aortic lymph nodes exihibited a larger accumulation of [125I]-Mab A7 compared to the contralateral popliteal and the pericolic lymph node (Table1).

Reductive effect of locally injected A7-NCS on tumor development.

To confirm that the local injection of A7-NCS can prevent tumor development, athymic nude mice bearing the SW1116 (Table 2) or KB cell (Table 3) but no palpable tumor were used in this study. The therapeutic effect of each preparation was evaluated by noting the ratio of mice which developed palpable tumor after the initiation of therapeutic treatment.

DISCUSSION

Antigen-specific monoclonal antibody can presumably retain a drug on the cancer cell surface by antigen-antibody interaction, inhibit the absorption of the drugs from the interstitial space into the blood and maintain a high concentration of the drug at the target area. In this study, the antigen-specific local retension property of Mab A7 was examined by injecting [125I]-Mab A7 peritumorally into the tumor-bearing mice and following the radioactivity of the tumor. The result showed that Mab A7 localized at the target tumor through antigen-antibody interaction to a greater extent in the peritumoral than in the systemic injection (Fig.1). Tumor localizaion of Mab in peritumoral injection may be observed when Mab is administered at the small tumor burden, particularly when cancer cells are scattered.

In human gastrointestinal cancer, lymphatic flow plays an important role in the spread of cancer and determines the prognosis of cancer patient to a considerable degree. This information has prompted many surgeons to prevent and eliminate lymphatic metastasis of cancer cell in gastrointestinal cancer therapy by additional adjuvant chemotherapy. In this study, we investigated the lymphatic delivery of Mab A7 in tumor free mice, with the aim of eliminating lymph node metastasis by using the monoclonal antibody–drug conjugate. The result showed that large amounts of locally injected Mab A7 reached regional lymph node in both injections (Table1). This high lymphatic delivery of antibody can be explained by the fact that lymph vessels have no continuous basement membranes and no endothelial lining that contain clefts between cells. The high efficacy of lymphatic delivery of monoclonal antibody will contribute to eliminating the lymphatic metastasis of cancer.

A single local injection of A7–NCS prior to palpable tumor formation exhibited a prominent inhibitory effect on tumor development, whereas the systemic injection of A7–NCS and the local injection of NCS did not show a markedly inhibitory effect. Simultaneous local injection of A7–NCS and large amount of free Mab A7 showed a higher ratio of tumor development than the local injection of A7–NCS alone (Table 2). In addition, single local injection of A7–NCS did not lead to a notable inhibitory effect on a tumor development in the antigen–negative tumor–bearing mice (Table 3). These findings suggest that a local injection of A7–NCS can contribute significantly in inhibiting a tumor growth initiated by scattered cancer cells, with antigen specificity. This animal model is comparable to a clinical setting in which a primary tumor has been surgically resected but a residual small tumor or scattered cancer cells are present.

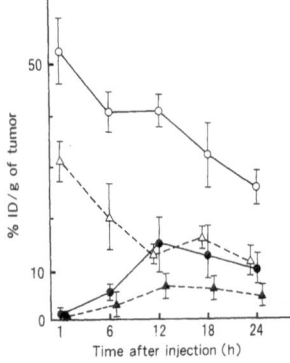

Fig. 1. Local retention of Mab A7:peritumoral injection. ^{125}I-Mab A7 or non-specific ^{125}I-IgG was administered to the site distal to the tumor grown on the thigh of athymic nude mice. As a comparison, the same amount of those labeled antibodies was injected i.v. into the mice. The mice were sacrificed 1, 6, 12, 18, and 24 h after antibody injection, and then the tumor was resected and weighed. The radioactivity of the tumor was measured in a gamma counter. Data were expressed as percent injected dose/g of tumor. ○, Mab A7, local; ●, Mab A7, i.v.; △, nonspecific IgG, local; ▲, nonspecific IgG, i.v. Bars, SE; n = 5.

Table 1 *Tumor development rates: antigen-positive*

A7-NCS equivalent to 5 units of NCS and 37 μg of Mab, 5 units of NCS, and saline alone were administered locally to the thigh near the site inoculated with SW1116 cells. The ratio of tumor development was calculated 7, 14, and 21 days after the treatment. To confirm the antigen specificity of A7-NCS i.t. treatment, A7-NCS with a 100-fold amount of free Mab A7 was administered locally to the mice in the same manner.

	7 days	14 days	21 days
A7-NCS i.t.	0/16	4/16	4/16
A-NCS + Mab A7 i.t.	8/15	8/15	11/15
A7-NCS i.v.	14/18	14/18	16/18
NCS i.t.	10/16	10/16	12/16
Saline i.t.	17/18	18/18	18/18

Table 2 *Tumor development rates: antigen-negative*

See Table 1.

	7 days	14 days	21 days
A7-NCS i.t.	2/15	7/15	10/15
NCS i.t.	8/15	11/15	13/15
Saline i.t.	16/16	16/16	16/16

REFERENCES

1. Goligher, J. Incidence and pathology of carcinoma of the colon and rectum. In:J.Goligher(ed) Surgery of the Anus, Rectum and Colon, Ed5, pp439–453, London:BailliereTindall, 1984.

2. Kitamura K, Takahashi T, Yamaguchi T, Noguchi A, Takashina K, Tsurumi H, Inagake M, Toyokuni T, Hakomori S (1991) Chemical engineering of the monoclonal antibody A7 by polyethylene glycol for targeting cancer chemotherapy. Cancer Res. 51:4310–4315

3. Kitamura K, Takahashi T, Kotani T, Miyagaki T, Yamaoka N, Tsurumi H, Noguchi A, Yamaguchi T (1992) Local administration of monoclonal antibody–drug conjugate: A new strategy to reduce the local recurrence of colorectal cancer. Cancer Res. 52:6323–6328.

4. Kitamura K, Miyagaki T, Yamaoka N, Tsurumi H, Noguchi A, Yamaguchi T, Takahashi, T(1993) The role of monoclonal antibody A7 as a drug modifier in cancer therapy. Cancer Immunol Immunother 36:177–184.

Preoperative ^{60}Co High Dose Rate Intraluminal Radiotherapy for Advanced Lower Rectal Cancer

Azusa Naito[1], Hisao Fujii[1], Saburo Sado[1], Masatoshi Yamamoto[1], Syusaku Yoshikawa[1], Hisashi Nakajima[1], Hiroshige Nakano[1], Hajime Ohishi[2], and Hitoshi Yoshimura[2]

[1]First Department of Surgery, [2]Department of Oncoradiology, Nara Medical University, Kashihara, Nara, 634 Japan

ABSTRACT

Twenty cases of adenocarcinoma of lower rectum were treated by ^{60}Co high dose rate intraluminal radiation(40Gy) combined the conventional external beam radiotherapy (30Gy),then radical surgery were performed within 2 or 3 weeks after completion of radiation therapy. Abdominoperineal resections were done in 17 patients,low anterior resections were done in 3.The effective radiation made the polypoid component flat.The average of reduction rate was 73.8 ± 18.6(%).The histological radiation effects according to Ohboshi-Shimosato's classificationwere excellent; 6 cases were in Grade IIa,11 cases were in Grade IIb,3 cases were in Grade III. In 7 patients(35%) perioperative and delayed complications occured.The administration of high doses(total dose 70Gy) of preoperative radiation makes excellent effects without increasing the complications.

KEY WORDS : Preoperative radiotherapy,Rectal cancer,Intraluminal radiotherapy

INTRODUCTION

In adjuvant irradiation therapy for advanced rectal cancer, radiation is generally administered from 30Gy to 50Gy using external beam technique [1,2] . However adenocarcinoma of the rectum is resistive for radiotherapy. So,high-dose radiotherapy is required.This study investigated the histologic effects and local control obtained high-dose rate preoperative radiotherapy .

PATIENTS AND METHODS

From January 1989 to December 1992,20 patients with rectal cancer tha had penetrated muscularis propria were treated with the preoperative radiation therapy and radical surgery. They were 16 males and four females.The mean age was 64.5 ± 9.1.As for gross features of the tumor before radiation,16 cases were ulcerative and localized,four cases were ulcerative and infiltrative .As for histological types on biopsy prior to radiotherapy, all cases except one were adenocarcinomas ("well differentiated" in seven cases,"moderately diff." in 10,and"poorly diff." in two).In one case biopsy failed, but moderately diff.adenocarcinoma was determined from the surgeal specimen. Radical surgery was performed out within apploximately 17days(10-28days) after radiothrapy. Abdominoperineal resections were performed in 17 cases,low anterior resection in three cases. Endoscopy, barium enema,CT and MRI were performed before and after radiatio to assess the therapeutic efficacy.

Table 1   Patient Details

Case No.	Sex	Age	Operation method*1	Histology before RD*2	RD Effect*3	Reduction rate(%)
1	M	64	APR	mod	IIB	75.5
2	M	76	APR	mod	IIB	80.4
3	M	71	APR	wel	III	100
4	F	61	APR	por	IIB	72.7
5	M	77	APR	wel	IIB	68.0
6	M	38	LAR	mod	III	100
7	F	74	APR	mod	IIB	70.0
8	M	53	APR	mod	IIB	100
9	M	69	APR	failed	IIA	62.3
10	M	72	APR	wel	IIB	100
11	F	62	APR	mod	III	81.3
12	M	66	APR	wel	IIA	63.6
13	M	71	APR	mod	IIA	50.0
14	M	57	APR	wel	IIB	42.9
15	M	64	APR	wel	IIA	93.9
16	M	57	APR	wel	IIA	**
17	M	64	LAR	mod	IIB	68.5
18	M	62	APR	por	IIA	76.7
19	F	72	LAR	wel	IIB	**
20	M	61	APR	wel	IIB	43.8

*1 APR:Abdominoperineal Resection

   LAR:Low Anterior Resection

*2 wel:well diff. adenocarcinoma

   mod:moderately diff. adenocarcinoma

   por:poorly diff. adenocarcinoma

*3 Ohboshi-Shimosato's

   classification

** not evaluated

Radiotherapy technique

Following external radiation with a lineal accelator (10MV X 30Gy/15F/3wks,whole pelvis), intraluminal irradiation with ^{60}Co remote automatic loading system(RALS) 40Gy/4F/2wks, (1.5cm from source) was administered to patients with lower rectal carcinoma .

Reduction rate

The reduction of the tumor was measured three dimensionally on the lateral view on barium enema.

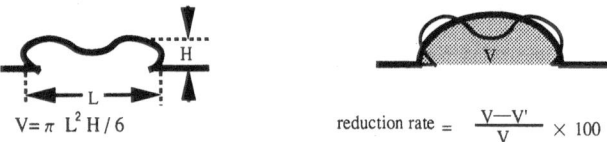

$$V = \pi L^2 H / 6$$

$$\text{reduction rate} = \frac{V - V'}{V} \times 100$$

Fig.1 before and after radiotherapy barium enema studies are performed,on the lateral view vertical extension(L) and height(H) are measured,volume(V) and reduction rate are calculated .

Histologic effects

The histologic effects of radiation were evaluated according to Ohboshi-Shimosato's classification.

Table 2 Ohboshi-Shimosato's classification

Grade 0 : No efficient
Grade I : There is no defect in tumor nests resulted from lysis of individual tumor cells.
Grade IIa : Destruction of tumor structure is mild ,and viable tumor cells are frequently observed.
Grade IIb : Destruction of tumor structure is sever ,and viable tumor cells are a few in number.
Grade III : Presumably non-viable tumor cells are present singly or in small clusters and viable cells are rarely seen.
Grade IV : No tumor cells.

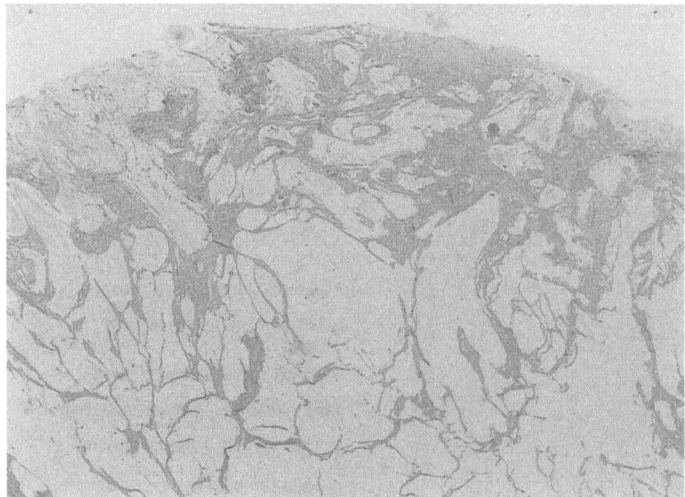

Fig.2 (Case No.3 , RD effect III, Reduction rate 100%) Acellular mucin extends,viable cells are rarely seen. (hematoxylin and eosin stain, x100)

Table 3 Perioperative and delayed morbidity

adhesion small-bowel obstruction	2
deep-vein thrombosis	1
delay of wound healing	6

RESULT

On barium enema and in gross appearance of surgical specimens,obvious reduction of the tumor was almost observed.The average of reduction rate was73.9$\pm$18.7%(Mean$\pm$MD).The effect radiation made the polypoid component flat, histologically tumor structures destroyed and tumor cells became nonviable.Regarding the histological criteria for the effects of radiation, six cases were in Grade IIa,11 cases were in Grade IIb,three cases were in Grade III.That is,three cases were classified into "markedly effective",while all others "moderately effective".In nine patients(45%) perioperative and delayed morbidity occured,there were no severe complications.the rate of complications was similar in a series of the patients treated with surgery only.

CONCLUSION

^{60}Co high -dose rate intraluminal radiation following conventional external beam radiation,total dose 70Gy allowed maximal focal dose,and excellent results were obtained without increasing complications or injuring adjacent structures.

REFERENCES

1.Cerald Marks MD;Mohammed Mohiuddin,MD;Arien Eitan,MD;Luigi Masoni,MD,Jan Rakinic, MD(1991) High dose Preoperative Radiation and Radical Shincter-Preserving Surgery for Rectal cancer.Arch-Vol 126:1534-1540
2.G.Newman,D.C.Calverley,B.D.Acker,M.Manji,J.HayandA.D.Flores(1992) The management of carcinoma of the anal canal by external beam radiotherapy,experience in Vancouver 1971-1988.Radoitherapy and Oncology,25:196-202

Histopathological Assessment in Rectal Carcinoma with Preoperative High-Dose-Rate Intraluminal Brachytherapy

HIDENORI YANAGI[1], MASATO KUSUNOKI[1], YOUICHIROU SAKANOUE[1],
MASAFUMI NODA[1], YASUTSUGU SHOJI[1], HIROKI IKEUCHI[1], NORIHIKO KAMIKONYA[2],
YOSHIO HISHIKAWA[2], TAKEHIRA YAMAMURA[1], and JOJI UTSUNOMIYA[1]

[1]Second Department of Surgery, [2]Department of Radiology, Hyogo College of Medicine, Nishinomiya,
Hyogo, 663 Japan

ABSTRACT

We investigated the histopathological effects of preoperative high-dose-rate
intraluminal brachytherapy (HDRIBT) in 76 rectal carcinomas to know whether pathologic
findings about the qualitive and quantitive assessment reflect local recurrence. The
down-staging of invasion after HDRIBT was shown in 27 tumors (36.0%). There was, however,
no significant difference about local recurrence rate between with and without down-
staging. The proportion of residual tumor nest to stroma, which was analyzed by image
analyzing system (IBAS-20, Zeis, Germany) could be better predictive factor of local
recurrence than qualitive assessment in our series. When the proportion of residual
tumors to stroma was less than 33%, a good local control for rectal cancer might be
achieved after preoperative HDRIBT.

INTRODUCTION

Preoperative radiotherapy has gained continually increasing a role in the treatment of
the rectal carcinoma. Several randomized trials have been indicated to improve survival
rates and decrease pelvic recurrence rates[1]. There have been, however, few reports
concerning predictive factor of local recurrence after radiotherapy. We attempted to
know whether pathologic findings about the quantitive and qualitive assessment reflect
local recurrence.

MATERIALS AND METHODS

Patients

From October 1986 to May 1992, 76 patients with rectal cancer were treated with remote
afterloading HDRIBT as adjuvant therapy prior to surgery at Hyogo College of Medicine.
Follow-up periods were ranged from 10.1 to 75.3 months (median value; 35.1 months). The
mean age of the patients was 59.9 y/o (ranged from 25 - 87 y/o). They were 52 men and
24 women. The tumors located 5.3 ±1.8 cm from the anal verge.

Radiation technique

All of the patients were treated with a remote afterloader RAL-303 (Toshiba, Tokyo). The
irradiation source was Cobalt-60 with an activity of 1.7Ci or 2.6Ci. Single doses ranged
from 4 to 80Gy, and total doses from 16 to 80Gy. In view of complication, standard
dose was determined at 30 - 40 Gy since July 1988 (59 patients). Doses at a point 5 mm
below the mucosa was calculated by using a medical computer (Varian-Ro7).

Operation

Operation performed regularly 14 - 16 days after HDRIBT in order to standardize the pathological examination of operative specimen, unless there was associate diseases which caused to prolong operation. Type of operation was shown in Table 1. Probable curative surgery was performed in 70 patients (92.1%). Sphincter preserving operation was performed in 58 patients (76.3%).

Table 1. Type of operation

No. of Patients		76
Operation	Method	
Sphincter preserving procedure 58 (76.3%)	LAR	7
	Coloanal	51
Permanent colostomy 18 (23.7%)	APR	15
	TPE	2
	Others	1

LAR:Low anterior resection, Coloanal:Coloanal anastomosis, APR:Abdominoperineal excision, TPE:Total pelvic excenteration

Table 2. Down-staging after Preoperative IBT

Depth of Invasion

Before IBT			After IBT		
		No residual	8	(10.5%)
0		Tis	0	(0.0%)
2	(2.6%)	T1	6	(7.9%)
21	(27.6%)	T2	17	(22.4%)
49	(64.5%)	T3	41	(53.9%)
4	(5.3%)	T4	2	(2.6%)

Depth of invasion: Tis (in situ), T1 (submucosa), T2 (muscularis), T3 (perirectal fat), T4 (adherence or invasion to adjacent organ)

Pathological examination

Surgical specimens were fixed by formalin and embedded in paraffin for hematoxylin-eosin staining. These section were selected from the area including the maximum diameter of each tumor along the longitudinal axis or the healed area in the case of grossly ablated tumor. The non-viability of residual tumor cells was determined according to the appearance of giant cells with atypical nuclei, nuclear karyorrhexis, coagulation necrosis of the tumor and acellular mucin lakes. These pathologic findings and transmural radiation fibrosis at the radial margin of the tumor verified the original tumor margin and the original depth of penetration. A qualitive assessment of pathological effect was indicated as down-staging of invasion depth. Pathological grading of invasion was made according to the UICC classification. A quantitive morphometric measure of the radiation effect was made on the resected specimens to determine the proportion of tumor nest to stroma. The proportion of residual tumor area to stroma was measured using the image analyzing system (IBAS-20, Zeis, Germany), which was composed of a microscope, RGB color monitoring system (2 CRT), digitizing tablet system, and a microprocessor. These proportion was taken as a percentage.

RESULTS

Table 2 shows depth of invasion of tumors before and after HDRIBT. The down-staging of invasion after IBT was shown in 27 tumors (36.0%).

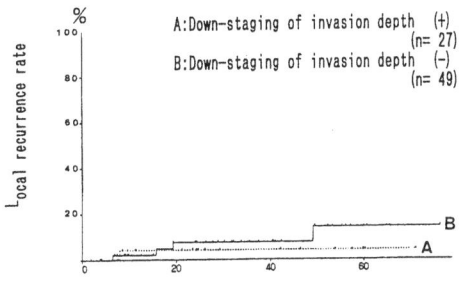

Fig. 1 Actuarial local recurrence rate by a qualitive analysis of radiation effect

There was no significant difference about local recurrence rate between with and without down-staging (Fig. 1).

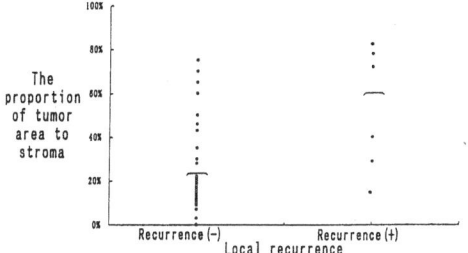

Fig. 2 Pathological effect after IBT and Local Recurrence

Fig. 2 shows the population of tumor area to stroma as a function of a local recurrence. These were 52.3 ± 29.1 (Mean ± S.D.) % in the group with local recurrence, which was higher than in the group without local recurrence (22.0 ± 22.1 %, p<0.01).

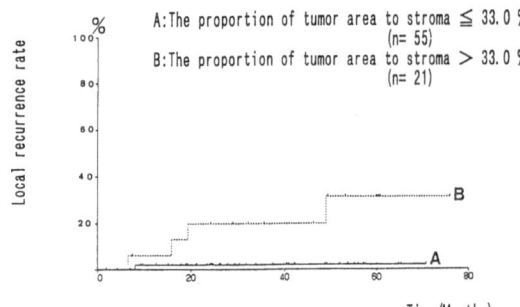

Fig.3 Actuarial local recurrence
rate by a quantitive analysis of
radiation effect

Fig. 3 shows cumulative local recurrence rate as a fuction of the proportion of tumor area to stroma. Local recurrence rate in the group with marked radiation effect histopathologically was lower than in the group without

DISCUSSION

Preoperative radiotherapy was ascertained to lead the reduction in both the size of the primary tumor and number of involved lymph nodes[1]. Down-staging after preoperative radiotherapy was proved at the several randomized control study[1-2]. It was, however, difficult to evaluate down-staging in each tumor because of a variety of histopathological findings after radiation. Recently it was reported that transrectal ultrasonography before and after preoperative radiotherapy could well predict down-staging after radiation[3]. The original margin of the tumors before radiation could be reproduced in the resected specimen by using their criteria of histopathological effect for radiation[3-4]. We evaluated down-staging of penetration as a qualitive assessment for radiation effect using similar criteria and the proportion of tumor nest to stroma as a quantitive measurement by image analyzing system. These quantitive analysis, which was a precise and objective method, could be better predictive factor of local recurrence than qualitive assessment in our series. When the proportion of residual tumors to stroma was less than 33%, a good local control might be achieved (Fig.3). It means that the histopathological grading system[5] of radiation effect can be also a well predictive factor of local recurrence after preoperative radiotherapy and surgery.

REFERENCES

1.Mendenhall WM, Bland KI, Rout WR, Pfaff WW, Millon RR, Copelland III EM (1987) Clinically resectable adenocarcinoma of the rectum treated with preoperative irradiation and surgery. Dis Col & Rectum 31:287-291
2.Kodner IJ, Shemish EI, Fry RD (1989) Preoperative irradiation for rectal cancer. Ann Surg 209: 194-9
3.Glaser F, Kuntz C, Schlag P, Herfarth C (1993) Endorectal ultrasound for control of preoperative radiotherapy pf rectal cancer. Ann Surg 217: 64-71
4.Schaldenbrand JD, Siders DB, Zainea GG, Thieme ET (1992) Preoperative radiation therapy for locally advanced carcinoma of the rectum. Clinicopathologic correlative review. Dis Colon Rectum 35: 16-23
5.The Japanese Research Society for Colorectal Cancer (In preparation) The general rules for colorectal cancer study.

Development of a Cisplatin Suppository for Regional Chemotherapy of Ano-Rectal Cancer

Osamu Kojima[1], Itoh Masahiko[1], Tamura Akitaka[1], Iizuka Ryouji[1], Kazuyoshi Ohnishi[1], Takashi Nishiue[1], Toshio Takahashi[1], Isao Hirata[2], and Hideki Kishimoto[2]

[1]First Department of Surgery, [2]Department of Pharmacy, Kyoto Prefectural University of Medicine, Kyoto, 602 Japan

ABSTRACT

Cisplatin has recently been evaluated as an anti-cancer agent for ano-rectal cancer. We have developed a cisplatin suppository with the aim of keeping cisplatin concentrations high in the rectum. The cisplatin suppository was completely released in vitro in 90 minutes. In a study using rabbits, a high concentration of cisplatin was detected in the rectal tissues. The cisplatin suppository group showed low concentrations in blood and renal tissue. These results indicate that the cisplatin suppository is an effective regional chemotherapeutic agent for ano-rectal cancer.

KEY WORDS: cisplatin suppository, ano-rectal cancer, local recurrence

INTRODUCTION

A major cause of the poor prognosis in case with ano-rectal cancer is local recurrence. Preventive methods of local recurrence includes (1) performing extended operation, (2) combined use of radiotherapy, and (3) combined use of chemotherapy. In order to prevent local recurrence of ano-rectal cancer, we have obtained favorable results with the following preoperative treatments for ano-rectal cancer, given in order: (1) administration of a 5-fluorouracil (5-FU) suppository, (2) radiotherapy, (3) combined therapy of 5-FU suppository administration and radiotherapy and (4) combined therapy of radiation, hyperthermia and 5-FU suppository [1,2,3]. Recently, cisplatin has been evaluated to be one of very effectable agent for rectal cancer [4]. However, when cisplatin was administered intravenously, the concentration of cisplatin was too low in the tumor. So, intra-arterial infusion, intratumoral injection of cisplatin caused the high concentration in tumors and the high rate of tumor response.
In order to keep the concentration in rectal cancers high, we developed the cisplatin suppository and investigated the concentration of cisplatin released from the suppository and the concentrations of cisplatin in some organs of rabbit after administration of the suppository.

METHODS

1. Preparation of the cisplatin suppository
The cisplatin powder (Japan Chemopharmaceutical Co. Ltd. Tokyo) (5 mg) was dissolved in polyethylene glycol 400 (700 mg). Polyethylene glycol 4,000 (90 mg) and polyethylene glycol 6,000 (700 mg) were then added to this mixture in a hot bath at 60°C while stirring. Each suppository was made from the homogenous mixture.
2. Release test of the cisplatin suppository in vitro
A suppository releasing test device (Fuji Industrial Co., Kyoto, Japan) was used for the release test of the cisplatin suppository. The saline solution (300 ml) was maintained at 37°C and 0.1 ml was put into the releasing phase. A milipore filter (pore size 3 μm) was placed between the cell phase and releasing phase and suppository was placed in the cell. A sample was collected from the releasing after a certain time.
3. Measurement of the cisplatin concentration
After treatment with the heparin, a blood sample was centrifuged at 3,000 rpm for 10 minutes to separate the serum. The serum was diluted with Trigon X-100 solution and then measured using a atomic absorption analyzer (Variant Techtron AA-40). The concentration of cisplatin in the tissue was measured as follows. After the addition of glass beads, 70% perchloric acid and nitric acid, the sample was heated and nitric acid was added.
This was followed by treatment with 1% hydrochloric acid and measurement of the total platinum levels by atomic absorption. The total platinum level in the plasma was expressed μg/ml and in tissues μg/g wet tissue.

4. Distribution of cisplatin in rabbits
Male rabbits weighing 2 kg were allocated into 10 groups consisting of 7 rabbits each. After
the cisplatin suppositories which contained 5 mg cisplatin were inserted, rabbits were sacrificed after 30 minutes, 1, 2, 6, and 12 hours and the total platinum concentration in blood,
rectal tissue and kidney was measured. In the control group, cisplatin (5 mg) was infused
intravenously. The rabbits were then sacrificed at the same time as the suppository group
and the concentration of total platinum was measured in blood, rectal tissue and kidney.
5. Statistical analysis
Statistical analysis was tested using an unpaired t-test and less than 0.05 P value was
statistically significant.

RESULTS

1. Release test for the cisplatin suppository in vitro
Figure 1 shows the results of the in vitro release test. The percentage of cisplatin released from the suppository was 41.3% after 15 minutes, 63.5% after 30 minutes, 81.7% after
45 minutes and 99.1% after 90 minutes.

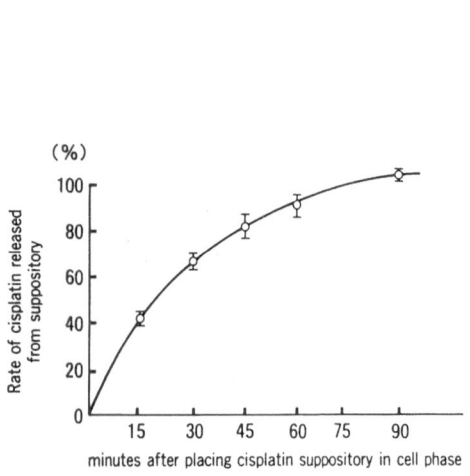

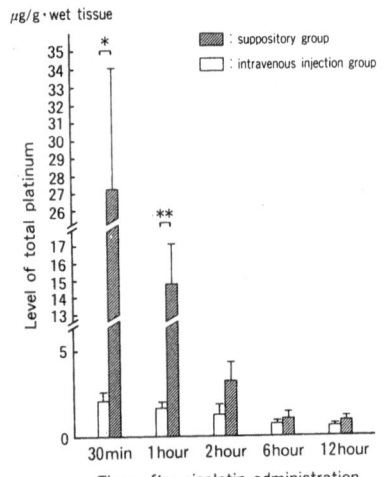

Fig. 1 Release test of cisplatin
suppository in vitro

Fig. 2 Comparison of total platinum level in rectal
tissue of cisplatin suppository group and
cisplatin intravenous injection group.
*: indicates p<0.01 and **: indicates p<0.005

2. Distribution of cisplatin in rabbit organs
The cisplatin suppository was dissolved macroscopically 30 minutes after administration.
1) Cisplatin concentration in serum
As Table 1, There was significant difference between the suppository group and the infusion
group after every time.

Table 1. Total platinum level in serum (μ g/ml)

	30 min*	1 hour*	2 hours*	6 hours**	12 hours*
Suppository group	0.55±0.14	0.27±0.04	0.21±0.11	0.26±0.06	0.18±0.16
Infusion group	1.08±0.36	0.57±0.10	0.46±0.14	0.43±0.15	0.47±0.11

*p<0.005, **p<0.025 (m±SD)

2) Cisplatin concentration in rectum and kidney
As Fig. 2, the concentration of total platinum in the rectal tissue was higher in the suppos-

itory group than in the infusion group after 30 min to 12 hours. The statistically significant difference between the suppository group and the infusion group was observed. Fig. 3 shows the concentration of total platinum in kidney. After 30 min to 12 hours, the concentration of total platinum was significantly lower in the suppository group than in the infusion group.

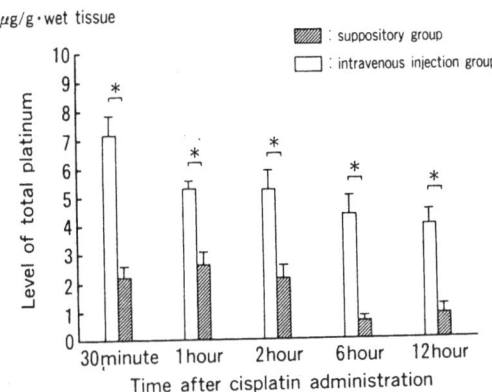

Fig. 3 Comparison of total platinum level in kidney of cisplatin suppository group and cisplatin intravenous injection group.
*: indicates p<0.005

DISCUSSION

Cisplatin, a platinum complex which has anti-tumor effects on the gastric cancer and ovarian cancer, is widely used. Moreover, it has also been reported that the combined administration of cisplatin and 5-FU is more effective than 5-FU alone for large bowel cancer [4]. We have also reported that the effects of cisplatin could be increased by hyperthermia in mice with tumor [5]. We devised a procedure incorporating intra-arterial infusion of cisplatin and 5-FU, hyperthermia and radiotherapy and performed trials on patients with recurring rectal cancer [2].
If the cisplatin suppository can be applied clinically and used in combination with the 5-FU suppository, further enhancements in the anti-rectal cancer effects may be expected. The results of this experiment confirmed that cisplatin suppository released cisplatin in vitro and in vivo. An in vivo study demonstrated the presence of high concentration of cisplatin in rectal tissue after 30 minutes. The ratio of the concentration in the rectal tissue to the concentration in blood was 23.5 in the suppository group and 3.2 in the intravenous injection group after 30 minutes. The ratio in the suppository group was higher than in intravenous injection group at all times. On the other hand, the concentration of cisplatin in kidney was significantly lower in the suppository group than intravenous injection group. These results indicated that because cisplatin could remain in the rectum at high concentration when the suppository was used, suppository administration might be superior to intravenous administration. Moreover, suppository administration was considered to be superior to the intravenous administration in terms of preventing side effect in the kidney.
When the cisplatin suppository was administered into the rectum, absorption of cisplatin from the rectal mucosa was confirmed. It has been reported that when cisplatin solution was administered into the stomach of rat, cisplatin inhibited the growth of tumors [6]. So, cisplatin can be considered to be absorbed from mucosa of the digestive tracts rectal mucosa. The present data indicate that the developed cisplatin suppository may be effective method for ano-rectal cancer.

REFERENCES

1. Takahashi T, Mizusawa H, Kato T, Yamaguchi T (1988) Preoperative irradiation and 5-fluorouracil suppository for carcinoma of the rectum. Am J Surg 156: 58-62
2. Kojima O, Takahashi T, Horie H, Itoh N, Nishiue T, Ohnishi K, Matsui M (1900) Combined therapy of hyperthermo-local chemotherapy for preventing of local recurrence and treatment of local recurrence cases in rectal cancer. J Jpn Surg Soc 91: 1283-1286
3. Kojima O, Suganuma Y, Tamura T, Ohnishi K, Nishiue T, Itoh M, Horie H, Sawai S, Takahashi T (1992) Clinical results of tumor shrinkage and evaluation of quality life in low rectal carcinoma after preoperative combined treatments. Jpn J Gastroenterol Surg 25: 2635-2639
4. Dy C, Gil A, Algarra SM, Aparicio LA, Clavo F, Herranz P (1986) Combination chemotherapy of cisplatin and 5-FU in advanced colorectal carcinoma. Cancer Treat Rep 70-465-468
5. Majima T (1988) Experimental studies of the combination therapy of hyperthermia and chemotherapy for cancer. J Kyoto Pref Univ Med 97: 13-23
6. Hasegawa Y, Morita M (1985) Antitumor effect of oral cisplatin on certain murine tumors. Chem Pharm Bull 33: 5511-5514

Radiological Findings of Minute and Small Depressed Colorectal Neoplasm

MASAAKI MATSUKAWA, MINORU KURIHARA, TATUYA TAKEMOTO, MASANAO HIRASIMA, and KAZUTO KIKUTI

Department of Gastroenterology, Toyosu Hospital, Showa University, Koto-ku, Tokyo, 135 Japan

ABSTRACT

We are required to detect colorectal cancer at the early stage in order to improve its prognosis. Minute cancers are an early cancer and are detected as a depressed lesion. We could demonstrate small and minute depressive cancers(4 lesions) and adenomas(6 lesions) emploing a new preparation of barium enema. This preparation consists of bisacodyl 15mg, massive isotonic citrated magnesium solution (25ml/b.w.kg), cysapride 15mg and a low-fat, low-residue meal. Ten depressed lesions (3 lesions ranging between 1 cm and 0.6 cm, 7 lesions of less than 0.6 cm) were demonstrated by double contrast method. Findings of those depressed lesions were demonstrated as a radiolucent area around a faint barium fleck.

KEY WORDS: minute depressed cancer, radiological findings, preparation

INTRODUCTION

There is recently an increasing incidence of colorectal cancer in Japan. We are expected to detect colo-rectal cancer at the early stage in order to improve its prognosis because the prognosis of early cancer is much better than advanced cancer. Almost of minute cancers are an early cancer and are detected as a depressed lesion. As the first step of mass-survey for detecting a colorectal cancer a fecal occult blood test is done. As the second step for a patient with positive reaction to occult blood test, examinaion of large bowel is done by either endoscopy or radiology. By a new endoscopic preparation of massive electrolytes intestinal lavage and an introduction of a new instrument(videoendoscope), we came to be able to detect many small lesions(plaque-like and depressed lesions) in large bowel. On the other hand, by a new preparation of barium enema, we have performed the examination of double contrast method in order to detect small/minute cancers. We could detected these lesios employing this preparation and analysed radiographic findings characteristric of these lesions. We can now detect many depressed lesions in terms of the above radiographic findings.

MATERIAL & METHOD

In our hospital, we have detected ten colorectal depressed neoplastic lesions by endoscopy and barium enema from Jan. 1992 to Dec. 1992.
Ten cases with a depressed leson (Table 1) is only man. The average age of the patients was 52.8 years, the ange being 44 to 64 yers.
There were 2 lesions in the transverse colon, 4 lesions in the descending colon and 4 lesions in the sigmoid colon.
A lesion less than 0.6cm in diameter is defined as a minute lesion and a lesion between 0.6 and 1.0cm in diameter as a small lesion. This study included 7 minute lesions and 3 small lesions. Early cancer consists of m cancer(defined as a lesion of cancerous involvement within the propria mucosa) and sm cancer (as a lesion of cancerous involvement until the submucosal layer).
We detected 4 cases with a cancer(m ca.:1, sm ca.:3) and 6 cases of an adenoma. Macroscopic forms of the depressed lesions were defined by findings of resected specimen, endoscopic and radiologic findings. A superficial depressed lesion is defined as type II c by macroscopic findings, a superficial elevation with a central depression as type II a+II c and a superficial elevation around a depressed area as type II c+II a. In this study depressed lesions included type II a+II c, type II c and type II a+II c.

Table-1. A list of cases with depressed colo-rectal neoplasm

Case	Age	Sex	Location	Size	Form	Histology
1.	44yr	M	Des	10mm	II a+II c	sm cancer
2.	53	M	Trans	10	II c+II a	sm cancer
3.	61	M	Sig	10	II a+II c	adenoma
4.	64	M	Sig	5	II a+II c	adenoma
5.	43	M	Des	5	II a+II c	m ca cancer
6.	52	M	Sig	5	II a+II c	sm cancer
7.	63	M	Trans	4	II a+II c	adenoma
8.	45	M	Des	4	II a+II c	adenoma
9.	55	M	Des	3	II c	adenoma
10.	47	M	Sig	3	II c	adenoma

1. A new preparation for barium enema

By this preparation(Fig. 1) for barium enema a examination of double contrast mrthod was performed 10 patients with a depressed lesion.

Fig. 1 A new preparation for barium enema
   the day before examination
      10:00   Please drink a glass of water.
      12:00   Please have a meal with a low-fat & low-residue.
      13:00   Please take Pursenid (15mg) & cisapride (7.5mg) with a glass of water.
      16:00   Please drink a glass of water.
      18:00   Please have a meal with a low-fat & low-residue,
               and take cisapride (7.5mg) with a glass of water.
      20:00   Please drink massive isotonic citrated magnesium solution (25ml/BW kg)
   the day of examination
      Intramuscular injection of anti-cholinergics 10 minutes before examination.

We have used about 220ml of 66% lukewarm barium suspension in examination.
We have taken 15 films in a patients by double contrast method.

RESULTS

1. Macroscopic form of the depressed lesions

Macroscopic form is decided by endoscopic, radiologic and macroscopic findings of the resected specimen. Minute or small depressed lesions are clearly recognized by dye-spraying method in endoscopy. Endoscopic findings are demonstrated by dye-spraying method is similar to radiological findings. A sm cancer of type II c+II a is a lesion with a mild elevation around a prominent central depression. A m cancer and adenoma are a lesion with a mild elevation around a faint depression.

2. Radiologic findings of the depressed lesions

A depressed lesion was recognized at radiographs which were demonstrated so-called fine network pattern on the colonic mucosa. A minute adenoma 0.3cm in diameter(by arrow) being in Fig. 2, adenoma and m cancer of the depressed pattern were more likely to show a faint barium fleck in mild elevation. Futhermore type II a+II c 1.0cm in diameter(arrow) and type II c+II a 1.0cm in diameter(arrow) being shown in Fig.3 and Fig.4 respectively, sm cancers of the depressed lesions were demonstrated as a mild elevation around a barium fleck by radiographic findings.

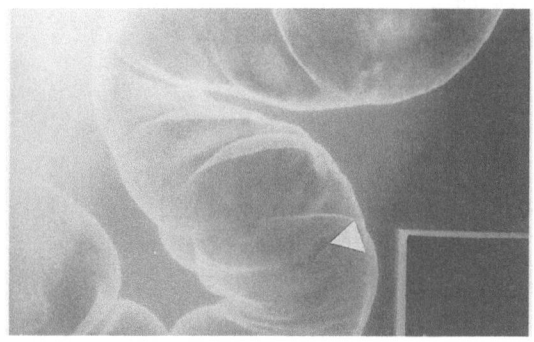

Fig.2 Radiographic findings showing
a minute depressed lesion (by arrow)
0.3cm in diameter in the sigmoid colon.
This lesion was resected by endoscopy and
adenoma by histologic findings.

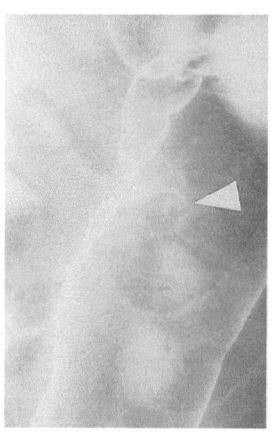

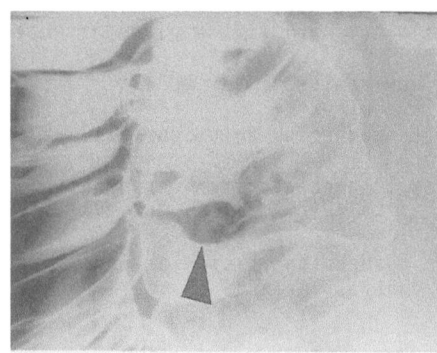

Fig.3 Radiographic findings showing a
small depressed lesion (by arrow) 1.0cm
in diameter in the descending colon.
This lesion was resected by operation and
sm cancer by histologic findings.

Fig.4 Radiographic findings showing a
small depressed lesion (by arrow) 1.0cm
in diameter in the transverse colon.
This lesion was resected by operation and
sm cancer by histologic findings.

DISCUSSiON

Ordinary preparation of barium enema has not been sufficient in order to remove
the fecal residue in the colon. In other words, the colonic mucosa cannot be
coated enough to visialize the fine network pattern with the method so far.
Radiological accuracy to detect lesions has been greatly improved depending on
the our new preparation of barium enema. We could successfully visialize depressed as a radiolucent area around barium fleck. Minute depressed lesions were
visialized as a faint barium spot in the radiolucent area. Small depressed lesions were visialized as a radiolucent area around barium fleck.

REFERENCE
1. Davis GR, Santa Ana CA, Morawski SG, et al:Development of a lavage solution
   associated with minimal water and electrolyte absorption or secretion.
   Gastroenterology 78:991-998, 1980

Liver

Comparative Epidemiology of Liver Cirrhosis and Liver Cancer in Japan

TAKESHI HIRAYAMA

Institute of Preventive Oncology, Shinjuku-ku, Tokyo, 162 Japan

ABSTRACT

A characteristic association was observed between the epidemic patterns of liver cirrhosis and liver cancer when mortality trends were compared by age groups. A 5 years time lag was commonly observed in each age group between the peak of the epidemic curve for liver cirrhosis and that for liver cancer of 5 years senior age. This is compatible with the conceived epidemiological model that HBV infection at birth is the common initiator for liver cancer while HCV infection is a strong promoter particularly in Japan together with alcohol drinking-liver cirrhosis-cigarette smoking sequence revealed by a large scale cohort study in Japan and heavy exposure to aflatoxin in selected areas.

KEY WORDS: liver cirrhosis, liver cancer, time trends, cigarette smoking, alcohol drinking

INTRODUCTION

Epidemiological characteristics of liver cirrhosis and liver cancer were compared in detail from the standpoint of both descriptive epidemiology and analytic epidemiology.

MATERIALS AND METHODS

Vital statistics in Japan, 1958-1990 were utilized for the study materials of descriptive epidemiology.

A large-scale cohort study conducted from 1965 to 1982 in Japan [1] was fully utilized as materials for the analytic epidemiology of both diseases.

RESULTS

1. Descriptive Epidemiology

Liver cancer mortality has been sharply increasing in recent years in Japan in men but not in women. For selected age groups in men, however, tendency of decline was also noticed (Fig. 1). When compared with similar graph for liver cirrhosis, it was observed clearly that such rise and fall in liver cancer mortality in each age group was preceded by the rise and fall in mortality for liver cirrhosis in the 5 year younger age groups (Fig. 2). In other words a 5 years time lag was commonly observed in each age group between the peak of the epidemic curve for liver cirrhosis and that for liver cancer of 5 years senior age (Fig. 1).

In addition to such close association of time trends between liver cirrhosis and liver cancer, a high correlation was observed in geographical distribution of both diseases and the correlation coefficient between age adjusted mortality rate for liver cirrhosis and liver cancer was highest when the rates for liver cirrhosis were compared with the rates for liver cancer of 5 years later year (Fig. 3).

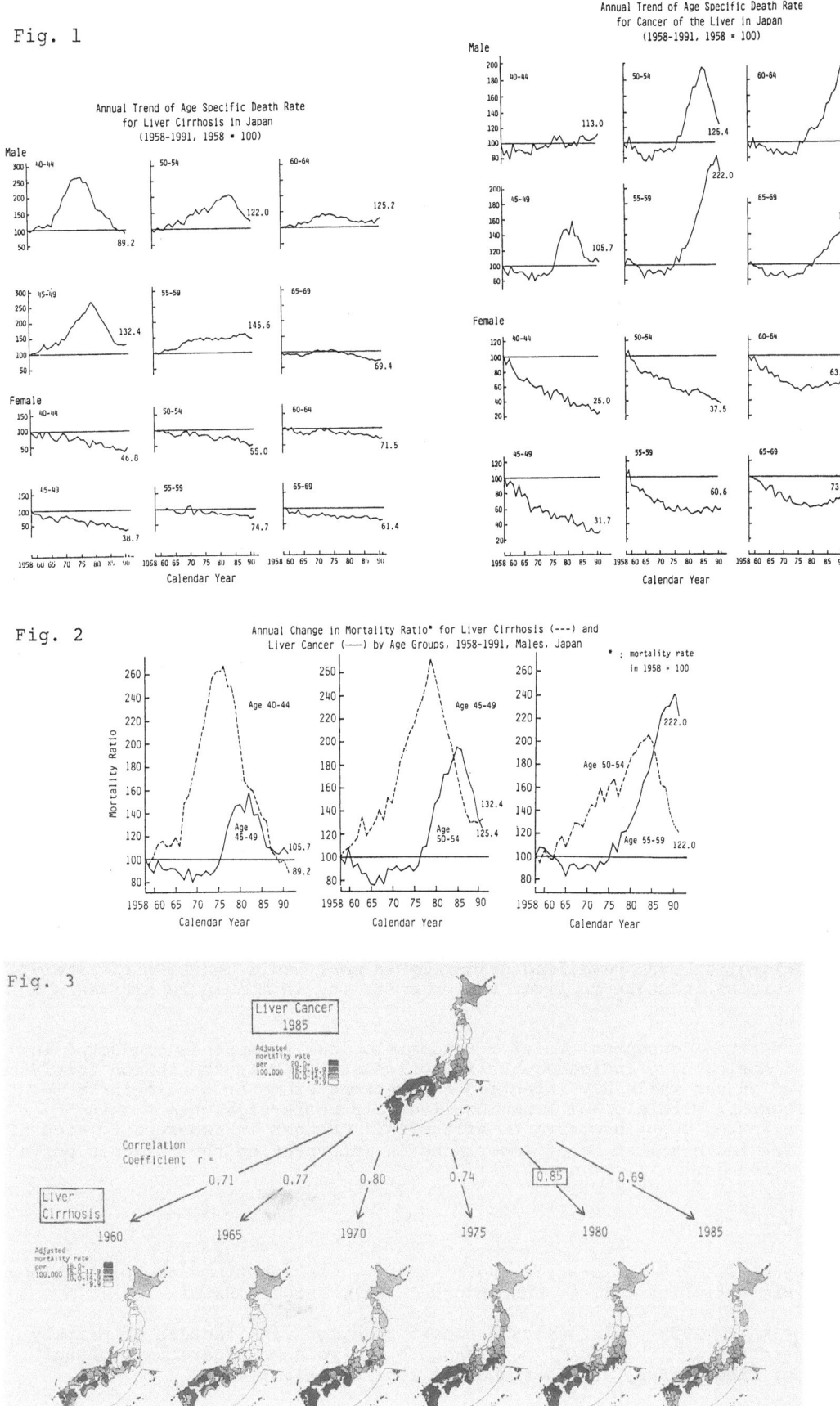

Fig. 1

Annual Trend of Age Specific Death Rate
for Liver Cirrhosis in Japan
(1958-1991, 1958 = 100)

Annual Trend of Age Specific Death Rate
for Cancer of the Liver in Japan
(1958-1991, 1958 = 100)

Fig. 2

Annual Change in Mortality Ratio* for Liver Cirrhosis (---) and
Liver Cancer (——) by Age Groups, 1958-1991, Males, Japan

Fig. 3

2. Analytic Epidemiology

A large-scale cohort study was conducted for 122,261(M) and 142,857(F) aged 40 and above in 29 Health Center Districts in six prefectures in Japan during 17 years follow-up period. Out of the 788(M) and 463(F) cases of liver cancer occurred during the 17 years of follow-up, 123(M) and 28(F) cases of primary liver cancer were detected. These cases were either diagnosed as such or developed in those with a clear-cut history of liver cirrhosis [2].

A striking dose-response relationship was observed with cigarette smoking and the risk of primary liver cancer, which is almost comparable to that for lung cancer. The relative risk(r.r.) for those smoking 30 or more cigarettes daily was 6.83 (3.56-13.10) for primary liver cancer, and 6.80 (5.51-8.41) for lung cancer compared to nonsmokers respectively.

For liver cirrhosis, daily alcohol drinking was observed to be of higher importance compared to daily cigarette smoking, r.r. being 1.82 (1.63-2.04) and 1.17 (1.00-1.36), respectively. For liver cancer, the risk for daily cigarette smoking was much higher than for daily alcohol drinking, r.r. being 3.14 (1.82-5.42) and 1.89 (1.40-2.55), respectively. The risk of developing liver cancer from liver cirrhosis was calculated therefore as 2.67 (1.49-4.79) for daily cigarette smoking and 1.00 (0.72-1.38) for daily alcohol drinking.

DISCUSSION

The possible reasons for liver cancer mortality increase in men in recent years in Japan would be as follows.

1. Advances in Liver Cancer Diagnosis : Owing to the rapid advances made in the diagnosis of liver cancer, more cases of liver cancer must have been detected in recent years. However, if this is the main reason for the mortality increase, such an increase should also appear in women.

2. Advances in Liver Cirrhosis Treatment : Owing to the advances made in medical care and treatment, the survival period of liver cirrhosis patients has been prolonged. This must have made the chances of developing liver cancer from liver cirrhosis much higher. But such an effect should also appear in women as well.

3. Hepatitis C virus Infection : Chronological seroepidemiological study revealed the infection of hepatitis C virus would likely be the reason for the recent increase in liver cancer mortality in Japan. But also in this case it would be necessary to clarify the reason why the increase is limited to men only.

4. Combined Effect of Smoking and Drinking : The combined effect of smoking and drinking, habits prevailing primarily in men, would be the most likely reason for the increase in liver cancer mortality in men in recent years in Japan.

5. A Summarized Conceptual Model : Epidemiological researches conducted in Asia and Africa have indicated HBV infection at birth as the common initiator for liver cancer while HCV infection as a strong promoter particularly in Japan together with alcohol drinking-liver cirrhosis-cigarette smoking sequence and/or heavy exposure to aflatoxin. Changes in exposure to each of these risk factors must be of importance in interpreting the epidemic curves of two diseases.

REFERENCES

1. Hirayama T (1990) Life-style and mortality. Contributions to Epidemiology and Biostatistics Vol. 6, Wahrendorf J (ed), Karger, Basel

2. Hirayama T (1989) A large-scale cohort study on risk factors of primary liver cancer, with special reference to the role of cigarette smoking. Cancer Chemotherapy and Pharmacology 23 (supple):S114-117

Prevalence of Hepatitis B, C and Delta Viral Markers in Turkish Patients with Hepatocellular Carcinoma

ÖZDEN UZUNALIMOGLU, ÖMER DÖNDERICI, ABDÜLKADIR DÖKMECI, NECATI ÖRMECI, EYÜP SELVI, and ŞÜKRÜ DUMLU

The Department of Gastroenterology, Faculty of Medicine, University of Ankara, Aukara, Turkey

ABSTRACT:

We have studied the prevalence of HBV, HCV and HDV in patients with hepatocellular carcinoma (HCC), referred to our unit, from 1983 to 1992. This study was carried out on 169 patients (149 men, 20 women, mean age 50.1, range 18-80) diagnosed by imaging procedures, confirmed by histopathology. Between 1983 and 1989, 110 of these patients were examined for hepatitis B virus' marker only. While between 1989 and 1992, 59 patients were tested for both HBV and HCV. Sera were tested for HBV markers by RIA (Abbott) and for anti HCV by ELISA (Abbott, second generation). In 110 patients studied from 1983 to 1989, seropositivity for HBsAg was detected in 66/110 (60.0 %); while in 59 patients who were studied from 1989 to 1992 the findings are 37/59 (62.7 %) seropositivity for HBsAg and 8/59 (13.6 %) seropositivity for anti HCV. Of these, 8 patients, 3 (5.1 %) were positive for both HBsAg and anti HCV. 14 cases (23.7 %) of the study group were negative for both HBsAg and anti HCV. In summary, no sigfnificant difference was found between patients with chronic liver disease and the study group for HBV and HCV status. Whereas the prevalence of anti-HDV (14.4 %) of those patients with HCC was less than that of patients with HDV in chronic liver disease.

KEY WORDS: Hepatitis B, Hepatitis C, Hepatitis Delta, Hepatocellular Carcinoma, Prevalence

INTRODUCTION:

Hepatocellular cancer (HCC) causing approximately 250.000 deaths per year world wide, has recently become one of the most interesting subject of hepatology. In spite of this great interest, disputation related to its etiopathogenesis keeps going on. The relation between HCC and chronic viral hepatitis also cirrhosis is well known today however the question about how they caused to cancer hasn't been brighten up yet.

The prevalence of chronic viral hepatitis causing HCC directly or indirectly the incidence of the tumour greatly affected by that and the ratio of viral hepatitis causing HCC varies widely from country to country. These epidemiological findings cast light on the subject HCC. In this article studying the serological markers of viral hepatitis, we aimed to participate to the disputation in a group of Turkish patient with HCC.

PATIENTS AND METHODS:

In this study 169 patients who are followed up between the years of 1983-1992 at our department were diagnosed by the imaging procedures (USG and BT) in which the diagnosis were supported also by alpha fetoprotein and liver needle biopsy specimen pathologically and cytologically examined. 149 of the patients were men (mean age 49.7) and 20 of the patients were women (mean age 53.3). Table I showing the age and sexual difference also illustrates to the facts that ratio of men to women is approximately 8/1, age distribution greatly varies between 18-80, women being older than men although not significant statistically (0.5>p>0.3).

Table I: The age and sexual difference In studying group

	n	%	Mean Age	Range
Male	149	88.2	49.7±11.2	27-80
Female	20	11.8	53.3±17.5	18-66
Total	169	100	50.1±14.2	18-80

The markers HBV (HBsAg, HBsAb, HBeAg, HBeAb), HDV (anti HDV) and HCV (anti HCV) were examined in patients. However in 110 patients, who applied before 1989 and whose serums were not stored, anti HCV couldn't be studied. HBV markers were studied by RIA (ABBOTT) and anti HCV marker by ELISA (ABBOTT second generation) technique. Statistically evaluation is made by t test, whereas mean values are given by means of: standard deviation. To determine the ratio of viral hepatitis to HCC 59 patients who underwent to the anti HCV study were also considered.

RESULTS:

Results were shown at Table II. The patients can be classified in to four groups.

Table II: The prevalence of viral markers In patients with hepatocellular carcinoma

Group	Marker		n	%	M/F	Mean Age	Range
B	HBsAg +	1983-89	66	60.0	64/2	47.8:12.1	29-71
		1989-92	37	62.7	34/3	55.2:13.5	18-80
C	Anti HCV +		5	8.5	4/1	60.0:9.2	43-70
BC	HBsAg +, Anti HCV +		3	5.1	2/1	60.0:3.0	56-63
NBNC	HBsAg -, Anti HCV -		14	23.7	11/3	55.0:11.3	36-68
	HBsAb +		7	11.9	5/2	60.0:8.9	40-68
	HBsAb -		7	11.9	6/1	50.0:11.1	36-66

GROUP B (HBsAg positive): HBsAg was positive in 66 patients (60 %) of 110 patients studied between the years 1983-1989, in 37 patients of 59 (62.7 %) patients studied between the years 1989-1992 and totally 103 (60.9 %) of 169 patients. If we compare the two different periods of time we see that the ratio of HBsAg positive patients do not differ which however it is striking that mean of age increases in time (47.8 to 55.2) and also men/women ratio decreases (32/1 to 11/1). In HBsAg positive patient group there were 98 men but only 5 women. Men/women ratio was 20/1. In contrast to the general patient group the mean age was 51.2 in men and while 36.4 women. In our study group of 59 patients, 9 patients (15.3 %) was determined anti HDV positivity. In 31 patients who were investigated HBe status, HBeAg was positive in 7 male patients (22.6%, mean age 58.6:13.3), while HBeAb was positive in 20 male (mean age 27.3:13.1) and 3 female (mean age 29.0:14.3) totally 23 (74.2 %) patients. Only in one male patient aged 43 (3.2 %) neither HBeAg nor HBeAb was positive.

GROUP C (anti HCV positive): Anti HCV was positive only in 5 patients (8.5 %) out of 59 who are evaluated after 1989. One of these patients was female (age 65) and four patients was male (mean age 57.8). The ages of the patients were among 43-70 and mean age was found 60.

GROUP BC (HBsAg and anti HCV positive together): Three of 59 patients (5.1 %) were both anti HCV and HBsAg positive. One of them was female (age 63), and two of them were male (age 56 and 61).

GROUP NBNC (HBsAg and anti HCV negative): In 59 patients investigated for anti HCV 14 (23.7 %) were neither HBV nor HCV carrier. Half of them was determined HBsAb positive (5 male, mean age 59.2 and 2 female mean age 61) while the other half (6 male mean age 47.3 and one female, aged 66) HBsAb negative. In this group, 11 of them were male (mean age 57.2) and 3 of them female (mean age 63.3). Ages vary 36 to 66 and mean age was found 55.

52 of 59 patients (88.1 %) HBV and/or HCV was positive. The results above illustrate that viral hepatitis is greatly responsible - HBV more than HCV- for HCC. In group B, male patients were more than female (0.05>p>0.01) and younger (0.2>p>0.1). Especially in this group the female patients are younger also (p<0.01).

In group B there were 37 liver cirrhosis, 2 chronic active hepatitis with cirrhosis and 2 normal patients diagnosed with liver needle biopsy. In BC group there were 2 cirrhosis, one cirrhosis with chronic active hepatitis, whereas in group C there were 3 cirrhosis, one cirrhosis with chronic active hepatitis and one chronic active hepatitis.

DISCUSSION:

The relationship between chronic viral hepatitis and cirrhosis was clearly pointed out by numerous prevalence studies. According to epidemiological investigations HCV prevalence doesn't differ much all over the world being 0.3-1.4 % approximately. On the other hand the ratio of HBV differs from 0.1 % to 15 % at different geographical regions of the world. That's why HCC incidence is greatly effected by the distribution of viral hepatitis in a country.

Three different countries as a sample is considered due to this general information above. The prevalence of HBV is the highest in South and Middle Africa, South-East Asia with 10-15 % approximately. In these endemic regions the infection is vertically transmitted from mother to baby and the chronicity is higher. HCC incidence is 50/100.000 to 200/100.000 per year. In these countries, HBV is predominant in HCC. In North America, North Europe and Australia the prevalence of HBV 0.1-0.5 % is low and the transmission is mostly horizontally during the young adulthood and young period. The incidence of HCC is correspondingly low below 5/100.000 per year in these countries. The difference between the distribution of HBV and HCV is not striking also. South Europe, North Africa, Middle-East and South America and the rest of Asia are the areas endemic countries, prevalence is 3-5 % and the infection is transmitted horizontally between the age of 1-5 in childhood. These parts of the world are transition regions for both viral hepatitis distribution in HCC and HCC incidence. In Italy, Spain and Japan like countries which is among the mean endemic regions, HBV only accounts for 1/4 of HCC patients being HCV most responsible for the tumour.

In Türkiye, HBV prevalence is considered 3.5-7 % and HCV prevalence is 0.3-0.8 %. The distribution of chronic liver disease except alcoholic, autoimmune and metabolic ones is 68 % in B, 19 % in C, 5 % BC and 8 % NBNC group, out of 327 patients. In our study the ratio of 60-62.7 % B, 8.5 % C, 5.1 % BC, 23.7 % NBNC are similar to the ratio of chronic liver disease and parallel also to the general population (Table III). Our country is in correspondence with the most Asian countries of high endemic areas for HBV infection.

Table III: Viral hepatitis prevalence in general population, chronic liver disease and HCC group.

	B	C	BC	NBNC
General Population	5.3	0.5	0.1	94.1
Chronic Liver Disease	68	19	5	8
HCC Studying Group	62.7	8.5	5.1	23.7

At this point the more important thing is the incubation period for HCC. In vertically transmitted Africa and Asia countries the mean age for HCC is 3rd decade whereas in horizontally transmitted West countries is 5th and 6th decades. Especially, the time needed for HCC formation in a HCV positive patient is 25-30 years (1) which means the prevalence we pointed out is a direct reflection of the prevalence of the society 20-30 years ago.

Our country Türkiye has developed a lot although we still have serious health problems. At least we don't use the same injector for vaccination in primary schools. The ratio of HBV carriers decreased from 9 % to 5 % among military donor between the years 1988 to 1991 (2). In Türkiye HCC viral distribution sample resembles much to those countries of higher endemic prevalence, and also HCV is which more common in chronic liver disease then HCC. Perhaps this results is strongly related with the long time for HCC to occur in a patient with chronic hepatitis. The time period for HCC formation is a strong evidence of HCC to turn out to be in the presence of chronic diffuse necroinflammatory disease or cirrhosis. However in our study in B group there were 2 patients with HCC with a normal histopathology of liver. This result also points out that there need not to be necessarily a cirrhotic development before HCC formation. The fact that even in seronegative HBV patients HDV DNA integration occurs (3), carcinogenic potential of HBV X gene protein (4,5) and tumour suppressed p 53 gene mutation (6) strongly supports that HBV is directly an oncogene virus.

In our study we have also seen that HDV ratio is statistically lower In HCC cases than the chronic liver disease patient (p<0.01). It may be suggested that HDV makes HBV progress rapidly and accelerates the transformation of HCC. But as the prognosis of HBV is worse the patient may die before HCC transformation, and this may reduce the incidence of HCC cases. More over the inhibitory effect of hepadnovirus helpers on replication phase may reduce the chance of HCC (7).

REFERENCES :

1. Kiyosawa K, Sodeyama T, Tanaka E et al (1990) 1990; 12:671-675
2. Alper A, Demiröz P (1991) IX. Ulusal Türk Gastroenteroloji Kongresi, 5-10 Kaslm 1991; ss102
3. Paterlini P, Gerken G, Nakajima E et al (1990) N Engl J Med 323:80-85
4. Spandau DF, Lee CH (1988) J Virol 62: 427-434
5. Seto E, Mitchell PJ, Yen TSB (1990) Nature 344: 72-74
6. Bressac B, Galvin KM, Liang TJ et al (1990) Proc Natl Acad Sci USA 87: 1973-1977
7. Purcell HR (1989) Cancer Detection and Prevention 14:203-207

Glutaminase and Glutamine Synthetase Activities During Azo-Dye Hepatocarcinogenesis in Rat

Iori Gotoh[1], Masahiro Ogawa[1], Hideo Ishizuka[1], Yasuyuki Arakawa[1], and Tetsuya Matsuno[2]

[1]The Third Department of Internal Medicine, Nihon University School of Medicine, Chiyoda-ku, Tokyo, 101 Japan
[2]National Institute of Health, Musashimurayama, Tokyo, 208 Japan

ABSTRACT

The activities of glutaminase and glutamine synthetase were determined in rats during induction of carcinogenesis by azo-dye. In the hepatoma tissue, the activities of phosphate-dependent glutaminase (PDG) and phosphate-independent glutaminase (PIG) significantly increased compared with those in normal appearing liver tissue. Increases of the two glutaminases were well correlated to serum alpha fetoprotein (AFP) levels. Furthermore, the difference of glutaminase isoenzyme form was demonstrated by electrophoresis using antibody to PDG extracted rat brain. On the other hand, glutamine synthetase activity was markedly decreased in the hepatoma tissue.

KEY WORDS: glutaminase, glutamine synthetase, α-fetoprotein, hepatoma, chemical carcinogenesis

INTRODUCTION

Glutamine is utilized as one of the major substrates for energy metabolism. At which time glutamine is hydrolized by glutaminase in mitochondria [1]. PDG (activated by phosphate) and PIG (activated by maleate) exist in this enzyme, but distinction of the roles between PDG and PIG is not clear. Previous studies [2] showed the activity of glutaminase was high in hepatoma cell lines, while the activity of glutamine synthetase (GS) was extremely low when compared with normal hepatic tissue, suggesting the importance of glutamine metabolism in transformation. It was, therefore, of interest to investigate these enzymes in vivo during hepatocarcinogenesis.

MATERIALS AND METHODS

Four-weeks-old male Donryu rats were used for the experiment. Experimental protocol is shown in Fig.1. Rats were divided into seven groups. Two control groups were fed with a normal diet, and five experimental groups were fed with a diet containing 0.06% 3'-methyl-4-dimethylamino-azobenzene (DAB). Further, the carcinogated liver was divided into two groups according to those macroscopical findings. One was the group of hepatoma tissue, designated "CA" group. The other one was the group of liver tissue surrounding hepatoma lesion, designated "CANC" group. Serum were collected at two weeks intervals from the 3rd week of initiating experiment. Serum AFP was determined by electrophoresis as described previously [3]. Rats were sacrified with ether, and livers were obtained. For measuring enzyme activities, tissues were immediately homogenized with cold physiological saline and supernatants were obtained after centrifugation at 3000rpm for 10min. Glutamine synthetase activity was assayed by the method of Matsuno et al [4]. The reaction mixture for glutaminase assay were performed according to the method of Matsuda et al [5], except that L-glutamine was replaced by [^{14}C]-glutamine(>250 mCi/mmol; Amersham, 0.2 μ Ci/tube). The reaction was carried out at 37 ℃ for 30min and terminated by adding cold ethanol. Specific radioactivity of ^{14}C trapped to DE81 paper(Whatman) was measured according to the method of Martin [6]. Protein was determined by the method of Smith et al [7] with bovine serum albumin as a standard. For the statistics, either unpaired t-test or Cochran-cox test was used. Electrophoresis of livers using antibody to PDG, extracted from rat brain was performed.

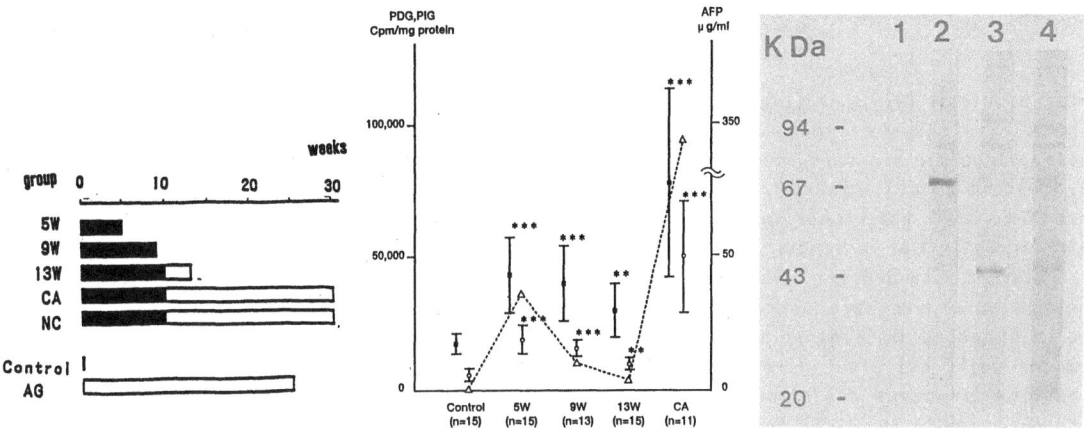

Fig. 1 Experimental protocol
　□ : a normal diet
　■ : a diet containing DAB
AG: Aging control,
CA: Carcinogenesis,
NC: no development of tumor

Fig. 2 PDG, PIG activities
and serum AFP during
hepatocarcinogenesis
(mean ± S.D.) ✻✻:p<0.01,
✻✻✻:p<0.001, ■ :PDG
○ :PIG , △ :AFP

Photo. 1 SDS-PAGE using
antibody to PDG extracted
from rat brain 1: liver of
"Control" 2: kidney of
"Control" 3: hepatoma
4: DAB-treated liver of "5W"

RESULTS

Glutamine metabolic enzyme activities during hepatocarcinogenesis is shown in Table 1. In hepatoma tissues, the activities of PDG and PIG significantly increased compared with those in the normal liver. The activities of PDG and PIG in hepatomas were approximately 4.5-fold and 8-fold higher than those in normal liver tissues, respectively. These activities in 5 (5W) and 9 week (9W) were slightly increased, while these activities were not observed significant change in liver tissues of "NC" group that did not develop hepatoma at 30th week. On the contrary, GS activity markedly decreased in hepatoma tissues. In 5(5W) and 9 week (9W), GS activities were slightly lower than those in normal control, while it was increased by 13 week (13W). GS activity in normal appearing tissues was higher than that in normal control. Fig. 2 shows the biphasal increase in the activities of the two glutaminases and serum AFP. First peak was seen in 5 week (5W), second peak was seen in the period of tumor development (CA). The enzymatic elevations were well correlated to serum AFP. SDS-PAGE four supernatants (normal liver of control, normal kidney of control, hepatoma, azo-dye-treated liver of "5W" group) was performed (Photo. 1). No apparent band was observed in normal liver tissue, but several bands were detected in hepatoma and liver treated with DAB for 5 weeks. Band were identical to those observed in kidney.

Table 1. PDG, PIG and GS activity during hepatocarcinogenesis
　　　　Values are mean ± S.D.. (versus control ✻:p<0.05, ✻✻:p<0.01, ✻✻✻:p<0.001)

Group (n:number of sample)		PD-glutaminase (cpm/mg protein)	PI-glutaminase (cpm/mg protein)	glutamine synthetase (U/mg protein)
Control	(n=15)	17824 ± 4153	6422 ± 1997	69.6 ± 13.7
Aging control	(n=15)	17713 ± 3712	5767 ± 1713	66.9 ± 8.6
5W	(n=15)	43040 ± 14114***	15500 ± 5685***	43.0 ± 9.7***
9W	(n=13)	36025 ± 10464***	11635 ± 3096***	44.7 ± 14.6***
13W	(n=15)	29524 ± 9797**	9756 ± 2684**	89.3 ± 17.7**
CA	(n=11)	76956 ± 34283***	50120 ± 21461***	6.0 ± 1.9***
CANC	(n=11)	23796 ± 6829*	10905 ± 4588*	84.2 ± 16.5*
NC	(n= 7)	27906 ± 13837	11794 ± 5202	81.8 ± 14.3

DISCUSSION

Glutamine is a key amino acid in the nitrogen metabolism as a nitrogen-doner for the biosynthetesis [8]. Glutamine is utilized as major respiratory substrate in malignant cell lines and transplantable tumors [1-2]. Glutamate, produced by the hydrolysis of glutamine, is catabolized via transamination in mitochondria for generating ATP [1]. At this time, glutamine is hydrolized by glutaminase in mitochondria. It was confirmed that the activity of this enzyme in hepatoma cells was higher than that in non-transformed cells [2]. Our results confirm that PDG and PIG activities in hepatoma were higher than those in normal liver. Furthermore, the activity in rats fed with DAB for 5 weeks were increased compared with those in normal controls and the enzyme activities were correlated to serum AFP. Pathology at the 5th week showed that oval cells appeared in liver acini, indicating that glutamine is catabolized and utilized not only cancer cells but also in rapidly proliferating cells like oval cells. Electrophoresis showed that the isoenzyme was altered to kidney type from liver type in hepatoma. Similar alteration was observed in the liver treated with DAB for 5 weeks. In previous study by Horowitz et al [9], it was proposed that PDG in the adult rat liver was different from that in kidney and other tissues. It is, however, well known that fetal liver consists of the kidney type. They further mentioned that a series of transplantable hepatomas may contain the kidney, rather than the liver, type of PDG, and that enzyme activities are well correlated to growth rate [10]. Similarly, the alterations of isoenzymes and enzyme activity appear to be closely correlated to cellular proliferation and immaturity produced by DAB. The ATP-dependent glutamine catalysis by glutamine synthetase is an important ammonia scavenger system in normal liver [2]. In the present study, GS activity was shown to be very low in hepatoma when compared to controls. In normal appearing tissue surrounding tumor, GS was higher than that in controls. We propose that the GS activity increase in normal tissue surrounding hepatomas might be a reflection of compensation for the increased metabolic demands from tumor cells which are unable synthesize glutamine. The present findings lead us to conclude that alterations in the glutamine metabolic enzymes also occur before neoplastic development, and that they closely relate to differentiation.

REFERENCES

1. Matsuno T, and Satoh T, Suzuki H (1986) Prominent glutamine oxidation activity in mitochondria of Avian transplantable hepatoma induced by MC-29 virus. J. Cell Physiol. 128:397-401

2. Matsuno T, and Hirai H (1989) Glutamine synthetase and glutaminase activities in various hepatoma cells. Biochem. Int. 19:219-225

3. Matsuno T, and Satoh T (1986) Glutamine metabolism in the Avian host bearing transplantable hepatomous growth induced by MC-29 virus. Int. J. Biochem. 18:187-189

4. Laurell CB (1966) Quantitative estimation of proteins by electro pholesis in agarose gel containing antibodies. Anal. Biochem. 15:45-52

5. Matsuno T, and Satoh T (1985) A sensitive assay for chicken glutamyltransferase. Int. J. Biochem. 17:1369-1371

6. Matsuda Y, Kuroda Y, Kobayashi K, and Katsunuma N (1973) Comparative study on glutamine, serine and glycine metabolism in ureotelic and uricotelic animals. J. Biochem. 73:291-298

7. Martin DW Jr. (1972) Radioassay for enzyme production of glutamate from glutamine. Anal. Biochem. 46:239-243

8. Smith PK, Krohn RI, Hermanson GT, Mallia AK, Gartner FH, Provenzano MD, Fujimoto EK, Goeke NM, Olson BJ, and Klenk DC (1985) Measurement of protein using bicinchoninic acid. Anal. Biochem. 150:76-85

9. Tata SS, and Meister A (1973) In: Glutamine metabolism, Prusiner E, and Stadtman ER (eds) Academic Press. New York, pp 75-85

10. Horowitz ML, and Knox WE (1968) A phosphate activated glutaminase in rat liver from that in kidney and other tissues. Enzymol. Biol. Clin. 9:241-253

11. Horowitz ML, Knox WE, and Morris HP (1969) Glutaminase activities and growth rates of rat hepatoma. Cancer Res. 29:1195-1199

Expression of the Antimetastatic Gene nm23 in Human Hepatocellular Carcinomas

Kaoru Nagahori, Masayuki Yamamoto, Hiroshi Kohno, Masatoshi Mogaki, Shingo Inoue, and Yoshiro Matsumoto

First Department of Surgery, Yamanashi Medical College, Tamaho-cho, Nakakoma-gun, Yamanashi, 409-38 Japan

ABSTRACT

Expression of nm23 messenger RNA was investigated by primer extension-reverse transcription and polymerase chain reaction method (RT-PCR) in patients with hepatocellular carcinomas (HCC). Relative density units (RDU) of the expression of nm23 (Mean ± S.D.) in non-cirrhotic liver, cirrhotic liver and HCC were 0.86 ± 0.26, 0.84 ± 0.24 and 0.56 ± 0.38, respectively. RDU in solitary HCCs less than 5 cm in diameter with no portal thrombus or capsular infiltration and multinodular HCCs in the whole liver were 0.74 ± 0.51 and 0.38 ± 0.26 ($p < 0.05$). Two years after gross resection of solitary HCCs, RDU in recurrent cases and in recurrence-free cases were 0.95 ± 0.57 and 0.49 ± 0.30, respectively ($p < 0.05$). These results suggest that the expression of nm23 decreases during progression of HCC. It may be a useful factor for predicting the risk of intrahepatic metastasis from HCC in individual cases at the time of initial surgical treatment.

KEY WORDS : hepatocellular carcinoma, nm23 gene, primer extension-reverse transcription and polymerase chain reaction method, metastatic potential

INTRODUCTION

In HCCs, clinicopathological analysis does not classify patients accurately into the risk groups[1]. In this study, we investigated the expression of antimetastatic gene, nm23[2], which encodes a potential tumor metastasis suppressor . Low expression of nm23 in human breast cancer significantly correlates with involvement of regional lymph nodes and decreased overall survival.[3] We investigated the association of nm23 with Staging of HCC[4] in HCC cancer specimens, to clarify its role as a prognostic indicator.

PATIENTS AND METHODS

Patients (Table 1)

Twenty nine patients with HCC and 4 patients without HCC received hepatectomy between Jan 1985 and Jan 1992 were examined (Table 1). In 16 Stage I and II patients (Group S) the tumors were solitary less than 5 cm in diameter, with no portal tumor thrombus or microscopic capsular infiltration. They were grossly removed. Ten Stage IV-A patients (Group M) had intrahepatic multiple nodules. The tumor-specimens in these patients were obtained from the main largest tumors. The nm23 expression was measured and compared in ; 1) non-tumorous non-cirrhotic liver (NL), cirrhotic liver (LC) and HCC of the Groups S and M, and 2) recurrent cases (n = 7) and recurrence-free cases (n = 9) after more than 2 years follow-up in Group S.

Preparation of RNA, Oligonucleotide primers, cDNA synthesis from RNA and PCR reactions

Resected liver and tumor tissues were obtained from surgical specimens. Specimens which were not macroscopically necrotic and not greatly influenced by the surgical procedures were frozen at $-80\,^{\circ}\mathrm{C}$ until use. Total cellular RNA was isolated from frozen tissue by acid guanidium thiocyanate, followed by density centrifugation in a cecium chloride gradient[5]. Primers specific for the nm23 cDNA sequence were designed based on the sequence reported[3].

5' − primer NMS2 : 5' − TATGGTCTGGGAGGGTCTGAAT − 3'
3' − primer NMA2 : 5' − ATGAATGATGTTCCTGCCAACT − 3'

Primers specific for the β-actin gene sequence were designed based on the gene sequence as follows[6] :

5' − primer BAS2 : 5' − AGGTCATCACCATTGGCAATGA − 3'
3' − primer BAA3 : 5' − GTCACACTTCATGATGGAGTTG − 3'

cDNA synthesis from RNA and PCR reactions were performed essentially according to the methods described by Okura et al[7]. Each amplified cDNA were electrophoresed through a polyacrylamide gel. The UV illuminated gels were photographed and densitometry was performed on the negative. The statistical significance of the differences in RDU was determined by two sample test with Welch's correction.

Table 1 patient characteristics

| | H C C | | L C | N L |
	solitary HCC (n=16)	multinodular HCC (n=10)	(n=13)	(n=4)
Median age (yr)	61.9	60.6	62.5	57.6
Sex (Men : Women)	12 : 4	9 : 1	11 : 2	4 : 0
Number of nodules	1	3.8		
Portal thrombus	0/16	7/10(70%)		
Capsular infiltration	0/16	8/10(80%)		
Size (cm)	3.4	4.8		

NL : non-cirrhotic liver
LC : cirrhotic liver
HCC : hepatocellular carcinoma

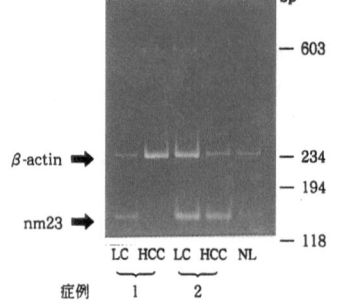

NL: non-cirrhotic liver
L : cirrhotic liver
H : hepatocellular carcinoma

Fig. 1 RT-PCR products of
nm23 and β-actin

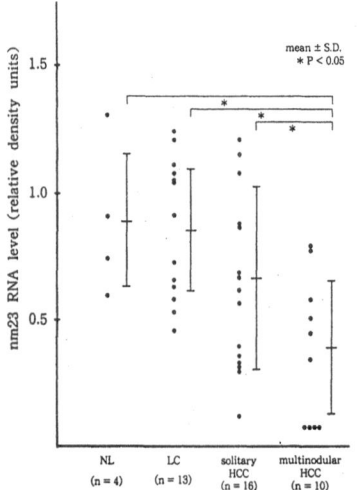

Fig. 2 nm23 expression in non-cirrhotic liver (NL),
cirrhotic liver (LC) and hepatocellular
carcinoma (HCC)

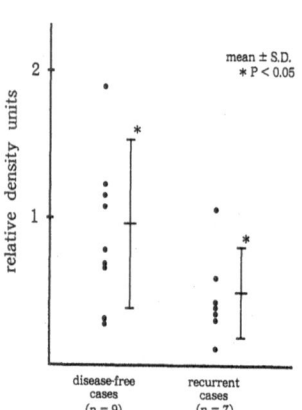

Fig. 3 nm23 expression in
solitary HCC

RESULTS

Fig.1 shows a UV photograph of the stained gel representing results of PCR coamplificaton of β-actin and nm23 performed on RNA isolated from LC and HCC. A 130 and a 239 bp fragment corresponded to the PCR products of nm23 and β-actin, respectively, as predicted. Several preliminary experiments were carried out to quality-control our semi-quantitative RT-PCR assay to determine the optimal PCR cycle numbers to yield informative data. The optimal cycle for discriminating RT-PCR expression was 25 cycles for both β-actin and nm23. RDU in NL, LC, HCC in Group S and HCC in Group M were 0.89 ± 0.26, 0.84 ± 0.24, 0.74 ± 0.54 and 0.38 ± 0.26, respectively (Fig. 2). The expression of HCC in Group M was significantly lower than that of NL, LC and HCC in Group S ($p < 0.05$). Within 2 years after hepatectomy in Group S 7 of 16 patients (43.7 %) had postoperative recurrence of HCC. RDU in the recurrent cases and in the recurrence-free cases were 0.95 ± 0.57 and 0.49 ± 0.30, respectively ($p < 0.05$) (Fig.3).

DISCUSSION

We investigated whether analysis of nm23 expression classifies patients accurately into the risk groups. In our present data, nm23 expression showed no significant association between NL, LC and HCC in the group S. In 10 matched samples of morphlogically cirrhotic liver and HCC, no significant association was shown. However, in HCC from Group M patients, the RDU was significantly lower than that in HCC from Group S patients. The Group M cases were classified as Stage IV-A, indicating advanced cancer. In Group S patients, all cases were single nodules without portal thrombus or capsular infiltration, indicating a relatively earlier stage. This data suggests that nm23 may be a suppressor gene in human HCC as in human breast cancer and that nm23 gene expression may be lost during tumor progression and differentiation. Sixteen patients in Group S were observed for possible recurrence for at least 2 years. The RDU in recurrent cases was slightly lower than that in disease-free cases. In conclusion, RDU in advanced HCC was significantly lower than that of earlier-stage HCC. These data are consistent with the hypothesis that reduced nm23 expression is associated with a high metastatic potential in primary HCC.

REFERENCES

1) Shirabe K, Kanematsu T, Matsumata T, Adachi E, Akazawa K and Sugimachi K (1991) Factors linked to early recurrence of small hepatocellular carcinoma after hepatectomy : univariate and multivariate analysis. Cancer 14 : 802 − 805.

2) Steeg PS, Bevilacqua G, Kopper L (1988) Evidence for a novel gene associated with low tumor metastatic potential. J Natl Cancer Inst 80 : 200 − 204

3) Hennesy C, Henry JA, May FEB, Westly BR, Angus B and Lennard TW (1991) Expression of the antimetastatic gene nm23 in human breast cancer : an associationwith good prognosis. J Natl Cancer Inst 83 : 281 − 285

4) American Jont Comittee on Cancer (1988) Manual for staging of cancer. Third edition. J.B.Lippincott Company, Philadelphia

5) Sambrook J, Fritsch EF and Maniatis T (1989) Molecular cloning, laboratory manual (second edition) C.S.H. Press, New York

6) Nakajima-Iijima S, Hamada S, Reddy P and Kakunaga T (1985) Molecular structure of the human cytoplasmic β-actin gene : interspecies homology of sequences in the introns. Proc Natl Acad Sci USA 82 : 6133 − 6137

7) Okura T, Kitani Y, Hamada S, Reddy P and Kakunaga T (1991) Quantitative measurement of extra-enal enin mRNA by polymerase chain reaction Biochem Biophys Res Commun 179 : 25 − 31

Decreased Frequency of Mitochondrial DNA Deletion in Hepatoma Developed from Cirrhotic Liver Detected by PCR Method

SHU FUKUSHIMA, KAZUO HONDA, MASAAKI AWANE, EIJI YAMAMOTO, RYOUJI TAKEDA, YOSHIO YAMAOKA, KEIICHIRO MORI, and KAZUE OZAWA

Second Department of Surgery, Faculty of Medicine, Kyoto University, Kyoto, 606 Japan

ABSTRACT

Using polymerase chain reaction (PCR) method, we analyzed the hepatic mitochondrial DNA deletion in relation to tumor, liver cirrhosis, age, sex, hepatitis B virus surface antigen and hepatitis C virus antibody. The 4977-bp deletion of mitochondrial DNA (mtDNA) was frequently detected in non-tumor specimens of adult liver, regardless of liver cirrhosis. However, none of the specimens obtained from cirrhotic liver of biliary atresia patients under 10 years old had that deletion of mtDNA. Ageing seems to be the main cause of deletion of mtDNA in non-tumor site of liver. The frequency of mtDNA deletion was decreased in hepatocellular carcinoma and other malignant tumors compared to non-tumor sites.

KEY WORDS: mitochondrial DNA, deletion, polymerase chain reaction, hepatocellular carcinoma, liver cirrhosis

INTRODUCTION

Recently, several types of deletions have been identified in the mtDNA of various tissues of old humans. Among these deletions, the 4977-bp deletion is the most prevalent one found in mtDNA of muscle, brain, heart, liver, lung, diaphragm and other organs [1-4]. In this study, we analyzed the 4977-bp mtDNA deletion of liver specimens in relation to tumor, liver cirrhosis, age, sex, HBs Antigen and HCV Antibody, using polymerase chain reaction (PCR) method to clarify the influence of the hepatic mitochondrial DNA deletion on post-operative clinical course of the patients.

MATERIAL AND METHODS

DNA Samples

The specimens are obtained from the patients who underwent hepatectomy from October 1991 to January 1993. Specimens were classified into 6 groups; 1) Hepatocellular carcinoma (HCC) with liver cirrhosis; 15 samples, 2) HCC without liver cirrhosis; 8 samples, 3) Metastatic liver tumor (without liver cirrhosis); 4 samples, 4) Other malignant tumors; 4 samples, 5) Benign tumors; 3 samples, 6) Liver cirrhosis (non-tumor site); 17 samples. 7) Normal; 29 samples. 8) Biliary atresia (Recipients of living-related liver transplantation); 12 samples.

DNA Purification and PCR analysis

Total DNA was extracted from each sample by standard methods. PCR analysis was carried out using standard buffers and Taq DNA polymerase (Perkin-Elmer Cetus). Two primers, encompassing the 4977-bp deletion, covered 7901-7920 and 13707-13729 of the Cambridge sequence [5], respectively.
To detect 5.83 kb PCR product from undeleted mtDNA, we performed the amplification cycle of 1 minute denaturation at 94 degree, 1 minute annealing

at 59 degree, and 5 minutes extension at 72 degree for 30 cycles in a Perkin-Elmer Cetus thermal cycler. In order to detect the shorter and rarer deleted mtDNA, we used the amplification cycle of 30 seconds at 94 degree, 20 seconds at 61 degree, and 15 seconds at 72 degree for 35 cycles. The amplified fragments were analyzed electrophoretically on agarose gel and the DNA bands were detected fluorographically after staining with ethidium bromide.

RESULTS

By using long PCR cycle time, we detected a product of 5.83 kb from all DNA samples. This result represents the amplification of the region between the primers in undeleted mtDNA. When using short PCR cycle time, we detected a product of 852 bp from some DNA samples, which represents amplification of the region between primers in mtDNA with 4977 bp deletion.
The 4977 bp deletion was detected in 6/15 samples (40%) of group 1, 0/8 (0%) of group 2, 1/4 (25%) of group 3, 1/4 (25%) of group 4, 3/3 (100%) of group 5, 11/17 (64.7%) of group 6. 23/29 (73.9%) of group 7, 0/12 (0%) of group 8 (Table 1). No deletion was found in any hepatic mtDNA of 12 patients under 10 years old (All of them underwent living-related liver transplantation for end-stage liver cirrhosis caused by biliary atresia). On the other hand 34 of 46 samples obtained from non-tumor site of patients over 20 years old (with or without liver cirrhosis) showed the 4977 bp mtDNA deletion (Table 2). Frequency of the deletion showed no significant relation to sex, HBs antigen and HCV antibody . Redox Tolerance Index (RTI), which indicates the changes of arterial ketone body ratio (acetoacetate/β-hydroxybutyrate), in response to 75g-OGTT (oral glucose tolerance test) [6], did not show any significant relationships with the deletion, either (Fig. 1).

Table 1 Frequency of mtDNA Deletion

	Cirrhosis (+)	Cirrhosis (−)	Total
HCC	6/15 (40%)	0/8 (0%)	6/23 (26.1%)
Metastasis *	−	1/4 (25%)	1/4 (25%)
Other Malignancy **	−	1/4 (25%)	1/4 (25%)
Benign Tumor ***	3/3 (100%)	−	3/3 (100%)
non-Tumor Site	11/17 (64.7%)	23/29 (79.3%)	34/46 (73.9%)
Biliary Atresia	0/12 (0%)	−	0/12 (0%)

    *   Liver metastasis of colorectal cancer
    ** Cystadenocarcinoma, Cholangiocarcinoma
    *** Angiomyolipoma, Hemangioma, Adenomatous Hyperplasia

Table 2 Relationship between Age and Frequency of mtDNA Deletion in non-Tumor Site

Age	Cirrhosis (+)	Cirrhosis (−)	Total
− 10 years	0/12 (0%)	−	0/12 (0%)
11 years −	−	−	−
21 years −	−	5/5 (100%)	5/5 (100%)
31 years −	−	1/2 (50%)	1/2 (50%)
41 years −	2/2 (100%)	7/8 (87.5%)	9/10 (90%)
51 years −	1/4 (25%)	2/5 (40%)	3/9 (33.3%)
61 years −	9/12 (75%)	5/5 (100%)	14/17 (82.4%)
71 years −	−	2/3 (66.7%)	2/3 (66.7%)

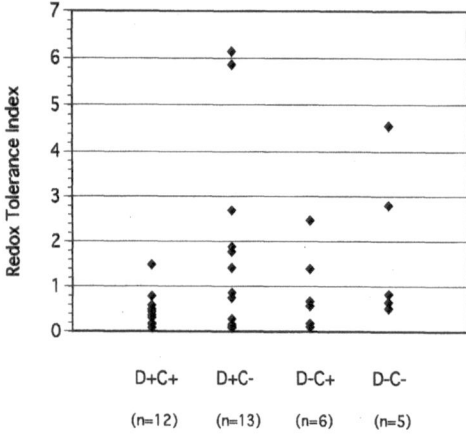

D+C+ : Deletion (+), Cirrhosis (+)

D+C- : Deletion (+), Cirrhosis (-)

D-C+ : Deletion (-), Cirrhosis (+)

D-C- : Deletion (-), Cirrhosis (-)

Fig. 1 Relationship between Redox Tolerance Index (RTI) and deletion of mtDNA with or without liver cirrhosis

DISCUSSION

A specific mutant mtDNA with a 4977-bp deletion was detected in liver and other various tissues of old humans and not observed in fetal tissues. In this study, we did not detect the 4977-bp deletion in cirrhotic liver of 12 pediatric patients with biliary atresia. On the contrary, mtDNA extracted from non-tumor site of adult liver samples showed high frequency of the deletion regardless of liver cirrhosis. So, it seems that ageing is the main cause of deletion of mtDNA in non-tumor site of the liver, whether cirrhosis is present or not, This study showed decreased frequency of mtDNA deletion of 4977 bp in HCC and other malignant tumors, compared to non-tumor sites. None of 8 samples obtained from HCC without liver cirrhosis showed the deletion of mtDNA. On the other hand, the deletion was found in 6/15 samples of HCC with liver cirrhosis. Deletion of mtDNA is supposed to diminish the ability of oxidative phosphorylation. So deleted mtDNA may be eliminated in the process of rapid proliferation and differentiation of tumor cells, such as "Bottle-neck effect". This may be one reason for decreased frequency of the mtDNA deletion in HCC and other malignant tumors.
As mitochondria play an important role in liver metabolism, accumulation of deleted mtDNA may lead to liver dysfunction. However Redox Tolerance Index, our pre-operative liver-functional index, failed to reveal any differences between the patients with the deleted hepatic mtDNA and the patients without deleted mtDNA. In this study, we only detected the existence of the deleted DNA, but could not determine its quantity and its rate to the undeleted DNA. So we are trying to determine these ratios, and investigate its clinical significance in post-operative course of hepatectomy.

REFERENCES

1. Cortopassi G.A, Arnheim N (1990) Nucleic Acids Res. 18: 6927-6933
2. Linnae A.W, Baumer A, Maxwell R.J, Preston H, Zhang C, Marzuki S (1990) Biochem. Int. 22: 1067-1076
3. Yen T.C, Su J.H, King K.L, Wei Y.H (1991) Biochem. Biophys. Res. Commun. 178: 124-131
4. Torii K, Sugiyama S, Tanaka M, Takagi K, Hanaki Y, Iida K, Matsuyama M, Hirabayashi N, Uno H, Ozawa T, (1992) Am. J. Respir. Cell Mol. Biol. 6: 543-549
5. Anderson S, Bankier A.T, Barrel B.G, de Bruijn M.H.L, Coulson A.R, Drouin J, Eperson I.C, Nierlich D.P, Roe B.A, Sanger F, Schreier P.H, Smith P.H, Staden R, Young I.G (1981) Nature 290: 457-465
6. Mori K, Ozawa K, Yamamoto Y, Maki A, Shimahara Y, Kobayashi N, Yamaoka Y, Kumada K (1990) Ann. Surg. 211: 438-446

The Significance of Biological Factors (DNA Ploidy Pattern, AgNOR Scores and Various Tumor Markers) in Cholangiocellular Carcinoma

Koichi Shimizu, Ryohei Izumi, Hideharu Tajima, Wataru Fukushima, Koya Sakamoto, Toru Ii, Masao Yagi, and Itsuo Miyazaki

The Second Department of Surgery, School of Medicine, Kanazawa University, Kanazawa, 920 Japan

ABSTRACT

DNA ploidy pattern and AgNOR (argyrophilic nucleolar organizer regions) scores of tumors, serum levels of tumor markers (CEA, HCG, and CA19-9) on diagnosis, and immunoreactivity of these tumor markers were examined in forty three cases of intrahepatic cholangiocellular carcinoma (CCC), with the relationship of these biological factors with clinicopathological factors and the prognostic significance being analyzed. Curative resection was performed in 14 cases, palliative resection in 10 cases, and no tumor was resected in 19 cases. Although no correlation was found between DNA ploidy patterns and the clinicopathological factors, the patients with DNA-diploid tumors had a significantly better prognosis than those with DNA-aneuploid tumors in curative resection patients. This result indicates that DNA ploidy pattern is an independent prognostic factor in CCC patients who underwent curative resection. Serum HCG is an indicator for the resectability of tumors. Patients with normal serum HCG had a relatively better prognosis than those with elevated serum HCG levels in all CCC patients. The good prognosis of the curative resection patients, when compared to the unresected cases, suggests that serum HCG reflects the degree of tumor growth.

KEY WORDS: intrahepatic cholangiocellular carcinoma, DNA ploidy pattern, AgNOR scores, tumor marker, prognostic significance

INTRODUCTION

Intrahepatic cholangiocellular carcinoma (CCC) is found in 5-6% of patients with primary liver cancer in Japan [1]. Because of its relative rarity, little is known about either the clinicopathological features of this tumor or the results of therapy.

Various biological parameters have been reported as the prognostic predictors of malignant tumors. Among other things, DNA ploidy pattern has been demonstrated to provide useful information about the prognosis for malignant tumors [2]. It has been reported that the number of argyrophilic nucleolar organizer regions (AgNOR) may reflect nuclear and cellular activities, and that they may act as an indicator of the degree of malignancy [3]. The use of tumor markers is useful in the follow-up of neoplastic patients, and some researchers propose the use of tumor markers as prognostic indices for different tumors [4,5].

The aim of this study is to evaluate the relationship of these biological factors with the clinical and pathological factors of intrahepatic CCC, as well as their prognostic significance.

MATERIALS AND METHODS

Forty three patients with a diagnosis of CCC were treated at the Second Department of Surgery, School of Medicine, Kanazawa University, during the period from 1970 to 1991. CCC was defined as an adenocarcinoma originating in the intrahepatic bile duct. Patients with hilar cholangiocarcinoma and bile duct cystadenocarcinoma were excluded from this study. Forty two patients had histologically proven CCC, and the remaining one patient was diagnosed as having CCC clinically and radiologically. There were 23 men and 20 women ranging in age from 32 to 78 with a mean age of 61 years.

In 28 cases, DNA ploidy patterns were analyzed using formalin-fixed and paraffin-embedded specimens by flow cytometry. DNA ploidy patterns were divided into diploidy and aneuploidy. The mean number of AgNOR per cell nucleus, or AgNOR scores, was determined in 28 cases by counting 100 nuclei directly on tissue sections at x400 magnification. The serum levels of carcinoembryonic antigen (CEA) in 36 patients, human chorionic gonadotropin (HCG) in 34, and carbohydrate antigen 19-9 (CA19-9) in 23 were measured by radioimmunoassey. In this study, the cut-off value was 5 ng/ml for CEA, 10 mIU/ml for HCG, and 37 U/ml for CA19-9. The production of these tumor markers in CCC were immunohistochemically examined: CEA in 33 cases, HCG in 28, and CA19-9 in 35.

For statistical analysis, the chi square test was used to get qualitative results. Survival was determined by Kaplan-Meier method and statistical differences were calculated by the generalized Wilcoxon's test.

RESULTS

The Stage of disease was determined according to UICC TNM classification [6]: two patients were in stage I, three in stage II, three in stage III, six in stage IV-A and 29 in stage IV-B. Thirty five patients (81%) presented with disease in an advanced stage (stage IV-A and IV-B). Intrahepatic metastases were found in 22 patients, peritoneal dissemination in seven, and distant metastases in four. Histologically, 31 patients had documented regional nodal metastases. Tumors were histologically categorized into three types according to the degree of cellular differentiation: well-, moderately-, and poorly-differentiated. Thirteen cases were classified as well-differentiated, 14 as moderately-differentiated, and 12 as poorly-differentiated.

Hepatic resection was performed with curative intent in 14 patients: bisegmentectomy with lymph node dissection for seven, segmentectomy with lymph node dissection for one, bisegmentectomy for two, segmentectomy for two, and subsegmentectomy for two. Palliative resection was performed in 10 patients. Sixteen patients had exploratory celiotomy and biopsy, and three did not undergo operation. Tumors in these patients were judged unresectable because of bilober multicentricity, major vascular invasion, peritoneal dissemination, or distant metastases.

Fifteen patients (53.6%) showed DNA-diploid tumors and 13 (46.4%) had DNA-aneuploid tumors. Sixteen patients (57.1%) had a tumor with low-AgNOR scores (under 3.0) and 12 (42.9%) had a tumor with high-AgNOR scores (above 3.0). DNA ploidy patterns and AgNOR scores did not correlate with the stage of disease, nodal metastases, intrahepatic metastases, peritoneal dissemination, histological grade of differentiation, and resectability of tumors. Serum CEA was high in 17 patients (47.2%), HCG was high in 13 (38.2%), and CA19-9 was high in 11 (47.8%). Statistical association was found between serum HCG and the resectability of tumors (p=0.0136). A trend was noticed between serum CEA and the resectability of tumors (p=0.0920). However, the serum levels of these tumor markers did not correlate with the stage of disease, nodal metastases, intrahepatic metastases, peritoneal dissemination, or histological grade of differentiation. Tumors with positive staining for CEA were found in 21 cases (63.6%), HCG-positive tumors in 12 (42.9%), and CA19-9-positive tumors in 20 (57.1%). No relationship was seen between the immunoreactivity of these tumor markers and clinicopathological factors, but a trend was found between HCG-immunoreactivity and the resectability of tumors (p=0.0986), and between CA19-9-immunoreactivity and histological grade of differentiation (p=0.0562).

Table 1 shows the survival rate of all patients and those who underwent curative resection, and the statistical significance. Among the patients who underwent curative resection, the patients with DNA-diploid tumors indicated a significantly higher survival rate than those with DNA-aneuploid tumors (p=0.0500). Any of AgNOR scores, the serum levels and the immunoreactivity of the tumor markers did not correlate significantly with the survival rate of either all patients or the curative resection patients, but the survival rate was relatively higher in the patients with normal serum HCG than in those with elevated serum HCG (p=0.0641).

Table 1. Univariate analysis of biological factors related to survival

| | | All patients | | | | Curative resection | | |
| | | Survival | | | | Survival | | |
	N	1-yr (%)	5-yr (%)	P	N	1-yr (%)	5-yr (%)	P
DNA ploidy								
diploidy	15	26.7	17.8	0.0598	4	75.0	75.0	0.0500
aneuploidy	12	8.3	0.0		4	25.0	0.0	
AgNOR scores								
under 3.0	12	41.7	10.4	0.1490	5	80.0	26.7	0.2630
above 3.0	15	6.7	6.7		3	33.3	33.3	
Serum CEA								
under 5ng/ml	17	35.3	14.1	0.1124	8	62.5	31.3	0.5934
above 5ng/ml	17	5.9	5.9		3	33.3	33.3	
Serum HCG								
under 10mIU/ml	20	30.0	12.0	0.0641	8	62.5	31.3	0.1766
above 10mIU/ml	12	0.0	0.0		2	0.0	0.0	
Serum CA19-9								
under 37U/ml	11	27.3	13.6	0.5987	6	50.0	25.0	0.8946
above 37U/ml	11	9.1	0.0		3	33.3	0.0	
CEA-immunoreactivity								
negative	11	27.3	9.1	0.5117	4	50.0	25.0	0.6925
positive	21	19.1	12.7		7	57.1	38.1	
HCG-immunoreactivity								
negative	14	14.3	0.0	0.2067	2	100.0	0.0	1.0000
positive	12	25.0	25.0		5	60.0	60.0	
CA19-9-immunoreactivity								
negative	14	21.4	7.1	0.7563	4	75.0	25.0	0.3336
positive	19	21.1	14.0		8	37.5	37.5	

DISCUSSION

Intrahepatic CCC is a relatively uncommon neoplasm. In spite of advances in diagnostic methods, the majority of the patients with intrahepatic CCC show the disease in a fairly advanced stage at the time of diagnosis. Curative resection, however, allowed some patients to survive for a relatively long period. In this study, we attempted to find out a prognostic factor after surgical treatment for CCC. A useful prognostic factor will allow us to perform a careful follow-up of patients and to decide what kind of adjuvant treatments is possible. DNA ploidy patterns showed a statistically significant correlation with the survival of the curative resection patients, while it did not indicate any statistical association with the stage of disease by UICC TNM classification, pathological factors, and the resectability of tumors. This result indicates that DNA ploidy patterns are an independent prognostic factor for CCC in curative resection patients. The patients with normal serum HCG had a relative better prognosis among all patients. A significant correlation between HCG levels and the resectability of tumors was found. The fact that curative resection patients had a good prognosis as compared to unresected patients suggests that HCG level reflects the degree of tumor growth.

REFERENCES

1. The Liver Cancer Study Group of Japan (1990) Ann Surg 211:277-287
2. Merkel DM, McGuire WL (1990) Cancer 56:1194-1205
3. Ploton D, Menager M, Jeannesson P, Himber G, Pigeon F, Adnet JJ (1986) Histochem J 18:5-14
4. Filella X, Molina R, Grau JJ, Pique JM, Garcia-Valdecasas JC, Astudillo E, Biete A, Bordas JM, Novell A, Campo E, Ballesta AM (1992) Ann Surg 216:55-59
5. Izumi R, Shimizu K, Kiriyama M, Hashimoto T, Urade M, Yagi M, Mizukami Y, Nonomura A, Miyazaki I (1992) J Surg Oncol 49:151-155
6. Hermanek P, Sobin LH (eds) (1987) UICC: TNM classification of malignant tumours, 4th edn. Springer, Berlin Heidelberg New York London Paris Tokyo

Diagnosis of Small Hepatocellular Carcinoma: Significance of Ultrasound and Tumor Markers

HIDEKAZU ITOH, HIDENORI NAKATA, HIROYA NAKATA, SHINYA KAWAGUCHI, TAKESHI HARA, YUKIHIRO YOKOYA, and SHINGO NISHIOKA

The Second Department of Internal Medicine, Wakayama Medical College, Wakayama, 640 Japan

ABSTRACT

Ultrasound (US) and tumor markers were used to examine 23 patients with small hepatocellular carcinoma (HCC) measuring less than 2 cm in diameter. US detected tumor echoes in 22 patients (96%). US patterns of internal echoes obtained from 22 patients with small HCC, included hypoèchoic patterns in 13 (59%), an isoechoic pattern in one (5%), hyperechoic patterns in seven (32%) and a mixed pattern in one (5%). These US findings were very different from those characteristic of large HCC that had been reported previously; few mosaic patterns, marginal hypoechoic zones (halo), lateral shadows or posterior echo enhancement were found. Alpha-fetoprotein (AFP) was positive, more than 21 ng/ml, in 65 percent of the patients, and protein induced by vitamin K absence or antagonist-II (PIVKA-II) was positive, more than 0.1 AU/ml, in 38 percent of the patients.

KEY WORDS: small hepatocellular carcinoma, ultrasound, alpha-fetoprotein, protein induced by vitamin K absence or antagonist-II

INTRODUCTION

With the recent advancement of imaging techniques and tumor markers, small hepatocellular carcinoma (HCC) is being detected more frequently than ever. Although small HCC had been traditionally defined based on various criteria, we defined HCC with a diameter of less than 2 cm, as small HCC, which was considered to be the severest criterion[1-3], for the purpose of this study. US patterns of HCC were reportedly characterized by a mosaic pattern of the internal echo of tumor, halo, a lateral shadow, posterior echo enhancement and others. This paper reports 23 patients with HCC measuring less than 2 cm in diameter which showed no above mentioned characteristic US patterns that had been traditionally stressed, but showed US findings peculiar to small HCC.

SUBJECTS AND METHODS

The subjects were 23 patients with less than 2-cm diameter small HCC that were diagnosed histologically in the Second Department of Internal Medicine, Wakayama Medical College, during a 10-year period from January 1983 to December 1992. There were 13 men and 10 women. Their ages ranged from 52 to 81 years, with a mean of 62 years. Ultrasonographic patterns of internal echoes of tumor were classified into four types:
1) hypoechoic: decreased echogenicity as compared to that of the hepatic parenchyma without cancer;
2) isoechoic: equal echogenicity;
3) hyperechoic: increased echogenicity; and
4) mixed echoic: a mixture of the these types (Fig. 1). Other findings studied, which had been reported previously as characteristic findings of HCC, included a mosaic pattern, a marginal hypoechoic zone (halo), a lateral shadow and posterior echo enhancement. Toshiba SSA-90A and SAL-77B and Aloka SSD-250, SSD-650 and SSD-670 were used as ultrasonic diagnostic devices for this study. Probes were used at 3.75 MHz and 3.5 MHz.

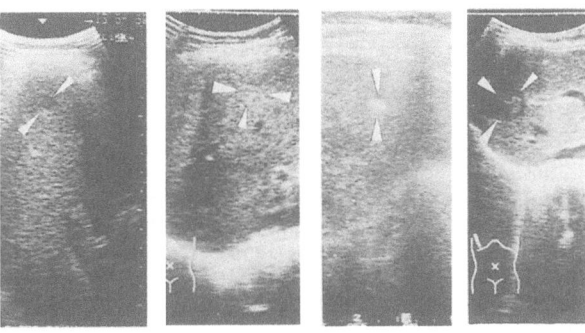

hypoechoic   isoechoic   hyperechoic   mixed

Fig. 1   Ultrasonographic pattern of hepatocellular carcinoma

Table 1   Clinical data of 23 patients with small hepatocellular carcinoma

No	Age	Sex	Associated liver disease	HBsAg/Ab	HCV Ab	AFP	PIVKA-II	Diagnostic clue
1	53	M	LC	+ / −	−	410	<0.06	US
2	61	M	LC	+ / −	−	8	<0.06	US
3	55	M	LC	− / −	+	9	<0.06	US
4	56	F	LC	− / −		940		AFP
5	67	F	LC	− / −		180		US
6	66	F	LC	− / −	+	19		US
7	55	M	LC	− / −	+	526	<0.06	AFP
8	74	M	LC	− / −		360		AFP
9	55	M	LC	− / −	+	37	<0.06	US
10	57	M	LC	− / +	+	75	<0.06	AFP
11	70	F	LC	− / −	+			US
12	59	M	LC	− / −		20	0.5	US
13	69	F	LC	− / +	+	63	1.49	US
14	54	F	CH	+ / −	−	11	1.17	US
15	75	F	CH	− / −	+	1730	0.17	AFP
16	54	M	LC	− / −		87		US
17	63	M	LC	− / −	+	22	<0.06	US
18	58	M	LC	− / −	+	45		US
19	61	F	LC	− / −	−	15	<0.06	US
20	52	M	LC	− / −	+	7	2.4	US
21	65	F	LC	− / +		51		US
22	81	M	LC	− / +		290		AFP
23	56	F	LC	+ / −		160		CT

Table 2   Ultrasonographic findings of 23 patients with small hepatocellular carcinoma

No	Tumor size (mm)	Internal echoes	Halo	Lateral shadows	Posterior echo enhancement	Location
1	8 × 9	hypoechoic	−	−	−	S5
2	12 × 12	hypoechoic	−	−	−	S6
3	12 × 14	hypoechoic	−	−	+	S6
4	14 × 15	hyperechoic	+	−	−	S4
5	14 × 15	hypoechoic	−	−	−	S5
6	15 × 15	hypoechoic	−	−	−	S8
7	14 × 17	hypoechoic	−	−	−	S4
8	16 × 16	hyperechoic	+	−	−	S4
9	15 × 18	hypoechoic	−	−	+	S6
10	16 × 18	hyperechoic	−	−	−	S8
11	17 × 17	hypoechoic	−	−	−	S6
12	16 × 20	hypoechoic	−	−	+	S4
13	17 × 19	isoechoic	+	−	−	S7
14	18 × 18	hyperechoic	−	−	−	S7
15	18 × 18	mixed	+	+	+	S8
16	18 × 20	hyperechoic	+	−	−	S2
17	18 × 20	hypoechoic	−	−	−	S2
18	19 × 19	hypoechoic	−	−	−	S6
19	19 × 20	hyperechoic	+	−	−	S7
20	20 × 20	hypoechoic	−	−	−	S8
21	20 × 20	hyperechoic	−	−	−	S6
22	20 × 20	hypoechoic	−	−	−	S2
23	20 × 20	(not observed)				S8

RESULTS

Twenty-three patients with less than 2-cm diameter small HCC had the following background. All of the patients had underlying chronic hepatic diseases; HCC did not develop from the normal liver. Of all patients, 21(91%) had liver cirrhosis (LC). The remaining 2 patients (9%) had chronic hepatitis (CH). Four (17%) of the 23 patients were HBs antigen-positive, and another four (17%) were HBs antibody-positive. Eight patients (34%) were infected with hepatitis-B virus. HCV antibody-positive patients were very frequently found—11 (73%) of the 15 patients—suggesting the close relationship between HCC and hepatitis-C virus. If alpha-fetoprotein (AFP) of 21 ng/ml or higher was evaluated as positive, the rate of positive tumor markers of small HCC was 65 percent. If the value of 0.1 AU/ml or higher was evaluated as positive, protein induced by vitamin K absence or antagonist-II (PIVKA-II) was positive in 38 percent of the patients. Served as a diagnostic clue was US in 16(70%) of the 23 patients and AFP in six (26%). Computed tomography (CT) was served as a diagnostic clue in only one patient (4%) (Table 1).

Table 2 shows US findings in 22 patients with less than 2-cm diameter small HCC. The shape of the tumor was round or oval in all patients. Thirteen patients (59%) showed hypoechoic patterns of internal echoes, one patient (5%) showed an isoechoic pattern, seven patients (32%) showed hyperechoic patterns, and one patient (5%) showed a mixed pattern. Uniform internal echoic patterns accounted for a great majority of the patients, 21 patients (95%). A mosaic pattern was found in only one (5%) of the patients. Six patients (27%) showed halo, which frequently appeared with hyperechoic patterns. A lateral shadow was observed in only one patient. Four patients (18%) showed posterior echo enhancement, which more frequently appeared with hypoechoic patterns of internal echoes.

DISCUSSION AND CONCLUSIONS

What policy is useful for early detection of small HCC? First, it is essential to monitor B and C types of chronic hepatic diseases carefully, particularly liver cirrhosis, which should be considered a high-risk group. Second, PIVKA-II is a useful tumor marker for small HCC. PIVKA-II was positive in only 38 percent of the patients with small HCC, but PIVKA-II was positive in three AFP-negative patients. This suggested that PIVKA-II was a good diagnostic indicator of small HCC.

US was unable to visualize a tumor which was detected by CT in one patient. This was because the tumor existed beneath the diaphragm dome in the Couinaud's S8—the liver segment—where a blind spot existed for US. US clearly visualized small HCC as a tumor echo in 22 patients except for the patient described above. US findings of HCC were characterized by mosaic pattern, halo, lateral shadow and posterior echo enhancement. However, only one patient (5%) with a less than 2-cm diameter small HCC showed all these features. Therefore, if US is used with the expectation of obtaining US findings characteristic of large HCC , US may not detect small HCC. In other words, small HCC shows very different US findings than those of ordinary sized HCC with a diameter of more than 2-cm. The most well defined feature of the US profiles obtained from 22 patients with small HCC was a uniform internal echo of the tumors. Indeed, 21(95%) of the 22 patients showed this feature. In sum, it is important for early detection of small HCC using US to conduct ultrasonically guided liver biopsy, paying close attention to internally uniform nodules without a halo, a lateral shadow or posterior echo enhancement.

REFERENCES

1. Kudo M, Tomita S, Tochio T, et al. (1992) Small hepatocellular carcinoma: Diagnosis with US angiography with intraarterial CO_2 microbubbles. Radiology 182: 155-160
2. Barbara L, Benzi G, Gaiani S, et al. (1992) Natural history of small untreated hepatocellular carcinoma in cirrhosis: A multivariate analysis of prognostic factors of tumor growth rate and patient survival. Hepatology 16: 132-137
3. De' Santis M, Romagnoli R, Cristani A, et al. (1992) MRI of small hepatocellular carcinoma: Comparison with US, CT, DSA and Lipiodol CT. J. Comput. Assisted Tomography 16: 189-197

Evaluation of Ultrasonically Guided Liver Biopsy for the Diagnosis of Small Hepatocellular Carcinoma

HIDEKAZU ITOH, JUN KAWAI, KENJI ARII, HIROSHI TOKUYAMA, TORU TANIDA, TETSUJI YAMANISHI, KIKUKAZU SAKATSUJI, KENICHI AIZAWA, and SHINGO NISHIOKA

The Second Department of Internal Medicine, Wakayama Medical College, Wakayama, 640 Japan

ABSTRACT

Ultrasonically (US)-guided percutaneous liver biopsies were carried out in 410 patients without postoperative complications. US-guided fine needle biopsies detected small hepatocellular carcinoma (HCC) with a diameter of 9 mm. As it is difficult to make a differential diagnosis of a small focal lesion in the liver using various imaging techniques and tumor markers, we recommend actively using a fine needle liver biopsy guided by US.

KEY WORDS: small hepatocellular carcinoma, liver biopsy, ultrasound

INTRODUCTION

With the recent widespread use of an ultrasound (US) diagnostic device, intrahepatic space occupying lesions are beginning to be detected accurately. A majority of the 22 patients were histologically diagnosed as having small hepatocellular carcinoma (HCC) with a diameter of less than 2 cm by US-guided liver biopsy carried out in the Second Department of Internal Medicine of Wakayama Medical College. This paper reports the practice of various techniques for liver biopsy and complications[1-3], evaluation of the ability of biopsy to hit the target tumor and an interesting case.

SUBJECTS AND METHODS

The subjects were 636 patients who had liver biopsies in the Second Department of Internal Medicine of Wakayama Medical College during 13 years from January 1980 to December 1992. Biopsies were conducted 226 times using 3-mm diameter thick Silverman needles[4] under laparoscopy, 172 times using 13 G Oku's Silverman-type needles guided by US, 132 times using 15 G Matsuda's True-cut type[5] needles, and 106 times using 21 G Majima's Aspiration type[6] fine needles. Figure 1 shows methods of collecting tissues for each liver biopsy technique.

RESULTS

Only one patient (0.4%) who had biopsy under laparoscopy developed hemobilia which needed blood transfusion. US-guided liver biopsies conducted in 410 patients caused no complications (Table 1). An analysis of the ability of a Majima fine needle to target intrahepatic small space occupying lesions with a diameter of less than 2 cm revealed that the needle tended to show a decreased ability to hit a distant target. As a whole, however, the needle showed a very high percentage of accuracy; it hit the target 43(75.4%) of the 57 times (Fig. 2).

CASE PRESENTATION

A 53-year-old man came to the Second Department of Internal Medicine of Wakayama Medical College regularly because of HBs Ag-positive liver cirrhosis B. He was diagnosed as having a 9-mm diameter hypoechoic lesion in the Couinaud's S5, the liver segment, by a US examination conducted at the out-patient clinic, and was hospitalized November 4, 1992. Laboratory

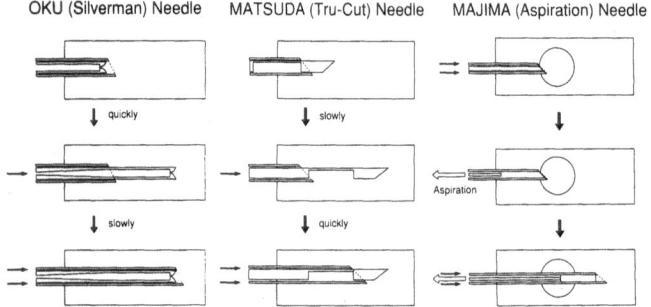

Fig. 1 Method of collecting tissues using various needles.

Table 1 Results and complications of liver biopsies conducted in the Second Department of Internal Medicine of Wakayama Medical College.

	name of inventors	type & diameter of needles	number of biopsies	complication
under laparoscopy	Silverman I.	Silverman ∅ 3 mm	226	1*
ultrasonically guided	Oku A. (Wakayama Med. College)	Silverman 13G	172	0
	Matsuda Y. (Ohtemae Hospital)	true-cut 15G	132	0
	Majima Y. (Kurume University)	aspiration 21G	106	0
		total	636	1

* hemobilia

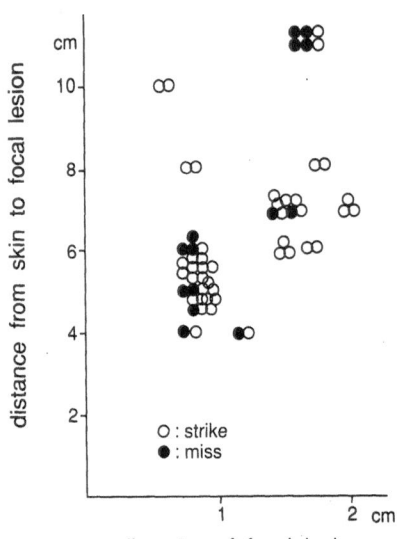

Fig. 2 Ability of the Majima's needle to target a less than 2-cm diameter space occupying lesion in liver.

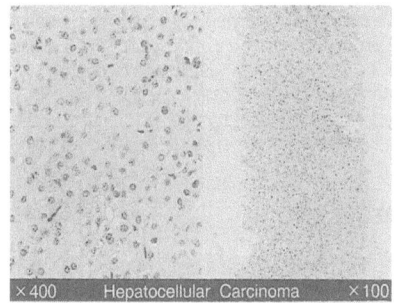

Fig. 4 Tissues for biopsy revealing hepatocellular carcinoma.

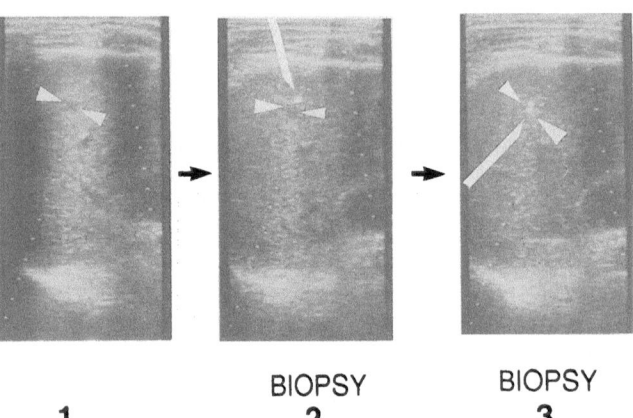

BIOPSY 1   BIOPSY 2   BIOPSY 3

Fig. 3 Short arrow indicating hypoechoic lesion in the Couinaud's S5 and long arrow demonstrating tip of a biopsy needle.

data showed RBC 405 × 10⁴, Hb 14.1, WBC 4000, platelet count 6.7 × 10⁴, PT
58 percent, T. Bil. 1.7 mg/dl, GOT 176 U/L, and ICG R15 25 percent. An
endoscopy revealed esophageal varix. A 21 G Majima fine needle punctured a
hypoechoic lesion of a tumor with a diameter measuring 9 mm 7 times. Six of
the seven tissues showed cancerous cells (Fig. 3 and 4).

DISCUSSION

Biopsy using a thick needle with a diameter of 3 mm under laparoscopy has
been conducted for a relatively long time. It is useful for histological
diagnosis of diffuse hepatic diseases, but may develop complications because
a thick needle is used. For this reason, recently this biopsy technique has
fewer opportunities to be used in the Second Department of Internal Medicine
of Wakayama Medical College. On the other hand, US-guided liver biopsy is
much safer than the above-mentioned technique for the following two reasons:
1) it uses a small diameter needle, 13G to 21G, and
2) it enables us to bypass risky parts of the liver while monitoring
   intrahepatic blood vessels and the bile duct at real time.
Even in US-guided liver biopsy, we try to control bleeding by padding the
operative field with oxydized cellulose-impregnated cotton when a little
large diameter needle, 13G or 15G, is used to diagnose a diffuse hepatic
disease.

We often use a 21G Majima type aspiration fine needle for the tumor biopsy
by hitting the target. The 21G Majima needle is characterized by its small
diameter, only 0.8 mm, the same diameter as that of a needle for intravenous
injection. The cross-sectional area of the Majima needle is less than 1/14
of that of the 3-mm diameter Silverman needle used under laparoscopy.
Because the Majima needle is fine and very safe, biopsy of small tumors can
be carried out many times, which helps to make diagnosis more accurate. For
biopsy of small tumor with a diameter of about one cm, we usually puncture
it five times to prevent any false negative results. We have not
experienced a disseminated tumor, and there are no reports that have been
written on it. Because this method provides a substantial amount of tissue,
as shown in Fig. 4, we have found no difficulties in making judgment on the
benignancy or malignancy of a tumor. Since aspiration biopsy using a fine
needle has lead to accurate diagnoses without any risk, we strongly
recommend using this technique for liver biopsy, allowing patients to be
treated before it is too late because of prolonged observation of the course
of an intrahepatic space occupying lesion without any particular reason.

REFERENCES

1. Buscarini L, Fornari F, Bolondi L, et al. (1990) Ultrasound-guided
   fine-needle biopsy of focal liver lesions: Techniques, diagnostic
   accuracy and complications. A retrospective study on 2091 biopsies.
   J. Hepatol. 11: 344-348
2. Jankovic G, Grbic R, Jesic R, et al. (1992) Ultrasonically guided
   fine-needle biopsy of liver hemangioma: Are there any risks? Arch.
   Gastroenterohepatology 11: 102-103
3. Lichtenstein DR, Kim D, Chopra S (1992) Delayed massive hemobilia
   following percutaneous liver biopsy: Treatment by embolotherapy. Am.
   J. Gastroenterol. 87: 1833-1838
4. Silverman I and Brooklyn NY (1954) Improved Vim-Silverman biopsy
   needle. J.A.M.A. 155: 1060-1061
5. Maharaj B and Pillay S (1991) "Tru-Cut" needle biopsy of the liver:
   Importance of the correct technique. Postgrad. Med. J. 67: 170-173
6. Ljubicic N, Bilic A, Lang N, et al. (1992) Ultrasonically guided
   percutaneous fine needle aspiration biopsy of the hepatic and
   pancreatic focal lesions: Accuracy of cytology in the diagnosis of
   malignancy. J.R. Soc. Med. 85: 139-141

The Significance of the Determination of AFP-Isoform in the Early Diagnosis of Hepatocellular Carcinoma (HCC)

Hideo Ishizuka, Hiroko Taga, Iori Gotoh, and Yasuyuki Arakawa

The Third Department of Internal Medicine, Nihon University School of Medicine, Chiyoda-ku, Tokyo, 101 Japan

ABSTRACT

AFP-isoform was determined retrospectively in 48 patients with HCC, and in 53 patients with liver cirrhosis(LC) prospectively using lectin electrophoresis by antibody-affinity blotting techinique. Results shows that (1)30% patients with HCC, HCC-type AFP-isoform had appeared 3 ~10 months before the graphic detection of HCC, and (2)60% patients with LC, whose AFP-isoform was similar, HCC developed within 1 year. Thus, the periodical determination of AFP-isoform in AFP positive patients with LC was considered very useful for the early diagnosis of HCC.

KEY WORDS:AFP-isoform, early diagnosis of HCC, sugar chain, lectin electrophoresis

INTRODUCTION

Serum alpha-fetoprotein(AFP)is the most useful tumor marker in detection of HCC. AFPs, however, also appear in patients with LC. AFP contains a small amount of sugar chain, and exhibits microheterogeneiety in its affinity to lectins(AFP-isoform). A sensitive electrophoretic techinique was established by Taketa et al [1]. The present study reports the successful earlier diagnosis of HCC by periodical AFP-isoform determination during the course of LC. It is thus possible that determination of AFP-isoform is helpful for differential diagnosis between LC and HCC.

MATERIALS AND METHODS

AFP-positive sera were collected periodically from 48 patients with HCC and 53 patients with LC at our hospital, and were stored at -80℃, until electrophoretic analysis. Lectin electrophoresis was performed accordingly to Taketa's method , using two lectins: Lentil lectin-A(LCA) and phytohemagglutinin-E_4 (PHA-E_4). Specimens were electrophoresed on the lectin agarose gel plates and the proteins were blotted on nitrocellulose membrane precoated with the specific horse antibody against human AFP. After electrophoresis, AFPs were blotted on the nitrocellulose membrane. The blotted AFPs were then detected by rabbit immunoglobulines to human AFP and horse radish peroxidase-labeled goat antibody to rabbit IgG , followed by color development with diaminobenzidine as the substrate for the peroxidase.

RESULTS

Figure 1 shows the typical patterns detected in the lectin electrophoresis of AFP with LCA and PHA-E_4. The pattern characterized by the retarding bands(L_3 in LCA or P_4, P_5 in PHA-E_4) was detected specificically in the patients with HCC(HCC-type isoform) and another pattern was mainly detected in the patients with LC(LC-type isoform).

Figure 1. Typical patterns of lectin electrophoresis of AFP in HCC and LC.

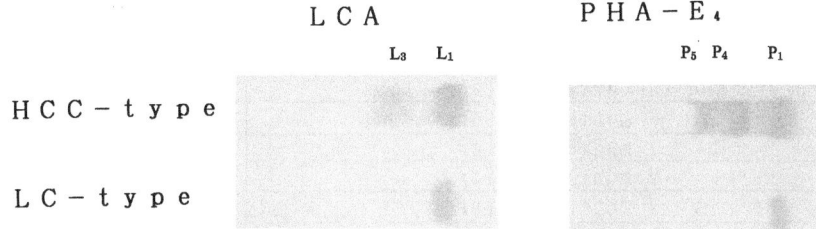

HCC-type AFP-isoform was detected in 44 out of 48 patients with HCC(92%). In 11 out of these 44 cases, AFP-isoform changed from LC-type to HCC-type during their courses. And in 3 out of those 11 cases, HCC-type isoform was detected 3～10 months before the graphic detection of HCC. Although the rates were not so high, the existense of such cases in which HCC-type isoform appeared earlier than the graphic detectin of HCC, suggested the posibility of the early diagnosis of HCC by the periodical detection of AFP-isoform, and led us to the prospective study in the patients with LC, the high-risk group of HCC.

Figure 2 shows the results of the periodical AFP-isoform determination in the patients with LC. HCC-type isoform was positive in 7 out of 53 patients with LC at the first determination, and in 9 out of remained 46 patients AFP-isoform changed from LC-type to HCC-type. Therefore, HCC-type isoform was detected in 16 out of 53 patients with LC during the observation term. And HCC developed in 9 out of these 16 patients within 1 year after the first detection of HCC-type isoform. Otherweise, HCC developed in 3 cases without the change of AFP-isoform.

Fig. 2. AFP-isoform in the patients with LC

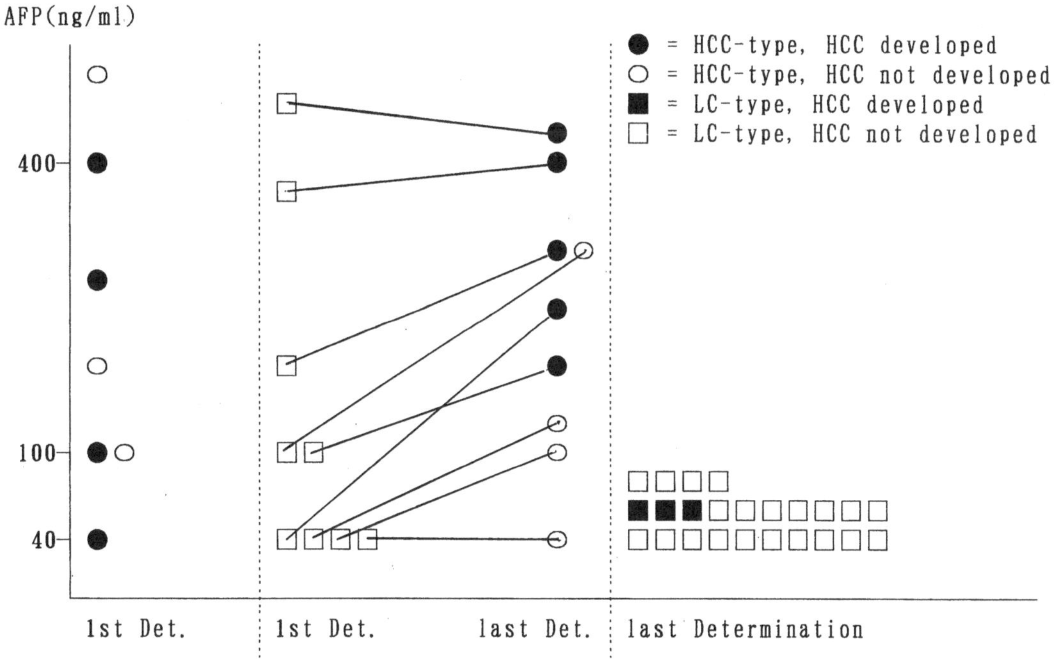

AFP(ng/ml)

● = HCC-type, HCC developed
○ = HCC-type, HCC not developed
■ = LC-type, HCC developed
□ = LC-type, HCC not developed

400—

100—

40—

1st Det.   1st Det.   last Det.   last Determination

Table 1 shows the summary of 9 cases of LC, found to have the HCC-type AFP-isoform and thereafter developed HCC. It was noticeable that in 4 cases indicated by ☆, the HCC-type AFP-isoform was detected 3 months or more before the first graphic diagnosis of HCC. Moreover, the fact that the size of tumor was below 20x20 mm in 3 out of these 4 cases, was impressible.

Table1. Summary of 9 cases of LC found to have the HCC-type AFP-isoform and thereafter HCC developed.

AFP level(ng/ml)	Relation between the detection of HCC-type isoform and the graphic diagnosis	Tumor size(mm)
383.0	☆ 6 months before	20x17
241.0	1 month after	20x18
103.0	2 months before	23x20
45.0	☆ 7 months before	diffuse
195.4	☆ 6 months before	20x20
483.0	3 months after	50x45
286.5	2 months after	45x35
150.0	6 months after	60x50
559.0	☆ 11 months before	20x20

DISCUSSION

According to the improvement of the assay system, AFP-positive cases increased in LC, on which almost all HCC superimposed. Then, it becomes important to differentiate between the AFPs appearing in sera of the patients with LC and HCC. Human AFP shows a single band in conventional electrophoresis, however, heterogeneiety has been demonstrated in its affinity to lectins(AFP-isoform)[2-6]. AFP contains 3-4%of sugars in its molecule and the structure of the sugar chain has caused the heterogeneiety. Many patients having small HCC do not show such high serum AFP, e.g., less than 200ng/ml. Therefore, specificity of AFP in the early stage of HCC is not enough high. This paper shows the usefulness of the qualitative follow-up of serum AFP with its isoform in the early diagnosis of HCC. It is surprising that isoform changed to HCC-type 3 months or more before the graphical detection of HCC in 4 out of 53 cases of LC, who were follow-uped at our hospital. Moreover, in 3 out of those 4 cases the sizes of tumors were less than 20mm in diameter supported the usefulness of the analyses of AFP-isoform in the early diagnosis of HCC. Antibody-affinity blotting techinique is very sensitive, however, this method requires much skill, lectins are considerably expensive, and serum concentraed is needed in cases having low levels of AFP(less than 50ng /ml). Development of the monoclonal antibody, sensible to the minimam change of sugar chains is optimal.

REFERENCES

1 Taketa K, Ichikawa E, Taga H, and Hirai H:Antibody-affinity blotting: A sensitive techinique for the detection of α-fetoprotein separated by lectin affinity electrophresis in agarose gel. Electrophoresis 6:492-495,1985.

2 Smith CJ, Kelleher PC: α-fetoprotein:qsaeparation of two molecular variants by affinity chromatography with concanavalin A-agarose. Biochim Biophys Acta 317: 231-235,1973.

3 Ruoslahti E, Engvall E, Pekkala A, Seppala A:Developmental changes in carbonhhydrate moiety of human alpha-fetoprotein. Int J Cancer 22:515-520,1978

4 Kerckaert J-P, Bayard B, Biserte G:Microheterogeneiety of rat, mouse and human α-frtoprotein as revealed by polyacrylamide gel electrophoresis and by crossed immunoaffinoelectrophoresis with different lectins. Biochim Biophys Acta 57 6:99-108,1979.

5 Breborowicz J, Mackewicz A, Breborowicz D:Microheterogeneiety of alpha:fetoprotein in patient serum as demonstrated by lectin affino-electrophoresis. Scand J Immunol 14:15-20,1981

6 Taketa K, Izumi M, Ichikawa E:Distinct molecular species of human α-fetoprotein due to differential affinities to lectins. Ann NY Acad Sci 417:61-68,1983

Intratumor Pressure in Hepatocellular Carcinoma

Tsuneo Tanaka, Eizo Okamoto, Naoki Yamanaka, Takeshi Oriyama,
Kazutaka Furukawa, Eisuke Kawamura, Fumihito Tomoda,
Nobutaka Ichikawa, Wataru Tanaka, and Chiaki Yasui

The First Department of Surgery, Hyogo College of Medicine, Nishinomiya, Hyogo, 663 Japan

ABSTRACT

Intratumor pressure and hepatic tissue pressure were measured intraoperatively in 50 patients with hepatocellular carcinoma. Changes in these pressure were monitored before and after individual occlusion of the proper hepatic artery and the portal vein. Our result indicated that intratumor pressure was regulated predominantly by hepatic arterial blood flow, and increased with tumor capsular formation. In contrast, hepatic tissue pressure was regulated predominantly by portal blood flow, and increased with portal vein pressure.

KEY WORDS: tumor pressure, hepatocellular carcinoma, hepatic tissue pressure, portal vein pressure

INTRODUCTION

We intraoperatively measured intratumor pressure in hepatocellular carcinoma and hepatic tissue pressure, and investigated the relationship between those pressures and tumor characteristics or hepatic circulation.

MATERIALS AND METHODS

Sixty patients who underwent hepatic resection for a liver tumor from June 1990 through December 1992 were included our study. Fifty patient had hepatocellular cartinoma (HCC), and ten patient had metastatic liver tumor. Patient age ranged from 45 to 70 years (average, 56 years), and the male-female ratio was 5:1. Intratumor pressure (TP) and hepatic tissue pressure (HTP) were measured by intraoperatively using a 21G needle filled with heparinized saline attached to a pressure trasducer (P23XL-1, NIHON KOHDEN), amplifier (RMP-6004M, NIHON KOHDEN), recorder (RJG4002, NIHON KOHDEN). The needle was inserted into tumor or non-tumor area under ultrasound guidance. In ten patient, TP and HTP were monitored before and after individual occlusion of the proper hepatic artery (PHA) and the portal vein (PV). Portal vein pressure (PVP) was obtained directly via the umbilical vein.

RESULTS

TP in patient with HCCs ($23.1 \pm 2.0 \mathrm{cmH_2O}$, mean$\pm$SE) was higher than HTP of them ($12.2 \pm 0.7 \mathrm{cmH_2O}$). HTP of cirrhotic liver ($12.2 \pm 0.7 \mathrm{cmH_2O}$) was higher than that of non-cirrhotic liver ($6.3 \pm 0.6 \mathrm{cmH_2O}$) (Fig. 1). TP in encapsulated HCCs ($25.9 \pm 2.3 \mathrm{cmH_2O}$, n=41) was higher than that of non-capsulated HCCs ($10.4 \pm 4.4 \mathrm{cmH_2O}$, n=9). Encapsulated HCCs with intracapsular necrosis induced by embolization before surgery had lower TP ($18.8 \pm 2.7 \mathrm{cmH_2O}$, n=10) as compared to those without necrosis ($28.2 \pm 2.7 \mathrm{cmH_2O}$, n=31) (Fig. 2). There was a significant correlation between HTP and PVP (Fig. 3). But there was no significant correlation between TP and PVP (Fig. 4). After occlusion of the PHA, TP dropped to 71%, PVP dropped to 87% and HTP remained at 97% of the preocclusion value. In contrast, PV occlusion resulted in a drop of PVP to 71%, HTP dropping to 82% while TP only declined to 94% (Fig. 5).

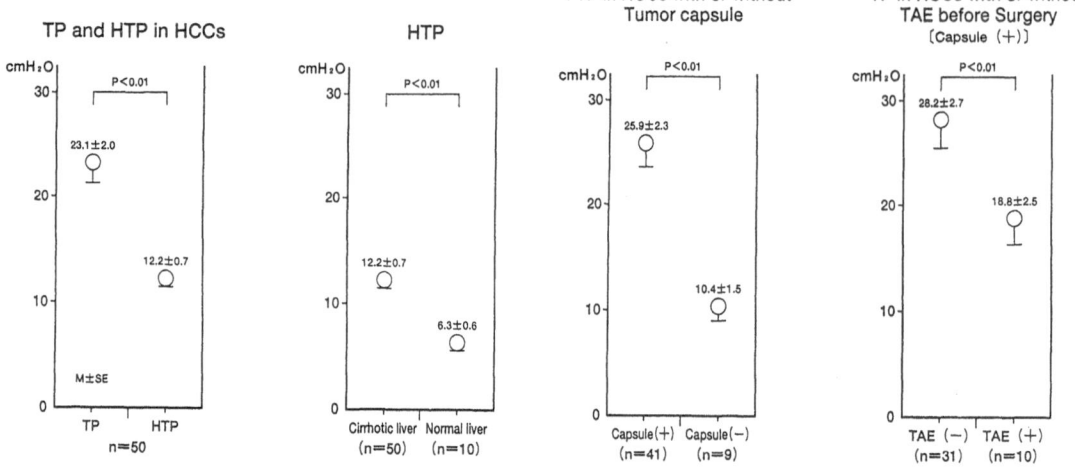

Fig. 1 Intratumor pressure (TP) in HCCs was signifcantly higher than hepatic tissue pressure (HTP) (P<0.01), and HTP in cirrhotic livers were higher than those of normal livers (P<0.01).

Fig. 2 TP in HCCs with tumor capsule was signicantly higher than that without capsule (P<0.01), and TP in HCCs treated with preoperative embolization (TAE) was higher than that without embolization (P<0.01).

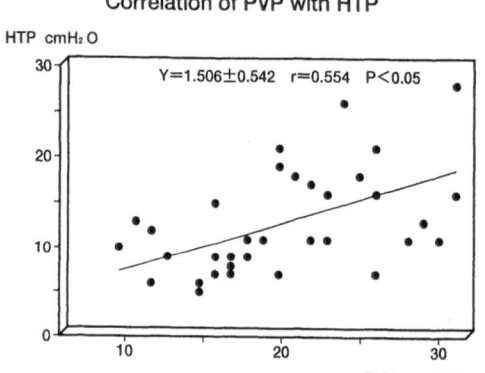

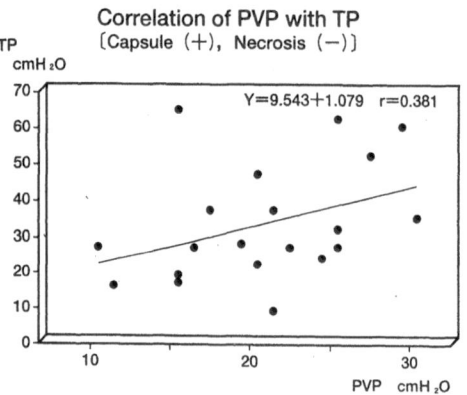

Fig. 3 HTP was significantly correlated with PVP (P<0.05).

Fig. 4 TP in HCCs had no significant correlation with PVP.

Change of each pressure
after occlusion of PHA and PV

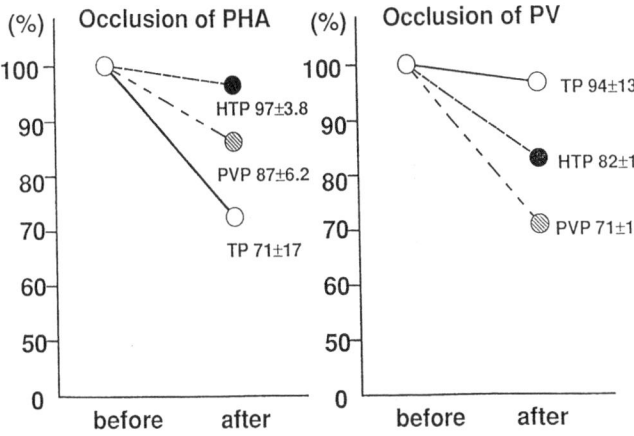

Fig. 5 After occlusion of the proper hepatic artery, TP in HCCs dropped to 71%, PVP dropped to 87%, HTP remained at 97% of the preocclusion value. In contrast, potal vein occlusion resulted in a dropped to 71%, HTP dropped to 82%, while TP only slightly declined to 94%.

DISCUSSION

Some previous studies showed a significant correlation between hepatic tissure pressure and portal vein pressure or wedged hepatic vein pressure.[1,2,3] However intratumor pressure and hepatic tissue pressure have not been investigated in relation to tumor regional characteristics and hepatic circulations. Intratumor pressure were significantly higher than those of hepatic tissue pressure. The pressure difference were minimal in the small sized HCCs in which tumor capsule was not formed or in the HCCs associating with tumor necrosis caused by preoparative embolization. In contrast, the differences were large in the HCCs with the tumor capsule formation. Regarding correlation of their pressure and hepatic circulation, pressure reductions following occlusion of the hepatic artery or the potal vein showed quite different pattern between the tumor part and the non tumor part. That was, the reduction in intratumor pressure was much greater following HA occlusion than following PV occlusion, while the reduction in hepatic tissue pressure showed the reverse following each vessel occlusion. Therefore, intratumor pressure had been influenced by tumor growth and vascularity, although it was partly influenced by the portal vein pressure.

REFERENCES

1. Vennes J (1966) Intrahepatic pressure: An accurate reflection of portal pressure. Medicine 45: 445–452
2. Boyer D, Triger D, Horisawa M, Redeker A, Reynolds T (1977) Direct transhepatic measurement of portal vein pressure using a thin needle. Gastroenterology 72: 584–589
3. Saito M, Ohnisi K, Saito M, Terabayashi H, Hayasaka, Iida S, Nomura F (1985) Measurment of intrahepatic pressure in patients with liver disease and its clinical significance. Acta Hepatologica Japonica 53: 1478–1486

Evaluation of Multislice Dynamic MRI of the Whole Liver by Turbo-FLASH Method

O. Satoh, M. Fujita, S. Naruse, T. Katsumori, T. Takahashi, and T. Maeda

Department of Radiology, Kyoto Prefectural University of Medicine, Kyoto, 602 Japan

ABSTRACT

We examined the whole liver by multislice dynamic MR using the Turbo-FLASH method in fifty-three patients with hepatocellular carcinoma(HCC).
We obtained slices of the whole liver during a 10-15 sec breath-hold. Small nodules which were not detected by CT or spin-echos, showed a high intensity on early phase. Residual or local recurrent lesions also showed a high intensity on early phase.
Multislice dynamic MR study is useful for diagnosis and follow-up of HCC.

KEY WORDS: Dynamic MRI,hepatocellular carcinoma

INTRODUCTION

Dynamic MR study has shown considerable utility in imaging hepatocellular carcinoma. Although dynamic study was commonly performed by 3-6 slices, hepatocellular carcinoma often causes multiple nodules in the liver. Therefore, multislice dynamic image covering the entire liver is necessary. Recently, the fast scan technique of MR image was developed ,and slices of the whole liver could be obtained during a 13-15 sec breath-hold using the Turbo-FLASH method. We evaluated dynamic images of the whole liver by Turbo-FLASH in patients with HCC.

MATERIALS AND METHODS

Patient Selection

Fifty-three patients with HCC were studied. Twenty two patients were evaluated before trans-arterial embolization(TAE), and 31 after TAE.

Equipment

MR imaging was performed on a 1.5T whole -body system (Magnetom,Siemens;Germany)
Imaging Protocols
Images with an 8mm slice thickness(gap:2mm) were obtained by spin-echo(SE) sequences: T1-weighted SE 500-600/15/4(TR/TE/excitations), T2-weighted SE 2000/20,80/2. Each acquisition matrix was 256x210 and 256x192.
Turbo-FLASH images,6.5/3/150/10(TR/TE/flip angle)were obtained,
follwing the slice thickness:10mm(no gap),acquisition matrix:128x128 and slices:13-15. Breath-holding interval was 13-15 seconds. Dynamic scan was performed after bolus injection of 0.1mmol/kg Gd-DTPA.

RESULTS

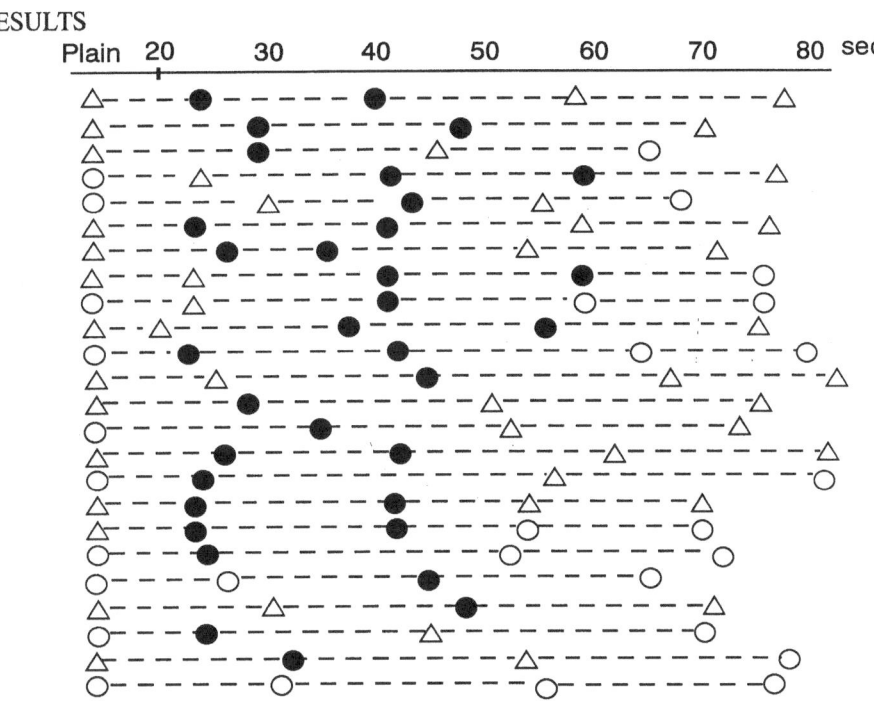

Hepatocellular carcinoma
(larger than 1cm)

○:low intensity △:isointensity ●:high intensity   n=26
Fig.1 The change of intensity of the tumor nodules

1) Except for 3 nodules, each lesion over than 10mm showed high intensity during the early phase after injection of Gadolinium,gradually turning to isointensity or low intensity.

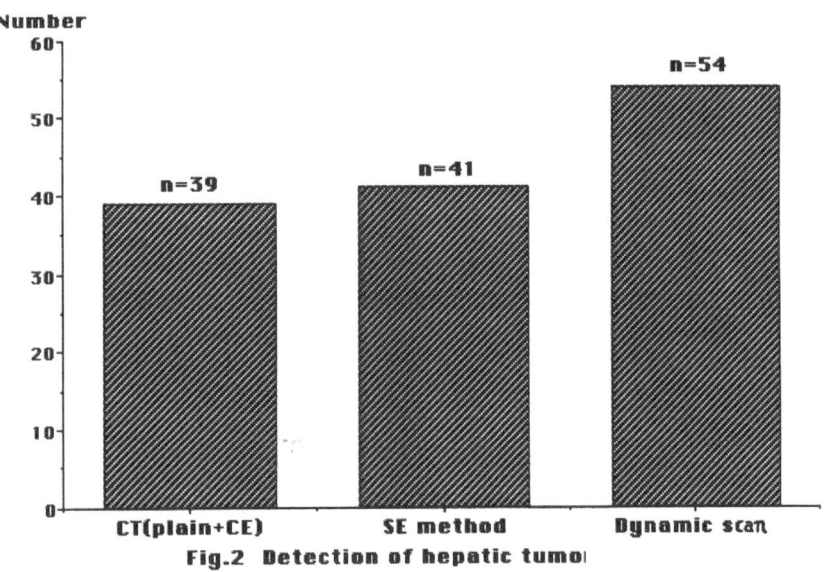

Fig.2 Detection of hepatic tumoı

2) Small nodules which were not detected by CT or the spin-echo method,showed high intensity on the early phase.

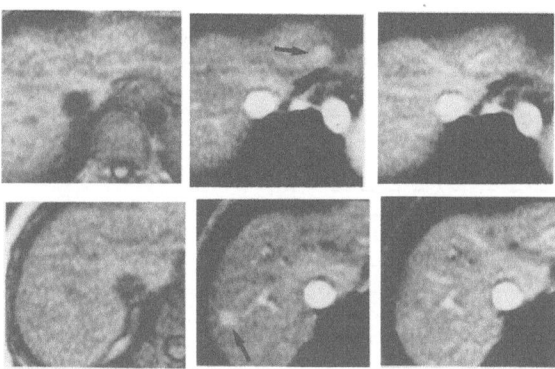

Fig.3 Hepatocellular carcinoma
A,B.pre-contrast, C,D.early phase, E,F.late phase of dynamic scan
The tumor in S2 is not detected by CT. Each nodule shows high intensity on the early phase, and changes to isointensity on the late phase.

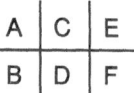

A	C	E
B	D	F

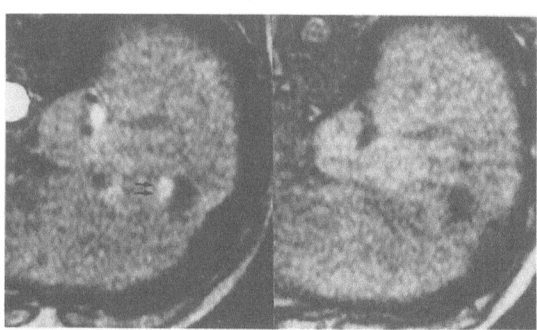

Fig.4 Hepatocellular carcinoma:
          local recurrence
A:pre-contrast, B:early phase of dynamic scan
On the early phase of dynamic scan, high intensity is found at the margin of the tumor.

A	B

3) Residual and local recurrent areas after TAE were enhanced on the early phase.

DISCUSSION

Using the Turbo-FLASH method, we can scan 13-15 slices during a 13-15 sec period and obtain a multislice dynamic image covering the entire liver. Hepatocellular carcinoma (HCC) generally shows a high intensity during the early phase of dynamic scans. Imaging the whole liver in the early phase after Gd-DTPA injection increases the changes for detection of hepatic tumors. This technique is also useful for diagnostic purposes because it can produce dynamic images of each lesion when there are other tumors in other segments of the liver.

REFERENCES

1.Edelman R R.,Siegel J B.,Singer A ,et al (1989) Dynamic MR imaging of the liver with Gd-DTPA:initial clinical results. AJR 153:1213-1219
2.Satoh O, Takahashi T, Naruse S, et al (1992) Evaliation of multislice dynamic MR imaging of the whole liver by inversion recovery snap shot FLASH method. NIPPON ACTA RADIOLOGICA 52:685-687

Non-Invasive Quantification of Human Liver Neoplasms by Positron Emission Tomography (PET) Using $C^{15}O_2$ Steady State Method

HIROKI TANIGUCHI, ATSUSHI OGURO, KAZUMI TAKEUCHI, KEIGO MIYATA, HIROSHI KOYAMA, HIROKI TANAKA, and TOSHIO TAKAHASHI

First Department of Surgery, Kyoto Prefectural University of Medicine, Kyoto, 602 Japan

ABSTRACT

Quantification of blood flow in hepatic tumors was successfully carried out by positron emission tomography using $C^{15}O_2$ steady state method, although this method has never been performed elsewhere. There was a significant difference between HCC blood flow and metastatic liver tumor blood flow ($p<0.01$). In addition, it was found that HCC blood flow was higher than liver blood flow while metastatic liver tumor blood flow was lower than liver blood flow. Because it is important to know tumor blood flow for diagnosis and treatment, PET measurement of the liver tumor is expected to become indispensable in the near future.

Key Words: hepatocellular carcinoma, metastatic liver cancer, blood flow, positron emission tomography (PET)

INTRODUCTION

Although the measurement of blood flow in human liver tumors has been attempted using many methods and instruments, the non–invasive, quantitative measurement of neoplastic blood flow has never been performed. There are some invasive methods, but they are only semi–quantitative, complicated, or not physiologically relevant. Therefore, it can be argued that all the present methods are only qualitative measurements. However, it is important for the diagnosis and treatment of liver tumors to measure the blood flow accurately and quantitatively. For example, hypertensive chemotherapy requires knowledge of increasing tumor blood flow, and the quantification of localized blood flow is necessary to evaluate the effects after transcatheter arterial embolization. We succeeded in quantifying human liver tumor blood flow using $C^{15}O_2$ steady state method positron emission tomography (PET). This method is simple, non–invasive, physiologically relevant, accurate, and can be replicated.

THEORY, PATIENTS and METHODS

Assuming that Kety's single compartment model can be applied and that a given hepatic neoplasm is supplied only from the hepatic artery, a hepatic PET using a steady state $C^{15}O_2$ method was performed to quantify the regional blood flow in the tumor. When Fick's theory is applied to the blood flow in the liver tumor, the rate of change of the concentration of a tracer in tissue at time t is related to Ft, Ca(t), and Ct(t) as shown in equation (1), where Ft is the blood flow in the tumor, Ca(t) is the concentration of the tracer in the arterial blood, Ct(t) is the tracer concentration in the tumor tissue, K is a an hepatic tumor – blood equilibrium partition coefficient for the tracer, and λ is the physical decay constant for the tracer. In this equation, the tumor tissue is perfused by blood flow Ft, which transports the tracer of concentration Ca(t) to the tissue. The transported tracer then mixes in the tissue to a concentration of Ct(t). The tracer is also cleared from the tissue by flow Ft, and its radioactivity reduced through physical decay.

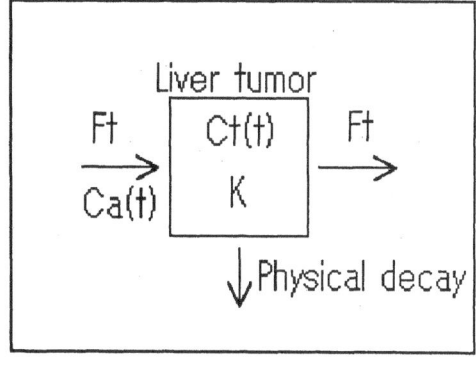

$$\frac{dCt(t)}{dt} = Ft \times Ca(t) - Ft \times \frac{Ct(t)}{K} - \lambda \times Ct(t) \cdots (1).$$

When a patient inhales $C^{15}O_2$, the $C^{15}O_2$ dissolves into the plasma and then changes into $H_2^{15}O$. Since continuous $C^{15}O_2$ inhalation is a steady state process, both sides of equation (1) do not change. Therefore, (1) becomes

$$\frac{dC(t)}{dt} = Ft \times Ca(t) - Ft \times \frac{Ct(t)}{K} - \lambda \times Ct(t) = 0 \cdots (2).$$

which can then be solved for Ft to yield

$$Ft = \frac{\lambda}{\dfrac{Ca(t)}{Ct(t)} - \dfrac{1}{K}} \cdots (3).$$

If Ct(t) can be measured by PET, then the flow Ft can be quantified.

A total of 19 patients were studied with their informed consent. Twelve patients (9 males and 3 females) whose ages ranged from 40 to 77 (mean: 63.0 years) with hepatocellular carcinomas were examined. There were also 6 males and 1 female with an age distribution of 39 to 74 (52.3 years) presenting 13 metastatic liver tumors. Of these 13 tumors, 6 were gastric cancer, 6 were colorectal cancer, and 1 was a leiomyosarcoma of the jejunum. PET measurement were performed with fasted patients in a recumbent position on the bed of a whole body PET scanner (HEADTOME III SET–120W, Shimadzu Co., Kyoto, Japan). After the confirmation of steady state following the $C^{15}O_2$ inhalation, the PET scanning was started. $C^{15}O_2$ gas was produced continuously by a medical cyclotron (BC–1710, Japan Steel Works, Muroran, Japan). Three PET scans, 10 mm in width and spaced at 15 mm intervals, were performed. ROIs were set on the liver tumors of the PET images, always referring to the X-ray computed tomographic images of on the same slices. Based on the PET images, the radioactive concentrations in the liver neoplasms were calculated; the blood flows in each was then determined by triplicate scans.

Blood samples were taken from the left brachial artery just before and after the PET measurements, and the radioactivity was measured immediately in a precalibrated well counter. The mean radioactivity of these two sample was substituted for Ca(t). In the current study, the specific gravity of the tumor and the hepatic tumor – blood equilibrium partition coefficient for water were assumed to be 1, and 0.34/min was used as the physical decay constant for ^{15}O.

RESULTS

The PET images revealed that the radioactivity concentration in the hepatocellular carcinoma was higher than in non-cancerous parts of the liver. However, the radioactivity of metastatic liver tumor was lower than in the normal liver, as shown in the photographs below. The calculated blood flows for the human liver tumors are summarized in Table. The blood flow in hepatocellular carcinomas ranged from 14.6 to 76.9 ml/100g/minutes (mean ± standard error: 44.7± 5.7 ml/100g/minutes). The blood flow in metastatic liver tumors ranged from 14.9 to 34.1 ml/100g/minutes (mean± standard error: 20.7±1.6 ml/100g/minutes). There was a significant difference in blood flow values between hepato-cellular carcinomas and metastatic liver tumors (p<0.01), but not between the various types of metastatic liver tumors.

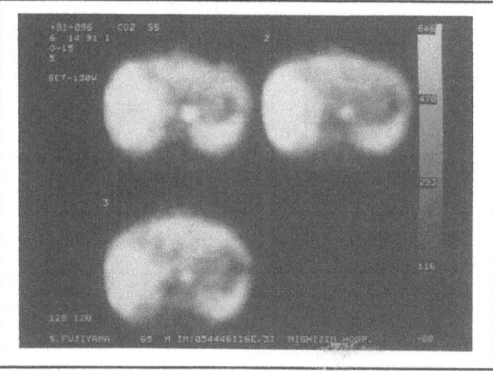

Hepatocellular carcinoma

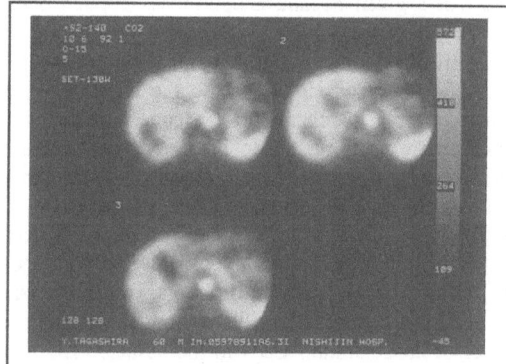

Liver metastases from gastric cancer

DISCUSSION

In PET theory, a positron which is administered to a patient collides with an electron and produces two X-rays with 0.51 MeV of energy in opposite directions. These X-rays are transmitted through the patient's body and can be detected by the PET scanner with simultaneous detection devices surrounding the patient. Thus, the radioactive concentration and the distribution of the positron can be ascertained. The sensitivity of this process is high and hence quantitative measurement is possible. Many interesting metabolic substrates can be studied with positron emitting radionuclides that are biologi-cally relevant. The biological radiotracer can be used to perform physiological measurement, and repeated measurements are possible. Furthermore, radiotoxicity is limited, as the positron which is made in a medical cyclotron has a short half-life[1]. The $C^{15}O_2$ inhalation steady state method had been established for measuring regional cerebral blood flow[2,3]. Inhaled $C^{15}O_2$ gas dissolves into the plasma, and then changes to $H_2^{15}O$ in the capillaries of the lungs. $H_2^{15}O$ is then transported systemically, and

Liver tumors	mean ± standard error (ml/100g/minutes) [range]
HCCs (n=12)	44.7 ± 5.7 [14.6–76.9]
metastatic liver tumors (n=13)	20.7 ± 1.6 [14.9–34.1]
gastric cancer (n=6)	18.3 ± 0.8
colorectal cancer (n=6)	21.1 ± 2.6
leiomyosarcoma (n=1)	32.2

thus the distribution of $H_2^{15}O$ is indicative of blood flow. Since there is a simple equilibrium between the concentrations of $H_2^{15}O$ in the tissues and in the blood under steady state, regional blood flow can be quantified simply [equation (3)]. In the current study, this method was applied for quantification of the blood flow in hepatic tumors. Since the tumor – blood equilibrium partition coefficient is not known, it was assumed to be 1. However, different hepatic tumors may require different values for this coefficient[4]. Therefore, the absolute value and magnitude of the tumor blood flow may be subject to some errors.

It has been reported that hepatic tumors are supplied only from the hepatic artery[5]. However, recently there have been reports that not only secondary hepatic cancers, but also primary liver cancers can have a dual blood supply from both the hepatic artery and the portal vein[6]. The current study was based on the assumption that the hepatic tumor receives its blood flow only from the hepatic artery. Therefore, the calculation of the tumor blood flow may include further errors due to this assumption. There are many methods for measuring the blood flow in the hepatic tumors, such as the hydrogen gas clearance method, reflectance spectrophotometry, and the laser doppler method[7].

However, these methods require laparotomy. Scintigraphy using radioactive colloids[8] or radioactive rare gases[9] can measure the blood flow, but only qualitatively or semi-quantitatively. Many methods have been attempted to quantify the blood flow in the human hepatic cancers, but all were invasive, non-physiological or qualitative. However, accurate knowledge of liver tumor blood supply is necessary for chemotherapy. For example, it is essential to know the amount of increased tumor blood flow during hypertensive chemotherapy. PET scanning is accurate, non-invasive, physiologically relevant, and replicable. The $C^{15}O_2$ continuous inhalation method is simple and does not require any injection. The combination of PET scanning and $C^{15}O_2$ inhalation gives a powerful tool not only for the diagnosis but also for the chemotherapeutic treatment of hepatic tumors.

REFERENCES

1. Coleman RE(1991): Single photon emission computed tomography and positron emission tomography in cancer imaging. *Cancer* 67: 1261–1270.
2. Frackowiak RSJ, Lenzi GL, Jones T, Heather JD (1980): Quantitative measurement of regional cerebral blood flow and oxygen metabolism in man using ^{15}O and positron emission tomography: Theory, procedure, and normal values. *J Comput Assist Tomogr* 4: 727–736.
3. Huang SC, Carson RE, Phelps ME (1982): Measurement of local blood flow and distribution volume with short-lived isotopes: A general input technique. *J Cereb Blood Flow Metabol* 2: 99–108.
4. Kairento Al, Brownell Gl, Schluederberg J (1983): Regional blood flow measurement in rabbit soft tissue tumor with positron imaging using $C^{15}O_2$ steady state and labeled microspheres. *J Nucl Med* 24: 1135–1142.
5. Ackerman NB (1972): Experimental studies on the circulatory dynamics of intrahepatic tumor blood supply. *Cancer* 29: 435–439
6. Taniguchi H, Daidoh T, Shioaki Y, Takahashi T (1993): Blood supply and drug delivery to primary and secondary human liver cancers studied with *in vivo* bromodeoxyuridine labeling. *Cancer* 71: 50–55.
7. Hemingway DM, Angerson WJ, Anderson JH, Goldberg JA, McArdle CS, et al (1992): Monitoring blood flow to colorectal liver metastases using laser doppler flowmetry: the effect of angiotensin II. *Br J Cancer* 66: 958–960.
8. Gyves JW, Ziessman HA, Ensminger WD, et al (1984): Definition of hepatic tumor microcirculation by single photon emittion computed tomography (SPECT). *J Nucl Med* 25: 972–977.
9. Sasaki Y, Imaoka S, Hasegawa Y, Nakano S, Ishikawa O, et al (1985): Distribution of arterial blood flow in human hepatic cancer during chemotherapy – Examination by short-lived ^{81m}Kr. *Surgery* 97: 409–413.222

Short-Term Results of Resection for Hepatocellular Carcinoma: A New Preoperative Combination Therapy

HITOSHI SEKIDO[1], AKIRA NAKANO[1], SHINGO FUKAZAWA[1], TADAO FUKUSHIMA[1], YASUHISA MOCHIZUKI[1], HIROSHI SHIMADA[1], KATSUAKI TANAKA[2], and SABURO NAKAMURA[2]

[1]The Second Department of Surgery, [2]The Third Department of Internal Medicine,
 Yokohama City University School of Medicine, Yokohama, 236 Japan

ABSTRACT

In order to reduce the postoperative recurrence, combination therapy of transecatheter arterial embolization (TAE) and percutaneous ethanol injection (PEI) were performed for hepatocellular carcinoma (TAE+PEI group). The patients who underwent no preoperative therapy (n-Tx group) or only TAE (TAE group) were entered in this study. Postoperative recurrence rate of TAE+PEI group was significantly lower than TAE group (P<0.05). It is concluded that preoperative combination therapy of TAE and PEI for HCC improves postoperative disease free survival rate, and the PEI has an occlusive effect of portal vein which may prevent intraportal implantation during surgical manipuration.

KEY WORDS: hepatocellular carcinoma, preoperative combination therapy, transcatheter arterial chemoembolization, percutaneous ethanol injection, hepatectomy

INTRODUCTION

Hepatocellular carcinoma (HCC) is one of the popular malignant tumor in Japan. Surgery is the only method potentially curative of HCC. However, the postoperative recurrence rate is very high. Furthermore, this recurrence cause poor prognosis of this disease. We performed preoperative combination therapy of transcatheter arterial embolization (TAE) and percutaneous ethanol injection (PEI) to prevent intraportal implantation during surgical manipuration. The purpose of this study is to evaluate if this new therapy is able to reduce a recurrence of HCC or not.

MATERIALS and METHODS

Patients

For the past 6 years (from January 1985 to December 1990), thirty three patients (23 men and 10 women) with HCC underwent hepatectomy in the second department of surgery. This study included twenty five patients (17 men and 8 women) of them. They were closely followed up for more than two years after hepatectomy. They were divided into three groups: (1) no preoperative treatment (n-Tx: n=8), (2) only TAE was performed before hepatectomy (TAE: n=11), (3) combination therapy of TAE+PEI before hepatectomy (TAE+PEI: n=6). The cases of absolute non-curative operation and post operative death caused by hepatic failure were excluded from this study.

Methods

TAE was performed with Seldinger's method. All cases were used chemoembolization that was injection of doxorubicin hydrochloride (Adriamycin), iodized oil (Lipiodol) and small pieces of gelatin sponge (Gelfoam). TAE+PEI: TAE was done and PEI was started at two weeks later. Absolute ethyl alcohol was injected two times a week (2-7times total) and total amount of ethanol administration was 12-63.8 (mean=31.3)ml. All HCC formed single nodule and all the patients were accompanied by cirrhosis of the liver and had class A lesions according to the Child's classification. The changes of blood chemistries before and after the preoperative treatment were assessed. Histological examination of resected specimens were also performed. Cumulative survival and disease free survival rates were calculated using Kaplan-Meier's method. Cox-Mantel's test and the generalized Wilcoxon test were used in statistical comparisons.

RESULTS

(1) Cumulative survival and disease free survival rates of all hepatectomy cases were as follows: one year survival rate, 80.2; five year survival rate, 49.7%; one year disease free survival rate, 60.9%; and two year disease free survival rate, 46.5%.
(2) There were no statistical significanses of clinical features among three groups, except necrosis rate of the tumor.
(3) There were no statistical significanses in survival rates among three groups.
(4) There was statistically significant between TAE+PEI group and TAE group in disease free survival rate (p<0.05, in Cox-Mantel's test and Generalized Wilcoxon test) (Fig. 1).
(5) Cut section of the resected specimen of TAE+PEI group showed massive necrosis of the tumor and fibrosis of the surrounding parenchyma which were confirmed by microscopic examination.

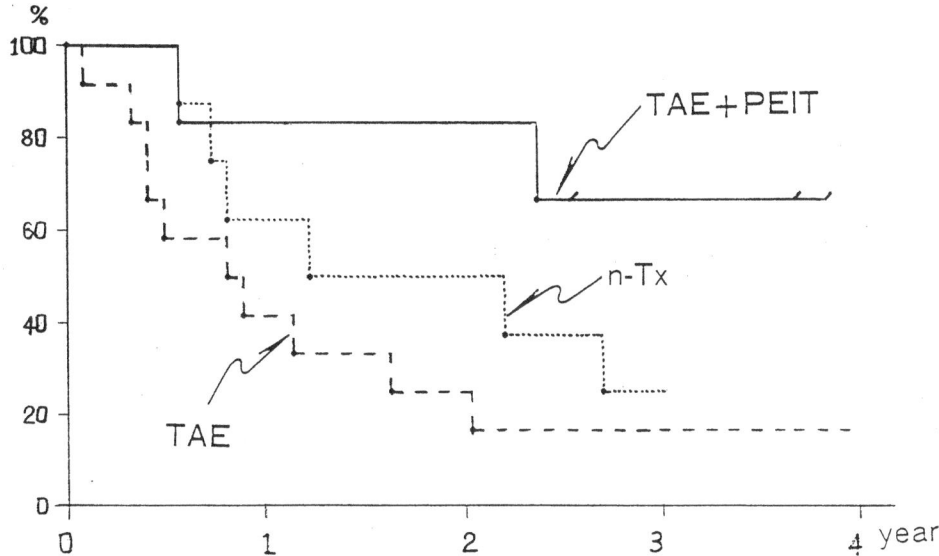

Fig. 1 Disease free survival rates of three groups are shown. There is statistical significance between TAE+PEI group and TAE group (p<0.05)

DISCUSSION

Recently, several therapeutic modalities for HCC have developed. Surgery is the potentially curative method for HCC. However, the postoperative recurrence rate is very high (1) and this recurrence cause poor prognosis of this disease. We performed a new preoperative combination therapy of TAE and PEI for HCC to prevent intraportal implantation during surgical manipulation and showed beneficial effect of this procedure.   We speculate on the mechanism of this effect (Fig. 2): surgical manipulation may induce tumor implantation, whereas the PEI has the occlusive effect of portal vein (2) and this occlusion may prevent intraportal implantation during surgical manipulation. In patients who have poor surgical risks, Tanaka et al. (3) described a combination therapy of TAE and PEI for HCC without surgery.

Nakamura (4) also described this combination therapy improved long-term survival compared with TAE. As surgical removal of the tumor is essentially curative method, the hepatectomy after this combination therapy will become a popular therapeutic modality for HCC.

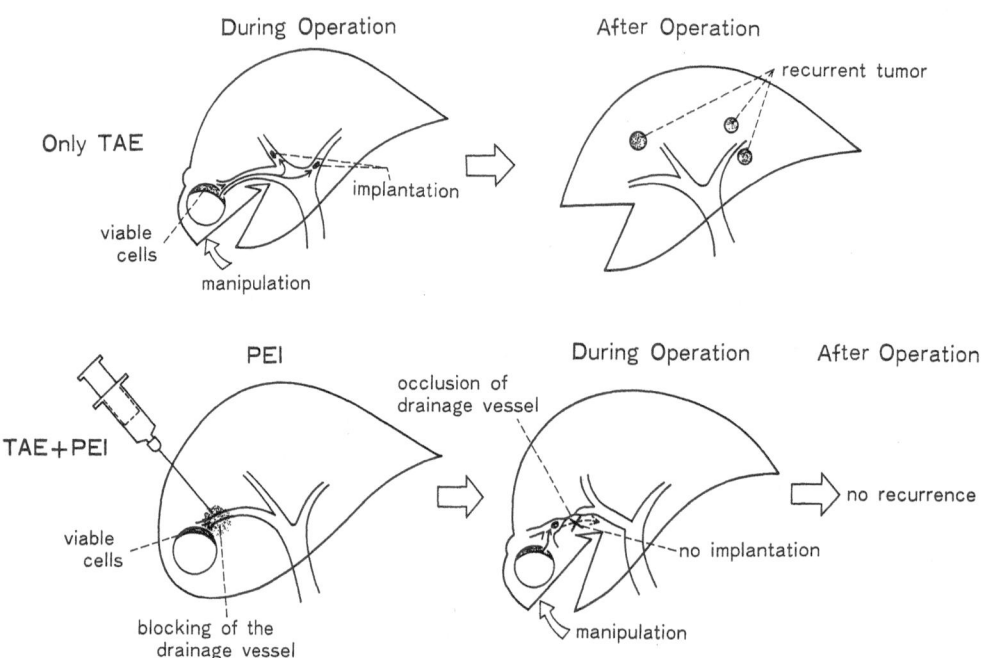

Fig. 2 Speculative beneficial effect of preoperative combination therapy is shown. The PEI has the occlusive effect of portal vein and it may prevent intraportal implantation during surgical manupulation

CONCLUSION

Preoperative combination therapy of TAE and PEI for HCC improved postoperative disease free survival rate. This PEI has the occlusive effect of portal vein and it may prevent intraportal implantation during surgical manipulation.

REFERENCES

1. Yamasaki S, Hasegawa H, Makuuchi M, Takayama T (1990) Acta Hepatologia Japonia 31: 558-564
2. Kinoshita H, Hirohashi K, Kubo S, Shuto T, Ikeda K (1992) Dagnostic Imaging of The Abdomen (in Japanese) 12: 206-212
3. Tanaka K, Okazaki H, Nakamura S, Endo O, Inoue S, Takamura Y, Sugiyama K, Ohaki Y (1991) Radiology 179: 713-717
4. Nakamura S (1993) The Yokohama Medical Journal (in Japanese) 44: 21-28

Factors Affecting Long-Term Survival and Recurrence of Hepatocellular Carcinoma (HCC) After Hepatic Resection

Kiyoaki Ouchi, Shuji Matsubara, Kenji Fukuhara, and Seiki Matsuno

Department of Surgery, Tohoku University School of Medicine, Sendai, 980 Japan

ABSTRACT

In order to elucidate prognostic factors affecting long-term survival and intrahepatic tumor recurrence, 56 patients with HCC who underwent hepatic resection in the past 10 years were studied. The actual survival rate of the patients excluding 9 hospital deaths was 65% at 3 years, and 43% at 5 years. Prothrombin time and size of tumor were the decisive factors that affected long-term prognosis. Nineteen patients had intrahepatic recurrence of HCC among 47 patients who were discharged from the hospital. Of the 19 patients with recurrence, 14 had multiple lesions, and 16 of the recurrences were detected within 3 years of surgery. Patients having multiple recurrent HCCs had larger sized tumors at the time of resection than those with a solitary recurrence. The survival rates after recurrence were significantly better in patients with a solitary recurrence, and those treated with transcatheter arterial embolization therapy (TAE). Hepatic resection for patients with functionally well-preserved livers, bearing small tumors correlates with long-term survival. Early detection as well as TAE for recurrent HCCs is necessary to improve long-term survival.

KEY WORDS: hepatocellular carcinoma, prognostic factors, intrahepatic recurrence

INTRODUCTION

In Japan, hepatocellular carcinoma (HCC) occurs predominantly in patients with cirrhosis. By following such patients regularly with serum α-fetoprotein measurements and various imaging techniques, small asymptomatic HCCs are frequently detected, and the surgical removal of small HCC has been successfully achieved [1]. It appears that hepatic resections are more frequently feasible but the long-term prognosis of the patients is not satisfactory. The high recurrence rate gives a poor prognosis for long-term survival. During the 10-year period from 1982 to 1991, 56 hepatic resections were performed at our institution. Based on these data, factors predictive of long-term survival and intrahepatic recurrence of HCC are analyzed, and recommendations for future improvement of the prognosis of HCC are made.

PATIENTS AND METHODS

The complete clinical records of all patients with histologically proven HCC treated between 1982 and 1991 were reviewed. Of the 56 patients who underwent resection, 47 patients were discharged from the hospital. Forty-three patients (77%) had liver cirrhosis. Limited hepatic resection (partial resection, subsegmentectomy, and segmentectomy) was carried out in 33 patients and major hepatic resection (lobectomy and extended lobectomy) in 14 patients. Of the 47 patients in the survival group, 9 survived more than 5 years (long-term survival group), and 12 died within 5 years (short-term survival group). During the follow-up period, 19 patients were diagnosed with recurrent HCCs in the liver remnant, and 12 were treated with transcatheter arterial embolization (TAE). Retrospective studies were made to search for significant prognostic indicators between the long-term survival group and the short-term survival group, and the recurrence-free group and the recurrent group.
Statistical analyses were made using Student's t test or the χ^2 test. Survival rates after hepatic resection and recurrence rates were obtained using the Kaplan-Meier method, and the comparison of survival was done using the generalized Wilcoxon test. A value of $p<0.05$ was significant.

RESULTS

Among various hepatic function tests measured preoperatively, only prothrombin time showed a statistically significant difference between the long-term survival group and the short-term survival group ($p<0.05$, Table 1).

There were no significant differences in the presence of capsular invasion or intrahepatic metastasis between the long-term survival group and the short-term survival group. The only prognostic indicator in tumor characteristics which affected long-term survival was the size of the tumor. Long-term survival patients were found to have smaller diameter tumors compared to the short-term survival patients (p<0.005). Neither extent of hepatic resection; major resection or minor resection nor margin-free tumor resection influenced the long-term survival of the patients.

Table 1. Preoperative hepatic function, tumor characteristics and operative intervention

	Prothrombin time (%)	Tumor size (cm)	Intrahepatic metastasis⊕ (%)	Capsular invasion⊕ (%)	Major resection (%)	Surgical margin⊕ (%)
Long-term survival group (n=9)	79 ± 16	2.4 ± 1.0	22	44	11	11
Short-term survival group (n=13)	69 ± 13^a	5.5 ± 2.8^c	23	77	31	15

values expressed as mean ± standard deviation   ⊕ means positive ^{a} p<0.05, ^{c} p<0.005

The long-term survival rates of 47 patients who were discharged from the hospital after hepatic resection were 65% and 43% at 3 and 5 years, respectively (Table 2). In addition, the disease-free survival rates were 44% and 28% at 3 and 5 years, respectively. Patients whose prothrombin time was 70% or greater had a better prognosis than those with prothrombin time less than 70% (p<0.01). Patients whose tumor size were 3 cm or less in diameter survived longer than those with tumors greater than 3 cm in diameter (p<0.05).

Table 2. Survival rate of patients with HCC after hepatic resection, excluding hospital mortality cases

survival rate	Overall (n=47)	Disease-free (n=47)	Prothrombin time ≧70% (n=31)	<70% (n=13)	Tumor size ≦3cm (n=18)	>3cm (n=29)
3-year (%)	65	44	81	41	86	55
5-year (%)	43	28	71	15^b	76	27^a

^{a} p<0.05, ^{b} p<0.01

At present, 19 patients are alive and disease-free, and 8 patients are alive with recurrent tumors. Causes of death were recurrent HCCs in 11 patients, hepatic failure in 5 patients, and unrelated causes to liver diseases in 4 patients. Thus a recurrence arising from the liver remnant was detected in 19 patients. Sixteen out of 19 patients had their recurrence detected within 3 years after surgery. Five of the 19 patients had a solitary tumor recurrence, while the remaining 14 had multiple or massive tumors at the time their recurrence was diagnosed. The survival rates of patients after a recurrent tumor was diagnosed were 47% and 16% at 3 and 5 years, respectively (Table 3). Patients with a solitary tumor recurrence had significantly higher survival rates than those with multiple tumors (p<0.05). Patients with a solitary tumor had a 5-year survival rate of 50%, whereas none of the patients with multiple tumors survived 4 or more years after the recurrence was diagnosed. In addition, patients who received TAE survived significantly longer than those who were not eligible for TAE (p<0.05). Among the factors which might influence

Table 3. Survival rate of patients with recurrent HCC following the detection of recurrent tumors

Survival rate	Overall (n=19)	Recurrent lesion Solitary (n=5)	Multiple (n=14)	Treatment for recurrence with TAE (n=12)	without TAE (n=7)
3-year (%)	47	100	31	74	0
5-year (%)	16	50	0^a	26	0^a

^{a} p<0.05

tumor recurrence, none of the following factors were associated with recurrence; hepatic function, tumor size, intrahepatic metastasis, capsular invasion, extent of hepatic resection, and surgical margins (Table 4). However, patients having a solitary recurrent tumor had a smaller sized primary tumor than those having multiple recurrent tumors (p<0.05).

Table 4. Factors affecting recurrence of tumor

	Tumor size (cm)	Intrahepatic metastasis⊕ (%)	Capsular invasion⊕ (%)	Major resection (%)	Surgical margin⊕ (%)
Recurrence-free group (n=28)	4.8 ± 3.3	14	39	32	18
Solitary recurrence group (n=5)	2.8 ± 1.4	20	20	0	40
Multiple recurence group (n=14)	6.2 ± 3.8^a	14	43	36	43

⊕ means positive   [a] $p < 0.05$

DISCUSSION

The prognosis of patients with HCC after hepatic resection is grossly determined by three main factors; the functional reserve of the liver bearing the HCC, the extent and characteristics of the tumor per se, and the operative intervention or radicality of the procedure used. Regarding functional reserve of the underlying liver disorders, the prothrombin time was the decisive factor that affected the long-term prognosis. Good preoperative liver function is an important factor in identifying long-term survivors. Nagorney et al [2] also reported decreased survival with prolonged prothrombin time. The actual survival rate at 5 years was 76% in patients with HCC smaller than 3 cm in diameter. The discovery of small HCC in mass screening in high-risk individuals results in significantly prolonged survival, and this favorable outcome has led to the general consensus that the size of the tumor is the most important factor influencing prognosis [3,4]. Although Hsu et al [5] reported that the significantly more favorable outcome of smaller HCC was related to the lower frequencies of liver invasion and intrahepatic metastasis, we could not prove these relationships. In addition, neither extent of operation nor margin-free resection affected the outcome of the patients.

The recurrence rate of HCC after resection is disappointingly high. In our series, the recurrence rate was as high as 40% in those who discharged from the hospital. The diagnosis of a recurrence was made within 3 years after hepatic resection in a majority of the patients. In addition, death within 2 years after hepatic resection was due mainly to a recurrence in the liver remnant. Patients having multiple recurrent tumor had larger sized primary tumors than those having a solitary recurrent tumor. These findings indicate that when multiple sites of recurrence occur, it is more likely the result of intraportal spread. Although tumor invasiveness or intrahepatic metastasis did not influence the recurrence risk, serial microscopic examination of the resected specimens may increase the detection of tumor spread. This study also did not demonstrate significant correlations among extent of hepatic resection, surgical margin and recurrence. The survival rate after the diagnosis of recurrent HCCs was significantly better in patients with a solitary recurrence than in those with multiple recurrence. In addition, although TAE was indicated for patients having a smaller extent of recurrent tumor spread and a better hepatic function, a better prognosis was achieved in patients treated with TAE than those without.

In conclusion, hepatic resection for patients with functionally well-preserved livers, bearing small tumors correlates with long-term survival. Early detection of any recurrence by close monitoring of the patients, combined with TAE for all treatable recurrences may improve the survival of patients with HCC.

REFERENCES

1. Okuda K (1980) Primary liver cancers in Japan. Cancer 45:2663-2669
2. Nagorney DM, van Heerden JA, Ilstrup DM, Adson MA (1989) Primary hepatic malignancy. Surgical management and determinants of survival. Surgery 106:740-749
3. Nagao T, Goto S, Kawano N, Inoue S, Mizuta T, Morioka Y, Omori Y (1987) Hepatic resection for hepatocellular carcinoma. Clinical features and long-term prognosis. Ann Surg 205:33-40
4. Yoshida Y, Kanematsu T, Matsumata T, Takenaka K, Sugimachi K (1989) Surgical margin and recurrence after resection of hepatocellular carcinoma in patients with cirrhosis. Further evaluation of limited hepatic resection. Ann Surg 209:297-301
5. Hsu H-C, Sheu J-C, Lin Y-H, Chen D-S, Lee C-S, Huang L-Y, Beasley RP (1985) Prognostic histologic features of resected small hepatocellular carcinoma (HCC) in Taiwan. A comparison with resected large HCC. Cancer 56:672-680

Indication Criteria of Hepatectomy for Hepatocellular Carcinoma Based on Long-Term Result

Naoki Yamanaka, Eizo Okamoto, Jiro Fujimoto, Takeshi Oriyama, Kazutaka Furukawa, Eisuke Kawamura, and Tuneo Tanaka

The First Department of Surgery, Hyogo College of Medicine, Nishinomiya, Hyogo, 663 Japan

ABSTRACT

The current study reports what patients with hepatocellular carcinoma can get a potential cure and good quality of life from hepatectomy based on the long-term results. 504 hepatectomized patients from 1973 through 1992 were used. The survival rate of curative resections was 24% at 10 years in contrast to 0% at 7 years. Crucial factors determining curability and prognosis were degree of portal invasion (Vp) and intrahepatic metastasis (IM), and nuclear DNA content (diploidy vs. aneuploidy). No Vp and IM were found in 72% of 66 patients who survived more than 5 years, and diploidy HCCs accounted for 89% of them. Single nodular type of HCC less than 5 cm in size and well reserved liver functions allowing a wide resection , in whom are definite indication of hepatectomy

Key Words: hepatocellular carcinoma, indication of hepatectomy, prognosis, nuclear DNA,

INTRODUCTION

In recent years when nonsurgical therapy of transcatheter arterial embolization (TAE) or ultrasonography guided percutaneous ethanol injection in addition to surgical therapy has been popularized for HCC patients, controversies over the selection of treatment have been arisen. The current study reports what patients can get benefit from hepatectomy.

MATERIALS AND METHODS

Between 1973 and the end of 1992, 540 patients underwent hepatectomy alone (n=504) or in combination with hepatic arterial ligation-cannulation (n=29) or intratumoral ethanol injection (n=27) for the intrahepatic metastases left unresected. The survival rates of 504 hepatectomized patients were calculated by the Kaplan-Meiyer method and compared by curability, nuclear DNA ploidy pattern, tumor size and tumor growth pattern. Curability of resection was determined based on the degree of portal vascular invasion (Vp), intrahepatic metastasis (IM), and completeness of resection (1). Curative resections (CR) was defined as the patients who had complete resection for the tumor in which macroscopic Vp was absent and IM was absent or confined to the same segment where the main nodule was located. Noncurative resections (NC) includes the patients who underwent apparently complete resections for HCC with macroscopic Vp or IM spreaded over the two segment or incomplete resections. The abbreviations used here are based on the General Rules for the Clinical and Pathological Study of Primary Liver Cancer (2).

RESULTS

Operative curability

The survival rate at 10 years was 13.9% for overall, 24% for CR and 0% for NC. Of the CR, the patients with single nodular type of HCCs (<5cm in diameter), no macroscopic Vp and no IM have achieved survival rate of 83% at 5 years and 45% at 10 years. There was no patients who survived more than 8 years in the NC (Fig .1).

Nuclear DNA ploidy

DNA content was determined on formal fixed resected specimens using flow cytometry. This flow cytometric analysis disclosed that 120 (53%) of DNA ploidy investigated cases were diploidy while the remaining 105 (47%) were aneuploidy. The survival rates of patients with diploidy HCCs were 62% at 5 years and 23% at 10 years in contrast to 20%

patients with diploidy HCCs were 62% at 5 years and 23% at 10 years in contrast to 20% and 15% for aneuploidy ones, respectively.   When the prognosis was compared by DNA ploidy pattern among the CR and the NC (Fig. 2), curative-diploidy group has achieved much more better survival rates than curative-aneuploidy group, which was nearly equivalent to the survival rate of NC-diploidy group, there was no difference in the prognosis between the diploidy HCCs and the aneuploidy ones at 5 years.   However, looking at 10 years in CR, there was no differnce between the prognosis of the two groups.   A similar superiority of diploidy over aneuploidy HCCs was obtained in their prognoses of the large sized tumors exceeding 10 cm in diameter.   No patients with aneuploidy and Vp positive HCCs survived more than one year.

Surgical distance from the tumor wedge and extent of resection

Survival rates were compared by a surgical distance from the tumor wedge (TW mm).   TW positive patients were defined as having resections with a surgical distance less than 10mm, and TW negative as 10 mm or more.   There was no significant difference in the prognosis between TW positive and negative patients in case of the advanced HCCs with Vp or IM (Fig. 3), while TW negative patients have shown significantly better survivals than Tw positive ones in case of the single nodular type (Fig. 4).   Extent of resection (large resection vs. small resection) also has strongly influenced on the survivals even in those with the HCCs of 2 cm or less in diameter (Fig. 5).

Tumor growth pattern

Tumor growth patterns of resectable HCC are classified into four types including single nodular type (A), multinodular type (B), single nodular type with extranodular spread (C) and multinodular fused type (D).   A type uneuivocally showed better survivals in contrast to the other types with extranodular spreads such as C or D (Fig. 6). Suprizingly, the prognosis of B type was exceeding that of A type.   Approximately 70% of all nodules in mutinodular cases, mostly treated with multiple resection, demonstrated well differentiated type of HCC, suggesting that these nodules developed in a fashion of multicentric growth.   This is probably the reason why multinodular cases had better survivals.

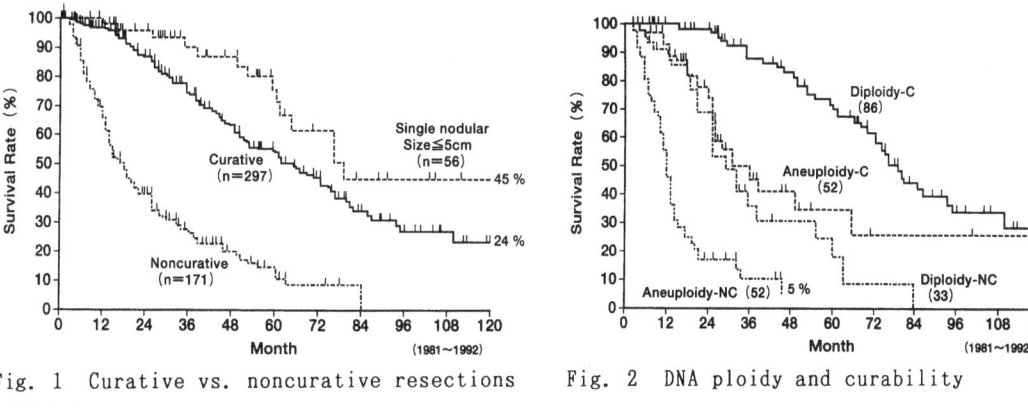

Fig. 1 Curative vs. noncurative resections   Fig. 2 DNA ploidy and curability

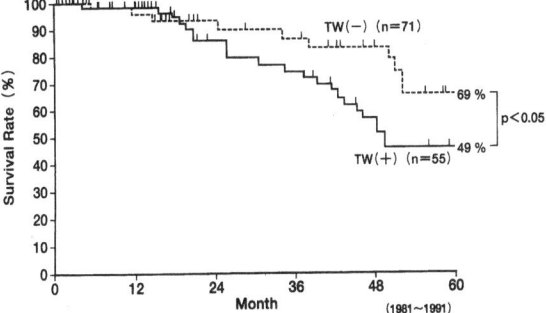

Fig. 3 TW (-) vs. TW (+)   Fig. 4 TW (-) vs. TW (+)
        in HCCs with extracapsular spread   in HCCs of single nodular type

642

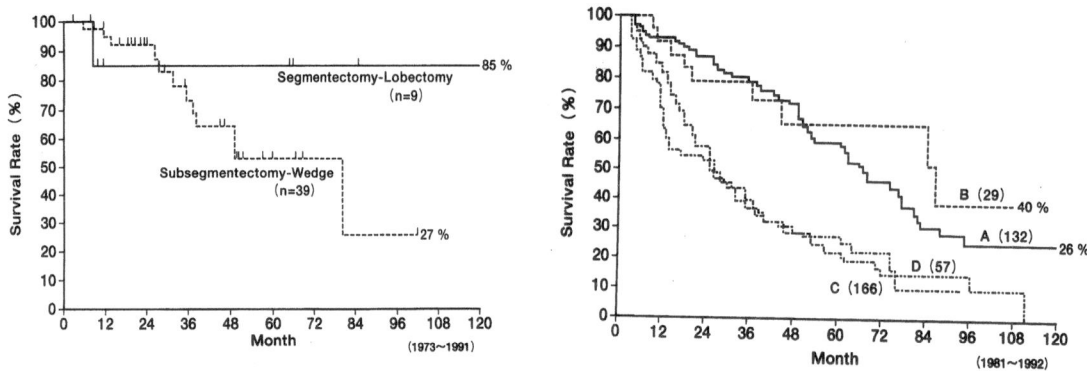

Fig. 5   Large resections vs. small resections
          in HCCs of 2cm or less in size

Fig. 6   Growth pattern

Clinicopathological features of patients surviving more than five year

There were 66 patients who survived more than 5 years following hepatectomy at the time
of July, 1992.   They accounted for 30% of the total 217 cases and 57% of 115 curative
ones, subjected to hepatectomy by July 1987.   The patients who survived 5 year with
tumor free state amounted to 39% (26) of 66.   The main characteristics of those are as
follows: 1) Well reserved hepatic functions. 2) No macroscopic Vp and IM in most
patients. 3) Diploidy HCCs in 89%. 4) Tumor size of 5 cm or less in 79%. 5) Extent of
resections are segmentectomy or lobectomy in 62%.

DISCUSSION

Important prognostic factors following hepatectomy are Vp, IM and nuclear DNA content
(3-5).The first two factors are also major criteria of determining a cure by resection.
Based on the long-term results and the clinocopathological features of long-term
survivors, hepatectomy can be absolutely indicated for HCC patients who can deserve a
potential cure within a safe limit of resection (6) in spite of DNA ploidy pattern and
largeness of HCCs.   Particularly in HCC patients with nodular type of growth and well
reserved liver functions allowing a wide resection, surgical complete removal is
unequivocally recommended, whatever its growth is unicentric or multicentric.   Because
only surgery can offer a chance to spend a good quality of life, tumor free, for an
acceptable period by single hospitalization.   What is important strategy for treatment
of HCC is as wider a resection as possible within a safe limit of resection before the
tumor shows extranodular spreads and changes to biologically more malignant character,
aneuploidy.

REFERENCES

1. Yamanaka N, Okamoto E, Toyosaka A et al (1989) Criteria of curability in the resection
   therapy for hepatocellular carcinomas. J Jpn Soc Cancer Ther 24: 1592-1599
2. Liver Cancer Study Group of Japan (1989) The general rules for the clinical and
   pathological study of primary liver cancer. J Surg 19: 98-129
3. Fujimoto T, Okamoto E, Yamanaka N et al (1991) Flow cytometric DNA analysis of
   hepatocellular carcinoma. Cancer 67: 2491-2501
4. Yamanaka N, Okamoto E, Toyosaka A et al (1990) Prognostic factors after hepatectomy
   for hepatocellular carcinoma: a univariate and multivariate analysis. Cancer
   65:1104-1110
5. Okamoto E, Yamanaka N, Fujimoto J et al (1991) The role of surgery in the treatment
   of hepatocellular carcinomas. Gann monograph on cancer research 38: 193-201
6. Yamanaka N, Okamoto E, Kuwata K et al (1984) A multiple regression equation for
   prediction of posthepatectomy liver failure. Ann Surg 200: 658-663

Results of Hepatic Resection for Small Liver Cancer

K. Takasaki, M. Yamamoto, M. Tsugita, T. Ohtsubo, H. Kobayashi, H. Sato, H. Katsuragawa, C. Maruyama, A. Saito, S. Kobayashi, and F. Hanyu

Institute of Gastroenterology, Tokyo Women's Medical College, Shinjuku-ku, Tokyo, Japan

ABSTRACT

Operative results of ninety-nine cases of small liver cancer were studied. These were classified into three types,based on the distribution of well-differentiated HCC area.Five-year survival were fairly good ,but these were many cases of recurrence. Causes of recurrence were two origins, i.e.multicentric and metastatic.Most of metastatic recurrence came in sight during three years ,multicentric recurrence also came in first two years after operation,but continue to come year after year.In type 1,all recurrences originated from multicentric recurrence.In type 2 and type 3, about 40% of recurrence were from multicentric recurrence.

KEY WORDS: Hepatic resection. Early liver cancer.Well differentiated HCC.

INTRODUCTION

Small liver cancer, i.e. less than two centimeters in diameter, is defined as early liver cancer in Japan. After resection a good prognosis has been expected, but the results were not always good because of a high incidence of recurrence. There are two causes of recurrence, one originating from metastatic nodules and the other from multicentric nodules. The role of surgical treatment is to prevent "metastatic recurrence." From a surgical point of view, it must be made clear whether it is metastatic or multicentric. This paper is concerned with the results after hepatic resection and the relationship between the pathological condition and the cause of recurrence

MATERIALS AND METHODS

Ninety-nine cases of small liver cancer among 623 cases of hepatic resection from 1982 through 1991 were studied. Among them, 61 cases were solitary tumors and 38 cases of multiple tumors. The latter was divided into two groups,i.e. 29 "multicentric" cases whose tumor were all arise from multicentric origin and 9 "multimetastatic" cases who have both primary and metastatic nodules.

Taking pathological findings into consideration, small liver cancer cases were classified into three types based on the distribution of well differentiated HCC areas. Type1,All part of tumor is consisted of well differentiated HCC. Type 2,Some area of moderate or poorly differentiated HCC inside the type1. Type3,Well differentiated HCC area is exist only at surrounding of tumor. Origin of recurrences were divided into two by pathological view or imaging diagnosis, i.e. "multicentric recurrence," and "metastatic recurrence." If a recurrent tumor is diagnosed as a primary tumor, it is decided to be a multicentric one.

Criteria for a primary tumor are as follow. 1) A well-differentiated HCC inside the tumor. 2) A negative enhancement recognized by angio-echography.(Note :that a well-differentiated HCC area is characteristic of "negative enhance" by angio-echography).

RESULTS and CONCLUSIONS

1,(Five-year survival) : Five-year survival rates after hepatic resection were fairly good, however these include many cases having recurrent tumors. Even in small liver cancer, the cancer free five-year survival rate was about 40%.(Fig 1).

2,(Dulation till recurrence) : Most of the "metastatic" recurrence appeared within three years following the operation. And strange to say,many of the "multicentric" recurrences also emerged during the first two years but these continued to surface year after year.(Fig 2).

3,(Pattern of recurrence in relation to the condition of a primary tumor) : There were good results in "solitary" and "multicentric" cases however there were many metastatic recurrences in "multi-metastatic" cases.(Fig 3).

4,(Type of primary tumor and recurrence) About half of the cases of all groups are alive with no recurrence. In type 1, all recurrences originated from "multicentric" recurrence. In types 2 and 3, about 40% of recurrence came from multicentric recurrence.(Fig 4)

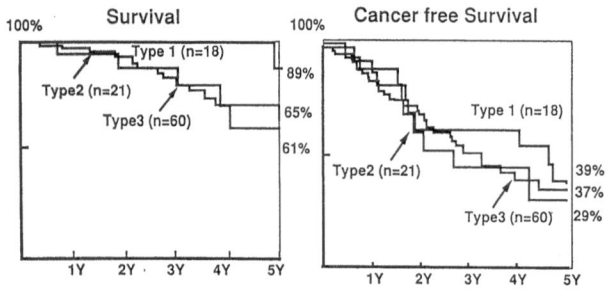

Fig 1,

Five-year survival and cancer free survival rates after hepatic resection.

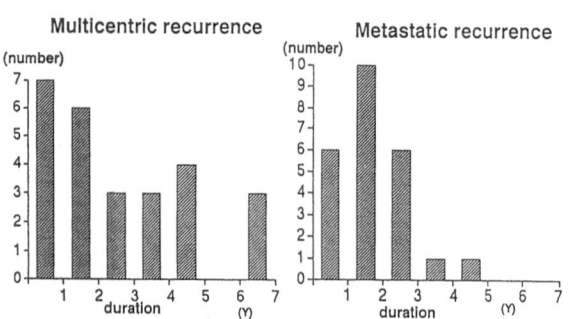

Fig 2,

Dulation till recurrence.

"Metastatic" recurrence and

"Multicentric" recurrences.

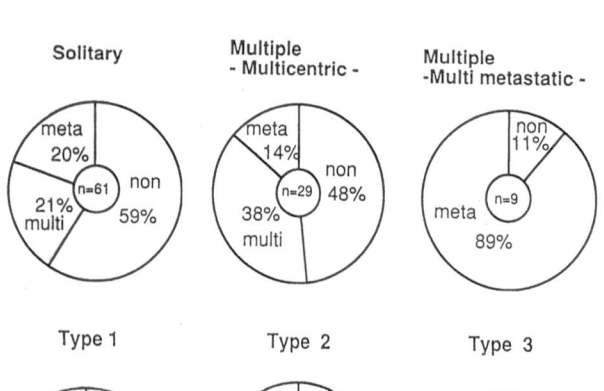

Fig 3,

Pattern of recurrence in relation to the condition of a primary tumor.

multi: multicentric recurrence

meta: metastatic recurrence

non : no recurrence

Fig 4,

Type of primary tumor and recurrence

Adverse Relationship Between Blood Transfusion and Survival After Hepatectomy for Hepatocellular Carcinoma Using Microtaze

KATSUYOSHI TABUSE, KAZUNARI MORI, SEIKI YAMAMOTO, MASAHIRO SAKAGUCHI, and NAKAHIRO SHIMOTSUMA

Department of Surgery, Osaka-Minami National Hospital, Kawachinagano, Osaka, 586 Japan

ABSTRACT

To evaluate the prognostic influence of blood transfusion in hepatocellular carcinoma patient, the survival rate of 122 hepatectomized cases using Microwave Tissue Coagulator during the years 1981 to 1990 were studied. Fifty-two patients(43%) had not been transfused and Kaplan-Meier estimate revealed the significant worsened prognosis in the transfused group ($p < 0.05$ for generalized Wilcoxon comparison of survival curve). This result couldn't be attributed to the differences in the backgrounds, i.e. maximum diameter of the tumor(ϕ), intrahepatic metastasis (IM), capsular formation (Fc), capsular invasion (Fc-inf), and K value of indocianine green test (KICG) between the transfused and non-transfused. Thus, the hypothesis that blood transfusions had an adverse effect on survival was supported by personal retrospective study.

KEY WORDS : blood transfusion, survival rate, hepatocellular carcinoma, Microwave Tissue Coagulator, Microwave Surgery

INTRODUCTION

Since 1978, Microwave Tissue Coagulator (Microtaze®), which was invented by the present author, has been used for the cases of hepatectomy [1.2]. Besides the advantage on surgical technique, excellent hemostasis, which is characteristic of this apparatus, might have the prognostic advantage for the cancer surgery. The immunosuppressive effect of homologous blood transfusions in kidney transplantation is well-known. And Gantt proposed that patients with malignant tumor who receive transfusions of whole blood were suppressed to the point where the malignant tumor has a better chance to survive [3]. So, for the hepatocellular carcinoma blood transfusions may effect the prognosis. In this paper, it is demonstrated that the adverse relationship between blood transfusion and survival after hepatectomy for hepatocellular carcinoma patients using Microtaze.

PATIENTS AND METHODS

Hepatectomy had been performed for the total 122 cases of hepatocellular carcinoma with the use of Microtaze® during the period from January 1, 1981 to August 31, 1990. In the 100 cases, complicated liver cirrhosis were present. Of the uncomplicated 22 cases, chronic hepatitis were present in 13 cases. One-hundred and four cases were men, while 18 cases were women. The average age in the cases was 58. As simultaneous concurrent operation, splenectomy was conducted in 4 cases, transesophageal transection and devascularization with splenectomy was performed for the esophageal varices in 5 cases, gastrectomy in 2 cases and cholecystectomy in 118 cases. On these operative cases, we examined 7 possible risk factors such as the method of atypical or typical resection (ATP/TYP), maximum diameter of the tumor(ϕ), surgical margin (TW), intrahepatic metastasis (IM), capsular formation (Fc), capsular invasion (Fc-inf), and K value of indocianine green test (KICG) as the prognostic factors in another study. Our own study revealed that the factors of ATP/TYP and TW hadn't affected the prognosis, but that the IM positive and Fc-inf positive had worsened the prognosis.
In this study, "transfused" was defined as transfusion (whole blood and packed red blood) given during the admission for operation and "non-transfused" was

defined as any case without "transfused". Exclusion criteria was the known palliative operation cases. Twenty-one out of 22 non-cirrhotic cases and 92 out of 100 cirrhotic cases were followed up and they were divided into two groups, respectively, one having received blood transfusion and the other not. The cumulative survival rates were compared between transfused group and non-transfused group. And, concerning to the cirrhotic cases, the ratio of above mentioned 7 factors were compared between the transfused and non-transfused groups to examine the uneven distribution in the background. The endpoint used was death related to cancer. The prognosis were determined by Kaplan-Meier estimate and significant difference test employed generalized Wilcoxon comparison of survival curves, χ^2 test and t-test.

RESULTS

The ratio of non-transfused cases was 64%(9 out of 14 cases)in partial resections, 45%(27 out of 60)in subsegmentectomy, 31%(9 out of 29)in segmentectomy and 37%(7 out of 19)in lobectomy. Collectively, 43%(52 out of 122 cases)didn't need perioperative blood transfusion. Median volume of intraoperative bleeding was 403 ml in partial resection, 800 ml in subsegmentectomy, 1300 ml in segmentectomy and 1,180 ml in lobectomy.
Figure 1 shows the cumulative survival rate after operation for hepatocellular carcinoma with liver cirrhosis, and figure 2 does it without liver cirrhosis. Survival rates were significantly higher in non-transfused groups than in transfused groups, no matter what the liver cirrhosis(p<0.05 for generalized Wilcoxon comparison of survival curve).

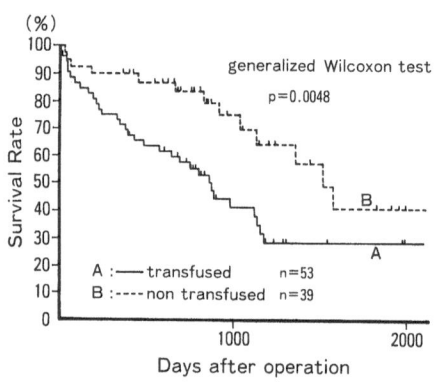

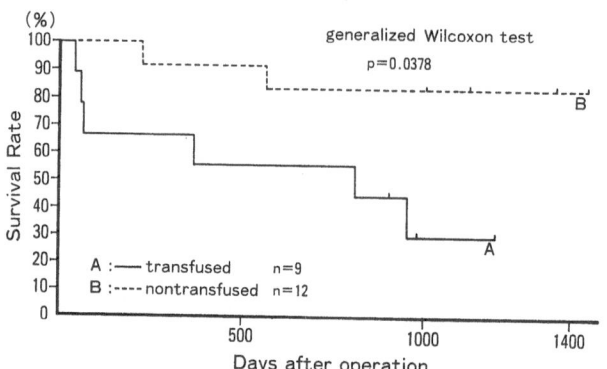

Fig.1 Cumulative survival rates after hepatectomy patients with and without perioperative blood transfusion for HCC with cirrhosis

Fig.2 Cumulative survival rates after hepatectomy patients with and without perioperative blood transfusion for HCC without cirrhosis

With regard to the background, there was no significant relationship found between transfusion and ATP/TYP, ϕ , TW, Fc, Fc-inf, or KICG, but blood transfusion was significantly more frequent in the intrahepatic metastasis(IM) positive cases. Then, the survival rate of the IM negative cases and the IM positive cases were examined respectively. Though there was no prognostic difference between transfused group and non-transfused group in the IM positive cases, in the IM negative cases the survival rate was significantly higher in the non-transfused group(Fig 3.4).

DISCUSSION

Except for the IM factor there was no significant difference in the background between transfused group and non-transfused group. Then furthermore, we examined the effect of blood transfusion limited to the IM positive or negative cases respectively. And it was found in the IM positive cases there was no prognostic difference between transfused and non-transfused, but that in the

IM negative cases survival rate was significantly higher in non-transfused group. Accordingly, at least the difference of the background concerning to the IM factor doesn't reverse our hypothesis that blood transfusion have an adverse effect on the survival.

Since 1978 we have performed hepatectomy using Microtaze® for a variety of about 300 cases of surgical liver disease such as metastatic hepatic cancer, biliary tract cancer, benign hepatic tumor, trauma of the liver, hepatolithiasis, etc. Excellent hemostasis, which is characteristic of this apparatus, has 3 important advantage.

(1) The parenchyma of the liver can be resected without ligating or blocking the trunk of the external portal vein, no matter whether it is controlled systematically or unsystematically.

(2) The influences on liver dysfunction, accompanied by the intraoperative blocking of the portal vein, can be avoided.

(3) The risk of recurrence of the tumor in the amputation stumps of the liver can be neglected.

In this paper we demonstrated that besides the advantage on surgical technique, prognostic advantage for the cancer is expected by this excellent hemostasis.

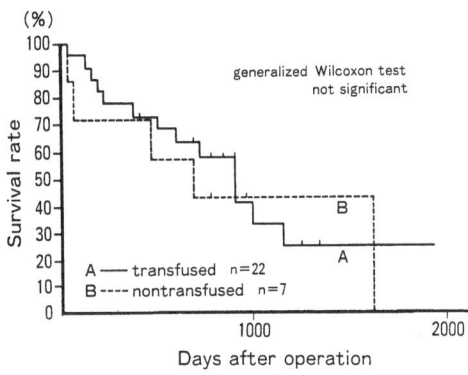

Fig.3 Cumulative survival rates after hepatectomy patients with and without perioperative blood transfusion for HCC with cirrhosis who have prognostic risk factor of intrahepatic metastasis(IM)

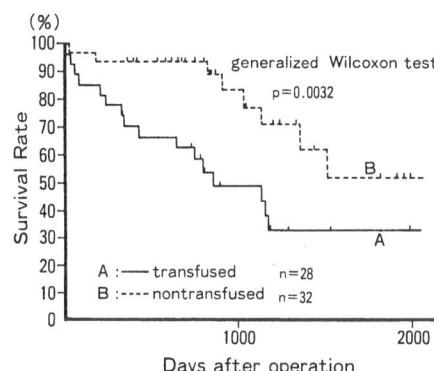

Fig.4 Cumulative survival rates after hepatectomy patients with and without perioperative blood transfusion for HCC without cirrhosis who have not prognostic risk factor of intrahepatic metastasis(IM)

REFERENCE

1. Tabuse K (1979) A new operative procedure of hepatic surgery using a microwave tissue coagulator. Arch Jpn Chir 48:160-173
2. Tabuse K, Katsumi M, Kobayashi Y. Noguchi H, Egawa H, Aoyama O, Kim H, Nagai Y, Yamaue H, Mori K, Azuma Y, Tsuji T (1985) Microwave surgery; hepatectomy using a microwave tissue coagulator. World J Surg 9:136-143
3. Gantt CL (1981) Red Blood cells for cancer patients. Lancet 2:363

Biliary Obstruction Due to Hepatocellular Carcinoma (HCC) — Report of Six Cases

Yasuyuki Shimahara[1], Yoshio Yamaoka[2], Mikiko Ueda[2], Nobuhiro Ozaki[2], Keiichiro Mori[2], Kazue Ozawa[2], and Nobuaki Kobayashi[1]

[1]The First Department of Surgery, Faculty of Medicine, Ehime University, Shigenobu-cho, Onsen-gun, Ehime, 791-02 Japan
[2]The Second Department of Surgery, Faculty of Medicine, Kyoto University, Kyoto, 606 Japan

ABSTRACT

We experienced 6 cases of hepatocellular carcinoma (HCC) with invasion to intrabiliary system in 542 cases of HCC operated at The Second Department of Surgery, Kyoto University between 1985 and 1992. Two cases out of 6 exhibited obstructive jaundice and received biliary drainage operatively by removing tumor thorombi from the bile duct. These cases, however, died of hepatic failure on the 10th and 66th postoperative day respectively. The other 4 cases exhibited no obstructive jaundice and received hepatic resection. One of these cases died of recurrence in the remnant liver, while other 3 cases survived longer than 19 months without any signs of recurrence. These results suggest that long term survival might be possible when hepatic resection can be performed, although this type of HCC often cocmbines also portal tumor thorombus and is considered to have poor prognosis. In this report, details of the 6 cases are demonstrated and the types of biliary invasion in HCC are summarized.

Key word: Hepatocellular carcinoma, Tumor thorombus, Obstructive jaundice

INTRODUCTION

It has been well known that HCC often combines tumor thorombus in portal and hepatic veins. Such vascular invasion is one of the factors which makes the treatment for HCC very difficult. On the other hand, biliary invasion by HCC has been considered relatively rare. However, this type of invasion in HCC sometimes causes obstructive jaundice and usually reveals very poor prognosis, since the stage of HCC is very advanced and the liver function is further deteriorated by icterus in addition to combined cirrhosis or chronic hepatitis. Although icteric HCC thus resists an ordinary therapy including liver resection, HCC with biliary invasion does not always exhibits obstructive jaundice and is often resectable. In this study, we analyzed the type of biliary invasion, choice of therapy, and survival period in 6 cases of HCC.

ANALYSIS OF THE PATIENTS

Table 1 shows the profiles, clinical symptoms and findings of the patients. The six patients were admitted with chief complaints of general malaise, epigastralgia and right hypochondralgia under the diagnosis of HCC. Two cases (Case 1 and 5) exhibited severe icterus.

Table 2 shows the laboratory data of these patients. Abnormalities were seen in the serum levels of GOT, GPT, Alkaline Phosphatase, γ GTP and LAP in some patients. In two patients with obstructive jaundice, the serum levels of total bilirubin were 21.3 and 17.5 mg/dl. In the other 4 patients, the bilirubin levels were within normal range. There were no tendencies in the levels of α fetoprotein and CA19-9 in these patients.

Table 1. PROFILES AND CLINICAL FINDINGS OF THE PATIENTS

CASE	AGE	SEX	CLINICAL SYMPTOMES AND FINDINGS
1	62	M	General Malaise, Icterus, Ascites
2	65	F	Epigastralgia
3	62	M	Epigastralgia
4	57	M	Right Hypochondralgia,
5	62	M	Genaral Malaise, Right Hypochondralgia, Icterus
6	44	M	Right Hypochondralgia

Figure 1 illustrates the localization of the tumors and modes of biliary invasion. In the patients with jaundice (Case 1 and 5), common bile duct was obstructed due to tumor thorombus. In the other 4 cases, tumor thorombi were seen only in the intrahepatic bile duct.

Table 3 shows the treatment, operation and outcome of the patients. In Case 1, PTCD was performed preoperatively but little effect was seen on the serum bilirubin level. Laparotomy revealed severe cirrhosis with large amount of ascites. Cholecystectomy, choledochotomy were performed and the tumor thorombus was removed from the common bile duct. There was uncontrollable bleeding from the common bile duct and right hepatic artery was ligated. The patient showed relatively well postoperative course for some time, however, died of hepatic failure caused by sudden GI bleeding due to AGML on the 66th postoperative day. Case 5 received also cholecystectomy, choledochotomy and removal of tumor thorombus. The right hepatic artery was ligated for the control of unresectable tumors. However, the patient died of hepatic failure on the 10th postoperative day. Other 4 cases received liver resections and could survive for relatively long period ranging from 16 months to 56 months.

Table 4 shows the pathological findings of the tumors. Histology was examined in the specimens of resected liver or removed tumor thorombi and hepatocellular carcinoma was ascertained in all cases. Portal tumor thorombus was seen in all cases. The main tumor tended to have no capsule formation.

DISCUSSION AND CONCLUSION

Tumorous invasion of the lumen of the bile duct is a mode of local extension which is relatively characteristic of hepatocelluar carcinoma. However, this mode of local extension is uncommon in comparison with that of portal and hepatic vein. In several studies including analysis of HCC by autopsy, the incidence of biliary invasion has been reported as 1-2 % (1, 2, 3). Lin et al reported that HCC with invasion into extrahepatic bile duct often developes to obstructive jaundice and called this type of HCC icteric type hepatoma (4). This type of hepatoma has generally very poor prognosis, since the stage of tumor is usually too advanced for an ordinary therapy including hepatic resection, TAE (transcatheter hepatic arterial embolization) etc. Also in our study, Case 1 and 5 could be categorised to this type and died of hepatic failure soon after the removal of tumor thorombi from the

Table 2. PREOPERATIVE LABORATORY DATA OF THE PATIENTS

CASE	GOT	GPT	T.BIL	ALP	γGTP	LAP	PLAT	AFP	CA19-9
1	106	89	21.3	1036	340	198	158000	8.5	470
2	29	14	0.7	82	230	218	90000	32	60
3	31	34	0.6	34	78	58	257000	15989	50.6
4	99	102	1.2	61	90	125	71000	11.6	?
5	66	73	17.5	119	213	380	250000	127	460
6	36	36	1.2	251	43	82	129000	92	17

GOT, GPT (IU/L), T.BIL:Total Bilirubin (mg/dl), ALP:Alkalinephosphatase(IU/L), γ GTP, LAP (IU/L), PLAT:Platelet (/mm3), AFP (ng/ml), CA19-9 (U/ml)

Figure 1.

LOCALIZATION OF THE MAIN TUMORS AND INVASION TO BILE DUCT

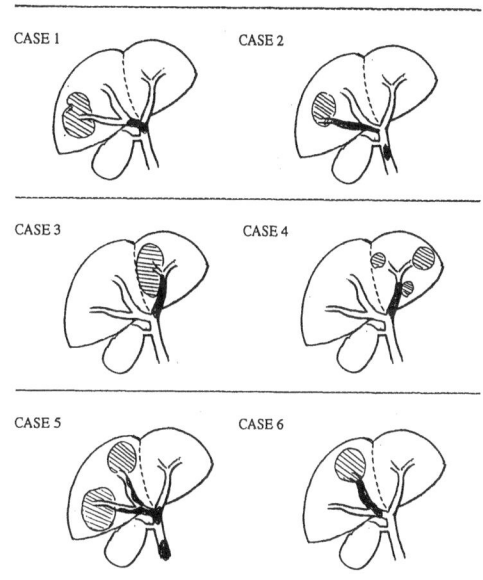

Table 3. TREATMENT, OPERATION AND OUTCOME OF PATIENTS

CASE	TREATMENT AND OPERATION	OUTCOME
1	PTCD, Cholecystectomy, Choledochotomy Removal of Tumor Thorombus Ligation of r-Hepatic Artery for Bleeding from bile duct	Died of Hepatic Failure (66POD)
2	Right Lobectomy	Died of Recurrence (16Months)
3	Extended Left Lobectomy, Choledochotomy Removal of Tumor Thorombus	Survive (56Months)
4	Extended Left Lobectomy, Choledochotomy Removal of Tumor Thorombus	Died of Apoplexy (19Months)
5	Cholecystectomy, Choledochotomy Removal of Tumor Thorombus Ligation of r-Hepatic Artery	Died of Hepatic Failure (10POD)
6	Right Lobectomy	Survive (24Months)

bile duct. This seems partially attributable to severe hepatic dysfunction due to persistent jaundice and combined portal tumor thorombus. As to removal of tumor thorombus from the bile duct, we have to be very careful for massive bleeding from the duct, because the tumor thorombus itself is also fed with hepatic arterial blood. On the other hand, HCC with biliary invasion but without obstructive jaundice has often indication of hepatic resection. In our series too, Case 2, 3, 4 and 6 received major hepatic resection and showed relatively long survial period. Two of these cases have no signs of recurrence for more than two years and one of them almost reaches at 5 years. In analysis of biliary invasion of HCC, the mode of extension might be classified into four types; Type I: Tumor thorombi are formed in peripheral bile ducts around the main tumor. This type is in an initial stage of biliary invasion of HCC and can be treated as other ordinary HCC (none of our series). Type II: Tumor thorombus invades first into the adjacent bile duct and cancer cells are disseminated in the bile duct and grow at different portions. This type forms a skip lesion in the main bile duct and often combines obstructive jaundice (Case 1 and 5 in our series). Type III: Tumor thorombus grows intraductally continuously connected with main tumors. This type possively developes to icteric hepatoma very fast in the near future (Case 3, 4, 6 in our series). Type IV: Tumor thorombus is once formed in an adjacent bile duct and detached from the main tumor followed by floating in the main bile duct. This type also has possibility to exhibit obstructive jaundice and should be differencially diagnosed from intraductal gallstone (Case 2). In conclusion, relatively long term survival could be expected by liver resection for HCC with intrabiliary invasion, when the lesion does not yet develop to obstructive jaundice. For this, careful preoperative image examinations are needed.

Table 4. PATHOLOGICAL FINDINGS OF THE TUMORS

CASE	Liver Resection	H	Fc	Vp	B	IM	Z	Edmondson
1	not resected	2	?	?	2	2	3	II
2	right lobectomy	2	(-)	2	2	2	1	II
3	ext. left lobectomy	2	(+)	0	1	1	1	III
4	ext. left lobectomy	1	(-)	2	1	2	1	II
5	not resected	2	?	3	2	2	2	II
6	right lobectomy	1	(-)	3	1	2	1	II

H: size of hepatic tumor, Fc: capsule formation, Vp: portal invasion, B: biliary invasion, Z: extent of cirrhosis , according to The General Rules for the Clinical and Pathological Study of Primary Liver Cancer by Liver Cancer Study Group of Japan.

REFERENCES

1. Okuda K, Peters RL: Hepatocellular carcinoma. (1976) New York, Wily Medical Publication.
2. Ihde DC, Sherlock P, Winarwer SJ, Fortner JG: Clinical manifestations of hepatoma. A review of 6 years experience at a cancer hospital. (1974) Am J Med 56: 83-91.
3. Edmondson HA: Tumors of the liver and intrahepatic bile ducts. In Atlas of tumor pathology. (1958) Washington DC, A. F. I. P. Section VII.
4. Lin TU, Chen KM, Chen UR: Icteric type haptoma. (1975) Med Chir Did 4: 267-270.

Comparison Between Portal Vein Branch Ligation and Embolization for Compensatory Hyperplasia of Unoccluded Hepatic Lobe

Minekatsu Nishida, Kazuma Yano, Kazuhisa Hiwaki, and Takashi Suzuki

Department of Surgery II, Yamaguchi University School of Medicine, Ube, Yamaguchi, 755 Japan

ABSTRACT

The effect on the liver of portal vein branch embolization was examined in rabbits by measuring the hepatic tissue blood flow and cellular kinetics using the bromodeoxyuridine labeling index, compared with that of portal vein branch ligation. The rabbit liver consists of three separate masses. In our experiment, the portal vein branch to the main lobe and caudate lobe (80.4 % of the total liver weight) were ligated or embolized just above the right posterior lobe(19.6 %), resulting in compensatory hyperplasia of the right posterior lobe together with atrophy of the main lobe and caudate lobe. 24 days after operation, the weight ratio of the right posterior lobe had reached 75.8 $\pm$ 5.6 % in the ligation group. In the embolization group, however, the increase in the weight ratio stopped six days after operation, resulting that it was about 40 % thereafter. During the first three days after operation, the blood flow ratio increased significantly in the both groups compared with the sham group. However, there were no significant difference between two groups. The labeling index of the ligation group still increased significantly compared to sham group until 12th day after operation. In the embolization group, however, there were no significant difference on the 12th days after operation compared to sham group. These results suggest that portal vein branch ligation was preferable to portal vein branch embolization with regard to compensatory hyperplasia for preoperative procedure in extensive hepatobiliary surgery.

Key words: portal vein embolization, portal vein ligation, compensatory hyperplasia

INTRODUCTION

It is generally agreed that occlusion of major branches of the portal vein induce atrophy of the corresponding part of the liver, while the remaining liver undergoes compensatory hyperplasia until the original hepatic mass has been restored(1-5) . Some studies have suggested that portal vein branch ligation succeeded by hepatectomy of the corresponding part was preferable to the one stage hepatectomy(2), since the remnant liver underwent compensatory hyperplasia. In recent times percutaneous transhepatic portal vein embolization has become a useful preoperative procedure in extensive hepatobiliary surgery in JAPAN(6). However, these studies neither detailed the course of hyperplasia and atrophy, nor demonstrated the differences between portal vein branch ligation and embolization. Moreover, the relationship between compensatory hyperplasia and blood flow is not understood. With this in mind, the authors have reevaluated the ligation of branches of the portal vein and portal vein branch embolization under rigidly controlled experimental conditions. Serial observations of hepatic blood flow and measurements of the cellular kinetics of compensatory hepatic regeneration using a monoclonal antibody to bromodeoxyuridine (BrdUrd) were carried out.

MATERIALS AND METHODS

Thirty female domestic rabbits (Seiwa Experimental Animals, Ltd., Japan) , weighing from 2.0 to 3.0 kg, were fed regular rabbit food (Oriental Yeast Co., Japan) throughout the experiments. The rabbit liver is lobulated, making it particularly well suited for experiments involving regional blood vessels and biliary drainage. The liver consists of two separate masses, each with its own vessels and ducts. In ten normal rabbis, the main lobe formed 75.6% of the total liver weight, the caudate lobe 4.8% and the right posterior lobe 19.6%. In our experiments the portal vein to the main lobe and caudal lobe were ligated or embolized just above the right posterior lobe, resulting in compensatory hyperplasia of the right posterior lobe together with atrophy of the main lobe. In case of a short distance between the caudate lobe and the right posterior lobe, a small part of the caudate lobe was resected first without disturbing portal blood flow to the right posterior lobe, and then the portal vein branch was ligated. Animals were fasted overnight before operation, but water was given ad libitum. Under anesthesia with 25 mg per kg body weight of ketamine given intramuscularly and 25 mg per kg body weight of pentoparbital sodium given intravenously, the abdomen was opened through a middle incision, and the gallbladder, which is susceptible to infection and buffers bile, was removed aseptically. Fifty milliliters of saline and 10 mg of minocycline were given intravenously during the operation. The rabbits were divided into the following three groups according to the operation performed.

Group 1 (n=10): Ligation of the branch of the portal vein to the main lobe (PBL group). Approximately a 1-cm segment of the portal vein to the main lobe was dissected free and doubly ligated with 4-0 silk without injury to adjacent structures, including the artery, bile duct, hepatic nerves and lyphatics.

Group 2 (n=10): Embolization of the portal vein branch to the main lobe (PBE group). 4 Fr. intravenous catheter (Atom Co., Japan) was inserted into the portal vein branch to the main lobe from a mesentery tributary, through which 80 mg/ml of fibrinogen and 250 units/ml of thrombin (Kaketsuken. Japan) were injected simultaneously until the branch was filled with fibrin clot. During injection, the portal vein branch just above the right posterior lobe occluded between the index finger and the thumb to prevent extension of the fibrin clot into the main portal vein.

Group 3 (n=10): Sham operation (sham group). A cholecystectomy and dissection of the bile ducts, hepatic artery and portal vein were done as all other groups. One, Three, six, 12 and 24 days after the initial operation, two rabbits from each group were weighed, and under intravenous anesthesia with pentobarbital sodium 25 mg per kg body weight, the abdomen was reentered, and the hepatic tissue blood flow of the main lobe and lobe mass were measured by laser Doppler flowmeter [Laserflo BPM 403A (TSI Co., U.S.A.)]. after the measurements were completed, all rabbits were sacrificed, and the livers were removed and weighed after blood and bile were allowed to drain by gravity. In order to obtain information about the proliferation of the unaffected hepatocytes , one hour before the rabbits were sacrificed, 5-bromo-2-deoxyuridine 3 mg per kg of body weight (Sigma Chemical Co., U.S.A.) was injected intravenously. The main lobe was fixed in 10% buffered formalin and stained with hematoxylin-eosin for histologic examination. The removed right posterior lobe was fixed in cold ethanol to determine the BrdUrd labeling index.

RESULTS

Changes in the liver weight ratio

The ratio of the weight of the right posterior lobe to the total liver was calculated, and regeneration was estimated on the basis of the change in the weight ratio. In ten normal rabbits, the average ratio was 19.6%. Twenty-four days after operation, the weight ratio of the right posterior lobe had reached $75.8 \pm 5.6\%$ in the PBL group. In PBE group, the increase in the weight ratio stopped six days after operation, presumably due to contraction of the fibrin clot; however the lobe mass weight had doubled by 12 days after operation (Fig. 3).

Changes in the blood flow ratio

The blood flow ratio was defined as the hepatic tissue blood flow to the right posterior lobe (ml/min/100 grams) divided by the hepatic tissue flow to the main lobe (ml/min/100 grams). In normal ten rabbits, average tissue blood flow in the main lobe was 11.3 ml/min/100 grams, and in the right posterior lobe 12.8 ml/min/100 grams(7). The absolute value of the tissue blood flow was not used for intergroup comparisons in this paper because it varied according to the level of anesthesia. However, in the PBL and PBE groups, the blood flow to the right posterior lobe after portal vein occlusion decreased approximately 30% of normal, while blood flow to the main lobe appeared to increase to 2 or 3 times normal. During the first three days after operation, the blood flow ratio increased significantly in the PBL and PBE groups compared to the sham group, yet, from six days after operation on, there were no significant differences between the groups (Fig. 4).

BrdUrd labeling index in the right posterior lobe

On the first day after operation, the labeling indices in the right posterior lobe had not increased significantly in any group. The highest values were found three days after operation in all groups except the sham group. The labeling index of the PBL group still was increased significantly compared to the sham group until 12th day after operation. In the PBE group, however, there were no significant differences on 12th day after operation compared to the sham group, which showed about one BrdUrd labeled hepatocyte per 1000 hepatocytes throughout the study period.

Histological findings

Fibrin clot, which is confirmed in the portal vein branch to the main lobe of the PBE, is contracted and floating in the portal vein (Fig. 1). Rabbits killed three days after PBL showed areas of necrotic1 foci throughout the main lobe, predominantly around the central veins. These foci were sharply demarcated, mostly devoid of nuclei and demonstrated monocyte accumulation. After 12 days, however, these necrotic foci had disappeared almost totally, and the lobules were small without fibrosis of Glisson's capsule(8). The PBE group showed similar histologic findings as in PBL group, despite the partial contraction of the fibrin clot in the portal vein (Fig. 2).

DISCUSSION

It is generally agreed that ligation of a branch the portal vein, if it involves a large enough region, induces compensatory hyperplasia in those region in which portal blood flow is maintained and atrophy of the affected areas(1-5). In our series, 24 days after operation, the weight ratio of the right posterior lobe which formed 19.6% of the total liver weight in sham group reached $75.8 \pm 5.6\%$

in the PBL group. However, from six days after operation on, the PBE group showed no more compensatory hyperplasia and the weight ratio was about 40 % thereafter. Histological findings showed that the fibrin clot was contracted and floating in the portal vein branch to the main lobe. These results suggest that portal blood flow to the main lobe was resumed and gradually increased according to the degree of the fibrin clot contraction. Portal blood flow to the main lobe, however, was not sufficient for restoring the main lobe because of blood flow disturbance by fibrin clot. Honjo et al. have discussed portal branch ligation as a treatment for patients with liver cancer in whom hepatic resection is not indicated(4). Recently, some surgeons in our country have suggested preoperative portal vein embolization causing hepatic regeneration might be useful as a kind of preparation for radical hepatectomy(6). These results suggest that portal vein branch ligation is preferable to portal vein branch embolization with regard to compensatory hyperplasia for preoperative procedure in extensive hepatectomy.

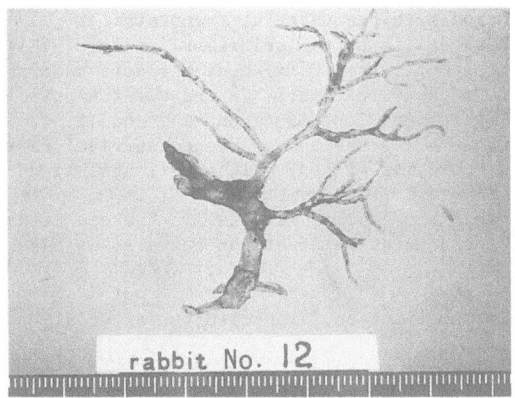

Fig.1 A fibrin mold of the portal vein branch to the main lobe

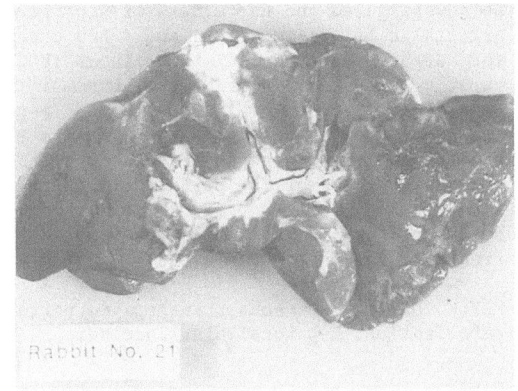

Fig. 2 Fibrin clot in the portal vein branch to the main lobe

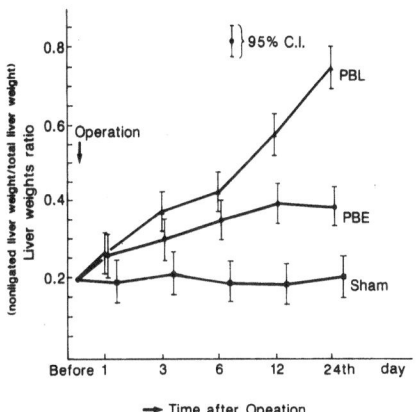

Fig. 3 Changes of nonoccluded lobes weight per total liver weight ratio

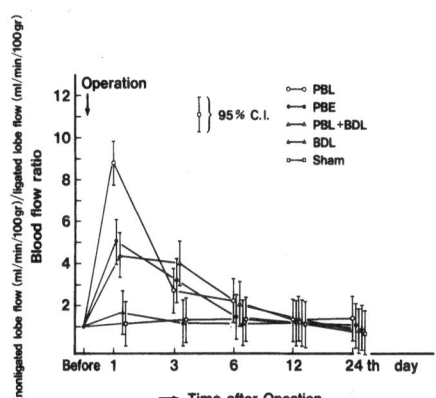

Fig. 4 Changes of blood flow ratio

REFERENCES

1. Lous P, Larimore LD. Relationship of the portal blood to liver maintenance. J Exp Med 1920;31: 609- 32
2. Kozaka S. Extensive hepatectomy in two stages. Arch Jap Chir 1963;32:99-123
3. Rozga J, Jeppsson B, Bengmark S. Portal branch ligation in the rat. Am J Pathol 1986;125:300-08
4. Honjo I, Suzuki T, Ozawa K. Ligation of a branch of the portal vein for carcinoma of the liver. Am J Surg 1975;130:296-302
5. Nishida M, Yano K, Murakami T, Suzuki T. Compensatory hepatic regeneration in rabbits: Effect of portal vein and/or bile duct branch ligation. Gastroenterology 1991; 100 : 1135-37.
6. Kinoshita H, Sakai K, Hirohashi K, Igawa S, Yamasaki O, Kubo S. Preoperative portal vein embolization for hepatocellular carcinoma. World J Surg 1986;10:803-08
7. Shepherd AP, Riedel GL, Kiel JW, Haumschild DJ, Maxwell LC. Evaluation of an infrared laser-Doppler Blood Flowmeter. Am J Physiol. 1987;252:G832-39
8. Kerr JFR. "Shrinkage necrosis" a distinct mode of cellular death. J Pathol 1971;105:13-20

Preoperative Portal Vein Embolization for Hepatocellular Carcinoma with Portal Thrombi

Shoji Kubo, Hiroaki Kinoshita, Kazuhiro Hirohashi, Ryutaro Iwasa, Nagahisa Fujio, and Kazuo Ikeda

Second Department of Surgery, Osaka City University Medical School, Osaka, 545 Japan

ABSTRACT

We investigated the usefulness of hepatic resection with preoperative transcatheter arterial embolization (TAE) and percutaneous transhepatic portal vein embolization (PVE) for advanced hepatocellular carcinoma (HCC) retrospectively. Fifty-nine patients underwent hepatic resection and had portal thrombi (vp). Of the 59 patients, 28 underwent hepatic resection only (group N), 20 underwent hepatic resection with TAE (group A), and 11 underwent hepatic resection with TAE and PVE (group AP). The nonrecurrence survival rate for the patients in group AP was higher than in the other groups. Eight patients had vp in the first branch of the portal vein (vp_3). Only two of these patients (both in group AP) survived long; in group AP, the vp was covered with the embolic material in the operative specimens. PVE seems to be useful not only as a preoperative treatment but also as one treatment for unresectable HCC.

KEY WORDS: percutaneous transhepatic portal vein embolization, transcatheter arterial embolization, hepatocellular carcinoma

INTRODUCTION

Hepatocellular carcinoma (HCC) can be symptomless, so we often see the patients with advanced HCC. The outcome of patients with advanced HCC is still poor because such HCC often invades the portal vein and forms portal thrombi (vp), an important factor in the prognosis [1,2]. We devised PVE and used it as one step in preoperative preparation [3,4]. We have reported that PVE strengthens the effect of TAE and extends surgical indications because PVE causes atrophy of the embolized part of the liver and hypertrophy of the nonembolized part [3,4]. In this paper, we investigated retrospectively the usefulness of liver resection with preoperative TAE and PVE for HCC with vp.

SUBJECTS AND METHODS

Our subjects were 59 patients who had HCC with vp, who underwent liver resection in the past 11 years. Fifty patients were men and nine patients were women. Patients were from 10 to 74 years old. Vp in operative specimens was identified histologically. Of the fifty-nine patients, 28 underwent hepatic resection only (group N), 20 underwent liver resection with preoperative TAE (group A), and 11 underwent liver resection with preoperative TAE and PVE (group AP). Laboratory test results and the classification of HCC by UICC criteria [5] are summarized in Table 1. There were no significant differences among the three groups in the values before treatment for the platelet count, prothrombin time, total protein, albumin, aspartate aminotransferase (AST), alanine aminotransferase (ALT), total bilirubin, or 15-min indocyanine green retention rate (ICGR-15). The number of patients in stages III plus IV in group AP was larger than that in the other groups. We compared the nonrecurrence survival rates of the three groups because the usual survival rate is affected by treatment after detection of the recurrence. The nonrecurrence survival rates were calculated by the Kaplan-Meier method and statistical analysis was done by the generalized Wilcoxson method and the Cox-Mantel method. Of the 59 patients, eight had vp in the right or left first branch of the portal vein (vp_3). We studied details of the clinical findings and the outcome in these eight patients. TAE was done by the method of Yamada et al. [6] two weeks before PVE. PVE was done as reported previously [3,4], 2 or 4 weeks before liver resection.

Table 1 Laboratory Test Results and Classification of Hepatocellular Carcinoma with Portal Thrombus

	Group AP	Group A	Group N
Platelets x 10^4/mm^3	17.3± 3.2	20.3± 5.3	16.2± 2.3
Prothrombin time, min	96 ± 7	95 ± 6	86 ± 4
Total protein, mg/dl	7.1± 0.1	6.7± 0.2	7.3± 0.2
Albumin, mg/dl	3.7± 0.1	3.7± 0.1	3.7± 0.1
Total bilirubin, mg/dl	0.8± 0.1	1.2± 0.5	0.8± 0.1
AST, IU	70.9±22.4	96.5±25.6	76.0±13.0
ALT, IU	74.3±18.7	105.5±57.8	7.6±11.5
ICGR-15 (%)	18.6± 1.8	15.4± 3.4	14.7± 2.4
Classification (UICC stage)			
II	3 (27%)	8 (38%)	13 (46%)
III	7 (64%)	10 (48%)	12 (43%)
IV	1 (9%)	3 (14%)	3 (11%)

RESULTS

Nonrecurrence survival rates in these three groups are compared in Fig. 1. The survival rate in group AP tended to be better than that in the other groups. Almost all of the recurrences in our patients were detected within three years of surgery. In group AP, the survival rate at 2 years after surgery was about 45% and that at 5 years and more was about 30%.

Table 2 Clinical Findings and Outcome in Cases of Hepatocellular Carcinoma with vp$_3$

Case	Age (yr) /sex	Group	Operation	Recurrence after surgery	Organ(s) with recurrence	Treatment after recurrence	Outcome
1	67/M	AP	rt lobectomy	1 yr 3 mo	Lung	Partial pneumonectomy	7 yr 3 mo, dead
				4 yr 7 mo	Liver	TAE, Liver resection	
2	54/M	AP	lt lobectomy	5 yr 1 mo	Liver	TAE, HAI	8 yr 4 mo, alive
3	63/M	AP	rt lobectomy	6 mo	Liver	Conservative	9 mo, dead
4	10/M	A	rt tri-segmentectomy	1 mo	Liver, Lungs	Conservative	1 yr 1 mo, dead
5	65/M	N	rt lobectomy	9 mo	Liver	Conservative	3 yr, dead
6	38/M	N	rt lobectomy	6 mo	Liver, Lungs	Conservative	11 mo, dead
7	69/F	N	rt lobectomy	1 mo	Lungs	Conservative	8 mo, dead
8	57/M	N	rt lobectomy	1 mo	Liver	Conservative	5 mo, dead

TAE, Trancatheter arterial embolization; HAI, hepatic arterial infusion chemotherapy.

Clinical findings and the outcome of the eight patients with vp$_3$ are summarized in Table 2. In all patients in groups A and N, recurrences were detected within 9 months after liver resection; the recurrence were in the liver in four of five patients and in the lungs in the three of five patients. In two of the three patients in group AP, the recurrences in the liver were detected 4 years and 7 months or 5 years and 1 month after liver resection. These two patients survived more than 7 years after surgery, and one of them is still alive.

We also examined anticancer effects of preoperative treatments by macroscopic inspection of operative specimens. The anticancer effects of TAE and PVE on the main tumor were stronger than those of TAE only. Almost all cancer cells in the vp in group AP were necrotic, but such an effect was seen in group A (Table 2). In group AP, the vp was covered with the embolic material used in PVE.

Table 3 Effects of Preoperative Therapies on Main Tumor and Portal Thrombi

Case	Group	Estimated necrotic change (%)	
		Main tumor	Portal thrombi
1	AP	50	90
2	AP	100	90
3	AP	90	90
4	A	50	0

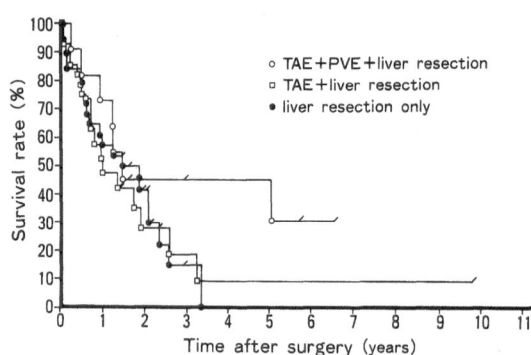

Fig. 1 Nonrecurrence Survival Rates of Patients after Different Therapies

DISCUSSION

It is generally accepted that dissemination by the portal vein is one main route by which HCC spreads [7]. We have already reported that PVE strengthens the anticancer effects of TAE, especially those on small intrahepatic metastases and portal thrombi, for which TAE is not effective. In this study, the nonrecurrence survival rates in group AP tended to be better than those in groups A and N. In the patients with vp_3 in groups A and N, recurrences in the liver were detected within a few months after liver resection, which means either that there had been small intrahepatic metastases at surgery or else that operative procedures spread cancer cells during surgery. Matsumata et al. [7] emphasized that it is important to establish a technique that prevents dissemination of cancer cells during operative manipulation. In operative specimens, the embolic material covered the portal thrombus in the patients with vp_3, which means that PVE may help to prevent the spread of cancer cells during surgery. Thus, PVE seems to be useful not only as a preoperative treatment but also as one treatment for unresectable HCC.

REFERENCES

1. Liver Cancer Study Group of Japan (1990) Primary liver cancer in Japan: clinicopathological features and results of surgical treatment. Ann Surg 211: 277-287
2. Yamanaka N, Okamoto E, Toyosaka A, Mitsunobu M, Fujihara S, Kato T, Fujimoto J, Oriyama T, Furukawa K, Kawamura E (1990) Prognostic factors after hepatectomy for hepatocellular carcinoma: a univarite and multivariate analysis. Cancer 65: 1104-1110
3. Kinoshita H, Sakai K, Hirohashi K, Igawa S, Yamasaki O, Kubo S (1986) Preoperative portal vein embolization for hepatocellular carcinoma. World J Surg 10: 803-808
4. Kinoshita H, Hirohashi K, Kubo S (1992) Preoperative portal vein embolization for hepatocellular carcinoma. In : Tobe T, Kameda H, Okudaira M, Ohto M, Endo Y, Mito M, Okamoto E, Tanikawa K, Kojiro M (eds) Primart liver cnacer in Japan. Springer-Verlag, Tokyo pp 283-290
5. UICC: International Union Against Cancer (1989) TNM atlas. Spiessl B, Beahrs OH, Hermanek P, Hutter RVP, Scheibe O, Sobin LH, Wagner G (eds). Springer-Verlag, Berlin pp 98-103
6. Yamada R, Sato M, Kawabata M, Nakatsuka H, Nakamura K, Takashima S (1983) Hepatic artery embolization in 120 patients with unresectable hepatoma. Radiology 148: 397-401
7. Matsumata T, Kanematsu T, Takenaka K, Yoshida Y, Nishizaki T, Sugimachi K (1989) Patterns of intrahepatic recurrence after curative resection of hepatocellular carcinoma. Hepatology 9:457-460

Therapeutic Strategy for Advanced Hepatocellular Carcinoma Using Systemic Interleukin-2 Infusion and Local Low-Dose Irradiation

T. Tsuchida[1], Y. Asano[1], J. Hiragushi[1], M. Nishiura[1], Y. Hyodo[1], K. Hiroishi[1], T. Koh[1], H. Iijima[1], S. Shimomura[1], Y. Amuro[1], K. Yamaguchi[1], T. Hada[1], K. Higashino[1], and Y. Hishikawa[2]

[1]The Third Department of Internal Medicine, [2]The Department of Radiology, Hyogo College of Medicine, Nishinomiya, Hyogo, 663 Japan

ABSTRACT

In two cases of unresectable HCC with multiple lesions, in which TAE was not indicated due to the vascular abnormality or allergy against iodide contrast medium, combination therapy with systemic low-dose IL-2 infusion and local low-dose tumor irradiation exhibited apparent anti-tumor effects such as the decrease of blood tumor marker level and the mass reduction judged by imaging diagnosis. Enhancement of NK and LAK cell killing, and the increased expression of IL-2R on NK cells were observed after the treatment. There were no serious side effects associated with the treatment.

KEY WORDS: hepatocellular carcinoma, immunotherapy, recombinant interleukin-2, low-dose irradiation,

INTRODUCTION

Hepatocellular carcinoma(HCC) is the second commonest cancer in South East Asia, which might correlate with high prevalence of hepatitis virus carriage, and is increasing recently also in Western countries. The progress of imaging diagnosis like ultrasonography and computed tomography(CT) enables earlier detection of small-sized HCC, which has increased the number of resectable cases. Consequently, the number of the patients surviving for longer periode after partial hepatectomy has increased recently. However, the prognosis of unresectable HCC including post-operative recurrence, is not yet satisfactory. The currently authorized treatments for unresectable HCC with multiple lesions, are transcatheter arterial embolisation(TAE) or intraarterial infusion of chemotherapeutic drugs. At present, radiotherapy is not considered as a first choice, because of possible radiotoxicity on cirrhotic liver,which are commonly associated with HCC, and generally low radiosensitive nature of adenocarcinoma. Immunotherapy utilizing adoptive transfer of lymphokine-activated killer (LAK) cells togehter with systemic recombinant interleukin-2(IL-2) infusion has been demonstrated to be partially effective for unresectable HCC . In this paper we report two cases of unresectable HCC with multiple lesions, who has been treated with low-dose IL-2 and local low-dose irradiation, because treatment requiring angiography was not indicated due to severe stenosis of common hepatic artery in the first case and to allergic responce against iodide contrast medium in the second case.

METHODS

IL-2 Administration

Human recombinant IL-2(Takeda,Japan) was administered through an indwelling central venous catheter by Deltek pump(Pharmacia,USA) over a period of 2 hours as a single dose of 1.6 mega JRU(1 Japan Reference Unit approximately corresponds to 2.6 IU) once a week. During IL-2 infusion, the patient received radiotherapy (20Gy/40 fraction/40 weeks).

Flowcytometric analysis of PBL subsets

Peripheral blood lymphocytes(PBLs) were separated from heparinised venous blood. Flowcytometric analysis was performed with FITC-conjugated monoclonal antibodies directed against T cells (OKT3), B cells(OKB20), NK cells(OKNK); Phycoerythrin(PE)-conjugated anti-IL-2 receptor(IL-2R) α chain antibody,; biotin-conjugated anti-IL-2R β chain antibody and PE-streptoavidin.

Measurement of NK and LAK cell activity

For the assay of direct killing activity of fresh PBLs(NK assay), ^{51}Chromium-labelled target cells,K562(NK sensitive)and

Daudi(NK resistant)tumor cell lines, were incubated with fresh PBLs for 4 hours with or without IL-2(final conc.1 nM). In order to induce LAK cells, PBLs were cultured with IL-2 for 7 days . LAK cell activity generated were assayed on Daudi cells in the same way as NK assay.

CASE PRESENTATION AND DISCUSSION

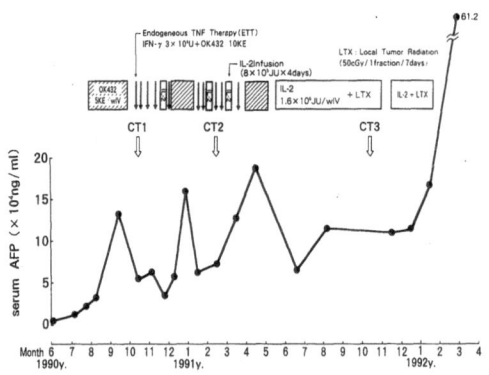

Fig. 1. Clinical Course of Case 1

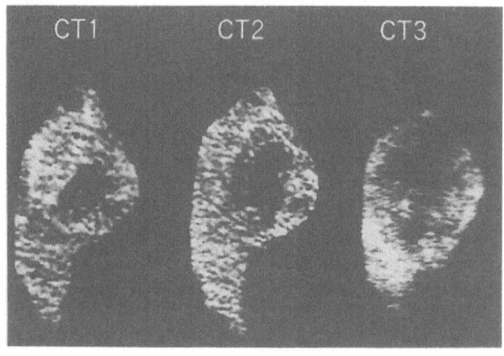

Fig. 2. Partially-enlarged CT showing Liver S6

[Case 1] The patient was a 59 year-old woman who was admitted to the hospital for the treatment of multiple HCC detected during angiography in a previous hospital. As common hepatic artery was severely stenosed due to the aneurysma possibly formed during selective catheterization in the previous hospital, TAE could not be carried out. Because of multiple tumor lesions in S1,S5 and S6, we gave up the idea of doing PEIT, and initiated immunotherapeutic regimen using sequential infusion of OK432(Chugai,Japan) and gamma-interferon for the purpose of endogenously induction of tumor necrosis factor(TNF)[1]. Three months later, serum alphafetoprotein(AFP) level decreased from 14×10^4 ng/ml to 3×10^4 ng/ml(Fig.1). Alternative treatment with endogenous TNF induction and systemic IL-2 infusion showed substantial anti-tumor responce. As the patient refused to take further treatment with hospitalization, we decided to change immunotherapeutic regimen from endogenous TNF induction requiring careful monitoring of severe hypotension, to intermittent IL-2 infusion on an outpatient basis.. Together with IL-2 we planned to use local tumor irradiation for the prophylaxis of portal vein tumor embolus. Two months later reincreased AFP decreased to 7×10^4 ng/ml and thereafter kept the constant level around 10^5 ng/ml for 5 months. Patient died of acute hepatic failure due to portal vein obstruction. Autopsy revealed the wide necrotic area in the tumor masses,which coincided with CT findings(Fig. 2), and the enormous clustering of cancer cells inside portal vein. Considering rapid doubling time(approx.27 days), it can be concluded that immunotherapy demonstrated cytostatic feasible effect in this case.

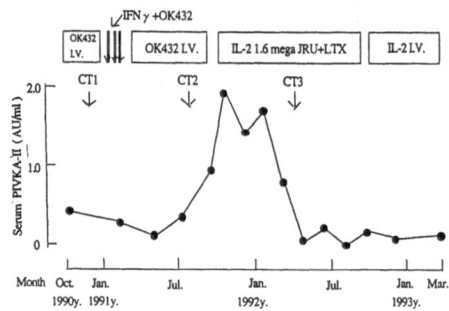

Fig. 3. Clinical Course of Case 2

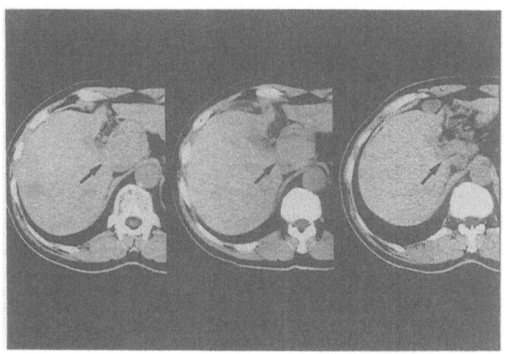

Fig. 4. Partially-enlarged CT showing Liver S1

[Case 2] The patient was a 60 year-old man who was admitted to the hospital for the precice examination of multiple hypoechoic masses in liver S1,S5,and S8. Biopsy revealed HCC of Edmondson type 1 . Blood chemistry revealed high level of plasma abnomal prothrombin (PIVKA-II) ,which correlated well with the growth of HCC. As the patient was allergic against iodide-containing contrast medium, TAE was not indicated. Consequently,we initiated immunotherapy using endogenous TNF induction. As shown in Figure 3, plasma PIVKA-II level decresed slightly. As the patient requested treatment on an outpatient basis, we started combination therapy with intermittent IL-2 infusion and local low dose irradiation by imitating the permissive result in the 1st case. Three months later, plasma PIVKA-II decreased rapidly and after next three months, plasma PIVKA-II finally fell below 0.05 AU/ml. Periodical examination of ultrasonograph and CT clearly indicated tumor mass reduction in whole liver. As shown in Fig. 4, tumor mass in S1 deacreased prominently. At present, 30 months after the beginning of immunotherapy the patient was treated only with IL-2 infusion after completing total radiation dose of 20 Gy. PIVKA-II level was kept within the range of 0.06 to 0.2 AU/ml and no significant alteration was shown radiographically.

In both cases, the patients did not have any serious side effects except mild flu-like symptoms such as mild fever, moderate malaise, slight headache, which are quite common with immunotherapy using IL-2. In terms of hepatic reserve function, prothrombin time or hepaplastin time improved significantly after treatment. We have measured several immunological parameters of PBL. As the tendency was similar in both cases, we have shown only the results of second case(Table 1). Tumoricidal activity of NK cells on K562 target cells increased almost 2-fold when assayed 6 months after the iniation of treatment. NK killing activity on NK-resistant Daudi cells was also high in the presence of IL-2(1 nM) ,suggesting endogenous induction of LAK cells in vivo. LAK cell activity induced even by low dose IL-2(100pM) in vitro showed apparent increase. Two color-flowcytometric analysis using the combination of anti-CD16 antibody and anti-IL-2R antibody, showed ten-fold increase of CD16-positive lymphocytes expressing IL-2R α chain, which means increased NK cells expressing high affinity IL-2 receptor, and it can explain the increased responsiveness to low dose IL-2.
Rosenberg first showed the effectiveness of high dose IL-2 infusion for the certain types of cancer like melanoma and renal cell cancer[2]. At present high-dose IL-2 therapy has been under reevaluation because of many toxic side-effects, high expenses and not so remarkable response-rate as expected. Recently German group has reported the good clinical effect using intermittent subcutaneous injection of low-dose IL-2 and alpha IFN,and their response-rate was equivalent to those of high-dose IL-2[3]. In murine tumor model other group has shown that intratumoral injection of low-dose IL-2 can be highly effective against metastatic cancer and without toxic side effects[4]. Studies in murine tumor model suggested that low-dose IL-2 therapy preferentialy activates tumor-specific T cells with immunological memory, while high-dose IL-2 therapy induces LAK cells[5]. Further investigations are needed in order to clarify the optimal IL-2 dose and delivery system. With regard to the role of local low-dose irradiation it can be speculated that local tumor irradiation might eliminate suppressor lymphocytes[6], or activate apoptotic mechanism in tumor cells[7]. Anyway, we don't have yet any direct evidence explaining about the mode of action. Recently several reports have demonstrated the synergism of immunotherapy and radiotherapy in animal[8] and clinical studies[9]. We are currently investigating the synergistic effect of systemic IL-2 infusion and local low-dose irradiation in murine hepatoma model. In conclusion we would like to emphasize that intermittent low-dose IL-2 infusion and local low-dose irradiation really exhibited the apparent clinical effectiveness in certain cases of advanced HCC without serious toxicities and by keeping high QOL.

Table 1.   Improvement of Immunological Parameters
after Treatment

	CD3	CD20	CD16	CD16 /α +1)	CD16 /β +1)	NK Killing 2) on K562	NK Killing 2) on Daudi	LAK Killing 3) on Daudi 100pM	LAK Killing 3) on Daudi 1nM
Pre	69	12	25	0.5	8	21(45)	1(14)	4	51
Post	76	15	27	5	8	41(82)	3(33)	49	74

1) Double-positive cells for anti-CD16Ab, and anti-IL-2R α chain or β chain Ab.
2) % killing at effector-to-target cell ratio 40 : 1
3) Natural killer assay was done with or without 1nM of IL-2. % killing in parentheses were data with IL-2. % killing at effector-to-target cell ratio 20 : 1

REFERENCES

1. Satoh M, Inagawa H, Shimada Y, Soma G-I, Oshima H, Mizuno D (1987) Endogenous production of tumor necrsis factor in normal mice and human cancer patients by interferons and other cytokines combined with biological response modifiers of bacterial origin. J Biol Response Mod 6:512-524
2. Rosenberg SA(1988) The development of new immunotherapies for the treatment of cancer using interleukin-2. Ann.Surgery 208:121-135.
3. Atzpodien J, Korfer A, Franks CR, Franks CR, Poliwoda H, Kirchner H (1990) Home therapy with recombinant interleukin-2 and interferon-alpha2b in advanced human malignancies. Lancet 335:1509-1513.
4. Maas R, Dullens HFJ, De Jong W, Den Otter W (1989) Immunotherapy of mice with a large burden of disseminated lymphoma with low-dose interleukin-2. Cancer Res 49:7037-7040.
5. Talmadge JE, Phillips H, Schneider J, Tribble H, Pennington R, (1987) Systematic preclinical study on the therapeutic properties of recombinant human interleukin 2 for the treatment of metastatic disease. Cancer Res 47:5725-5730.
6. Mills C, North R. (1983) Expression of passively tranferred immunity against an established tumor depends on generation of cytolytic T cells in recipient ;Inhibition of suppressor T cells. J Exp Med 157:1448-1460.
7. Cohen J. (1991) Programmed cell death in the immune system. Advances in Immunology 50:55-85.
8. Cameron R, Spiess P, Rosenberg S. (1990) Synergistic antitumor activity of tumor-infiltrating lymphocytes, interleukin 2 and local tumor irradiation. J Exp Med 171:249-263.
9. Mukai M, Morita S, Tsunemoto H.(1992) Combination therapy of local administration of OK-432 and radiation for esophageal cancer. Int J Radiation Oncology Biol Phys 22:1047-1050.

Fundamental Studies on Direct Injection of Ethanol (Et)+Polyethylene Glycol (PEG) Mixture into Hepatocellular Carcinoma (HCC) in Rats

Shozo Miyawaki, Yukihiko Adachi, and Toshio Yamamoto

Second Department of Internal Medicine, Kinki University School of Medicine, Osaka-Sayama, Osaka, 589 Japan

[Abstract]
To improve the therapeutic effect of percutaneous ethanol injection therapy (PEIT), mixtures of Et with polyethylene glycol 400 (PEG) as injection materials were evaluated for tumor shrinkage and necrosis rate. The Et,PEG-Et mixtures or PEG was injected into the subcutaneously produced rat hepatoma (AH109A) in rats.A significant decrease (P<0.05) in tumor size was found in the 2 PEG+Et groups,and a significant increase (P<0.05) in degenerative necrosis was found in the PEG+Et(Et66%) group in comparison wiht the Et group. From these results, the use of PEG-Et(Et66%) will be most effective in improving therapeutic effect of PEIT.

Key Words :hepatoma , ethanol , polyethylene glycol 400 ,percutaneous ethanol injection therapy (PEIT)

[Introduction]
In the treatment of hepatocellular carcinoma (HCC) 2 cm or smaller in size, percutaneous ethanol injection therapy (PEIT)[1-3] has been used clinically. To increase the local retention of ethanol, and to enhance the therapeutic effect of PEIT, we made a mixture of ethanol and polyethylene glycol 400 (average molecular weight: 400, PEG), a material with a large molecular weight which is harmless to the human body and is generally used as a solvent for drugs. The mixture was injected into the subcutaneously produced rat hepatoma, and its tumor-necrotizing effect was evaluated.

[Methods]
We used AH109A rat hepatoma cells provided by Dr. Fukushima, Faculty of Pharmacology, Kumamoto University. AH109A was subcultivated in ascites, and 0.5 ml of a solution containing 4×10^6 cells/ml was injected subcutaneously into each of male Donryu rats of 6-8 weeks old. In 7-10 days, tumors of 2-3 cm in diameter developed in the subcutaneous tissue. The rats were divided into the following four groups each consisting of 6-7 animals: Group to receive 1 ml of ethanol [ethanol concentration 99.5% (here in after referred to as Et group)], group to receive 1 ml of PEG + ethanol [PEG 34%, ethanol 66% (referred to as PEG-Et66)], group to receive 1 ml of PEG + ethanol [PEG 54%, ethanol 46% (referred to as PEG-Et46)], and group to receive 1 ml of PEG [referred to as PEG]. The solution was injected into the tumor in the animal.
Seven days after injection, changes in tumor size were checked, and the ratio of the size before injection against the size before injection was calculated. At the same time, measurement was made of the rate of degenerative necrosis in the largest slice of the tumor.

In another set of Et, PEG-Et66, and PEG-Et46 groups, ^{14}C-ethanol was used instead of ethanol. In this experiment, the tumor was taken out 30 minutes after injection. Its tissue was then dissolved in Soluene-350, and ^{14}C-radioactivity retained in the tumor was measured.

In one more set of two groups, one to receive ^{14}C-ethanol at 50 ul/100 g body weight and the other to receive a mixture of PEG and ^{14}C-ethanol (66%). The solution was intravenously given, and disappearance of ^{14}C-radioactivity from the blood was observed.

[Results]

PEG-Et66 group (average 17.8%) and PEG-Et46 group (average 47.4%) each showed a significant shrinkage (P<0.05) in the ratio of tumor sizes in comparison with Et group (average 217.9%) (Fig.1). However, no significant difference was seen between PEG-Et66 group and PEG-Et46 group. There was no significant difference in the ratio of tumor sizes between Et group and PEG group. However, the ratio tended to be higher in Et group.

The rate of degenerative necrosis in Et group was 55.7% on average, and only PEG-Et66 group showed a significant increase (P<0.05) in degenerative necrosis(average 82.6%) (Fig.2). PEG-Et46 group showed no significant difference against Et group. In comparison between Et and PEG groups, there was no significant difference, though the rate of degenerative necrosis tended to be higher in Et group. Fig.3 shows typical histopathological picture of each group. As for the rate of ethanol retention in tumor at 30 minutes after injection of ^{14}C-ethanol, PEG-Et66 group (average 56.2%) and PEG-Et46 group (average 62.5%) each showed a significant increase compared with Et group (average 45.5%) (P<0.01) (Fig.4). Although no significant difference was seen between PEG-Et66 and PEG-Et46 groups, higher PEG concentration tended to show a better ethanol retention rate.

In comparison of intravenous administrations of ^{14}C-ethanol and PEG-^{14}C-ethanol (66%), the mixture containing PEG showed a better retention in the blood (Fig.5).

[Discussion]

As shown in Fig.1, PEG-Et66 group and PEG-Et46 group both exhibited a more remarkable suppression of the tumor growth in comparison with Et group.

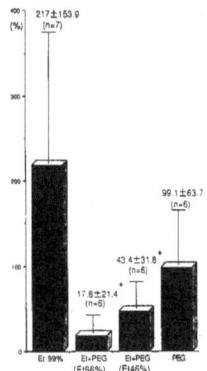

FIG.1 Volume ratio (after/before treatment) 7 days after injection. *: p<0.05 comparared with the Et group.

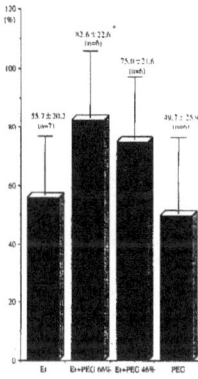

FIG.2 Necrosis rate 7 days after injection. *: p<0.05 comparared with the Et group.

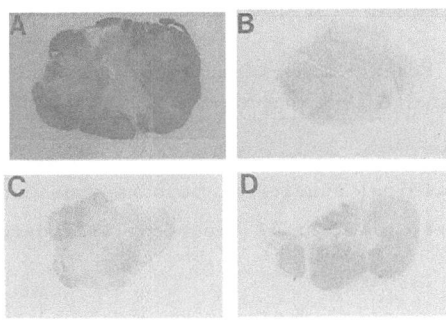

FIG.3 Macroscopic finding of the subctaneous tumor (AH109a) 7 days after injection. (H-E stain)
A:Et group B:Et+PEG(Et66%) group
C:Et+PEG(Et46%) group D:PEG group

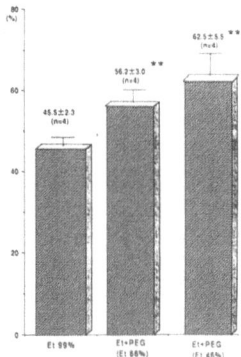

FIG.4 ^{14}C-Radioactivity retained in the tumor 30 minutes after ^{14}C-ethanol injection. **:p<0.01 comparared with the Et group.

And only PEG-Et66 group with a high ethanol concentration showed a significant increase in the rate of degenerative necrosis (Fig.2).

Therefore, in the treatment of HCC, the use of PEG-Et66 will be most effective in improving therapeutic effect.

Retained ^{14}C-radioactivity was more when ^{14}C-ethanol was injected into the tumor with higher concentration of PEG (Fig.4). This indicates that higher concentration of PEG may help tumor retention of ethanol. Higher retention of ^{14}C-ethanol in blood after intravenous injection of PEG-^{14}C-ethanol (66%) (Fig.5) also suggests a possibility that ethanol is retained with PEG in the tissue as in the blood.

Viscosity of PEG at 25°C is 80-110 cps, which is far higher than that of ethanol (99.5%, 1.00-1.19 cps). PEG is well miscible with ethanol. Besides, there is a report that, when applied to the skin, it sticks to the tissue[4].

The terminal hydroxyl group of PEG readily combines with fatty acid to form an ester that has a surfactant effect, an effect which possibly helps retain ethanol in the tissue. From these, the mixture of ethanol with PEG will increase the viscosity of the injection
solution, and thereby will increase the retention of ethanol in the tissue. The LD$_{50}$ of PEG 400 in rats is 43.6g/kg and its toxicity is very low[5]. Taking all of these into account, it will be promising to use a mixture of ethanol with PEG in the PEIT.

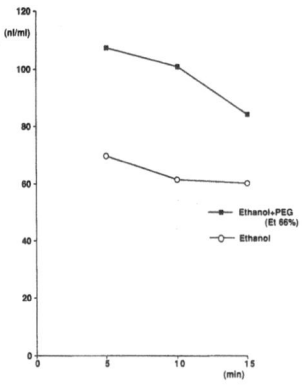

FIG.5 Plasma disappearance of ^{14}C-Radioactivity after injection of ^{14}C-ethanol.

[References]

1. Shinagawa T, Ukaji H, Iino Y, Isomura S, Yamaguchi H, Ishizuka S, Sugiura N, Ohto M (1985) Intratumoral injection of absolute ethanol under ultrasound imaging for treatment of small hepatocellular carcinoma. Kanzo 26:99-105

2. Majima Y, Tanikawa K (1987) Percutaneous Ethanol Injection Therapy. Medicina 24:1616-1618

3. Fuzimoto T (1988) The experimental and clinical studies of percutaneous ethanol injection therapy(PEIT) under ultrasonography for small hepatocellular carcinoma. Kanzo 29:52-59

4. Ishidate M, Momose M, Shimomura T, Uno M, Suzuki I (1986) An explanation on the eleventh revision of the Japanese Pharmacopoeia. Hirokawa Press. Tokyo, D913-D918

5. Smith H F JR, Carpenter C P, Weil C (1950) The toxicology of the polyethylene glycols. J.Am.Pharm.Assoc.39:349-354

Segmental/Subsegmental Hepatic Arterial Embolization
— A New Therapy for Hepatocellular Carcinoma

Masato Fujita, Tetsuya Katsumori, Osamu Satoh, Takeshi Takahashi, Syoichi Akimoto, Kazumi Akimoto, Koji Ohno, Yuji Miyamoto, Yasuhiko Nakano, and Tomoho Maeda

Department of Radiology, Kyoto Prefectural University of Medicine, Kyoto, 602 Japan

ABSTRACT

We carried out segmental Lipiodol-TAE in 114 patients with HCC in order to preserve hepatic function and to reinforce the anticancer effect. It was performed by advancing the catheter into the subsegmental or segmental hepatic artery feeding the tumor and by superselective injection of Lipiodol mixed with the anticancer drug and gelatin sponge particles. In non-resected 100 patients with HCC, the cumulative survival rates were 94.1% at 1 year and 63.8% at 3 years Segmental Lipiodol-TAE is one of the best therapies for HCC when the tumor is localized within one segment.

KEY WORDS: TAE, Hepatic segmental catheterization, Lipiodol, HCC

INTRODUCTION

Transcatheter arterial embolization(TAE) is widely accepted as an effective therapy for hepatocellular carcinoma(HCC)1. Improved catheterization techniques have enabled us to embolize a localized target area in the liver. The embolized range should change according to the spread of tumor and hepatic function. Recently, segmental Lipiodol(oily contrast medium)-TAE is performed to reinforce the anticancer effect and to preserve hepatic function2. The therapeutic outcome of segmental Lipiodol-TAE is comparable to that of surgical resection. We describe the therapeutic results of segmental Lipiodol-TAE in 114 patients with HCC with particular emphasis on differences in dose of Lipiodol, tumor size and hepatic function.

MATERIALS AND METHODS

Segmental Lipiodol-TAE was performed in 114 patients with HCC, including 14 patients who were treated surgically after TAE. The tumors were confined to one segment in solitary nodule or three subsegments in two nodules. Segmental Lipiodol-TAE was performed by advancing the catheter into the segmental or subsegmental hepatic artery feeding the tumor. Then, Lipiodol mixed with the anticancer drug(Adriamycin or Farmorubicin) and gelatin sponge particles were injected superselectively. The patients were classified into two groups by plain radiograph obtained immediately after TAE:Seg-TAPE(group A)---51 patients with Lipiodol retention in both the tumor and the portal vein branches close to the tumor and Seg-TAE(group B)---63 patients with Lipiodol retention only in the tumor(Fig. 1). The non-resected patients were also classified into three groups by tumor size:group 1---32 patients with tumors less than two cm($\Phi \leqq 2$), group 2 ---45 patients with tumors between 2 cm and 5 cm(2< Φ <5) and group 3---23 patients with tumors more than 5 cm(5 $\leqq \Phi$).

RESULTS

There was no significant difference in patient background between groups A and B
(Table 1). Average volume of injected Lipiodol was 5.97 ±2.74 ml in group A and
4.29±2.99 ml in group B. This was statistically significant. In the non-resected
100 cases, the cumulative survival rates were 94.1% at 1 year, 68.1% at 2 years a
nd 63.8% at 3 years. In group A(45 patients) , 92% at 1 year and 87.1% at both 2
and 3 years and in group B(55 patients), 95.8% at 1 year, 58.8% at 2 years and
53.5% at 3 years(Fig.2). The difference in survival rates between groups A and B
was not significant. The cumulative non-recurrence rates were 71.8% at 1 year
and 41.6% at 2 years in group A and 26.7% at 1 year in group B. This difference
was significant(Fig.3). Local control was better in group A than in group B.
Fourteen patients underwent surgical resection after segmental Lipiodol-TAE. In
seven cases, complete necrosis of the tumor was histologically verified. In four
of the six resected cases in group A, complete necros was found. Concerning tumor
size, the cumulative survival rates were 96.8% at 1 year and 74% at both 2 and 3
years in group 1, 97% at 1 year and 68% at both 2 years and 3 years in group 2
and 84% at 1 year and 58% at 2 years in group 3. There was no significant
difference between groups. Concerning hepatic function, the cumulative survival
rates were 100% at 1 year, 85.8% at 2 years and 78% at 3 years in Child's A(60
patients), 92% at 1 year and 44.6% both at 2 yearsand 3 years in Child's B(29
patients) and 68.6% at 1 year and 51.4% at2 years in Child's C(11 patients).
There were significant differences between Child's A and the other
classifications. In all patients, fever and pain after embolization was easily
controlled.

DISCUSSION

The mixture of Lipiodol and anticancer drug injected through an intraarterial
catheter flows into the portal branches close to the tumor as well as the tumor
vessels3. An anticancer effect from the portal as well as the arterial side can
be expected and may attack the marginal tumor areas supplied by portal blood
flow. Because Lipiodol retention both in the arterial and portal branches also
affects non-tumor areas, Lipiodol-TAE of the whole liver should be avoided.
Therefore, Segmental Lipiodol TAE should be performed for HCC localized within
one segment. In this study, the therapeutic results of segmental Lipiodol-TAE
were comparable to those of surgical resection. Since the cumulative survival
rates relative to tumor size did not significantly differ, larger tumors can be
treated by this method than can be treated by PEIT(percutaneous ethanol
injection therapy). Seg-TAPE should be performed when hepatic function is
sufficient for segmental Lipiodol retention. Seg-TAE should be performed when
poor hepatic function makes segmental Lipiodol retention unacceptable. However,
there was no significant difference in patient backgrounds between groups A and
B. Average volume of injected Lipiodol was larger in group A than that in group B.
The case with which Lipiodol stasis occurs varies by individual. However,
better local control in group A than in group B was proven by histological study
in the resected cases and the non-reccurrence rates. The differencein survival r
ates of group A and B were not significant. The difference may not be obvious
because the follow up period was short. However, it is true that the survival
rates do not reflected local control only. In patients with HCC, the tumor is
multicentric and usually accompanied by liver cirrhosis. In this study, the
cumulative survival rates were better in patients with good hepatic function
(Child's A). Segmental TAE is preferable in preserving hepatic function of non
embolized areas. However, TAE is one of the best conservative therapies for HCC.
Segmental Lipiodol TAE is one of the best local therapies for HCC as well as
surgical resection and PEIT.

CONCULUSION

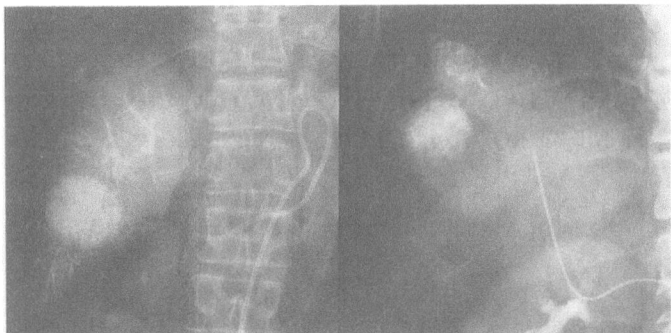

Fig. 1 Plain radiograph immediately after TAE:Left, Seg-TAPE. Right, Seg-TAE

Table 1. background factors of the patients

	Stage				T				IM				Vp				size			Child's		
	1	2	3	4	1	2	3	4	0	1	2	3	0	1	2	3	2cm≧	2< <5	5cm≦	A	B	C
group A	5	33	6	7	5	33	6	7	39	7	5	0	50	1	0	0	15	22	14	36	9	6
group B	13	30	15	5	13	30	15	5	44	10	9	0	61	2	0	0	19	30	14	36	21	6

A(51 patients):male 38, female 13, age 60.6±10.5 B(63 patients):male 40, female 23, age 61.4±8.7

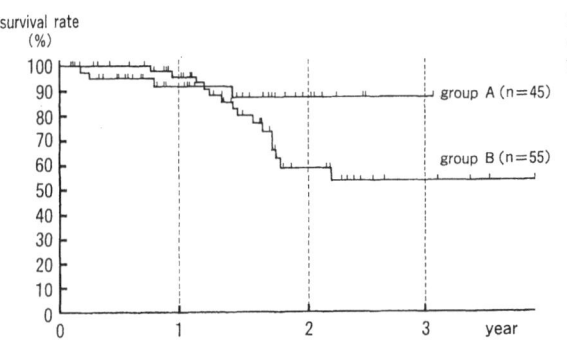

Fig. 2 The cumulative survival rates in non-resected cases after embolization.

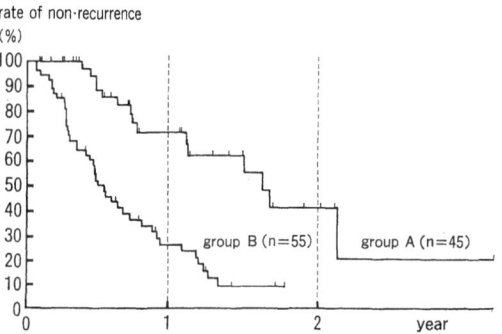

Fig. 3 The cumulative rates of non-recurrence in non-resected cases after embolization.

Segmental Lipiodol-TAE is one of the best therapies for HCC when the tumor is localized within one segment. The anticancer effect increases in relation to the amount of Lipiodol infused.

REFERENCES

1. Yamada R, Sato M, et al:Hepatic artery embolization in 120 patients with unresectable hepatoma. Radiology 148:397-401, 1983
2. Uchida H, Ohishi H, et al:Transcatheter hepatic segmental arterial embolization using Lipiodol mixed with an anticancer drug and gelfoam particles for hepatocellular carcinoma.
3. Nakamura H, Hashimoto T, et al:Iodized oil in the portal vein after arterial embolization. Radiology 167:415-417, 1988

Factors Involved in the Resistance to Repeated Transcatheter Arterial Embolization for Hepatocellular Carcinoma

Koji Umeshita[1], Morito Monden[1], Mitsukazu Gotoh[1], Masato Sakon[1], Toshio Kanai[1], Yasunori Hasuike[1], Hiroshi Nakano[1], Taro Marukawa[2], Hironobu Nakamura[2], Chikazumi Kuroda[2], Jun Okamura[1], and Takesada Mori[1]

[1]Department of Surgery II, [2]Department of Radiology, Osaka University Medical School, Osaka, 553 Japan

ABSTRACT

In this study, we investigated the relationship between TAE frequency and its effectiveness. TAE was ineffective in 11 of 15 patients who underwent TAE 4 times or more, although earlier TAE had been clearly effective in all of them. Two different patterns of resistance to TAE were observed, i.e. collateral arterial supply (epicholedochal plexus in most cases) and conversion of an expanding tumor to an infiltrating tumor. To avoid the former, it is important not to cause intimal injury in the proximal arteries during TAE procedures. In the latter case, use of new anti-cancer drugs may be effective.

KEY WORDS: resistance to transcatheter arterial embolization, hepatocellular carcinoma, collateral, epicholedochal plexus, massive growth

INTRODUCTION

Transcatheter arterial embolization (TAE) has been widely employed as a therapeutic tool for hepatocellular carcinoma (HCC), not only in unresectable cases but also as a part of multidisciplinary treatment [1, 2]. However, it is known that tumors acquire resistance to TAE after repeated procedures. In this study, we investigated the relationship between TAE frequency and its effectiveness.

MATERIALS AND METHODS

This study included 243 consecutive patients who underwent TAE for HCC at Osaka University Hospital from November 1979 to December 1988. There were 203 males and 40 females, the age was between 30 and 94 (mean: 59), and the mean follow-up period was 24 months.

A total of 366 TAE procedures were performed on them. After the patency of the portal trunk was confirmed by arterial portography, the celiac axis was cannulated and an arteriogram was taken to define the anatomy. Next, the catheter was positioned in an appropriate artery (in most cases the right or left hepatic artery, and in selected cases the proper hepatic artery or more peripheral artery). TAE was performed with anti-cancer agent, iodized oil, and embolic material. Doxorubicin or epirubicin was used as the anti-cancer agent in most cases, but mitomycin C or cisplatinum was occasionally used. Iodized oil has been routinely used since 1984. The embolic material was gelfoam cube of about 1 mm^3. Gelfoam powder or mitomycin C microcapsule was used in only a small number of patients.

The serum levels of alphafetoprotein (AFP) were frequently measured after TAE. Computed tomography (CT) was taken one week after and one month after each TAE. TAE was judged effective if: 1) AFP continued to decrease for 1 month; 2) tumor size in CT decreased by more than 25% at 1 month; or 3) iodized oil uniformly accumulated in the tumor for more than 1 month. TAE was repeated when recurrence was suspected based on AFP or CT.

RESULTS

Table 1 shows the frequency of TAE procedures in the 243 patients. Fifteen of them underwent TAE 4 times or more. The last TAE was ineffective in 11 of the 15 patients (73%), although the earlier TAE had been clearly effective (Table 2). There were two different patterns of resistance to repeated TAE which are presented below with description of typical cases.

Case reports

Case 1. A 60-year-old male was admitted to Osaka University Hospital in December 1986. Hepatic arteriography revealed a nodule of 8 cm in diameter in the anterior segment and multiple small nodules in both lobes of the liver. A catheter was positioned in the proper hepatic artery and TAE was performed with doxorubicin, iodized oil, and gelfoam cubes. Follow-up CT revealed tight accumulation of iodized oil in the small nodules, but partial wash-out of iodized oil from the main nodule. The second TAE was performed from the right hepatic artery three months later, and follow-up CT demonstrated uniform accumulation of iodized oil in all the nodules. The third TAE was performed with cisplatinum, iodized oil, and gelfoam cubes in October 1987. At the time of the fourth TAE in March 1988, the right hepatic artery was completely occluded and collateral arterial supply through the epicholedochal plexus was observed. The collateral could not be embolized due to technical reasons. The main nodule in the anterior segment continued to grow despite oral administration of a 5-fluorouracil-derivative and several arterial infusions of anti-cancer drugs through the implanted port. The patient expired in September 1989. This patient was categorized in the "collateral" group (group 1: Fig. 1).

Case 2. A 60-year-old male was referred to Osaka University Hospital for HCC in May 1984 with a tumor, 1 cm in diameter, located deep in the posterior segment. As the patient refused surgical resection, the first TAE was performed in July 1984, and AFP decreased from 120 to 9 ng/ml. The second and third TAE were performed in March and November 1985, respectively, and both were judged effective from the decrease in AFP. The fourth TAE in February 1986 could not suppress AFP, although no collaterals were seen on the arteriogram. Follow-up CT demonstrated rapid growth of the tumor, and subsegments 7 and 8 were resected in May 1986. In the resected specimen, there was an original encapsulated tumor and spread of invasive tumor beyond the capsule was observed. This indicated that previous "nodular" type HCC had been converted into "massive" type HCC. It was speculated that most of the original tumor was controlled by TAE, but those tumor cells which were resistant to TAE survived, and grew beyond the capsule. Soon after the operation, intrahepatic metastases and distant metastasis to the humerus were found. The patient died in November 1986. This patient was categorized in the "massive conversion" group (group 2: Fig. 2).

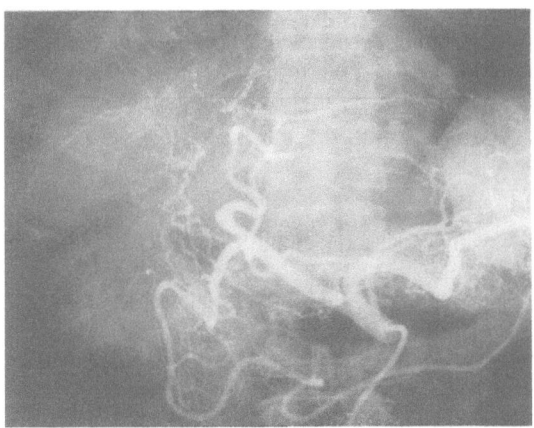 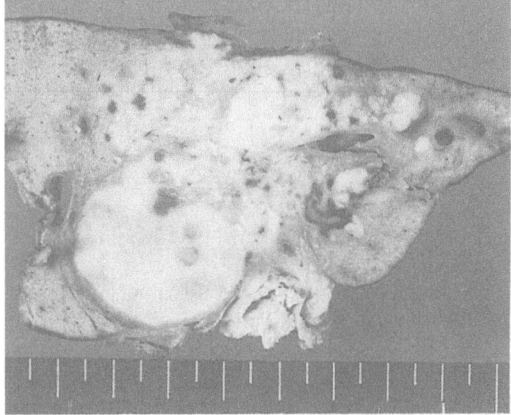

Fig. 1 Group 1. Right hepatic artery is occluded and collateral through the epicholedochal plexus is seen.

Fig. 2 Group 2. An infiltrative tumor extends from an original encapsulated tumor.

Of the 11 TAE-resistant patients, six were in group 1 and five were in group 2 (Table 2). In group 1, four patients had collateral through the epicholedochal plexus, one had it through the left gastric artery, and one had both of them. All these patients had relentless downhill courses and died within a short period.

Table 1. Number of TAE procedures and number of patients

1	176
2	34
3	18
4	10
5	3
6	1
7	1

Table 2. Effectiveness of TAE in 15 patients who underwent TAE 4 times or more

Effective	4		
Ineffective	11		
Collateral		6	
Epicholedochal plexus			4
Left gastric artery			1
Both			1
Massive conversion		5	

DISCUSSION

TAE has been widely employed as a useful therapeutic tool for hepatocellular carcinoma. The cumulative survival rates at 1, 3, and 5 years after TAE for unresectable HCC were 65%, 30%, and 16%, respectively [3]. TAE does improve the prognosis of patients with unresectable HCC, but has proved to be ineffective for certain types of HCC. It has been reported that the "nodular" type of HCC with a circumferential capsule is sensitive to TAE, whereas the "massive" type of HCC is resistant [4].

In our series, TAE was ineffective in 11 of the 15 patients who underwent TAE 4 times or more. In all these 11 patients, the tumors had clear capsules and were classified as the "nodular" type at the time of the first TAE. All patients responded to TAE. However, at the time of the last TAE, the tumors had changed into the "massive" type in 5 of the 11 patients and did not respond to TAE. Probably this was because those tumor cells resistant to anoxia and anti-cancer drug survived, became prominent, and grew aggressively beyond the capsule. Use of other anti-cancer agents might be effective in such patients.

Michels reported that there are at least 26 possible different routes of collateral blood supply to the liver [5]. There have been reports that the arterial circulation of the liver is re-established within a short time after ligation of the hepatic artery [6,7]. Since TAE occludes more peripheral arteries, the probability of collateral formation is lower, but in this series, tumors did receive a blood supply from collaterals after repeated TAE. Successful TAE through these collaterals is possible in some cases [8-11], but collaterals along the choledochus (epicholedochal plexus) is technically difficult to treat. As the epicholedochal plexus was always accompanied by proximal interruption of the hepatic artery in this series, it is speculated that the cause of epicholedochal plexus formation after repeated TAE is not TAE per se but incidental intimal injury in the proximal arteries. Therefore, to avoid the formation of collateral through the epicholedochal plexus, care should be taken to prevent intimal injury in the proximal arteries.

REFERENCES

1. Yamada R, Sato M, Kawabata M, Nakatsuka H, Nakamura K, Takashima S (1983) Radiology 148: 397-401
2. Okamura J, Horikawa S, Fujiyama T, Monden M, Kambayashi J, Sikujara O, Sakurai M, Kuroda C, Nakamura H, Kosaki G (1982) World J Surg: 352-357
3. Monden M, Sakon M, Gotoh M, Kanai T, Umeshita K, Wang KS, Sakurai M, Kuroda C, Okamura J, Mori T (1992) Cancer Chemother Pharmacol 31: S38-S44
4. Kuroda C, Sakurai M, Monden M, Marukawa T, Hosoki T, Tokunaga K, Wakasa K, Okamura J, Kozuka T (1991) Cancer 67:81-86
5. Michels N (1953) Cancer 6: 708-724
6. Bengmark S, Rosengren K (1970) Am J Surg 119: 620-624
7. Koehler RE, Korobkin M, Lewis F (1975) Radiology 117: 49-54
8. Soo CS, Chuang VP, Wallace S, Charnsangavej C, Carrasco H (1983) Radiology 147: 45-49
9. Nakamura H, Hashimoto T, Oi H, Sawada S (1987) Am J Roentgenol 148: 626-628
10. Ohtomo K, Furui S (1988) Radiat Med 6: 157-158
11. Duprat G, Charnsangavej C, Wallace S, Carrasco CH (1988) Acta Radiologica 29: 427-429

A New Approach to the Treatment of Hepatocellular Carcinoma with Intrahepatic Metastases — Transarterial Immuno-Embolization (TIE) with OK-432 and Fibrinogen

Toshio Kanai[1], Morito Monden[1], Masato Sakon[1], Mitsukazu Gotoh[1], Koji Umeshita[1], Yasunori Hasuike[1], Takushi Monden[1], Takumichi Murakami[2], Hironobu Nakamura[2], and Takesada Mori[1]

[1]Department of Surgery II, [2]Department of Radiology, Osaka University Medical School, Osaka, 553 Japan

ABSTRACT

In this study, we analyzed the results of a new therapy for hepatocellular carcinoma (HCC) : transarterial immuno-embolization (TIE) with OK-432 and fibrinogen. Of 19 patients with advanced HCC in which other treatments were ineffective, 14 (74%) were surviving at 2 to 16 months after TIE. Serum levels of the tumor markers decreased in all patients and a marked reduction of tumor size was observed in 6 patients after TIE. High fever was observed in all patients. However, deterioration of liver function seemed to be negligible. Histological examination of resected specimens following TIE showed massive infiltration of mononuclear cells around tumor cell nests of the main tumor and intrahepatic metastases.

KEY WORDS: transarterial immuno-embolization (TIE), OK-432, hepatocellular carcinoma (HCC), intrahepatic metastasis

INTRODUCTION

The prognosis for HCC has improved due to recent advances in three therapeutic modalities, i.e., surgical resection, transcatheter arterial embolization (TAE) and percutaneous ethanol injection therapy (PEIT). However, the prognosis of patients with multiple HCC is still poor even after treatment by these methods (1). Therefore, we devised a new therapy of transarterial immuno-embolization (TIE) with OK-432 and fibrinogen, which has been reported to enhance not only the systemic immunological potential but also local cytotoxicity against colorectal cancer (2). In the present study, we analyzed our preliminary results on the clinical effects and side effects of TIE for HCC.

PATIENTS AND METHODS

TIE therapy was performed a total of 28 times on 25 patients with HCC at Osaka University Hospital between September 1991 and March 1993. We applied the treatment to 19 patients with advanced HCC who had been treated several times previously by other methods and had proven to be insensitive to the conventional treatment in the first series. The biological response modifiers used were OK-432 which is a penicillin-treated lyophilized powder of the avirulent Su strain of Streptococcus pyogenes(3) and a commercially available fibrin glue which contains Factor-XIII. TIE was done according to our protocol. Double catheters consisting of a balloon catheter and an S-P catheter were inserted into the tumor-feeding artery as shown in Figure 1. OK-432 (2.5 KE/ml), fibrinogen (60 mg/ml) and thrombin (1 U/ml) were mixed together. Under this condition, conversion of fibrinogen into fibrin occurred about 2.5 min after mixing at room temperature. Lipiodol was also added to the mixture at the ratio of 1: 4. Approximately

5-10 ml of the mixture was injected through the S-P catheter after the hepatic artery flow had been decreased by the blowing up of the balloon. No anti-cancer drugs were used. The serum level of the tumor markers, alpha-fetoprotein (AFP) and des-gamma-carboxy prothrombin (PIVKA II), the size of the tumor in the CT scan, and liver function were serially examined. Histological examination was performed in resected cases after TIE.

RESULTS

The clinical response and side effects of TIE were investigated in 19 inoperable patients with multiple HCC. Four patients died of the carcinoma at 4, 8, 16, and 17 months after TIE. One patient died of an unrelated cause. The remaining 14 patients (74%) are surviving; Four patients were alive at 14, 14, 16 and 16 months (Table 1). All patients with a high serum level of tumor markers showed a decrease immediately after TIE. Furthermore, a marked reduction of tumor size was observed in six patients after TIE. The incidence of side effects after TIE was summarized in Table 2. High fever was seen in all cases, and abdominal pain and appetite loss were also observed. White cell count in peripheral blood increased to over 20,000 /ul after TIE in two cases, and serum GOT level increased to more than 400 U/l after TIE

Table 1. Results of TIE in inoperable patients with advanced HCC

Case	Age · Sex	Location of tumor	Initial treatment	Date of TIE	Initial AFP (ng/ml)	Outcome
1 MT	60 M		subsegmentectomy(S₈) TAE (3)	1991. 9. 10 1991. 9. 17	20193	dead (17M)
2 SO	50 M		TAE (3)	1991. 11. 8	98	alive (16M)
3 AI	62 M		lateral sementectomy TAE (1)	1991. 11. 22	12279	alive (16M)
4 TY	47 M		posterior segmentectomy LAK · TAE (1)	1992. 1. 8 1992. 4. 24	11	alive (14M)
5 IT	59 M		subsegmentectomy(S₈) TAE (2)	1992. 1. 29	2250	dead (14M)
6 KS	67 M		TAE (2)	1992. 2. 4	10	alive (14M)
7 ND	71 M		TAE (2)	1992. 4. 23	428	alive (11M)
8 MI	67 M		TAE (3)	1992. 7. 17	45	alive (8M)
9 YK	51 M		subsegmentectomy(S₈) TAE (1)	1992. 7. 31 1993. 1. 29	2326	dead (8M)
10 YK	74 M			1992. 8. 26	392	dead (7M)
11 MO	44 M		TAE (1)	1992. 9. 4	174	alive (7M)
12 NY	54 M		partial resection (S₈) TEA (1)	1992. 9. 11	282	alive (7M)
13 MI	60 M		TAE (2)	1992 9. 16	32	alive (7M)
14 TY	66 F		TAE (4)	1992. 10. 30	3093	alive (5M)
15 YU	57 M		TAE (1)	1992. 11. 6	12	dead (4M)
16 YT	66 M			1992. 11. 11	11	alive (4M)
17 SF	61 F		TAE (2)	1992. 12. 18	2580	alive (3M)
18 MN	77 F		TAE (2)	1993. 1. 12	91	alive (3M)
19 YY	38 M		TAE (1) PEIT (1)	1993. 1. 27	236	alive (2M)

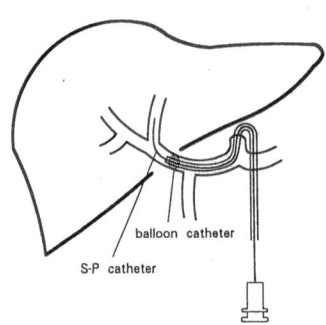

Fig. 1. Schema of TIE procedure

Table 2. Incidence of side effects after TIE

Side effects	No. of patients(%)
Symptomatic:	
Fever	18/18 (100%)
Abdominal pain	7/18 (39%)
Appetite loss	6/18 (33%)
Nausea	2/18 (11%)
Vomiting	2/18 (11%)
Laboratory data:	
GOT (>400 U/l)	3/13 (23%)
T. Bil (>2.0 mg/dl)	3/13 (23%)
BUN (>30mg/dl)	2/14 (14%)
WBC (/ul)	
10000-20000	10/15 (67%)
>20000	2/15 (13%)
Platelet (/ul)	
<50000	5/15 (33%)

in three cases. However, these values decreased to pretreatment levels within one week. No disturbance of the coagulation-fibrinolysis system was observed in all patients. The influence on other liver functions seemed to be negligible.

After confirmation of the safety of this method, we started a second series of study on six other patients. All underwent hepatic resection following TIE. Histological examination performed using six resected-tumor specimens on day 6, 6, 14, 20, 23, 48 post-TIE showed massive infiltration of mononuclear cells focused on destroyed tumor cell nests. Furthermore, lytic necrosis as well as coagulation necrosis was observed in the main tumor and the intrahepatic metastases in two cases. These findings were quite different from those observed with conventional TAE.

DISCUSSION

In recent years, the remarkable progress in imaging modalities has made it possible to detect HCC at an early stage. Furthermore, improvement in assessment of the function of the liver remaining after resection has led to a high increase of the resectability rate of HCC. However, the long-term survival rate of the patients with multiple HCC is not yet satisfactory and of a limited efficacy regardless of the extent of the hepatic resection or the other treatment modalities (1).

Our results show that TIE with OK-432 and fibrinogen induced a marked decrease in serum AFP level and a marked reduction of tumor size in inoperable patients. In addition, histological findings clearly show that TIE is quite effective against the main tumor and small intrahepatic metastases, which are believed to the key factors in determining the prognosis.

OK-432 has been widely used as a biologic response modifier (BRM) in Japan (3). Normal peripheral blood mononuclear cell treated with OK-432 showed cytotoxic activity against various tumor cell lines (4). In humans, it has been reported to improve survival and response rates in some forms of cancers (5). In addition, the antitumor effect of OK-432 on colorectal carcinoma was found to be greatly augmented when it was injected intratumorally in conjunction with fibrinogen. This immunotherapy seemed to induce the antitumor effect of OK-432 most efficiently by changing the fibrin metabolism in cancer stroma (2). Alternatively, fibrinogen might be easily delivered into the tumor vessels and more diffusely distributed throughout the liver as compared with gelatin particles. OK-432 encapsulated in an insoluble fibrin clot may be gradually released from this clot into the tumor tissue.

In conclusion, our results indicate that TIE is a safe and effective therapy for HCC patients with intrahepatic metastases. We believe that TIE is one of the promising modalities for HCC.

REFERENCES

1. Monden M, Sakon M, Gotoh M, Kanai T, Umeshita K, Wang KS, Sakurai M, Kuroda C, Okamura J, Mori T(1992) Selection of therapeutic modalities for hepatocellular carcinoma in patients with multiple hepatic lesions. Cancer Chemother Pharmacol 31: 38-44.
2. Monden T, Morimoto H, Shimano T, Yagyu T, Murotani M, Nagaoka H, Kawasaki Y, Kobayashi T, Mori T (1992) Use of fibrinogen to enhance the antitumor effect of OK-432. 69: 636-642.
3. Okamoto H, Shoin S, Kashimura S, Shimizu R(1976) Studies on the anticancer and streptolysin S-forming abilities of hemolytic streptococci. Jap J Microbiol 11: 323-336.
4. Wakasugi H, Oshimi K, Miyata M, Morioka Y(1981) Augmentation of natural killer(NK) cell activity by a streptococcal preparation, OK-432, in patients with malignant tumors. J Clin Immunol 1:154-162.
5. Watanabe Y, Iwa T(1984) Clinical value of immunotherapy for lung cancer by the streptococcal preparation, OK-432. Cancer 53:248-253.

Effect of Intra-Arterial Injection of Mitoxantrone-Lipiodol Emulsion on Hepatocellular Carcinoma

Wataru Ichikawa, Zenro Nihei, Toshiki Yamashita, Hiroyuki Uetake, Shigeo Sawai, Yasuyuki Kawachi, Renzo Hirayama, and Yoshio Mishima

The Second Department of Surgery, Tokyo Medical and Dental University, Bunkyo-ku, Tokyo, 113 Japan

ABSTRACT

The effect of intra-arterial injection of mitoxantrone emulsified with ethiodized oil was investigated in 24 patients with hepatocellular carcinoma. After treatment, 6 of the patients underwent hepatectomy. In 18 unresected cases, there were 8 (44%) partial responses, which had continued 2 to 10 months (mean, 7.4 months). In the remaining 6 resected cases, the necrotic areas in the main nodules accounted for 65% (mean, 85%) of the nodule, with complete necrosis in three cases. The results in this preliminary study are encouraging to further study.

KEY WORDS: mitoxantrone, chemolipiodolization, hepatocellular carcinoma

INTRODUCTION

Mitoxantrone (MIT) (Novantrone®, Lederle Ltd., Tokyo, Japan) is an anthraquinone anticancer agent with structural similarities to doxorubicin [1]. We previously reported MIT emulsified with ethiodized oil in a mixture with iohexol, a nonionic water-soluble contrast medium [2]. This current study was undertaken to investigate the effect of hepatic arterial chemolipiodolization using MIT without embolization.

MATERIALS AND METHODS

Patients

Twenty-four patients with hepatocellular carcinoma (HCC) were eligible from October 1990 to March 1992. Characteristics of the patient population are shown in Table 1. According to the Manual for Staging of Cancer [3], 2 cases were classified as Stage I (4.2%), 12 as Stage II (50.0%), 6 as Stage III (25.0%), and 4 as Stage IV (8.4%), respectively. All patients were treated with chemolipiodolization using MIT. There were 18 unresectable cases, due to underlying cirrhosis and/or tumor spread. On the other hand, hepatic resection was performed in the remaining 6 of the 24 patients (25.0%).

Table 1. Clinical Characterisics of the patients with hepatocellular carcinoma

Average age in yr (range)	58(36-78)
Sex (male:female)	16 : 8
T-bilirubin level (mg/ml)	1.2±0.8
Albumin level(g/dl)	3.6±0.6
AST level (U/l)	58.6±25.7
Stage I:II:III:IV	2:12:6:4
Resection	6 (25.0%)

Response Criteria

In unresected cases, the clinical response to treatment was assessed objectively by changes in tumor size. Response criteria were based on the Criteria for the Evaluation of the Clinical Effects of Solid Cancer Chemotherapy [4].
In the resected cases, the specimens were cut into serial slices of 5 mm in thickness, after fixing them with formalin. Histologic examinations of all samples of resected specimens were carried out using hematoxylin and eosin staining.

Chemolipiodolization of Mitoxantrone

MIT was prepared as previously reported [2]. In brief, to make the specific gravity equal to Lipiodol Ultra Fluide® (LPD) (ethiodized oil, Laboratories Gerber, Aulnay-sous-Bois, France), MIT was dissolved with iohexol (Omnipaque 300®, Daiichi Pharmacy, Tokyo, Japan) at the following doses: MIT, 2 mg; iohexol 2 ml. This solution was mixed with 2 ml to 4 ml of LPD by the pumping method. MIT emulsion (MIT-LPD) is stable in the form of water-in-oil.
Following conventional hepatic angiography, a vascular catheter was inserted superselectively into the hepatic artery feeding the tumor. MIT-LPD was slowly given through the catheter.

RESULTS

Treatment

A total of 58 courses of MIT-LPD injections were performed (mean, 2.4 courses per patient; range, 1 to 8 courses). A catheter was selectively positioned at the hepatic artery in 11 patients (45.8%) and in the appropriate segmental hepatic artery in 13 patients (54.2%). The dose of MIT administrated ranged from 2.0 to 10.0 mg (mean, 3.6 mg per course), to obtain full accumulation of LPD in the tumor vessels. The duration of therapy was 0.9 to 6.2 months (mean, 3.2 months).

Responses

All 18 patients without operation were evaluated for response. According to the response criteria, there were 8 (44.4%) partial responses, which have continued for 2.0 to 10.0 months (mean, 7.4 months), and 7 (38.9%) minor responses. There were no change in 3 cases (16.7%), and no progressive disease (Table 2).

Table 2. Responses to therapy in 18 patients who could be examined.

Stage	CR	PR	MR	NC	PD	Total
I	0	1	0	0	0	1
II	0	4	3	0	0	7
III	0	1	3	3	0	7
IV	0	2	1	0	0	3
Total	0(0%)	8(44.4%)	7(38.9%)	3(16.7%)	0(0%)	18

Note:CR;complete response:PR;partial response:MR;minor response:NC;no change;PD;progressive disease.

In histopathological examinations, three of six main tumors were completely necrotic. The other three cases had nests of viable cancer cells, but the necrotic areas accounted for over 65% in the main nodules. Regarding accessory lesions, five of the patients had daughter nodule, capsular invasion and/or tumor embolus. In these patients, except for the patient No. 3 with tumor emboli in the portal veins, the necroic area was greater than 50% (Table 3).

Table 3. Histopathological findings in resected tumors

No.	Tumor Size(cm)	Main nodule	Doughter nodule	Capsular invasion	Tumor embolus
1	3.5x3.2	100%	(-)	CN	(-)
2	2.6x2.0	65%	viable	viable	viable
3	4.4x3.5	100%	CN	(-)	(-)
4	2.3x1.9	95%	(-)	(-)	(-)
5	5.4x3.2	80%	partially viable	minutely viable	(-)
6	2.7x2.9	100%	minutely viable	(-)	(-)

Note:CN;complete necrosis:partially viable;it is >50% and
<90%:minutely viable;it is >90%

Side effects

There were no serious complications such as hepatic failure and renal failure.
The major side effect observed after MIT-LPD injection was abdominal pain
(40.0%), which disppered within a few days. The values of serum AST and total
bilirubin were elevated in about 50% of patients, but they returned to pre-
therapeutic levels within 2 weeks. Neither myelosuppression nor cardiotoxicity
was observed.

DISCUSSIONS

MIT demonstrated antitumor activity for HCC in various clinical trials. Dunk et
al.[5] reported a 27% response rate in a phase II trial of systemic
administration to 40 patients with previously untreated HCC. Anticancer activity
was confirmed by Shepherd et al.[6], who reported a 26% response rate via
hepatic arterial infusion in 23 patients.
Since Nakamura et al. reported chemolipiodolization for HCC [7], anticancer
agents such as doxorubicin and cisplatin have been applied exclusively in
combination with LPD. It has been found that LPD was selectively deposited not
only in main tumors but also in daughter nodules, and anticancer agents were
slowly released from collected LPD in the tumor [7,8].
There have been no other studies of MIT-LPD for HCC. We employed two parameters
for the assessment of anticancer effect: tumor size and histopathological
finding. Tumor size decreased to less than 50% of the pre-treatment size in 44%
of the treated patients. However, it is still unclear whether this pronounced
tumor regression will result in the prolongation of survival, because the
duration of follow-up is too short. Sasaki et al. [8] complete necrosis was
obtained in about 50% of patients treated in combination with embolization. In
this study, to evaluate the effect of MIT-LPD, we used no embolic materials. It
is of interest to note that complete necrosis of the main tumor occurred in 3
out of 6 cases.
These results are encouraging to further study. This treatment might be the
therapy of choice not only for unresectable cases but also for resectable
cases.

REFERENCES

1. Murdock KC, Child RG, Fabio PF, Angier RB (1979) Antitumor agents:1.4-
bis[(aminoalkyyl)amino]-9,10-anthracenediones. J Med Chem 22:1024-1030
2. Ichikawa W, Nihei Z, Sawai S, Yamashita T, Uetake H, Kawachi Y, Hirayama R,
Mishima Y, Tamaru H (1992) Successful preparation of mitoxantrone emulsion
containing non-ionic contrast medium. Jpn J Cancer Chemotherapy 19:1550-1552
(with English abstract)
3. American Joint Committee on Cancer. Liver (including intrahepatic bile
ducts). (1988) In: Manual for Staging of Cancer, ed.3. JB Lippincott,
Philaderphia, pp 87-89
4. Japan Society For Cancer Therpy. Criteria for evaluation of direct effects of
solid cancer chemotherapy. (1986) In: Criteria for the Evaluation of the
Clinical Effects of Solid Cancer Chemotherapy, J Jpn Soc Cancer Ther 21:925-953
(in Japanese)
5. Dunk AA, Scott SC, Johnson PJ, Melia W, Lok ASF, Murray-Lyon I, Williams R,
Thomas HC (1985) Mitoxantrone as single agent therapy in hepatocellular
carcinoma. J Hepatol 1:395-404
6. Shepherd FA, Evans WK, Blackstein ME, Fine S, Heathcote J, Langer B, Taylar
B, Habal G, Pritchard KI (1987) Hepatic arterial infusion of mitoxantrone in the
treatment of primary hepatocellular carcinoma. J Clin Oncol 5:635-640
7. Nakamura K, Tashiro S, Hiraoka T, Uemura K, Konno T, Miyauchi Y (1983)
Studies on anticancer treatment with an oily anticancer drug injected into the
ligated feeding hepatic artery for liver cancer. Cancer 52:2193-2200
8. Sasaki Y, Imaoka S, Kasugai H, Fujita M, Kawamoto S, Ishiguro S, Kojima J,
Ishikawa O, Ohigashi H, Furukawa H, Koyama H, Iwanaga T (1987) A new approch to
chemoembolization therapy for hepatoma using ethiodized oil, cisplatin, and
gelatin sponge. Cancer 60:1194-1203

Treatment of Unresectable Hepatocellular Carcinoma by Intra-Arterial Infusion of THP-Adriamycin Under Occlusion of Hepatic Arterial Flow

Yoshie Une, Junichi Uchino, Mitsuo Yasuhara, Kazuhito Misawa, Toshiya Kamiyama, Tsuyoshi Shimamura, Naoki Sato, Yasuaki Nakajima, and Yoshinobu Hata

The First Department of Surgery, Hokkaido University School of Medicine, Sapporo, 060 Japan

ABSTRACT

Recently, we developed an intrahepatic artery catheter and device attached with an implantable double lumen reservoir which can be used for repeated intra-arterial infusion chemotherapy (IAIC) in out patients clinic. Eight patients with unresectable hepatocellular carcinoma(HCC) were treated by infusion of THP-Adriamycin with this method. Combined administration of carboplatin was done in two patients. The catheter was inserted into proper hepatic artery under laparotomy. The occlusion balloon was attached to the common hepatic artery, and catheters were connected to subcutaneous double lumen reservoir. Six out of eight patients were survived more than 2 years. Compared with the results of the previous conventional IAIC group, the more favorable survival rates were obtained by using this method.

KEY WORDS: hepatocellular carcinoma, balloon occluded intra-arterial infusion chemotherapy, THP-Adriamycin

INTRODUCTION

IAIC under the occlusion of hepatic arterial flow causes augmentation of intra-hepatic drug concentration which is expected to have higher response rates than conventional arterial infusion methods 1). Recently, we developed an intrahepatic artery catheter and device attached with an implantable double lumen reservoir 2). 4'-0-tetrahydropyranyladriamycin (THP-ADM) was reported to be superior to ADM in its weaker cardiotoxicity and has faster cellular uptake 3)4). In the present study, we report the clinical results of IAIC by THP-ADM using this device in the patients with unresectable hepatocellular carcinoma.

PATIENTS AND METHODS

From July 1989 to July 1991, twenty six consecutive patients with unresectable hepatocellular carcinoma(HCC) were treated at IAIC in The First Department of Surgery, Hokkaido University Hospital. Eight patients out of 26 patients were treated with IAIC by THP-ADM under occlusion of hepatic arterial flow using our new technique. The device consists of three parts; intra-arterial catheter, double lumen reservoir and a cylinder like device with a small silicone balloon on its inner part. The catheterization was done under laparotomy, inserted into proper hepatic artery via gastroduodenal artery. The occluder was attached to the common hepatic hepatic artery. Intra-arterial and balloon catheters were connected to subcutaneous double lumen reservoir (Fig. 1). A few quantity (0.5 ml average) of distilled water injected through the one port of double lumen reservoir inflated the balloon compressing the artery within the cylinder like occluder 2). THP-ADM 30 mg was infused intra-arterially via the other part of the double lumen reservoir by this method every 2 weeks. Carboplatin 250 to 450 mg was injected alternately in 2 patients. Survival curves after insertion of the catheter were estimated by Kaplan-Meier method and analyzed by generalized Wilcoxon's method.

RESULTS

Three to seven times of repeated infusions were possible without any severe side effects. This treatment was easy to perform in the out-patient clinic. The characteristics of the patients in group A and group B showed no differences (Table 1). The more favorable survival rates were obtained in group A compared with group B. Three out of eight patients were survived more than

2 years. Two year survival rates were 51.6 % in group A,while 13.9 % in group B, which were statistically significant (Fig.2).

DISCUSSION

Balloon occluded arterial infusion is an expecting and widely accepted method for augmentation of the intrahepatic tissue level of anticancer drugs 1). Repeated intra-arterial chemotherapy in particular combined with occlusion of arterial flow without disturbing patients quality of life is expected for more excellent therapeutic method which causes an anticancer drug to efficiently act on the affected site. This subcuatneously implantable device is highly accepted by the patients because of its small size and easy to provide a repeated occlusions and infusions. IAIC by THP-ADM for HCC under occluding blood flow using this device promises to be a more convenient and more effective method.

Table 1. Patients profiles treated by intra-arterial infusion of THP-adriamycin under occlusion of hepatic arterial flow (Group A) and patients treated by Adriamycin without occlusion (Group B)

Varieties		Group A	Group B
Age		67.4±5.8	61.4±8.6
Sex	male	7	18
	female	1	0
Stage	1	0	0
	2	0	3
	3	0	1
	4 A	7	14
	4 B	1	0
Clinical stage	1	4	13
	2	3	4
	3	1	1
no cirrhosis		1	0
with cirrhosis		7	18
HBsAg	positive	1	6
	negative	5	12
	unknown	2	0
HCV antibody	positive	2	2
	negative	1	2
	unknown	5	14

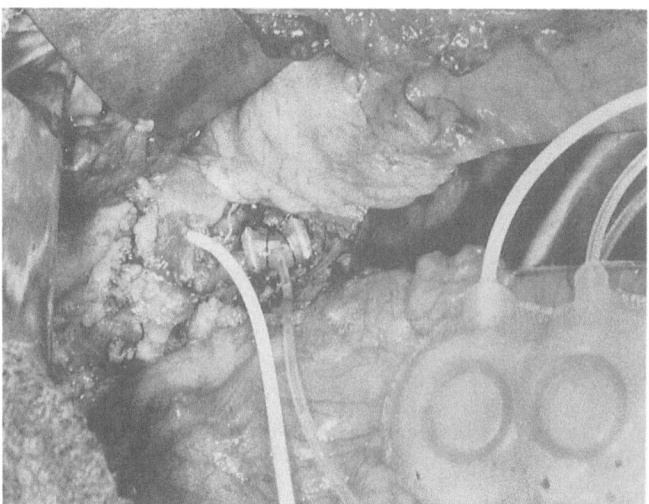

Figure 1. Method of intra-arterial cannulation and attachment of occluder

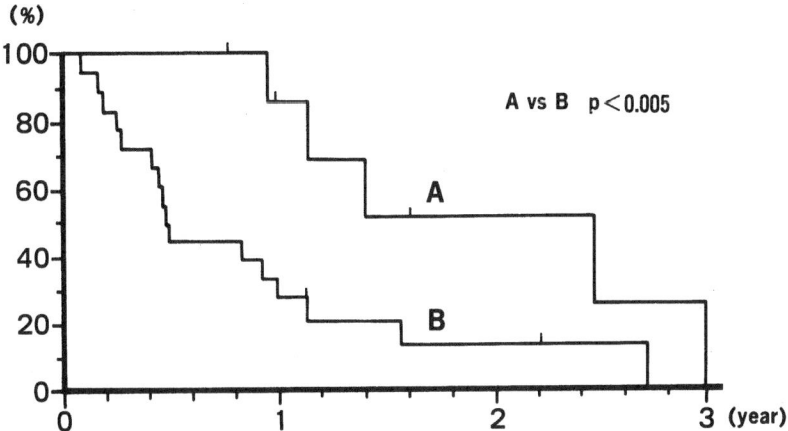

Figure 2. Survival rates of group A and group B
        Group A: Patients treated by double lumen reservoir
        group B: Patients treated by conventional IAIC

REFERENCES

1. Lise M, Cagol PP, Nitti D, Feltrin G, Fosser V, Cecchetto A, Rubaltelli L, Pucciarelli S (1980) Temporary Occlusion of the Hepatic Artery Plus Infusion and Systemic Chemotherapy for Inoperable Cancer of the Liver, International Surgery 65: 315-323.
2. Une Y, Kamiyama T, Nagabuchi E, Ogasawara K, Tamura M, Sato N, Nakajima Y, Uchino J (1989) Intra-arterial infusion chemotherapy under flow occlusion using double lumen reservoir. Jpn J Cancer Chemother 16(8) : Part-Ⅱ, 3081-3086.
3. Umezawa H, Takahashi Y, Kinoshita M, Nagasawa H, Masuda T, Ishizuka M, Tatsuta K, Takeuchi T (1979) Tetrahydropyranyl derivatives of daunomycin and adriamycin. J Antibiotics 32: 1082-1084.
4. Rougier P, Munck JN, Eoias D (1990) Intra-arterial hepatic ;chemotherapy with pirarubicin. Am J Clin Oncol 13(Suppl. 1): s1-s4.

Combination of Hepatic Arterial Infusion Chemotherapy and Portal Vein Occlusion for Unresectable Hepatocellular Carcinoma

Shoji Kubo, Hiroaki Kinoshita, Kazuhiro Hirohashi, Nagahisa Fujio, Ryutaro Iwasa, and Hiroki Nakamura

Second Department of Surgery, Osaka City University Medical School, Osaka, 545 Japan

ABSTRACT

We tried a combination of percutaneous transhepatic portal vein embolization (PVE) or portal vein ligation (PVL) and hepatic arterial infusion chemotherapy (HAI, with or without a reservoir) or transcatheter arterial embolization (TAE) for five patients with hepatocellular carcinoma (HCC) in whom the tumors were not resected. The patients were from 50 to 70 years old, and all had cirrhosis. The tumors were classified as being in stage III or IV by the UICC classification. Three of the five patients underwent PVE and the other patients underwent PVL. Adriamycin (ADR), epi-Adriamycin (epi-ADR), mitomycin C (MMC), or mitoxantrone (MIT), or some combination was used during HAI. These combinations of therapy was effective for hepatic tumors in all patients, as judged by decreases in tumor size and serum levels of α-fetoprotein (AFP) after treatment. The combination of HAI and portal occlusion may be effective for unresectable HCC.

KEY WORDS: hepatic arterial infusion chemotherapy, portal vein embolization, portal vein ligation, transcatheter arterial embolization, hepatocellular carcinoma

INTRODUCTION

Despite progress in diagnostic imaging and screening of high-risk groups, hepatocellular carcinoma (HCC) is still often detected only when advanced. Most of the patients with HCC have liver cirrhosis, which decreases operability [1]. We devised percutaneous transhepatic portal vein embolization (PVE) and used it before liver resection. We have reported that PVE causes atrophy of the embolized part of the liver and hypertrophy of the nonembolized part. We have also reported that PVE strengthens the anticancer effect of transcatheter arterial embolization (TAE), extends surgical indications for HCC, and makes liver resection safer [2,3]. Recently, we tried the combination of portal vein occlusion by PVE or portal vein ligation (PVL) and transarterial treatment with hepatic arterial infusion chemotherapy (HAI), TAE, or both for unresectable HCC. This paper reportes the results of this treatment.

SUBJECTS AND METHODS

Subjects were from 50 to 70 years old and all were men. All patients had liver cirrhosis. Three tumors were classified as being in stage III and the others were in stage IV-A by the UICC classification [4]. The tumors were not resected because of the advanced HCC, poor liver function and reasons other than medical ones, or some combination of these reasons. Three of the five patients under went PVE and the other patients underwent PVL. All patients also underwent HAI with or without TAE. In HAI, Adriamycin (ADR), epi-Adriamycin (epi-ADR), mitomycin C (MMC) or mitoxantrone (MIT), or some combination were used. Effectiveness was evaluated by the tumor size measured on computed tomograms (CT) or sonograms and by serum levels of α-fetoprotein (AFP).

RESULTS

Results of treatment are summarized in Table 1.

Table 1. Patients undergoing portal occlusion and transarterial therapy

Case	Age (yr), sex	Stage	Associated liver disease	Treatment	Outcome
1	70, M	IV-A	Cirrhosis	TAE (4 times), PVE (3 times), Surgery (cholecystectomy), HAI (7 times)	Survived, 7.0 yr
2	58, M	III	Cirrhosis	TAE, PVE, HAI (2 times)	Alive at, 5.4 yr
3	51, M	III	Cirrhosis	TAE, PVE, Surgery (cholecystectomy, reservoir), HAI (7 times), Oral chemotherapy	Survived, 1.6 yr
4	50, M	III	Cirrhosis	TAE, Surgery (PVL, chole-cystectomy, wrapping of right lobe), HAI (9 times)	Alive at, 1.2 yr
5	52, M	IV-A	Cirrhosis	Surgery (PVL, cholecystectomy, wrapping of right lobe, resec-tion of lymph nodes), HAI (2 times)	Survived. 0.5 yr

Case 1. The main tumor and intrahepatic metastases were in the right lobe of the liver. At first PVE and TAE were done three times each. The tumor size and the volume of the right lobe decreased gradually. We tried to resect tumor, but it was impossible because of liver cirrhosis and an intrahepatic metastasis in the left lobe. Then HAI using a reservoir and HAI by the Seldinger method after removal of the reservoir were done. TAE was repeated. The tumors in the right lobe were well controlled, but the tumor in the left lobe enlarged. The patient died 7 years after the first treatment. Case 2. We tried to resect the tumor in the right lobe, but it was impossible. We did HAI twice with ADR, MMC, and epi-ADR. The tumor size and volume of the right lobe decreased greatly (Fig. 1). The levels of AFP also decreased (Fig. 2). The patient is alive 5 years and 4 months after the first treatment.

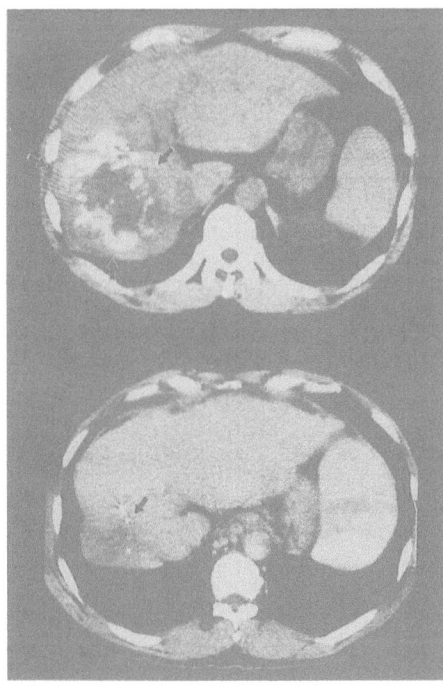

Fig. 1 Computed tomograms in case 2. Upper, before treatment; lower, 5 years after treatment.

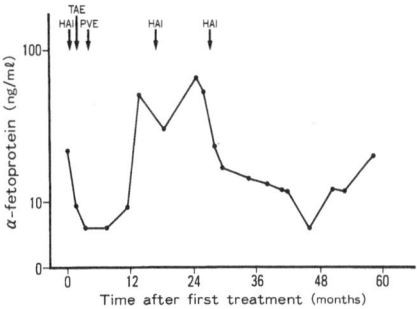

Fig. 2 Changes in serum levels of AFP in case 2

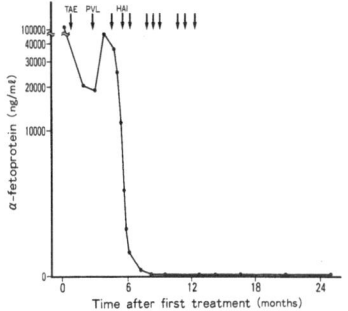

Fig. 3 Changes in serum levels of AFP in case 4

Case 3. The tumor with an intrahepatic metastasis was in the right lobe. There was a portal thrombus. We did TAE and PVE as preoperative preparation. However, liver resection was not done because the patient had severe liver cirrhosis. Cholecystectomy was done, and an infusion tube inserted from the gastroduodenal artery up to the proper hepatic artery was connected with a reservoir. HAI using MIT was done 6 times. The serum level of AFP was well controlled during the period when HAI was repeated. However, the level increased rapidly after the removal of the reservoir because of obstruction of the catheter. The patient died 1 year and 7 months after the first treatment. Case 4. We did PVL, cholecystectomy, and wrapping the right lobe with a Goatex sheet to prevent blood supply from the surrounding tissues to the tumor. Then, a reservoir was put into place. We did HAI with MIT 9 times. The tumor size decreased. The levels of AFP decreased greatly after the start of HAI (Fig. 3). The patient is alive 1 year 7 months after the first treatment. Case 5. The tumor was in the right lobe and medial segment, and a portal thrombus and an intrahepatic metastasis were detected. The lymph nodes along the aorta and hepatic artery were involved. To lengthen survival, we did PVL, wrapping the right lobe with Goatex, and cholecystectomy, and resected the lymph nodes when possible. HAI using epi-ADR was done twice after the operation. The tumor size in the liver decreased gradually, but the size of the lymph nodes increased. The patient died 6 months after the first treatment.

DISCUSSION

TAE and HAI are the most effective treatments for unresectable HCC. However, it is difficult to cause complete necrosis of tumors tissue, especially small intrahepatic metastases and portal thrombi [2,3]. Ligation of the portal branch results in atrophy of the affected hepatic lobe and hypertrophy of the opposite lobe [5]. Other investigators showed that ligation of the portal branch supplying the tumor-bearing lobe caused regression of the size of the hepatic tumor [6]. Honjo et al. [7] reported that portal ligation was effective in some patients with liver cancer. Recently we devised PVE, and are using it as a preoperative treatment. In this paper, we report the results of combination therapy with PVE or PVL and transarterial treatment (TAE and HAI) in five patients with unresectable HCC. In spite of the advanced HCC, all tumors in the liver were well controlled; the size of the tumors decreased in some patient, and the serum levels of AFP decreased in some. One of the five patients survived for 7 years. In two of other patients, the serum levels of AFP are very low, and the patients are still alive. The reasons for the effectiveness of this treatment are not known. One reason might be that portal occlusion blocks the outflow of the anticancer agents injected through the hepatic artery, giving high concentrations of the agents in the liver and tumor. We need to investigate what kind of anticancer agents is most effective against HCC.

REFERENCES

1. Liver Cancer Study Group of Japan (1990) Primary liver cancer in Japan: clinico-pathological features and results of surgical treatment. Ann Surg 211:277-287
2. Kinoshita H, Sakai K, Hirohashi K, Igawa S, Yamasaki O, Kubo S (1986) Preoperative portal vein embolization for hepatocellular carcinoma. World J Surg 10:803-808
3. Kinoshita H, Hirohashi K, Kubo S (1992) Preperative portal vein embolization for hepatocellular carcinoma. In: Tobe T, Kameda H, Okudaira M, Ohto M, Endo Y, Mito M, Okamoto E, Tanikawa K, Kojiro M (eds) Primary liver cancer in Japan. Springer-Verlag, Tokyo, pp 283-290
4. UICC: International Union Against Cancer (1989) TNM Atlas. Spiessl B, Beahrs OH, Hermanek P, Hutter RVP, Scheibe O, Sobin LH, Wagner G (eds). Sprtinger-Verlag, Berlin, pp 98-103
5. Rous P, Larimore LD (1920) Relation of the portal blood to liver maintenance: a demonstration of liver atrophy conditional on compensation. J Exp Med 31:609-632
6. Kraus GE, Beltran A (1959) Effect of induced infarction on rat liver implanted with Walker carcinoma 256. AMA Arch Surg 79:769-774
7. Honjo I, Suzuki T, Ozawa K, Takasan H, Kitamura O, Ishikawa T (1975) Ligation of a branch of the portal vein for carcinoma of the liver, Am J Surg 130:296-302

Tumor Marker Doubling Time of Liver Metastases from Stomach and Colonic Cancer and Its Clinical Significance

Yutaka Takahashi[1], Masayoshi Mai[1], and Satoru Kusama[2]

[1]Department of Surgery, Cancer Research Institute, Kanazawa University, Kanazawa, 921 Japan
[2]Department of First Surgery, Tokyo University School of Medicine, Bunkyo-ku, Tokyo, 113 Japan

ABSTRACT

The growth rate of liver metastases from stomach cancer and colonic cancer as investigated with tumor markers. Tumor doubling time calculated from CT or Echo was hardly different from tumor marker doubling time in each cases. Tumor marker doubling time of 48 cases with liver metastases from stomach ranged from 12 to 50 days, with a mean of 27.7 ± 10.3 (SD) days. On the other hand, that of 34 cases with liver metastases from colonic cancer ranged 10 to 130 days, with a mean 59.7 ± 29.5 days. There is significant difference between that of stomach and colon. Moreover, postoperative survival was found to be significantly correlated with the tumor marker doubling time in individual cases.

KEY WORDS: liver metastases, stomach cancer, colonic cancer, growth rate, tumor marker

INTRODUCTION

It is well known that tumor growth rate has a substantial influence upon survival time [1-3]. Although some fragmentary information on growth rate may be obtained by measuring recurrent or metastatic lesions, in general it is difficult to ascertain the growth rate of human tumors. In recent years, tumor markers have been found, not only experimentally but also clinically, to show exponential growth that has a good correlation with the increase in tumor volume [4,5]. In this paper, we calculated the doubling time of liver metastases from the changes in tumor marker levels and studied the clinical significance of tumor marker doubling time.

MATERIAL AND METHODS

Out of the patients who suffered from liver metastases at the Department of Surgery, Cancer Research Institute, Kanazawa University, 48 patients with stomach cancer and 34 patients with colonic cancer showed increased levels of serum alpha-fetoprotein (AFP) or carcinoembryonic antigen (CEA). Pre-treatment serum tumor marker level was logarithmically on the ordinate (Y) and plotted against time (days) on the abscissa (X) for linear regression analysis according to the equation, $Y = aX + b$, by which tumor marker doubling time, defined as $\log 2/a$, was obtained. In addition, the relationship between tumor marker doubling time and tumor doubling time calculated by CT or Echo; clinicopathological factors, including sex, age, histological type; the postoperative survival, were investigated.

RESULT

Comparison between Tumor Marker Doubling Time and Tumor Doubling Time

As shown in Fig.1, tumor marker doubling time was found to be significantly correlated with tumor doubling time calculated by CT or Echo in 24 cases expressed by the formula $Y = 0.95X + 1.82$. Thus, tumor marker doubling time obtained AFP or CEA was almost the same as the tumor doubling time.

Comparison of Tumor Marker Doubling Time between Stomach and Colonic Cancers

Tumor marker doubling time of 48 cases with liver metastases from stomach ranged from 12 to 50 days, with a mean of 27.7± 10.3 (SD) days. On the other hand, that of 34 cases with liver metastases from colonic cancer ranged 10 to 130 days, with a mean of 59.7± 29.5 days. There is significant difference between that of stomach and colon. Namely, the growth rate of liver metastases from stomach cancer was approximately twice that of metastases from colonic cancer (Fig.2).

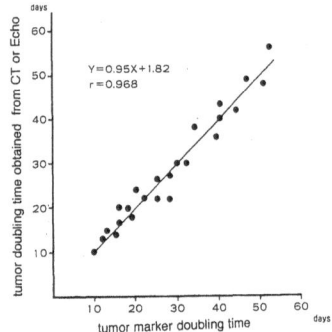

Fig.1 Comparison between tumor marker doubling time and tumor doubling time obtained from imaging (CT or Echo)

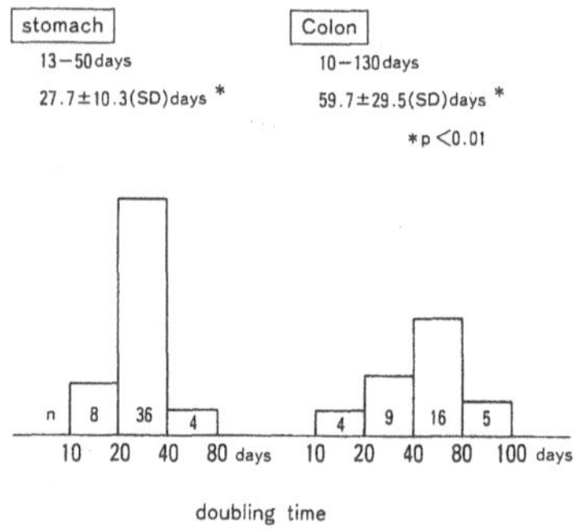

Fig.2 Comparison of the tumor marker doubling time of liver metastases between stomach and colonic cancers

Clinicopathological Factors Related to Tumor Marker Doubling Time

In 48 patients with stomach cancer, the mean tumor marker doubling time was 30.5± 12.3 days in the male group (n=30) and 25.6± 9.8 days in the female group (n=18). The mean tumor marker doubling time was 26.3± 10.5 days in patients under 60 (n=22) and 29.7± 12.1 days in those 60 or older. There were no significant differences between these two values. Although mean tumor marker doubling time in patients with poorly differentiated adenocarcinoma (23.6± 8.3 days) and papillary adeno-carcinoma (24.2± 8.3 days) was shorter than in those with well differen-tiated adenocarcinoma (35.7± 13.8 days) or moderately differentiated adenocarcinoma (30.5± 8.7 days), no significant difference was noted too. In 34 patients with colonic cancer, the mean tumor marker doubling time was 61.8 ± 24.5 days in the male group (n=21) and 51.4 ± 16.8 days in the female group (n=13). The mean tumor marker doubling time was 56.3 ± 18.5 days in patients under 60 (n=22) and 59.2± 22.1 days in those 60 or older. There were no significant differences between these two values as same as stomach cancer. In contrast, the mean tumor marker doubling time was 18.5± 7.2 days in patients with poorly differentiated adenocarcinoma, was significantly shorter than in those with well defferentiated adenocarcinoma (78.7 ± 25.6 days) or moderately differentiated adenocarcinoma (62.5 ± 23.7 days).

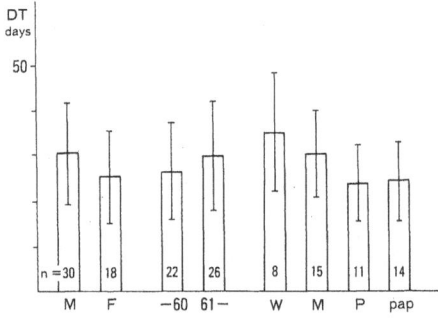

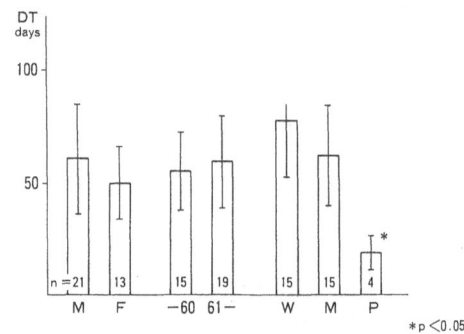

Fig.3 Clinicopathological factors related to tumor marker doubling time in patients with stomach cancer

Fig.4 Clinicopathological factors related to tumor marker doubling time in patients with colonic cancer

Correlation between Tumor Marker Doubling Time and Postoperative Survival

Of the 24 patients with stomach cancer whose postoperative survival could be confirmed,we excluded 12 patients who received hepatectomy or/and effective chemotherapy.
In the remaining 12 patients, a significant correlation was observed between tumor marker doubling time and postoperative survival(Fig.5). The other 12 patients showed longer survival than theoretical survival calculated by tumor marker doubling time.

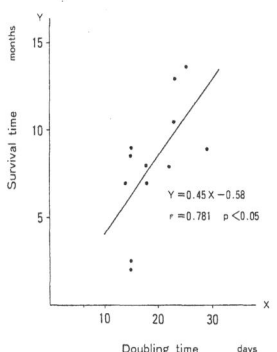

Fig.5 Correlation between tumor marker doubling time and post-operative survival in patients who don't received any therapy

DISCUSSION

From the standpoint of cancer biology, we have been pointing out that in discussing the degree of a cancer malignancy, the growth rate of the cancer is as important as clinicopathological findings such as invasive growth or metastatic growth of the cancer [3,5]. In the past, however, the growth rate of cancer could be studied only in limited kinds of tumors, because determination of the growth rate requires monitoring of the tumor size on two or more different occasions by direct measuring. On the other hand, the tumor markers used in this study can be easily measured, furthermore, even lesions so small that they can not be detected by imaging can often be revealed by the level of tumor marker.
In this study, we showed that the doubling time obtained from imaging as almost the same as the doubling time obtained from tumor markers. This findings indicated that we can determine the growth rate quite easily and quickly from measuring any of tumor markers.
Clinicopathological analysis to determine the influence factors for the tumor marker doubling time revealed significant difference between stomach and colon, among histological type in colonic cancer. We showed the growth rate of stomach cancer was approximately twice that of colonic cancer, and growth rate of poorly differentiated adenocarcinoma in histological type was faster than that of the other histological differentiation. These findings suggest that a kind of common opinion concerning growth rate was proved for the first time by the tumor maker doubling time.
A significant correlation was observed between the tumor marker doubling time and postoperative survival in spite of large differences in individuals background factors including systemic condition, size or number of metastatic lesions, etc. This finding is considered to indicate a very important role of the growth rate in evaluation the degree of cancer malignancy.

REFERENCE

1.Collins VP, Loeffler RK and Tivey H (1956) Observations on growth rate of human tumors. Am J Roentgenol 76:988-1000
2.Spratt JS and Spratt TL (1964) Rates of growth of pulmonaly metastases and host survival. Ann Surg 159:161-171.
3.Kusama S, Spratt JS, Donegan WL, Watson FR (1972) The gross rates of growth of human mammary carcinoma. Cancer 30:594-599
4.Stabb HJ, Anderer FA, Hornung A, Stumpf E and Fischer R (1982) Doubling time of circulating CEA its relation to survival of patients with recurrent colorectal cancer. Br J Cancer 46:773-781
5.Takahashi Y, Mai M, Akimoto R and Kusama S (1985) Growth rate of liver metastases from stomach and colonic cancer by tumor marker. Jpn J Gastroenterolo Sur 18:927-931

Prognosis of Liver Metastases from Colorectal Cancer After Hepatectomy

TOSHIYUKI FUKUOKA, YOSHIYUKI NAKAJIMA, MUNEAKI MATSUMOTO,
HIROMICHI KANEHIRO, HISAO FUJII, SABURO SADO, and HIROSHIGE NAKANO

The First Department of Surgery, Nara Medical University, Kashihara, Nara, 634 Japan

ABSTRACT

Seventy-five patients with liver metastases from colorectal cancer received surgery from 1983 to 1992, and 35 were hepatectomized. Hepatectomy improved the prognosis on condition that extrahepatic disease was completely resected. The 5-year survival of 30 hepatectomized without extrahepatic disease was 28.5% and that of 23 unhepatecotmized was 12.4%. On the other hand, there were no 3-year survivors in the 22 with extrahepatic disease indifferently whether hepatectomized or not. Tumor resection with minimal margin was proved to be a sufficient surgery to removed hepatic metastases, and had similar prognostic contribution as major hepatectomy that may cause major postoperative complications.

KEY WORDS: colorectal liver metastases, hepatectomy

INTRODUCTION

The liver is one of the most frequent site of metastases from colorectal cancer, and hepatectomy is the most effective treatment for patients suffering from colorectal secondaries. However, reliable criteria for resection of hepatic metastases from colorectal cancer remain controversial. We reviewed our experience of recent 10 years in a consecutive series of patients with colorectal liver metastases in order to determine the prognostic aspect in applying hepatectomy.

PATIENTS AND METHODS

Seventy-five patients with liver metastases from colorectal cancer received surgery from 1983 to 1992 at the First Department of Surgery, Nara Medical University. In the same period, 391 patients with colorectal cancer received colorectal surgery. Fifty-five of the whole 75 patients had synchronous liver metastases and the other 20 had metachronous liver metastases. Thirty-five patients were hepatectomized, which included 9 patients with hepatic lobectomy or more, 12 with hepatic segmentectomy, and 14 with partial hepatectomy. Although one of the hepatic segmentectomies resulted in an incomplete resection of the liver metastases, the other 34 hepatectomies could successfully remove hepatic tumors and were regarded as potentially curative hepatectomy. The 34 patients with potentially curative hepatectomy included 18 synchronous liver metastases and 16 metachronous liver metastases. The extrahepatic disease was curatively resected in 53 of the whole 75 patients, while the extrahepatic disease remained in the other 22 patients. Thirty of the 53 patients without extrahepatic disease received potentially curative hepatectomy, but the other 23 carried remaining liver tumors. Among the 30 patients who received potentially curative surgery for both the liver metastases and the extrahepatic disease, 19 patients received major hepatectomy (more than hepatic segmentectomy with ample margin from the liver tumor) or tumor resection with ample margin and the other 11 patients received tumor resection with minimal surgical margin (less than 1cm). Four of the 22 patients with remaining extrahepatic disease received potentially curative hepatectomy, and the other 18 carried remaining liver tumors.

Survival and tumor-free survival were estimated by means of the Kaplan-Meier product limit method. Statistical significance between survival curves was determined by the Wilcoxon log-rank test.

RESULTS

The 3- and 5-year survival rates of the whole 75 cases were 26.3% and 16.4%, respectively. In the 53 patients without remaining extrahepatic disease, the 3- and 5-year survival of 30 patients who received potentially curative hepatectomy were 42.7% and 28.5%, respectively and were significantly higher than those of 23 patients with remaining liver tumors (24.8% and 12.4%, respectively). On the other hand, there were no 3-year survivors in the 22 patients with remaining extrahepatic disease indifferently whether they received potentially curative hepatectomy or not (Fig.1).

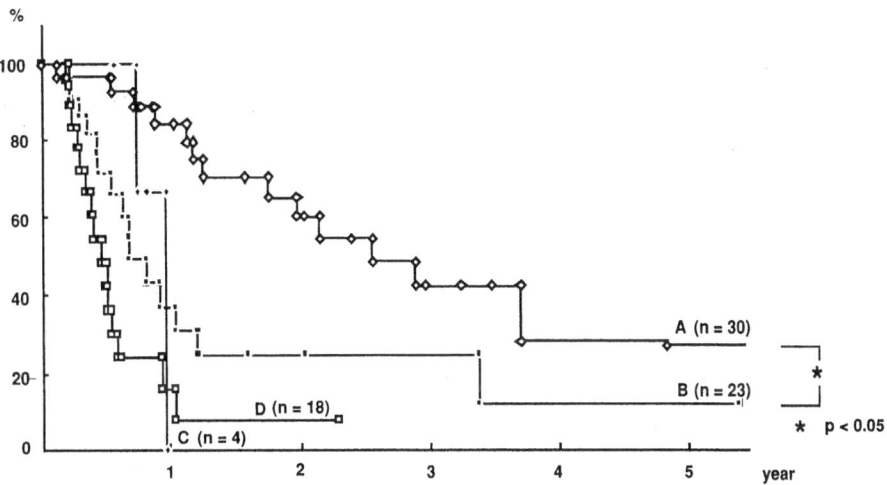

Fig.1 Survival of 75 colorectal liver metastases after surgery
(A:both the intra- and extra-hepatic tumors resected, B:only the extrahepatic tumor resected, C:only the intrahepatic tumor resected, D:both the tumors remaining)

In the 34 patients who received potentially curative hepatectomy, 16 metachronous liver metastases showed significantly better prognosis than the other 18 synchronous liver metastases. The 3- and 5-year survival of the metachronous cases were 70.1% and 46.8%, respectively. The 3-year survival of the synchronous cases was 9.7%, and there were no 5-year survivors. As for the background, 15 of 18 synchronous cases had positive lymph node metastases (classified as Dukes C), while only 9 of 16 metachronous cases had positive node. Four synchronous cases had multiple liver metastases affecting both the hepatic lobes, while only one metachronous case had such an advanced liver metastases. With respect to extent of hepatectomy, prognosis was analyzed in 30 patients who received potentially curative surgery for both the liver metastases and the extrahepatic disease. Eleven patients who received tumor resection with minimal surgical margin showed similar prognosis as 19 patients who received major hepatectomy or tumor resection with ample margin. The 5-year survival and tumor-free survival of hepatectomy with ample margin were 23.2% and 39.0%, respectively and those with minimal margin were 38.1% and 26.5%, respectively. Twelve of 19 patients hepatectomized with ample margin experienced tumor recurrence. The liver was involved in 7 cases, and 2 relapsed only in the liver. These 7 cases consisted of 4 multiple recurrences affecting both the hepatic lobes and 3 solitary recurrence adjacent to the hepatectomized site. Seven of 11 patients hepatectomized with minimal margin had relapse, and the liver was involved in 6 cases (3 relapse only in the liver). These 6 cases consisted of 5 multiple recurrences and one solitary recurrence distant from the hepatectomized site. Major postoperative complications such as gastrointestinal bleeding, vena caval thrombosis, or multiple organ failure were experienced in 4 patients with major hepatectomy (more than hepatic segmentectomy), but none in patients with tumor resection.

DISCUSSION

Hepatectomy is surely the most effective therapy for liver metastases from colorectal cancer, and there seems no superior therapeutic alternative that is currently available[1-5]. However, the selection criteria for resection of hepatic metastases remains controversial. Is there any chance of better prognosis by hepatectomy in patients with extremely advanced intrahepatic and concomitant extrahepatic disease? It is also required to determine the contraindication to hepatic resection, and it would be of great benefit to elucidate what type or extent of hepatectomy should be employed for a metastatic tumor when hepatectomy is indicated.

Our institutional experience supports the increasing acceptance of hepatic resection as the preferred treatment of colorectal liver metastasis. As long as extrahepatic disease had been curatively resected, patients who received potentially curative hepatectomy showed significantly better prognosis than those with remaining liver tumors. However, patients with remaining extrahepatic disease showed poor prognosis indifferently whether they received curative hepatectomy or not. This may describe the contraindication to hepatectomy as remaining extrahepatic disease that was also postulated by others[1]. Patients with synchronous liver metastases showed worse prognosis than those with metachronous metastases. As synchronous cases included many advanced intrahepatic or extrahepatic cancers, the chronological difference of prognosis was supposed to be caused by the difference of the background of the patients.

The amount of liver to resect is also controversial. Some advocate wedge resection, others formal hepatic resection, and still others favor segmentectomy[2]. In our experience, patients who received tumor resection with minimal margin showed similar prognosis as those with ample margin. The liver was involved with tumor relapse, however, it was not the only site of recurrence after hepatectomy as reported by others[3-5]. Moreover, most intrahepatic recurrence in our series were multiple recurrence affecting both the hepatic lobes, and there were no cases in which insufficient surgical margin of hepatectomy was regarded as a cause of intrahepatic recurrence. As for major postoperative complications, some occurred in major hepatectomy but none in tumor resection. These facts suggests that hepatectomy with minimal margin is sufficient and rather favorable surgery for colorectal liver metastases.

In conclusion, hepatectomy improves the prognosis of patients with colorectal liver metastases on condition that extrahepatic disease is completely resected. Tumor resection with minimal surgical margin is a sufficient surgery to removed hepatic metastases, and has similar prognostic contribution as major hepatectomy that may cause major postoperative complications.

REFERENCES

1. Scheele Johannes, Stangl Richard, Alendor-Hofmann Annelore, Gall Franz P (1991) Indicators of prognosis after hepatic resection for colorectal secondaries. Surg 110: 13 - 29

2. Lind D Scott, Parker George A, Horsley J Shelton, Kornstein Michael J, Neifeld James P, Bear Harry D, Lawrence Walter (1992) Formal hepatic resection of colorectal liver metastases. Ann Surg 215: 677 - 684

3. Bozzetti F, Bignami P, Montalto F, Doci R, Gennari L (1992) Repeated hepatic resection for recurrent metastases from colorectal cancer. Br J Surg 79: 146 - 148

4. Hohenberger P, Schlag P, Schwarz V, Herfarth C (1990) Tumor recurrence and options for further treatment after resection of liver metastases in patients with colorectal cancer. J Surg Oncol 44: 245 - 251

5. Fortner JG (1988) Recurrence of colorectal cancer after hepatic resection. Am J Surg 155: 378 - 382

Hepatic Metastasectomy of Colorectal Cancer: Evaluation of 8 Years Result

M.M. Rahman, K. Ouchi, Y. Katayose, T. Htwe, and S. Matsuno

First Department of Surgery, Tohoku University School of Medicine, Sendai Japan

ABSTRACT

There were 108 cases of hepatic metastases from various primaries during 8 year period. Among the 26 resectable cases 24 (92.4%) were colorectal in origin. The 5 year survival following hepatic resection was 44.4%. Among 4 long -term survivors all had solitary metastatic tumors. There was no significant difference in the survivability between synchronous and metachronous or between solitary and multiple hepatic metastasis. Long term survival was not influenced by lymph node involvement or lymphatic or venous invasion and Dukes classification.

KEY WORDS : Colorectal carcinoma. Hepatic metastases. Hepatic metastasectomy. Survival.

INTRODUCTION.

The discovery of metastatic deposits in the liver means to most clinicians that cancer has spread beyond a hope of cure. But this is not true in all cases of liver metastases, mainly in the context of metastatic colorectal cancer. The natural history of colorectal liver metastases showed that there were no survivors beyond 5 years and over 80% died within 2 years of diagnosis[1]. Several studies confirm this fact and have focussed on the importance of prognostic variables in case selection for safe and effective resection [2].

Low mortality rates (i.e.5%) and 5 year survival figures ranging from 15% to 50% encourage aggressive surgical treatment in patients with potentially operable disease [3]. Prospective randomized trials have been suggested but for obvious ethical reasons no prospective study comparing resection of liver metastases versus no treatment can be undertaken. The aim of the present study is to evaluate the possible prognostic factors and to study the factors that influence the survivability after hepatic metastasectomy in 24 patients out of 66 cases of liver metastases from colorectal primary treated by one surgical team.

PATIENTS AND METHODS.

108 patients with hepatic metastases from various primaries were seen from January 1983 to December 1990 at the First Dept. of Surgery, Tohoku University School of Medicine. 66 patients had colorectal adenocarcinoma, out of which 24 underwent curative hepatic resection. The extent of liver involvement and the site and number of metastases were assessed by computed tomography (CT), selective hepatic angiography, pre-operative and intra-operative ultrasonographic examination (US) and magnetic resonance imaging (MRI). The resections were considered curative as no gross residual disease was evident within or outside the liver and at least 1 cm of normal liver tissue surrounding the tumor was resected and there were no microscopic invasion of the resected margins. 12 patients underwent synchronous resection of the liver together with primary colorectal cancer and another 12 patients had metachronous resection. Types of resection offered to these patients were as follows: there were 2 cases with multiple secondaries in one lobe in whom we did extended right hepatectomy in one and partial resection in the other. In the remaining 22 cases there was only one solitary secondary and right lobectomy was done in 6, left lobectomy in 4, lateral segmentectomy in 3 and partial resection in 9 patients.

FOLLOW UP AND STATISTICAL EVALUATION

Follow up consisted of physical examination, carcino-embryonic antigen determination, liver function test and abdominal ultrasonography.Abdominal CT and US were done if recurrence is suspected. No patients were lost in follow up and tumor status can be define in all. Survival was calculated by Kaplan-Meier method and statistical comperison of survivals was done by Wilkoxon rank-sum test. A value of $p < 0.05$ was defined as statistically significant

RESULTS

There were no operative mortality nor major post-operative complications, The overall 5 year survival rate was 44.4%. Of the 42 patients without surgery none survived more than 2.5 years (figure 1). Out of 44 cases with synchronous hepatic metastases only 12 (27.3%) underwent resection, whereas in 22 patients with metachronous lesions we could do resection in 12 (54.0%), which was statistically significant (P<0.05 Table 1).

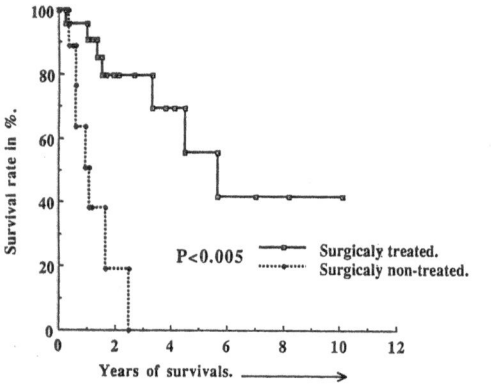

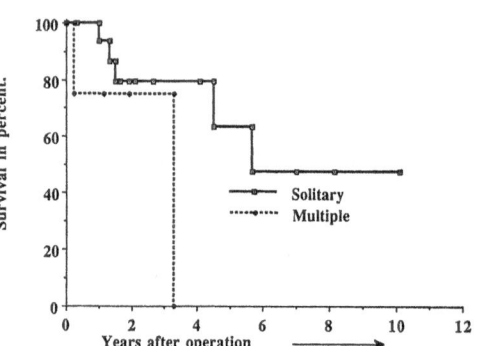

Fig. 1 Comparison of survival rates between surgically treated and surgically nontreated patients

Fig. 2 Comparison of survival rates between solitary and multiple hepatic secondaries.

Table 1. Synchronous and metachronous lesions, the resectibility is significantly higher in metachronous cases.

	Liver metastases	Liver resection
Synchronous	44	12 (27.3%)
Metachronous	22	12 (54.0%) *
Total cases	66	24

* P<0.05

No significant difference in the survivability between synchronous versus metachronous or between solitary versus multiple hepatic metastases were seen. (figure 2) . But hepatic metastasectomy [HM] cases with multiple metastases did not survive more than 3.5 years. (figure 3). There were 4-5 year survivors after HM and all had solitary metastases with sizes vary from 2X2 to 7X7 cm..There were 2 Dukes C and 2 Dukes A cases and 2 died at 5 years and 8 month and the other at 5 years and 11 months. The remaining 2 is still living up to now(Table 2).

Table 2. Characteristics of long term survivors. NC indicates the lesion was not confirmed.

Time	Node	Venous	Lymphatic	Dukes	Size	Survival time
Metachronous	0	1	1	A	3X3cm	8Y-2M (Alive)
Metachronous	1	NC	NC	C	7X7cm	7Y (Alive)
Synchronous	0	0	1	A	5X4cm	5Y-11M (Dead)
Synchronous	1	2	2	C	2X2cm	5Y-8M (Dead)

DISCUSSION

Colorectal cancer has the propensity to metastasize preferentially to the liver. As response rate to radio-therapy and chemotherapy is low surgical resection offers the only hope of cure to these patients . We could select only 24 patients undergoing resection out of 66 cases with hepatic metastases. Low mortality (0 - 5%) and the morbidity rate following hepatic metastasectomy encourages surgeons in many center to attempt hepatic resection. Our 5 year survival rate following hepatic resection was 44.4% and 4 patient survived more than 5 years. All of them had various sizes of solitary lesion in the liver. It was found that resectability is significantly high in metachronous cases. Major determinants of good prognosis derived from treated patients are also known nowadays [4]. Pre-operative and intra-operative evaluation can determine the resectability of the metastatic tumor but occult extra hepatic tumor metastases need better techniques for imaging combined with biologic markers [5]. As only some patients (44.4% in our series) are beneficial to hepatic metastasectomy, better case selection with these methods will definitely improve 5-year survival figures.

REFERENCES

1.Foster JH,Berman MM (1977) Solid Liver Tumors, Major Problem in Clinical Surgery.Philadelphia: WB Saunders, pp 1-342.
2 . Scheele J,Stangl R,Altendorf-Hofmann A, (1990) Hepatic metastases from colorectal carcinoma: Impact of surgical resection on the natural history. Br.J.Surg.;77: 1241-1246.
3. Asbun HJ,Hughes KS. 1993,73 no.1. Colorectal cancer. Surgical Clinics of North America.Philadelphia.W>B> Saunders pp145-166.
4. R.Doci, L.Gennari,P.Bignami,F.Montalto,A.Morabito and F. Bozzetti. (1991) One hundred patients with hepatic metastases from colorectal cancer treated by resection: Analysis of prognostic determinants. Br.J.Surg 78, 797-801.
5. L.C.Barr,A.I.Skene and J.M.Thomas. (1992) Metastasectomy.Br.J.Surg.79,1268-1274.

Extensive Surgery for Carcinoma Recurrence After Initial Hepatectomy for Liver Metastasis of Colorectal Carcinoma

Satoshi Nakamura[1], Yoshihiro Yokoi[1], Raisuke Nishiyama[1], Atsushi Serizawa[1], Yoshiro Nishiwaki[1], Hiroyuki Konno[1], Shozo Baba[1], and Kenzo Yasui[2]

[1]The Second Department of Surgery, Hamamatsu University School of Medicine, Hamamatsu, Shizuoka, Japan
[2]The Department of Surgery, Aichi Cancer Center, Nagoya 464 Japan

ABSTRACT

Since 1978, we have performed extensive resection for recurrent carcinoma after initial hepatectomy for liver metastasis of colorectal carcinoma. Twenty-five patients had recurrence of carcinoma, and 14 of them had a resectable metastatic tumor. Eight patients with hepatic metastases underwent repeat hepatectomy on 11 occasions, and 8 patients, who had lung metastases underwent partial pulmonary resection on 11 occasions. Two patients underwent brain resection on 3 occasions, and one patient underwent right adrenalectomy combined with grafting of a 4.5-cm segment of the inferior vena cava. Results after surgery were compared with those obtained in 11 patients with nonresectable recurrent carcinoma. There were no operative deaths. The 5-year survival rate after initial hepatectomy in patients undergoing repeat hepatectomy, and pulmonary resection was 42.9 % and 37.5 %, respectively. Thus, surgical treatment of recurrence after hepatectomy achieved a significant improvement of survival compared with patients who had nonresectable recurrence (p<0.01).

KEY WORDS: colorectal carcinoma, hepatic metastasis, repeat hepatectomy

INTRODUCTION

The 5-year survival of patients with recurrent carcinoma after hepatectomy for liver metastasis of colorectal carcinoma is very poor, although cancer chemotherapy has improved survival of patients with carcinoma. When patients develop recurrent carcinoma after initial hepatectomy, it is still unclear which treatments are effective for hepatic metastases and/or lung metastases. We have performed extensive surgery for recurrence of carcinoma after hepatectomy for liver metastasis of colorectal carcinoma. The results of surgery are reported and the value of such surgery is discussed in this article.

PATIENTS AND METHODS

Patients

Since March 1978, 42 patients underwent hepatectomy for liver metastasis of colorectal carcinoma at our department. Excluding two patients dying within 30 days postoperatively, 25 of the 40 patients had recurrence of carcinoma after initial surgery. Fourteen of these 25 patients had resectable tumors (mean age: 56 years; range: 29-75 years; 8 men and 6 women). Eleven of the 25 patients had nonresectable tumors and their survival was compared with the 14 patients having resectable tumors. The remaining 15 patients are presently alive without recurrence after the first hepatectomy.

Methods

Of the 14 patients who had recurrence of carcinoma, 5 underwent complicated operations on 2-5 occasions. Eight patients underwent repeat hepatectomy on 11 occasions, 8 underwent partial pulmonary resection on 11 occasions, 2 underwent brain resection on 3 occasions, and one underwent right adrenalectomy (Table 1). In all 8 patients having hepatic metastases, partial hepatic resection was performed and 3 of them underwent a third hepatectomy procedure. One patient underwent segmental resection of the inferior vena cava and insertion of a 4.5-cm ringed expanded polytetrafluoroethylene graft combined with partial hepatectomy and right adrenalectomy.

690

Table 1. Patients undergoing resection of recurrent carcinoma after hepatectomy

		Organs resected				Survival after	Present
Pts. No.	1st	2nd	3rd	4th	5th	initial hepatectomy	status
1.	Liver	Lung	IVC,liver,adrenal	Lung	Lung	94 m	DOD
2.	Liver	Lung	Liver	Lung		37 m	DOD
3.	Brain	Brain	Lung			52 m	AWD
4.	Liver	Lung				69 m	DOD
5.	Liver	Liver				54 m	NED
6.	Lung					25 m	DOD
7.	Liver					28 m	DOD
8.	Liver					71 m	DOD
9.	Liver					15 m	DOD
10.	Liver					13 m	DOD
11.	Lung					33 m	DOD
12.	Lung					11 m	DOD
13.	Lung					10 m	DOD
14.	Brain					18 m	DOD

DOD: dead of disease, AWD: alive with disease, NED: no evidence of disease.

RESULTS

The morbidity rate was 56 % after hepatectomy and 27 % after pulmonary resection, respectively, but there were no operative deaths. Complications included posttransfusion hepatitis in two patients, hemothorax in 2, pleural effusion in 1, massive bleeding in 1, biliary fistula in 1, and mediastinitis in 1, respectively. The 5-year survival rate after the first time of detection of cancer recurrence in the 8 patients who underwent repeat hepatectomy was 50 % (Fig. 1), and the 5-year survival after detection of recurrence in the 8 patients who underwent pulmonary

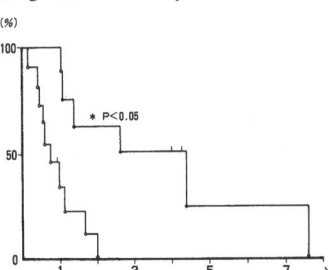

Fig. 1 Survival from the time of detection of carcinoma recurrence after initial hepatectomy in 8 patients undergoing repeat hepatectomy (•) and 11 with nonresectable recurrent tumors (○). *: p< 0.01

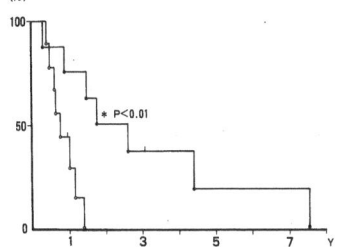

Fig.2 Survival from the time of detection of carcinoma recurrence after initial hepatectomy in 8 patients undergoing pulmonary resection (•) and 11 having nonresectable tumors (○). *: p<0.05

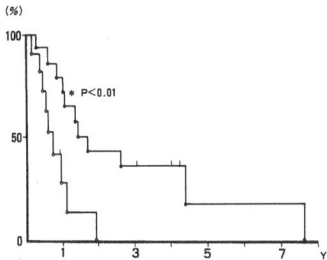

Fig. 3 Survival from the time of detection of carcinoma recurrence after initial hepatectomy in 14 patients undergoing the resection of recurrent tumors (•). *: p<0.01

resection was 37.5 % (Fig. 2). The 5-year survival of the 14 patients who had resectable recurrent carcinoma was 30.7 % (Fig. 3). Consequently, the 2-, 3- and 5-year survival rates after initial hepatectomy in the original 40 patients undergoing hepatectomy for liver metastases were 83, 67, and 48.5 %, respectively.

DISCUSSION

The median survival of patients with untreated hepatic metastases has been reported to range from 3.4 to 24 months depending upon the extent of liver involvement (1). Liver metastases are likely to exert a major influence on survival, and liver resection has recently been performed as the best available treatment. However, the reported results of hepatectomy for colorectal metastases are not yet satisfactory. In addition, 5-year survival following regional chemotherapy for hepatic metastases of colorectal carcinoma is rare (2). Therefore, in the treatment of metastatic liver and/or lung cancer, repeat resection has been recognized as an effective treatment in selected patients.

Our experience suggests that approximately two-thirds of patients undergoing hepatectomy for liver metastases develop recurrence of carcinoma, and that two-thirds of them have resectable recurrent tumors. Although the morbidity rate of repeat surgery was high in our series, there were no operative deaths. Since operative and postoperative massive bleeding may occur and may cause hepatic failure, the selection of candidates and operative procedures and the assessment of coagulation factors which are produced by the liver should be done carefully.

There have been nine reports (3) concerning the results of second liver resection procedures. In the present study, the survival after the detection of recurrence following initial hepatectomy for liver metastases was compared between patients with resectable and unresectable recurrent tumors. Our results were good compared with the previously reported survival periods. The survival of our patients who underwent repeat hepatectomy and/or pulmonary resection was significantly better than that of patients with unresectable recurrence. Consequently, in 40 patients undergoing hepatectomy for liver metastases of colorectal carcinoma, the overall 5-year survival rate after initial hepatectomy was 48.5 %, which is good compared with the results reported in the literature (4). Thus, extensive resection of recurrent tumors after hepatectomy for liver metastases of colorectal carcinoma significantly improves the survival of patients with hepatic and/or pulmonary metastases. Furthermore, in order to increase survival further, a careful check for other distant metastases, para-aortic metastases, and intrapelvic recurrence should be performed before planning lung resection or hepatectomy.

REFERENCES

1. Nakamura S, Sakaguchi S, Nishiyama R, Suzuki S, Yokoi Y, Baba S, Muro H (1992) Aggressive repeat liver resection for hepatic metastases of colorectal carcinoma. Jpn J Surg 22:260-264
2. Balch CM, Urist MM, Soong S-J, McGregor M (1983) A prospective phase II clinical trial of continuous FUDR regional chemotherapy for colorectal metastases to the liver using a totally implantable drug infusion pump. Ann Surg 198:567-73
3. Griffith KD, Sugarbaker PH, Chang AE (1990) Repeat hepatic resections for colorectal metastases. Surgery 107:101-104
4. Stone MD, Cady B, Jenkins RL, McDermott WV, Steele GD Jr (1990) Surgical therapy for recurrent liver metastases from colorectal cancer. Arch Surg 125:718-722

Prognostic Comparison of Hepatic Resection of Liver Metastases and Chemotherapy via the Portal Vein with Liposome-Entrapped Adriamycin for Unresectable Liver Metastases on Gastric Cancer

I. Mizuno[1], T. Yotsuyanagi[2], T. Ichino[1], Y. Akamo[1], T. Yamamoto[1], M. Nagata[2], T. Yasui[1], K. Kobayashi[1], S. Shibata[1], N. Tanimoto[1], S. Usami[1], and J. Yura[1]

[1]First Department of Surgery, Medical School, [2]Faculty of Pharmaceutical Sciences, Nagoya City University, Nagoya, 467 Japan

ABSTRACT

The prognoses of hepatic resection of the liver metastases on the gastric cancer were compared with those by chemotherapy via the portal vein with liposome-entrapped adriamycin for unresectable liver metastases. Seven cases of hepatic resection in liver metastases were operated from 1988 to 1992. Postoperative mean survival times were 15.6 months in Hr0(L), 12.7 months in Hr1(L) and 35.4 months in Hr2(AP). To date, 7 cases of unresectable liver metastases have been evaluated via the potal vein with Lipo-ADM(20-30mg/every 2 weeks/body). There were no side effects via the portal vein with Lipo-ADM. As compared with survival time of hepatic resection and unresectable cases with Lipo-ADM for liver metastases, statistically there were no differences between hepatic resection and unresectable cases in the survival time.

KEY WORDS: Gastric cancer, Liver metastasis, Hepatic resection, Chemotherapy, Liposome-entrapped adriamycin

INTRODUCTION

Postoperative prognosis in gastric cancer has mainly been concerned with recurrences of hepatic metastases, local lymph nodes metastases and peritoneal metastases.
For the purpose of improvement in these postoperative prognosis, the strategies of prophylactic and therapeutic management have been urgently required.
Recently, hepatic resection of liver metastasis can be performed safely according to the advances of various diagnotic techniques(tumor makers, arteriography, ultrasound, radioisotope imaging, computed tomography etc). However, there were few opportunities of hepatic resection because of multiple metastases.
In our groups, for the therapy of liver metastases, We attached great importance to the metastatic route via the portal vein and have studied the administration of various anti-cancer agents. Furthermore, in contact with our Fuculty of Pharmaceutical Sciences, we have studied the effects of liposome-entrapped adriamycin(Lipo-ADM) administered via the portal vein and the clinical application of this treatment in the therapy of unresectable liver metastases. This Lipo-ADM administration was confirmed to be safe and revealed a decrease in the heart toxicities compared with free adriamycin. There were no liver dysfunction, bone marrow suppresion or other side effects where Lipo-ADM was administered(Jpn. J. Cancer Res. 81,1052-1056, 1990).
We report that the prognoses of hepatic resection of liver metastases on gastric cancer were compared with those by chemotherapy via the portal vein with Lipo-ADM for unresectable liver metastases.

MATERIALS AND METHODS

Preparetion of freeze-dried Lipo-ADM
ADM supplied as a freeze-dried form containing 10mg of ADM and 100mg of lactose per vial was reformulated to a freeze-dried form of egg lecithin-ADM mixture under aseptic conditions. A required amount of egg lecithin and cholesterol mixture(molar ratio, 2:1; hexane-ethanol (95/5) stock solution) was taken into a sterilized round-bottomed flask and the solvent was removed using a rotary evaporater. The resulting lipid thin film was dissolved in ether, to which an appropriate amount of water for injection containing mannitol was added. The mixture was vortexed for about 5 min to give a W/O emulsion and the solvent was removed accord-

ing to the reverse-phase evaporation method. The resulting liposome suspension was distributed into ADM vials, and vortexed until the original freeze-dried cake was completely dissolved. Each vial contains 75 mg of lecithin, 12mg of cholesrerol and 10 mg of ADM in 3 ml. The content was freeze-dried and stored at 4°C until use. Liposomes were reconstituted for use by adding water for injection to the dried cake through a rubber cap, and sonicated using a ultrasonic apparatus(UD-200, Tomy Seiko Co.Ltd., Tokyo) equipped with a cup horn-type irradiation unit. The unit was employed to reduce the particle size of the suspension in the vial without contamination, during which process the temperature of the unit was controlled by water circulation. The reconsutituted liposomes were further extruted through 0.45μm nucleopore filters prior to experiments. The mean particle size was measured by dynamic light scattering(DLS-700,Otsuka Electronics Co.Ltd.,Osaka).

Clinical details of cases in hepatic metastases
Among the cases treated in our department during the 5-year period between January 1988 and December 1992, there were 14 cases of hepatic metastases are listed in Table 1 and Table 3. In 7 cases of hepatic resection in liver metastases(6 cases of synchronous metastases,1 case of metachronous metastases) were operated. On the other hand, 7 cases of unresectable liver metastases(4 cases of synchronous metastases, 3 cases of metachronous metastases) have been evaluated via the portal vein using a subcutaneously implanted the reservoir with Lipo-ADM (20-30mg/every 2 weeks/body) to date.

Statistical analysis
The statistical significances of differences was determined by using the generalized Wilcoxon test(Table 3).

RESULTS

Characterization of freeze-dried Lipo-ADM
The size distribution of liposome preparations after reconstitution with water and sonication in the cup horn was investigated. The liposomes had a mean diameter of 256.2 nm before filtration and 219.6nm after. The ADM content of liposomes was $32\pm6\%$ and the prepared Lipo-ADM was endotoxin-free as assayed using the Toxicolor Test(Seikagaku Kogyo, Tokyo).

Treatment and prognoses of hepatic resection
Postoperative suvival times were from 170 days to 1227 days. Mean survival times of 7 cases in hepatic resection were 600 days. Mean survival times of hepatic resection were 15.6 months in Hr0(L)(2 cases),12.7 months in Hr1(L)(3 cases), and 35.4 months in Hr2(AP)(2 cases) (Table 2)

Treatment and outcome of Lipo-ADM
Survival times with Lipo-ADM were from 128 days to 879 days. Mean suvival times of 7 cases were 362 days. Postoperative mean survival times of unresectable cases with Lipo-ADM were 19.4 months in metachronous metastases and 6.6 months in synchronous metastases.
There were no livr dysfunction, bone marrow suppression and other side effects via the portal vein with Lipo-ADM. (Table 1)

Case	Age Sex	Degree of metastases	Total dosage of Lipo-ADM	Survival (days)	Response rate (Method)
1	64 M	H_3	360 mg	879	CR (CT, US)
2	72 F	H_3	300 mg	223	NC (CT)
3	47 M	H_3	900 mg	620	PR (CT, US)
4	65 M	H_3	340 mg	247	NC (CT)
5	53 M	H_3	280 mg	213	PR (CT)
6	78 F	H_3	100 mg	128	NC (CT)
7	60 M	H_3	80 mg	224	NC (CT)

Prognoses of treatment (mean months)			Prognoses of operation (mean months)	
Resectable cases	synchronous (6 cases)	16.5	Hr 0 (L) (2 cases)	15.6
	metachronous (1 case)	40.5	Hr 1 (L) (3 cases)	12.7
Unresectable cases	synchronous (4 cases)	6.6		
	metachronous (3 cases)	19.4	Hr 2 (AP) (2 cases)	35.4

Table 1   Summary of treatment and outcome of unresectable liver metastases.

Table 2   The prognostic comparison of treatment and operation on the liver metastases.

Survival rate of cases in hepatic metastases
As compared with survival time of hepatic resection and unresectable cases with Lipo-ADM for
liver metastases, statitically there were no differences between hepatic resection and unresectable cases in survival time.

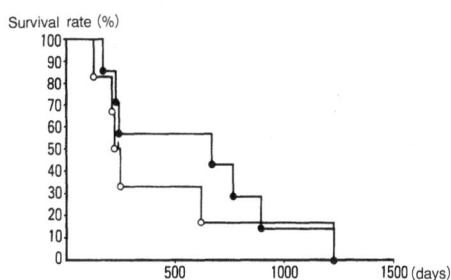

Table 3 Comparison of survival rate on resectable and unresectable cases.
● — ● resectabl cases.   ○ — ○ unresectable cases.

DISCUSSION

Postoperative prognosis of the advanced gastric cancer has mainly been concerned with recurrences of peritoneal metastases, lymph nodes metastases and hepatic metastases.
Hepatic resections of liver metastasis rarely have been performed at the gastric operation.
However, there were few opportunities of hepatic resection because of multiple metastases in
many cases. The prognoses of liver metastases in gastric cancer are relatively poor compared
with colonic cancer. For the purpose of improvement in these postoperative prognosis, experimentally we have stuidied the effects of Lipo-ADM administered via the portal vein and the
clinical application of this treatment in the therapy in contact with our Fuculty of Pharmaceutical Sciences. We examined the distribution in tissues and antitumor effect of freeze-
dried Lipo-ADM administered via the portal vein to rabbits bearing VX2 tumors.
The liver concentration of ADM increased after delivery and cardiac uptake decreased compared with free ADM treatment. The in vivo antitumor effect of Lipo-ADM was determined in
rabbits inoculated with VX2 tumor. Repeated injection of free ADM via the portal vein prolonged the life span of tumor-bearing rabbits. The life span was further prolonged by Lipo
-ADM treatment compared with the control group and the free ADM group. Histological examination revealed that the damage to the liver caused by Lipo-ADM administered via the portal
vein did not differ from that obseved in animals treated with free ADM. These results indicate that portal vein administration of Lipo-ADM may be more effective in dealing with liver
metastases than treatment with free ADM and may be therapeutically useful without toxic side
effects(Jpn.J. Cancer Res.81, 1052-1056,1990).
Consequently from these experimental data and clinical outcome, these results suggest that
chemotherapy via the portal vein for unresectable metastases with Lipo-ADM may improve the
survival time, and furthermore this administration is also expected in prophylaxis of the
postoperative liver metastases.

REFERENCES

1. Ichino T,Yotsuyanagi T,Mizuno I,Akamo Y,Yamamoto T,Saito T,Kurahashi S,Tanimoto N,Yura J.
   (1990) Antitumor Effect of Liposome-entrapped Adriamycin Administered via the Portal Vein.
   Jpn.J.Cancer Res. 81,1052-1056.

2. I.Mizuno, T.Yotsuyanagi, T.Ichino, Y.Akamo, T.Yamamoto, T.Yasui, Y.Itabashi, T.Saito,
   S.Kurahashi, N.Tanimoto, S.Usami, J.Yura. (1991) Chemotherapy via the Portal Vein with
   Liposome-Encapsulated Adriamycin on Inoperable Metastatic Liver Cancer.   Proceedings of
   ASCO VOL.10 MARCH

3. Ichino T,Mizuno I,Akamo Y,Yamamoto T,Itabashi Y,Yasui T,Saito T,Kurahashi S,Tanimoto N.
   (1992) Effect of liposome-entrapped adriamycin administered to rats via the portal vein
   on tissue cytotoxicity. Nagoya Medical Journal, 36(3·4):205-214.

Management of Metastatic Liver Cancer

HIROKI TANIGUCHI[1], YOSHIYUKI SHIMAMURA[2], and TOSHIO TAKAHASHI[1]

[1]First Department of Surgery, Kyoto Prefectural University of Medicine, Kyoto, 602 Japan
[2]Department of Surgery, National Matsudo Hospital, Matsudo, Chiba, 272 Japan (National Cancer Center Hospital East at Present)

ABSTRACT

One hundred and twenty-four patients with metastatic liver cancer were treated in National Matsudo Hospital between June 1980 and December 1987. They received multi-disciplinary treatment and 40 of them underwent hepatectomy. The survival rate after hepatectomy for metastatic liver cancer was better than without hepatectomy, but there was no significant difference in the prognoses of gastric and colorectal cancer liver metastases after hepatectomy. The prognosis after hepatectomy was similar between synchronous metastases and metachronous metastases and the survival rate after liver resection was the same for solitary and multiple lesions. These results suggest that surgical reduction of liver metastases is a good treatment. In addition, there was no significant difference between the survival rate of patients with unresectable liver metastases who were treated with transcatheter arterial embolization and with hepatic arterial infusion of an anticancer agent emulsified in a lipid contrast medium.

Key Words: Metastatic liver cancer, hepatic resection, transcatheter arterial embolization, lipid contrast medium

INTRODUCTION

The most common cause of death in cancer patients is metastasis. The liver is a common site of metastasis from not only gastrointestinal malignancies but also from other malignant sites. Recently, hepatic resection for metastatic liver cancer has been performed with good prognosis and low operative mortality. However, many patients died from the recurrence of hepatic metastases, and there are many patients with unresectable liver metastases. Thus, it is important to clarify the prognosis after hepatectomy for liver metastases and that of non-surgical treatment of unresectable hepatic metastases. This report shows the results of our treatment against metastatic liver cancers.

PATIENTS AND METHODS

This study was based on 124 patients (male:84, female 40) with metastatic liver tumors who were treated at National Matsudo Hospital between June 1980 and December 1987. Hepatic resection was performed on patients with metachronous metastasis who had had curative organ surgery and had neither local recurrences nor distant metastasis other than in the liver. Patients with synchronous metastasis underwent hepatic resection one to two months after curative organ surgery except for cases with small solitary liver metastasis. These patient had hepatic resection at the same time as curative organ surgery. After the hepatic resection carcinoembryonic antigen (CEA) tests and abdominal echograms were taken every month, and an abdominal computed tomography (CT) scan was performed every three months. If a recurrence was detected in a patient after hepatectomy, transcatheter arterial embolization (TAE), or transcatheter hepatic arterial infusion of anticancer agents (HAI)(mainly, 5-fluorouracil [5-FU], mitomycin C [MMC], doxorubicin [ADM] and/or cis-platin [CDDP]) and/or ADM emulsified in Lipiodol (a lipid contrast medium, Lipiodol Ultra-Fluid, Laboratoire Guerbet, Paris, France) was administered (L-HAI) under Seldinger's procedure every three months. Patients with unresectable hepatic metastases had the same treatment. Survival rates were analyzed using the Kaplan-Meier method and the generalized Wilcoxon test.

RESULTS

Characteristics of patients are shown in Table 1. There was only one case of operative death (2.5%), where operative death refers to death within one month after surgery. Fourteen cases were synchronous metastases and 22 were metachronous metastases. Because four cases had had organ surgery at an other institute, whether they were synchronous or metachronous is unknown. Minor resections were performed on 19 patients and 12 underwent major resection. Nine patients underwent combined resection. Nineteen patients had solitary metastasis, seven cases had two metastases, and 12 patients had more than three metastases.   There was no significant difference between survival of patients who had hepatectomies for gastric cancer liver metastases (6 patients) and that of cases with hepatectomies for metastases from colorectal cancer (29 patients)(Fig.1).   There was no significant difference in survival after hepatic resection between patients with synchronous (14 patients) and metachronous liver metastases (22 patients).   There was no significant difference in survival after hepatectomy between cases with solitary (19 patients) and multiple hepatic metastases (19 patients).   After hepatectomy five patients (23.8%) died from the recurrence of liver metastases (Table 2).   This rate is similar to the rate of patients without hepatectomy (24.3%). Of 84 patients who were unable to receive hepatectomies, 18 were not treated at all, 7 were treated with a hepatic arterial infusion of anticancer agents emulsified in Lipiodol (L-HAI) and 26 underwent transcatheter arterial embolization (TAE) therapy with or without L-HAI.   Primary locations of patients with liver metastases treated with these methods are shown in Table 3.   There was no significant difference between the survival of patients who received L-HAI, and TAE with or without L-HAI (Fig.2).

Table.1 Characteristics of patients (%)

	all	with hepatectomy	without hepatectomy
Mean age	59.6 yr	55.9 yr	61.4 yr
Primary site			
stomach	24 (19.4)	6 (15.0)	18 (21.4)
small intestine	1 (0.8)	0	1 (1.2)
large intestine	63 (50.8)	29 (72.5)	34 (40.5)
biliary or			
pancreas	17 (13.7)	2 (5.0)	15 (12.6)
breast	1 (0.8)	0	1 (1.2)
lung	10 (8.1)	3 (7.5)	7 (8.3)
other	7 (5.6)	0	7 (8.3)
unknown	1 (0.8)	0	1 (1.2)
First method of detection			
tumor marker	11 (8.9)	9 (22.5)	2 (2.4)
echogram	34 (27.4)	6 (15.0)	28 (33.3)
x-ray CT	29 (23.4)	8 (20.0)	21 (25.0)
angiogram	1 (0.8)	0	1 (1.2)
organ surgery	9 (7.3)	5 (12.5)	4 (4.8)
Hepatic distribution at time of primary organ surgery			
H(-)	44 (35.5)	22 (55.0)	22 (26.2)
H(+)	8 (6.5)	6 (15.0)	2 (2.4)
H(++)	36 (29.0)	8 (20.0)	28 (33.3)
not operated	14 (10.9)	0	14 (16.7)
unknown	22 (17.7)	4 (10.0)	18 (21.4)
Total	124	40	84

H(-) indicates no liver metastasis
H(+) indicates unilober metastases
H(++) indicates bilober metastases

Table 2. The cause of death

	No. of patients (%)		
	all	with hepatectomy	without hepatectomy
Liver	22 (24.2)	5 (23.8)	17 (24.3)
Peritoneal	8 (8.8)	3 (14.3)	5 (7.1)
Local	4 (4.4)	1 (4.8)	3 (4.8)
Lymphnodes	1 (1.1)	0	1 (1.4)
Other	6 (6.6)	1 (4.8)	5 (7.1)
Combined	38 (41.8)	7 (33.3)	31 (44.3)
Other disease	9 (9.9)	3 (14.3)	6 (8.6)
Operation	3 (3.3)	1 (4.8)	2 (2.9)
Total	91	21	70

Table 3. Characteristics of patients with liver metastases undergoing interventional therapy

Primary location	No. of patients (%)		
	untreated	TAE	L-HAI
Stomach	4 (22.2)	7 (26.9)	0
Small bowel	0	1 (3.8)	0
Large bowel	7 (38.9)	12 (46.1)	4 (57.1)
Biliary or			
pancreas	2 (11.1)	5 (19.2)	1 (14.3)
Lung	1 (5.6)	1 (3.8)	1 (14.3)
Other	4 (22.2)	0	1 (14.3)
Total	18	26	7

TAE: Transcatheter Arterial Embolization,   L-HAI: Hepatic Arterial Infusion of an anticancer agent emulsified in Lipiodol

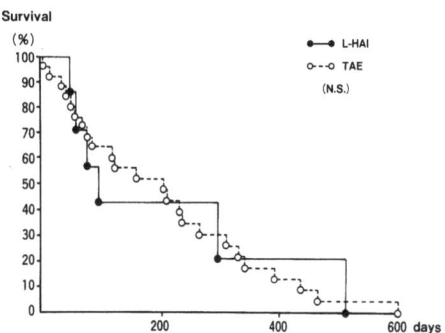

Fig.1

Fig.2

DISCUSSION

Although the resectability of all hepatic metastases in the current study was 32%, that of colorectal liver metastasis was 46%, higher than the reports of many authors[1]. This appears to be the result of our policy of aggressive hepatectomy against metastatic liver cancer. However, half of cases (22/44) with metachronous metastases and a quarter of patients (2/8) with unilobar synchronous metastases were not resectable (Table 1). The examination of serum tumor markers[2], commonly CEA, was the most important as a first method of detection of hepatic metastases with a detection rate of 22.5% in patients with hepatectomy but only 8.9% in patients without hepatectomy. In spite of the improvement of imaging instruments, frequent examinations with CEA are still necessary. In this study, numbers of minor resections and major or combined resections were about the same. Although the prognosis of patients with more than three metastases is not greatly improved after hepatectomy according to many reports[3], we performed hepatectomy on patients with more than three metastases. More than a quarter of the cases with hepatectomy had more than three tumors. Although many liver resections for colorectal metastases have been carried out in many institutes, there were few reports of hepatectomy for gastric cancer liver metastases and they all reported poor prognosis after hepatectomy against liver metastases from gastric cancer[4]. Liver resections for gastric cancer hepatic metastases were performed for six patients, and the present study would suggest a trend that is not verifiable that the survival of patients who had hepatectomy for gastric liver metastases was poor. However the difference between survival time of patients who had hepatic resection for gastric cancer and patients without liver resection who had gastric cancer liver metastases without extrahepatic cancer, was smaller than the difference between survival time of cases who had hepatectomy for colorectal cancer liver metastases and cases without liver resection who had colorectal hepatic metastases but not extrahepatic metastases. Many published studies[3,4] have shown that the prognosis after hepatectomy for synchronous liver metastases was similar to that of metachronous metastases. We had the same results in our cases including colorectal cancer patients. In several reports[3], survival rates after hepatectomy against more than three or four metastases was poor. In this study, there was no significant difference between the survival after hepatectomy for a solitary and multiple metastases. The prognosis of patients after hepatectomy who had more than three metastases was better than those without liver resection, but the difference was not significant. It is very important to clarify the cause of death of patients who underwent hepatectomy for metastatic liver cancer, because if most cases after hepatectomy die from liver metastases, hepatic resection is wasteful. In the current study, death from liver metastasis only formed about 24% of patients after hepatectomy, the same as patients without hepatectomy. Twenty-four per cent is not so large, but it is disappointing that the mortality from liver metastases after hepatectomy is the same with or without liver resection. Although it is a problem if the prognosis after hepatectomy is not better than without hepatectomy, the length of survival after hepatic resection for metastatic liver cancer clearly improved. Therefore, we will perform hepatectomy for liver metastasis aggressively from now on. However, we must note that more than 20% of patients after hepatectomy died from other causes than recurrence to the liver. Ideally the rate of death from other disease should be 100%. Patients who only have liver metastases should be operated on after they are identified to have neither local recurrence nor other distant metastasis. We must examine in detail whether a patient has any metastases and recurrence other than in the liver before hepatic resection[3]. We compared patients who cannot have hepatectomies and so were treated by L-HAI and TAE. Ackerman and associates[5] reported that metastatic liver tumors had arterial blood supplies, and therefore TAE is widely performed against primary and secondary liver tumors[6]. Recently, anticancer agents emulsified or suspended in an ethiodized oil have been infused into the hepatic artery for metastatic liver cancers (L-HAI)[7]. This therapy is an application of the phenomenon that an oil infused into the hepatic artery is retained in the tumor tissue[7,8], and liver damage is little and anticancer drugs are in contact with the cancer tissue for long time[7]. From the present study the effectiveness of TAE is not better than that of L-HAI. Because TAE damages the liver, L-HAI should be used for metastatic liver cancer, rather than TAE. As we reported[8], even if hepatic arterial blood supply is interrupted, the portal vein still supplies blood to the metastatic liver tumor and so it is thought that therapy using anticancer agents is better than TAE.

REFERENCES

1. Liotta LA (1987): Overview of biology of cancer invasion and metastases. In Rosenberg SA (ed.), Surgical treatment of metastatic cancer. Philadelphia, J.B.Lippincott, pp1-51.
2. Registry of Hepatic Metastasis (1988): Resection of the liver for colorectal carcinoma metastases: A multi-institutional study of indication for resection. *Surgery* 103: 278- 288.
3. Roh MS (1989): Hepatic resection for colorectal liver metastases. *Hematol/Oncol Clin North Am* 3: 171- 181.
4. Foster JH (1987): Survival after liver resection for secondary tumors. *Am J Surg* 153: 389- 394.
5. Ackerman NB, Hechmer PA (1980): The blood supply of experimental liver metastasis. *Am J Surg* 140: 625- 631.
6. Tan YO (1989): Non-surgical management of liver metastases. *Ann Academy Med* 18: 28- 31.
7. Taniguchi H, Takahashi T, Yamaguchi T, Sawai K (1989): Intraarterial infusion chemotherapy for metastatic liver tumor using multiple anticancer agents suspended in a lipid contrast medium. *Cancer* 64: 2001-2006.
8. Taniguchi H, Shioaki Y, Daido T, Takahashi T (1993): Blood supply and drug delivery to primary and secondary human liver cancer studied with in vivo bromodeoxyuridine labeling. *Cancer* 71: 50-55.

A Study of Prophylactic Arterial Infusion Chemotherapy for Remnant Liver in Case of Resected Liver Metastasis from Colorectal Cancer

Akihiko Tsuchida, Kozaburo Kimura, Yasuhisa Koyanagi, Tatsuya Aoki, Atsushi Nakajima, Koichiro Kato, Toshiaki Aoki, Daikichi Yasuda, Takashi Ozawa, and Hikaru Ozawa

Department of Surgery, Tokyo Medical College, Shinjuku-ku, Tokyo, 160 Japan

ABSTRACT

We performed the prophylactic arterial infusion chemotherapy for remnant liver in cases with resected liver metastasis from colorectal cancer in order to prevent the hepatic recurrence. Patients with intra-arterial infusion chemotherapy (IAC) showed good survival rate and disease free survival rate when compared with the patients without IAC. No severe complication that could not be managed conservatively was observed.

KEY WORDS: arterial infusion chemotherapy, hepatic recurrence, colorectal cancer

INTRODUCTION

Increased indication for resection of hepatic metastasis has recently improved the outcome of treatment for colorectal cancer. However the rate of recurrence in the remaining liver is still high [1], suggesting that potential metastasis might exist in other parts of the liver even after the apparent metastasis was resected [2]. We report the results of prophylactic arterial infusion chemotherapy for remnant liver after resection in order to prevent the recurrence of residual metastasis.

MATERIAL & METHOD

Forty cases were evaluated among 43 patients who underwent hepatectomy for liver metastasis from colorectal cancer. Patients were randomized to one of two treatment as follows: IAC group (22 cases): 5-FU 167mg/m^2/day, 2 weeks in hospital, and thereafter that 5-FU 334 mg/m^2/day, once a week, non-IAC group (18 cases): 5-FU 200mg/day (orally), or 5-FU 250mg/week (intravenously) (Table 1). We evaluated the background, operative procedure, recurrence in the remaining liver and survival rate in these groups. Survival curves were established using the Kaplan-Meier method, and these results were compared by generalized Wilcoxon test.

Table 1. Protocol of chemotherapy after hepatectomy for hepatic metastasis from colorectal cancer

---

IAC Group   (n=22): 5-FU 167mg/m^2/day (2 week) → 5-FU 334mg/m^2/day, once a week
               in hospital

non-IAC Group (n=18): 5-FU 200mg/day (orally) or 5-FU 250mg/week (intravenously)

RESULTS

The male to female ratio was 17:5 in the IAC group, and 12:6 in the non-IAC group. The median age was 58.3 year old (range 46-68) in the IAC group, and 59.4 (range 41-71) in the non-IAC. The synchronous to metachronous ratio was 11:11 in the IAC group, and 12:6 in the non-IAC. Histological types were tub$_1$:11, tub$_2$:10, por:1 in the IAC group, and tub$_1$:9, tub$_2$:9, por:0 in the non-IAC. Operative procedures employed partial or tumorectomy:15, systemic resection:7 in the IAC, and partial or tumorectomy:10, systemic resection 8 in the non-IAC. Histological findings preoperatively showed that 3 of 15 cases with systemic resection had micro-metastasis which was not detected preoperatively (Fig. 1). There were no difference between the 2 groups (Table 2).

With respect to the recurrence of remnant liver, there were 9 (40.9%) IAC cases which underwent partial or tumorectomy (8 cases) and systemic resection (1 case). The average duration of recurrence was 12.7 months. In the non-IAC group the recurrence of remnant liver was observed in 12 (66.7%) cases, which underwent 6 partial or tumorectomy and 6 systemic resection. The mean recurrent time was 10.1 months. Concerning the relation between the number of resected metastases and the recurrent rate, 5 (38.5%) of 13 IAC cases and 9 (69.2%) of 13 non-IAC cases with the isolated metastasis showed recurrence. In cases with multiple metastases, recurrence was observed in 4 (44.4%) of 9 IAC cases and 3 (60.0%) of 5 non-IAC (Table 3).

The overall survival showed that one year survival rate was obtained in 95% of the IAC group and in 70% of the non-IAC group, and 3 year survival rate was in 68% and in 28%, respectively. The survival period of IAC group was significantly longer than non-IAC group (P=.04) (Fig. 2).

The IAC group was significantly longer disease free survival period than the non-IAC group (P=.04) (Fig. 3). In cases with isolated metastasis the IAC group was significantly longer than the non-IAC (P=.02) (Fig. 4), though there was no significant difference in cases with multiple metastases. In the cases of systemic resection, the IAC group showed significantly better results than the non-IAC group (P=.05) (Fig. 5), though there was no significant difference in the cases of partial or tumorectomy.

Table 2. Patient characteristics according to treatment arm

Characteristic	IAC	non-IAC
Male:female	17:5	12:6
Median age (range)	58.3 (46 - 68)	59.4 (41 - 71)
Synchronous:metachronous	11:11	12:6
Number of metastasis isolated:multiple	13:9	13:5
Histological type well differentiated adeno ca. (tub_1)	11	9
moderately differentiated adeno ca. (tub_2)	10	9
poorly differentiated adeno ca. (por)	1	0
Operative procedure Partial or tumorectomy	15	10
Systemic hepatectomy	7	8

Table 3. Characteristics of the recurrence in the remnant liver

Characteristic	IAC	non-IAC
Number of recurrence (%)	9/22 (40.9%)	12/18 (66.7%)
isolated:multiple	5:4	9:3
Average duration of recurrence (month)	12.7	10.1
Operative procedure partial or tumorectomy	8	6
systemic resection	1	6

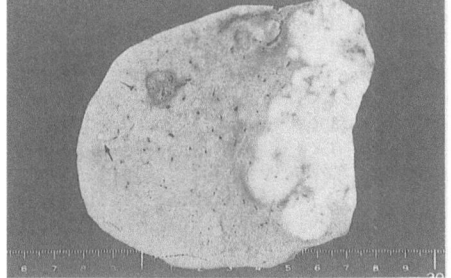

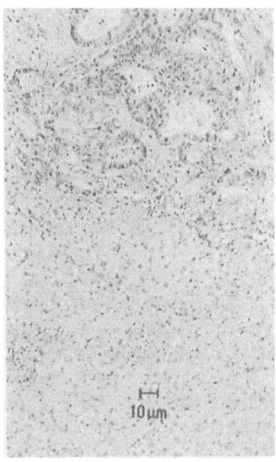

Fig. 1 Macroscopic and Histological finding (H.E stain, x100) of micro-metastasis

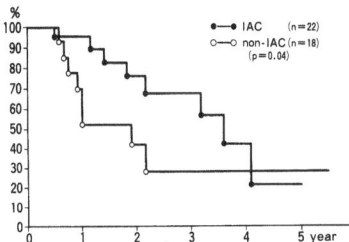

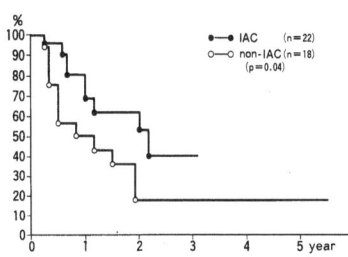

Fig. 2 Overall cumulative survival rate for IAC group and non-IAC group

Fig. 3 Overall disease free survival rate for IAC group and non-IAC group

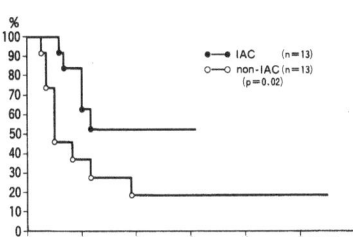

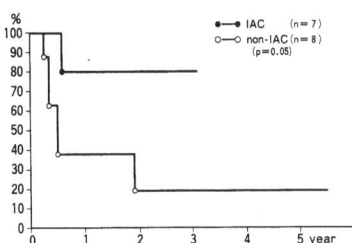

Fig. 4 Disease free survival of patients with isolated metastasis for IAC group and non-IAC group

Fig. 5 Disease free survival of patients with systemic hepatectomy for IAC group and non-IAC group

DISCUSSION

The multidisciplinary treatment which includes conservative and surgical therapies has been improving outcome of treatment for liver metastasis from colorectal cancer. Our results showed that 3 year comulative survival of the patients with hepatic resection was approximately 55%, although it was less than 10% in the patients who had unresectable hepatic metastasis [3]. Nevertheless, the most important problem is to identify the best way to prevent recurrence in the remaining liver because the hepatic recurrence is most frequently observed after surgery.

In this study intra-arterial infusion chemotherapy group obtained significantly better results for overall and disease free survival rates when compared with non-IAC group. The results of the recurrence in the remaining liver suggested that the patients with isolated metastasis had less possibility of potential micro-metastasis which was not detected by image analysis and intra-arterial infusion chemotherapy could prevent its progression. On the other hand it is supposed that intra-arterial infusion chemotherapy was not efficient for the patients with multiple metastases because they had already had some volume of micro-metastasis. Concerning the operative procedure, systemic resection could remove the potential micro-metastasis which surrounded main lesion, indicating that it is better than partial or tumorectomy. In conclusion, the prophylactic arterial infusion chemotherapy after hepatectomy is able to prevent the recurrence in the remaining liver especially for isolated metastasis which underwent systemic resection.

REREFENCES

1. Hughes KS (1986) Resection of the liver for colorectal carcinoma metastases: A multi-institutional study of patterns of recurrence. Surgery 100:278-284
2. Nishida O (1989) Extended operation for colorectal cancer metastatic to the liver. Jpn J Gastroenterol Surg 21:1061
3. Yasuda D, Kimura K, Koyanagi Y, et al. (1990) A study of low-dose intermittent intra-arterial infusion chemotherapy for liver metastasis in colorectal cancer. Jpn J Cancer Chemothe 17:1670-1673

Hepatic Arterial Infusion Therapy with Leucovorin and 5-Fluorouracil for Liver Metastasis of Gastric and Colorectal Cancer

Toshiro Konishi, Kazuhiko Shinohara, Mamoru Hiraishi, Yoshio Ushirokouji, Syun-ichi Yumoto, Haruhiro Nishina, and Yasuo Idezuki

The Second Department of Surgery, University of Tokyo, Bunkyo-ku, Tokyo, 113 Japan

ABSTRACT

We conducted a biochemical modulation with leucovorin (LV) and 5-fluorouracil (5-FU) through hepatic arterial infusion (HAI) for metastatic liver tumors. Eight patients of hepatic metastasis of adenocarcinoma from the gastrointestinal tracts (3 from gastric cancer and 5 from colorectal cancer) received HAI treatment of LV 20mg/m2 and 5-FU 425mg/m2 for the consecutive 5 days, repeated every 4 weeks. Tolerable leukocytopenia, nausea and vomiting, diarrhea, anorexia, and stomatitis were seen. Response rate of 50% (2 CR and 2 PR) without severe adverse effect indicates the high efficacy of this biochemical modulation via HAI against liver metastatic tumors.

KEY WORDS: biochemical modulation, leucovorin, 5-fluorouracil, hepatic arterial infusion, metastatic liver tumor

INTRODUCTION

For metastatic liver tumor a hepatic arterial infusion (HAI) has the advantage of getting high doses of drugs with hopefully less systemic toxicity [1]. Biochemical modulation, a newly developed multidrug chemotherapy, involves the use of a modulating agent (modulator) to enhance pharmacokinetics or pharmacodynamics of a cytotoxic agent (effector). A modulator of Leucovorin (LV) enhances the cytotoxic effect of 5-fluorouracil (5-FU) from increasing formation of the stable ternary complex consisting of 5-fluorodeoxyuridylate (FdUMP), 5,10-methylene tetrahydrofolate, and thymidylate synthetase (TS), resulting in blockage of DNA synthesis in tumor cells. Although many trials have showed the intravenous LV and 5-FU improved chemotherapeutic efficacy in treating advanced colorectal cancer [2], only a few reports on HAI with any kind of biochemical modulation therapy has published previously [3]. Patt et al.coinfusedfloxuridine (FUDR) and folinic acid through HAI and response rate of 58% (14/24) was achieved [4]. We conducted HAI therapy with LV and 5-FU for metastatic liver tumors to investigate efficacy and toxicity of the treatment.

METHODS AND PATIENTS

Hepatic arterial infusion of d, l-LV 20mg/m2 and 5-FU 425mg/m2 for the cosecutive 5 days was repeated via an implanted access every 4 weeks, according to the reported method of systemic intravenous injection for the advanced colorectal carcinoma [5]. Eight patients were entered into this protocol. Three patients had hepatic metastases from the gastric cancer (2 post-operative recurrent metastases and one simultaneous metastasis with unresectable gastric cancer). Other 5 patients had recurrent metastasis after surgery of the colorectal cancer. A HAI with 5-FU and LV was performed to 7 patients, except one patient who underwent the subselective intra-aortic infusion to treat both unresectable primary gastric cancer and metastatic liver tumors. Resected specimen of 7 patients showed 5 of well differentiated type and 2 of moderately differentiated type of tubular adenocarcinoma. One tubular adenocarcinoma of stomach was diagnosed from endoscopic biopsy.

In 4 patients the dose of 5-FU was reduced to the two thirds of the previous dose without reduction of the dose of LV, since moderate adverse effects (2 with leukocytopenia, one with alopecia and another with general malaise) were seen after the initial treatment.

Toxicity of LV and 5-FU via HAI

	grade 1	2	3	4	Total
Leukopenia				2	2/8 (25%)
Thrombocytopenia	1		1		2/8 (25%)
Nausea, Vomitus	2		3		5/8 (62.5%)
Diarrhea		1	1	1	3/8 (37.5%)
Stomatitis	1	1			2/8 (25%)
Alopecia	1				1/8 (12.5%)

Table 1. Most severe toxicity was leukocytopenia
and diarrhea Nausea and vomiting was not
severe. Any liver dysfunction were not seen.

Response of LV and 5-FU via HAI

Case	Total courses	Response	Response duration	Survival	death cause
1	6	CR	4m	11m dead	pulmonary liver peritoneum
2	22	PR	13m	2y9m alive	
3	8	NC		1y4m dead	liver
4	4	PD		7m dead	liver
5	5	NC		1y2m dead	liver peritoneum
6	4	PR	2m	8m dead	liver
7	2	PD		5m dead	liver pulmonary
8	9	CR	8m (PR 2m CR 6m)	1y2m dead	lymph node

Table 2. Response rate was 50% (2 CR and 2 PR).

RESULTS

Table 1 displays toxicity associated with this treatment, categorized with the WHO classification. Most severe toxicity was grade 4 leukocytopenia occurred in 2 patients and diarrhea in one patient. Although nausea and vomiting was most frequently seen (5/8), its grade was not severe like the grade of stomatitis. Any liver dysfunction or toxic death were not seen in this study.

The characteristics and response data of all patients are presented in Table2. There are 2 CR and 2 PR (both one in each gastric and colorectal cancer) and response rate of 50% was obtained.
All of the 4 responders are mentioned below.

Case 1(CR). Multiple liver tumors were found in 40-year-old female two years after the resection of sigmoid colon (Figure 1, upper). Although the grade 4 leukopenia (WBC 600) and diarrhea, and the grade 3 thrombocytopenia and nausea had been seen after the initial HAI treatment, CT examination revealed disappearance of liver tumors (Figure 1, lower). The treatment of modified dose was repeated on 5 more courses and response period of 4 months was achieved. She died from pulmonary metastasis associated with peritoneal dissemination and regrowing of liver metastasis 11 month after the beginning of the treatment.

Case 2 (PR). PR was obtained in a 75-year-old male, treated for the metastatic liver tumors recurred after resection of rectal cancer (Figure 2). PR had continued during 13 month duration and although he is well and alive now, the liver tumors are enlarging again while repeated 22 courses of HAI.

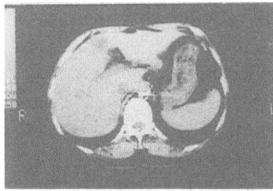
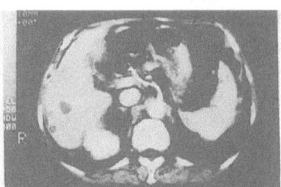

Figure 1. Case 1 (CR)

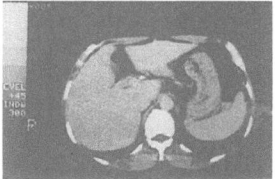
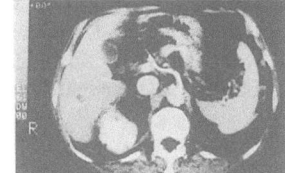

Figure 2. Case 2 (PR).

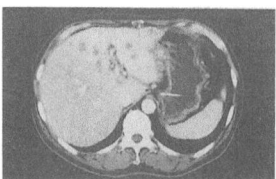

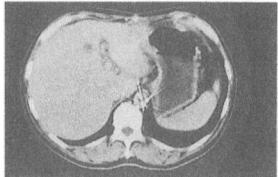

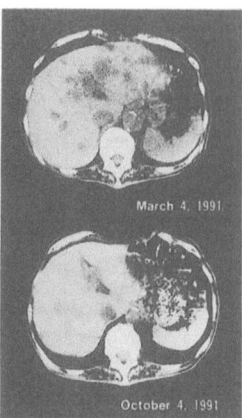

Figure 3. Case 6 (PR).   Figure 4. Case 8 (CR).

Case 6 (PR). For the liver metastasis associated with unresectable advanced gastric cancer the intra-aortic subselective HAI was started in a 48-year-old male (Figure 3, upper). A PR in liver tumors was revealed after the initial course (Figure 3, lower). The duration of response was 2 month period and after 8 months he died from liver metastasis.

Case 8 (CR). Multiple liver metastasis were detected in 69-year-old female one and a half year after surgery of gastric cancer (Figure 4, upper). After 5 courses of the HAI, the liver tumors showed PR, and CR was gained after 7 courses (Figure 4, lower). The response on the liver tumors continued during 8 months while the repeated HAI of 9 courses. She died from the obstructive jaundice caused with enlargement of lymph nodes around the hepatic hilum.

DISCUSSION

Response rate of 50% without severe adverse effect obtained by a biochemical modulation with LV and 5-FU via HAI indicates the high efficacy of this biochemical modulation against liver metastases from gastric and colorectal cancer. It was revealed from our study that this treatment was tolerable and its toxicity is less severe than the systemic administration of the treatment. With reduction of doses this treatment can be continued safely at the outpatient section. Chemical hepatitis frequently seen in the long term FUDR HAI [1] were not seen in this treatment. A PR patient shows intra-aortic subselective infusion also effective to those lesions. However, since death causes of the responders to this treatment were extrahepatic lesions like pulmonary metastasis or lymph nodes enlargement, a combined treatment with this HAI should be explored for getting longer survival duration.

REFERENCES

1. Kemeny N (1992) Seminars in Oncology 19(2) Supple 3(April): 155-162
2. Zhang ZG, Harstrick A, Rustum YM (1992) Seminars in Oncology 19(2) Supple 3(April): 10-15
3. Suga T, Takahashi Y, Ogino T, Mai M (1991) Jpn J Cancer Chemother 18:1962-1964 (in Japanese)
4. Patt YZ, Roh M, Chase J, Levin B, Hohn D (1990) Proc Am Soc Clin Oncol 9:118
5. Poon MA, O'Connell MJ, Moertel CG, Wieand HS, Cullinan SA, Everson LK, Krook JE, Mailliard JA, Laurie JA, Tschetter LK, Wiesenfeld M (1989) J Clin Oncol 10:1407-1418

The Therapeutic Effects of Liposomal Adriamycin Pretreated with Lentinan

Hiroyuki Konno, Yuji Maruo, Tatuo Tanaka, Satoshi Nakamura, and Shozo Baba

Second Department of Surgery, Hamamatsu University School of Medicine, Hamamatsu, Shizuoka, 431-31 Japan

ABSTRACT

To enhance the therapeutic effects of liposomal adriamycin (Lip-ADM) for cancer treatment, lentinan (LNT), which is known to increase the permeability of vessels, was administered peritumorally prior to systemic administration of Lip-ADM and the therapeutic effects of Lip-ADM with LNT were investigated by using a xenotransplanted human colon cancer strain. The ADM levels of the tumor tissue in mice treated by the Lip-ADM with LNT were significantly higher than in those without LNT. The significant therapeutic effects of Lip-ADM with LNT were demonstrated by the evaluation of the tumor growth curve and actual tumor weights.

KEY WORDS: Liposome, Lentinan, Adriamycin

INTRODUCTION

One of the major advantages of the liposomal system is that drugs entrapped in liposomes can remain in circulation longer without inactivations more than unentrapped drugs. This suggests us that in the liposomal system the concentrations of antineoplastic drug in tumors would be increased and the cytotoxic effects would be enhanced if the permeability of the tumor vessels can be increased before the administration of liposomes. Lentinan (LNT) was reported to increase the permeability of vessels, when it was administered locally [1].
In the present study, we prepared adriamycin (ADM) entrapped in liposomes (Lip-ADM) and investigated experimentally whether the ADM levels in the tumor increase by the local pretreatment with LNT prior to the systemic administration of Lip-ADM, and whether the therapeutic effects of Lip-ADM can be enhanced by the pretreatment.

MATERIALS AND METHODS

Preparation of ADM entrapped in liposomes (Lip-ADM)
ADM was encapsulated by the modified remote loading procedure, previously described by Mayer et al. [2,3]

Tissue distribution studies on ADM
Eight BALB/c nu/nu male mice were inoculated subcutaneously with small pieces (5-6 mm^3) of TK3, which was maintained with subcutaneous inoculation into the mice. The mice were divided randomly into two groups, when the estimated tumor weights (calculated as 1/2 x length(mm) x width(mm)^2) reached approximately 500 mg. Saline solution or 1mg/kg of LNT were peritumorally injected at 5 or 6 points into the mice, 1 hr prior to systemic administration of Lip-ADM (7.5 mg/kg of ADM concentration). At 6 hr after injection of Lip-ADM, the animals were sacrificed, and the tumor, heart, liver were excised immediately, and stored at -80 °C for the measurement. The organs were homogenized and the levels of ADM in the supernatant were determined by high performance liquid chromatography (HPLC)

Therapeutic effects of Lip-ADM with LNT

As described above, 16 mice were inoculated subcutaneously with TK-3. When the estimated tumor weight reached 300-500 mg (about 10-14 days after inoculation), the mice were divided randomly into four groups. Each group of mice received three injections at 4-day intervals through the tail vein of saline, LNT (1mg/kg), or Lip-ADM (7.5mg/kg) pretreated with saline or LNT (1mg/kg) (LNT was injected 1 hr prior to Lip-ADM). After the sacrifice of the mice (3 weeks after the intial treatment), the therapeutic effects of Lip-ADM with LNT were evaluated by tumor growth curve and actual tumor weights. The statistical significances were examined by means of Student's t-test.

RESULTS

The tissue distribution of ADM

ADM levels in the tumor were significantly higher in the group injected with Lip-ADM pretreated with LNT, as compared to the group injected with Lip-ADM pretreated with saline solution. The local pretreatment of LNT made the ADM levels lower in the liver and higher in the heart as compared to the group without the pretreatment of LNT, however, the differences were not significant.

Table 1. Adriamycin levels in the tumor, heart and liver
(μg/g tissue)

	tumor	heart	liver
Lip-ADM with LNT	0.91+0.335	2.36+0.768	12.7+4.62
Lip-ADM without LNT	0.51+0.123	1.34+0.391	20.3+1.26

Therapeutic effects of Lip-ADM with LNT

In the inhibition of tumor growth, Lip-ADM with LNT showed the highest therapeutic effects. The lowest ratios of relative mean tumor weight (relative mean tumor weight; the ratio of estimated tumor weight at given time to that at the start of the treatment) of each teatment group to that of control group were 37.2 % in Lip-ADM with LNT, 56.8 % in Lip-ADM with saline solution, and 93.4 % in LNT group, respectively. The actual tumor weights after each treatment were as follows: 1711.4 ± 349.4 (SD)mg in control, 1422.5 ± 709.8mg in LNT alone, 1206.7 ± 362.5mg in Lip-ADM with saline solution, and 781.7 ± 328.5mg in Lip-ADM with LNT. The significant difference of Lip-ADM with LNT group from Lip-ADM with saline solution group was observed (p<0.05).

DISCUSSION

Liposomal adriamycin have been attracted since it can decrease the adverse effects of adriamycin, especially the cardiotoxicity, which is one of the most undesirable adverse effects in its clinical use [4,5]. Previously, we reported that the therapeutic effect of 5 mg/ kg of ADM (free ADM) on a human colon cancer strain could not be evaluated because of its high toxicity to mice, recognized as a severe decrease in body weight [6]. On the other hand, the body weight loss of mice treated with 7.5 mg/kg of Lip-ADM were not observed in the present study.
LNT is BRM which is widely used as a treatment for gastric or colon cancers. However, in the present study, LNT was used to increase of permeabilities of tumor vessels. The results of tumor growth curve revealed that in the present experimental protocol the local injection of LNT could not show the cytotoxic effects on TK-3 as a BRM and that the increase of the permeability induced by LNT enhance the thepaeutic effects of Lip-ADM.

In order to improve the Lip-ADM with LNT system, additional experiments concerning about the timing of LNT pretreatment, or the optimal size and composition of liposomes should be performed.
In conclusion, the combination therapy of Lip-ADM and LNT can be used as an excellent treatments against digestive organ cancers, although optimal dosage and timing of administrations should be examined.

REFERENCES

1. Maeda YY, Watanabe ST, et al. (1984) T-cell mediatede vascular dilation and hemorrhage induced by antitumor polysaccharides. Int J Immunopharmac 6, 493-501

2. Mayer LD, Balley MD, et al. (1985) Uptake of antineoplastic agents into large unlammellar vesicles in response to a membrane potential. Biochem Biophys Acta 816, 294-302

3. Mayer LD, Balley, MD, et al. (1986) Uptake of adriamycin into large unilamellar vesicles in response to a pH gradient. Biochim Biophys Acta 857, 123-126

4. Forssen EA and Tokes ZA (1981) Use of anionic liposomes for the reduction of chronic doxorubicin-induced cardiotoxicity. Proc Natl Acad Sci USA 78, 1873-1877

5. Gabizon A, Dagan A, et al.(1982) Liposomes as in vivo carriers of Adriamycin: reduced cardiac uptake and preserved antitumor activity in mice. Cancer Res 42, 4734-4739

6. Maruo Y, Konno H, et al. (1992) Therapeutic effects of liposomal adriamycin in combination with tumor necrosis factor-α. J Surg Oncol 49, 20-24

Continuous Hepatic or Splenic Arterial Infusion of Recombinant Interleukin-2 (rIL-2) and Cyclophosphamide (CY) in Patients with Liver Metastasis of Colorectal Carcinoma and Hepatobiliary Carcinoma

KAZUHIRO HAYAKAWA, DAI SEITO, TAKAYUKI MORITA, and MITSURU KONN

The Second Department of Surgery, Hirosaki University School of Medicine, Hirosaki, 036 Japan

ABSTRACT

Patients with unresectable liver metastasis of colorectal carcinoma or hepatobiliary carcinoma were treated with the continuous arterial infusion of low dose rIL-2 (n=9) or that with low dose CY (n=3) for 2-6 weeks. One of the patients treated with rIL-2 alone was estimated as MR. All the patients treated with rIL-2 and CY responded and reduced tumor markers and tumor size in a short period. There were no differences of immunological parameters but apparent differences of therapeutic effects between the infusion of rIL-2 alone and rIL-2 with CY. This protocol should be valuable for the patients with metastatic liver tumors.

KEY WORDS: arterial infusion, recombinant interleukin-2 (rIL-2), cyclophosphamide, liver metastasis

INTRODUCTION

Interleukin-2 has been used with and without lymphokine-activated killer (LAK) cells or activated tumor-infiltrating lymphocytes (TILs)[1]. It is obvious that rIL-2 is useful for the patients with some kinds of malignant tumors like melanoma and renal cell carcinoma. Rosemberg et al. reported preliminary success with high dose administration of rIL-2 alone in vivo, although with a low response rate[2]. LAK or activated TIL therapy needs experienced staffs and is expensive, though the response rate is small. Patients do not easily tolerate diffuse capillary leak syndrome like interstitial lung edema in high doses of rIL-2. They need high doses of rIL-2 in intravenous bolus administration but it is difficult to keep a certain serum level of rIL-2 in tumor site continuously because rIL-2 has a short half life in serum and is diluted to the level under detection by blood quickly. At first, we made the protocol of splenic arterial infusion of rIL-2 for the purpose of activating splenic lymphocytes on standby and TILs in metastatic liver tumors. In this protocol, patients were not administered high doses of rIL-2 because they could get enough concentration of rIL-2 in local site continuously. In addition, we made other protocols of continuous hepatic arterial infusion of rIL-2 with CY to delete suppressor T cell function in local site.

PATIENTS AND METHODS

Patients

Patients were eligible for this treatment, if they had failed all standard chemotherapy or had disease for which no effective therapy was available. Twelve patients with liver tumors, including eight men and four women were treated in the ward of the second department of surgery. Their ages ranged from 39 to 77 years old. Five patients had colorectal carcinoma, three had hepatoma, three had bile duct carcinoma, and one had gall bladder carcinoma. In these patients, two with hepatoma had not received prior operations and the others were operated to resect the primary tumors. They showed the presence of measurable intrahepatic lesions for the evaluation.

Methods

The catheter for the infusion was placed in the left thoracico-acromial artery, and the tip was located in splenic or hepatic artery. Continuous infusion was done with automatic infusion pump (SP-10, Nipro, Tokyo). For the patients receiving rIL-2 infusion alone, low dose rIL-2 (S-6820, Shionogi, Tokyo) (7×10^5U/m^2/day) was administered for 10-14 days. When done with CY, low dose of CY (70mg/m^2/day) was administered 2 days prior to rIL-2 administration. This protocol was done 3 times repeatedly, if possible. When serious side effects appeared, the administration was discontinued. Each patient received $1-7 \times 10^7$U rIL-2 totally. Tumor markers (CEA, CA19-9) were checked every 2 weeks. Basic phenotypic analysis (CD3, CD4, CD8, CD16, CD25, and HLA-DR) of peripheral blood lymphocytes (PBLs) in each patient was performed at the same time. Computed tomographic (CT) scans of the abdomen were performed before and after the therapy at one month intervals.

Assessment of Treatment
CT scans were used to assess the therapies A complete response (CR) was defined as the disappearance of all measurable tumor for at least one month; a partial response (PR) as a decrease of at least 50% in the sum of the products of the perpendicular diameters of all measurable lesions for at least one month; a minor response (MR) as a 25% to 49%

708

reduction; no response (NR) as less reduction than MR, a progressive disease (PD) as a progression in the course of therapy.

RESULTS

Response to Therapy in Continuous Splenic Arterial Infusion of rIL-2

Nine patients were treated in this protocol, including three colorectal carcinoma, three bile duct carcinoma, and three hepatoma. In this study, we administered low doses of rIL-2 , usually 1×10^6U/day. Three patients received increased amounts of rIL-2 for the purpose of further effectiveness. No PRs were observed among them. One MR, three NRs, and Four PDs were observed, and one patient was discontinued this protocol because of high fever and unconsciousness caused by hepatic failure(Table 1.). Some patients showed increases in CD3 and CD4, however all patients showed increases in NK activity, LAK activity, CD25 and HLA-DR expression(Table 2.). Tumor markers decreased after the therapy temporally, even when they didn't show any responses in CT scans.

Toxicity of Therapy in Continuous Splenic Arterial Infusion of rIL-2

Six patients complained high fever , six had slight appetite loss. All the patients had enormous eosinophilia. Though, no significant side effects appeared except one patient who showed unconsciousness from hepatic failure. The patient had severe hepatic failure and strong jaundice prior to the therapy. There were no serious side effects resulting in extravasation of intravascular fluids leading to weight gain, dyspnea, and hypotension.

Response to Therapy in Continuous Splenic or Hepatic Arterial Infusion of rIL-2 and CY

Three patients were treated in this protocol, including two rectal carcinoma and one gall bladder carcinoma. All three patients showed PR in this therapy(Table 1). Patient no.10 sustained a 85% reduction in all measurable lesions for 2 months after the continuous hepatic arterial infusion of rIL-2 and CY (Fig.1). This patient was a 58-year-old woman who received in extended cholecystectomy one year prior to her symptom of severe jaundice, and the tumor occupied almost 30% of her liver volume. In the course of this therapy, jaundice subsided quickly. CT scans were performed before the therapy, before the end of the protocol, and thereafter. CEA in serum level decreased from 1600 ng/ml to 3.2 ng/ml in a month. One month later, CEA increased up to 1000 ng/ml without any increase of the tumor size on CT scans. The therapy was performed again. After the second administration, she had trans-arterial embolization (TAE) of the tumors with lipiodol resulting in the formation of a liver abcess. Patient no.11 sustained a 60% reduction of the tumor for more than three months. This patient was 53-year-old woman who received a rectal operation three years before this therapy. rIL-2 and CY was administered from the proper hepatic artery. CEA decreased from 32ng/ml to 5.6 ng/ml in one month. Patient no.12 was 65-year-old man who sustained a 60% reduction of the liver tumor. The therapy was repeated twice. CEA decreased from 31.6 ng/ml to 9.7 ng/ml. At last, after the assessment of the therapy by CT scans, the patient received the operation of tumor resection. There was necrosis, infiltration of enormous lymphocytes, fibrinoid degeneration, and no tumor cell detected in the specimen on pathologic findings.

Toxicity of Therapy in Continuous Splenic or Hepatic Arterial Infusion of rIL-2 and CY

There were no serious side effect except patient no.11. He had a liver abcess formation after TAE.

Table 1. Therapy and Results

Patient No.	Age	Sex	Original Disease	rIL-2 ($\times 10^4$U) day dose	Total dose	Infusion route	Result
Continuous arterial infusion of rIL-2							
1	51	F	Sigmoid colon carcinoma	100	3000	splenic artery	NR
2	77	F	Ascending and Sigmoid colon carcinomas	100-200	7000	splenic artery	PD
3	71	M	Rectal carcinoma	100-200	5000	splenic artery	PD
4	70	M	Common bile duct carcinoma	100	3000	splenic artery	MR
5	56	M	Common bile duct carcinoma	100	1100	splenic artery	NE
6	46	M	Common bile duct carcinoma	100-250	6800	splenic artery	PD
7	58	M	Hepatoma	100	6000	splenic artery	NR
8	67	M	Hepatoma	100	3000	splenic artery	NR
9	39	M	Hepatoma	100	3000	splenic artery	PD
Continuous arterial infusion of rIL-2 and CY							
10	58	F	Gall bladder carcinoma	100	2500	hepatic artery	PR
11	53	F	Rectal carcinoma	100	2000	hepatic artery	PR
12	65	M	Rectal carcinoma	100-200	2700	splenic artery	PR

Table 2. Characteristics of Patients' PBLs Before and After Therapy

Patients' condition	Surface marker (%)						Cytotoxocity (%)	
	CD3	CD4	CD8	CD16	CD25	HLA-DR	NK	LAK
Infusion of rIL-2 (n=9)								
Before therapy	73±2.5	52±3.6	20±3.7	11±2.2	1.8±0.3	24±3.8	20±4.8	2.2±0.4
After therapy (14th day)	76±4.6	56±5.2	20±3.5	11±1.8	7.8±2.2	29±2.5	32±6.4	6.8±2.1
After therapy (28th day)	64±4.0	46±4.3	17±3.5	14±1.8	7.5±1.6	28±3.4	57±8.6	14±4.6
Infusion of rIL-2 and CY (n=3)								
Before therapy	58±6.0	30±6.0	27±4.8	15±2.5	3.2±0.6	21±1.6	18±2.5	2.5±0.8
After therapy (14th day)	71±8.9	40±4.4	28±2.9	10.3±1.1	5.4±1.5	30±4.9	42±8.6	12±2.3
After therapy (28 th day)	68±5.4	35±5.3	31±4.1	13.6±2.6	3.8±0.2	29±3.6	38±6.2	14±3.8

All the phenotypes were checked using FACS.
NK activity is the cytotoxicity against K-562 cells and LAK is against Daudi cells in 4-hour Cr assay.

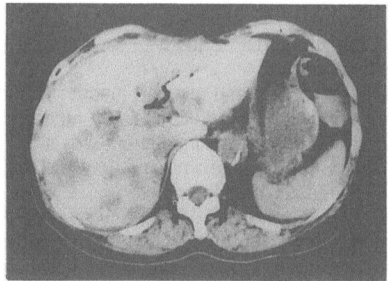 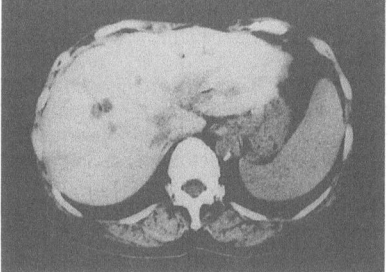

Fig.1 Patient no.10 (1) before therapy   (2) after therapy
Tumors were almost disappeared after therapy.

DISCUSSION

At first, we designed this continuous splenic arterial infusion of rIL-2 as a method of in vivo induction and activation of LAK cells in spleen on standby. There may be a possibility of activation of TILs in local site. It was certain that a small amount of rIL-2 was detected in portal vein during the period of splenic arterial infusion. NK and LAK activities of PBLs in the patients increased after the therapy. Nevertheless, the results were one MR, three NRs, and four PDs. For the purpose of increased effectiveness, another protocol was designed. CY was reported to delete suppressor T cells [3], and we have found the same result in murine model. CY augmented cytotoxic T lymphocyte (CTL) activity of tumor bearing mouse with the administration of rIL-2, but it did not augment enough CTL activity of non tumor bearing mouse even with rIL-2. Hepatic arterial infusion was designed as a better approach to activate TILs in liver tumors. Three patients were treated with continuous hepatic or splenic arterial infusion of rIL-2 and CY. All of them responded and were evaluated as PRs. There was no difference of the tendency of phenotypes, NK activity, and LAK activity in PBLs between the infusion of rIL-2 alone and rIL-2 with CY(Table 2). The results suggest that, for the most part, PBLs are not involved in antitumor immunity in tumor sites. Although it was difficult to check the cytotoxicity of PBLs or TILs to autologous tumor cells in these protocols, the pathologic finding seen in the specimen of patient no.12 indicated CTL activation of TILs in tumor sites. Though the number of patient is not large enough for statistical significance, this protocol should be valuable for the patients with metastatic liver tumors.

REFERENCES

1. Grimm EA, Mazumder A, Zhang HZ, Rosemberg SA (1982) Lymphokine activated killer cell phenomenon. Lysis of natural killer-resistant fresh solid tumor cells by interleukin-2-activated autologous human peripheral blood lymphocytes. J Exp Med 155: 1823
2. Rosemberg SA, Lotz MT, Muul LM, Chang AE, Avis FP, Leitman S, Linehan WM, Robertson CN, Lee RE, Rubin JT, Seipp CA, Simpson CG, White DE (1987) A progress report on the treatment of 157 patients with advanced cancer using lymphokine-activated killer cells and interleukin-2 or high-dose interleukin-2 alone. N Engl J Med 316: 889
3. Rollinghoff M, Starzinski-Powitz A, Pfizenmaier K, Wagner H (1977) Cyclophosphamide-sensitive T lymphocytes suppress the in vivo generation of antigen-specific cytotoxic T lymphocytes. J Exp Med 145: 455

Effects of Serial Transarterial Infusion Chemotherapy Combination with Multi-BRM for Metastatic Liver Tumor

MOTOHISA KATO, KIICHI MIYA, and SHIGETOYO SAJI

Second Department of Surgery, Gifu University School of Medicine, Gifu, Japan

ABSTRACT

In order to improve therapeutic efficacy for metastatic liver tumor, serial transarterial infusion of anticancer drugs in combination with multi-BRM(Biological Response Modifier) was performed by use of reservoir apparatus. A total of 19 patients were treated according to the following schedule: 10mg of ADM(or MMC) were administered at day 0, 0.5KE of OK-432 on day 1 and 4×10^5JRU of recombinant interleukin 2 (rIL-2)on day 4,7 and 11. The above therapy was repeated at every two weeks as long as possible. In terms of direct antitumor effect and decrease of tumor markers, the overall response rate was 38.9% and 70.6%,respectively.

KEY WORDS : metastatic liver tumor, transarterial infusion therapy, BRM, LAK

INTRODUCTION

The adoptive immunochemotherapy using LAK(lymphokine activated killer) cells induced from peripheral blood mononuclear cells(PBMC) of cancer patients was considered to be not so effective as expected. In present investigation, the most effective methods to induce endogenous LAK or CTL (cytotoxic T lymphcyte) which were induced by serial administration of OK-432 and IL-2 in combination with anticancer drugs into local regions of cancer were examined. The main purpose of preadministration of anticancer drugs such as mitomycin C or adriamycin was to suppress cancer cell growth and to induce antigen presentation.

MATERIALS AND METHODS

A total of 19 patients(9 cases of gastric cancer, 5 of colon cancer, 2 of pancreatic cancer, 1 of gallbladder cancer, 1 of breast cancer and 1 of biliary carcinoid) were treated in accordance with the schedule shown in Fig.1. Before the schedule, a implantable drug delivery system was settled into common hepatic artery by open surgery or Seldinger method. The schedule was continued at every two weeks(one cycle) as long as possible. In terms of grades of liver metastasis(H), H1, H2 and H3 were 12 cases(63.2%), 3 cases(15.8%) and 4 cases(21.1%), respectively. 12 cases(63.2%) had extrahepatic cancer lesions. As for performans status, 4,3,2,1 and 0 were 1 case, 1 case, 5 cases , 8 cases and 4 cases, respectively. As for nutritional state, the average of PNI(Onodera's prognostic nutritional index)value was 43.0(24.0-53.2). The average treatment times was 8.5(2-24)cycles. Average given BRM dosage of OK-432 and rIL-2 were 6.2(1.2-24)KE and 57.7(9-240)$\times 10^5$JRU, respectively and average given anticancer drugs dosage of MMC or ADM(terarubicin, epirubicin) was 96(34-290)mg. In cases of colon cancer, 5-FU was used simultaneously due to its positive drug sensitivity(Table 1).

Fig.1 The schedule of serial transarterial infusion therapy combination with multi- BRM and anticancer drugs for metastatic liver tumor

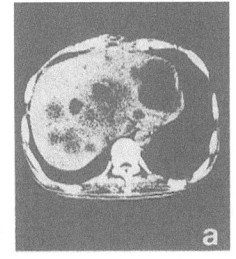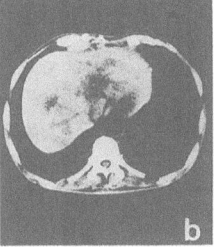

Fig.2 The CT findings of the liver in case 2 at pre-(a) and post-(b)treatment.

Table 1.Summary of the serial transarterial infusion chemotherapy in combination with multi-BRM for metastatic liver tumor

case age sex			primary focus	grades (liver meta)	extrahepatic focus	times of therapy	therapeutic effect				survival days	result (cause of death)
							liver	tumor marker	extrahepatic focus	PS		
1	55	M	g. c.	H2	P2	6	NC	CEA↑		→	389	(perit. dissem.)
2	68	M	g. c.	H3	—	22	PR	CEA↓		↑	310	(liver meta.)
3	53	F	g. c.	H3	—	3	PR	CEA↓		→	488	(liver meta.)
4	57	M	g. c.	H3	P3, lung	24	PR	CEA↓	lung.meta.↓↓	↑	318	(malnutrition)
5	45	M	g. c.	H3	pf	6	NC	CEA↓		↓	364	(perit. dissem.)
6	58	M	g. c.	H3	—	3	(NE)	(NE)		→	282	(liver meta.)
7	56	M	g. c.	H3	—	6	PD	CEA↑		↓	126	(liver meta.)
8	59	M	g. c.	H3	P	15	NC	AFP↓	ascites↓	↑	349	(liver meta.)
9	64	F	g. c.	H1	N4	4	MR	CEA↓		→	170	survival
10	80	F	c. c.	H2	—	2	MR	(NE)		→	95	(liver meta.)
11	43	F	c. c.	H3	lung	5	NC	CEA↓		→	1,105	unknown
12	70	M	c. c.	H3	lung	7	NC	CEA↓		→	171	(liver meta.)
13	55	F	c. c.	H1	—	6	PD	CEA↑		↓	428	(perit. dissem.)
14	63	F	c. c.	H1	bone	8	NC	CEA↓		→	290	survival
15	56	M	p. c.	H3	pf, P3, bone	8	PR	CA125↓	ascites↓↓	↑	246	(pleural dissem.)
16	68	F	p. c.	H3	pf	10	MR	(NE)		→	444	(perit. dissem.)
17	65	F	gb. c.	H1	pf, N4	10	PR	CA19-9↑		↓	352	(perit. dissem.)
18	42	F	b. car.	H2	—	8	PR	CEA↓		→	906	survival
19	53	F	br. c.	H3	P, bone	8	PR	CEA↓	ascites↓↓	↑	197	(perit. dissem.)
average						8.5					370	

abbreviation : g. c.(gastric cancer), c. c.(colon cancer), p. c.(pancreatic cancer), gb. c.(gallbladder cancer)
b. car.(billiary carcinoid), br. c.(breast cancer), pf (primary focus),

(1992. 4. 30)

RESULTS

(1)The direct effect of liver metastasis: CR,PR,MR,NC and PD were 0,7,3,6 and 2 cases, respectively (one case was unestimable), and the overall response rate was 38.9%(more than PR) or 55.6%(more than MR). (2)The primary focus: the response rate of gastric cancer, pancreatic cancer, gallbladder cancer, billiary carcinoid, breast cancer and colon cancer were 33.3%(3 of 9), 50%(1 of 2),100%(1 of 1),100%(1 of 1),100%(1 of 1) and 0%(0 of 5),respectively. (3)The grades of liver metastasis of the responder cases: H1,H2 and H3 were 25% (1 case),33.3%(1 case) and 41.7%(5 cases) respectively.The response rate had no reference to the grades of metastasis. (4)Tumor marker:In 12 of 17 cases(70.6%), they reduced and showed normal value in 3 cases. (5)The extrahepatic foci: 1 case of lung metastasis and 3 cases of ascites due to peritoneal dissemination were diminished or disappeared. (6) Performance status was improved in 5 cases(26.3%). 50% survival days, one year survival rate and two years survival rate were 349 days, 33.4% and 13.4%,respectively. The survival curves of the treatment group was significantly higher than the systemic chemotherapy group in gastric cancer(Fig.3). The H,P(peritoneal dissemination) and N(lymphnode metastasis) factor of the two groups had no significant differences, but as for S(serosal invasion) factor, the latter group had more advanced cancer cases . (8)In some cases ,second look operation was performed and partial hepatectomy was possible. Moreover,it was found that the fibrous changes and bloody necrosis of the liver metastasis were observed by HE stain, and CD4, CD8 positive monocytes and slight CD20 positive cells were infiltrated around cancer cells by immunochemical stain, while there were no CD56 positive cells(Fig.4).

SIDE EFFECTS

Fever in all cases, general fatigue that continued to the next day at the administration of OK-432 and/or rIL-2 in 7 cases(37%), appetiteloss in 4 cases(21%), nausea and abdominal pain in 3 cases(16%) and leucocytopenia and vomitting in 2 cases(11%) were recognized, while there was no severe side effect which needed special treatment.

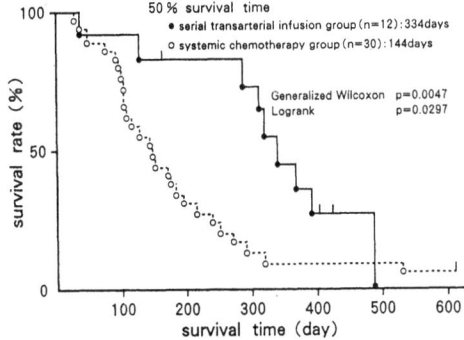

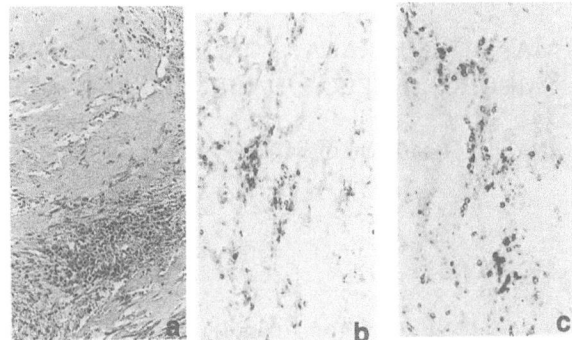

Fig.3 Comparison of survival curves between the the transarterial infusion therapy group and the systemic chemotherapy group in gastric cancer

Fig.4 HE stain(a) and immunochemical stain CD4(b) and CD8(c) in the metastatic liver specimen obtained from operation

DISCUSSION

For the success of immunotherapy, most effective BRM have to be used and given into cancer region where some kinds of effector cells may be located. From this point of view, the liver has many immunocompetent cells and is considered as the appropriate target organ for locoregional immunotherapy. Ogata and others reported that the number and LAK activity of intrasinusoidal LGL(large granular lymphcyte) in rats increased after injection of OK-432 and IL-2[1]. Our investigation also proved that the therapeutic effect of the treatment group showed more exellent results than the systemic chemotherapy group in human, the models of rats experimental tumor and rabbits metastatic liver tumor[2] [3] (these are not shown in this meeting). We appreciate the transarterial infusion chemotherapy in combination with multi-BRM at the points of
(1)prolongation of administration time by the decrease of single dose of anticancer drug
(2)direct antitumor effect of BRM to the tumor resistant to anticancer drug
(3)the therapeutic effect to extrahepatic foci by antitumor effect through host.
According to our speculation, MMC or ADM might react not only as anticancer drug but as immunomodulator, and cancer cells may be modified and expressed their antigen presentation. Otherwise, OK-432 induce multicytokines(IL-1,TNF and IFN etc.) around cancer cells to present IL-2 receptor on pre-T cell and induce LAK or CTL-like cell by IL-2 stimulation. Sakamoto and others reported that administration of a little dose of MMC suppressed the production of suppressor T-cell and increased NK activity[4]. In our responder cases, fibrous changes and bloody necrosis were observed at metastatic liver foci and the infiltration of many CD-4 or CD-8 positive cells were noted around it. While NK activity of PBMC reduced significantly soon after transarterial infusion of OK-432 or rIL-2. Above findings may suggest that actirvated NK cells were accumulated at cancer foci of the liver. Moreover, the infiltration of CD-56 positive NK cell was not revealed in the liver tissue at hepatectomized specimen. It was suggested that CD-56 positive cells might mobilized to local region soon after transarterial infusion and might be differenciated into LAK or CTL.

REFERRENCES

1.Ogata H, Tanaka M,Shimada M and Tanigawa K(1989) Effect of OK-432 and IL-2 on rat liver sinusoidal large granular lymphcyte. Biotherapy 3:42-45
2.Kawai M, Saji S, Kaneda N, Kashizuka T, Takahashi H, Sugiyama Y, Miya K and Tanemura H(1991) Characterization of endogenously activated spleen cell by intrasplenic administration of OK-432 and rIL-2,and its antitumor effects for metastatic liver tumor.Biotherapy 5:1080-1085
3.Kaneda N, Saji S, Azuma S, Miya K, Kawai M and Kashizuka T (1992) Experimental studies of efficacy of transarterial infusion immunochemotherapy for metastatic liver tumor using rabbits. Jpn J Gastroentero Surg 25:1764
4.Sakamoto K, Ohtsuki S, Hasegawa M, Shimizu M, Sako M, Yuri H, Nishiwaki Y and Yokogawa S (1985) Selective intraarterial infusion of OK-432 to advanced malignancies. J Jpn Soc Cancer Ther 20:84-93

A Simple New Method of Hyperthermo-Chemo-Hypoxic Isolated Liver Perfusion for Hepatic Metastasis

MASATO HORIKAWA, YOSHIYUKI NAKAJIMA, MICHIYOSHI HISANAGA, KIYOSHI KIDO, SAIHO KO, KAZUO OHASHI, and HIROSHIGE NAKANO

The First Department of Surgery, Nara Medical University, Kashihara, Nara, 634 Japan

ABSTRACT

A simple new method of isolated liver perfusion (hyperthermo-chemo-hypoxic) was designed as a regional therapy for hepatic metastasis. This paper describes a technique for in vivo isolated liver perfusion for 30min without oxygenation through the portal vein. Experimentally, all dogs survived without hepatic insufficiency and systemic toxicity. All clinical cases could well tolerate the liver perfusion. AKBR returned quickly. GPT and ALP levels were observed mild elevation, and returned to the normal range within 14days. Amylase, BUN and Creatinine were not changed. These results indicate that the simple new system of isolated liver perfusion can be accomplished with relative ease and low morbidity for hepatic metastasis.

KEYWORDS: metastatic liver cancer, liver perfusion, hyperthermo-chemotherapy, hypoxia

INTRODUCTION

The conventional administration of cytotoxic drugs is limited by the systemic side effects. While, isolated liver perfusion technique has been suggested to be supplied with high doses of cytotoxic drugs to the liver and to prevent systemic side effect. Moreover, hyperthermia may increase anti-tumor effect of cytotoxic drugs. Such methods have been described, but those were complicated and needed high costs. We have therefore developed a simple new method of isolated liver perfusion (hyperthermo-chemo-hypoxic) as a regional therapy for hepatic metastasis. In the present study, the influence of this method on the normal hepatic tissue and other organs was experimentally evaluated, and we applied it to clinical cases.

MATERIALS AND METHODS

Experimental

The four beagle dogs were used in this study. The animal was intubated under anesthesia and the abdomen was opened through a midline incision. After liver was isolated, a cannula was putted into the portal vein and infra hepatic vena cava. Supra-, infra-hepatic vena cava and hepatic artery were clamped. The isolated liver was perfused in vivo for 30 min through the portal vein by gravity 70cmH2O under the V-V bypass. Lactate Ringer's solution warmed to 43°C was used as the perfusate. Cisplatin (CDDP) was added to the perfusate in a dose of 2ng/ml. At the end of the perfusion, the clamp of supra-hepatic vena cava was removed after unclamping the hepatic artery and the portal vein and infra hepatic vena cava were repaired. Temperature of the liver and esophagus were observed. Blood chemical analysis and histological examination were performed.

Clinical

Two patients underwent the liver perfusion just same as experimental cases, after they had

714

Table 1. Clinical cases of hyperthermo-chemotherapy

Case	Primary cancer location & tomor extension His.	Liver metastasis	location & size (cm)	Hepatectomy
1	stomach SS,N0,P0,M0 leiomyosarcoma		S -5,8 3.5 x 2.8 cm 2.3 x 2.8 cm 2.8 x 2.6 cm	partial resecsion
2	rectum SS,N2,P0,M0 moderate		S -7 1.0 x 1.3 cm 0.3 x 0.3 cm	partial resecsion

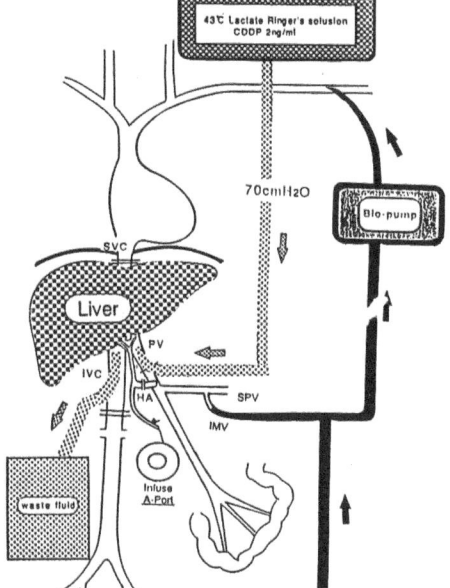

Fig.1 Schema of Hypertthermo-chemotherapy

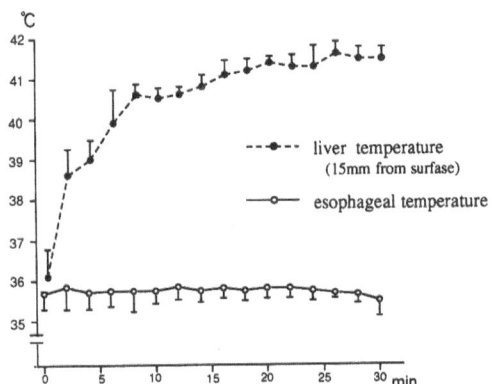

Fig.1 Schema of Hypertthermo-chemotherapy

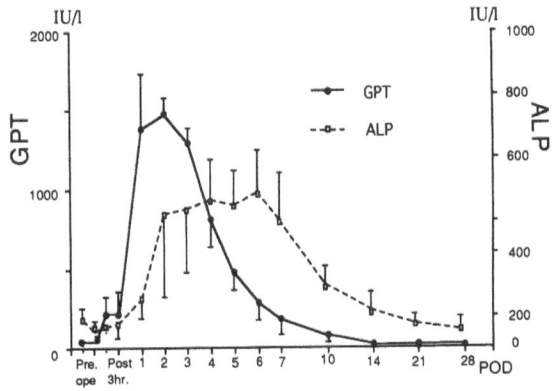

Fig.3 Changes of GPT and ALP (experimental n=4)

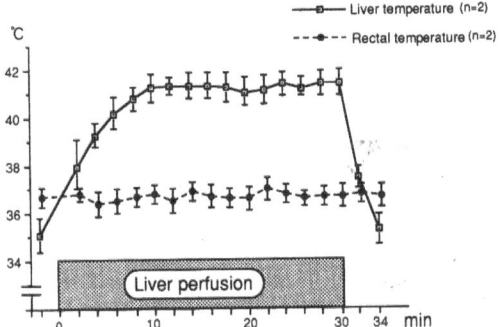

Fig.4 Changes of Liver and Rectal Temperature (clinical n=2)

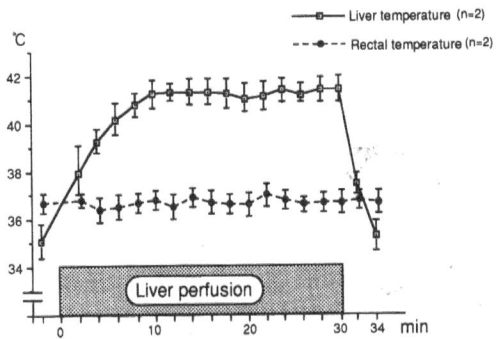

Fig.4 Changes of Liver and Rectal Temperature (clinical n=2)

been removed the primary tumor and performed hepatectomy for the liver metastasis (Table 1). After this procedure, a infuse-A-port was putted into the gastroduodenal artery for the postoperative chemotherapy(Fig. 1). During the perfusion, temperature of the liver and rectum were observed. Serum drug levels were assessed. Blood chemical analysis and histological examination were performed.

RESULTS

Experimental

All dogs survived without hepatic insufficiency and systemic toxicity. Temperature in the liver reached to 41-42℃ within 10 min. after starting the perfusion but in the esophagus was not changed during it(Fig.2). Arterial ketone body ratio (AKBR) returned quickly to the normal level after liver perfusion. Elevated levels of GPT and ALP after the perfusion were restored within two weeks(Fig. 3). Amylase, BUN, and Creatinine were not changed. The histologic picture was normal on 14th day.

Clinical

The human livers cloud well tolerate the perfusion. During the perfusion temperature in the liver was kept at above 41℃, but in the rectum was not changed(Fig. 4). Leakage of the cytotoxic drug to the systemic circulation was not observed during and after the perfusion. AKBR was restored same as experimental cases. GPT and ALP levels were elevated, and returned to the normal range within 14days （Fig.5). Amylase, BUN, and Creatinine were not changed. All patients can be diseased free after the therapy(case1-6months, case2-5months).

DISCUSSION

Some methods have been described for perfusing the isolated liver, and could be effectable for the hepatic malignancy [1,2] . However they were probably complicated and needed high costs. We designed a simple new system of isolated liver perfusion (hyperthermo-chemo-hypoxic) as a regional therapy for hepatic metastasis. In the perfusion without oxygenation , there were some hepatocellular damage. The damage, however, seemed to return to the normal range within 14days. The temperature of the liver tissue (above 41℃) has a selective lethal effect on tumor cells [3] . Therefore, high doses of cytotoxic drugs should be more effective on tumor cells. In this study, there was no sign of systemic toxicity. These experimental and clinical results indicate that the isolated liver perfusion method used in this study can be accomplished with relative ease and low morbidity for hepatic metastasis, although in order to prove tumor cidal effect of this method , further clinical observations must be performed.

REFERENCES

1. Radnell M, Jeppsson B, Bengmark S, (1990) A technique for isolated liver perfusion in the rat with survival and results of cytotoxic drug perfusion on liver tumor growth. J.Surg.res. 49:394-399
2. Skibba JL, Quebbeman EJ, (1986) Tumoricidal effects and patient survival after hyperthermic liver perfusion. Arch.Surg. 121:1266-1271
3. Giovanelli BC, Stehlin JS, Morgan AC, (1976)Slective lethal effect of supranormal temperatures on human neoplastic cells. Cancer Res. 36:3944-3950

Prophylactic Effects of Doxorubicin on Hepatic Recurrence of Colonic VX2 Cancer Lesions

Yoshiki Tabuchi[1], Masayoshi Sakane[2], Yasuyuki Tada[2], Shiro Nakae[2], Hiroyuki Deguchi[2], Takeshi Nakamura[2], and Yoichi Saitoh[2]

[1]School of Allied Medical Sciences, Kobe University, Kobe, 654-01 Japan
[2]The Department of Surgery, Kobe University School of Medicine, Kobe, 650 Japan

ABSTRACT

The prophylactic effects of doxorubicin (ADR) on hepatic recurrence following resection of colonic VX2 cancer lesions were examined by varying the injection doses, routes and time, using 43 rabbits. The colonic cancer lesions without metastasis were resected 14 days after implantaion of the cancer cells, and the animals were autopsied 14 days after resection. The efficacy of ADR was evaluated by the rate, size and number of hepatic recurrences at the time of autopsy. The results suggest that postoperative portal injection or an appropriate combination of preoperative peripheral and postoperative portal injection of ADR is effective for prophylaxis, but that inappropriate peripheral plus portal injection can promote hepatic recurrence.

KEY WORDS: liver recurrence, doxorubicin, adjuvant chemotherapy, VX2 cancer

INTRODUCTION

In spite of extensive studies, no reliable prophylactic chemotherapy for liver recurrence in colorectal cancer patients has been found, although few reports have shown some positive findings [1]. In the present study, the prophylactic effects of doxorubicin (adriamycin, ADR) on the recurrence according to different injection doses, routes and time were examined, using a colon VX2 cancer model with reliable liver recurrence and high sensitivity to ADR [2].

MATERIALS AND METHODS

Implantation of VX2 Cancer Cells in Experimental Animal Groups

VX2 cancer cells were maintained by successive transplantaion into the muscle of Japanese white rabbits. Immediately after sacrifice of the donor rabbits by intravenous anesthesia, the VX2 cancer was aseptically stripped and minced mechanically with scissors in cold physiological buffered saline. As previously reported by us [2,3], viable cells were finally adjusted to a concentration of 1×10^7 cells/ml.

Forty-three Japanese white rabbits were used. Under intravenous anesthesia, laparotomy was performed, and 0.1 ml (1×10^6 cells) of the suspension was implanted using a needle into the subserosa and/or proper muscle layers of the ascending colon. Immediately after implantation, a minute nodule formed, and the aperture was closed by a clamp, then ligated with surgical silk. Primary colon cancer lesions were resected 14 days after implantation at a distance of 3 cm from the edge of the tumor, followed by the formation of a proximal colostomy and closure of the distal colon. The rabbits were divided into nonchemotherapeutic (control) and chemotherapeutic groups, which consisted of 5 and 38 rabbits, respectively. The latter group was subdivided into the 3 groups: a portal group, to which an ADR dose of 1.0 or 0.5 mg/kg was injected into a mesenteric vein immediately after resection; a peripheral group, to which the same doses as the portal group were injected into the auricular vein after resection; and a peripheral plus portal group, to which an ADR dose of 0.5 mg/kg was peripherally injected 0 (1 hour), 1 or 2 days prior to resection, followed by a portal injection of ADR 0.5 mg/kg after resection. All of the animals were sacrificed 14 days after resection.

Examination of Specimens and Statistical Analysis

The lungs and abdominal organs were resected from each autopsied animal.
After macroscopic observation of all the specimens, followed by the measurement and recording of cancer lesions as they were found, the specimens were
fixed in 10% formalin solution. The colonic lesions and lymph nodes were
histologically examined by studying four sections. The examination process
for each liver and lung began with slicing 5-mm-thick sections. When cancer
lesions were found, the number and diameter of the lesions were recorded.
Two sections were obtained from the tissues with cancer lesions, and another
two sections were taken from the tissues without lesions. Every section was
examined histologically. The data were analyzed by Student's t test and the
chi-square test.

RESULTS

Macroscopic and microscopic findings of the colonic cancer lesions in the
chemotherapeutic group were almost the same as those in the control group.
The mean diameter of the lesions was 8.0 - 8.4 cm in the control and three
chemotherapeutic groups. Venous and lympatic invasion was found in almost
all of the animals in these four groups.
  Cancer recurrence was found in the liver and lymph nodes. The recurrence
rate in the nodes was 60% (3/5), 40% (4/10), 40% (4/10) and 67% (12/18) in
the control, portal, peripheral, and peripheral plus portal groups, respectively. No significant difference was found among them. In the liver, the
recurrent nodules were scattered sporadically. Microscopically, they were
mainly found in the perilobular areas, always accompanied by cancer emboli
in the interlobular veins or inlet venules. The hepatic recurrence rate and
mean number and diameter of the recurrent nodules are summarized in Table 1.

Table 1. Number of animals with hepatic recurrence, and mean number and
diameter of recurrent nodules in the liver

Experimental group(day[a])		Dose of ADR (mg/kg)	Hepatic recurrence		
			No.(rate)	Nodule[b]	Diameter[b](mm)
Control		0.0	5/5(100%)	57 ± 60	3.2 ± 0.4
Portal		1.0	0/5(0%)*	–	–
		0.5	3/5(60%)	18 ± 17	2.7 ± 1.2
Peripheral		1.0	3/5(60%)	68 ± 26	6.0 ± 2.2
		0.5	5/5(100%)	141 ± 88	10.2 ± 2.9**
Peripheral	(2)	0.5 + 0.5	0/6(0%)*	–	–
plus	(1)	0.5 + 0.5	6/6(100%)	125 ± 109	5.3 ± 2.3
portal	(0)	0.5 + 0.5	4/6(67%)	81 ± 109	6.0 ± 2.5

[a]Day in parenthesis indicates the day of peripheral ADR (0.5 mg/Kg) injection prior to resection. [b]Mean ± SD. *Significant difference from the
control, peripheral (0.5 mg/kg) and peripheral plus portal(1) groups
(P<0.05). **Significant difference from the control group (P<0.05).

Although liver recurrence was found in all of the animals of the control
group, recurrence was not confirmed in any animal macro- or microscopically
in the portal (1.0 mg/kg) and preoperative peripheral plus portal (2)
groups. The recurrence rates in the latter groups were significantly lower
than that in the control group. However, no significant difference was found
in the rates between the other chemotherapeutic and control groups (Table
1). The mean number and diameter of hepatic nodules in the peripheral (0.5
mg/kg) and preoperative peripheral (0 and 1) groups were greater than those
seen in the control group. Although the mean diameter of the nodules in only
the peripheral (0.5 mg/kg) group was significantly larger than that in the

control group, no significant difference was found in the number and diameter between the chemotherapeutic and control groups (Table 1).

DISCUSSION

In general, hepatic recurrence has been thought to originate mainly from two sources; (1) postoperative growth of preoperative micrometastasis in the liver and (2) occurrence of hepatic metastasis on the basis of entry of cancer cells or clusters into the portal vein at the time of operation [2,4,5]. These events seem to play an important role in the formation and also extension of liver recurrence, because the recurrent nodules have been mainly found in the perilobular areas, and were always accompanied by cancer emboli in the interlobular veins or inlet venules in the present study. As previously reported by us, micrometastases and entry to portal branches in the liver are considered to occur during a very short period, between 10 and 14 days after implantation, in this animal model [5].

In the present study, hepatic recurrence was found in every animal of the control group. The suppressive or prophylactic effects of ADR on the recurrence varied greatly according to the different injection routes, doses and time. The results clearly indicated that postoperative portal injection or an appropriate combination of preoperative peripheral plus postoperative portal injection was more effective for prophylaxis of hepatic recurrence than postoperative peripheral injection alone. The prophylactic mechanism seems to be mainly related to the sensitivity of cancer cells, the concentration of ADR, and the microcirculation of micrometastases or cancer clusters in the liver. VX2 cancer has high sensitivity to ADR [2]. The concentration of ADR has been demonstrated to be significantly higher after portal than peripheral injection [2]. Micrometastases or clusters of cancer cells depend mainly on the portal circulation, becoming more dependent on the arterial than the portal circulation as they grow [6]. Thus, recurrence is thought to be more effectively suppressed by portal than peripheral injection. The additive effect of peripheral plus portal injection seems to act on the primary lesions and retard the metastases. In the present study, it is also suggested that inadequate doses and inappropriate timing of peripheral injection can promote liver recurrence. The mechanism is unclear, but cancer cells in the liver seem to be promoted by depression of the host defense mechanism against cancer induced by ADR itself.

Although our results in the VX2 animal model with high sensitivity of ADR may not necessarily be applicable to humans, postoperative portal injection or an appropriate combination of preoperative peripheral plus postoperative portal injection of anticancer agents including ADR may be useful as adjuvant chemotherapy for the prophylaxis of liver recurrence in recently clarified patients with high risk of hepatic recurrence, as well as for patients undergoing resection of liver metastatic or recurrent nodules. However, preoperative systemic injection of anticancer agents as adjuvant chemotherapy should be carefully performed with caution, because adverse effects may occur.

REFERENCES

1. Taylor I, Machin D, Mullee M, Trotter G, Cooke T, West C (1985) A randomized controlled trial of adjuvant portal vein cytotoxic perfusion in colorectal cancer. Br J Surg 75:359-363
2. Tabuchi Y, Nakae S, Nakamura T, Saitoh Y (1990) Prophylactic effects of intraportal administration of mitomycin C(MMC) and adriamycin(ADR) on experimental liver metastases. Bull Allied Med Sci(Kobe) 6:7-13
3. Tabuchi Y, Nakamura T, Saitoh Y (1991) Liver metastases induced by implantation of VX2 cancer into the gastrointestine. J Surg Res 50:216-222
4. Fisher ER, Turnbull RB (1955) The cytogenetic demonstration and significance of tumor cells in the mesenteric venous blood in patients with colorectal carcimona. Surg Gynecol Obstet 100:102-108
5. Tabuchi Y, Sakane M, Tada Y, Nakamura T, Saitoh Y (1992) Induction of experimental model with a high frequency of liver metastases and recurrence from colonic VX2 cancer lesions. Bull Allied Med Sci(Kobe) 8:49-60
6. Guilem EB, Varona AA, Vanaclocha FV (1989) Selective implantation and growth in rats and mice of experimental liver metastasis in acinar zone one. Cancer Res 49: 4003-4010

Effect of OK-432 for Prevention of Spontaneous Metastasis in the Liver

KEITARO KAN, HISAKAZU YAMAGISHI, KOUJI OHMORI, MASAO KOBAYASHI, HIROTAKA KOMICHI, YOSHIYUKI TANAKA, YUJI UEDA, TAKASHI HAYASHI, TAKANOBU UEKI, and TAKAHIRO OKA

The Second Department of Surgery, Kyoto Prefectural University of Medicine, Kyoto, 602 Japan

ABSTRACT

C57BL/6 murine reticulum cell sarcoma M5076 was injected into the left footpad to induce spontaneous metastasis in the liver and other organs. The preventive effect of OK-432 was assessed with this spontaneous metastasis model. Hepatic colony incidence and number were reduced in OK-432-treated mice compared with untreated. In LATA, spleen cells obtained from treated mice showed significantly higher antitumor effects than those from untreated. The survival time of treated mice was significantly longer than that of untreated. These findings suggested that the treatment by intrasplenic administration with OK-432 had cytotoxicity against metastatic tumor cells in the liver.

KEY WORDS : hepatic metastasis, OK-432, M5076 mouse tumor

INTRODUCTION

Metastasis of cancer cells is a characteristic of malignant cancer. Therefore, the prevention and treatment of metastasis is an important factor affecting the prognosis of cancer. In particuler, the liver is a frequent organ of distant metastasis of various cancers such as digestive tract, lung, and breast cancers. M5076 tumor, spontaneously developed reticulum cell sarcoma derived from the mouse overies, is characterized by spontaneous metastasis mainly to the liver and also to other organs such as the spleen, kidneys, and lungs. We produced a spontaneous hepatic metastasis model that is closer to clinical metastasis using this characteristic and evaluated the preventive effects of OK-432 on liver metastasis.

MATERIALS AND METHODS

Animals

Male C57BL/6 (Japan ELC Ltd.) aged 6 weeks (body weight : 20−24 g) were used.

Tumor cells

M5076 tumor cells, reticulum cell sarcoma cells that spontaneously developed in the ovaries in the same strain were used. These cells are characterized by spontaneous metastasis to organs such as the liver, spleen, kidneys, lungs, and overies irrespective of the tumor implantation route [1].

Production of a model of spontaneous hepatic metastasis

M5076 tumor cells (1×10^6 cells/0.05 ml) were inoculated into the mouse footpad. The mice were serially killed and examined for the presence or absence of hepatic metastasis, the number of macroscopic hepatic tumor nodules, the liver weight, and extrahepatic metastasis. In addition, the tumor-bearing limb was serially amputated. The animals were killed 21 days after amputation, and similar examination was performed.

Treatment

a. Drug and administration route
OK-432 (Chugai Pharmaceutical Co.) was used.
The spleen was subcutanously relocated and fixed,
and the drug was percutaneously injected into the
spleen.
b. Drug administration schedule (Table 1)
The mouse spleen was subcutaneously relocated
with pedicles and fixed on Day-14. On Day 0, the
tumor $(1 \times 10^6$ cells/0.05 ml) was implanted into the
footpad. From Day 7, the mice were intrasplenically
injected with 1 KE of OK-432 (OK-432-treated
group) or physiological saline (untreated group)
for 7 days. The tumor-bearing limb was amputated
on Day 14, and the mice were killed and examined
on Day 35.

In vivo tumor-neutralizing activity of spleen cells

Table 1. Schedule for antitumor effect of OK-432

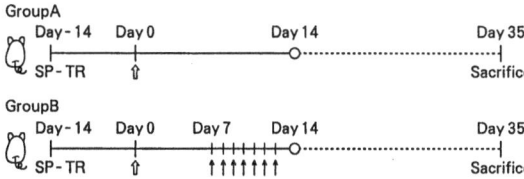

SP-TR : Spleen translocation
⇑ : M5076 1×10^6 cell/0.05ml implantation to foot pad
↑ : OK-432 IKE/0.1ml injection to spleen
—O⋯ : foot amputation performed

1) The spleen of the mice in Groups A and B was implanted in the left
lateral subcutis on Day-14.(SP-TR : Spleen translocation)
2) 1×10^6 M5076 tumor cells were inoculated into the left footpad of
both groups of mice on Day 0.
3) Group A mice were injected with 1KE of OK432 in the spleen from
Day 7 to Day 13, and Group B with saline for the same duration.(↑)
4) In both groups, the tumor-bearing leg was amputated on Day 14
and the mice were killed on Day 35 to enumerate liver colonies.

Spleen cell activity was assessed by local adoptive transfer assay (LATA). Effector cells were prepared
from spleens in each group mice. 1×10^6 effector cells and 1×10^4 M5076 tumor cells (E/T ratio=100:1) were
admixed and inoculated subcutis into native syngeneic mice. Tumor sizes were measured in mean tumor
diameters (mm±S.E.) 21 days after inoculation.

Survival rate

The survival rate in the two groups was evaluated. The period of observation was 70 days after inoculation
of tumor.

RESULTS

Influence of the primary tumor upon the formation of gross metastases

On about Day 21 (the mean tumor diameter in the primary lesion, 9.5 mm), hepatic metastasis was observed
in 5 of the 10 mice and splenic metastasis in 1. On Day 25 (mean tumor diameter in the primary lesion, 10.1
mm), hepatic metastasis was observed in all mice. Death of cancer occurred from Day 28, and most mice
(7/10) died of cancer by Day 35. About this time, kidney and lung metastasis in addition to splenic metastasis were observed.

Pathological findings

Fig. 1 shows the liver, spleen, kidneys, and lungs removed from the mice killed on Day 35. The liver had
been replaced by tumor tissue with nearly fused nodules and markedly swollen. The other organs also
showed swelling and many tumor nodules. The micrograph shows HE staining of a liver section from the
mice killed on Day 14. In the resected liver, no gross metastatic nodule was observed, but formation of a
metastatic focus, probably micrometastasis, was demonstrated by microscopy.

Effect of tumor-bearing time upon the metastases formation

Hepatic metastasis was observed in 1 of the 10 mice after resection of the tumor on Day 4, 3 after resection
on Day 7, 7 after resection on Day 14, and all 10 after resection on Day 18 or later.

Treatment effects

In the OK-432-treated group, the rate of metastasis to the liver was 2/10 (20%), and the average incidence of metastasis was 0.2. On the other hand, in the untreated group, the rate of metastasis to the liver was 8/10 (80%), and the average incidence of metastasis was 26. OK-432 was effective in the prevention of metastasis to the liver (P<0.01).

Spleen cell activity

The tumor size 21 days after inoculation of the tumor cells was 6.5±0.5 mm in the OK-432-treated group and 9.4±0.2 mm in the untreated group. These results showed that spleen cells with significantly higher antitumor neutralization activity were induced in the treated group than in the untreated group.

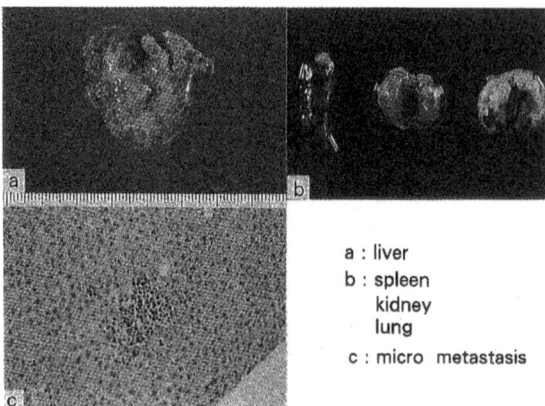

a : liver
b : spleen
    kidney
    lung
c : micro metastasis

Fig. 1   Pathological findings

Survival rate

In the OK-432-treated group, the mean survival time was 68.3±1.0 days, and in the untreated group, the time was 58.5±2.9 days. The difference in survival time was significant.

DISCUSSION

Development of the liver metastasis after operation is an important factor affecting the prognosis. In particuler, in patients treated by curative resection of digestive tract cancer, liver metastasis markedly affects the prognosis, and its prevention and treatment are major problems. In patients showing recurrence of hepatic metastasis after curative resection, hepatic micrometastasis may have already been present at the time of operation. We consider that metastasis can be prevented and inhibited, if it is at this micrometastasis stage, by administering a BRM with anti-tumor action to the tumor-bearing host. We previously evaluated the preventive effects of OK-432 on metastasis using MCA-38 tumor, colon adenocarcinoma in the same strain, in an artificial liver metastasis model [2]. In this study, we produced a spontaneous liver metastasis model that is closer to clinical metastasis and evaluated the preventive effects of OK-432 on metastasis. As the administration route, intrasplenic administration was performed because this route was the most effective in the artificial hepatic metastasis model. The results in the OK-432-treated group were as follows : 1) the rate as well as incidence of liver metastasis were reduced, 2) splenic cells with marked tumor neutralizing activity were induced, 3) the survival rate increased. These findings suggested the effectiveness of preoperative intrasplenic OK-432 administration in the tumor-bearing host. Further studies are planned with changes in the administration route, time, and dose of OK-432 to determine the administration method most appropriate for clinical application.

REFERENCES

1. Ian R. Hart, James E. Talmadge, Isaiah J. Fidler (1981) Metastatic Behavior of a Murine Reticulum Cell Sarcoma Exhibiting Organ-specific Growth. Cancer Reserch 41 : 1281−1287
2. Ohmori K, Yamagishi H, Kan K (1992) Experimental Study on Effects of BRM on Artifical Liver Metastasis. BIOTHERAPY 6 (5) : 759−761

Effects of Continuous Venous or Portal Administration of Carboplatin Against VX$_2$ Tumor Metastasizing to the Liver

KAZUMI TAKEUCHI, HIROKI TANIGUCHI, ATSUSHI OGURO, YASUO UESHIMA, KEIGO MIYATA, HIROSHI KOYAMA, HIROKI TANAKA, and TOSHIO TAKAHASHI

First Department of Surgery, Kyoto Prefectural University of Medicine, Kyoto, 602 Japan

ABSTRACT

To prevent the liver metastases induced by inoculating 1×10^6 VX2 cells into the mesenteric vein of rabbits, carboplatin (7 mg/kg) was administered continuously for 7 days via either the portal or jugular vein with mini osmotic pump. On 14 days after inoculation, untreated rabbits had 126.2 ± 19.2 (mean±s.e.) metastatic colonies on the surface of their livers, whereas those receiving the carboplatin via the mesenteric or jugular vein had substantially fewer with only 22.8 ± 9.5 and 50.4 ± 6.3 colonies, respectively. These results suggest that the continuous venous administration of carboplatin (especially via the portal vein) may be an effective means for treating liver metastases arising from colorectal cancers.

Key words: Liver metastasis, Mini osmotic pump, Continuous administration, Carboplatin, VX2 tumor

INTRODUCTION

The incidence of colorectal cancer is increasing recently in Japan. Even though postoperative results have improved, deaths due to recurrent tumor growth, particularly metastasis in the liver, after curative surgery are fairly common. The majority of these liver metastases were probably present at the time of surgery, but remained occult to pre- or intra-operative investigation. In some cases the tumor cells probably disseminated into the portal circulation at the time of surgery. The micrometastases thus formed, are initially maintained by portal blood flow until new capillaries are able to sprout from the hepatic artery. Thus, it is logical to assume that the chemotherapeutic agents administered by the portal venous route would help prevent the establishment of live metastases in the postoperative period. To verify this suggestion we administered carboplatin into the portal vein of rabbits with a mini-osmotic pump for 7 days after having injected VX2 cancer cells into the mesenteric vein.

MATERIALS AND METHOD

White rabbits weighing 2.5–2.8 kg were used in this experiments.
A rabbit transplantable experimental tumor, the VX2 carcinoma cell line, was maintained by successive transplantation of 0.3 mg of these cells into subcapsular parenchyma of the spleen with an 18-gauge needle bimonthly. Two weeks after inoculation the tumors were isolated under sterile conditions, minced with scissors, and gently stirred in Hank's solution. After filtration through a stainless steel filter 1×10^6 VX2 cells were injected into the mesenteric vein through a midline laparotomy in pentobarbital sodium (30 mg/kg, i.v.) anesthetized rabbits.

Experiment 1; Administration of carboplatin after tumor implantation

After tumor implantation, the rabbits were separated into the following three groups.
Control (5 rabbits). Not treated after tumor implantation.
Group 1 (5 rabbits). Immediately after the VX2 carcinoma cell injection, a catheter tube was inserted into the mesenteric vein. Carboplatin (7 mg/kg) was administered continuously for 7 days using a mini osmotic pump (ALZET, model 2ML1)
Group 2 (5 rabbits). Immediately after the VX2 carcinoma cell injection, a catheter tube was inserted into the left external jugular vein. Carbopaltin was administered as in Group 1.
On day 14, the livers of the rabbits were removed and weighed, and the number of metastatic colonies on the surface was counted.

Experiment 2; Quantitative analysis of platinum concentration in organs and plasma

On 14 days after portal implantation of VX2, rabbits were used to assess the platinum concentrations in various organs after 4 days of continuous infusion of carboplatin (7 mg/kg) into the portal (n=5) or jugular (n=5) vein using mini osmotic pump.   Through a laparotomy performed under pentobarbital sodium anaesthesia, liver metastases, normal liver, heart, lung, kidney, femoral muscle samples, as well as blood from portal vein and abdominal aorta, were taken.   The blood was centrifuged and plasma was ultrafiltrated for 20 min with an Amicon Centrifree micropartition system provided with YMT membranes (Amicon, Oosterhout, The Netherlands).   Platinum concentrations in these organs, plasma, and plasma ultrafiltrate (free Pt) were determined by flameless atomic absorption spectrometry.

The nominal performance of the mini osmotic pump used in this study at 37°c is as follows: Pumping rate, 10.0 l/hr; Duration, 7 days; Reservoir volume, 2000 μl.

RESULTS

1.The numbers of metastatic colonies

On 14 days after implantation of VX2, metastatic colonies, 2–5 mm in diameter were detected macroscopically on the surface of the liver (Fig 1).   The number of macroscopic metastatic colonies counted on the surface of livers of carboplatin treated rabbits was substantially less than in untreated rabbits.   Rabbits that received carboplatin via the portal vein (group 1) had significantly fewer colonies than those treated through the jugular vein (Fig 2).

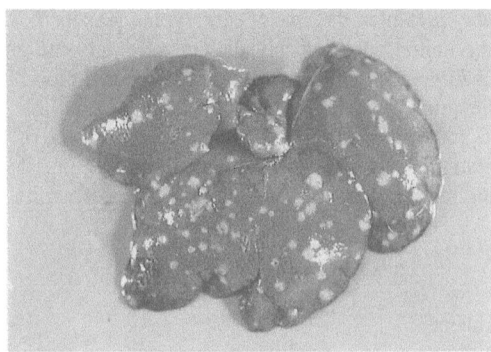

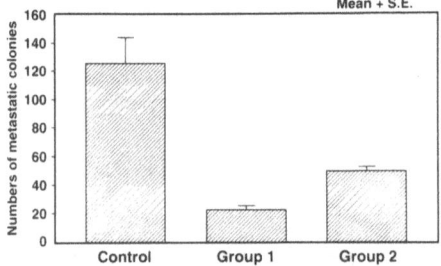

Fig.1   Macroscopic   metastatic   colonies   were detected on the surface of the liver on 14 days after VX2 carcinoma cell implantation.

Fig.2   The number of metastatic colonies of treated rabbits (Group 1 and Group 2) was substantially less than in control group. (P<0.01)   Portal administration group had significantly fewer colonies than jugular administration group.   (P<0.01)

2.Platinum concentrations

The platinum concentrations in various organs after 4 days of continuous carboplatin treatment are shown in Fig 3. Administration of the drug via the portal vein resulted in significantly higher accumulations of platinum in the metastatic colonies, normal liver tissue and kidney than in heart, lung, and femoral muscle. With those rabbits receiving carboplatin via the jugular vein the platinum concentrations were similar in all tissues with the exception of kidney which had substantially higher amounts of the metal.   With the two routes of administration were compared no significant differences were noted in the platinum concentrations in the heart, lung, kidney, and femoral muscle. However, the levels of platinum were significantly greater in the metastatic colonies and normal liver when the drug was administered via the portal vein.

The concentrations of platinum in the plasma and plasma ultrafiltrate (free Pt) of portal and arterial blood samples were essentially the same for either route of administration (Fig. 4).

However, a significantly higher portal plasma platinum concentration was noted in rabbits receiving drugs via the portal vein when compared to the jugular route of administration.

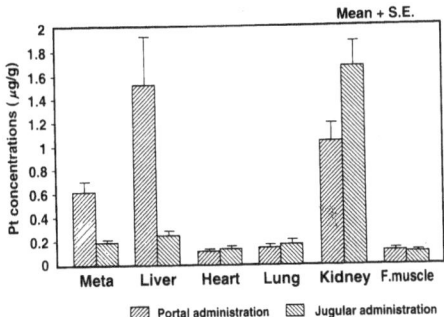

Fig.3 Pt concentrations in organs after continuous
administration of carboplatin.

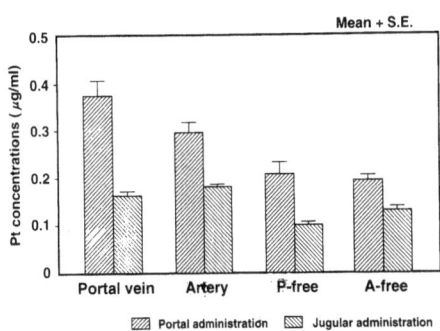

Fig.4 Pt concentrations in the plasma and plasma
ultrafiltrate after continuous administration of
carboplatin.

DISCUSSION

With this study we tested the hypothesis that continuous venous administration of carboplatin would reduce the incidence of liver metastasis. In addition, we investigate the accumulation of platinum in various organs following portal or jugular administration of the drug. Although it has been reported that the cells responsible for metastatic development arrive via the hepatic artery [1], other have suggested that the portal vein might be more important in seeding micrometastases [2]. From these considerations the administration of drugs into the portal vein may be more useful for treating early stage metastases before they develop into cancer nodules. In fact Taylor and coworkers [3] have shown that the administration of 5-Fluorouracil into the portal vein reduced the incidence of hepatic metastasis following surgical removal of colorectal cancers. Our results show that the accumulation of platinum in the liver probably contributes to the substantial reduction in the number of metastatic colonies. Since the amount of platinum that accumulates in other organs was similar following portal or jugular vein infusion of carboplatin the side effects of this drug are probably independent of the route of administration.

Recent studies with low dose cisplatin and continuous infusion of 5-FU chemotherapy have been encouraging [4,5]. In fact, the study of Cantrell and coworkers [5] suggests that continuous infusion of 5-FU with weekly treatments of cisplatin was more effective for metastatic colorectal cancer than expected. Since carboplatin, a second generation platinum coordination complex, has significantly less toxicity than cisplatin [6], it may be useful to consider continuous infusion of the carboplatin instead of the weekly low dose cisplatin. As a follow up to the present study we are presently examining the efficacy of continuous portal infusion of 5-FU and carboplatin in preventing VX2 metastasis in the liver of rabbits.

REFERENCES

1. Breedes, C., and Young, G. (1954) The blood supply of neoplasms in the liver. AJR 30:969–985
2. Daido, R., Okanishi, S., Tamura, T., et al, (1973) Experimental studies of the liver metastasis induced by VX2. J. Kyoto Pref. Univ. Med., 82:361–366
3. Taylor, I., Machin, D., Mullee, M., et al, (1985) A randomized controlled trial of adjuvant portal vein cytotoxic perfusion in colorectal cancer. Br. J. Surg. 72:359–363
4. Burton, GV., Grant, JP., Bedrosian C. (1987) Cisplatin and continuous infusion 5-FU chemotherapy in metastatic colon cancer. Proc Am Soc Clin Oncol 6:85
5. Cantrell Jr, JE., Hart, RD, Taylor, RF., (1987) Pilot trial of prolonged continuous infusion 5-fluorouracil and weekly cisplatin in advanced colorectal cancer. Cancer Treat Rep 71:615–618
6. Mulder, POM., De Vries, EGE., et al, (1990) Pharmacokinetics of carboplatin at a dose of $750 mgm^{-2}$ divided over three consecutive days. Br. J. Cancer 61:460–464

Experimental Study on the Efficacy of Intrahepatic Arterial and Portal Venous Infusion of Anticancer Drugs to Inhibit the Growth of Portally Inoculated VX-2 Carcinoma

Masami Hoshino, Yoshihisa Koyama, Wataru Igarashi, Toshiyuki Ono, Yuichi Hatakeyama, and Rikiya Abe

Second Department of Surgery, Fukushima Medical College, Fukushima, 960-12 Japan

ABSTRACT

To evaluate the efficacy of intraarterial and portal venous infusion of anticancer drugs to inhibit the growth of portally inoculated VX-2 tumor cells (1×10^7), adriamycin (1mg/kg) was administered into the hepatic artery (HA) and portal vein (PV) at 3'rd, 5'th, 7th days (group 1), immediately, 2'nd, 4'th days (group 2) after tumor cell inoculation respectively, and no adriamycin was administered as the control group. The number of tumor nodules on the whole liver surface at three weeks after tumor inoculation in the control, HA. group 1, PV. group 1, HA. group 2 and PV. group 2 was 409 ± 138.5, 46.3 ± 42.4, 130.7 ± 77.7, 0.0 ± 0.0, and 10.5 ± 5.7 respectively.

KEY WORDS: VX-2 liver cancer, hepatic arterial infusion, portal venous infusion, adriamycin

INTRODUCTION

Large hepatectomy are now successfully performed with little risk, including metastatic liver cancer. A 5-year over-all survival rate of the hepatectomized patients with metastatic colorectal cancer achieved about 25%. However, Alberto et al[1] reported that 26 of the 35 hepatectomized patients (74%) had recurrent disease after a mean follow up 25.8 months, and the site of recurrence was the residual liver of 23 patients (83%). Therefore, to inhibit the growth of the cancer cells within the residual liver is the most essential to prevent recurrence. The experimental study was carried out to compare the efficacy of either hepatic arterial or portal venous infusion of anticancer drugs, for preventing the recurrence of the residual liver after hepatectomized patients.

MATERIALS AND METHODS

Tumor Inoculation

The VX-2 tumor was maintained through serial inoculating into the hind limb muscle of Japan white rabbits. The tumor fragments of VX-2 carcinoma excised, were minced and passed through 40 micrometer nylon mesh. Tumor cells were suspended in physiological saline (1×10^7 cells/5ml) and tumor cell suspension was inoculated through the portal vein to the liver. At three weeks after inoculation of VX-2 tumor cells, a large number of the multiple nodules of VX-2 carcinoma were appeared on the liver.

Hepatic arterial and Portal venous infusion

Animals used in the experiment were 23. The laparotomy was carried out through midline incision under the general anesthesia by intravenous injection of penthobarbital sodium (39mg/kg). A polyethylene catheter with 0.61 mm diameter(PE10, Becton) was inserted through the gastroduodenal artery to the hepatic artery or a 3Fr, polyethylene catheter through the ileocaecal vein to the portal vein and tightly fixed. The catheters outside of the peritoneal cavity were kept between the skin and muscle layer, led to the posterior neck, and brought out through the skin. The drug infusions were postoperatively performed through this catheter to hepatic artery or portal vein.

Adriamycin (ADR, 1mg/kg) dissolved in physiological saline was infused to the liver as following four methods. Group 1A: via HA at 3'rd, 5'th and 7th days, Group 1P: via PV at the same time as group 1A, Group 2A: via HA at immediately, 2'nd and 4th days and Group 2P: via PV at the same time as group 2A after tumor inoculation. No ADR was injected in the control group. At three weeks after tumor inoculation, rabbits were sacrificed and the number of the tumor nodules on the whole liver surface were counted.

Data was analyzed by student's t test. A p-value of <0.05 was interpreted as statistically significant.

RESULTS

The number of the tumor nodules on the whole liver surface was 409.8 ± 138.5 in the control group, 46.3 ± 42.4 in the group 1A, 130.7 ± 77.7 in the group 1P, 0.0 ± 0.0 in the group 2A and 10.5 ± 5.7 in the group 2P. Hepatic arterial or portal venous infusion of ADR were performed at the same time in the group 1A and 1P, or in the group 2A and 2P respectively. The administration of ADR reduced significantly the number of the VX-2 tumor nodules on the liver surface, comparing with that in the control group ($p=0.01$ or $p<0.05$). Hepatic arterial infusion of ADR tended to decrease the number of the tumor nodules more than portal venous infusion on any time of ADR administration (group 1P>group 1A, $p<0.1$). The tumor growth was more strongly inhibited in the animals of ADM was administered earlier after the tumor inoculation (group 1) than in the group 2(group 1P>group 2P, $p=0.05$). On group which ADM administration was done through intrahepatic artery immediately after the tumor inoculation, no tumor growth were observed on whole liver surface (Table 1).

Fig. 1, Fig. 2 shows macroscopic appearance of the liver in the group 1 and 2 respectively

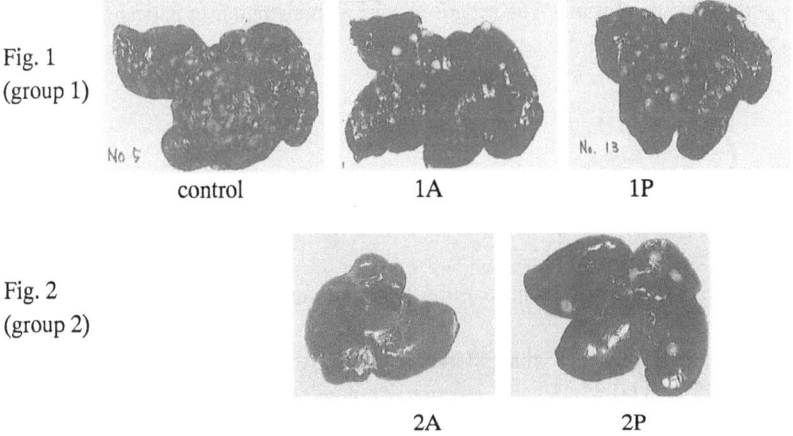

Fig. 1
(group 1)

control   1A   1P

Fig. 2
(group 2)

2A   2P

Table 1 Number of the tumor nodules on the liver surface in the control and each groups

Group	injectional route	time to start injection	number of tumor nodules
Control(n=6)			409.8 ± 138.5
1A(n=4)	H.A	third days	46.3 ± 42.4
1P(n=4)	P.V	third days	130.0 ± 77.7
2A(n=3)	H.A	immediately	0.0 ± 0.0
2P(n=4)	P.V	immediately	10.5 ± 5.7

DISCUSSION

It has been reported that the liver metastasis is occurred in 10 to 25 percent of patients with colorectal carcinoma[2]. Surgical resection is chosen as the most effective treatment for patient with hepatic metastasis and the reported 5-year survival rate have ranged from 21 to 52%[3][4]. However, More than half of these hepatectomized patients will ultimately develop a recurrent diseases. More than 40% of recurrence after hepatectomy are confined to the liver alone and 20% involve both the remaining liver and extrahepatic organs. Therefore, adjuvant chemotherapy is thought to be important to prevent the recurrence after hepatectomy. The liver metastases are theoretically separated to synchronous and metachronous metastases by the detection time of the disease. Although metachronous metastases have been thought resulting from scattering of the tumor cells to the portal vein at the operating procedure, recently the hypothesis that early microscopic detectable metastases (micrometases) is already present in the liver at the time of primary operation is also reported[5]. Therefore, following two studies are required to evaluate the method of adjuvant chemotherapy for preventing metachronous metastases, 1)how to inhibit the growth of tumor cells scattered to the portal vein at the time of operating procedure, 2) how to inhibit the growth of micrometastases. Tumor cells were observed to invade to the liver tissue through vessel wall at 24 hours after tumor cells inoculation into the portal vein. In our experiment, micrometastases are present in the liver at 3'rd days after tumor inoculation to the portal vein. The number of tumor nodules on the liver surface was decreased by ADR administration, irrespective of whether the injectional route or the time. Especially hepatic arterial injection immediately after tumor inoculation was the most effective to inhibit the tumor growth than another injectional methods. If microscopic liver metastases might occur by means of portal vasculization[6], drug infusion via the portal vein is thought be the most appropriate. However, depends upon the neovascularization accompanying tumor growth within the liver, the portal supply may be obliterated and the hepatic arterial supply then becomes predominant at the stage of small, detectable disease[7]. In our experiment, more remarkable decrease of the number of tumor nodules by the hepatic arterial administration of ADR was obtained than by the portal venous infusion. The hepatic arterial administration of anticancer drugs as soon as possible after hepatectomy was the most effective way to decrease the rate of recurrence in the remaining liver.

REFERENCES

1. Holom A, Bradley E, Aldrete J (1988) Hepatic resection of metastasis from colorectal carcinoma. Ann Surg 209:428–434

2. Bestsson G, Corlson G, Hafstrom L et al (1981) Natural history of patients with untreated liver metastases from colorectal. Cancer 141:585–598

3. Iwatsuki S, Shan BW Jr, Starzl TE (1983) Experience with 150 liver resection. Ann Surg 197:245–253

4. Avguse DA, Sugarbaker PH, Ottow RT et al (1985) Hepatic resection of colorectal metastases: Influence of clinical factors and adjuvant intraperitoneal 5–fluorouracil via Tenkhoff catheter on survival. Ann Surg 147:554–559

5. Liotta LA, Stevenson WGS (1989) Principles of molecular cell biology of cancer: cancer metastases. In Cancer, Principles and Practice of Oncology (ed. by Devita Jr. Vt., Hellman S. and Rossenberg SA), 3rd Edition, Lippincot, Philadelphia, pp.98–115

6. Ensminger WD, Gyves JW (1983) Clinical pharmacology of hepatic arterial chemotherapy. Semin Oncol 10:176–182

7. Daly JM, Kemeny N, Sigurdson E, et al (1987) Regional infusion of colorectal hepatic metastase– a randmized trial comparing the hepatic artery with portal vein. Arch Surg, 122:1273–1277

Anti-Angiogenic Agent, AGM-1470 Inhibited Liver Metastasis of VX2 Carcinoma in Rabbits

Yasushi Suganuma, Toshio Takahashi, Hiroki Taniguchi, Kazumi Takeuchi, Yasuo Ueshima, and Hiroki Tanaka

First Department of Surgery, Kyoto Prefectural University of Medicine, Kyoto, 602 Japan

ABSTRACT

AGM-1470 (TNP-470), exhibits inhibitory activity on endothelium. The agent inhibits DNA synthesis of endothelium. In tumor tissue, the agent inhibits proliferation of tumor induced endothelium then causes anti-tumor effect. The activity was studied on a VX2 carcinoma metastasized to the liver in rabbits. VX2 carcinoma cells were injected into the spleen to cause liver metastasis via the portal vein. AGM-1470 was administrated intravenously. The number of metastasized tumor on the liver in administrated group was less than in the control group.($p<0.05$) We concluded that AGM-1470 suppresses the tumor cell growth inhibiting tumor neovascularization.

KEY WORDS: AGM-1470 (TNP-470), anti-angiogenesis, liver metastasis, VX2 carcinoma

INTRODUCTION

Tumors induces neovascularization for its growth (1). Inhibition of angiogenesis has a potency of anti-tumor effect (2). At an early phase of tumor metastasis, angiogenesis plays an important role for its growth. Prophylactic action for tumor metastasis is expected of anti-angiogenic agent. Ingber et al. reported a novel angiogenesis inhibitor, fumagillin, a natural product of Asprgillus fumigatus (3). They so showed that AGM-1470(O-(chloroacetyl-carbonyl)fumagillol), the new synthetic analog of fumagillin, exhibit potent inhibitory activity on endothelial cell and solid tumor (4). The anti-angiogenic activity of this product inhibits tumor growth. This activity will inhibits growth of malignant neoplasm and its metastasis. The inhibitory activity of this product was explored on a VX2 carcinoma metastasized to the liver in rabbits.

MATERIALS AND METHODS

Anti-angiogenic agent. AGM-1470(O-(chloroacetyl- carbonyl)fumagilol):synthetic analog of fumagillin which is a natural product of Aspergillus fumigatus obtained from Takeda chemical Industries, Ltd. (Osaka, Japan)

Animals and tumor. Fourteen Japanese white rabbits weighing 2.5 to 3.0 kg were used for this study. VX2 carcinoma was obtained fresh from a donor rabbit and minced in Hank's balanced salt solution (HBSS), filtering it through a mesh stainless gauze. The cells were suspended in HBSS to a concentration of 4.0×10^6 per ml.

Tumor cell inoculation. Rabbits were anesthetized by an intravenous injection of pentobarbital sodium (30 mg/kg) and laparotomy was performed. The 1.0×10^6 cells of VX2 carcinoma in HBSS suspension was injected via a 24-gauge needle into the subcapsular parenchyma of the spleen to cause liver metastasis via portal route (5).

Administration of the agent. Fourteen rabbits were classified into 2 groups: Group A (7 rabbits): 5.0mg of AGM-1470 was administrated intravenously every two days from the second day of tumor inoculation(day 2) to the tenth day(day 10). Group C (7 rabbits): No agent was administrated for control.

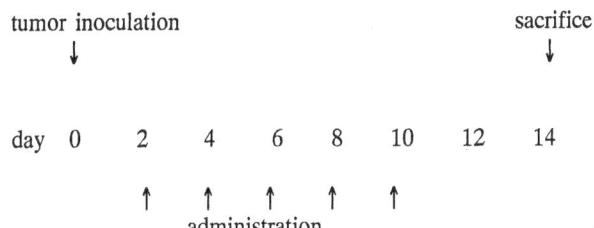

729

Evaluation of the effect of the agent. On the day 14, rabbits were sacrificed and then the number of the tumor metastasized on the surface of the liver was counted macroscopically. The number was used for the evaluation.
Statistical analysis. In each group, results of the 2 rabbits of which metastasis is the most and the least were excluded and the average of 5 results were used for the statistical analysis. Student's t-test was used for the analysis.
Evaluation of the effect of the agent. On the day 14, rabbits were sacrificed and then the number of the tumor metastasized on the surface of the liver was counted macroscopically. The number was used for the evaluation.Student's t-test was used for the analysis.

RESULTS

Number of the tumor metastasized to the liver

Administrated	89.6±70.2	*
Control	226±59.0	

mean±SD   * p<0.05 versus the control

Although the macroscopic examination was performed to look for metastasis in the inner area of the liver, all tumor was located at subcapsular parenchyma of the liver.

DISCUSSION

Neoplasm induces neovascularization for growth (1). The angiogenesis also contributes to growth of metastatic tumor. In avascular environment, for example the anterior chamber of the eye, metastatic growth of retinoblastoma is restricted (6). The concept that "tumor growth is angiogenic dependent" was first proposed in 1971 by Folkman et al.(2). The supporting evidences for this hypothesis have been reported (7-9). The hypothesis is also applied to metastatic tumor. A decreased rate of tumor angiogenesis associated with a decreased rate of metastasis (10). If angiogenesis is suppressed in early phase of tumor metastasis, growth of metastatic tumor will be inhibited. From this perspective, prophylactic action for tumor metastasis is expected in angiogenic inhibition.

Anti-tumor effect of anti-angiogenic agents were previously reported, for example heparin, steroids (11), polysaccharide (11-12), tetracycline (12-13) or antibody targeting (14). AGM-1470(molecular weight: 401.89) is a synthetic analog of fumagillin. Fumagillin was derived from *Aspergillus fumigatus* as an anti-fungal drug (15). Ingber *et al.* found its anti-angiogenic effect (3). After then, AGM-1470 was synthesized as an anti-angiogenic drug. AGM-1470, also fumagillin has a clear and simple anti-angiogenic effect on the endothelium itself and an effective anti-tumor action unlike other anti-angiogenic drugs previously reported (3-4). In vitro, AGM-1470 inhibits [^{3}H]-thymidine uptake of endothelial cell at the concentration of suppressing cell proliferation. In vivo, AGM-1470 decreases the BrdU labeling index of endothelial cell belongs to the tumor more than of tumor cell itself. From these distinctive pharmacokinetics, AGM-1470 inhibits neovasularization to suppress tumor growth. AGM-1470 has a low molecular weight and inhibits specific an endothelium, not tumor tissue.

We made up the liver metastasis model of rabbits. In this model, the"primary" lesion is implanted tumor on the spleen and the metastasis is caused via the portal vein. We think this model is physiological. In this experimental model, AGM-1470 inhibits VX2 liver metastasis. This result suggests AGM-1470 suppressed endothelial cell proliferation at the site of metastasis to inhibit its growth. This findings support the hypothesis that the anti-angiogenic action of AGM-1470 inhibited the neovascularization to suppress the tumor cell growth in its early phase.

A metastatic tumor from the primary lesion located in an organ that is drained into the portal system tends to induce a complex vasculature composed of arterial and portal circulation (16-18). The metastatic liver tumor is supplied by both arterial and portal systems but this agent will inhibit neovascularization of both systems, arteries and portal veins. So this agent is expected to have no specificity on the route of administration. A prophylactic treatment of cancer metastasis has not been established. If we can inhibit the growth of cancer in its early phase, a radical treatment of cancer metastasis will be established. Compare with other anti-tumor drugs, AGM-1470 is a novel anti-tumor agent for prophylactic treatment in following points.

1) The agent has no cytotoxic or cytostatic effect except on the newly forming vasculature. 2) The agent is expected to have no specificity on any cancer because the target of the agent is the endothelium of tumor vessels not tumor cell itself. AGM-1470 has a potency to be a clue to the prophylactic cancer treatment. We must make further examination for dose, drug delivery system and side effect of AGM-1470 to provide this agent has the potency.

REFERENCES

1) Wood, S., Jr.(1958) Pathogenesis of metastasis formation observed in vivo in the rabbit ear chamber
Arch. Pathol. *66*: 550-568

2) Folkman, J. (1971) Tumor angiogenesis: Therapeutic implications.
N. Engl. J. Med. *285*: 1182-1186

3) Ingber, D., Fujita, T., Kishimoto, S., Sudo, K., Kanamatsu, T., Brem, H., and Folkman, J. (1990) Synthetic analogues of fumagillin that inhibit angiogenesis and suppress tumor growth
Nature *348*: 555-557

4) Kusaka, M., Sudo, K., Fujita, T., Shogo, M., Itoh, F., Ingber,D., and Folkman, J. (1991) Potent anti-angiogenic action of AGM- 1470: comparison to the fumagillin parent
Biochem. Biophys. Res. Commun. *174*: 1070-1076, 1991

5) Tsukuda, N., Taniguchi, H., Daidoh, T., Itoh, A., Oguro, A., Sawai, K. and Takahashi, T.
Antitumor effect of intra-arterial injection of sclerosing agents against VX2 tumor metastasizing to the liver
Reg. Cancer Treat. *4*: 132-135, 1991

6) Starkey J. R, Crowle P. K. and Taubenberger, S. Mast-cell- deficient W/Wv mice exhibit a decreased rate of tumor angiogenesis.
Int.J.Cancer *42*: 48-52,1988

7) Teicher, B. A., Sotomyor, E. A. and Zhen D. H. Antiangiogenic agents potentiate cytotoxic cancer therapies against primary and metastatic disease
Cancer Res. *52*: 6702-6704, 1992

8) Tanaka, N. G., Sakamoto, N., Inoue, K., Kadoya, S., Ogawa, H.and Osada, Y. Antitumor effects of an antiangiogenic polysaccharide from an arthobactor species with or without a steroid.
Cancer Res. *49*: 6727-6730, 1989

9) Tamrgo, R. J., Bok, R. A. and Brem, H. Angiogenesis inhibition by minocycline.
Cancer Res. *51*: 672-675, 1991

10) Burrows, F. J., Watanabe, Y. and Thorpe, P.E., A murine model for antibody-directed targeting of vascular endothelial cells in solid tumor
Cancer Res. *52*: 5954-5962, 1992

11) Yamamoto, T., Kusaka, M., Sudo, K., Fujita, T.,

Biotherapy *6*: 501, 1992

12) Taniguchi, H., Daidoh, T., Shioaki, Y. and Takahashi, T. Blood supply and drug delivery to primary and secondary human liver cancers studied with in vivo bromodeoxyuridine labeling.
Cancer *71*: 50-55, 1993

13) Ackerman, N. B. The blood supply of experimental liver metastasis. IV. Changes in vascularity with increasing tumor growth.
Surgery *75*: 589-596, 1974

14) Healy, J. E., Jr. Vascular patterns in human metastatic liver tumors.
Surg. Gynecol. Obstet. *120*: 1187-1193, 1955

Anticancer Effects of an Angiogenesis Inhibitor (TNP-470) After Arterial Injection in Rabbits Bearing VX-2 Carcinoma

Hiroaki Okada, Shigeo Yanai, Yuji Kuge, Kazuhiro Saito, Yayoi Inoue, Shigeru Kamei, and Hajime Toguchi

DDS Research Laboratories, Pharmaceutical Research Division, Takeda Chemical Industries, Ltd., Osaka, 532 Japan

ABSTRACT

TNP-470, an angiogenesis inhibitor, is a new type of anticancer drug that inhibits tumor neovascularization which is critical to tumor growth. Chemoembolization using TNP-470 microspheres prepared with a biodegradable polymer provided striking regression of the tumor, but growth was again observed 1 week after injection. TNP-470 dissolved in Lipiodol (a liquid lymphographic agent) or MIGLYOL 812 (medium-chain triglycerides) caused persistent suppression of the tumor growth for 2 or 3 weeks after a single intraarterial injection due to sustained drug release from the preparation. Coadministration of TNP-470 and a conventional chemotherapeutic agent resulted in enhanced antitumor effects.

KEY WORDS: TNP-470, angiogenesis inhibitor, chemoembolization, rabbit VX-2 carcinoma, medium-chain triglycerides

INTRODUCTION

The angiogenesis inhibitor TNP-470, 6-O-(N-chloroacetylcarbamoyl)-fumagillol (Fig. 1), is a new type of anticancer drug that inhibits the neovascularization which is critical to tumor growth and blocks the supply of nutrients to the tumor [1-3]. Chemoembolization is a useful cancer treatment which combines chemotherapy and tumor devascularization by intraarterial (i.a.) injection of an chemotherapeutic agent together with an embolizing material. This treatment achieves strong antitumor activity with less severe systemic side effects due to the regional increase in drug concentration in the tumor and the blockage of the nutrient supply. For enhanced antitumor activity, we combined the physical blockage of the nutrient supply achieved by embolization with chemical blockage of the nutrient supply using TNP-470. In a previous study, we found that chemoembolization using TNP-470 microspheres (msp.) prepared with a biodegradable polymer, poly(DL-lactic/glycolic acid) (PLGA), caused striking tumor regression in rabbits bearing VX-2 squamous cell carcinoma after a single injection into the femoral artery running to the tumor [4, 5]. In present study, the antitumor effects of i.a. injection of TNP-470 dissolved in several injectable oils were examined in the rabbit tumor model. The antitumor activity of TNP-470 coadministered with conventional chemotherapeutic agents, doxorubicin hydrochloride (ADM) or mitomicin C (MMC), was also evaluated.

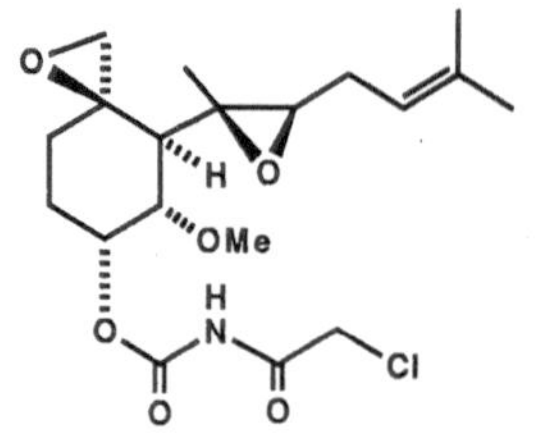

Fig. 1   Chemical structure of TNP-470

MATERIALS AND METHODS

Preparation of Microspheres and Oil Solution

TNP-470 was synthesized in the Production Research Laboratories of Takeda Chemical Ind. Microspheres were prepared using PLGA (lactic/glycolic ratio=3/1, m.w.=6800; purchased from Wako Chemical Ind.) by an in-water drying method as previously described [5]. Microspheres with a diameter of 53 to 125 μm were used. Lipiodol (LPD, Gurbert Lab., Aulnay-Sous-Bois, France), sesame oil (Takemoto Yushi, Aichi, Japan) and MCT (caprilic and capric acid triglycerides, MIGLYOL 812, Huls A.G., Marl, Germany) were utilized for the oil based preparations.

In vitro Release Test

The amount of TNP-470 remaining in msp. (50 mg) and oil preparations (1 ml) was determined after dispersion in pH 7.0 phosphate buffer (5 ml) containing 0.05% Tween 80 (Kao, Tokyo, Japan) at 37 °C. The initial TNP-470 content was 1 mg for each preparation. After centrifugation at 3000 rpm, the remaining drug in the preparations was analyzed by HPLC [4] after dissolving in acetonitrile.

Tumor Inoculation

A female rabbit bearing VX-2 carcinoma and male rabbits (Kbl, JW) weighing around 2.0 to 2.5 kg were purchased from Funabashi Farm (Chiba, Japan) and Kitayama LABES (Kyoto, Japan), respectively. Male rabbits were inoculated subcutaneously with VX-2 carcinoma cell suspension (10%, 0.5 ml, about 10^7 cells) at a position on the inside of the right leg just below the knee. Two weeks after inoculation, when the tumors had grown to 1 to 2 cm in length, treatment was started. The VX-2 carcinoma cell line was maintained by successive inoculation of untreated control rabbits.

Antitumor Effects

The msp. (50 mg) and oil preparations (LPD, sesame oil: 1 ml; MCT: 0.5 ml) containing TNP-470 at different concentrations were injected into the femoral artery through polyethylene tubing (PE-50, Clay Adams, NJ) under pentobarbital anesthesia. After administration the blood flow in the femoral artery was reopened by inserting the tubing upward into the artery. Control rabbits were either untreated or given an i.a. injection of placebo msp. or placebo oil preparations by the same cannulation method. For combination therapy, 1 mg of ADM or MMC was suspended in the TNP-470 oil solutions. Furthermore, the TNP-470 MCT preparation was injected three or four weeks after inoculation to determine the anticancer effect on well-developed tumors.

RESULTS AND DISCUSSION

In vitro Drug Release

The drug release from the msp. after dispersion in the buffer was relatively rapid, lasting only 3 to 5 days, even though the msp. remained lodged in a lung artery, the model used to represent the tumor artery, for 2 to 3 weeks after injection [4]. The drug was found to be very stable in the MCT solution, and the release of the drug from the preparation was sustained for 2 weeks. The release from the sesame oil solution was more rapid than that from the msp. The release profiles were attributed to the stability of the drug in the preparation bases and the partition between the buffer and the bases. The oil based preparation could be observed in the tumor arteries by X-ray angiography one week after i.a. injection. TNP-470 was sustainedly released from the MCT prepara-

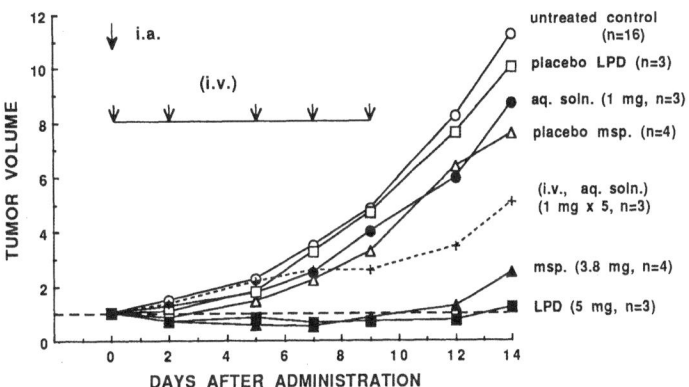

Fig. 2 Antitumor activity of TNP-470 in PLGA microspheres and LPD solution in rabbits bearing VX-2 carcinoma after i.a. injection

tion locating around the tumor and suppressed the neovascularization essential for tumor growth (to be published).

I.A. Injection of the Msp. and LPD Solution [4, 5]

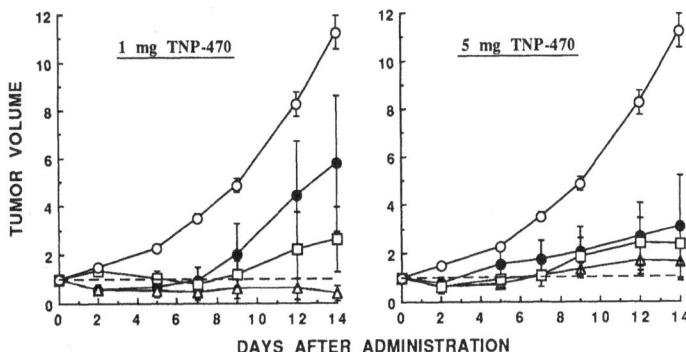

Fig. 3 Antitumor activity of TNP-470 in sesame oil (1 ml) in rabbits bearing VX-2 carcinoma after i.a. injection (mean±SE)

    —○— untreated control (n=16),   —●— TNP-470 alone (n=3),
    —△— + 1 mg ADM (n=3),   —□— + 1 mg MMC (n=3)

The tumor in the untreated control rabbits gradually grew to about 12 times the initial volume (Fig. 2). TNP-470 strongly inhibited the tumor growth after injection at a dose of 1 mg, i.v. (Fig. 2) and 5 mg, s.c. 5 times at 2 or 3 days intervals. The placebo PLGA msp. and LPD not containing TNP-470 scarcely suppressed the tumor growth after i.a. injection, whereas i.a. injection of the PLGA msp. and LPD solution containing TNP-470 (3.8 mg for msp. and 5 mg for oil preparation) caused striking regression of the tumor. In the group receiving the TNP-470 msp., regrowth of the tumor occurred 1 week after injection following the end of drug release from the msp. The TNP-

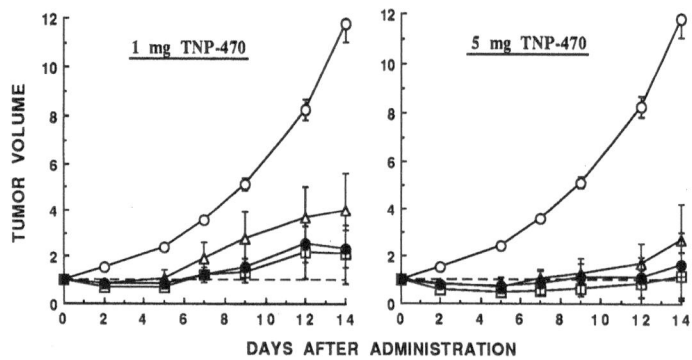

Fig. 4 Antitumor activity of TNP-470 in MIGLYOL 812 (0.5 ml) in rabbits bearing VX-2 carcinoma after i.a. injection (mean±SE)

—○— untreated control (n=22),   —●— TNP-470 alone (n=6),
—△— + 1 mg ADM (n=3),   —□— + 1 mg MMC (n=3)

470 LPD solution caused regression of the tumor for a long period, over 2 weeks.

I.A. Injection of the Sesame Oil and MCT solutions

Figure 3 shows the antitumor activity in the rabbit tumor model after i.a. injection of the TNP-470 sesame oil solution with and without ADM or MMC. Dose-dependent suppression of the tumor growth was observed after a single injection of the oil preparation. The suppression was slightly less than that with the LPD solution. Coadministration of TNP-470 and 1 mg of ADM or MMC in the oil solution resulted in greatly enhanced antitumor activity, and the combination of ADM and TNP-470 caused the strongest suppression of the tumor growth for the 2 weeks following injection. TNP-470 dissolved in MCT (MIGLYOL 812) after i.a. injection exerted a more persistent tumor regression than the sesame oil preparation, compared with LPD solution (Fig. 4). In this preparation, coadministration of conventional chemotherapeutic agents had barely enhancement in the antitumor activity. The reason for this phenomena is now obscure.

Antitumor Activity upon Injection 3 or 4 Weeks after Tumor Inoculation

We determined the antitumor activity of these formulations on well-developed tumors, i.e. 3 or 4 weeks after tumor inoculation. Figure 5 shows the activity for the 3 weeks following i.a. injection of 5 mg of the drug in various formulations 3 weeks after tumor inoculation. In the case of msp., marked rebound tumor growth occurred after transient initial regression. The oil preparations however provided persistent suppression of the tumor growth with the MCT solution causing regression of the tumor for the entire 3-week period following a single injection. These differences in antitumor activity can be explained by the *in vitro* release profiles as above described. From these results, we decided to use the MCT preparation for i.a. injection of TNP-470. The preliminary evaluation of the antitumor effect upon i.a.

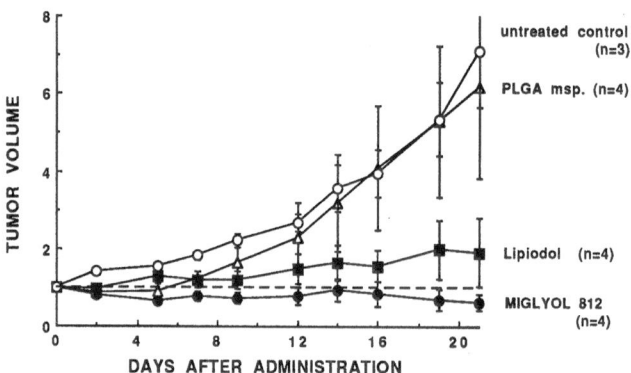

Fig. 5 Antitumor activity of TNP-470 (5 mg) in rabbits bearing VX-2 carcinoma following i.a. injection of various formulations 3 weeks after tumor inoculation (mean±SE)

injection of the TNP-470 MCT solution using tumor bearing rabbits 4 weeks after tumor inoculation showed dramatic activity: the tumor volume was reduced to less than one-fifth in two cases, and the tumor disappeared in one case. In conclusion, arterial injection of the MCT solution of the angiogenesis inhibitor TNP-470 should offer promising and reliable anticancer therapy due to long lasting blockage of the supply of nutrients to the tumor.

REFERENCES

1. Marui S, Itoh F, Kozai Y, Sudo K, Kishimoto S (1992) Chemical modification of fumagillin. I. 6-O-acyl, 6-O-sulfonyl, 6-O-alkyl, and 6-O-(N-substituted-carbamoyl) fumagillols. *Chem. Pharm. Bull.* **40**:96-101
2. Ingber D, Fujita T, Kishimoto S, Sudo K, Kanamaru T, Brem H, Folkman J (1990) Synthetic analogues of fumagillin that inhibit angiogenesis and suppress tumour growth. *Nature* **348**:555-557
3. Kusaka M, Sudo K, Fujita T, Marui S Itoh F, Ingber D, Folkman J (1991) Potent anti-angiogenic action of AGM-1470: Comparison to the fumagillin parent. *Biochem. Biophys. Res. Commun.* **174**:1070-1076
4. Okada H, Kamei S, Yoshioka T, Inoue Y, Ogawa Y, Toguchi H (1992) Anticancer effects of chemoembolization using microspheres of an angiogenesis inhibitor (TNP-470) in rabbits bearing VX-2 carcinoma. *Drug Delivery System* **7**:97-102
5. Kamei S, Okada H, Inoue Y, Yoshioka T, Ogawa Y, Toguchi H (1993) Antitumor effects of Angiogenesis inhibitor TNP-470 in rabbits bearing VX-2 carcinoma by arterial administration of microspheres and oil solution. *J. Pharmacol. Exp. Ther.* **264**:469-474

Liposomes Coated with Molecular Recognition Site Are Useful for Active Targeting Chemotherapy on Cancer Cells

Tohru Segawa[1], Masayuki Yamamoto[1], Katsuro Ichinose[1], Katsuya Takasu[1], Shunichi Matsukawa[1], Kunihide Izawa[1], Tsukasa Tsunoda[1], Takashi Kanematsu[1], and Junzo Sunamoto[2]

[1]Second Department of Surgery, Nagasaki University School of Medicine, Nagasaki, 852 Japan
[2]Department of Polymer Chemistry, Faculty of Engineering, Kyoto University, Kyoto, 606 Japan

ABSTRACT:

We investigated the antitumor effects of adriamycin (ADM) encapsulated in 3 types of liposomes using rat hepatoma cells (AH66) in vitro and in vivo. Liposomes were coated with cholesterol pullulan (CHP) and 1-aminolactose conjugated to CHP (lactose CHP) as a molecular recognition site for cancer cells. Antitumor activity of ADM encapsulated in lactose CHP was the most effective compared to that of liposomes alone or CHP on AH66 cells assyed by MTT test in vitro. Furthermore, growth of the tumor (AH66 cells) implanted into BALB/c mice was markedly inhibited by the treatment with ADM in lactose CHP-coated liposomes. Thus, lactose CHP-coated liposomes are an effective drug carrier for active targeting chemotherapy on cancer cells.

KEY WORDS: liposome, 1-aminolactose, active targeting chemotherapy

Since Bangham and co-workers[1] demonstrated vesicle of a closed bilayer structure (liposome), liposomes have been employed as a drug carrier. Liposomes in drug delivery system have advantages of biocompatibility, biodegradability, low cytotoxicity, low immunogenecity and possibility to encapsulate both hydrophilic and hydrophobic drugs in large quantity. Liposomes, however, are the structural instability and low cell specificity. To overcome these, Sunamoto et al.[2)3)] carried out chemically modification of polysaccharides with the palmitoyl chain to tightly bind polysaccharides and liposomal membranes and succeeded in assembling an artificial cell wall comprised of pullulan cholesterol (CHP) derivatives on the outermost surface of liposomes. CHP-coated liposomes were stable even in the presence of blood serum and plasma compared with conventional liposomes without polysaccharide-coating. In practical use of liposomes as drug delivery system, CHP-coated liposomes could be available for systemic administration. Furthermore, 1-aminolactose was introduced to liposomes coated with polysaccharides in order to utilizes this sugar as a molecular recognition site against target cancer cells.

Egg phosphatidylcholine (egg PC) was isolated and purified from fresh egg yolk according to the method described by Singleton et al.[4] with some modifications. Forty mg of egg PC were dissolved in 5 ml of chloroform, and the solvent was removed by evaporation. Ten mg of ADM in 1.5 ml of saline was added to the dried lipid film, and multilamellar vesicles were prepared by vortex dispersion. The liposomes were further sonicated into smaller vesicles with the sonicator, and the uncapsulated ADM was removed by gel filtration on a Sephadex G-50 column (equilibrated with saline).

In vitro: AH66 cells (4×10^5 cells/well) were incubated with ADM (4 µg/ml) entrapped in each liposomes (conventional, CHP-coated, lactose CHP-coated) for 3 hours. Antitumor activity of ADM in liposomes coated with lactose CHP on AH66 cells was the most effective compared to others by MTT assay[5].
In vivo: Eight weeks old BALB/c nude mice received subcutaneously 2×10^5 cells of AH66 which had been previously cultured in vitro. Mice whose tumor growth became a small finger tip size at 2 weeks were begun to treat for this experiment. The growth of the tumor inplanted to nude mice was markedly inhibited by the treatment with ADM in lactose CHP-coated liposomes compared with other groups which had recieved the same dose of ADM that was free or CHP-coated liposomes.

Drug delivery system using liposomes as carriers of anticancer agents is one of the attempts to obtain full efficacy of chemotherapy against malignant tumor. Liposomes in drug delivery system have two serious obstacles as mentioned above, one is structural instability another low cell specificity. To attain increased stability of liposomes, polysaccharide-coated liposomes which were protected against chemical and physicochemical stimuli were developed[2)3)]. Gabizon et al.[6)] reported that hydrogenated phophatidylinositol containing liposomes showed a characteristic long circulation time in plasma. Targeting of drugs to cancer cells is another important problem for liposomes as carriers. Active targeting is attained by molecular recognition through the specific interaction between the recognition site on the surface of drug carrier and the cell membrane of the cancer cells. Interaction between liposomes and cancer cells is thought to several mechanisms such as non-specific or specific adsorption, endocytosis and fusion. Monoclonal antibody has been conjugated to liposomes to target drugs to a lesion[3)7)]. Monoclonal antibody, however, has immunogenecity in vivo system. 1-aminolactose was conjugated with liposomes as a molecular recognition site. In this study, we investigated the specific interaction of lactose CHP-coated liposomes to cancer cells (AH66), which could serve as drug carriers in active targeting chemotherapy.

References:

1) Bangham AD, Horne RW (1964) Negative staining of phospholipids and their structural modification by surface-active agents as observed in the electron microscope. J Mol Biol 8:660-668
2) Sunamoto J, Iwamoto K (1986) Protein-coated and polysaccharide-coated liposomes as drug carriers. CRC Crit Rev Therapeutic Drug Carrier Systems 2:117-136
3) Sunamoto J, Sato T, Hirota M, Fukushima K, Hiratani K, Hara K (1987) A newly developed immunoliposome - An egg phosphatidylcholine liposome coated with pullulan bearing both a cholesterol moiety and an IgMs fragment. Biochem Biophys Acta 898:323-330
4) Singleton WS, Gray MS, Brown ML, White JL (1964) Chromatographically homogenous lecithin from egg phospholipids. J Am Oil Chem Soc 42:53-56
5) Maehara Y, Kusumoto T, Kusumoto H, Anai H, Sugimachi K (1988) Sodium succinate enhances the colorimetric reaction of the in vitro chemosensitivity test: MTT assay. Oncology 45:434-436
6) Gabizon A, Shiota R, Papahadjopoulos D (1989) Pharmacokinetics and tissue distribution of doxorubicin encapsulated in stable liposomes with long circulation times. J Natl Cancer Inst 81:1484-1488
7) Konno H, Suzuki H, Tadakuma T, Kumai K, Yasuda T, Kubota T, Ohta S, Nagaike K, Hosokawa S, Ishibiki K, Abe O, Saito K (1987) Antitumor effect of adriamycin entrapped in liposomes conjugated with anti-human α-fetoprotein monoclonal antibody. Cancer Res 47:4471-4477

Augmentation of Uptake of Mitomycin C in the Tumor Tissue After Infusion of Plasma Treated with Protein A: A Model Study of Metastatic Liver Tumor Using Rabbits Bearing Vx2 Carcinoma

M. FUNATSUKA, T. YAMAMOTO, K. TAMURA, and A. NAKASE

First Department of Surgery, School of Medicine, Shimane Medical University, Izumo, Shimane, 693 Japan

ABSTRACT

Vx2 carcinoma cells were injected into the portal vein of Japanese white rabbits. Uptake of Mitomycin C (MMC) was studied in animals with an infusion of protein A-treated plasma (PA plasma: 25 ml) on day 21-22. Tissue levels of MMC were elevated by 7 folds when animals received PA plasma 3-4 days prior to MMC injection (0.168 ug/ml vs. 0.024 ug/ml in animals with an infusion of non-treated plasma). Survival days of animals with MMC (2mg/injection) were 39 in animals with MMC and PA plasma plus MMC on day 3 of plasma infusion, while the days were 32 in those with MMC and non-treated plasma and MMC.

KEY WORDS: Mitomycin C, Protein A, Vx2 carcinoma, Liver metastasis

INTRODUCTION

The antitumor response observed after infusion of protein A (PA)-treated sera or plasmas has been reported to be clinically beneficial [1,2]. However, response rates (less than PR) of only 36% in patients with advanced breast adenocarcinoma and 15% in patients with cancer originated in colo-rectum were achieved in multi-institutional study [3]. The purpose of the present study is to explore the possibility of a combined use of the plasma therapy and chemotherapy for the betterment of the response rate.

MATERIALS AND METHODS

Animals, tumor and plasmas

Japanese white rabbits, male, weighing 3 kg, received an intra-portal injection of Vx2 carcinoma cells as a model of liver metastasis of carcinoma originated in the digestive tract. Briefly, Vx2 tumor was minced, pushed through a 350 um stainless screen mesh and suspended in Hanks' balanced salt solution containing 200 U/ml of penicillin G. Under an anesthesia with pentobarbital sodium (30 mg/kg), the animals received laparotomy and 0.2 ml of 1.0 % tumor suspension (approx. 1×10^6 tumor cells) was injected into a mesenteric vein using a 24G needle. 14-16 days after the injection of the Vx2 tumor suspension, 30-40 nodules (0.5-1.0 cm in diameter) were formed in the liver. Plasmas were obtained, throughout the present study, before the tumor inoculation by phlebotomy using a 50 ml syringe which contained 5 ml of CPD. After a centrifugation (800g x 15 minutes), formed elements were resuspended in saline and returned to the animals. Plasmas were kept frozen at -20 ℃ until use. In all experiments, autologous plasma was returned to the animals after PA treatment or without PA treatment.

Ex-vivo modulation of plasma with protein A.

Protein A immobilized to silica matrix (IMURÉ Corporation, Seattle, U.S.A), in an amount of 0.8mg, was packed in a cylindrical column (1 cm diameter x 4cm long). At experiments, the column was washed with 500ml of saline before use. Fresh-thawed plasmas (approx. 30 ml for each perfusions including CPD) were put through the column by gravity (30ml/30 minutes). After passage of the plasma, the column was washed with additional 20 ml of saline. The collected plasma and saline was drip infused to the animals (50ml/60 minutes). Mitomycin C dissolved in saline was injected intravenously in amount of 2mg for studies on survival periods and 4mg for studies on tissue uptake.

Determination of tissue levels of Mitomycin C

MMC (4mg) was given before an injection of pentobarbital sodium (30mg/kg). Sample tissues were obtained 15 and 30 minutes after the injection of MMC. Tissues were weighed and homogenized in 1/15 mol phosphate buffer (pH 7.2), and 10 % suspension of the tissue was heated at 100 ℃ for 1 minutes. The supernatant obtained after a spinning at 800g for 10 minutes was kept at -20 °C for MMC determination. Concentrations of MMC was determined by a bioassay method[4].

Studies on survival periods

     For the study on survival days, animals were divided into 6 groups and received a return of the plasma on day 7 after the injection of the tumor suspension. MMC was given in amount of 2 mg at each injection. Control Vx2 animals received a Vx2 injection and a plasma return without the modulation with PA nor MMC injection. Test animals received the following treatments.

Group 1: A return of PA-treated plasma.

Group 2: MMC, 3 hours prior to the return of non-treated plasma.

Group 3: MMC, 3 hours prior to the return of PA-treated plasma.

Group 4: MMC, 96 hours after the return of PA-treated plasma.

Group 5: MMC, 3 hours prior to and 74 hours after the return of PA-treated plasma.

Group 6: MMC, 3 hours prior to and 74 hours after the return of non-treated plasma.

Statistics

     The mean were compared by Student's t test; P values less than 0.05 were significant. The method of Kaplan-Meier was used to calculate the survival curves and the difference were analyzed using generalized Wilcoxon test.

RESULTS

     Levels of MMC in Vx2 tumor tissue, when given on days 3 and 4 of the return of PA-treated plasma, were elevated to levels 7 times higher than the control levels (0.168 $\pm$0.013 ug/ml vs. 0.024$\pm$0.002 ug/ml), while given on days 1,2 or 7 post plasma return, no elevation of MMC uptake was observed. (Fig.1)

     Animals which received the return of PA-treated plasma lived for 34.14$\pm$1.35 days (group 1), achieving a prolongation of the survival period by 5 days in comparison with the control animals (29.07$\pm$1.03 days)(P<0.05), but no prolongation was observed in those animals which received a combination of MMC and non-treated plasma (group 2: 29.80$\pm$1.25 days). (Fig.2)

     Animals with MMC and PA-treated plasma (group 3: 34.14$\pm$1.86 days) lived only as long as those with PA-treated plasma alone (group 1), while animals PA-treated plasma plus MMC on day 4 after plasma infusion (group 4: 36.14$\pm$1.77 days) lived longer by 7 days (P<0.01).(Fig.3)

     Animals with MMC and PA-treated plasma plus MMC on day 3 post infusion (group 5: 39.13 $\pm$0.99 days) survived longer than animals with MMC and non-treated plasma plus MMC (group 6: 31.90$\pm$0.64days).(Fig.4)

DISCUSSION AND SUMMARY

     Terman et al. described that, in dogs with spontaneous mammary adenocarcinoma, combined use of cytosine arabinoside and plasma perfusion procedure over Staphylococcus aureus Cowan I achieved antitumor effect which exceeded the algebraic sum of effects expected with each modality alone [5]. Recently Fradji et al. reported clinical trials of combined use of plasma therapy and chemotherapy [6]. Rationale for the use of different modalities in combined manner, in general, stands on an expectation to achieve a synergistic antitumor effect with minimum adverse effects.

     The initial damage caused by (the host response after) an infusion of PA-treated plasma has been reported to be disruption of the continuity of the tumor cell membrane [2]. Our study with electron microscopy (Vx2 tumor and PA perfusion) has revealed this membrane disruption begins 3-6 hours after a return of the ex-vivo treated plasma, while nuclei of tumor cells remained rather unaffected [7]. MMC has been reported to be incorporated to nucleal DNA and RNA, thus, causing damages in DNA and RNA synthesis, the actions being diffrent from those reported with PA plasma therapy.

     We summarized the results presented here as follows: (1) uptake of MMC was augmented by 7 folds when combined with infusion of PA-treated plasma; However, (2)the augmentation of uptake of MMC was achieved only when the MMC was given on day 3 or 4 of post infusion, but not right after or 1 week after the return of PA-treated plasma, and (3) a combined usage of plasma perfusion procedure and chemotherapy on day 3 or 4 after plasma perfusion, have successfully achieved a significant prolongation of the survival days of animals with intra-portally implanted tumor of Vx2. These data suggest, in conclusion, that a proper combination of plasma therapy and chemotherapy may achieve more benefits than expected when each modalities are applied alone.

Tissue levels of MMC after 4 mg i.v.

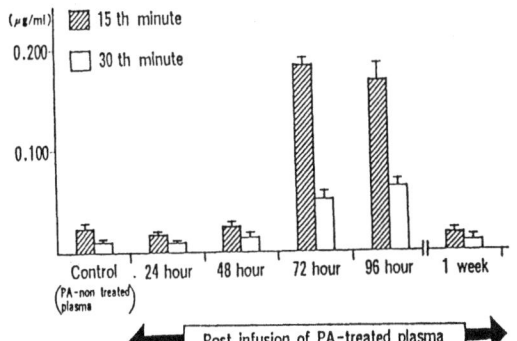

Fig.1
Tissue up-take of MMC reached, when given on day 3 or 4 of post return of PA-treated plasma, to levels 7 times higher than those in non-treated animals (0.168±0.013ug/ml vs. 0.024±0.002 ug/ml), while given on days 1,2 or 7 post return of PA treated plasma, no elevation of MMC uptake was observed. (P<0.05)

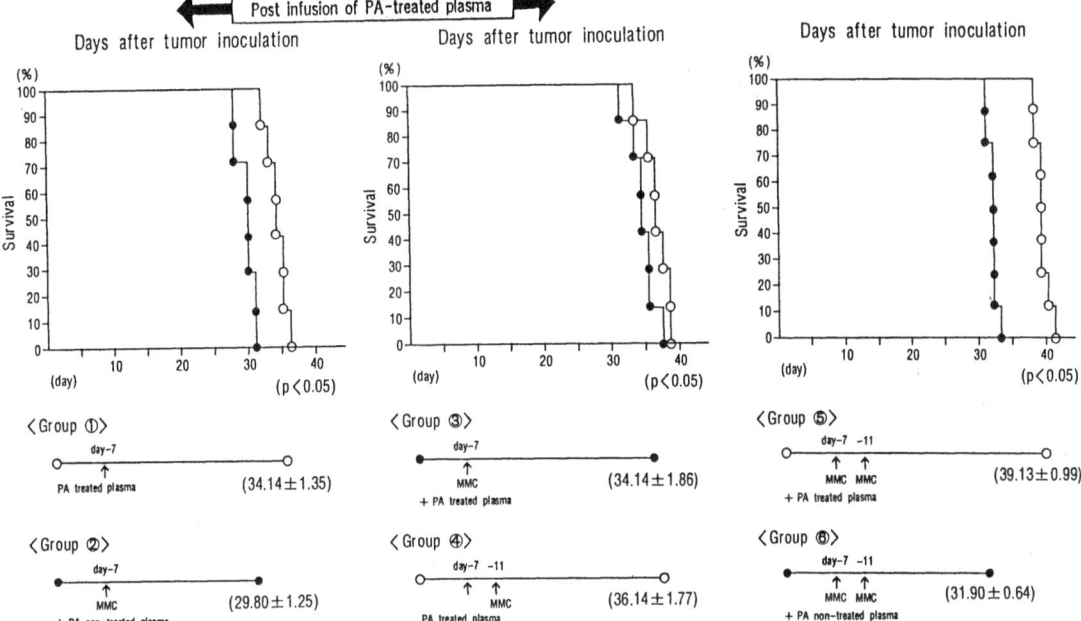

Fig.2 The return of PA-treated plasma achieved a prolongation of the survival period by 5 days (Group 1), but no prolongation was observed in those with a a combination of MMC (2mg) and non-treated plasma (group 2). (P<0.05)

Fig.3 Animals with MMC plus PA-treated plasma (group 3) lived only as long as those with PA-treated plasma alone (group 1), while animals with MMC and PA-treated plasma lived longer by 2 days (group 4). (P<0.05)

Fig.4 Animals with MMC and PA-treated plasma plus MMC on day of 3 post PA-treated plasma (group 5) survived 2 days longer than those with MMC and non-treated plasma plus MMC (group 6). (P<0.05)

REFERENCES

[1] Bansal,S.C, et al: Ex Vivo removal of serum IgG in a patient with colon carcinoma. Some biochemical, immunological and histological observations, Cancer,42:1-18, 1978.

[2] Terman,D.S, et al: Extensive necrosis of spontaneous canine mammary adenocarcinoma after extracorporeal perfusion over staphylococcus aureus Cowans 1. Description of acute tumoricidal response: Morphologic, and serologic findings, J.Immunol.,795-805 124:1980.

[3] Messerschmidt,G.L,et al: Protein A immunoadsorption in the treatment of malignant disease, J.Clin.,6:203-212,1988.

[4] Miyamura,T, et al: Genomic structure of human polyoma virus JC:nucleotide sequence of the region containing replication origin and small T-antigen gene.J.Virol.45:73-79: 1983.

[5] Terman,D.S.,et al: Tumoricidal response induced by cytosine arabinoside after plasma perfusion over Protein A ; Science, 209:1257-1259,1980.

[6] Fradji,A,et al: A randmized study of combined 5-fluorouracil and plasma perfusion over protein A-Sepharose in human advanced colorectal carcinoma,Biotherapy,2:87-94,1990.

[7] Okada,T, et al: A Sequential Histological and Ultra structural Study on the Acute Anti-tumor Response after Infusion of Plasma Perfused over Immobilized Protein A. J.Jpn.Soc,Cancer Ther,11.2394-2401:1991

Metastases Models of Human Colon Cancer in Congenitally Athymic Mice

Kazuhiko Yoshida, Tohru Fujikawa, Akihiko Tanabe, and Kenji Sakurai

First Department of Surgery, The Jikei University School of Medicine, Minato-ku, Tokyo, 105 Japan

ABSTRACT

Although current limits in the treatment of metastases from colorectal carcionoma require the understanding of biology and new therapeutic approaches, few metastases models of human colorectal carcinoma (HCC) have been reported. We demonstrated reproducible murine models of hepathic, pulmonary and peritoneal metastases from HCC in congenitally athymic mice. Ninety−eight percent (88/90) of mice developed hepatic metastases approximately 4 weeks after intrasplenic injection of 4×10^6 HT−29LMM HCC cells. Sevently percent (7/10) of mice also produced pulmonary metastases after tail vein injection of HT−29LMM cells. One hundred percent (10/10) of mice developed peritoneal metastases after intraperitoneal injection of HT − 29LMM cells. Macro and microscopic findings of hepatic, pulmonary and peritoneal metastases were very similar to those in the human being. Those reproducible models provide useful tool for the evaluation of the biology and new therapeutic approaches for colorectal metastases in vivo.

KEY WORDS: colon cancer, metastasis, nude mouse

INTRODUCTION

Colorectal carcinoma, is one of the most frequent malignant diseases and incidence of this diseases has been increasing in Japan. By the time many colorectal carcinomas are diagnosed and surgically excised, macro and micrometastases are already present in the liver, peritoneum, lung and other organs(1). Colorectal metastases which are potentially curable by second-look surgery are uncommon. Additionally, systemic and loco-regional chemotherapy in the management of metastases is also of limited value(1). It is clear that alternative approaches to the treatment of colorectal metastases are required. Most metastases models have been developed from animal cell lines in mice, rats and guinea pigs. However, these models are not suitable for the evaluation of the biology and expeimental therapies to human tumor. This study was undertaken to determine the reproducibity and suitability of hepatic, pulmonary and peritoneal metastases models after each intrasplenic, tail vein and intraperitoneal injection of HT-29LMM human colorectal carcinoma (HCC) cells in nude mice.

MATERIALS AND METHODS

Mice
Specific pathogen − free athymic BALB/c female mice 3 to 4 weeks of age were cared for at the animal facility in the Jikei University School of Medicine. Mice were kept under sterile conditions in a laminar flow room in cages with filter bonnets and were fed sterilized water.

Prepatation of Cell line for Injection
The HCC cell line HT−29LMM was established from multiple tumors grown in the liver after intrasplenic injection of HT−29 cells in nude mice and was kindly provided by Dr. Fidler (M.D. Anderson Hospital, Houston, TX, U.S.A.) The cell line was grown and maintained under humidified conditions in the presence of 5% carbon dioxide in Dulbecco's modified minimum essential medium supplemented with 10% fetal bovine serum (GIBCO, Grand Island, NY, U.S.A.).

Development of Hepatic Metastases
The mice were anesthetized with intraperitoneal pentobarbital (12 µg /gram body weight) and placed in the right lateral decubitus. The abdomen was prepared in a sterile fashion. A small incision was made at the left flank through the skin and peritoneum, exposing medial aspect of the spleen. Injection of 3-4 × 10^6 HT-29LMM cells in volume of 0.05 ml beneath the splenic capsule was made with 30-gauge needle so as to raise a visible pale wheal. No significant bleeding or extravasation was encountered. The spleen was returned to the abdominal cavity, and the wound was closed in one layer with wound clips.

Development of Pulmonary Metastases
The mice were fixed on the table. Injection of 6 − 8 × 10^6 HT-29LMM cells in volume of 0.1 ml into the tail vein was made.

Development of Peritoneal Metastases
Injection of 3-4 × 10^7 HT-29LMM cells in volume of 0.5 ml into the peritoneal space was made.

RESULTS

Development of Hepatic Metastases
Ninety-eight (88/90) of mice developed hepatic metastases approximately 4 weeks after intrasplenic injection of HT - 29LMM cells. Macroscopically, hepatic metastases were multiple irregular gray-white nodules of varying size were evenly distributed in both lobes. Some nodules demonstrated scarring and retraction producing and umbilicated appearance. Microscopically, hepatic metastases revealed moderately differentiated adenocarcinoma of human colon, with no change from the primary splenic tumors evident of light microscopy. Hepatic metastases were demonstrated to form distinct nodules and to displace hetatocytes. However, areas of necrosis were rarely present in the center of the nodules (Figure; left). Some foci which consisted of proliferative tumor cells in portal tributaries and periportal area were observed. These pathological findings appeared similar to hepatic metastases in the human.

Development of Pulmonary Metastases
Seventy percent (7/10) of mice produced pulmonary metastases approximately 6 weeks after tail vein injection of HT - 29LMM cells. Macroscopically, a few lung metastases were present in both lung and were irregular gray-white nodules. Microscopically, lung metastases demonstrated to displace alveoli (Figure; middle). Some foci were found in the pulmonary arteries.

Development of peritoneal Metastases
One hundred percent (10/10) of mice developed peritoneal metastases approximately 3 weeks after intraperitoneal injection of HT - 29LMM cells. Some mice produced peritonitis carcinomatosa. Peritoneal metastases were gray-white nodules which were evenly distributed in the peritoneum. Microscopically, peritoneal metastases reveal tumor nodules on the peritoneum (Figure; right)

DISCUSSION

Since the first report on the successful use of the athymic (T-cell-deficient) nude mouse for growing xenografted human tumors (2), the availability of this model has provided a most valuable tool for examining many aspects of human tumors in vivo (6-8). Most human neoplasms growing in nude mice maintain their morphological and biochemical characteristics (3) and the response of such xenografts to chemotherapeutic and immunotherapeutic agents frequently is predictive of the clinical response (4). The similarities between the behavior of the tumor in the natural host and in the nude mouse demonstrates the potential value of this model system for studies on human tumors.
It is frequently stated that malignant human tumors metastasize only rarely in nude mice (5). The relatively brief life span of nude mice compared with human being may explain why. However, many other factors do influence this process in a more profound manner. First, the majority of human neoplasms xenografted into nude mice have been implanted subcutaneously, and anatomical site that bears little relevance

to the organ of origin in the neoplasm (6). Second, the metastatic capacity of human tumor cells implanted subcutaneously in nude mice has been correlated with invasion of the body wall(5).

The injections of cancer cells into the spleen, tail vein and peritoneum represent advantageous routes to development of hepatic, pulmonary and peritoneal metastases and are physiologically comparable to the metastatic process in HCC. Although these tumor cells do not go through the initial step of metastases as the separation from pimary neoplasm, all the subsequent steps in the metastatic process such as survival in the blood or peritoneum, invation and growth in the liver, lung and peritoneum must occur for metastases to become established.

The reproduciblity of liver metastases after intrasplenic injection and pulmonary metastases after tail vein injection of primary HCC cell lines has been reported in the past to be low (7). The ability of HCC of cells to produce metastases is not due to simple trapping in the liver, lung and peritoneum. The formation of metastases is a selective process. Choosing appropriate metastatic cells and host conditions (i.e. young healthy mice) is essential for high reproducibility of metastases in nude mice.

It is clear that new and more effective approaches to the treatment of metastases are required. These models provide a useful tool for the evaluation of biology and the experimental therapy for colorectal metastases.

LEGEND

Figure: Microscopic findings of the metastases in liver (left; HE × 40), lung (middle; HE × 10) and peritoneum (right; HE × 10).

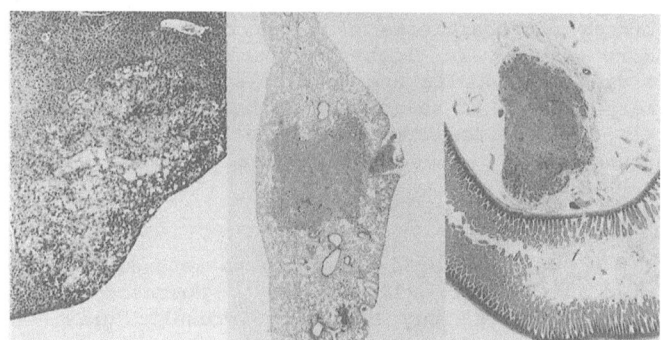

REFERENCES

1. August DA, Ottow RT, Sugarbaker PH (1984) Clinical perspectives of human colorectal cancer metastases. Cancer Met Rev 3:303 − 325
2. Rygaard J, Povlsen CO (1969) Heterotransplantarion of a human malignant tumor to nude mice. Acta Pathol Microbiol Scan 77:758 − 760
3. Povlsen CO, Jacobsen GK (1975) Chemotherapy of a human malignant melanoma transplanted in the nude mouse. Cancer Res 35:2790 − 2796
4. Giovanella BC, Stehlin JS Jr, Williams LJ Jr, Lee S, Shepard RC (1978) Heterotransplantation of human cancers into nude mice. Cancer 42:2269 − 2281
5. Sharkey FE, Fogh J (1979) Metastases of human tumors in athymic nude mice. Int J Cancer 24:733 − 738
6. Hart IR (1982) "Seed and soil" revisited: mechanisms of site - specific metastases. Cancer Met Rev 1:5 − 17
7. Giavazzi R, Campbell DE, Jessup JM, Cleary K, Fidler (1986) Metastatic behavior of tumor cells isolated from primary and metastatic human colorectal carcinomas implated into different sites in nude mice. Cancer Res 46:2269 − 2281

Adhesion of Human Cancer Cells to Vascular Endothelium Mediated by a Carbohydrate Antigen, SPan-1

Nobuya Yamada, Yong-Suk Chung, Yoshito Yamashita, Naoyoshi Onoda, Kiyoshi Maeda, Yasuyuki Kondo, Itsuo Nakanishi, Tetsuji Sawada, Masahiro Okuno, and Michio Sowa

The First Department of Surgery, Osaka City University Medical School, Osaka, 545 Japan

A new human extrahepatic bile duct carcinoma cell line (OCUCh-LM1) and a new human colon cancer cell line (OCUC-LM1) were established from respective hepatic metastases in our laboratory. Cells of both lineages express various carbohydrate antigens such as sialyl Lewis[x] and SPan-1. Recent studies have shown a cell adhesion molecule called ELAM-1, which is expressed on vascular endothelium, to be capable of recognizing sialyl Lewis[x] as a ligand. In this report, we demonstrate that carbohydrate antigen SPan-1, which has a different epitope from sialyl Lewis[x], plays a significant role in the adhesion of human cancer cells to endothelial cells.

KEY WORDS: OCUCh-LM1, OCUC-LM1, Carbohydrate antigen, SPan-1, HUVECs

INTRODUCTION

Recently the cell adhesion molecule called ELAM-1 which is expressed on vascular endothelium, was reported to recognize sialyl Lewis[x] as a ligand [1-4], and such carbohydrate antigens expressed on the surface of cancer cells may be involved in the process of adhesion between cancer cells and endothelial cells. However, it is a likely possibility that another carbohydrate antigen can serve as a ligand for ELAM-1. In order to ascertain whether or not SPan-1 antigen, which has a different epitope from sialyl Lewis[x], contributes to the adhesion of human cancer cells to vascular endothelium, the adhesion assay using HUVECs was undertaken. Here we report that SPan-1 antigen plays a significant role in the adhesion of human cancer cells to endothelial cells.

MATERIALS AND METHODS

Cell lines and Antibodies

A new human extrahepatic bile duct carcinoma cell line (OCUCh-LM1) and a new human colon cancer cell line (OCUC-LM1) were established from respective hepatic metastases and have been maintained in DMEM supplemented with 10% fetal calf serum (Table 1). These cell lines grow in a monolayer pavement-like cell arrangement on phase contrast microscopy and express various carbohydrate antigens such as sialyl Lewis[x], CA19-9, and SPan-1. The anti-sialyl Lewis[x] antibody (FH6, murine IgM) and anti-SPan-1 antibody (murine IgM) used in the assay were kindly supplied by Otsuka Assay Laboratories, Tokushima, Japan and Dainabot Co. Ltd., Tokyo, Japan, respectively.

Adhesion assay using HUVECs

HUVECs (Human Umbilical Vein Endothelial Cells, obtained from Kurabou Co. Ltd., Osaka, Japan) were stimulated with 1ng/ml of recombinant interleukin-1β (rIL1β, The Central Research Laboratory of Otsuka Pharmaceutical Co., Tokushima, Japan) for 4 hours in 96-well microplates. OCUCh-LM1 and OCUC-LM1 (1.0×10^6/ml) cells, which were pretreated with monoclonal anti-sialyl Lewis[x] or anti-SPan 1 antibody (50μg/ml), were added to HUVECs and incubated for 30 minutes at room temperature with shaking. A short incubation time and continuous shaking were employed to minimize possible nonspecific bindings of cancer cells to endothelial cells. After incubation for 30 minutes, the microplates were gently washed with PBS(-) and the adhering cells were detected by incubating with 0.5mg/ml MTT for 3 hours at 37°C. The crystals were measured with an automated microplate reader.

RESULTS

Carbohydrate antigens secreted into the spent media after 5-day cultivation of OCUCh-LM1 and OCUC-LM1 cell suspensions of 1.0×10^5/ml concentration are summarized in Table 2.

Table 1. Background of Cell lines

cell lines	Patient age/sex	Origin	Histology
OCUCh-LM1	61 / M	cholangioma	tub.ad.ca.
OCUC-LM1	40 / M	rectal ca.	tub.ad.ca.

Table 2. Carbohydrate antigens secreted into the spent media

cell lines	CA19-9 (U/ml)	SLX (U/ml)	SPan-1 (U/ml)
OCUCh-LM1	85	32.3	67.2
OCUC-LM1	1669	40.4	281.2
control	<5	<5.0	<3.0

Both OCUCh-LM1 and OCUC-LM1 cells expressed various carbohydrate antigens such as sialyl Lewis^X, CA19-9, and SPan-1. The adhesion of OCUC-LM1 cells to HUVECs was seen only when HUVECs were activated by rIL1β, while OCUCh-LM1 cell adhesion to HUVECs was seen irrespective of whether HUVECs were preincubated with rIL1β or not. When cancer cells were pretreated with anti-sialyl Lewis^X antibody, adhesion of only 13.0% of OCUC-LM1 cells and 19.7% of OCUCh-LM1 cells to HUVECs was inhibited. On the other hand, when cancer cells were pretreated with anti-SPan-1 antibody, adhesion of 78.4% of OCUC-LM1 cells and 58.4% of OCUCh-LM1 cells to HUVECs was inhibited. Thus the adhesion of OCUCh-LM1 and OCUC-LM1 to HUVECs was inhibited to a greater extent by treatment with anti-SPan-1 antibody than with anti-sialyl Lewis^X antibody (Fig.1). The inhibition pattern of the adhesion of OCUC-LM1 cells to rIL1β-activated HUVECs is shown in Fig.2.

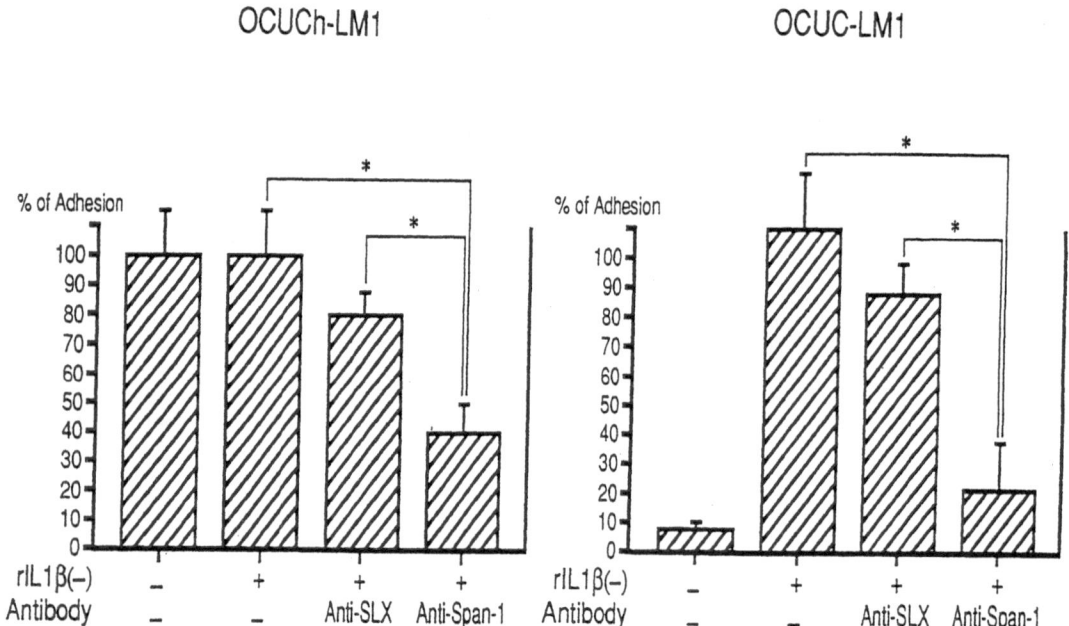

Fig.1 The effect of anti-SLX and anti-SPan-1 antibodies on the adhesion of OCUCh-LM1 and OCUC-LM1 cells to HUVECs. *P<0.01

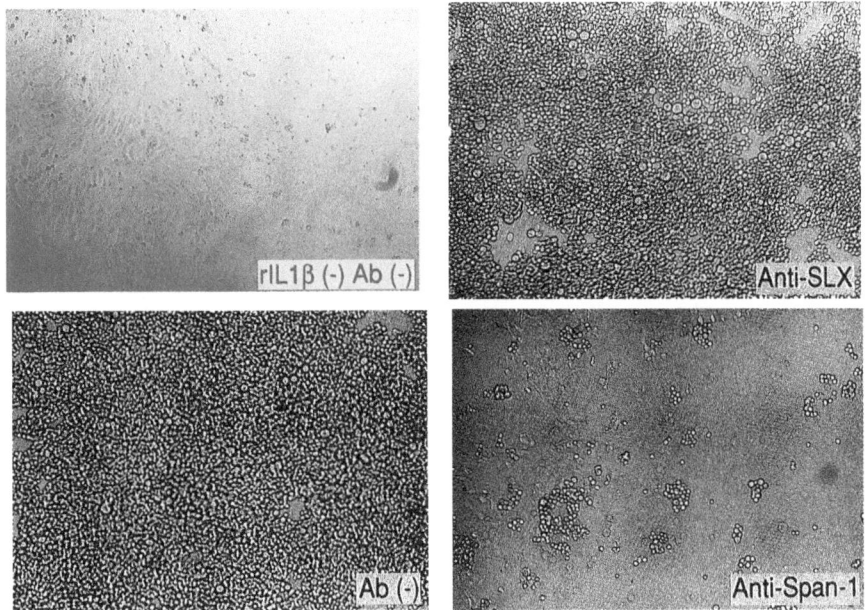

Fig.2 The inhibition pattern of the adhesion of OCUC-LM1 cells to rIL1β-activated HUVECs by treatment with anti-SLX and anti-SPan-1 antibodies.

DISCUSSION

Most of cancer cells adhered to HUVECs when HUVECs were activated by cytokines such as, IL1β, TNFα and INFγ, but a few did adhere to HUVECs not preincubated with cytokines [5]. OCUC-LM1 cells were adherent to HUVECs only when the latter cells were preincubated with rIL1β, whereas OCUCh-LM1 cells were adherent to HUVECs irrespective of preincubation with rIL1β. Thus OCUCh-LM1 and OCUC-LM1 cells showed different patterns of adhesion to HUVECs. The murine monoclonal antibody SPan-1 was produced against the human pancreatic cancer cell line SW1990. SPan-1 antibody is IgM and was purified from spent hybridoma culture media. The carbohydrate structure of SPan-1 antigen remains yet unclear, but SPan-1 antigen belongs to Type I carbohydrate and the terminal structure is sialylated [6,7]. The adhesion of OCUCh-LM1 and OCUC-LM1 to HUVECs was more markedly inhibited by treatment with anti-SPan-1 antibody than with anti-sialyl Lewis[x] antibody. These findings suggest that SPan-1 antigen plays a significant role in the adhesion of OCUCh-LM1 and OCUC-LM1 cells to endotherial cells.

REFERENCES

1. Lowe JB, Stoolman LM, Nair RP, Larsen RD, Berhend TL, Marks RM (1990) ELAM-1-dependent cell adhesion to vascular endothelium determined by a transfected human fucosyltransferase cDNA. Cell 63:475-484
2. Phillips ML, Nudelman EG, Gaeta FCA, Perez M, Singhal AK, Hakomori S, Paulson J (1990) ELAM-1 mediates cell adhesion by recognition of a carbohydrate ligand, sialyl-Le[x]. Science 250:1130-1132
3. Waitz G, Aruffo A, Kolanus W, Bevilacqua M, Seed B (1990) Recognition by ELAM-1 of the sialyl-Le[x] determinant on myeloid and tumor cells. Science 250:1132-1135
4. Tiemeyer M, Swiedler SJ, Ishihara M, Moreland M, Schweingruber H, Hirtzer P, Brandley BK (1991) Carbohydrate ligands for endothelial-leukocyte adhesion molecule 1. Proc Natl Acad Sci USA 88:1138-1142
5. Takada A, Ohmori K. Yoneda T, Tsuyuoka K, Hasegawa A, Kiso M, Kannagi R (1993) Contribution of carbohydrate antigens sialyl Lewis A and sialyl Lewis X to adhesion of human cancer cells to vascular endothelium. Cancer Res 53:354-361
6. Chung YS, Ho JJL, Kim YS, Tanaka H, Nakata B, Hiura A, Motoyoshi H, Satake K, Umeyama K (1987) The detection of human pancreatic cancer-associated antigen in the serum of cancer patients. Cancer 60:1636-1643
7. Ho JJL, Chung YS, Fujimoto Y, Bi N, Ryan W, Yuan S, Byrd JC, Kim YS (1988) Mucin-like antigen in a human pancreatic cancer cell line identified by murine monoclonal antibodies SPan-1 and YPan-1. Cancer Res 48:3924-3931

Pancreas

Extended Pancreatectomy for Locally Advanced Pancreatic Cancer Involving the Portal Vein — Indications and Limitations

Osamu Ishikawa, Hiroaki Ohigashi, Shingi Imaoka, and Takeshi Iwanaga

Department of Surgery, The Center for Adult Diseases, Osaka, 537 Japan

ABSTRACT

A retrospective study was made to determine the indications and limitations of extended pancreatectomy for locally advanced carcinoma of the pancreas, in terms of postoperative prognosis. An extended pancreatectomy with portal vein and/or superior mesenteric vein (PV/SMV) resection and regional lymphadenectomy was performed for 44 patients out of 66 consecutive patients whose cancers extended into the retroperitoneal spaces involving the PV/SMV. The 3-year survival rate was 61% in 22 selected patients whose PV/SMV invasions had been angiographically both hemicircular or less and 1.3 cm or less in length, and 0% in the remaining 24 patients whose PV/SMV invasions were either beyond hemicircular or more than 1.3 cm in length ($p<0.02$). As the latter result was even worse than that of the 22 non-resectable patients, it can be concluded that the degree of PV/SMV invasion on angiography is a good indicator for aggressive surgery for locally advanced pancreatic cancer.

KEY WORDS: pancreatic carcinoma, portal vein

INTRODUCTION

During the surgery for adenocarcinoma of the pancreas, we frequently encounter a locally advanced tumor which directly extends into the retroperitoneal spaces and involves the portal vein and/or superirior mesenteric vein (PV/SMV). For such cases, many previous authors have abandoned curative pancreatectomy, while we have tried to resect it in combination with both PV/SMV resection and lymphatic and connective tissue clearance [1]. Thus, the present paper is designed to detect more reliable indicators which can predict the differentiation between the long-term survivors and the patients with early postoperative disease-failure.

PATIENTS and METHODS

During the period from 1984 to 1991, surgical laparotomy was performed on 66 consecutive patients with locally advanced adenocarcinoma of the pancreatic head and body, at the Center for Adult Diseases, Osaka. Though distant metastasis was not detected in any case, their primary tumors directly involved the PV/SMV. An extended pancreatectomy with PV/SMV resection and lymphatic and connective tissue clearance was performed for 44 patients, and abandoned for the other 22 patients whose cancer invasions were still more severe. In 44 resected specimens, the degrees of PV/SMV invasion, tumor size, and nodal involvement were investigated, and compared with the postoperative patients' prognosis. Prior to laparotomy, all patients had received the SMA- angiography with the aid of Prostaglandin E1 to delineate the SMV and PV. The pattern of PV/SMV narrowing was classified as reported previously [2], and its length was divided by 1.2 (magnification rate).

RESULTS

After pancreatectomy, three patients died of complications within 30 post-operative days. Within 2 post-operative years, two patients died of other diseases and four are alive without disease recurrence. Excluding these 8 patients, the other 35 patients were classified according to whether they survived 3

748

years (Group A, n=10) or not (Group B, n=25). When the backgroud factors were compared between these two subgroups, age, sex, tumor location, nodal involvement and major artery invasion did not differ significantly(Table 1). However, the incidene the PV/SMV invasion was semicircular or less was 100% in Group A, which was significantly higher than that of Group B (p<0.02). Also, the length of PV/SMV invasion was 1.6±0.5 cm (range 0.8-2.0 cm) and 2.5±1.0 cm (range 1.0-5.4), respectively (p<0.01).

Table 1. Background factors in association with patints' survival

Background factors	Patient's Survival Period		p-value
	Group A > 3-yr (n=10)	Group B < 3-yr (n=25)	
Age (yr)	64±5	62±8	NS.
Sex (M/F)	6/4	16/9	NS.
Pancreatectomy			
Whipple's procedure	6 (60%)	16 (64%)	
Caudal pancreatectomy	2 (20%)	2 (8%)	NS.
Total Pancreatectomy	2 (20%)	7 (28%)	
Nodal Involvement	9 (90%)	23 (92%)	NS.
Major Artery Involvement	0 (0%)	6 (24%)	NS.
PV/SMV invasion			
Semicircular or less	10 (100%)	13 (52%)	<0.02
Maximum length (cm)	1.6±0.5 (0.8-2.0)	2.5±1.0 (1.0-5.4)	<0.01

In order to know whether the degrees of PV/SMV invasion can be predicted by preoperative angiography, the pattern of PV/SMV invasions were compared between histology and angiography in the 44 patients who underwent resection. Among 28 patients whose PV/SMV invasions were semicircular or less in histology, normal/smooth shift patterns were seen in 15(54%), unilateral narrowing patterns in 11(39%), and bilateral narrowing patterns in 2(7%). Among 16 patients whose PV/SMV invasions were beyond semicircular in histology, bilateral narrowing patterns were observed in 12 (75%), and other patterns were observed in 4 (25%). With regard to the length of PV/SMV invasion, the following formula was obtain from the comparison between histology and angiography:

$y=0.72x-0.13$ (x:length in histology, y=length in angiography) (r=0.755, p<0.05)

For instance, y equals 1.3 when x is 2.0 (the maximum value in the Group A).

Table 2. Comparison of PV/SMV Invasion Between Histology and Angiography

PV/SMV Invasion on Histology	Narrowing Patterns on Angiography		
	Normal or Smooth Shift	Hemilateral Narrowing	Bilateral Narrowing
Semicircular or less (n=28)	15 (54%)	11 (39%)	2 (7%)
Beyond semi-circular (n=16)	1 (6%)	3 (19%)	12 (75%)

Figure 1a shows the cumulative survival rates in the resected group (n=44) and the nonresected group (n=22). The former group had significantly higher rates at 2, 3, 4 and 5 years. The resected group was classified into two subgroups, based on the narrowing pattern and its length on angiography: normal- hemilateral narrowing patterns and 1.3 cm or less in length (n=20); and bilateral narrowing pattern or longer than 1.3 cm in length (n=24). The former subgroup had significantly higher rates at 1-5 years (Fig. 1b), and the result of the latter subgroup was still worse than that of non-resected group(Fig. 1a).

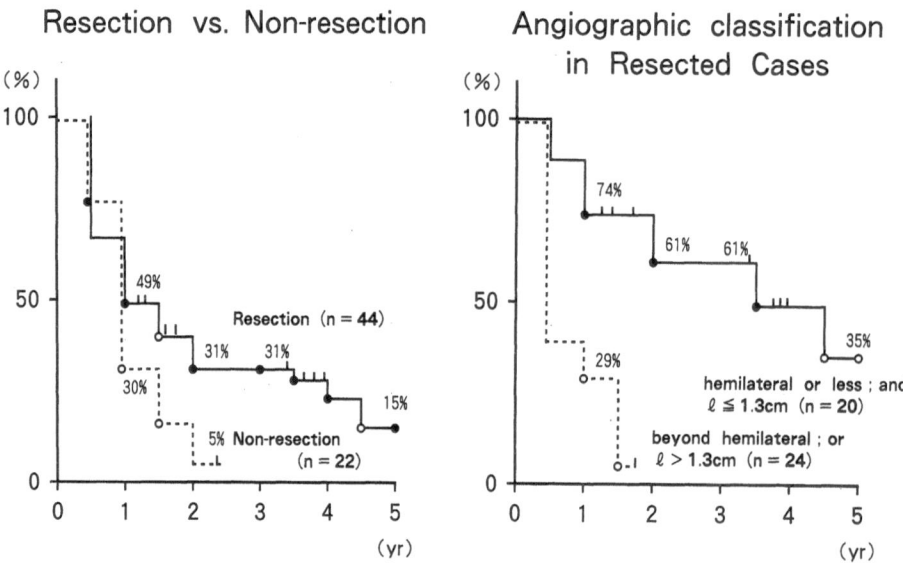

Fig 1. Cumulative survival rates. Comparison between resected and non-resected cases (a). Comparison between the two subgroups classified on the angiographic findings(b). A significant difference is observed in each comparison.

DISCUSSION

Many authors have abandoned pancreatectomy as a treatment for locally advanced pancreatic cancer involving the PV/SMV. However, with a wide range of lymphatic and connective tissue clearance, PV/SMV resection combined with pancreatectomy produced long-term survivors. This beneficial effect was limited to the patients whose PV/SMV invasions were normal-hemilateral and shorter than 1.3cm on the routine angiographic findings. By using this indicator, we can avoid both losing the chance of cure by surgery and the useless laparotomy.

REFERENCES

1. Ishikawa, O., Ohigashi, H., Sasaki, Y., et al.(1988) Practical usefulness of lymphatic and connective tissue clearance for the carcinoma of the pancreas head. Ann Surg. 208:215-220.
2. Ishikawa, O., Ohigashi, H., Imaoka, S., et al.(1992) Preoperative indications for locally advanced pancreas cancer involving the portal vein. Ann Surg. 215:231-236.

Indications for Extended Radical Whipple Operation for Ductal Adenocarcinoma of the Head of the Pancreas

M. Suzuki, F. Hanyu, T. Imaizumi, T. Nakasako, and N. Harada

Department of Gastroenterological Surgery, Tokyo Women's Medical College, Shinjuku-ku, Tokyo, Japan

ABSTRACT

The aim of this study is to investigate indications of extended radical Whipple operation for patients with ductal adenocarcinoma of the head of the pancreas. The postoperative survival rates at one year, 3 and 5 years were 100%, 60%,and 60% ,respectively among the patients in whom CT scan and abdominal angiography showed no tumor invasion to the retroperitoneum, the portal vein, and major abdominal artery. Among the patients who had massive tumor invasion to the retroperitoneum and the portal vein and the major abdominal artery, the survival rates were 5% at one year, and no patients survived more than 3 years. Indications for extended radical Whipple operation should be determined by using CT scan and abdominal angiography.

KEY WORDS: Indication, Whipple operation, Pancreatic cancer, CT scan, Abdominal angiography

INTRODUCTION

Majority of patients with ductal adenocarcinoma of the head of the pancreas have extrapancreatic tumor invasion. Standard Whipple operation without regional lymphadenectomy and dissection of the retroperitoneal connective tissues did not provide long-term survivors. Extended radical Whipple operation is necessary to obtain pathologically curative resection in patients with ductal adenocarcinoma of the head of the pancreas. Even extended radical Whipple operation,however, did not produce survival benefits in patients with too advanced tumor. Selection of the patients for extended radical operation is important. Using modern imaging techniques such as CT-scan or selective abdominal angiography, it has been possible to determine whether a patient has massive tumor invasion to the major abdominal vessels or to the retroperitoneal tissues. The aim of this study is to establish indications for extended radical Whipple operation for ductal adenocarcinoma of the head of the pancreas.

MATERIALS AND METHODS

From 1968 to 1992 December, 224 patients underwent Whipple operation for ductal adenocarcinoma of the head of the pancreas at our hospital. Among the 224 patients, 64 patients who had CT-scan and abdominal angiography preoperatively were selected for this study. Those patients who had liver metastasis or distant metastasis were excluded.The 64 patients were divided into four groups (Clinical Stage 1 to 4), on the basis of the grades of tumor invasion to the retroperitoneal connective tissues (Rp0 to Rp3), to the portal vein (PV0 to PV3), to the major abdominal artery (A0 to A3) Figure 1,3.

Figure 1. Grades of Tumor Invasion to the Retroperitoneum Diagnosed by CT Findings

Rp0   :Peripancreatic fatty plane is normal.
Rp1   :Mild spiculation in peripancreatic fatty plane.
Rp2   :Moderate spiculation in peripancreatic fatty plane.
Rp3   :Massive tumor invasion to the extrapancreatic organs.

Figure 2. Grades of Tumor Invasion to the Major Abdominal Vessels Diagnosed by Abdominal Angiography.
Portal system(Portal vein,Superior mesenteric vein,and Splenic vein)
PV0   :No abnormality is noted in the portal vein.
PV1   :Mild irregularity of the portal vein.
PV2   :Moderate irregularity
PV3   :Severe irregularity with collateral vessels formation.

752

Figure 3.   Major Abdominal Artery   (Hepatic artery, Superior mesenteric artery)
            A0   :No abnormality is noted in artery.
            A1   :Mild displacement or rigidity
            A2   :Moderate displacement or rigidity
            A3   :Stenosis of the artery.

Clinical stage was categorized into 4 groups on the basis of CT scan and abdominal angiography findings. Patients with Rp0,Pv0,and A0 were classified to CS1. Patients with Rp1,PV1,and A0 were CS2. Patients with Rp2,PV2,and A0 were CS3. Patients with Rp3,PV3,or A1 to A3 were classified as CS4.Figure 4

Figure 4. | Clinical stage | Retroperitoneal invasion | Portal invasion | Arterial invasion |
| --- | --- | --- | --- |
| CS1 | Rp0 | PV0 | A0 |
| CS2 | Rp1 | PV1 | A0 |
| CS3 | Rp2 | PV2 | A0 |
| CS4 | Rp3 | PV3 | A1~3 |

CS1 included 6 patients and all the 6 patients obtained curative resection which was confirmed by histopathological study. CS2 included 14 patients and 86% of the 14 patients obtained curative resection. 31 patients were graded as CS3 and curability was 55%. No one obtained curative resection in 13 patients with CS4.Figure 5

Figure 5. | Clinical stage | Number of patients | Curability |
| --- | --- | --- |
| CS1 | n= 6 | 100% |
| CS2 | n=14 | 86% |
| CS3 | n=31 | 55% |
| CS4 | n=13 | 0% |

The postoperative survival rates in the patients with CS1 were 100% at one year, 60% at 3 years, 60% at 5 years. In the patients with CS2, 3 and 5 years survival rates were 26%. One year survival rate in the patients with CS3 was 55% and it was 15% at 2 years. No patients survived more than 3 years in the patients with CS3 or CS4. The survival rates in the patients with CS4 were extremely poor.Figure 6

Figure 6. Survival curves after extended radical Whipple operation for adenocarcinoma of the head of the pancreas.

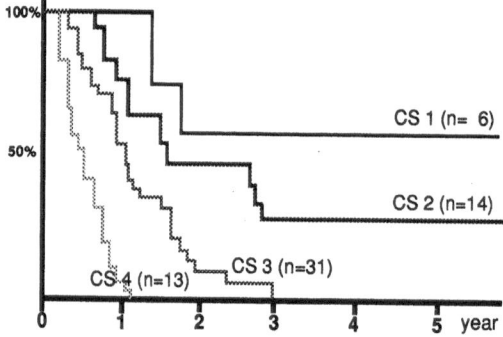

SUMMARY

Those data show that extended radical Whipple operation could produce long-term survival in patients with ductal adenocarcinoma of the head of the pancreas. But even extended radical Whipple operation did not provide survival benefits for the patients who had massive tumor invasion to the retroperitoneum or major abdominal artery. Indications for extended radical Whipple operation should be determined by clinical staging using CT scan and abdominal angiography.

Simultaneous Intraoperative Interstitial Hyperthermia and Intraoperative Electron Beam Radiation Therapy for Pancreatic Carcinoma

TAKESHI MORIMOTO, MITSUNORI YASUE, KENZO YASUI, and SEIICHI MIYAISHI

Department of Gastroenterological Surgery, Aichi Cancer Center, Nagoya, 464 Japan

ABSTRACT

To improve local control of pancreatic carcinoma, a new trial of simultaneous intraoperative interstitial hyperthermia (IOHT) and intraoperative electron beam radiation therapy (IORT) was initiated as a pilot study. After surgical exposure, metal catheters were implanted into pancreatic carcinoma for IOHT. Then the patient was given IOHT. At the midpoint in time during 30 minutes of steady state temperature of 43 °C, 25Gy of IORT was delivered using high-energy electrons(12-16 MeV). There were no critical side effects or complications such as bleeding or pancreas fistula after surgery. This pilot study has proven the clinical feasiblity of these 2 simultaneous treatment modalities.

KEY WORDS: hyperthermia, radiation therapy, pancreatic carcinoma

INTRODUCTION

The cure rate for patients with pancreatic carcinoma remains low [1-5]. In our previous study, conventional intraoperative radiation therapy (IORT) for pancreatic carcinoma has been shown to improve survival a little [6], but it remains unsatisfactory and not very effective in our ten years' experience with 109 cases of IORT. Building on our prior experience with patients having locally advanced pancreatic carcinoma, we initially treated these patients with simultaneous intraoperative interstitial hyperthermia (IOHT) and intraoperative electron beam radiation therapy (IORT) as a pilot study to potentially improve local control [Fig 1].

MATERIALS AND METHODS

This simultaneous IOHT-IORT was initiated in February 1992 for patients with pancreatic carcinoma diagnosed histologically. Six patients were treated, four were not resected, and two were resected after simultaneous IOHT-IORT. Interstitial hyperthermia treatment is delivered by a MINERVE hyperthermia system (Odam Co. Ltd, France). After surgical exposure, three to four pairs of metal catheters are implanted into the pancreatic carcinoma under ultrasonic

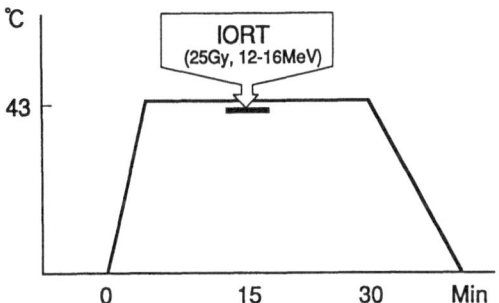

Fig. 1 At the midpoint in time during 30 minutes of steady state temperature of 43 'C, 25Gy of IORT was delivered using high-energy electrons(12-16 MeV).

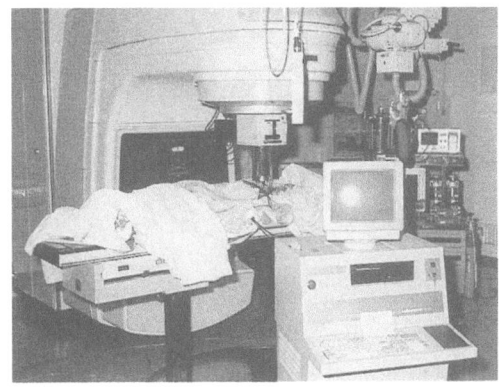

Fig. 2 The patient is under the linear accelerator beside the MINERVE system.

tomography for IOHT. Then the patient is moved under the linear accelerator beside the MINERVE system [Fig 2]. For non-resectable patients, the position of the implanted metal catheters is examined by intraoperative CT scanning. Under the linear accelerator, electrodes with minerve thermometer are inserted into the metal catheters in pancreatic carcinoma [Fig 3], and the cone for IORT is positioned over the treatment field [Fig. 4]. At the midpoint in time during 30 minutes of steady state temperature at 43°C, 25Gy of IORT is delivered using high-energy electrons (12-16 MeV). After completion of IORT and IOHT, the IORT cone system is disengaged and the hyperthermia electrodes are removed. After removal of each metal catheter, the Z or U sutures are placed and tightened to prevent back bleeding and leakage of pancreatic secretions into the abdomen. Then for unresected patients, fibrin glue is sprayed on the sutured field and gastrojejunostomy and/or hepatico-duodenostomy are performed. For resectable cases pancreaticoduoden-ectomy with regional lymphnodes dissection is performed.

RESULTS and DISCUSSION

Six patients underwent the simultaneous IOHT-IORT treatment. Four were unresected and two were resected cases. In resected cases, the purpose of this therapy prior to resection is to prevent intraportal dissemination to the liver during manipulation of pancreas resection.

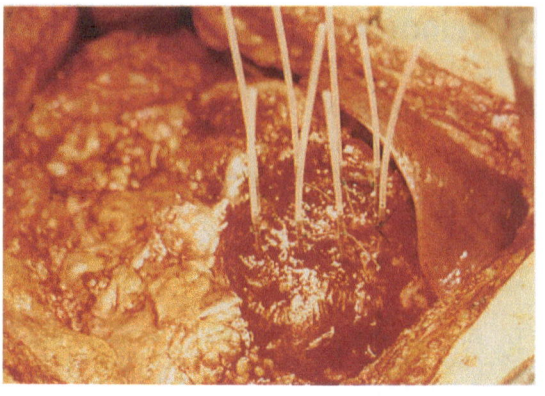

Fig. 3 Four pairs of metal catheters are implanted into the pancreatic carcinoma for IOHT

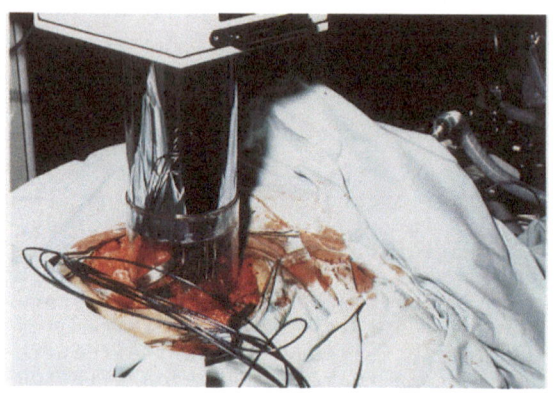

Fig. 4 The cone for IORT is positioned over the treatment field.

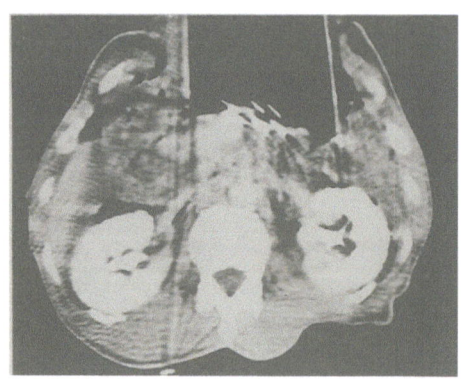

intraoperative CT

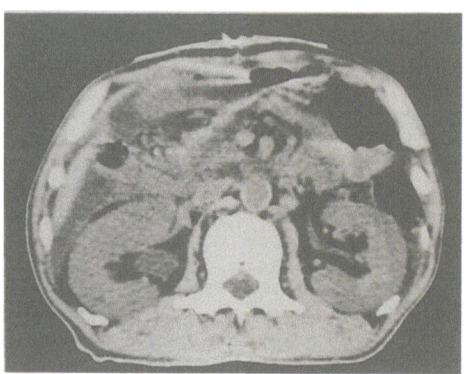

CT at 3 weeks after operation

Fig. 5 The presence of a CT-documented decrease in the size of the primary tumor mass.

The advantage of this method is simultaneous use of two effective modalities for local tumor control. Overgaard reported his experiment in which the thermal enhancement ratios for tumors were higher after simultaneous treatment than when heat and radiation were given in immediate succession. And he showed there is a log-linear relationship between thermal enhancement ratio and temperature, 1.2 at 41°C, 2.0 at 42°C, 2.5 at 42.5°C, 4.0 at 43°C and 5.4 at 43.5°C [7]. In our clinical trial 43.0°C 30 min heat and 25 Gy radiation were applied at exactly the same time. Evaluation of local control was

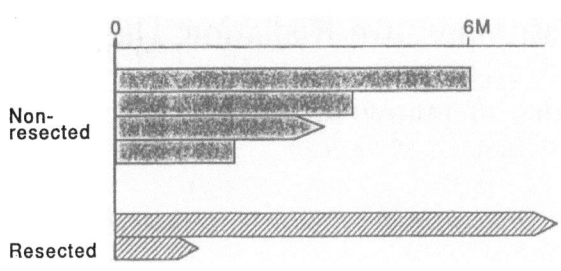

Fig. 6 Survival of patients treated by simultaneous intraoperative interstitial hyperthermia (IOHT) and intraoperative electron beam therapy (IORT).

attempted with CT scanning at 3-4 weeks and three months. In two unresected cases, the presence of a CT-documented decrease in the size of the primary tumor mass was noted [Fig 5]. Survival was shown in Fig. 6 in the figure. In four unresected cases, one lived for 3 months, and the others were survived 6, 4, and 2 months, respectively. Two resected cases given IOHT-IORT before resection have lived for 7 months and one month now. In the six cases under study, there were no critical side effects or complications such as bleeding [8] or pancreas fistura after surgery. Mild bleeding and/or small leakage of pancreatic secretion from a hole of the metal catheter were noted from almost all holes after removal of catheters. Treatment for such leakage by the prescribed methods during operation completely prevented any oozing. The safe clinical course were confirmed after operation. This pilot study has been proven that simultaneous IOHT and IORT are safe and clinically feasible forms of treatment.

REFERENCE

1. Tepper JE, Noyes D, Krall JM, Sause WT, Wolkov HB, Dobelbower RR, Thomson J, Owens J, Hanks GE (1991) Intraoperative radiation therapy of pancreatic carcinoma: A report of RTOG-8505. Int J Radiation Oncology Biol Phys 21 1145-1149
2. Gastrointestinal Tumor Study Group (1987) Futher evidence of effective adjuvant combined radiation and chemotherapy following curative resection of pancreatic cancer. Cancer 59:2006-2010
3. Jeekel J, Treurniet-Donker AD (1991) Treatment perspective in locally advanced unresectable pancreatic cancer. Br J Surg 78:1332-1334
4. Michelassi F, Erroi F, Dawson PJ, Pietrabissa A. Noda S, Handcock M, Block GE (1989) Experience with 647 consecutive tumor of the duodenum, ampulla, head of pancreas and distal common bile duct. Ann Surg 210:544-556
5. Dobelbower RR, Konski AA, Merrick III HW, Bronn DG, Schifeling D, Kamen C (1991) Intraopgerative electron beam radiation therapy (IOEBRT) for carcinoma of the exocrine pancreas. Int J Radiation Oncology Biol Phys 20:113-119
6. Yasue M, Sakamoto J, Yasui K, Morimoto T, Kurimoto K, Kuno N, Morita K (1992) A randomized trial of intraoperative radiation therapy (IORT) vs IORT plus chemotherapy (MTX-5FU) for adenocarcinoma of the pancreas. Proc Am Soc Clin Oncol 11:161
7. Overgaard J (1980) Simultaneous and sequential hyperthermia and radiation treatment of an experimental tumor and its surrounding normal tissue in vivo. Int J Radiation Oncology Biol Phys 6:1507-1517

Resection of Remote Metastases from Pancreatic Cancer in Patients Previously Treated with Radical Resection Combined with Intraoperative Radiation Therapy

Hiroshi Takamori, Takehisa Hiraoka, Keiichirou Kanemitsu, and Yoshimasa Miyauchi

First Department of Surgery, Kumamoto University School of Medicine, Kumamoto, 860 Japan

ABSTRACT

Since 1984, we have performed extended radical resection combined with extended intraoperative radiation therapy (IORT) for pancreatic cancer. This approach has provided a dramatic improvement in long-term survival and control of local recurrence. Among patients with this combined therapy, two patients without local recurrence underwent resection for remote metastases. They are still alive over 6 years, and 2 years and 5 months after the first operation, respectively. These two cases suggest that surgical approach for the removal of remote metastases may result in long-term survival of pancreatic cancer.

KEY WORDS: pancreatic cancer, liver metastases, extended radical resection, intraoperative radiation therapy

INTRODUCTION

Even after radical resection of pancreatic cancer, a high proportion of patients have local recurrence and hepatic metastases at autopsy. In order to control local recurrence after radical resection, we have performed extended radical resection combined with extended intraoperative radiation therapy (IORT) since 1984. We have had a dramatic improvement in long-term survival and control of local recurrence compared with other approaches [1,2]. However, although local recurrence are uncommon, most patients died of remote metastases. In two patients without local recurrence after the combined therapy, we performed resections of remote metastases. Surgical approaches for remote metastases after radical resection for pancreatic cancer has not previously been reported.

CASE REPORTS

Case 1

A 70-year-old man was admitted with a 1 month history of painless jaundice, pruritus, and light colour stool. He had lost 3 Kg in 1 month. Tumour markers (elastase-1; 300 ng/dl and CA19-9 ; <6 u/ml) were within normal limits. Computed tomographic (CT) scan revealed a 4 cm low density mass in the head of the pancreas. Endoscopic retrograde cholangiopancreatography showed disruption of the main pancreatic duct of the head of the pancreas and stenosis of the intrapancreatic common bile duct. Endoscopic retrograde biliary drainage was achieved preoperatively. Visceral angiography showed that the posterior superior and anterior superior pancreatoduodenal artery were not visualized; and the pancreatic segment of the portal vein was only slightly narrowed. These imaging studies revealed no liver metastases. He underwent operation and a 6 cm tumour was identified on the neck of the pancreas. This tumour appeared to be directly invading the portal vein. The retroperitoneal surface of the pancreas appeared to be intact but there was tumour involvement of the juxta-regional lymph nodes adjacent to the pancreas. Hepatic metastases and metastases in other organs were not detected. A radical extended total pancreatectomy with resection of the pancreatic segment of the portal vein was performed. The juxta-regional and regional lymph nodes together with the connective tissue around the aorta extending from the diaphragm above to the inferior mesenteric artery below was dissected. Following dissection and vascular reconstruction, a dose of 30 Gy with 9 MeV of electron beam was administered to the operative field including the paraaortic area from the diaphragm to the inferior mesenteric artery using a special applicator that could be varied in size to accommodate the operative field on an individual basis. The bile duct was kept outside of the irradiation field [2]. Histopathological findings showed a moderately differentiated tubular adenocarcinoma of stage III (pT2, pN1, pM0) according to the TNM classification. At the resection margin of the resected specimen, cancer cells were found histologically. This operation was identified as a nonradical operation. He was discharged 4 months later. For adjuvant chemotherapy, he was treated with Tegafur (N_1-(2'-tetrahydrofuryl)-5-fluorouracil) 600 mg per day orally. A CT scan 29 months later revealed a 3 cm low density area enhanced by contrast medium in the S_6 segment of the liver. Visceral angiography showed the same sized tumour stain as that of CT scan. Ultrasonography revealed isoechoic area surrounded by a low echoic band in the same area. No local recurrence was detected and he underwent partial resection of the liver. Pathological diagnosis was well differentiated tubular adenocarcinoma with invasion into Glisson's sheath. A CT scan 17 months after the hepatic resection revealed a 3 cm low density area in the remnant S_6 segment of the liver. Visceral angiography, and ultrasonography suggested it was metastatic tumour. Operative findings showed that this tumour invaded into the right kidney, ascending colon, and right diaphragm. We performed partial resection of the liver combined with partial resection of the right kidney, ascending colon, and right diaphragm. Pathological findings showed well differentiated tubular adenocarcinoma, indicating metastasis from the pancreatic cancer. After the operation, fractional external beam radiation with a dose of 50 Gy was administered to the resected area. He has recovered with an excellent performance status. He is still alive over 6 years after the first operation.

Case 2

A 58-year-old man was admitted complaining of epigastric pain, back pain, and jaundice. Tumour markers were elevated (CA 19-9; 24640 u/ml, SPAN-1; 48.4 U/ml, elastase-1; 876 ng/dl). Abdominal ultrasonography revealed a 3.5 cm irregular solid mass in the head of pancreas. CT scan revealed that the head of the pancreas was enlarged, and the main pancreatic duct in the body and tail of the pancreas was dilated. Percutaneous transhepatic cholangiography showed complete obstruction of the

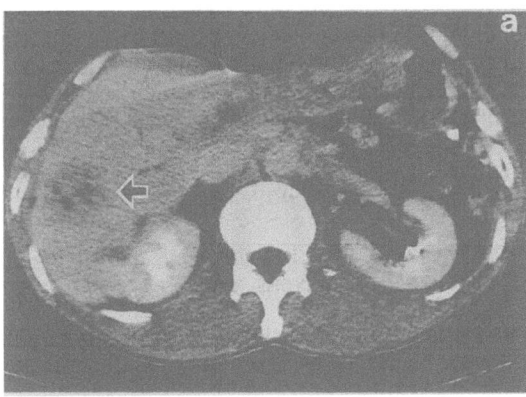
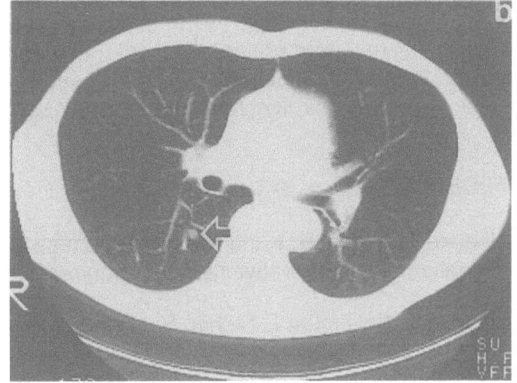
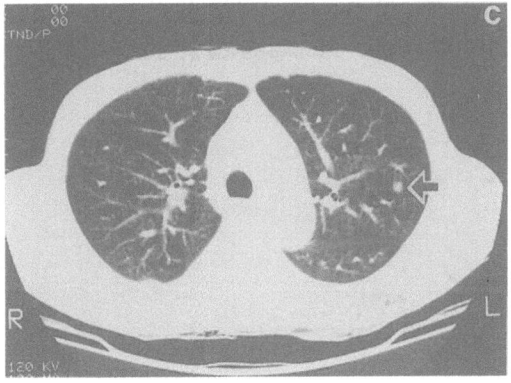

Fig. 1 Metastatic tumour (arrow) in the liver (a), and right lung (b), respectively as seen by computed tomography one year and 9 months after the extended radical resection. A left lung metastases as seen by CT 2 months after resections of metastatic lesions of the liver and right lung. (arrow, c)

intrapancreatic common bile duct, and percutaneous transhepatic biliary drainage was performed preoperatively. Visceral angiography showed that the anterior and posterior superior pancreatoduodenal artery had irregular encasement. These imaging studies revealed no liver metastases. At surgery a tumour of 5 x 3 x 3 cm with involvement of the juxta-regional lymph nodes was identified on the head of the pancreas. No metastases were detected in the liver. A radical extended pancreatoduodenectomy was combined with intraoperative radiation therapy, using the same parameters as in case 1. Histopathological findings showed a moderately differentiated tubular adenocarcinoma of stage III (pT2, pN1, pM0). This operation was histologically nonradical because of cancer cells at the resection margin of the specimen. After discharge, he was treated with adjuvant chemotherapy of Tegafur 600 mg per day orally. One year and 9 months after his resection CT scans showed a low density area of 2 cm in diameter in the S_6 segment of the liver, and a coin lesion in the S_6 segment of the right lung (Fig. 1 (a, b)). For hepatic metastases, he underwent percutaneous ethanol injection therapy three times, but the size of the tumour increased. There was no local recurrence at that time, so a radical partial resection of the liver and the right lung was performed. Pathological findings showed moderately differentiated tubular adenocarcinoma. A CT scan 2 months later, however, showed a coin lesion in upper lobe of the left lung (Fig. 1 (c)), so he underwent a radical partial resection of the left lung. He is still alive over 2 year and 5 months after the first operation.

DISCUSSION

Despite recent advances in diagnostic and surgical techniques for pancreatic cancer and improvements in operative and perioperative management, many reports have demonstrated that not only the rate of resectability but the long-term results after resection have been disappointing [3]. Traditionalists believe that is no reason to study cancer of the pancreas, because 1) the patients all die, anyway; 2) palliative procedures are of no benefit; 3) symptomatic treatment is unsatisfactory; 4) biopsy is too risky; and 5) early diagnosis is impossible; 6) there are no clusters of patients to study [4]. Since 1984, however, we have performed IORT with a dose of 30 Gy with 9 MeV following extended operation on 14 patients. The 5 year cumulative survival rate of these cases was 33.3%. Four autopsies showed no local recurrences in three cases. Control of local recurrence was improved by introduction of extended operation combined with extended IORT [1]. Although the two cases presented here had macroscopically complete tumour clearance, cancer cells were found at the resection margin of the specimen microscopically. Local recurrence, however, was not detected clinically after the combined therapy indicating the effectiveness of the intraoperative radiation. Therefore, we could perform surgery for metastatic lesions from pancreatic cancer in these two cases and get survival for over 6 years and 2 years and 5 months, respectively. These cases suggest that even in patients with pancreatic cancer, it is possible to perform surgical resections of metastatic lesions, and achieve long term survival.

REFERENCES

1. Hiraoka T, Uchino R, Kanemitsu K, Toyonaga M, Saitoh N, Nakamura I, Tashiro S, Miyauchi Y (1990) Combination of intraoperative radiation with resection of cancer of the pancreas. Int J Pancreatol 7:201-207
2. Hiraoka T, Nakamura I, Tashiro S, Miyauchi Y (1989) Intraoperative radiation therapy for pancreatic cancer in Japan. Dobelbower RR and Abe M, eds., Intraoperative Radiation Therapy. CRC, Boca Raton, FL 181-193
3. Watanapa P, Williamson RCN (1992) Surgical palliation for pancreatic cancer: developments during the past two decades. Br J Surg 79:8-20
4. Douglass HO Jr (1987) Pancreatic cancer: Nihilism is obsolete! Pancreas 2:230-232

A Quantitative Analysis of Gastrointestinal Motility After Intraoperative High Dose Irradiation to Paraaortic Lymph Nodes in Dogs

Masanao Ito, Yoshihiro Asanuma, and Kenji Koyama

The First Department of Surgery, Akita University School of Medicine, Akita, 010 Japan

ABSTRACT

The effect of high dose intraoperative radiation therapy (HDIORT) around the root of superior mesenteric artery (SMA) on gastrointestinal motility was studied in conscious dogs. Four strain-gauge force transducers were implanted on the antrum and jejunum. HDIORT caused diarrhea within 2 weeks after irradiation, in conjunction with the modulation of gastrointestinal motility such as increase of rate and duration of phase II of antral IMC, changes of hourly peak of postprandial motility of antrum and jejunum. The bowel habit gets normalized 1 month after irradiation, and the changes of gastrointestinal motility assessed by force transducer is almost normalized 1 year later.

KEYWORDS: intraoperative radiation therapy, gastrointestinal motility, radiation injury, pancreatic cancer, strain-gauge force transducer

INTRODUCTION

Of pancreatic cancer, perineural and lymphatic invasions around the root of SMA is one of the prognostic factors. Extensive cleaning of the regional lymph nodes had been widely applied in Japan, however the prognosis had not been improved, moreover patients suffer from severe diarrhea postoperatively. Intraoperative irradiation to paraaortic lymph nodes is to be effective for cancer invasion, however cytocidal effect can not be expected at the present dose of 25 to 30Gy. The dose increase may result in the radiation injury such as stenosis of SMA or degeneration of celiac ganglions, which can cause the disturbance of gastrointestinal motility. The purpose of this study is to evaluate the change of gastrointestinal motility for up to 1year after HDIORT.

MATERIALS AND METHODS

Experiments were performed on twelve healthy mongrel dogs, each weighting 10-15kg. In six dogs using for acute effect study, three in control group and three in HDIORT group, four strain-gauge force transducer were implanted on the antrum (A) and the jejunum at 10 (J1), 60 (J2), 110 (J3) cm from the ligament of Treitz under general pentobarbital anesthesia (25mg/kg) to record circular muscle contractions. The conducting wires were brought out through the skin and dogs were fitted with protective jacket to cover wires. The dogs were allowed 14 days to recover from surgery. Each dog served as its own control. After an overnight fast, interdigestive recordings were made for 24h before the dogs were fed. After the end of IMC in J3, each dog were fed a 30kcal/kgBW solid meal with 400ml water. The postprandial recordings lasted for 8h. The dogs then underwent laparotomy under general anesthesia, so that intraoperative irradiation of 80Gy was performed using 7MeV electrons with a dose rate of 3.0Gy/minute with 35x45 mm rectangular cone. Three dogs used as the control underwent only laparotomy. Another six dogs using for chronic effect study, three in control group and three in HDIORT group, four strain-gauge force transducers were implanted 1 year after irradiation. The recordings were carried out in the same way as the acute effect study, starting at 14 day after implantation. Gastrointestinal motility was recorded in conscious dogs and analysed at 1, 2, 3, 4 weeks and 1 year after irradiation in both the fasted and fed state. The recordings were made on a 4-channel recorder. The signals were transferred to a NEC computer for sampling at

100ms, A-to-D conversion, storage, and analysis. Of gastrointestinal motility, IMC and postprandial pattern were analysed. Four phases of IMC of antrum was identified visually and measured on the recording paper. Motor complexes which migrated from A to J3 were recognized as the IMC. IMCs originated only in jejunum were distinguished as intestinal IMC (I-IMC) from gastrointestinal IMC (GI-IMC). Of postprandial contractions, the integrated area of the curve (MI:motility index) of A and J1 was calculated in every 1h by the computer and the hourly changes of MI were investigated. The amplitude of each contraction was expressed in grams of force, therefore hourly MI was expressed in gram-hours. Nature of feces, body weight, serum albumin were also evaluated. All values are expressed as the mean ± SEM. Comparisons were made by Student-t test. A p value less than 0.05 was considered statistically significant.

RESULTS

Clinical Symptoms and Laboratory Data

None of the dogs had diarrhea before laparotomy. In the control group, no diarrhea was observed. After 80Gy irradiation, diarrhea took place in 2 out of 3 dogs, but improved within 4 weeks. Body weight decreased by 10% at 1 week in both group and its recovery was delayed in HDIORT group. Serum albumin at 1 week after operation decreased by 9% (2.75 ± 0.25 to 2.5 ± 0.1 g/dl) in control group and 12% (3.0 ± 0.16 to 2.6 ± 0.12 g/dl) in HDIORT group compared to the value before operation. In control group, it was recovered (3.0 ± 0.20 g/dl) at 4 weeks, whereas it could not recover (2.7 ± 0.23 g/dl) in HDIORT group.

Effects of HDIORT on Gastrointestinal Motility

Table 1. Mean cycle duration and the components of IMC of HDIORT group

	Phase I (%)	Phase II (%)	Phase III (%)	Phase IV (%)	IMC Cycle(min)
p r e	43.3± 4.0	33.8± 4.4	16.8± 1.6	6.1± 2.3	103.6± 9.4
1 W	47.7± 8.7	*42.3± 9.8	*8.6± 1.5	*1.4± 0.5	*198.0± 44.7
2 W	34.4± 5.5	*44.6± 6.3	16.4± 2.2	4.6± 1.0	122.0± 16.8
3 W	43.2± 6.8	39.5± 6.9	12.7± 1.2	4.6± 0.9	121.0± 11.9
4 W	43.1± 3.9	32.5± 3.2	16.4± 1.4	8.0± 1.6	101.7± 6.7
1 Y	*72.0± 2.5	*15.3± 2.6	*10.1± 0.5	2.6± 0.3	120.5± 6.0

*p< 0.05

Table 2. Incidence of I-IMC

	CONTROL %I-IMC	HDIORT %I-IMC
p r e	16.7± 6.8	15.1± 6.8
1 W	16.7± 6.8	*45.0± 8.5
2 W	19.4± 8.2	17.8± 7.9
3 W	15.0± 6.2	27.3± 3.2
4 W	12.2± 5.2	15.1± 3.2
1 Y	26.1± 3.2	23.2± 4.4

*p< 0.05

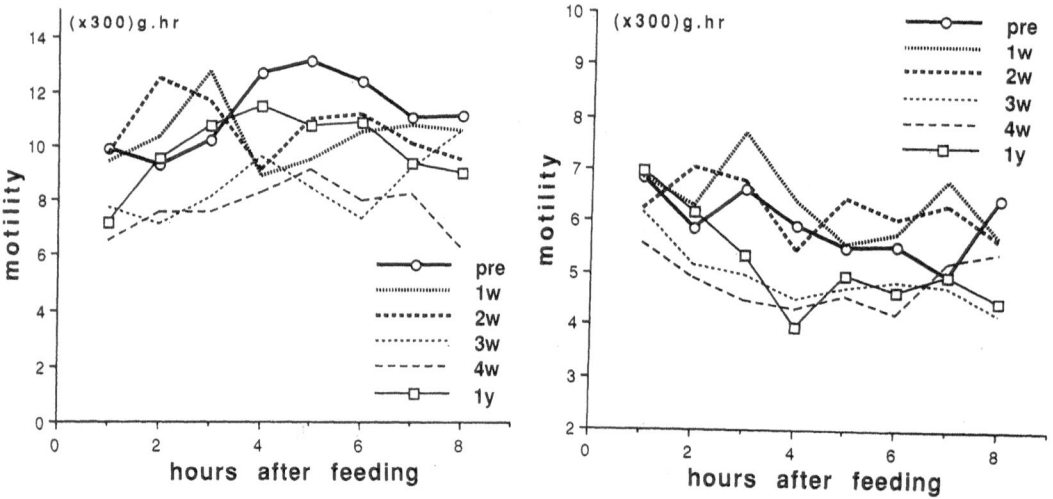

Fig. 2 Changes in hourly MI of antrum(left) and jejunum(right) of HDIORT group

Table 1 shows the characteristics of IMC of antrum in HDIORT group. In control group, there was no significant difference at any stage. In HDIORT group, the duration of phaseII increased after radiation, thus the rate of phaseII in IMC cycle also increased by 8.5-10.8% at 1,2 week. Average IMC cycle was elongated up to 190% at 1 week. Another striking feature was the consistency of the duration of phase III and IV of the complex. At 1 year, the duration and rate of phaseII were almost the same among control group and radiation group. Table 2 shows the mean incidence of I-IMC (%I-IMC:100 x No. of I-IMC / total No. of IMC). In HDIORT group, I-IMC occurred frequently at 1 week. After feeding, hourly changes of MI of the antrum and jejunum were analyzed (Fig.2). At any stage of control group, the hourly changes of MI were not different. In control group, the peak of hourly MI of antrum occurred 4-5h after feeding. But in radiation group the peak occurred earlier (2-3h) at 1,2 week. The peak of MI of jejunum located within 1h after feeding, therefore the MI tended to decrease gradually in control group. But in radiation group, the MI had its peak in 2-3h after feeding at 1,2 week. At 1 year in HDIORT group, MI was normal except for hypokinetics in early phase of antrum.

DISCUSSION

The advantage of intraoperative radiation therapy is controllability of irradiated area and depth. But if the dosage is less than cytocidal dose of cancer cell, we can not take advantage of irradiation. Furthermore, if the side effects with the increase of radiation dose occur severely, we can not increase the dose. Marlett and Code (1) reported that celiac and superior mesenteric ganglionectomy, causes the temporal irregularity of the cycles of the IMC from the myoelectrical activity. They reported that the variability of the duration of the cycles was increased 2-5 times after the ganglionectomy. They also found that the duration of phase III was unaltered by the ganglionectomy. These phenomenons in the acute stage after the ganglionectomy are so similar to our experimental results. Therefore it is presumed that HDIORT may cause transient dysfunctions of the ganglions. The hypokinetics of antrum observed in late stage of our experiment may be the late effect of HDIORT. Otterson et al (2,3) reported the effect of external beam radiation therapy on small intestinal motor activity. They documented that IMC cycle persisted during fractionated irradiation and that the side effect such as diarrhea and vomiting may be related to the giant migrating contractions and retrograde giant contractions. In this study, small intestine had never been irradiated, therefore the giant contractions were not observed. But the changes of the hourly peak of postprandial motility of antrum and jejunum seemed to reflect the rapid transit and cause the change of nature of feces. So one of the factors that may alter the characteristics of gastrointestinal motility was likely to the dysfunction of the ganglions. Another factor that can change the intestinal motility was mesenteric blood flow. Fioramonti et al (4) concluded that in the conscious dog the blood flow profile in a mesenteric artery is associated with the motor profile of the segment. In conclusion, HDIORT caused diarrhea within 3 weeks after irradiation in conjunction with the modulation of gastrointestinal motility such as the increase of duration and rate of phaseII of antral IMC, changes of hourly peak of postprandial motility of antrum and jejunum. Summers et al (5) emphasized that total abdominal irradiation produced profound functional abnormalities in intestinal muscle even though the morphology was minimally altered. The mechanisms by which gastrointestinal motility can be modulated after HDIORT has to be investigated hereafter.

REFERENCES

1. Marlett JA, Code CF (1979) Effects of celiac and superior mesenteric ganglionectomy on interdigestive myoelectric complex in dogs. Am J Physiol 237:432-436
2. Otterson MF, Sarna SK, Moulder JE (1988) Effects of fractionated doses of ionizing radiation on small intestinal motor activity. Gastroenterology 95:1249-1257
3. Otterson MF, Sarna SK, Lee MB (1992) Fractionated doses of ionizing radiation alter postprandial small intestinal motor activity. Dig Dis Sci 37:709-715
4. Fioramonti J, Bueno L (1984) Relation between intestinal motility and mesenteric blood flow in the conscious dogs. Am J Physiol 246:108-113
5. Summers RW, Flatt AJ, Prihoda MJ, Mitros FA (1987) Effect of irradiation on morphology and motility of canine small intestine. Dig Dis Sci 32:1402-1410

Immunohistological Expression of Pancreatic Cancer Associated Mucin Antigen and Radioimmunodetection in Pancreatic Cancer

Yong-Suk Chung[1], Yasuyuku Kondo[1], Tetsuji Sawada[1], Akimasa Inui[1], Kwang-Sa Kim[1], Yoshito Yamashita[1], Masahiro Okuno[1], Hironobu Ochi[2], Jenny J.L. Ho[3], Young S. Kim[3], and Michio Sowa[1]

[1]The First Department of Surgery, [2]Division of Nuclear Medicine, Osaka City University Medical School, Osaka, Japan; [3]VA Medical Center, University of California, San Francisco, CA, USA

ABSTRACT

Nd2 is a murine monoclonal antibody produced against a mucin fraction purified from pancreatic cancer cell line SW1990 and the antigen recognized has been clarified to be a non-circulating antigen. In this study the specificity of Nd2 and clinical significance of ^{111}In-Nd2 in radioimmunodetection for pancreatic cancer were evaluated. Immunohistochemical analysis revealed the presence of the Nd2 antigen in pancreatic cancer tissues with high incidence but not in tissues of normal pancreas and chronic pancreatitis. Distinct immuno-scintigrams of corresponding tumors in patients with pancreatic cancer were obtained by administration of ^{111}In-Nd2 and positive rate of radioimmunodetection was over 70% with no false positives.

KEY WORDS: Nd2, pancreatic cancer, radioimmunodetection

INTRODUCTION

Reports of successful radioimmunodetection (RAID) with monoclonal antibodies (MoAb) have increased steadily for a number of malignancies [1-3]. However, only a few MoAb have been described for pancreatic cancer. Nd2 is a murine MoAb produced against mucins purified from xenografts of a human pancreatic cancer cell line SW1900 and the antigen recognized by Nd2 has been clarified to be non-circulating antigen [4,5]. In this study we evaluated the specificity of Nd2 for tissues of pancreatic cancer and RAID in nude mice bearing pancreatic cancer, and the possibility of application of RAID in which Nd2 is applied as a carrier to tumors in patients with pancreatic cancer.

MATERIALS AND METHODS

Immunohistochemical Investigation

The intraoperatively obtained tissue samples from pancreatic cancer, chronic pancreatitis including tumor forming pancreatitis, pancreatic cyst and normal pancreas were fixed in formalin and embedded in paraffin. Immunoperoxidase staining of tissues was performed by the avidin-biotin-peroxidase complex method. A specimen was considered positive if at least 5% of the optical field was stained. Effects of various treatments such as neura-minidase, trypsin and NaIO4 on Nd2 antigenicity were also evaluated.

Radioimmunodetection

Nd2 hybridomas were injected i.p. into Balb/c mice and Nd2 was purified from ascites of mice by affinity chromatography on protein A columns. For RAID, ^{111}In labeled Nd2 was prepared as follows. A 10 molar ratio cyclic DTPA was conjugated to Nd2, and unconjugated DTPA was removed by gel filtration on a Sephadex G-25 column. DTPA-conjugated Nd2 was labeled with ^{111}In by simple incubation at room temperature, and the labeling efficiency was more than 90% without any further purification steps. The specific activity of ^{111}In-labeled Nd2 was 1mCi(37MBq)/mg protein. Fifty μ Ci of ^{111}In-labeled Nd2 was injected intravenously to nude mice bearing the SW1990 xenograft, and immunoscintigraphy was performed with a gamma camera equipped with a pinhole collimator on the 4th day after injection. The clinical trial of RAID by ^{111}In labeled Nd2 was reviewed and approved by the Institutional Review Board of Osaka City University, Medical School. Eleven patients who were initially diagnosed to have pancreatic cancer prior to resection were injected with ^{111}In labeled Nd2 (2mCi/2mg protein in 100ml normal saline solution with 2% human albumin). Scintigraphy was obtained on the 3rd day after injection.

RESULTS

Immunohistochemistry

Normal pancreatic tissues did not express any of the Nd2 antigen except a few ductules whose staining intensity was very faint. Nd2 did not react with acini, ducts or islet cells. In chronic pancreatitis including tumor forming pancreatitis, the expression of Nd2 antigen closely resembled that of normal pancreatic tissue in terms of staining distribution. Nd2 stained the majority of pancreatic cancer tissues, and Nd2 antigen was expressed in both apical membrane and cytosol of positive cells, furthermore in stromal tissues in some cases. Well and moderately differentiated cancer had much higher Nd2 reactivity compared to poorly differentiated cancer (Table 1). Nd2 antigenicity of cancer tissues was not reduced by the treatment with neuraminidase and NaIO4, and trypsin tended to increase the expression immunohistologically.

Table 1. Immunohistochemical expression of Nd2 in pancreatic diseases

Tissues	positive No./tested No.	positive ratio (%)
Pancreatic cancer	34 / 41	82.9%
well	15 / 16	93.8%
moderate	14 / 16	87.5%
poor	5 / 9	55.6%
Chronic pancreatitis	0 / 18	0%
Pancreatic cyst	0 / 4	0%
Normal pancreas	0 / 26	0%

Immunoscintigraphy

When a nude mouse bearing the SW1990 xenograft was scanned on the 4th day after administration of ^{111}In-labeled Nd2, tumor imaging was detected distinctly. However, non-specific accumulation in the liver was seen. Table 2 shows the characteristics of the patients studied and the results of RAID. RAID by ^{111}In-labeled Nd2 visualized tumors in six of 8 patients (75%) with pancreatic cancer, and there were no false positive cases and specificity was very high (100%) in this series. Fig. 1 shows a case with positive tumor imaging.

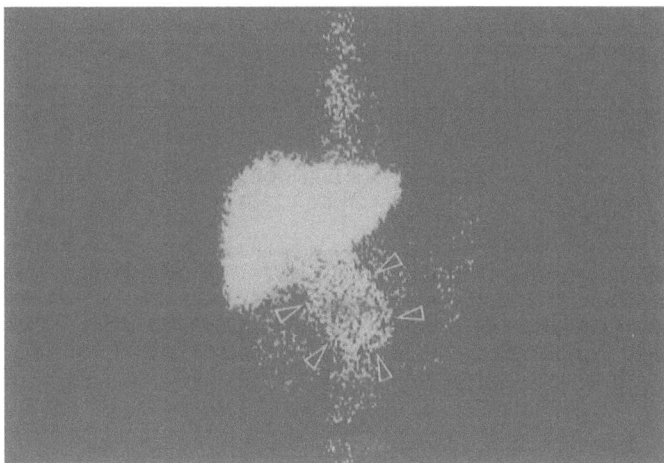

Fig.1 Anterior view scintigraphy of a patient (No.10 in Table 2) with pancreatic cancer show uptake of ^{111}In-Nd2 by the tumor.

Table 2. Patients and Radioimmunodetection

patients	age/sex	final diagnosis	RAID
1	39 / F	TFP	N
2	59 / M	PC. recurrence	P
3	59 / M	PC. metastasis	P
4	69 / M	PC	P
5	46 / F	PC	N
6	45 / M	islet cell ca.	N
7	50 / M	PC	P
8	61 / M	PC	N
9	35 / F	NED	N
10	68 / M	PC	P
11	60 / M	PC	P

TFP: tumor forming pancreatitis, PC: pancreatic ductal cell carcinoma
NED: no evidence of disease, P: positive image, N: negative image

DISCUSSION

In spite of modern diagnostic procedures and highly developed concervative and surgical therapeutic strategies in oncology, pancreatic carcinoma of ductal origin is still almost invariably an incurable disease. A characteristic tumor biology with regard to growth behavior, metastatic mode, and unspecific symptoms in the initial stage are responsible for this poor prognosis. The introduction of the hybridoma technique has enable us to produce MoAb directed against the cell surface and intracellular antigen of cancer cells. So far, several pancreatic cancer associated tumor markers such as CA19-9 and SPan-1 whose antigenetic determinants are carbohydrate structures, have been reported by employing the MoAb technique. Those markers show a high sensitivity in the diagnosis of pancreatic cancer. However they have some problems due to a relatively high false positive rate. Differentiation of pancreatic cancer from benign pancreatic disease is also, difficult sometimes. Therefore, new methods to detect pancreatic cancer are required, and monoclonal antibodies with high specificity for pancreatic cancer is needed. In this study, we showed that MoAb Nd2 has considerable specificity for pancreatic cancer, and this MoAb was considered to be suitable for application to detect pancreatic cancer. The antigen recognized by Nd2 has been clarified to be a non-circulating antigen which suggests that it can not be used as a serum marker. However, the characteristics of Nd2 are ideal as a carrier for radioimmunodetection [4,5]. When this kind of MoAb is injected to patients, MoAb does not make a complex with the antigen in sera, so that it can arrive at the tumor cells effectively without trapping. By means of labeling techniques, radiopharmacons can be coupled to MoAbs, and these conjugates are known to be of some value in the diagnosis of several tumors. Previous attempts of reports of RAID in pancreatic cancer have not been successful. We initiated a diagnostic RAID study employing Nd2 MoAb in patients with pancreatic cancer, and they showed clear tumor localization with high incidence and no false positives. These findings indicate that Nd2 has high specificity for pancreatic cancer tissues and ^{111}In-Nd2 has clinical usefullness in diagnosis and tumor localization of pancreatic cancer.

REFERENCES

1. Winzelberg GG, Grossman SJ, Rizk S, Joyce JM, Hill JB, Atkinson DP, Sudina K, Anderson K, McElwain D, Jones AM (1992) Indium-111 monoclonal antibody B72.3 scintigraphy in colorectal cancer. Cancer 69:1656-1663.
2. Krishnamurthy S, Morris JF, Antonovic R, Ahmed A, Galey WT, Duncan C, Krishnamurthy GT (1990) Evaluation of primary lung cancer with indium 111 anti-carcinoembryonic antigen (Type ZCE-025) monoclonal antibody scintigraphy. Cancer 65:458-465.
3. van Dongen GAMS, Leverstein H, Roos JC, Quak JJ, van den Brekel MWM, van Lingen A, Martens HJM, Castelijns JA, Visser GWM, Meijer CJLM, Teule GJJ, Snow GB (1992) Radioimmunoscintigraphy of head and neck cancer using 99mTc-labeled monoclonal antibody E48F(ab')2. Cancer Res 52:2569-2574
4. Ho JJL, Bi N, Yan P, Yuan M, Norton KA, Kim YS (1991) Characterization of new pancreatic cancer-reactive monoclonal antibodies directed against purified mucin. Cancer Res 51: 371-380
5. Sawada T, Chung YS, Kondo Y, Sowa M, Umeyama K, Ochi H, Ho JJL, Kim YS (1991) Radioimmunodetection of human pancreatic cancer using 111In-labeled monoclonal antibody Nd2. Antib Immunoconjug and Radiopharm 4:493-499

Biodistribution and Imaging of Chimeric Fab Fragment of Anti-Carcinoembryonic Antigen (CEA) Monoclonal Antibody in Nude Mice Bearing Pancreatic Carcinoma Xenografts

T. Kamigaki[1], M. Yamamoto[1], Y. Saitoh[1], H. Ohyanagi[2], T. Kaneda[3], T. Ohmura[3], and K. Yokoyama[3]

[1]First Department of Surgery, Kobe University School of Medicine, Kobe, 650 Japan
[2]Department of Surgery II, Kinki University School of Medicine, Osaka-Sayama, Osaka, 589 Japan
[3]Central Research Laboratories, The Green Cross Corporation, Hirakata, Osaka, 573 Japan

ABSTRACT

We tested radiolocalization of pancreatic carcinoma xenografts in nude mice with recombinant mouse/human chimeric Fab fragment (chimeric Fab) of A10 anti-CEA monoclonal antibody (MAb). When compared to the parental A10 MAb, we obtained higher tumor to normal tissue labeling ratios and clearer tumor detection using chimeric Fab. No significant difference in tumor to normal tissue ratio was observed between the chimeric Fab and murine Fab fragment prepared from the A10 MAb. Our results indicate that chimeric A10 Fab may be a potential candidate for localization of pancreatic carcinoma studies.

KEY WORDS:chimeric Fab fragment, monoclonal antibody A10, pancreatic carcinoma

INTRODUCTION

Murine monoclonal antibodies (MAbs) and their fragments are being employed in the diagnosis and therapy of human malignancies. We have previously shown that the murine anti-CEA MAb A10 reacted specifically with various gastro-intestinal carcinomas [1]. However, the use of murine antibodies in humans is limited by the development of human anti-mouse antibodies after frequent injections. In an attempt to reduce the immunogenecity of A10 MAb, we prepared chimeric mouse/human Fab fragment (Fab) and tested them in tumor localization studies in nude mice bearing antigen-positive pancreatic carcinoma xenografts.

MATERIALS AND METHODS

Preparation of Chimeric Fab Fragments

The recombinant mouse/human chimeric A10 Fab was expressed in *Escherichia coli* E101/pING3204, constructed at Xoma Corp.(Santa Monica.CA.). The chimeric A10 Fab was purified by ion-exchange chromatography from culture supernatants of *E.coli* grown in a mini-jar fermentation plant. A10 MAb were prepared by standard hybridoma technology as previously described [1]. Murine A10 Fab was obtained from parental murine MAb by papain digestion.

Pancreatic Cancer Cell Line and Xenografts

The human pancreatic carcinoma cell line, BxPC-3 which synthesizes CEA [2], was grown in RPMI 1640 medium supplemented with 10% FCS. Congenitally athymic 5-week old female nude mice were injected subcutaneously with approximately 2×10^7 BxPC-3 cells, and were utilized in biodistribution experiments four weeks later.

Biodistribution Study of Radiolabeled Chimeric A10 Fab

Chimeric A10 Fab, murine Fab and MAb were radiolabeled with ^{125}I using the solid-state lactoperoxidase method (0.6mCi/mg). Mice bearing BxPC-3 xenografts were given injection with each radiolabeled fragment or MAb (2.3μg/mouse) into the tail vein. At 3, 24 and 48hr after infusion, the tumor-bearing mice were sacrificed and radiolabel uptakes of tissues including tumor were determined. The results were expressed as %ID/g (percentage of injected dose per tissue gram) and as the ratio of %ID/g in the tumor relative to that in normal tissue. The tumor was imaged by thin-slice whole-body autoradiography of mice 24hr after radiolabeled antibody administration.

RESULTS

Biodistribution of Chimeric A10 Fab in Mice Bearing BxPC-3 Xenografts

For mice infused with chimeric Fab, the tumor uptakes were significantly greater than the uptakes in normal tissues (except for the kidney and lung at 3hr post-injection) (p<0.045). However, %ID/g of chimeric Fab in tumors was lower as compared to murine MAb (Table 1). The tumor to other normal tissues (except kidney) uptake ratios of chimeric Fab were significantly greater in contrast with murine MAb at 24hr post-infusion (p<0.040). In particular, the ratio of tumor to blood in mice injected with chimeric Fab was fifteen-fold higher than the ratio of murine MAb 24hr after antibody administration (p<0.001). However, ratios for chimeric Fab were equivalent to murine Fab. The tumor to kidney ratio for chimeric Fab, murine Fab and MAb were 8.6, 8.4 and 7.5 respectively (Fig.1).

Table 1. Comparative biodistribution of chimeric A10 Fab (ch-Fab) and murine MAb (m-MAb) in mice bearing human pancreatic carcinoma BxPC-3 xenografts. The mice were euthanized at the indicated times and the uptakes in tissues were calculated. The data are mean ± SEM and shown as %ID/g.

| Tissue | Time after administration (hr) | | | | | |
| | 3 | | 24 | | 48 | |
	ch-Fab	m-MAb	ch-Fab	m-MAb	ch-Fab	m-MAb
Tumor	5.28±1.02	6.96±0.93	1.05±0.07	25.18±3.34	0.56±0.06	22.79±5.03
Blood	2.20±0.22	11.34±0.44	0.02±0.00	7.80±0.31	0.01±0.00	5.57±0.66
Liver	1.64±0.17	6.92±0.93	0.06±0.01	4.32±0.38	0.04±0.01	3.02±0.72
Spleen	2.08±0.21	4.84±0.31	0.04±0.01	3.26±0.28	0.04±0.01	1.86±0.35
Pancreas	2.68±0.39	1.39±0.28	0.02±0.01	1.48±0.10	0.02±0.00	1.02±0.26
Kidney	5.71±0.99	4.95±0.43	0.12±0.01	3.36±0.27	0.06±0.01	2.61±0.35
Lung	3.07±0.22	7.17±0.24	0.08±0.02	4.38±0.12	0.06±0.02	3.74±0.34

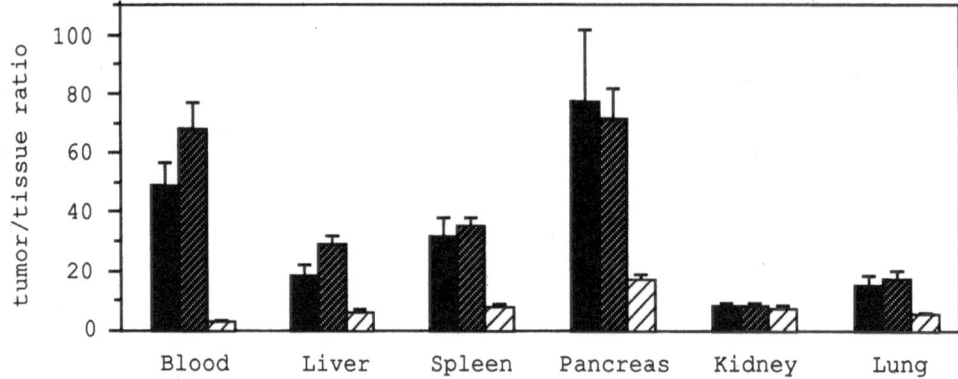

Fig. 1 Tumor to normal tissues ratios in biodistribution studies at 24hr after injection. The ratios for chimeric Fab (■) were compared with murine Fab (▨) and MAb (▱). The vertical bars indicate SEM.

Whole-body Autoradiography Study

Chimeric Fab allowed clear tumor imaging without visible accumulation in normal tissues (Fig.2a), whereas murine MAb showed higher distribution of radiolabeled antibodies in normal organs (Fig.2b).

a   b

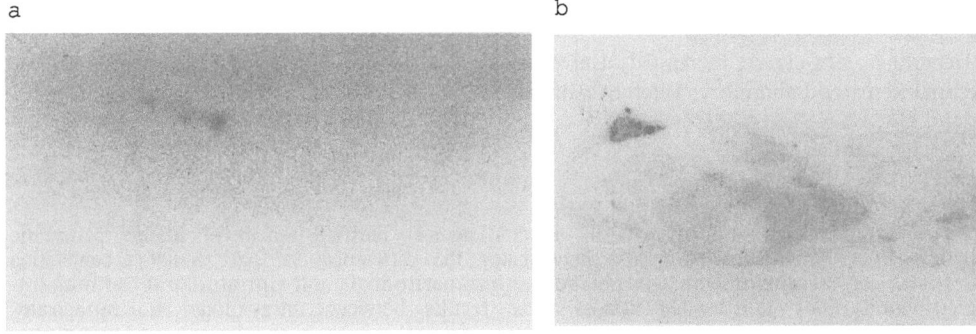

Fig. 2 Whole-body autoradiography of mice given a) chimeric Fab and b) murine MAb at 24hr post-injection

DISCUSSION

Recently, bacterial systems for the direct expression of functional chimeric antibody fragment removed the need to produce these fragments from intact MAb by proteolytic digestion [3]. In present studies, we prepared a recombinant murine/human chimeric Fab using variable regions of anti-CEA MAb A10, and expressed it in *E.coli*. We tested the radiolabeling kinetics of chimeric Fab in a nude mouse model of pancreatic carcinoma xenografts. Biodisribution studies showed significant greater uptakes of radiolabeled chimeric Fab in the BxPC-3 tumors than in normal tissues, although %ID/g of chimeric Fab in tumors was lower compared with murine MAb. Furthermore, the ratios of tumor to normal tissues (with the exception of kidney) for mice injected with chimeric Fab were substantially greater than in mice injected with murine MAb. There were no notable differences between chimeric and murine Fab fragments for the tumor to normal tissues ratios. Murine Fab fragment had been reported to give excellent tumor imaging in an animal model compared to murine whole IgG [4]. However, some investigators showed that Fab fragments were not always suitable for tumor localization because of greater non-specific accumulation in the kidney, as compared to MAbs [5,6]. The present study showed lower uptakes of chimeric A10 Fab in the kidney at 24 and 48hr post-injection. In addition, chimeric Fab showed lower normal tissue distribution than MAb in whole-body autoradiography imaging at 24hr post-infusion. These results indicate that chimeric Fab could potentially be a better reagent than murine MAb for localization of pancreatic carcinoma.

REFERENCES

1.Soyama N, Yamamoto M, Ohyanagi H, and Saitoh Y (1989) Comparative studies on monoclonal antibody KM10 and anti-CEA monoclonal antibodies. J Jpn Surg Soc 90:1834-1839 (in Japanese)
2.Tan MH, Nowak NJ, Loor RM, Ochi H, Sandberg AA, Lopez C, Pickren JW, Berjian R, Douglass HO and Chu TM (1986) Characterization of a new primary human pancreatic tumor line. Cancer Invest 4:15-23
3.Better M, Chang CP, Robinson RR and Horwitz AH (1988) *Escherichia coli* secretion of an active chimeric antibody fragment. Science 240:1041-1043
4.Wilbanks T, Peterson JA, Miller S, Kaufman L, Ortendahl D and Ceriani RL (1981) Localization of mammary tumors *in vivo* with ^{131}I-labeled Fab fragment of antibodies against mouse mammary epithelial (MME) antigens. Cancer 48:1768-1775
5.Wahl RL, Parker CW and Philpott GW (1983) Improved radioimaging and tumor localization with monoclonal F(ab')$_2$. J Nucl Med 24:316-325
6.Khaw BA, Strauss HW, Cahill SL, Soule HR, Edgington T and Cooney J (1984) Sequential imaging of Indium-111-labeled monoclonal antibody in human mammary tumors hosted in nude mice. J Nucl Med 25:592-603

Biodistribution of Monoclonal Antibody Nd2 Following Administration of Several Routes

YASUYUKI KONDO[1], YONG-SUK CHUNG[1], TETSUJI SAWADA[1], MICHIO SOWA[1], AKIMASA INUI[1], YOSHITO YAMASHITA[1], and YOUNG S. KIM[2]

[1]The First Department of Surgery, Osaka City University Medical School, Osaka, 545 Japan
[2]Gastrointestinal Research Laboratory, Veterans Administration Medical Center, University of California, San Francisco, CA, USA

ABSTRACT

Nd2 is a murine monoclonal antibody (MAb) directed against purified mucin of human pancreatic cancer cell line SW1990. In this study we investigated the differences of Nd2 tumor accumulation rate with routes of administration; intravenous, intraperitoneal and intratumoral administration. Biodistribution study resulted in almost same results between intravenous and intraperitoneal administration of Nd2. Intratumoral administration exhibited high degree and long-term retention of Nd2 in tumor, compared with a control group (non-specific IgG$_1$ intratumorally administered). The results indicated usefulness of intratumoral administration of Nd2 for the treatment of human pancreatic cancer.

KEY WORDS: mouse monoclonal antibody Nd2, pancreatic carcinoma, intratumoral administration

INTRODUCTION

MAbs directed against tumor-associated antigen(TAA) have been utilized in the imaging and therapy on various diseases. But it was reported that proportional accumulation dose at the tumor site, was so low compared with total injected dose that effective antitumor effect using MAbs could not be expected[1]. In this study, we investigated how tumor accumulation rate differed depending on route of administration of Nd2 to SW1990-bearing nude mice. A previous biodistribution and radioimmunoimaging study of Nd2 (Sawada et al.[2]) demonstrated that the tumor accumulation rate of Nd2 was excellent and that apparent positive images of xenografts could be obtained using In-111-labeled Nd2.

MATERIALS AND METHODS

Monoclonal antibody and cell line

The antibody used in this study was a murine MAb of the IgG$_1$ isotype, Nd2, directed against purified mucin[3] from human pancreatic cancer cell line SW1990[4]. Nd2 hybridoma was kindly provided by Dr.Kim, GI Research Laboratory, VA Medical Center, CA, USA. Nd2 hybridoma was cultured under the condition described below. SW1990 cell line was established in 1978 from a human pancreatic adenocarcinoma. SW1990 cell line was also provided by Dr.Kim. SW1990 cells were cultured in DMEM medium supplemented with 5% fetal calf serum in ϕ 100mm Falcon tissue culture dishes. When confluent, cells were harvested by using 0.06% trypsin in 0.02% EDTA solution, washed with medium, and resuspended in tissue culture medium.

Radiolabeling

Chloramine-T method was adopted for Nd2 iodination (I-125). After the conjugation of Nd2 with I-125, free I-125 was removed by gel permeation. The radioactivity of Nd2 was adjusted to approximately 40-60 MBq-I-125/mg-protein.

Xenograft

A total of 5X10^6 SW1990 cells were inoculated subcutaneously into the left flank of balb/c nude mice. SW1990-bearing nude mice were used in this studies two weeks after inoculation.

Routes of administration

I-125-labeled Nd2 (7.5 μCi/5.0 μg) was administered to SW1990 bearing nude mice intravenously (i.v.group), intraperitoneally (i.p.group) and intratumorally (i.t.group). There were four mice respectively. As a control for the i.t.group, I-125-labeled non-specific mouse IgG1 was also administered intratumorally. 12 hours, 1 day, 3 days and 7 days after the administration of radiolabeled Nd2 and non-specific IgG₁, nude mice were sacrificed to measure radioactivity of organs. Radioactivity of I-125 was measured with a well-type scintillation counter.

RESULTS

Biodistribution

1. Intravenous administration

Intravenously injected I-125-Nd2 accumulated in the SW1990 xenograft in the following fashion. The %ID/g in the tumor was shown in table 1. Tumor accumulation rate increased with time until 3 days after administration. On the other hand, I-125 radioactivity in blood and other organs was gradually decreasing. The T/B ratios at 3 days and 7 days were especially high. The T/B ratios of organs other than the tumor were not more than 1 at any time point of measurement.

2. Intraperitoneal administration

The %ID/g in the tumor was 7.3% at 12 hrs, 13.4% at 1 day, 40.8% at 3 days and 44.9% at 7 days. There were no significant differences between the i.v.group and i.p.group in either %ID/g or T/B ratio.

3. Intratumoral administration

The %ID/g in the tumor was extraordinary high as shown in table 2. Much of the dose of I-125-Nd2 remained in the tumor even 7 days after intratumoral administration. The values of %ID/g in blood were much lower than those for the i.v.group. On the other hand, in the group administered non-specific IgG1 intratumorally as a control for the Nd2 i.t.group, the values of %ID/g in the tumor were much less than those for the I-125-Nd2 i.t.group. In non-specific IgG₁ i.t.group, I-125-IgG₁ rapidly disappeared from the tumor. Most of the urinary excretion of intratumorally administered I-125-Nd2 was accomplished by 1day after administration.

Table 1. Percentages of injected dose of I-125-Nd2 per gram of tissue
in I-125-Nd2 i.v.group

organs＼time	12 hrs	1 day	3 days	7 days
tumor	6.5	16.8	45.0	37.8
blood	35.9	19.7	14.2	7.3
urine	23.1	21.5	5.4	3.5
stomach	5.2	3.0	1.6	0.9
spleen	8.1	7.1	3.5	1.7
bone	6.0	4.0	2.8	1.4

Table 2. Percentages of injected dose of I-125-Nd2 per gram of tissue
in I-125-Nd2 i.t.group

organs＼time	12 hrs	1 day	3 days	7 days
tumor	850.8	1200	1074	642.7
blood	1.1	7.4	8.8	4.0
urine	24.1	10.2	7.1	2.9
stomach	0.7	1.0	1.8	0.8
spleen	0.5	1.8	1.9	1.0
bone	0.4	1.3	1.5	1.0

DISCUSSION

Methods for the diagnosis of malignant diseases are not particularly tumor-specific and qualitative diagnosis can be sometimes difficult to achieve with their use. Diagnostic methods utilizing MAbs directed against TAAs are to some extent tumor-specific and may therefore prove diagnostically in respect other than those for the techniques noted above. In recent years, radioimmunodetection(RAID) using radiolabeled MAb has come into clinical use for qualitative diagnosis and tumor localization. Concerning pancreatic cancer, results have not always been satisfactory. The hypovascularity of pancreatic cancer may be one of the reasons for this. MAb Nd2 is a murine MAb, which Ho et al.[5] have already reported to possess a high degree of specificity to human pancreatic cancer. In immunohistochemical studies of human pancreatic cancer specimens, approximately 83% have been found to be positive for Nd2 and In-111-labeled Nd2 resulted in a clear positive image on SW1990-bearing nude mouse. On the other hand, there are drawbacks associated with the use of MAbs recognizing TAA. One is that accumulation in tumor is small compared with total dose of administration since most of administered MAb is excreted in the urine. In this study, we attempted to determine routes of administration yielding higher rates of accumulation of Nd2 in tumor. A biodistribution study including several routes of administration, i.p. administration of Nd2 was associated with no improvement in accumulation in tumor. I.t. administration resulted in abundant retention of Nd2 in tumor 12 hrs after administration and even by the 7th day after administration the amount accumulated had diminished only slightly. The %ID/g in the blood remained at a low level, indicating that outflow of Nd2 into the blood from the tumor was small compared with that noted for the group administered i.t.non-specific IgG_1. Since non-specific IgG_1 rapidly disappeared from the tumor and correspondingly increased in level in blood and urine, retention of Nd2 in the tumor appears probably to have been the result of a specific antigen-antibody reaction. The %ID/g in the tumor in Nd2 i.t.group was about 17 times higher than that noted in another report[6]. It seems quite reasonable that %ID/g in tumor in the group subjected to i.t.administration was high; however, given that in the non-specific IgG_1 i.t.group, radioisotope disappeared rapidly from tumor, Nd2 retention in the tumor would appear to have been due to tumor specificity. Intratumoral administration using MAb, as a drug or radioisotopic conjugate, can be expected to result in a strong antitumor effects due to long-term retention in the tumor. Therefore, intratumoral administration using Nd2 may be a practically applicable method for the treatment of pancreatic cancer. Intratumoral administration was found to result in long-term and high-degree retention of Nd2 in tumor. This finding suggests that it may be usable as a method for the treatment of patients with inoperable or incurable pancreatic cancer.

CONCLUSION

A study of the biodistribution of murine MAb Nd2 following intravenous administration demonstrated excellent tumor localization and low background. Intratumoral administration of Nd2 resulted in much of the dose being retained in the tumor even on the 7th day after administration; the degree of retention was much larger than was the case for intravenous administration. The result of this biodistribution study suggests that the intratumoral administration of Nd2 may be useful as a carrier of antitumor agent in the treatment of pancreatic cancer.

REFERENCES

1. Vaughan ATM, Bradwell AR, Dykes PW, Anderson P (1986) Illusions of tumour killing using radio-labeled antibodies. Lancet June 28: 1492-1493
2. Sawada T, Chung YS, Kondo Y, Sowa M, Umeyama K, Ochi H, Ho JJL, Kim YS (1991) Radioimmuno-detection of human pancreatic cancer using ^{111}In-labeled monoclonal antibody Nd2. Antibody Immunoconj Radiophar 4: 493-499
3. Nardelli J, Byrd JC, Ho JJL, Fearney FJ, Tasman-Jones C, Kim YS (1988) Pancreatic cancer mucin from xenografts of SW1990 cells: isolation, characterization, and comparison to colon cancer mucin. Pancreas 3: 631-641
4. Kyriazis AP, McCombs III WB, Sandberg AA, Kyriazis AA, Sloan NH, Lepera R (1983) Establishment and characterization of human pancreatic adenocarcinoma cell line SW1990 in tissue culture and the nude mouse. Cancer Res 43: 4393-4401
5. Ho JJL, Bi N, Yan P-S, Yuan M, Norton KA, Kim YS (1991) Characterization of new pancreatic cancer-reactive monoclonal antibodies directed against purified mucin. Cancer Res 51: 372-380
6. Rowlinson-Busza G, Bamias S, Krausz T, Epenetos AA (1991) Uptake and distribution of specific and control monoclonal antibodied in subcutaneous xenografts following intratumor injection. Cancer Res 51: 3251-3256

Enhanced Antitumor Effect of Neocarzinostatin Conjugated to Monoclonal Antibody A7 on Human Pancreatic Carcinoma Grafted in Nude Mice

Eigo Otsuji, Toshiharu Yamaguchi, Nobuki Yamaoka, Tatsuya Kotani, Makoto Kato, Katsunori Taniguchi, Kazuya Kitamura, and Toshio Takahashi

The First Department of Surgery, Kyoto Prefectural University of Medicine, Kyoto, 602 Japan

ABSTRACT

Recent research has been directed toward the use of monoclonal antibody–drug conjugates for solid tumors. In this study, we used the monoclonal antibody A7 to target the antitumor drug neocarzinostatin (NCS) to pancreatic cancer cells. The in vivo localization of the radiolabeled MAb A7 was investigated using pancreatic carcinoma grafted nude mice. Mab A7 localized in the tumor at a tissue/blood ratio of 2.04. Moreover, A7–NCS was administered to the nude mice with pancreatic carcinoma xenografts. A7–NCS showed a greater antitumor effect than free NCS.

Key Words: monoclonal antibody A7, immunoconjugate, targeting chemotherapy

INTRODUCTION

The development of hybridoma technology by Köhler and Milstein offered the possibility of an effective means to deliver chemotherapy specifically to cancer cells. A number of monoclonal antibodies (MAb) have been linked to various antitumor drugs, cytotoxines and enzymes in an attempt to increase the effectiveness of chemotherapy[1]. However, there have been few reports of the clinical application of monoclonal antibody–drug conjugates to human pancreatic carcinomas. We have previously produced the MAb A7 and conjugated it with the antitumor drug, neocarzinostatin (NCS)[2,3]. A7–NCS was then used clinically for the treatment of patients with colonic carcinomas. We describe here the in vivo antitumor effect of A7–NCS conjugate on the growth of pancreatic carcinoma cells as a basic study to assess the potential usefulness of this conjugate in the patients with pancreatic cancer.

MATERIALS AND METHOD

Cell Line and Tumor Xenograft

The human pancreatic carcinoma cell line, HPC–YS[4], was used in this study. Cultured HPC–YS cells were harvested by treatment with EDTA, washed in phosphate buffered saline (PBS) and resuspended in PBS. Approximately 1×10^7 viable cells were injected s.c. into the left flank of thymus–deficient, 8–week–old male mice (BALB/C, nu–nu) (SLC Co., Shizuoka, Japan) weighing approximately 22 g. A tumor mass was detected in all mice injected with the HPC–YS cells 7 days after inoculation.

Monoclonal Antibodies and Preparation of Radiolabeled MAbs

MAb A7 was produced from the spleen cells of a mouse immunized against human colonic carcinoma as described previously[2]. MAb A7 reacts with 73 % of the human pancreatic carcinoma cell lines tested in addition to human colonic carcinoma and does not react immunohistochemically with normal pancreatic tissues as reported previously[5]. Normal mouse IgG was purchased from Boehringer Mannheim Biochemical (Mannheim, F.R.G.). Radiolabeling of MAb A7 with ^{125}I (Amersham Japan, Ltd., IMS 30, Japan) was performed by the chloramine–T method. Mab A7 and normal mouse IgG were labeled with ^{125}I to specific activities of 4.5 µCi/µg and 4.0 µCi/µg, respectively.

Neocarzinostatin Conjugation to MAb A7

MAb A7 was conjugated to NCS with SPDP (N–succinimidyl–3–(2–pyridyldithio)–propionate) as described previously by Fukuda[3]. The conjugation ratio used was 2 mol of NCS per mol of MAb A7, i.e., 7.5 mg of MAb A7 was bound to 1 mg of NCS.

771

In Vivo Reactivity of Radiolabeled MAB A7

The nude mice with HPC–YS tumor xenografts were injected intraperitoneally with 0.7 μCi of either ^{125}I–labeled MAb A7 or or normal mouse IgG. Eight days later, the mice were killed and dissected. After dissection, tumor, blood and normal organ tissues were weighed. The radioactivity in the tissues was then measured using a gamma scintillation counter (Packard). The tissue/blood ratios of the radioactivity on a weight basis were calculated from these data. Statistical significance of differences was determined by Student's t–test. Significant difference was set at P less than 0.05.

In Vivo Antitumor Effect of A7–NCS and Tumor Localization of NCS after Intravenous Administration of A7–NCS

The in vivo antitumor effect of A7–NCS was investigated using nude mice bearing HPC–YS tumors. Once small tumors were detected in the mice (seven days after inoculation), they were divided into three groups: seven received the A7–NCS conjugate in PBS (A7: 1.5 mg/Kg, NCS: 500 units/Kg), seven received only NCS in PBS (500 units/Kg), and seven received only PBS as a control. All treatments were done by intravenous injection into the tail vein in 100 μl of PBS. The drug solution was administered twice a week for three weeks. The tumors were measured (maximum length and width) twice a week until Day 32. The tumor volume (V) was calculated using the formula, $V=(a^2 \times b)/2$, where a was the maximum width and b was the maximum length. To standardize the variation in tumor volume, the relative tumor volume (RV) was calculated using the formula, $RV=V_2/V_1$, where V_1 was the initial tumor volume and V_2 was the tumor volume at any given time. The data are presented as the mean±standard error (S.E.). Nude mice bearing 14 day old HPC–YS tumors were intravenously injected with the A7–NCS conjugate (500 unit/Kg) in a volume of 100 μl. The mice were killed four days after injection, and the tumors were cut into frozen sections. The immunoperoxidase staining was performed by the avidin–biotin peroxidase complex technique. Normal rabbit serum was used for control staining.

RESULTS

In Vivo Reactivity of Radiolabeled MAB A7

Figure 1 shows the tissue / blood ratios of ^{125}I–labeled MAb A7 and ^{125}I labeled normal mouse IgG on Day 8. The MAb A7 tumor tissue / blood ratio of reached 2.04±0.2. In contrast, those of normal organs ranged from 0.11±0.02 to 0.38±0.03. MAb A7 remained localized in the tumor even on Day 8. In contrast, the normal mouse IgG tumor tissue / blood ratio was 0.34±0.02. The differences between these two groups was statistically significant.

In Vivo Antitumor Effect of A7–NCS and Tumor Localization of NCS after Intravenous Injection of A7–NCS

Figure 2 shows the results for the mice which received A7–NCS and free NCS. The relative tumor volume in these mice was 3.5±0.4 for the A7–NCS treated group and 5.8±0.5 for those receiving free NCS. The antitumor effect of A7–NCS was significantly greater than that of free NCS and PBS on Day 32 (P<0.05).
With immunoperoxidase staining using antibody against NCS, NCS was detected in the HPC–YS tumor tissues of the mice which received A7–NCS.

DISCUSSION

With the development of tumor immunology many antibodies have been used as carriers of cytotoxic agents. We chose the antitumor drug NCS and the MAb A7 for two reasons. First, NCS can be covalently joined to an antibody without destroying the activity of either[6]. Second, it was reported that 12 percent of patients with pancreatic cancer had tumor reduction after the administration of NCS alone and did not experience severe side effects[7,8]. In this study, the relative tumor volumes in the A7–NCS or free NCS treated groups were approximately 40 percent or 66 percent, respectively, of that in the PBS control group. Because its activity was significantly greater than that of free NCS,

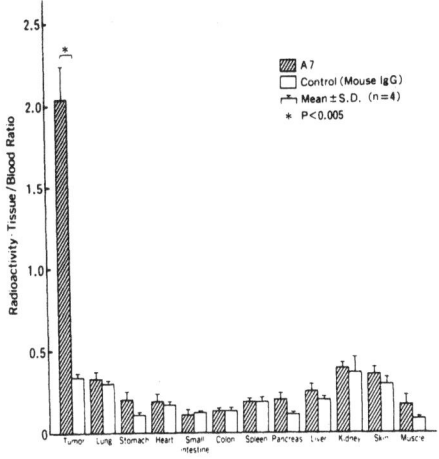
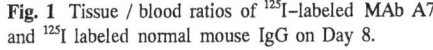

Fig. 1 Tissue / blood ratios of ^{125}I-labeled MAb A7 and ^{125}I labeled normal mouse IgG on Day 8.

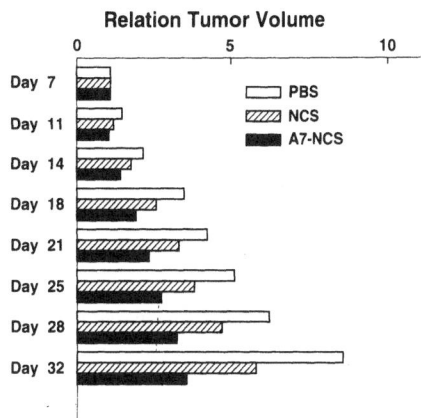

Fig. 2 In vivo antitumor effect of A7-NCS and free NCS.

the conjugation of NCS to MAb A7 enhanced the antitumor activity of NCS. In the immunohistochemical experiments, NCS was detected in the tumors from mice which were treated with the A7-NCS conjugate. These results suggest that the antitumor activity of NCS can be expected to persist for more than four days after the administration of the A7-NCS solution, while the clearance of free NCS may be very rapid, as previously reported[8]. To be useful as a carrier of antitumor agents, the monoclonal antibody requires high in vivo specificity, i.e., it should bind to pancreatic tumor cells and not to normal tissue cells. To address this issue, we studied the distribution of MAb A7 in nude mice harboring human pancreatic carcinoma xenografts. The ^{125}I-labeled MAb A7 tumor / blood ratios were approximately 6.2 times greater than that using ^{125}I labeled normal mouse IgG, on Day 8. However, the ^{125}I-labeled MAb A7 and normal mouse IgG normal tissue / blood ratios were low and similar to each other. These results suggest that localization of MAb A7 to the pancreatic carcinoma was due to specific binding. A number of monoclonal antibodies have been conjugated to anticancer drugs, cytotoxins, and enzymes to increase their therapeutic efficacy. MAb A7 has been covalently linked to NCS, and this conjugate has been used to treat patients with colorectal cancer. Some of the patients who have been treated with this conjugate have had at a potential regression of their tumor. Since NCS has some efficacy against human pancreatic carcinoma, we believe that the MAb A7-NCS conjugate might be more effective than chemotherapy alone for pancreatic cancer patients.

REFERENCES

1. Hurwitz, E., Levy, R., Maron, R., Wilchek, M., Arnon, R., and Sela, M. The covalent binding of daunomycin and adriamycin to antibodies, with retention of both drug and antibody activities. Cancer Res., 35: 1175-1181, 1975.

2. Kotanagi, H., Takahashi, T., Masuko, T. A monoclonal antibody against human colon cancers. Tohoku J. Exp. Med., 148: 353-360, 1986.

3. Fukuda, K. The study of targeting chemotherapy against gastrointestinal cancer. Akita J. Med., 12: 451-468, 1985.

4. Yamaguchi N, Yamamura Y, Koyama K, et al.: Characterization of new human pancreatic cancer cell lines which propagate in a protein-free chemically defined medium. Cancer Res 50: 7008-7012, 1990.

5. Otsuji, E., Yamaguchi, Y., Yamaguchi, N., Koyama, K., Imanishi, J., Yamaoka, N., Takahashi, T. Expression of the cell surface antigen detected by the monoclonal antibody A7 in pancreatic carcinoma cell lines. Surg. Today 22, 351-356 (1992).

6. Kimura, I., Ohnishi, T., Tsubota, T., Sato, Y., Kobayashi, T., and Abe, S. Production of tumor antibody neocarzinostatin conjugate and its biological activities. Cancer Immunol. Immunother., 7: 235-242, 1980.

7. Jung, G., Kohnlein, W., Luders, G. Biological activity of the antitumor protein neocarzinostatin coupled to a monoclonal antibody by N-succinimidyl 3-(2-pyridyldithio)-propionate. Biochem. Biophys. Res. Commun., 101: 599-606, 1981.

8. Fujita, H., Nakayama, N., Sawabe, T., Kimura, K. In vivo distribution and inactivation of neocarzinostatin. Jpn. J. Antibiotics, 23: 471-478, 1970.

TNF-α, IFN-α and Tegafur Combination Therapy for Advanced Pancreatic Cancer

Noriaki Tanaka, Hiromasa Kasino, Akira Gouchi, Akio Hizuta, Yoshio Naomoto, Luis Fernando Moreira, Hiromi Iwagaki, Jiroh Ohida, Tuyoshi Matuno, and Kunzo Orita

First Department of Surgery, Okayama University Medical School, Okayama, 700 Japan

ABSTRACT

Eighteen patients with advanced adenocarcinoma of the pancreas were treated with a combination of natural human tumor-necrosis factor-α, natural human interferon-α, and tegafur. Complete and partial response was observed in one and two patients respectively(17% response rate). Seven patients (39%) showed stable disease. The median survival period for the overall population of patients treated is 209 days. Patients with evidence of tumor response or with apparent disease stabilization had a median survival of 313 days, while patients with progressive disease lived 154 days.

KEY WORDS: pancreatic cancer, tumor necrosis factor-α, interferon-α, tegafur

INTRODUCTION

A current strategy in chemotherapy using 5-FU for the treatment of advanced gastro-intestinal cancer is based upon the ability of some drugs such as folinic acid to modulate the cytotoxic effect of 5-FU. Two randomized trials found a modest improvement in survival in patients with advanced colorectal carcinoma[1]. Recently, synergistic action between IFN and 5-FU has been shown against different cancer cell lines. Although the use of nHuIFN-α2a combined with 5-FU may produce a response rate (26%) in patients with colorectal cancer, it was not substantially superior to alternative 5-FU programs[2].
On the other hand, we have reported a synergistic antineoplastic activity of IFN-α and TNF-α in vitro[3] and in vivo[4] experiments. Using a mixture of high-purity natural human IFN-α (nHuIFN-α) and natural human TNF-α (nHuTNF-α) derived from the BALL-1 cell line, we have conducted a phase II trial, with an over all response 12.5% (14/112)[5]. Based on the encouraging results, we have employed a trials of nHuIFN-α, nHuTNF-α and tegafur in patients with inoperable pancreatic cancer. This reports describes results of this trial, and make an addition of a preceding case study using the cytokines and 5-FU.

PATIENTS AND STUDY DESIGN

Between April 1989 and June 1992, 20 patients were entered this trial. Patients were diagnosed histologically and imagiologically as pancreatic cancer that was not considered suitable for surgery or radiotherapy. Patients were eligible for the treatment if there were no factors such as serious physiological or hematological abnormalities, active infections, or recent chemotherapy. A leukocyte count of 4,000/μl and a platelet count of 100,000/μl or more were required before initiation of the course. Informed consent was obtained from all patients and/or their families. The clinical characteristics of the subjects are found in Table 1.
Patients received UFT (Tegafur 100 mg plus uracil 224 mg/tab, Taiho Lab., Tokyo, Japan) by mouth at a dose of 4 tab/day for continuous period as long as the patients could be tolerable. nHuIFN-α and nHuTNF-α was administered twice a day intravenously at a maintenance dose of 2×10^6 IU and 2 μg respectively for consecutive days as long as patients could afford.

RESULTS

Of the 20 patients entered in this study, 18 were evaluated for response. One patient rejected to continue in this study due to fatigue and anorexia. Another one patient dropped out because of his request for discontinue the treatment without apparent reason. The regimen was generally well tolerated. Anorexia was frequent during first month of the treatment. Nausea and vomiting were less common and readily controlled with anti-emetic therapy. Fever and chill were the most common findings. Almost all patients complained of fatigue. Neurotoxic or psychiatric symptom were not presented. Skin rash was shown in only one patient. Leukocytopenia was observed in 5 patients. This alteration was reversible by discontinuing or reducing the IFN and TNF dose. Three of 18 patients (17%) showed CR (1 case) or PR(2 cases). Seven patients (38.9%) had SD and 8 patients (44.4%) progressed during treatment. Patients showing objective response achieved it within 3 months of treatment. Six patients, those with CR and PR (3 cases) and 3 others with SD, had a reduction in their elevated value of CA19-9. The median survival period for the overall population of patients treated is 209 days. Patients with evidence of tumor response or with apparent disease stabilization had a median survival of 313 days, while patients with progressive disease lived 154 days (P<0.05) (Table 2).

Table 1 Patient Characteristics

No. entered	20
No. evaluable	18
male: female	13:5
Primary tumor site	
Head	7
Head + Body	2
Body + Tail	9
Facotrs of non-resectable	
Peritoneum	5
Liver	5
Bone	1
Retroperitoneum	18
Portal invasion	14

Table 2 Response and Survival

	Number of case	(%)	Median survival(days)
CR	1	(5.6)	
PR	2	(11.1)	313
SD	7	(38.9)	
PD	8	(44.4)	154
	18		209

CR: complete response, PR: partial response
SD: stable disease, PD: progressive disease

CASE REPORT

A 48-year-old woman was admitted to the hospital in April of 1987 complainig of abdominal tumor in the right hypochondrium. She had lost 5kg in weight during four months before admission. Physical examination revealed mild tenderness and a hard tumor mass in the epigastrium. CA19-9 was 2600U per ml and CEA was 1.9ng per ml. An abdominal computerized tomographic(CT) scan showed 6.3 x 6.2cm tumor mass at the head of the pancreas which involved the portal vein, the duodenum and the retroperitoneal soft tissue. The patient underwent exploratory laparotomy which confirmed unresectability of this lesion due to its envelopment of the portal vein and the superior mesenteric vessels. Gastro-jejunostomy and multiple biopsies of the tumor were performed. Pathologic examination of the tumor revealed tubular adenocarcinoma with squamous metaplasia. After recovery from operation, the patient was scheduled to receive the cytokines (IFN-α plus TNF-α) and 5-FU combined therapy by the following protocol: intravenous daily administration of the cytokines two times a day and 5-FU (250mg/day) for 7 months. The cytokines was a mixture of 1 x 10^6U of nHuIFN-α and 2μg of nHuTNF-α dissolved in 5% human albumin solution. One month later, the CA19-9 decreased to 1350U/ml from the maximum value (3600u/ml). The patient felt well, and noticed relief of abdominal pain. The CA19-9 furthermore decreased thereafter, and dropped to 330U/ml in September. On clinical examination, the tumor shrinks in size, and a CT scan also showed decrease of tumor size to 4.2 x 3.8cm (Fig.1). Since partial response was confirmed 1 month later, the patient underwent re-exploration at December. The tumor was revealed to be resectable and removed in continuity with the head of the pancreas, duodenum, and gastric antrum. A Roux-en-Y pancreaticojejunostomy, choledochojejunostomy and gastrojejunostomy were performed.

Microscopic examination revealed th_t the tumor was composed of adenocarcinoma and squamous cell carcinoma. A moderate-differentiated adenocarcinoma was mainly situated in the center of the tumor in the pancreas and several nests of a moderate-differentiated squamous cell carcinoma are located at the periphery of the tumor in the duodenal muscle layer.

Patient recovered uneventfully from surgery, and discharged at January. However, she readmitted at February, complaining general fatigue and appetiteloss. In spite of 5-FU-cytokine combined therapy, laboratory examination showed a steep elevation of CA19-9, and she expired one month later.

DISCUSSION

IFN inhibits malignant cell growth and cause cytostasis by the inhibition of cell cycle progression, with partial block either the transition from G_0-G_1 to S_1, progression through S_1 or even generalized inhibition[6]. We previously reported that the combination of nHuIFN-α and nHuTNF-α bring a marked recruitment of cells to the S-phase combined with S-G_2/M block[7]. Therefore, it has been postulated that they should be used in combination with other cytotoxic agents specific for S-phase such as 5-FU. In the recent experimental study using nude mice transplanted with a human colon cancer cell line, we observed that combined administration of nHuIFN-α, nHuTNF-α, and 5-FU elevated labeling index by BrdU, decreased mitotic index, and increased 5-FU concentration in the tumor tissue, which resulted in marked reduction of the tumor weight (data not published). In this study, the dose of nHuIFN-α, nHuTNF-α, which was determined on the basis of the previous combination therapy for cancer patients, resulted in acceptable toxicity. Mild to moderate degree of leukocytopenia was detected in 5 of 18 patients, and quickly reversed by discontinuing therapy or by reducing the dose. Anorexia was seen in all our patients, probably due to TNF-α. This study in advanced pancreatic cancer has provided a response rate of 17%, with a 7 month median survival for all cases. Three out of 18 cases (17%) have lived 1 year or longer. Two of the responders remained alive for 23 and 34 months. Although the response rate in this study was similar to those rate observed in the previous trials using FSM regimen, our patients showing PR and ST could show a mean survival of 10 months, which is longer than that of responders in FSM[8]. In this study, responder and non-responder with SD could survive longer than non-responders with PD. However, the increased survival could not be a direct result of this regimen, because there were differences in the possible prognostic variable such as initial performance status or extent of metastatic disease between two groups.
It is our belief that nHuTNF-α, nHuIFN-α and UFT regimen should be used as therapy for pancreatic adenocarcinomas as well as an adjunct to radiotherapy for treatment of less advanced disease.

REFERENCES

1. Arbuck SG (1989) Overview of clinical trials using 5-fluorouracil and leucovorin for the treatment of colorectal cancer. Cancer 63 (6): 1036-1044.
2. Kemmey N, Younes A, Seiter K, Kelsen D, Sammarco P, Adams L, Derby S, Murray P, Houston C.(1990) Interferon alpha-2a and 5-fluorouracil for advanced colorectal carcinoma. Cancer 66 (12): 2470-2475.
3. Matsubara N, Fuchimoto S, Orita K.(1991) Antiproliferative effects of natural human tumor necrosis factor-α, interferon-α, and interferon-γ on human pancreatic carcinoma cell line. Int J Pancreatol 8 (3): 235-243.
4. Naomoto Y, Tanaka N, Orita K.(1989) Antitumor effect of natural human tumor necrosis factor-α in combination against human cancer transplanted into nude mice. Acta Med Okayama 43 (4): 211-221.
5. Orita K, Fuchimoto S, Kurimoto M, Ando S, Minowada J. (1992) Early phase study of interferon-α and tumor necrosis factor-α combination in patients with advanced cancer. Acta Medica Okayama 46(2):103-112.
6. Tamm I, Jasny BR, Pfeffer LM.(1987) Antiproliferative action of interferons. In: Pfeffer LM (eds) Mecahanisms of interferon actions, Vol. 2, Boca Raton, FL: CRC Press, Inc., pp25-58.
7. Muro M, Naomoto Y, Kunzo O.(1991) Mechanism of the combined anti-tumor effect of natural human tumor necrosis factor-α and natural human interferon-α on cell cycle progression. Jpn J Cancer Res 82 (1): 118-126.
8. Martin W, Gray R, Panasci L, Perry MC.(1986) Chemotherapy for advance pancreatic cancer; A comparison of 5-fluorouracil, adriamycin, and Mitomycin (FAM) and 5-fluorouracil, Streptozocin, and Mitomycin (FSM). Cancer 57 (1): 29-33.

Differential Diagnosis of the Cystic Lesion of the Pancreas

Nobuhiko Harada, Toshihide Imaizumi, Mamoru Suzuki, Toshiaki Nakasako, and Fujio Hanyu

Department of Gastroenterological Surgery, Tokyo Women's Medical College, Shinjuku-ku, Tokyo, 162 Japan

ABSTRACT

To obtain the differential diagnosis of the cystic lesion of the pancreas, histological records of seventy-eight patients who underwent resection of the cystic lesion of the pancreas were reviewed. Sixteen patients who had received CT-scan, ERP and endoscopic ultrasonography(EUS) preoperatively were selected for this study to evaluate the detectability of internal structure of the cystic lesion. This study suggests that the cystic lesion 3cm or more in diameter with solid component or septum could be diagnosed as having neoplastic cysts. EUS is also useful to detect the internal structure of the cystic lesion of the pancreas.

KEY WORDS: pancreatic cyst, pancreatic cystadenocarcinoma, differential diagnosis, endoscopic ultrasonography

INTRODUCTION

The cystic lesion of the pancreas has been easily diagnosed by recent imaging diagnostic techniques. However, it is sometimes difficult to differentiate between the patients with neoplastic cysts and non-neoplastic ones on the clinical grounds without histologic confirmation[1,2]. The aim of this study is to clarify differential diagnosis in the cystic lesion of the pancreas and to evaluate the detectability of the internal structure by imaging techniques.

MATERIALS AND METHODS

Seventy-eight patients who underwent resection of the cystic lesion of the pancreas were selected for this study. The patients were divided into two groups on the basis of the histological findings; neoplastic group in 25 patients (cystadenocarcinoma 13, cystadenoma 12) and non-neoplastic group in 53 patients (retention cyst 18, pseudocyst 35). The size of the cystic lesion in diameter, solid component formation and septum formation in the cystic lesion were compared in the two groups of the patients.

Of the 78 patients, sixteen patients who had received CT-scan, ERP and EUS preoperatively and underwent resection of the cystic lesion were reviewed; 8 patients with cystadenocarcinoma and 8 patients with retention cyst. Detectabilities of solid component and septum in the cystic lesion were studied comparing diagnostic abilities of imaging techniques.

RESULTS

1. Size (Fig. 1)

The mean size of the cystic lesion in diameter was 6.7cm(range; 3.0 to 11.0cm) in cystadenocarcinoma, 7.6cm (range; 1.5 to 18.0cm) in cystadenoma, 3.9cm(range; 0.7 to 10.0cm) in retention cyst and 3.9cm(range; 1.1 to 16.0cm) in pseudocyst.

2. Solid component formation (Table 1)

Incidence of the patients who had solid component was 92% in cystadenocarcinoma, 83% in cystadenoma, 6% in retention cyst and 3% in pseudocyst.

3. Septum formation (Table 2)

Incidence of the patients who had septum was 85% in cystadenocarcinoma, 75% in cystadenoma, 27% in retention cyst and 6% in pseudocyst.

4. Size, Solid component formation, and septum formation (Table 3)

Incidence of the cystic lesion 3cm or more in diameter with solid component or septum in it were 92% in the patients with neoplastic cysts(cystadenocarcinoma, cystadenoma) and 9% in those with non-neoplastic cysts(retention cysts, pseudocysts).

5. Diagnosis of solid component and septum formation by CT-scan, ERP, and EUS (Table 4, 5)

The sensitivity, specificity and overall accuracy of the solid component were 60%, 90%, 80% in CT-scan, 100%, 75%, 85% in ERP, and 80%, 73%, 75% in EUS. And those of the septum were 100%, 80%, 93% in CT-scan, 63%, 80%, 69% in ERP, and 100%, 100%, 100% in EUS.

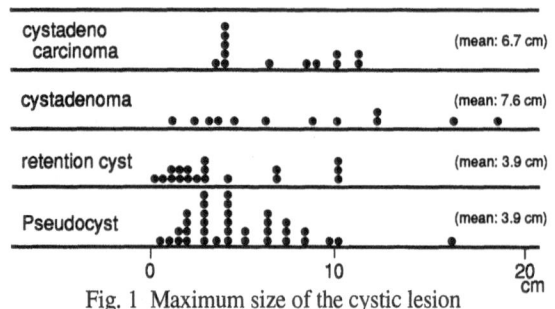

Fig. 1 Maximum size of the cystic lesion

Table 1. Solid component Formation

cystadeno carcinoma(n=13)	92%	neoplasma 88%
cystadenoma (n=12)	83%	
retention cyst (n=18)	6%	non-neoplasma 4%
pseudocyst (n=35)	3%	

Table 2. Septum Formation

cystadeno carcinoma(n=13)	85%	neoplasma 80%
cystadenoma (n=12)	75%	
retention cyst (n=18)	27%	non-neoplasma 13%
pseudocyst (n=35)	6%	

Table 3. Incidence of the cystic lesion 3cm or more with solid component or septum

cystadeno carcinoma(n=13)	100%	neoplasma 92%
cystadenoma (n=12)	83%	
retention cyst (n=18)	22%	non-neoplasma 9%
pseudocyst (n=35)	6%	

Table 4. Detection rates of Solid component

	CT (+)	CT (−)		ERP (+)	ERP (−)		EUS (+)	EUS (−)
histology (+)	3	2	(+)	5	0	(+)	4	1
histology (−)	1	9	(−)	2	6	(−)	3	8

sensitivity	60%	100%	80%
specificity	90%	75%	73%
overall accuracy	80%	85%	75%

Table 5. Detection rates of Septum

	CT (+)	CT (−)		ERP (+)	ERP (−)		EUS (+)	EUS (−)
histology (+)	10	0	(+)	5	3	(+)	11	0
histology (−)	1	4	(−)	1	4	(−)	0	5

sensitivity	100%	63%	100%
specificity	80%	80%	100%
overall accuracy	93%	69%	100%

SUMMARY

These data suggest that the cystic lesion 3cm or more in diameter with solid component or septum could be diagnosed as having neoplastic cysts. It is still difficult to determine whether the cystic lesion of the pancreas is benign or malignant. EUS is also useful to detect the internal structure of the cystic lesion.

REFERENCES

1. Talamini MA, Pitt HA, Hruban RH, Boitnott JK, Coleman JA, Cameron JL (1992) Spectrum of cystic tumors of the pancreas. Am J Surg 163:117-124

2. Nakasako T, Hanyu F, Imaizumi T (1990) Differential Diagnosis of Cystic Disease of the Pancreas. J. Bil. Panc. 11:53-60

Adjuvant Therapy Following Resection
of Pancreatic Head Carcinoma According to the Histopathological
and Biological Features

P. Vaidya, S. Isaji, K. Kato, K. Tanigawa, K. Okamura, Y. Ogura,
T. Noguchi, Y. Kawarada, and R. Mizumoto

First Department of Surgery, Mie University School of Medicine, Tsu, 514 Japan

ABSTRACT

The purpose of this study was to find appropriate adjuvant therapy
following resection of pancreatic head carcinoma according to the
histopathological and biological features. There was a significant
correlation between histological tumor spread and biological factors. When
all three biological factors, proliferating cell nuclear antigen (PCNA),
epidermal growth factor (EGF), and tenascin (TN) were positive, the
incidence of liver metastases was 78.6%, while it was only 7.1% when all
three were negative. With the results of these factors and posterior
surgical margin of the resected tumor (ew) we have proposed a protocol for
adjuvant therapy following resection of the pancreatic head carcinoma.

KEY WORDS: proliferating cell nuclear antigen, epidermal growth factor,
tenascin, intrahepatic arterial infusion chemotherapy, radiation therapy.

INTRODUCTION

Inspite of extended radical resection of pancreatic head carcinoma,
prognosis of patients with this disease has not been improved
significantly. This is mainly due to the fact that recurrence in the liver
and / or retroperitoneal space often develop during the early postoperative
period. Therefore, adjuvant therapy is helpful to improve the prognosis.

MATERIAL AND METHOD

Among 57 patients with resection for ductal cell carcinoma of the
pancreatic head, 35 were evaluated and divided in two groups: long-term
(Group L) and short-term (Group S) survivors. Group L consisted of 8
patients who survived 3 or more years after resection. Group S consisted of
27 patients who died of tumor recurrence within two years. The
histopathological study was performed according to the General Rules for
the Study of Cancer of the Pancreas proposed by Japan Pancreas Society
(1986). As for biological factors, immunohistochemical staining of cancer
cells was performed by avidin-biotin peroxidase complex method for PCNA,
EGF and TN. Tumors were scored as positive for PCNA, EGF when the
percentage of positively stained cancer cells were 30% or more by counting
1000 cancer cells. Staining for tenascin was determined as positive when
clear stromal staining was observed in a 30% or greater area of the cancer
cell nest. Combined analysis of these three biological factors was
performed to find out the high risk group of early recurrence, and a
protocol for adjuvant therapy was proposed and tried.

RESULTS

In the analysis of histopathological factors, the patients in Group S
demonstrated a significantly higher incidence of poorly to moderately
differentiated carcinoma, positive venous (v) and neural invasion (ne), and
positive tumor spread such as lymph node involvement (n) and portal vein
invasion (pv), compared with those in Group L. In biological factors, the
patients in Group S had a significantly higher incidence of tumors staining
positive for PCNA, EGF, and TN. All 35 patients in Groups L and S were

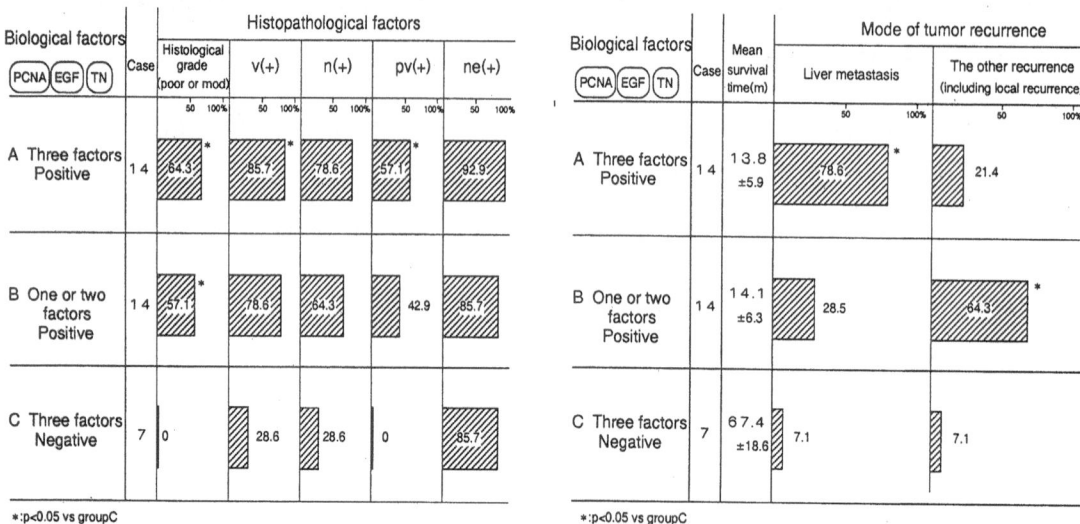

Fig.1 Correlation between Combined Biological
and Histopathological Factors

Fig.2 Correlation between Combined Biological
Factors and Mode of Tumor Recurrence

also classified into three groups A, B and C according to the number positive of three factors, PCNA, EGF and TN (Fig 1). The incidence of poor or moderate histological grade, v, n, and pv was higher in Groups A and B than in Group C. Mean survival time demonstrated a significant difference between Groups A and B vs. Group C (Fig 2). The incidence of liver metastasis was highest in Group A. In contrast, the incidence of recurrence at the other sites was highest in Group B. In Group C, the recurrance rate was very low. With these results and histological result of posterior surgical margin (ew), we have proposed a new protocol of adjuvant therapy following radical resection of pancreatic head carcinoma (Table 1).
Case reports: Case 1 is a 62-year old male who underwent total pancreatectomy with portal vein resection. The histopathological report of the resected specimen was poorly differentiated adenocarcinoma, v(-), n(-), pv(+), ne(+) and ew(-). All three biological factors were positive. Thus intrahepatic arterial (IHA) continous infusion of 5FU was started postoperatively to prevent liver metastasis. Unfortunately, despite our best effort, the patient developed multiple liver metastasis 8 months after operation. Case 2 is a 63-year old female who underwent pancreatico-duodenectomy with portal vein resection. The histopathological report was moderatly differentiated adenocarcinoma, v(+), n(+), pv(+), ne(+) and ew(+) and the biological results were PCNA(+), EGF(-), TN(+). An afterloading catheter was inserted for 192-Ir brachytherapy intraoperatively because ew was positive. Extra-abdominal radiation therapy and brachytherapy (total dose: 61 Gy) were administered to the local site and thereafter continous infusion of 5FU was given. The patient was discharged and is doing well 4 months after surgery.

DISCUSSION

The prognosis of pancreatic head carcinoma is extremely poor, despite the radical operative procedures with extended lymph node dissection and with or without resection of portal vein. It has been reported that this is due to the early postoperative hepatic metastases and residual tumor in the surgical margin (1). As this carcinoma is unlikely to be cured by a radical operative procedure alone, combined therapy, consisting of radical resection with radiation therapy and chemotherapy, is being used more frequently and it is seen that these combination therapy has improved the prognosis (2). The problem still remains to find out which patients are most likely to have liver metastases and/or recurrence in the other sites so that appropriate therapy can be administered to the proper site. However, there are no guidelines as yet on how to choose the high risk patients for recurrence in one or both sites so that proper adjuvant

Table 1 Postoperative Adjuvant Therapy According to Histopathological and Biological Features of the Tumor

Biological factors PCNA, EGF, Tenascin	ew*	Postoperative adjuvant therapy
Three factors Positive	(-)	IHA continuous infusion (reservoir)
	(+)	Radiation therapy + IHA continuous infusion (reservoir)
One or two factors Positive	(-)	IHA single injection + Intravenous chemotherapy
	(+)	Radiation therapy + IHA single injection + Intravenous chemotherapy
Three factors Negative	(-)	Intravenous chemotherapy
	(+)	Radiation therapy + Intravenous chemotherapy

★ew : posterior surgical margin

therapy can be concentrated at the particular site without risking the patients to unnecessary and harmful therapy. Our results show that the three biological factors, PCNA, EGF, and TN, are significantly correlated to the histopathological tumor characteristics, the mode of tumor recurrence and survival period. For patients with pancreatic carcinoma, it is well recognized that intraoperative dissection of the pancreas may result in tumor dissemination and implantation with the subsequent development of peritoneal metastases. Therefore, we also chose the histological result of posterior surgical margin (ew) as an important factor for selection of adjuvant therapy. When the three biological factors are positive, we concentrate our therapy on the liver, and when one or two factors are positive, because of the high incidence of recurrence in the other sites we stress our treatment of giving intravenous chemotherapy. In all the groups, when ew is positive, radiation therapy is added to our protocol. With this protocol, we expect to improve the prognosis in patients with this disease.

REFERENCES

1. Cristopher G. Willett, Kent Lewandrowski, Andrew L. Warshaw, James Efird, and Carolyn C. Compton (1993) Resection Margins in Carcinoma of the Head of the Pancreas. Ann Surg 217: 144-148
2. Hideo Ozaki, Keiichi Hojo, Taira Kinoshita, Sunao Egawa and Kiyozo Kishi (1988) Multidisciplinary treatment for resectable pancreatic cancer. Int J Pancreatol 3: 249-260

Nuclear DNA Content and Short-Term Survival Analysis in Carcinoma of the Pancreas: A Study Using Flow Cytometry

SEON HAHN KIM, BUM-HWAN KOO, and SAE MIN KIM

Department of Surgery, College of Medicine, Korea University, Seoul 152-050, Korea

ABSTRACT

The nuclear DNA contents were analyzed using flow cytometry from formalin-fixed, paraffin-embedded specimens for 36 carcinomas of the pancreas, of which 30 specimens obtained from pancreatic resection and 6 specimens from biopsy. Thirty-six percent (n=13) had an aneuploid DNA pattern, and 64% (n=23) were diploid. A multivariate analysis using log-lineal regression model demonstrated that the pattern of nuclear DNA ploidy was an independent prognostic factor as strong as or stronger than the type of surgery (resection or palliative surgery). The survival time of diploid tumor was approximately two times longer than that of aneuploid tumor (p<0.05).

KEY WORDS : pancreatic cancer, flow cytometry, DNA ploidy, survival

INTRODUCTION

The experience with measurement of DNA content for many human cancers has shown that a biologic and clinical significance of DNA ploidy is diverse according to the origin of tumors [1]. At the year of 1987, Weger and his colleagues [2] proposed DNA analysis of ductal carcinoma of the pancreas yielded important additional information for prognosis and for treatment planning. Joensuu et al [3] in 1989 found that resectable pancreatic cancers formed a highly selected subgroup often with diploid DNA, a low S phase fraction, and less aggressive biological behaviour. Thus they insisted that treatment recommendations based on survival data from non-randomized, retrospective series were likely to be grossly misleading, and that the superiority of "curative" over palliative surgery or biopsy should be interpreted with great caution. Warshaw [4] in 1991 suggested that the reason on rising of cure rates after pancreatoduodenectomy (adjusted for surgical mortality and stage at presentation) in recent reports may be related to the changes in the nature of pancreatic cancer such as the pattern of ploidy or proliferative index. The aim of the present study was to investigate the prognostic and biological value of nuclear DNA content and cell-cycle analysis by flow cytometry in pancreatic carcinoma, of which the incidence has been rising in Korea.

MATERIALS AND METHODS

This retrospective study is based on clinical follow-up data of 36 pancreastic cancer patients. The patients were treated surgically from 1983 to 1991, and followed up for a period of 12.5 ± 1.7 months (mean± SE). Thirty patients had a resection and 6 patients had a bypass or an explorative laparotomy and biopsy only. The patients who died within 30 postoperative days or died without cancer during the follow-up period were excluded. Samples for flow cytometry were prepared from formalin-fixed, paraffin-embedded blocks. Fifty-μm-thick section were cut, deparaffinized, and treated with pepsin and trypsin. The cell suspension was stained with propidium iodide fluorescence dye. The DNA distribution and cell cycle were measured on a flow cytometer FACScan (Becton & Dickinson Immunocytometry Systems, San Jose, CA) using CellFIT Cell-cycle analysis version 2.0. A histogram was considered to be diploid if its DNA distribution showed a single G1 peak. Any additional G1 peak was considered as aneuploidy. Statistical evaluation was carried out using the SAS package program. A multivariate analysis was performed using log-lineal regression model to estimate the relative importance of prognostic factors.

RESULTS

Table 1 shows the correlations between DNA ploidy patterns and clinico-histologic parameters. DNA ploidy was related significantly to histologic grade (p=0.014), and tumors which were located in the body &/or tail were associated with aneuploidy as compared with the head (p=0.028).

Table 1. Correlations between DNA ploidy patterns and clinico-histologic parameters

Parameters		DNA ploidy		% of aneuploid	p value*
		Diploid	Aneuploid		
Age	≤40	3	2	40	NS
	>40	20	11	36	
Sex	Male	16	10	38	NS
	Female	7	3	30	
Location	Head	20	7	30	0.028
	Body &/or tail	3	6	67	
T stage**	T1	5	4	44	
	T2	11	4	27	NS
	T3	7	5	42	
Lymph node	Negative	12	4	25	NS
	Positive	11	9	45	
Grade	1	10	1	9	
	2	10	5	33	0.014
	3	3	7	70	

* Chi-squared test
** T1: limited to the pancreas, T2: extended to duodenum, bile duct, or peripancreatic tissues,
   T3: extended to stomach, spleen, colon, or adjacent large vessels

Figure 1 shows the Kaplan-Meier survival curves for the 23 patients with diploid and the 13 patients with aneuploid pancreatic carcinoma : One-year survival rates and mean ($\pm$ SE) survival times were 66% and 19.7$\pm$3.0 months in diploid and 38% and 11.9$\pm$3.1 months in aneuploid, respectively.

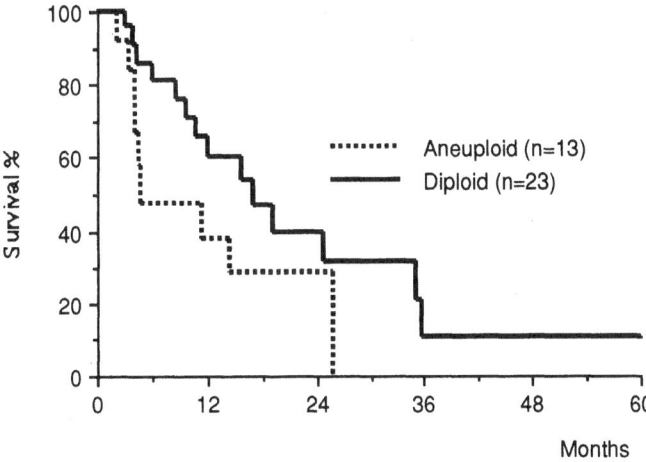

Fig. 1. Kaplan-Meier survival curves for the 23 patients with diploid and the 13 patients with aneuploid pancreatic carcinoma

Multivariate analyses using log-lineal regression models demonstrated that ploidy pattern, tumor growth status, nodal involvement, and the type of surgical treatment (resection or palliative surgery) were statistically significant prognostic factors (Table 2).

Table 2. Results of multivariate analysis by log-lineal regression model

Panels*	Variables	Regression coefficient	p value	Effect to survival time**=exp$^{(RC)}$
1	Resection vs palliative	1.0004	0.0024	2.72
	Aneuploid vs diploid	-0.6242	0.0343	0.54
2	T1 vs T3	1.4829	0.0001	4.41
	T2 vs T3	0.6381	0.0156	1.89
	Aneuploid vs diploid	-0.7502	0.0024	0.47
3	Nodes negative vs positive	0.6233	0.0631	1.87
	Aneuploid vs diploid	-0.6654	0.0380	0.51
4	Resection vs palliative	0.2390	0.5400	1.27
	Nodes negative vs positive	-0.1997	0.5776	0.82
	T1 vs T3	1.4305	0.0016	4.18
	T2 vs T3	0.4792	0.1551	1.61
	Aneuploid vs diploid	-0.6689	0.0333	0.51
	PI $\leq$ 15.1 vs $>$ 15.1	0.1817	0.6164	1.20

* Each panel represents a separate multivariate model
**The effect to survival time was calculated as a value of exp $^{(regression coefficient)}$

DISCUSSION

The present investigation shows that nuclear DNA assessments through flow cytometry can provide additional prognostic information for conventional clinico-histologic predictors in pancreatic carcinoma as in other studies [1,4-7]. As shown in table 2, the patients with diploid tumor survived two times longer than ones with aneuploid, even after adjustment for the type of surgery, tumor growth status, or lymph node involvement, respectively. We also investigated a survival difference between resected aneuploid tumor and unresected diploid tumor, which was not shown in this paper. The result revealed that there was no statistically significant difference in survival. Therefore, we concluded that the pattern of nuclear DNA ploidy was an independent prognostic factor as strong as or stronger than the type of surgical treatment. The Hopkins group [1] observed that a subset of patients with "large" (>2.5cm) aneuploid cancers were identified who had uniformly poor survivals even after "curative" resection, and proposed carefully the hypothesis of abandoning resection in therse subgroup But in this study, the size of tumor was not a significant prognostic factor. In summary, aneuploid tumors were associated with poor histological differentiation, and tended to be more frequent in the body and/or tail than in the head. It may be concluded that DNA ploidy pattern appears to be one of the most important predictors of survival in patients with carcinoma of the pancreas and diploid carcinoma are associated with longer survival than aneuploid ones.

REFERENCES

1. Allison DC, Bose KK, Hruban RH, Piantadosi S, Dooley WC, Boitnott JK, Cameron JL (1991) Pancreatic cancer cell DNA content with long-term survival after pancreatectomy. Ann Surg 214:648-656
2. Weger AR, Graf AH, Askensten U, Schwab G, Bodner E, Auer G, Mikuz G (1987) Ploidy as prognostic determinant in pancreatic cancer. Lancet 2:1031
3. Joensuu H, Alanen KA, Klemi PJ (1989) Doubts on "curative" resection of pancreatic cancer. Lancet 1:953-954
4. Warshaw AL (1991) Implications of malignant-cell DNA content for treatement of patients with pancreatic cancer. Ann Surg 214:645-647
5. Alanen KA, Joensuu H, Klemi PJ, Nevalainen TJ (1990) Clinical significance of nuclear DNA content in pancreatic carcinoma. J Pathol 160:313-320
6. Eskelinen M, Lipponen P, Marin S, Haapasalo H, Makinen K, Puittinen J, Alhava E, Nordling S (1992) DNA ploidy, S-phase fraction, and G2 fraction as prognostic determinants in human pancreatic cancer. Scand J Gastroenterol 27:39-43
7. Weger AR, Falkmer UG, Schwab G, Glaser K, Kemmler G, Bodner E, Auer GU, Mikuz G (1990) Nuclear DNA distribution pattern of the parenchymal cells in adenocarcinoma of the pancreas and in chronic pancreatitis. Gastroenterology 99:237-242

Long Term Prognosis and DNA Ploidy Pattern After Pancreatoduodenectomy for Cancer of the Head of the Pancreas

HIDEKI YASUDA, TADAHIRO TAKADA, KATSUHIRO UCHIYAMA, HIROSHI HASEGAWA, and TATSUSHI IWAGAKI

First Department of Surgery, Teikyo University School of Medicine, Itabashi-ku, Tokyo, 173 Japan

ABSTRACT

We investigated a long-term survival after surgical resection of carcinoma of the head of the pancreas and DNA ploidy pattern. 17 cases out of 34 had diploid patterns and 17 cases had aneuploid patterns. Out of 25 curative cases, cumulative survival rates for diploid pattern were 85% after 1 year, 68% after 3 years, and 50% after 5 years, which were significantly better than those for aneuploid pattern. Among 9 non-curative cases, there was no significant difference between two groups in terms of prognosis. In conclusion, DNA ploidy pattern is useful as an indicator for evaluating prognosis after surgical resection of carcinoma of the head of the pancreas.

Key Words: pancreatic carcinoma, DNA ploidy pattern, pancreatoduodenectomy, survival rate

INTRODUCTION

In recent years, quantity of nuclear DNA has been utilized as a prognostic factor for malignant tumors. In this paper, we analyzed the amount of nuclear DNA in surgically resected specimens of carcinoma of the head of the pancreas by flow cytometry, and investigated relations between DNA ploidy pattern and post operative long term survival.

MATERIAL

34 cases with carcinoma of the head of the pancreas were studied between August 1981 and December 1991. In all these cases, DNA was quantified and their prognosis was followed up.

METHODS

In order to investigate nuclear DNA ploidy pattern in surgically resected specimens of carcinoma of the head of the pancreas, thin sections of 50 μm were prepared from paraffin embedded trimmed cancerous tissue block first. Next, deparaffinization of carcinoma tissue sections was performed in Xylene according to Schutte's method (1). Then, after trypsinization, sections were stained by Propidium Iodide. The amounts of nuclear DNA from 10000 cells were measured by flow cytometry and their patterns were grouped into diploid and aneuploid.

RESULTS

(1) DNA ploidy pattern in resected specimens of carcinoma of the head of the pancreas:
DNA ploidy patterns in 34 resected specimens of carcinoma of the head of the pancreas were 17 diploid (50%) and 17 aneuploid (50%).
(2) DNA ploidy pattern and cumulative survival rates:
In 17 cases with diploid pattern, one-year survival rate was 76%, three-year survival was 56%, and five-year survival was 41%. In 17 cases with aneuploid pattern, one-year survival rate was 58%, three-year survival was 18%, and five-year survival was 12%. Aneuploid pattern had a significantly ($p < 0.05$) poorer prognosis than diploid pattern. (Fig. 1)
(3) Curability and DNA ploidy pattern:
Out of 34 cases who underwent surgical resection of carcinoma of the head of the pancreas, 25 cases were cured and 9 cases were not cured. Ploidy patterns of 25 curative cases were as follows; diploid patterns: 14 cases, & aneuploid pattern: 11 cases. Ploidy patterns of 9 non-curative cases were as follows; diploid patterns: 3 cases, & aneuploid pattern: 6 cases. There was no significant difference in the proportion of ploidy patterns among curative and non-curative cases. (Fig. 2)

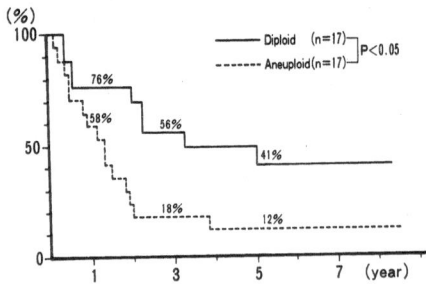

Fig 1 : DNA ploidy pattern and Cumulative survival rate

	Diploid	Aneuploid	
curative	14	11	n.s.
non-curative	3	6	

Fig 2 : Curability and DNA ploidy pattern

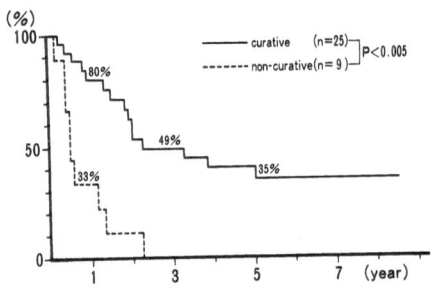

Fig 3 : Curability and Cumulative survival rates

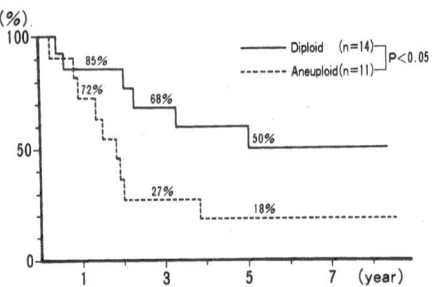

Fig 4 : Prognosis of culative cases and DNA ploidy pattern

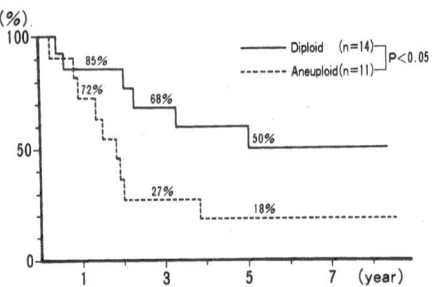

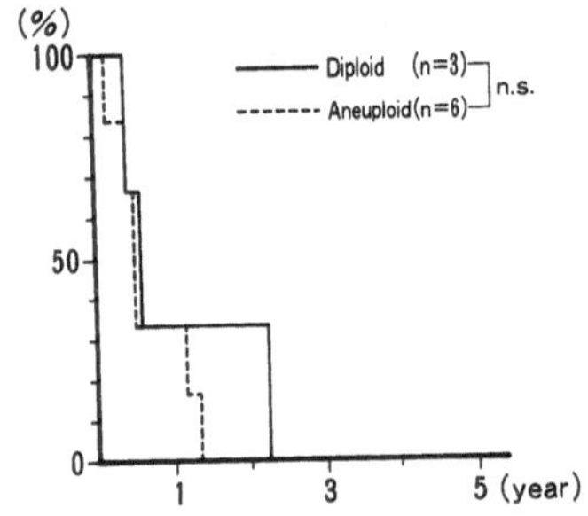

Fig 5 : Prognosis of non-culative cases and DNA ploidy pattern

	Diploid	Aneuploid
Stage I	7	1
Stage II	5	2
Stage III	1	2
Stage IV	2	12

—P<0.05—

Fig 6 : Stage classification and DNA ploidy pattern

(4) Curability and cumulative survival rates:

Cumulative survival rates in 25 curative cases were as follows; one-year survival: 80%, three-year survival: 49 %, and five-year survival: 35%. On the other hand, one-year survival of 9 non-curative cases was 33%, and no cases survived beyond 3 years. Cumulative survival rates in curative cases were significantly better than those in non-curative cases. (Fig. 3)

(5) Prognosis of curative cases and DNA ploidy pattern:

Relations between prognosis and DNA ploidy pattern were studied in 25 curative cases. Cumulative survival rates in 14 diploid cases were as follows; one-year survival: 85%, three-year survival: 68%, and five-year survival: 50%. Cumulative survival rates in 11 aneuploid cases were as follows; one-year survival: 72%, three-year survival: 27%, and five-year survival: 18%. Diploid pattern had a significantly ($p < 0.05$) better prognosis than aneuploid pattern. (Fig. 4)

(6) Prognosis of non-curative cases and DNA ploidy pattern:

In 9 non-curative cases, no significant difference in survival rates was seen between diploid pattern (3 cases) and aneuploid case (6 cases). (Fig. 5)

(7) Stage classification and DNA ploidy pattern:

Macroscopic progression of the disease (Stage classification) was evaluated in 34 subjects according to general rules for cancer of the pancreas by Japan Pancreas Society (2) and the results were as follows. Stage I: 8 cases, Stage II: 7 cases, Stage III: 3 cases, and Stage IV: 14 cases. Diploid cases were significantly better than aneuploid cases in terms of stages. On the contrary, aneuploid cases had poorer stages. (Fig. 6)

DISCUSSIONS

Diagnosis of pancreatic cancer has been remarkably improved by the development of image analysis such as ultrasound examinations and CT examinations. However, in this country, prognosis of pancreatic cancer after surgeries was extremely poorer than other intestinal cancer as evidenced by one-year survival of 51% and three-year survival of 23%. Prognostic factors in surgically resected pancreatic cancer cases have been primarily focused on image analysis or pathological findings. TNM classification by UICC employed post-surgical histo-pathological classificaion in addition to pre-treatment clinical classification which was bases on pre-surgical iamge analysis. However, prognosis varied remarkably even if CT findings, pathohistological findings and staging were similar. Therefore, analysis of nuclear DNA quantity was introduced as new prognostic factors.

In 1983, Hedley et al reported that quantitative measurements of nuclear DNA using paraffin-embedded pathological material made a prognostic evaluation possible (3). In 1985, Shutte et al further improved Hedley's method by intensifying fluorescence (1). In this paper, we investigated a long-term survival after surgical resection of carcinoma of the head of the pancreas and DNA ploidy pattern using Schutte's method. In this study, we found that 17 cases out of 34 had diploid pattern and 17 cases had aneuploid pattern. We compared cumulative survival rates in two groups. Diploid pattern were significantly better than aneuploid pattern in terms of survival, i.e., one-year survival of 76%, three-year survival of 56%, and five-year survival of 50%. However, we found no significant difference in cumulative survival rates of diploid and aneuploid pattern among non-curative cases. Namely, when cumulative survival rates were studied among curative cases after surgical removal of carcinma of the head of the pancreas, diploid pattern had a significantly better prognosis than aneuploid pattern. Thus, DNA ploidy pattern may be a useful indicator for evaluating prognosis of pancreatic cancer after curative surgeries.

REFERENCES

1. Shutte B, Reynder MMJ, Bosman FT, et al (1985) Flow cytometric determination of DNA ploidy level in nuclei isolated from paraffin embedded tissue. Cytometry 3:26-30.
2. Japan Pancreas Society (1991) Report nation-wide investigations of registered pancreatic cancer patients.
3. Hedley DW, Friedlander MT, Taylor TW, et al (1983) Method for analysis of cellular DNA content of paraffin-embedded pathological material using flow cytometry. J. Histochem Cytochem. 31:1333-1335.

Role of O-Linked Oligosaccharides and Sialic Acids in Pancreatic Cancer Cell Interaction with Extracellular Matrix

Tetsuji Sawada[1,2], Jenny J.L. Ho[1], Yong-Suk Chung[2], Michio Sowa[2], and Young S. Kim[1]

[1]Gastrointestinal Research Laboratory (151M2), Veterans Affairs Medical Center, University of California, San Francisco, CA 94121, USA
[2]First Department of Surgery, Osaka City University Medical School, Osaka, 545 Japan

Human pancreatic cancer cell, SW1990 produce high mucin which have predominantly O-linked oligosaccharides. SW1990 cell also have high levels of in vitro invasiveness and high in vivo liver metastatic potential. Treatment of SW1990 cells with neuraminidase, O-linked oligosaccharide synthesis inhibitor (Bz-GalNAc) and sialyl transferase inhibitor (NM8110) reduced in vitro invasion. Treatment with Bz-GalNAc and NM8110 decreased the total activity of secreted metalloproteinase, but slightly increased the level of urokinase plasminogen activator. Cell adhesion to matrigel was enhanced after these treatments and adhesion to specific extracellular matrix proteins, laminin and collagen type IV, was also increased particularly with neuraminidase treatment. These results suggests that alteration of sialylated O-linked oligosaccharides affect the interaction with the extracellular matrix and thus may play a role in tumor cell invasion and metastasis.

KEY WORDS: pancreatic cancer, extracellular matrix, sialic acid, O-linked oligosaccharide

INTRODUCTION

Sialic acids and mucin production on cancer cell surface have been reported to be correlated with the cell's metastatic potential [1]. Tumor cell interaction with extracellular matrix (ECM) has also shown to be dependent upon cell surface carbohydrates [2,3]. In this study, to investigate the relationship between mucin production and invasiveness or metastatic potential in pancreatic cancer we used three cell lines, SW1990, CAPAN-2 and PANC-1. Both SW1990 and CAPAN-2 produce high mucin, glycoprotein which have predominantly O-linked oligosaccharides, while PANC-1 does not [4]. Furthermore, to elucidate the role of cell surface O-linked oligosaccharides and sialic acids in cell-ECM interaction we used an O-linked oligosaccharide synthesis inhibitor (benzyl-α-N-acetyl galactosamine, Bz-GalNAc) [5], an inhibitor of sialyl transferase (NM8110) [6] and neuraminidase. We measured in vitro invasiveness through basement membrane (matrigel), secreted proteolytic activity (metalloproteinase and urokinase-type plasminogen activator) and adhesiveness to matrigel, laminin and collagen type I, IV.

MATERIALS AND METHODS

Cell Lines and Culture

Human pancreatic adenocarcinoma cell line SW1990, CAPAN-2 and PANC-1 were grown in Dulbecco's modified Eagle's medium (DMEM) containing 10% fetal calf serum (FCS), penicillin (100U/ml), streptomycin (100μg/ml). Cultures were maintained at 37°C in a humidified 5% CO_2 atmosphere.

In Vitro Invasion Assay and In vivo Liver Metastasis Assay

Transwell cell culture chambers (8.0 μm pore filter, 6.5 mm diameter) (Costar, USA) were used for this assay. Cell suspension, 7.5×10^4 cells/filter in DMEM containing 10% FCS were seeded on filter coated with matrigel (111μg/filter). After incubation for 48 hr, the number of invasive cells was estimated by 3-(4,5-dimethylthiazol-2yl)-2,5 diphenyl-2,4 tetrazolium bromide (MTT, Sigma, USA). For metastasis assay a small left flank incision was made in athymic nude mice and the spleen was exteriorized through a incision. After ligating vessels at upper pole of spleen, 7×10^5 cells in 0.1 ml SFM were slowly injected into spleen and splenectomy was performed 1 min after injection. Mice were sacrificed 5 weeks later and liver metastasis were estimated by metastatic nodules.

SW1990 Cell Treatment with Neuraminidase, Bz-GalNAc and NM8110

$1×10^6$ cells were incubated in phosphate beffer saline (PBS) with 100 mU/ml neuraminidase from clostridium perfringens (Sigma) for 30 min at 37°C. Control cells were incubated in only PBS. In case of Bz-GalNAc and NM8110 treatment, cells were incubated with medium containing 2 mM Bz-GalNAc (Sigma) or 0.2 mM 5-fluoro-2',3'-isopropyl-idene-5'-O-(4-N-acetyl-2,4-dideoxy-3,6,7,8-tetra-O-acetyl-1-methoxycarbonyl-D-glycero-α-D-galactooctapyranosyl) uridine (NM8110) (provided by MECT Co., Tokyo, Japan) in the presence of 10% FCS for 48 hr. Bz-GalNAc and NM8110 have been previously shown to inhibit O-mucin glycosylation and sialylation in these conditions [1,3,6].

Metalloproteinase (MMP) Assay and Urokinase-Plasminogen Activator (u-PA) Assay

After SW1990 cells were treated with Bz-GalNAc or NM8110 for 48 hr, the spent medium was collected and used for assay. Total MMP activity was measured using a thiopeptolide substrate (Ac-ProLeuGly-S-Leugly-OC_2H_5, Bachem. USA) assay as previously descrived [7]. As urokinase plasminogen activator activity produced by cells was determined by a method of Zimmerman et al. [8] using gly-gly-arg-AMC (Bachem).

Adhesion Assay

96-well plates were coated with Matrigel (8μg/well), laminin (4μg/well), collagen type I, IV (8μg/well). After the plates were left at 4°C over night and washed 2 times with SFM, cells treated with neuraminidase, NM8110 and Bz-GalNAc were suspended to $7.5×10^5$ cells/ml in DMEM containing 0.2 mg/ml BSA. To each well, 100 μl of these cell suspension were seeded and cells were allowed to attach for 1 hr at 37°C. The plates were then washed gently twice with PBS to remove unattached cells. The number of adherent cells were also estimated by MTT colorimetric assay. Cells were incubated with 0.5 mg/ml MTT for 1 hr at 37°C.

RESULTS

SW1990 cells showed the highest invasiveness and metastatic ability in liver colonization assay compared with two other pancreatic cancer cell lines, CAPAN-2 and PANC-1 (Table 1).

Table 1. Invasive and metastatic abilities of pancreatic caner cell line

Cell line	% of invasion	Number of metastasis bearing mice
SW1990	22.6±1.7[a]	5/6[b] (83.3%)
CAPAN-2	17.9±0.7	0/5 (0 %)
PANC-1	7.3±1.3	0/3 (0 %)

[a] Values are the represent mean±SD of triplicate.
[b] Macroscopic liver colonization 5 week after intrasplenic injection.

Removal cell surface sialic acids by neuraminidase and treatment of SW1990 cells with Bz-GalNAc and NM8110 significantly reduced SW1990 invasion (Fig.1). The total activities of metalloproteinase secreted by SW1990 cells treated with Bz-GalNAc and NM8110 were reduced to 80.9 and 70.8% of untreated cells although the difference was not significant. In contrast, the activity of urokinase-plasminogen activator was seen to be slightly increased (Fig.2A,B).

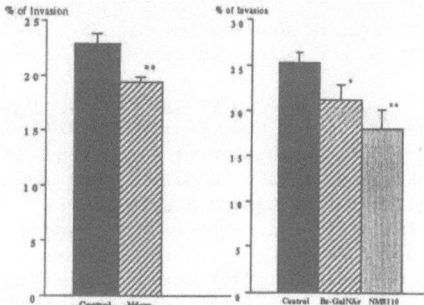

Fig.1 Effect of neuraminidase (100 mU/ml), Bz-GalNAc (2 mM) and NM8110 (0.2 mM) on SW1990 invasion assay. *P<0.05, **P<0.01

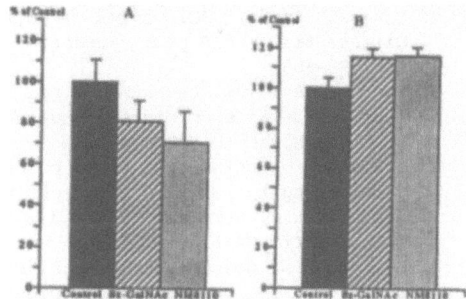

Fig.2 Effect of Bz-GalNAc and NM8110 on MMP (A) and u-PA assay (B).

Neuraminidase and NM8110 treatment showed a similar effect on adhesion to ECM. There was an increased adhesion to matrigel, laminin and collagen type IV, but no effect was observed on adhesion to collagen type I (Fig.3A,B). Bz-GalNAc treatment increased cell adhesion to matrigel and collagen IV, but not to laminin and collagen type I (Fig.3C).

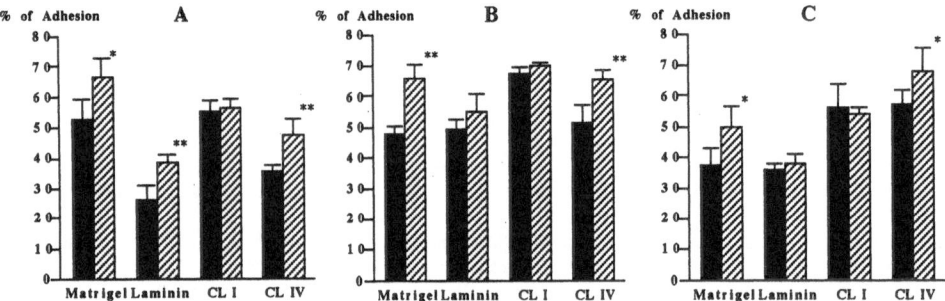

Fig.3 Effect of neuraminidase (A), NM8110 (B) and Bz-GalNAc (C) on SW1990 cell adhesion to matrigel, laminin, CL I (collagen type I) and CL IV (collagen type IV). *P<0.05, **P<0.01 control (■), treated cell (▨)

DISCUSSION

The relationship between mucin and metastatic ability have previously been reported [1-3]. The current findings are consistent with these reports. SW1990 pancreatic cancer cells produce a large amount of mucins [4] and we have shown these cells to be highly invasive and metastatic. Removal of sialic acids or inhibition of sialylation and O-glycosylation all reduced SW1990 invasiveness. NM8110 (an inhibitor of sialylation) or Bz-GalNAc (an inhibitor of O-glycosylation) both reduced MMP activity somewhat but not u-PA activity. A similar effect on MMP activity has been reported in a mucin producing colonic cancer cell line [3]. The present study also showed that treatments with neuraminidase, NM8110, and Bz-GalNAc enhanced SW1990 cell adhesion to matrigel, laminin and collagen type IV. It has been reported that adhesion to ECM may induce cell differentiation and contact inhibition and reduce the mobility [2]. Thus in our study increased adhesion may also contribute to the reduced invasiveness of SW1990 cells after treatment. Adhesion to laminin, fibronectin and collagen type IV have been previously reported to be increased by treatment with neuraminidase [2,9]. This effect was thought to be due to sialic acids masking or hindering specific receptors for these substrates. Our results with SW1990 cells may be explained by a similar mechanism. Thus alterations of sialic acids and O-linked oligosaccharides may affect cell interactions with the ECM in at least two ways: altering the levels of proteolytic activity and cell adhesiveness. In these way sialylated O-linked oligosaccharides may play an important role in pancreatic tumor cell invasion and metastasis.

REFERENCES

1. Bresalier RS, Niv Y, Byrd JC, Duh QY, Toribara NW, Rockwell RW, Dahiya R, Kim YS (1991) Mucin production by human colonic carcinoma cells correlates with their metastatic potential in animal models of colon cancer metastasis. J clin invest 87: 1037-1045
2. Dennis J, Waller C, Timp R, Schirrmacher V (1982) Surface sialic acid reduces attachment of metastatic tumour cells to collagen type IV and fibronectin. Nature 300:274-276
3. Schwartz B, Bresalier RS, Kim YS (1992) The role of mucin in colon-cancer metastasis. Int J Cancer 52:60-65
4. Yonezawa S, Byrd JC, Dahiya R, Ho JJL, Gum JR, Griffiths B, Swallow DM, Kim YS (1991) Differential mucin gene expression in human pancreatic and colon cancer cells. Biochem J 276:599-605
5. Kuan SF, Byrd JC, Basbaum CB, Kim YS (1989) Inhibition of mucin glycosylation by aryl-N-acetyl-α-galactosaminides in human colon cancer cells. J Biol Chem 264:19271-19277
6. Suda IK, Miyamoto Y, Toyoshima S, Itoh M, Osawa T (1986) Inhibition of experimental pulmonary metastasis of mouse colon adenocarcinoma 26 sublines by a sialic acid: nucleoside conjugate having sialyltransferase inhibiting activity. Cancer Res 46:858-862
7. Weingarten H, Martin R, Feder J (1985) Synthetic substrates of vertebrate collagenase. Biochemistry 24:6730-6734
8. Zimmerman M, Quigley JP, Ashe B, Dorn C, Goldfarb R, Troll W (1978) Direct fluorescent assay of urokinase and plasminogen activators of normal and malignant cells: Kinetics and inhibitor profiles. Proc Natl Acad Sci USA 75:750-753
9. Acheson A, Sunshine JL, Rutishauser U (1991) NCAM polysialic acid can regulate both cell-cell and cell-substrate interaction. J Cell Bio 114:143-153

Biliary

UICC and Japanese Stage Classifications for Carcinoma of the Gallbladder

Makoto Sasaki, Toshifumi Eto, Tsukasa Tsunoda, and Takashi Kanematsu

Second Department of Surgery, Nagasaki University School of Medicine, Nagasaki, 852 Japan

ABSTRACT

UICC stage classification (UICC-SC) for carcinoma of the gallbladder was compared with its Japanese stage classification (JPN-SC), using 75 patients undergoing resectional surgery. The 5-year survival rates according to the clinical stages I, II, III and IV were 68, 73, 17, and 6% by the UICC-SC, and 80, 15, 23, and 9% by the JPN-SC, respectively. In the postoperative cumulative survival rates, the UICC-SC showed a significant difference among the corresponding stages except between stage I and II, and III and IV, respectively. It is concluded that the UICC-SC more accurately reflected the prognosis of the patients with gallbladder carcinoma than that of JPN-SC, because grading of the T factor was well correlated with the extent of histopathological progression of the tumor.

KEY WORDS: carcinoma of the Gallbladder, UICC stage classification, Japanese stage classification, prognosis

INTRODUCTION

The UICC stage classification (UICC-SC)[1] for gallbladder cancer was based on T, N and M factors. Japanese Society of Biliary Surgery proposed a more detail stage classification system (JPN-SC)[2] that includes several pathological factors. Stage classification for carcinoma should accurately reflect the prognosis of pateints after the treatment. In this study, surgical results were compared in terms of each classification.

PATIENTS AND METHOD

Seventy-five among the 132 patients with carcinoma of the gallbladder underwent resectional surgery at the Second Department of Surgery, Nagasaki University School of Medicine, during the last 22 years. The charts of these patients were reviewed. The correlation between stage of the disease and distribution of patients, and postoperative cumulative survival curves and rates according to the clinical stage were assessed in terms of each UICC-SC and JPN-SC. Furthermore, postoperative cumulative survival curves at each grade of T factor by UICC-SC, and positive rate of the histopathological elements in each grade of T factor were analyzed. The stages of UICC-SC and JPN-SC are shown in Table 1.

Table 1. The stage grouping of UICC-SC and JPN-SC

		UICC-SC						JPN-SC						
STAGE	0	Tis	N0	M0		STAGE	I	S0	Hinf0	H0	Binf0	P0	N0	S: serosal invasion
STAGE	I	T1	N0	M0		STAGE	II	S1	Hinf1	H0	Binf1	P0	N1	Hinf: hepatic invasion
STAGE	II	T2	N0	M0		STAGE	III	S2	Hinf2	H0	Binf2	P0	N2 or 3	H: liver metastasis
STAGE	III	T1	N1	M0		STAGE	IV	S3	Hinf3	Any H	Binf3	Any P	N4	Binf: invasion to the
		T2	N1	M0										hepatoduodenal ligament
		T3	Any N	M0										P: disseminating metastasis
STAGE	IV	T4	Any N	M0										to the peritoneum
		Any T	Any N	M1										N: lymph node metastasis

Table 2 shows correlation between two stages and distribution of patients.

Table 2. Correlation between two stages and distribution of patients

	JPN I	JPN II	JPN III	JPN IV	Total
UICC I	11	0	0	0	11
UICC II	<u>11</u>	5	0	1	17
UICC III	1	3	10	<u>14</u>	28
UICC IV	0	0	3	16	19
Total	23	8	13	31	75

Stage corresponded in the two staging systems in 42 of the 75 patients (56%). Eleven out of 17 patients in stage II by UICC-SC belonged to stage I by JPN-SC because of no serosal invasion. Fourteen out of 28 patients in stage III by UICC-SC were classified into stage IV by JPN-SC. The PCS curves and rates according to the clinical stage by UICC-SC and JPN-SC are shown in Figures 1 and 2.

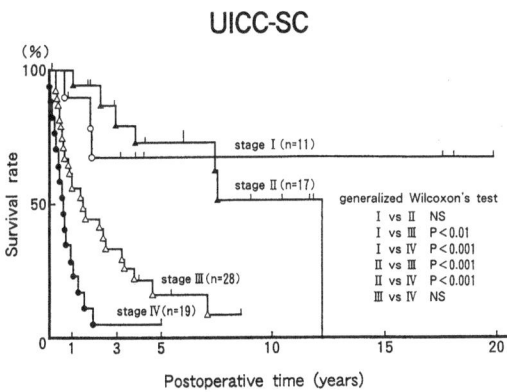

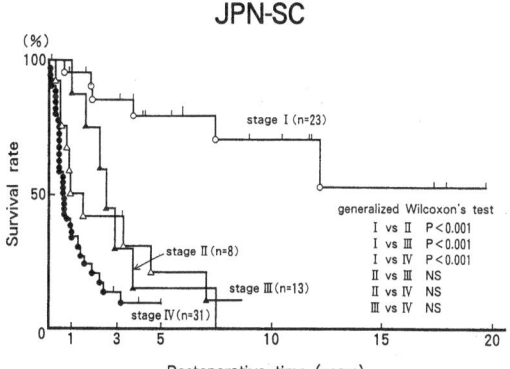

Fig.1 The postoperative cumulative survival
curves according to the clinical stage
by UICC-SC

Fig.2 The postoperative cumulative survival
curves according to the clinical stage
by JPN-SC

The 5-year survival rates according to the stages I, II, III and IV were 68, 73, 17, and 6 % by the UICC-SC, and 80, 15, 23, and 9% by the JPN-SC, respectively. Statistically significant difference was evident in UICC-SC among the corresponding stages except between stage I and II, and III and IV in the survival curves and 5-year survival rates, while by the JPN-SC, no significant difference was noted between the stages II and III, II and IV, and III and IV, respectively. The postoperative cumulative survival curves at each grade of T factor are shown in Figure 3 and positive rates of the histopathological elements in each grade of T factor are summarized in Table 3.

Table3. Positive rates of histopathological elements in each grade of T factor

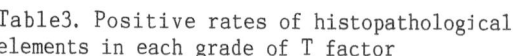

	T1 (n = 11)	T2 (n = 29)	T3 (n = 16)	T4 (n = 19)
n	0* (0)	41.4 (12)	68.8 (11)	89.5 (17)
binf	0 (0)	6.9 (2)	37.5 (6)	63.2 (12)
ly	9.1 (1)	79.3 (23)	93.8 (15)	94.7 (18)
v	9.1 (1)	31.0 (9)	68.8 (11)	63.2 (12)
pn	0 (0)	31.0 (9)	37.5 (6)	78.9 (15)

* Expressed in %, Parenthesis : number of patients, n : metastasis to the regional lymph node, binf : invasion to the hepatoduodenal ligament ly : lymphatic invasion, v : venous invasion, pn : perineural invasion * : $p < 0.05$, ** : $p < 0.01$

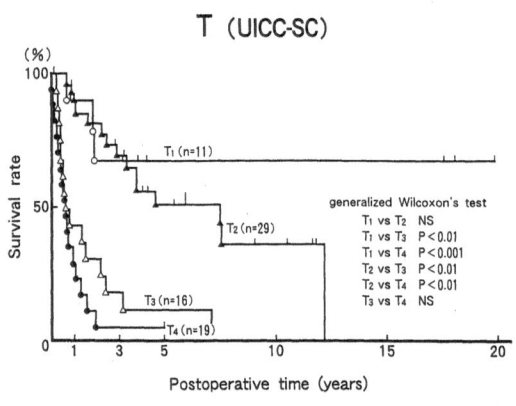

T (UICC-SC)

generalized Wilcoxon's test

T1 vs T2	NS
T1 vs T3	P < 0.01
T1 vs T4	P < 0.001
T2 vs T3	P < 0.01
T2 vs T4	P < 0.01
T3 vs T4	NS

Fig.3 The postoperative cumulative survival curves at each grade of T factor

A significant difference was observed in the survival curves among the corresponding stages except between T1 and T2, and T3 and T4. In Table 3, only one patient in T1 had lymphatic invasion (ly) and another patient in T1 showed venous invasion (v). Positive rates of lymph node metastasis (n), ly, and perineural invasion (pn) in T2 were significantly higher than those in T1. A significant difference was observed between T2 and T3 according to positive rates of invasion to the hepatoduodenal ligament (binf) and venous invasion (v).

DISCUSSION

Stages for carcinoma of the gallbladder are classified based on the depth of invasion. [3][4]UICC-SC also includes the factor of the depth of invasion in the T factor. Grading of the T factor is well correlated with the extent of histopathological progression of the tumor. Our surgical results are suggestive taht prognosis of patients with gallbladder carcinoma is more reflected by UICC-SC than JPN-SC.

REFERENCES

1. UICC (1987) TNM classification of malignant tumors, 4th ed. Springer-Verlag

2. Japanese Society of Biliary Surgery (1986) General rules for surgical and pathological studies on cancer of biliary tract, 2nd ed. Kanehara Publishing, Tokyo (in Japanese)

3. Nevin JE, Morgan TJ, Kay S, King R (1976) Carcinoma of the gallbladder; Staging, treatment and prognosis. Cancer 37:141-148

4. Yamaguchi K, Enjoji M (1988) Carcinoma of the gallbladder. A clinicopathology of 103 patients and a newly proposed staging. Cancer 62:1425-1432

Clinicopathologic Factors Influencing Survival of the Patients with Bile Duct Carcinoma: A Multivariate Statistical Analysis

Md. Mukhlesur Rahman Bhuiya, Yuji Nimura, Junichi Kamiya,
Satoshi Kondo, Masato Nagino, and Naokazu Hayakawa

The First Department of Surgery, Nagoya University School of Medicine, Nagoya, 466 Japan

Key words: Bile duct cancer, Prognostic factors, Multivariate analysis

ABSTRACT

To evaluate the influence of various clinicopathologic factors on survival of the patient with bile duct carcinoma, a computer analysis was performed on 70 resected cases of bile duct cancer. Significant prognostic factors using univariate analysis including location of primary lesion, pancreatic invasion, duodenal invasion, macroscopic and microscopic vascular involvement, perineural invasion, lymphatic vessel involvement, lymph node metastasis, histologic type of lesion, and depth of cancer invasion. However, when an interactive effects of these factors were taken into account, the pancreatic invasion and perineural invasion were selected as two most prognostic factors in a multivariate analysis using Cox stepwise proportional hazard model.

INTRODUCTION

With the recent improvement of surgical techniques in hepatobiliary surgery, a curative surgical resection of bile duct carcinoma can be accomplished with reasonable morbidity and mortality [1, 2]. However, the prognosis of this patient is frustrating particularly in case of carcinoma of the hepatic hilus, although it is small, slow growing and metastasizes late [3]. Resection of these difficult lesions offers the best hope of survival [4, 5]. Previously Tompkins et al [6] demonstrated the prognostic factors affecting survival of the patient with bile duct carcinoma, however they did not use the Cox proportional hazard model [7] for analysis. In this article, an effort was made to evaluate the influence of various clinicopathologic factors on survival of patient with bile duct carcinoma by using the Cox proportional hazard model.

MATERIALS AND METHODS

This study was conducted on 70 resected cases of bile duct carcinoma, who were treated at the First Department of Surgery, Nagoya University Hospital from January 1979 through September 1990. All the lesions were resected at operation after preoperative precise diagnosis. The resected specimens were examined and the relationship between clinicopathologic findings and patients survival was studied. Average follow-up time was 66.5 months (range 21 to 133 months) after surgery.

Variables: The following clinicopathologic variables were considered for prognostic effect: age, sex, location of primary tumor (upper, middle and lower bile duct carcinoma), size of the tumor, macroscopic type of lesions (papillary, nodular, nodular infiltrating and infiltrating), serosal invasion (present or absent), lymph node metastasis (present or absent), hepatic infiltration (present or absent), pancreatic invasion (present or absent), duodenal invasion (present or absent), macroscopic vessels involvement (present or absent), microscopic vessels involvement (present or absent), lymphatic vessels involvement (present or absent), perineural invasion (present or absent), resected proximal margin of the bile duct (cancer positive or negative), resected distal margin (cancer positive or negative), exposed surgical margin (cancer positive or negative), histologic type of lesion (papillary adenocarcinoma, well differentiated adenocarcinoma, moderately differentiated adenocarcinoma, poorly differentiated adenocarcinoma and adenosquamous cell carcinoma), and depth of cancer invasion (invasion limited to fibromuscular layer, invasion limited to adventitia and subserosal layer, and invasion to and beyond the serosal layer).

Analysis. Independent variables were first analyzed by univariate methods. Statistical significance of the variables were determined by Student - t test and chi-square test. Survival for each variable was estimated by the method of Kaplan and Meier, and the significance of survival was determined by generalized Wilcoxon method. Only the variables which were statistically significant by univariate analysis were included in a multivariate analysis. The multivariate results were confirmed using the Cox stepwise proportional hazard model.

RESULTS

Clinical findings: Of the 70 resected cases, 48 were men and 22 were women. Average age at the time of operation was 57.5 years, with a range from 32 to 82 years. Of these, 52 (74.3%) were upper bile duct cancer, 8 (11.4%) were middle bile duct cancer and 10 (14.3%) were lower bile duct cancer patient. All the lesions were resected at operation. Curative resection was done for 51 patients and non-curative for 19 patients. Bile duct resection was done in 2 patients, hepatectomy with bile duct resection in 46, pancreatoduodenectomy in 18, and hepatopancreatoduodenectomy [8] in 4 patients.

Overall survival:

Univariate analysis. The 5- year survival rate for all patients was 25%. Nineteen clinicopathologic factors were analyzed and the prognosis was significantly related to 10 of the 19 variables analyzed by univariate method. The significant variables were : location of primary tumor, microscopic type of tumor, depth of cancer invasion, perineural invasion, macroscopic and microscopic vessels involvement, lymphatic invasion, lymph node metastasis, duodenal invasion and pancreatic invasion. Whereas, the following factors were not significantly associated with prognosis: age, sex , size of the primary lesion, macroscopic type of tumor, hepatic infiltration, serosal invasion, resected surgical margin (proximal and distal), and exposed surgical margin.

Multivariate analysis: Multivariate analysis using the Cox proportional hazard model involving the 10 significant factors determined by univariate analysis identified two most prognostic variables (Table 1). These were the pancreatic invasion and the perineural invasion.

Table 1. Relative values of two prognostic variables derived from Cox stepwise proportional hazard model.

Variable	β	Standard error	Chi-square	P	Hazard ratio	95% Confidence interval
Pancreatic invasion	0.89	0.33	7.01	0.008	2.4	(1.22- 4.75)
Perineural invasion	1.01	0.44	5.25	0.02	2.76	(1.16- 6.55)

Model chi-square = 13.28   (P = 0.001)

Pancreatic invasion and survival: Pancreatic invasion was observed in 14 (20%) of the total 70 cases of bile duct carcinoma. It was observed in 6 of 10 (60%) of the lower bile duct cancer, 4 of 8 (50%) of the middle bile duct cancer, and 4 of 52 (8.3%) of the upper bile duct cancer. Pancreatic invasion was the first prognostic variable detected by the cox stepwise proportional hazard model (Table 1). The 3- year and 5- year survival rates for patients with negative pancreatic invasion were 52% and 36% respectively. Whereas, no 5- year survivors could be seen in patient with positive pancreatic invasion (Figure 1). A statistically significant difference of the survival could be observed between the patient with positive and negative pancreatic invasion (P< 0.005). The death risk for patient with positive pancreatic invasion was 2.4 times greater than the patient with negative pancreatic invasion.

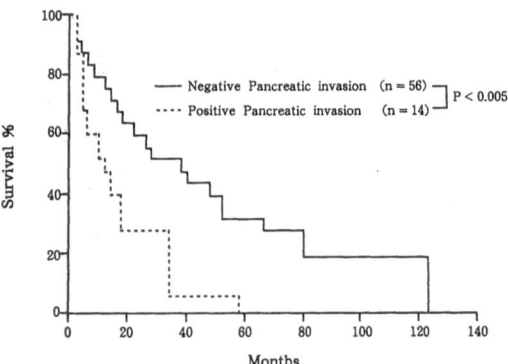
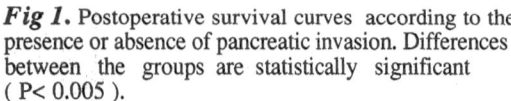
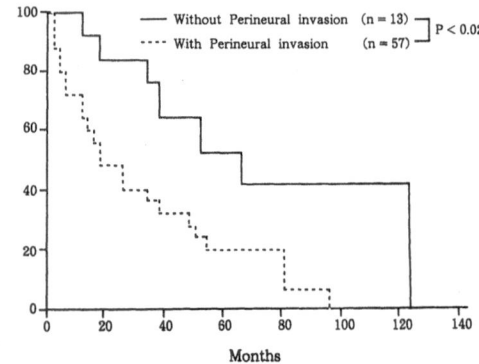

Fig 1. Postoperative survival curves according to the presence or absence of pancreatic invasion. Differences between the groups are statistically significant (P< 0.005).

Fig 2. The survival curves of the bile duct cancer according to the presence or absence of perineural invasion. A statistically significant difference of survival could be seen between the two groups (P<0.02).

Perineural invasion and survival: The perineural invasion was seen in 82.8% of the cases of bile duct cancer. Multivariate analysis showed a statistically significant difference of survival between positive perineural invasion and negative perineural invasion groups (P<0.02). The 3- and 5-year survival rates for the negative perineural invasion patients are 84% and 52%, whereas, the positive perineural invasion patients showing 40% and 19%, respectively (Fig 2). The Cox stepwise proportional hazard model detected the perineural invasion as the 2nd prognostic variables for bile duct cancer patients (Table 1). The positive perineural invasion patients had a 2.76 times greater death risk than the negative perineural invasion patients.

Pancreatic invasion and Perineural invasion versus location of primary lesion: Pancreatic invasion was significantly   correlated with the location of primary lesion (P=0.001) (Table 2). It was observed significantly in the lower and middle bile duct cancer. However, the perineural invasion was not significantly associated with the location of primary lesion. Therefore, the perineural invasion was the independent prognostic factor irrespective of location of primary lesion.

Table 2. Pearson   Correlation Coefficients Among   Variables   Coefficients   Value (Probability Value).

Variable	Location of primary lesion
Perineural invasion	-0.201016
	0.0806
Pancreatic invasion	0.38419
	0.001

DISCUSSION

With the continual progress of diagnostic and surgical techniques in biliary surgery, a good number of biliary cancer can be resected with a reasonable morbidity and mortality [1]. The local recurrence of bile duct cancer is relatively more even after curative resection of this lesion. Therefore, a suitable surgical procedure should be considered for preventing the undesirable outcome.

It is important to know what prognostic factors relating to the survival of the patient with bile duct cancer. Until now, no reports have appeared in the world literature using Cox stepwise proportional hazard model to identify the best prognostic variables in patients with bile duct carcinoma. Tompkins et al [7] analyzed the prognostic variables of bile duct cancer patient, however, they did not use the Cox proportional hazard analytic method. This Cox stepwise proportional hazard analysis identified the two independent prognostic variables of bile duct cancer patient.

The pancreatic invasion is the first prognostic variable. The patients with negative pancreatic invasion survived significantly better than the patients with positive pancreatic invasion after resecting the lesion. Our finding showed that the 5- year survival rate for the patients with negative pancreatic invasion was 46%, whereas 0% for the patient with positive pancreatic invasion. This might be due to the fact that when the bile duct cancer invade the pancreatic tissue, then it behaves like a primary pancreatic cancer and leads to worst prognosis. Perineural invasion was determined as the second prognostic variable by the multivariate analysis. We studied extensively the clinicopathologic significance of perineural invasion previously [9]. The result of the present study substantiated the previous findings. The negative perineural invasion group showed significantly better prognosis than the positive perineural invasion group.

The patient with lower bile duct cancer survived favorably after resection than the patient with middle and upper bile duct cancer. This finding substantiated the finding reported by the others [7]. However, the patient with upper bile duct cancer showing relatively good postoperative survival comparing to the middle bile duct cancer, this finding differs from the previous authors. The preoperative precise diagnosis and appropriate hepatic segmentectomies [1] may be the reason for better survival of our patient with upper bile duct cancer.

The depth of cancer invasion limited to fibromuscular layer group showed significantly better postoperative survival than the patient with cancer invasion to or beyond the adventitial layer group. Moreover, the depth of cancer invasion to or beyond the serosal exposure group showing the worst prognosis. Beazly et al [5] and Topmkins et al [7] demonstrated several factors responsible for favorable outcome of their patients with bile duct carcinoma. However, they did not mention the pancreatic and the perineural invasion as prognostic factors. According to White et al (10) blood vessels invasion and perineural invasion were not the prognostic factors for survival of the patient with bile duct carcinoma. We and many authors [9,11], however, have pointed out a significant correlation between perineural invasion and postoperative survival.

Findings from this study showed that prognosis of the patient with bile duct cancer was significantly associated with pancreatic invasion, perineural invasion, location of primary lesion, histologic type of the lesion, macroscopic and microscopic vessels involvement, depth of cancer invasion, lymphatic invasion, lymph node metastasis and duodenal invasion. However, the age, sex, size of the lesion, macroscopic type of lesion, serosal invasion, exposed surgical margin and resected surgical margin were not significantly associated with survival.

According to this study the patient with positive pancreatic invasion showed worst prognosis and the pancreatic invasion is the first most prognostic factor in bile duct cancer. However, it was observed significantly in the lower and middle bile duct cancer. The perineural invasion is the second most prognostic factor in bile duct cancer and the patient with positive perineural invasion implied hopeless prognosis. It was the unfavorable prognostic factor irrespective of site of lesion. Moreover, the death risk for patient with both positive pancreatic and perineural invasion was 6.65 times greater than the patient with both negative pancreatic and perineural invasion.

REFERENCES

1. Nimura Y, Hayakawa N, Kamiya J, Kondo S, and Shionoya S. : Hepatic segmentectomy with caudate lobe resection for bile duct carcinoma of the hepatic hilus. World J. Surg. 14: 535, 1990
2. Pinson CW, Rossi RL. : Extended right lobectomy, left lobectomy, and skeletonization resection for proximal bile duct cancer. World J. Surg. 12: 52, 1988
3. Klatskin G. : Adenocarcinoma of the hepatic duct at the bifurcation within the porta hepatis. An unusual tumor: Distinctive clinical and pathological features. Am. J. Med. 38:241, 1965
4. Cameron JL, Pitt HA, Zinner MJ, Kaufman SL, Coleman J. : Management of proximal cholangiocellular carcinomas by surgical resection and radiotherapy. Am. J. Surg. 159 : 91, 1990
5. Beazly RM, Hadjis N, Benjamin IS, Blumgart LH. : Clinicopathological aspects of high bile duct cancer. Experience with resection and bypass surgical treatments. Ann. Surg. 199 : 623, 1984
6. Tompkins RK , Thomas D, Wile A, Longmire WP Jr. : Prognostic factors in bile duct carcinoma; analysis of 96 cases. Ann. Surg. 194:447, 1991
7. Cox DR. Regression models and life tables. : JR. Stat. Soc. 34:187, 1972
8. Nimura Y, Hayakawa N, Kamiya J, Maeda S, Kondo S, Yasui A, Shionoya S. : Hepatopancreatoduodenectomy for advanced carcinoma of the biliary tract. Hepato-Gastroenterol. 38:170, 1991
9. Bhuiya MMR, Nimura Y, Kamiya J, Kondo S, Fukata S, Hayakawa N, and Shionoya S. : Clinicopathologic studies on perineural invasion of bile duct carcinoma. Ann. Surg. 215:344, 1992.
10. White TT.: Skeletization resection and central hepatic resection in the treatment of bile duct cancer. World J. Surg.12: 48, 1988
11. Geopfert H, Dichtel WJ, Mediana JE, Lindberg RD, Luna MD.: Perineural invasion in squamous cell skin carcinoma of the head and neck. Am. J. Surg. 148:542, 1984

Gallbladder Cancer Associated with Anomalous Junction of the Pancreaticobiliary Ductal System Without Bile Duct Dilatation

Koki Tanaka, Akihiro Nishimura, Kazuhiko Yamada, Ryohei Ishibe, Naoki Ishizaki, and Akira Taira

Second Department of Surgery, Kagoshima University Faculty of Medicine, Kagoshima, 890 Japan

ABSTRACT

The purpose of this study is to delineate some clinical features and prognosis of gallbladder cancer associated with pancreaticobiliary maljunction without bile duct dilatation. A retrospective study of our seven cases is presented. Resection of the tumor was performed in five cases and only tumor biopsy was performed in two. Only one case undergone curative operation is still alive four years after operation. The other six cases died of original disease within a period between three to 30 postoperative months.
In conclusion, patients with this anomalous junction and absent bile duct dilatation should have prophylactic cholecystectomy preventing development of malignant lesion.

KEY WORDS: pancreaticobiliary maljunction, gallbladder cancer, prophylactic cholecystectomy

INTRODUCTION

Pancreaticobiliary maljunction (PBM) is a congenital anomaly defined as a union of the pancreatic and biliary ducts that is located outside of the duodenal wall. Two directional regurgitations may occur because the action of the sphincter muscle (Oddi) does not functionally affect the union. Accordingly, various pathological conditions such as cholangitis, gallstone, biliary cancer, pancreatitis and pancreatolithiasis can be occurred[1].
Recently, attention has been paid to the high incidence of biliary tract cancer in this anomaly[2]. Especially in PBM without bile duct dilatation, the high incidence of gallbladder cancer is noted. The purpose of this study is to delineate some clinical features and prognosis of gallbladder cancer accompanying this anomaly.

MATERIAL AND METHOD

For the past 15 years, between January 1977 and December 1991, 32 adult cases of PBM were treated in our department. Of those patients, seven cases had gallbladder cancer without bile duct dilatation. They were retrospectively reviewed.
The diagnosis of this maljunction was made on the basis of both long common channel and anomalous form of junction according to the diagnostic criteria of PBM[1]. The mean age was 60.7 years, ranging from 43 to 77. There were two males and five females. The staging of the tumor was classified according to the Japanese society of biliary surgery[3].

RESULTS

The majority of the patients were first seen with abdominal pain. The cholangiopancreatograms are shown in Figure 1. The mean length of common channel was 26.7mm ranging from 20 to 35. There were no gallstones in any cases. The amylase level in the bile, which was determined in four cases, was extremely high. Serum carcinoembryonic antigen (CEA) levels were abnormally high in two cases.

The clinicopathological findings of the tumor are summarized in Table 1. In only one case, the tumor was limited to the gallbladder wall without lymph node involvement. The tumor was resected in five cases. For the other two patients with stage IV, only laparotomy and tumor biopsy were performed. Curative resection was done in only two cases. Lymph node involvement was present in five cases (71%). Only one case undergone curative operation is still alive four years after operation. The other six cases died of original disease within a period between three to 30 postoperative months.

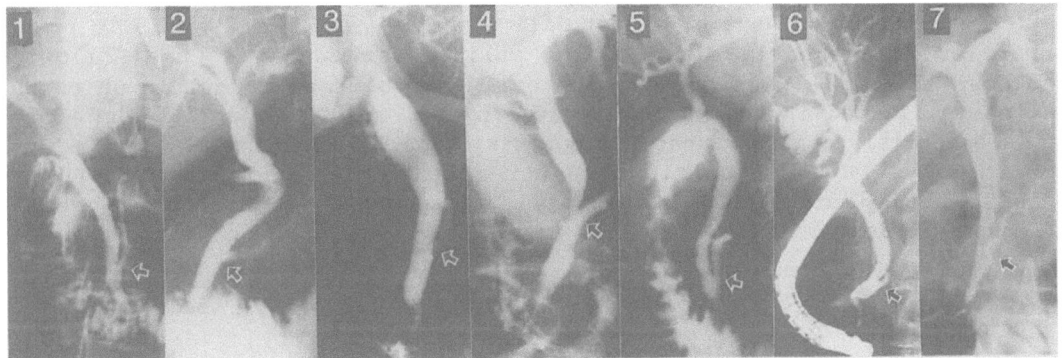

Figure 1. Direct cholangiopancreatogram of gallbladder cancer associated with PBM without bile duct dilatation. The arrows indicate the junction of the pancreatic and biliary duct.

Table 1. Clinicopathological findings of the tumor

No.	Age	Sex	Tumor Size (mm)	Location	Stage	Operation	Curability	Histological findings	Outcome
1	43	F	60 × 67	Gnb	II	Chole	None	por se n(-)	11 mo died
2	72	F	40 × 60	Gfbn	II	Chole	None	tub₂ ss n(+)	12 mo died
3	55	F	50 × 60	Gbfn	IV	PD HR	None	tub₁ se n(+)	11 mo died
4	53	M	30 × 44	Gb	III	PD HR	Curative	pap se n(+)	30 mo died
5	77	M	25 × 10	Gnb	I	Chole WHR	Curative	tub₂ ss n(-)	48 mo alive
6	63	F		Gbfn	IV	expl lapa	—	tub₁ si n(+)	3 mo died
7	58	F		Gbfn	IV	expl lapa	—	por si n(+)	6 mo died

G n.b.f; location of the tumor in the neck, body, and fundus of the gallbladder; chole, cholecystectomy; PD, pancreaticoduodenectomy; HR or WHR, subsegmental or wedge shape hepatic resection; pap, papillary adenocarcinoma; tub₁, tub₂ or por, well, moderately or poorly differentiated adenocarcinoma; depth of invasion: ss, tumor limited to the subserosal layer; se, exposed to the serosa; si, invaded another organ; n(+) or n(-), with or without lymph node matastasis.
(Tanaka K et al: British Journal of Surgery in press. reference number 4. Used by permission.)

DISCUSSION

Aoki et al[2] collected 569 cases with PBM in Japan. Dilatation type occurred in the majority (84%) of this anomaly, and no dilatation type occurred in only 80 cases (15%). A total of 131 cases (23%) were accompanied by biliary tract cancer; 93 cases gallbladder, 31 cases bile duct and seven unknown origin. There were some characteristic features on the difference of the age of the patient and shape of the bile duct. Under 30 years of age, the incidence of no dilatation type was only from 1.2 to 5.2% of this anomaly. However, the incidence gradually increased after age 30 and reach to 31% at age 60's.

Of 253 cystic dilatation type, only 30 cases (12%) were accompanied by biliary tract cancer. However, of 80 no dilatation type, 49 cases (61%) had biliary tract cancer.

In our previous bibliographical study on Japanese literature, 61% of the gallbladder cancer in this category are classified as stage IV, even at the time when their initial diagnosis were made[4]. Only two cases survived more than three years after operation. This dismal prognosis is largely depend on delayed diagnosis of the gallbladder cancer. The incidence of gallstones in patients with PBM without bile duct dilatation is very low[2]. This is really a barrier to get early diagnosis of gallbladder cancer. Cure following cholecystectomy is possible only in early gallbladder cancer in which the lesion is limited in the mucosal or the proper muscle layer[5]. Therefore, it is essential to make an early diagnosis of gallbladder cancer.

Accordingly, it is a judicious requirement to the patients with PBM to receive prophylactic cholecystectomy even under the condition of absent malignant lesion.

REFERENCES

1. The Committee of Diagnostic Criteria of the Japanese Study Group on Pancreaticobiliary Maljunction (1991) Diagnostic criteria of pancreaticobiliary maljunction. Syokaki Geka 14: 654-655
2. Aoki H, Sugaya H, Shimazu M (1987) A clinical study on cancer of the bile duct associated with anomalous arrangements of pancreaticobiliary ductal system. Analysis of 569 cases collected in Japan. Tan to Sui 8: 1539-51
3. Japanese Society of Biliary Surgery (1986) General rules for surgical and pathological studies on cancer of biliary tract. Kanehara Shuppan Inc. Tokyo p33.
4. Tanaka K, Nishimura A, Yamada K, Ishibe R, Ishizaki N, Yoshimine M, Hamada N, Taira A. Cancer of the gallbladder associated with anomalous junction of the pancreatobiliary duct system without bile duct dilatation. Br J Surg in press
5. Mizumoto R, Ogura Y, Matsuda S, Kusuda T, Taoka T, Kaneda M, Yazima Y, Tabata M (1990) Cooperative survey of surgical treatment for carcinoma of the biliary tract in Japan. Tan to Sui 11: 869-882

Detection and Surgical Treatment of Gallbladder Cancer Operated for Cholelithiasis

Hiroshi Isozaki, Kunio Okajima, and Hitoshi Hara

Department of Surgery, Osaka Medical College, Takatsuki, Osaka, 569 Japan

ABSTRACT

Clinical problems of gallbladder cancer operated for cholelithiasis were studied in 9 such patients out of 53 patients with gallbladder cancer. The diagnosis of cancer was made during operation only in 1 case, but by postoperative pathological examination in 8. Gross type of cancer was flat type in 6 and elevated type in 3, as early cancer in 5 and advanced cacner in 4. Advanced cancer was frequently observed in gallbladder showing marked inflammation. Two patients with advanced cancer who underwent simple cholecystectomy died of recurrent cancer. When a diagnosis of advanced cancer is made after operation, local resection of liver and regional lymph node dissection by prompt reoperation is recommended.

KEY WORDS: gallbladder cancer, cholelithiasis.

INTRODUCTION

Many of gallbladder cancer are detected before operation by imaging studies which developed in recent years. However, there are the patients with gallbladder cancer who underwent operation for cholecystolithiasis and diagnosed as with gallbladder cancer during or after operation. Clinical problems of such patients with gallbladder cancer were studied in this study.

SUBJECTS

Subjects consist of 9 patients with gallbladder cancer operated for cholelithiasis from August, 1978 to December, 1992 in the Department of Surgery, Osaka Medical College (17.0% of 53 patients with gallbladder cancer, 0.8% of 1,137 patients with cholelithiasis).

RESULTS

Table 1 shows 9 cases with gallbladder cancer operated for cholelithiasis.

Preoperative imaging studies
Cholecystogram was positive in 4 cases and negative in 5 cases. Echogram detected the thickness of wall in 4 cases. Cancer was not suspected in these preoperative studies.

Type of stones
All of the patients included cholesterol type.

Time of diagnosis as cancer
The diagnosis of cancer was made by intraoperative frozen sections in 1 case but by postoperative pathological examination in 8 cases.

Gross type of cancer
Macroscopically, there were flat type of cancer in 6 cases and elevated type in 3 cases.

Depth of cancer invasion and inflammation of cholecyst
The deepest layer of cancer invasion were mucosa in 3 cases, muscularis propria in 2 cases, subserosa in 3 cases and slight invasion to the liver in 1 case.
Advanced cancer which invades beyond muscularis propria was frequently observed in gallbladder showing severe inflammation (Fig. 1)

Table 1 Cases of gallbladder cancer operated for cholelithiasis

Case (age, sex)	Cholecystogram	Echogram of wall	Type of stone	Diagnosis as cancer	Gross type of cancer	Depth of invasion	Histology	Inflammation of cholecyst	Operative method	Long-term outcome
1 (73yo, M)	P	no elevation	cholesterol	after operation	elevated	mucosa	well diff. ad. ca.	no	cholecystectomy	alive (12ys)
2 (76yo, M)	P	no thickness	cholesterol	after operation	flat	mucosa	well diff. ad. ca.	chronic (slight)	cholecystectomy	alive (4ys)
3 (54yo, F)	P	no elevation	cholesterol	during operation	elevated	mucosa	well diff. ad. ca.	no	cholecystectomy, LND	alive (3ys)
4 (65yo, F)	N	no thickness	cholesterol	after operation	flat	muscularis propria	well diff. ad. ca.	chronic (slight)	① cholecystectomy ② LR, LND	alive (10ys)
5 (69yo, F)	P	slight thickness	cholesterol	after operation	flat	muscularis propria	mod. diff. ad. ca.	chronic (slight)	cholecystectomy	alive (4ys)
6 (59yo, F)	N	thickness	cholesterol	after operation	flat	subserosa	mucinous ad. ca.	acute (severe)	cholecystectomy	died of cancer (2ys 2m)
7 (87yo, F)	N	thickness	cholesterol	after operation	flat	subserosa	mod. diff. ad. ca.	chronic (severe)	cholecystectomy	died of cancer (1y 3m)
8 (71yo, M)	N	localized thickness	cholesterol	after operation	elevated	subserosa	well diff. ad. ca.	chronic (severe)	① cholecystectomy ② LR, LND	alive (3ys)
9 (57yo, F)	N	unclear	cholesterol	after operation	flat	slight invasion to the liver	papillary ad. ca.	chronic (severe)	① cholecystectomy ② LR, LND	alive (3ys)

P, positive; N, negative; ①, first operation; ②, second operation;
LND, regional lymph node dissection; LR, local liver resection

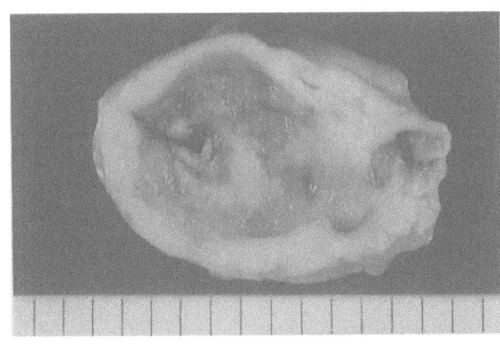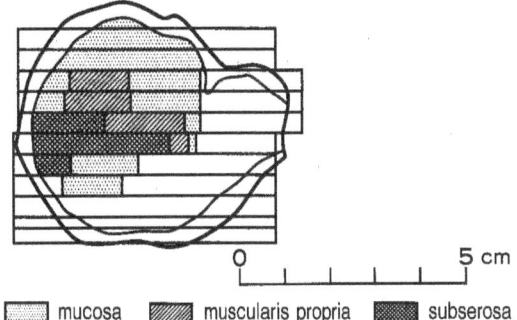

Fig. 1 Resected gallbladder and schema of cancer lesion (case 7). Thickness of the wall
and erosion of the surface was observed. The defect of tissue was artificial.

Operative method
Cholecystectomy was performed in all patients. In one patient (case 3) who diagnosed during
operation, regional lymph node dissection was performed. Three (cases 4, 8, 9) out of 8
patients underwent reoperation which consisted of local liver resection and regional lymph
node dissection. In patients who underwent lymph node dissection, no lymph node metastasis
was detected histologically.

Long-term results
Two patients with advanced cancer (case 6, 7) who underwent simple cholecystectomy died of
recurrent cancer, but the others have survived to date.

DISCUSSION

Gallbladder cancer is frequently associated with cholelithiasis [1]. The low diagnostic rate
of gallbladder cancer before operation was reported [2]. The development of imaging studies
have brought about an increase in preoperative diagnostic rate (70%) of gallbladder cancer,
but 30% of the patients with gallbladder cancer diagnosed during or after operation for
cholelithiasis in Japan [3]. In this study, many of the gallbladder cancer operated on
with a preoperative diagnosis of cholelithiasis were of flat type and were difficult to
diagnose macroscopically. Especially in cases showing severe inflammation, paticular attention should be paid to the presence of gallbladder cancer, and intraoperative pathological
examination should be made. Concerning the surgical treatment, 2 of 4 patients with advanced
cancer, both patients underwent simple cholecystectomy, died of recurrent cancer. When
a diagnosis of advanced gallbladder cancer is established after operation, resection of
local liver and regional lymph node dissection by prompt reoperation is recommended.

REFERENCES

1. Piehler JM, Crichlow RW (1978) Primary carcinoma of the gallbladder. Surg Gynecol Obstet
   147:929-942
2. Hamrick RE, Liner FJ, Hastings PR, Cohn I (1982) Primary carcinoma of the gallbladder.
   Ann Surg 195:270-273
3. Uchimura M, Waki S, Kida E, Kanda K, Sato T, Narita K (1989) The surgical treatment of
   carcinoma of the gallbladder. J Biliary Tract Pancreas 10:1575-1580 (In Japanese)

Resection with Preoperative Radiation Therapy for Cancer of the Extrahepatic Bile Duct

SHOICHI HISHINUMA and YOSHIRO OGATA

Department of Surgery, Tochigi Cancer Center, Utsunomiya, 320 Japan

ABSTRACT

In an attempt to enhance local control and survival, nine patients with bile duct cancer received preoperative radiation therapy to a dose of 40.6 to 58.4 Gy. All patients underwent resection within 5 weeks of completing radiotherapy. Two patients had positive margins. According to the histological grading of Shimosato and Oboshi, irradiation effect was judged to be Grade I, IIa, and IIb. Four patients had major complications and three of them died perioperatively. Three patients died of cancer with local failure. Two patients are alive without evidence of disease at 50 and 17 months. Further study is necessary to determine the effectiveness of this combined therapy.

KEY WORDS: bile duct cancer, preoperative radiation therapy, adjuvant, surgery

INTRODUCTION

Surgical resection has been advocated for cancer of the extrahepatic bile duct, but many patients undergoing resection succumbed to local recurrence. Tsuzuki suggested that cancer cells in the connective tissue of the hepatoduodenal ligament may play a major role in local recurrence [1]. Local recurrence may also be attributed to perineural invasion which is considered one of the main routes of extension of bile duct cancer [2]. Surgical resection alone is unlikely to improve the current treatment results. We should expect adjuvant therapy to improve local control and survival. However, the magnitude of the operation has prevented many patients from receiving postoperative adjuvant therapy. Because of the poor results with conventional therapy, we undertook this study consisting of preoperative radiation therapy and resection for cancer of the extrahepatic bile duct. The objectives of this study were to determine the feasibility of radical resection following preoperative radiation therapy, to document the pathologic response to irradiation, and to determine whether preoperative radiation therapy can enhance local control and survival.

MATERIALS AND METHODS

Between January 1988 and December 1992, nine patients with cancer of the extrahepatic bile duct received preoperative radiation therapy. Criteria for patient selection included absence of metastatic disease and having a performance status of 0 to 2. Patients with tumor confined to the lower third of the extrahepatic bile duct were excluded. There were eight male and one female patients, ranging in age from 58 to 77 years with a median age of 67. Staging studies included chest roentgenography, ultrasonography, computed tomography, percutaneous or endoscopic cholangiography, and angiography. All patients began to receive radiation therapy during the period of correcting obstructive jaundice. The radiation dose ranged from 40.6 to 58.4 Gy (Table 1). The radiation field included the primary tumor with a margin of 2 to 6 cm covering the proximal bile duct, entire extrahepatic bile duct, and lymph nodes in the hepatoduodenal ligament. No patient received concurrent chemotherapy. Following restaging, surgery was performed between 18 and 35 days after completion of radiation therapy. Surgery consisted of resection of the bile duct in five patients, resection of the hepatic hilum with caudate lobectomy in one, right trisegmentectomy in one, and pylorus-preserving pancreaticoduodenectomy in two. Eight of the nine patients received intraoperative radiation therapy (IORT) to a dose of 6 to 18 Gy with 6 to 12 MeV(Table 1). The intraoperative radiation field included the tumor bed and stumps of the bile ducts. According to the histological criteria and grading of therapeutic effects defined by Shimosato and Oboshi [3], the irradiation effects were evaluated in terms of cytologic changes and the amount of viable tumor cells remaining.

RESULTS

Only one patient experienced a delay in correcting jaundice. No patients were found to have distant metastases. Four patients had a combined resection of vessels. Patient No.5 and 6 underwent a combined resection of the right proper hepatic artery without vascular reconstruction. Patient No.4 had a wedge resection of the portal vein. Patient No.7 had a segmental resection of the portal vein. Patient No.5 did not receive IORT, because the tumor extended up into both lobes along the intrahepatic bile ducts. Patient No.8, whose frozen section of the distal and proximal ends of the divided bile duct was positive for cancer, underwent palliative resection and receivedIORT with the radiation field covering the tumor bed, distal, and proximal stumps of the bile duct, because her tumor had spread beyond the limit of resection.

Table 1. Characteristics of patients undergoing resection following preoperative radiation therapy

PT #	Tumor Origin	Preop. (Gy)	Interval (day)	Surgical Procedures	IORT Gy (MeV)	Complications	p-TNM Stage	Effect Grade	Effect on pn	Surgical Margins	Sites of Failure	Outcome / Survival
1	Hilum	42.0	18	Resection of hepatic hilum with caudate lobectomy	18 (9)	Biliary fistula Bleeding Liver abscess	IVA	IIa	++	(−)	No evidence of disease	Died of Liver failure / 8 mo.
2	Middle Third	40.6	23	Pylorus - preserving PD	12 (6)	(−)	II	IIa	−~+	(−)	Local, liver, lung peritoneum	D O C / 35 mo.
3	Middle Third	50.4	21	Resection of CBD, CHD, and GB	16(12)	(−)	II	IIa	Pn(−)	(−)	No evidence of disease	Alive / 50 mo.
4	Upper Third	55.0	27	Resection of HD, CHD, CBD, and GB Wedge resection of PV	6 (9)	(−)	IVA	IIb	++	(−)	Local, liver peritoneum	D O C / 18 mo.
5	Middle Third	58.4	29	Resection of CHD, CBD, and GB Combined resection of r-HA	(−)	(−)	II	I	+	(+)	Loca , liver	D O C / 5 mo.
6	Middle Third	55.2	26	Pylorus - preserving PD Combined resection of r-HA	16(12)	Pancreatic anastomotic leak Bleeding	II	IIa	+	(−)	No residual tumor (at autopsy)	D O S / 10 days
7	Hilum	57.8	35	Rt - trisegmentectomy Segmental resection of PV	14(9)	Billiary anastomotic leak liver failure	II	IIb	++	(−)	No residual tumor (at autopsy)	D O S / 19 days
8	Upper Third	55.8	26	Resection of HD, CHD, CBD, and GB	16(9)	(−)	II	IIb	++	(+)	No evidence of disease	Alive / 17 mo.
9	Hilum	50.4	32	Resection of HD, CHD, CBD, and GB	9 (9)	Myocardial infarction	II	IIa	+	(−)	No residual tumor (at autopsy)	D O S / 19 days

HD = Hepatic duct, CHD = Common hepatic duct, CBD = Common bile duct, IHBD = Intrahepatic bile duct ,Pn = Perineural invasion
GB = Gall bladder, HA = Hepatic artery, PV = Portal vein, PD = Pancreaticoduodenectomy,
DOS = Died of surgical complication, DOC = Died of cancer, ++=Marked effect, +=Moderate effect, −~+=Minimal effect,

Major complications (Table 1)

Major complications occurred in four patients and three of them died perioperatively. Patient No.1 had a biliary fistula in the immediate postoperative period, but cholangiography via the biliary stent tubes did not reveal leakage. On postoperative day 10, massive intestinal hemorrhage occurred. Angiography revealed a pseudoaneurysm of the right proper hepatic artery rupturing into the Roux loop. Bleeding was controlled by embolization of the artery. Thereafter this patient repeated liver abscesses and died of liver insufficiency at 8 months. Patient No.6 had an intraabdominal hemorrhage due to a pancreatic anastomotic leak, which necessitated reexploration on postoperative day 6, and died of multiple organ failure on postoperative day 10. Patient No.7 died of hepatic insufficiency on postoperative day 19, and a biliary anastomotic leak was found at autopsy. Patient No.9 died of a myocardial infarction on postoperative day 19 without evidence of a biliary anastomotic leak at autopsy.

Pathological Findings (Table 1)

Stage classifications based on pTNM factors are listed in Table 1. Patient No.1 and No.4 had microscopic metastases to the lymph nodes in the hepatoduodenal ligament. The tumors of Patient No.1 and No.4 involved the liver parenchyma and portal vein, respectively. Patient No.7 undergoing a segmental resection of the portal vein showed no tumor invasion of the portal vein. In patient No.5 and 6, the resected right hepatic arteries were not involved microscopically. All but two (No.5 and No.7) had negative surgical margins. All resected specimens showed histologic evidence of tumor cell injury. Irradiation effect was judged to be Grade I in one patient, Grade IIa in five, and Grade IIb in three. Eight patients showed perineural invasion. Four of the eight patients showed marked irradiation effect on perineural invasion, three patients moderate effect, and one patient only minimal effect. In patient No.4, all cancer cells recognized in the wall of the resected portal vein were nonviable.

Sites of Failure and Survival (Table 1)

Patient No.3 and 8 are alive without evidence of disease 50 and 17 months after surgery, respectively. Patient No.1 died of hepatic insufficiency without known recurrence at eight months. Three patients (patient No.2,4,and 5) died with both local failure and distant metastases 35, 18, and 5 months after surgery. Patient No.5 with positive margins died of liver failure resulting from extensive cancer spread along the intrahepatic bile ducts. Patient No.2 died with recurrence at the bilioenteric anastomosis which were confirmed by endoscopy. In patient No.4, autopsy revealed no tumorous mass in the hepatic hilum, but microscopic examination revealed viable cancer cells in the connective tissue around the bilioenteric anastomosis.

DISCUSSION

Surgery remains the main treatment modality for cancer arising at or near the bifurcation of the hepatic ducts. Even though a potentially curative resection is performed, the majority of patients will have local recurrences, providing the rationale for adjuvant radiation therapy. It is conceivable that devitalization of the tumor by preoperative irradiation might decrease the number of viable cells entering circulation during surgical manipulation of the tumor. A high percentage of patients show infiltration along the bile duct wall with spread to regional lymphatics or perineural invasion. Preoperative radiation therapy might sterilize these microdeposits of tumor and reduce the incidence of local failure. Radiation therapy can be delivered during the period of biliary decompression that the majority of patients with bile duct cancer require before surgery.

One of the objectives of this study was to determine whether radical resection can be performed with an acceptable morbidity and mortality following radiation therapy. Unfortunately, major complications occurred in four patients and three of them died perioperatively. However, we can never be sure of the possible relationship between these complications and preoperative radiation therapy. We experienced two major hemorrhages, one of which resulted in death. These hemorrhages with a biliary fistula or pancreatic anastomotic leak occurred in the immediate postoperative period. Irradiated arteries seemed to be rather easily eroded if an anastomotic leak once occurred.

No patients demonstrated a complete pathologic response in the resected specimens. Therefore, surgical resection can be warranted as an integral part of the radical strategy against bile duct cancer. Four patients showed marked irradiation effect on perineural invasion. The all patients showing a radiation effect of Grade IIb received more than 55 Gy. However, Patient No.4 showing both Grade IIb and marked irradiation effect on perineural invasion failed locally. Although determination of the effectiveness of this combined modality therapy, as measured by patient survival and local control, awaits further recruitment of patients and follow-up, our results show encouraging features. No patient showed distant metastases, and only two patients had microscopic lymph node metastases. Seven of the nine patients could have tumor-free surgical margins. These facts suggest that preoperative radiation therapy may help control locoregional disease and allow a potentially curative resection.

It can be proved only by a large scale trial whether preoperative irradiation can significantly enhance local control and survival. Entering patients into multi-institutional randomized trials is needed.

REFERENCES

1. Tsuzuki T, Kuramochi S, Sugioka A, Ueda M, Iida S, Nakanishi I (1991) Postresectional autopsy findings in patients with Cancer of the main hepatic duct junction. Cancer 67:3010-3013
2. Qualman SJ, Haupt HM, Bauer TW, Taxy JB (1984) Adenocarcinoma of the hepatic duct junction: A reappraisal of the histologic criteria of malignancy. Cancer 53:1545-1551
3. Shimosato Y, Oboshi S, Baba K (1971) Histologic evaluation of effects of radiotherapy and chemotherapy for carcinomas. Jpn J Clin Oncol 1:19-35

Radiation Therapy in the Treatment of Bile Duct Cancer

Jun-ichi Tanaka, Yasuhiko Sato, Akiko Umezawa, Yujiro Kato, Kenichi Miyasaki, Yoshihiro Asanuma, and Kenji Koyama

Department of Surgery, Akita University School of Medicine, Akita, 010 Japan

ABSTRACT

A total of 48 patients with bile duct cancer were treated with resection at the Akita University School of Medicine between 1985 and 1992. Seventeen patients were treated with resection only, and 8 patients died of cancer within 27 months after surgery. 28 patients out of 31 patients who received adjuvant radiotherapy were postoperatively treated with intracavitary irradiation via bile duct with remote afterloading system (RALS) including two patients treated with additive external radiation. Three patients with lower bile duct cancer received intraoperative radiation therapy in combination with pancreatoduodenectomy. Of 28 patients treated with RALS, nine patients received curative resection and 19 patients received non-curative resection. Additionally, 5 out of 24 patients with cancer of the hepatic duct confluence received RALS via inferior vena cava for caudate lobe irradiation. Survival rates of 28 patients at 12, 24 and 60 months were 71%, 58% and 26%, respectively. There were no mortalities within 30 days after surgery nor serious postoperative complications.

KEY WORDS: bile duct cancer, radiation therapy, remote afterloading system (RALS)

INTRODUCTION

Extrahepatic bile duct cancer is associated with a poor prognosis because the majority of patients are at an advanced stage with low resectability in spite of recent advances in diagnostic imaging modalities such as computed tomography(CT) and ultrasound(US). Even if curative resection were performed, the incidence of recurrence is high. Although an extended radical operation would be feasible, high mortality and morbidity have been reported. Therefore, it is necessary to perform additive treatments combined with surgical removal of the tumor. The present study evaluated the potential benefit of adjuvant radiotherapy in the surgical treatment of bile duct cancer.

PATIENTS, MATERIALS AND METHODS

From April, 1985 through December, 1992, a total of 72 patients with bile duct cancer were treated at the Akita University School of Medicine. Of 48 patients who received resection, 28 (58 %) patients received postoperative radiation therapy and 3 patients with lower bile duct cancer received intraoperative radiation therapy. Table 1 summarizes the patients of the present study. 25 patients didn't receive tumor resection. 17 patients underwent internal or external biliary drainage including one patient treated with intracavitary irradiation. Only when the curative resection was expected, hepatic lobectomy or combined extended resections were performed. Table 3 shows the summary of the radiation therapy. Intracavitary irradiation with RALS was carried out once a week and the pellet of ^{60}Co of 3 curie was utilized as a radiation source. Radiation dose was measured at a site 1cm apart from the center of the source. All the patients of the present study were followed up and the cumulative survival rate was evaluated using the Kaplan-Meier method.

Table 1 Overview of the patients with bile duct cancer

Treatment Procedure	Patients (n)
Tumor resection	<u>48</u>
Alone	17
with RALS[a] (via bile duct)	21
with RALS (via bile duct and IVC)	5
with RALS + ERT[b]	2
with IORT[c]	3
No tumor resection	<u>24</u>
Palliative operation (Drainage, Endoprosthese)	12
PTBD[d]	7
No resection	4
PTBD with RALS	1
Total	72

[a]:Remote afterloading system, [b]:External radiation therapy,
[c]:Intraoperative radiation therapy, [d]:Percutaneous transhepatic biliary drainage

Table 2 Operative procedure

Operative procedure	Patients (n)
Hepatic hilar resection	20
Pancreatoduodenectomy	16
Hepatic lobectomy	4
HHR[a] + PD[b]	4
Hx[c] + PD	1
Bile duct resection	3
Total	48

[a]Hepatic hilar resection,
[b]Pancreatoduodenectomy,
[c]Hepatic lobectomy

Table 3 Radiation therapy

	Patients (n)	Radiation dose
Intracavitary irradiation		
RALS via RTBD[a]	28	33.6* (16 ~ 92)Gy
RALS via IVC[b]	5	16,16,16,16,24 Gy
RALS via PTBD[c]	1	29 Gy
External radiation	2	50, 50 Gy
Intraoperative radiation	3	24, 25, 25 Gy

[a]Retrograde transhepatic biliary drainage,*mean, see Figure 1,
[b]Inferior vena cava, [c]Percutaneous transhepatic biliary drainage

Figure 1 Patient distribution in RALS treatment

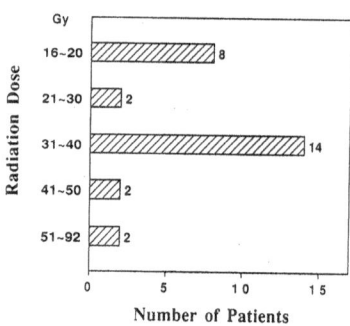

Figure 2 Survival of proximal bile duct cancer

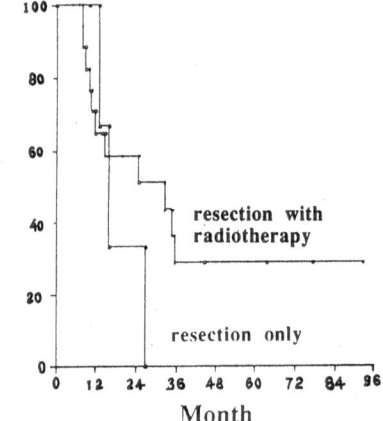

Table 4 Cumulative survival rate of bile duct cancer
-Kaplan Meier-

	n	1-	2-	5-year(%)	Wilcoxon test
Overall	72	60.5	41.4	22.9	
Resection	48	73.5	54.2	30.0	W/SQRT=4.202
No Resction	24	22.9	0.0	0.0	0.005<P<0.01
Proximal BDC*					
Resection only	4	100	33.3	0.0	W/SQRT=0.352
Resection with RT**	19	65.1	51.8	29.6	NS
Distal BDC					
Resection only	10	70.0	50.0	50.0	W/SQRT=0.879
Resection with RT	12	90.0	67.5	27.0	NS

*Bile duct cancer, **Radiation therapy

RESULTS

Overall survival of the patients with bile duct cancer is shown in Table 4. The cumulative 1-year, 2-year and 5-year survival rate was 60.5, 41.4, and 22.9%, respectively. While the patients without tumor resection died within 14 months after diagnosis, the patients who received tumor resection survived longer with 30.0% of 5-year survival. A significant difference was found between the two groups (p<0.01, generalized Wilcoxon test) as shown in Table 4. Concerning the operative procedures undergone for the patients with bile duct cancer as shown in Table 2, the frequent operative procedure was hepatic hilar resection for the proximal bile duct cancer and pancreatoduodenectomy for distal bile duct cancer.

Of 23 patients with proximal bile duct cancer, Table 4 compares the survival data for those patients who underwent resection with or without adjuvant radiotherapy. Of 4 patients treated with tumor resection only, three patients died 13, 16, or 27 months after the operation. Nineteen patients who underwent resection with adjuvant radiotherapy, mainly intracavitary irradiation, had 12 months of the median survival and 32 months of the mean survival. Then, 5-year survival was 29.6%. A significant difference was not found statistically between patients who underwent tumor resection only and those who underwent tumor resection with adjuvant radiotherapy. However, the additive radiotherapy for patients with proximal bile duct cancer who underwent tumor resection could be feasible.

Among the patients with distal bile duct cancer, there was no significant difference between patients who received resection only and those who received resection and radiotherapy.

DISCUSSION

It has been reported to be difficult to perform curative resection for bile duct cancer since hepatic hilar bile duct cancer is commonly associated with hepatic infiltration and lower bile duct cancer with pancreatic infiltration. Our previous study showed that the prognostic factors of the proximal bile duct cancer were remnant carcinoma at the surgical dissection, cancerous invasion into the lymphatics, veins, perineural spaces around the intrahepatic bile ducts and caudate lobe of the liver [1]. In order to control these factors and improve the prognosis of the proximal bile duct cancer, we have proposed a new strategy consisting of the hepatic hilar resection, specific chemotherapy focused on the cancer invasion to the periductal lymphatics, and intracavitary irradiation by the RALS through the bile duct focused on the periductal infiltration of the carcinoma and through the inferior vena cava focused on the caudate lobe of the liver [2]. Although a randomized clinical trial for the analysis of the feasibility of radiation therapy would be desirable from a theoretical point of view, the small number of the patients and the variation in treatments will make it extremely difficult to carry out a randomized clinical trial with fully informed patients' consent. In the present study no randomized control study was carried out and some of the patients were studied retrospectively, however analysis of the data has indicated that those patients who received adjuvant radiotherapy may have a greater chance of survival than those who did not receive radiotherapy.

REFERENCES

1. Koyama K, Tanaka J, Kato S, Asanuma Y (1989) New strategy for treatment of carcinoma of the hilar bile duct. Surg Gynecol Obstet 168: 523-530
2. Koyama K, Tanaka J, Sato Y, Kato Y, Asanuma Y, Kato T (1991) Intracavitary irradiation treatment via the inferior vena cava for caudate lobe invasion in hepatic hilar bile duct cancer. Hepato-Gastroenterol 38:422-426

Differentiation Therapy for Human Bile Duct Cancer

JUN-ICHI TANAKA, AKIKO UMEZAWA, YUJIRO KATO, KENICHI MIYASAKI, YASUHIKO SATO, and KENJI KOYAMA

Department of Surgery, Akita University School of Medicine, Akita, 010 Japan

ABSTRACT

The effect of dibutyryl cyclic adenosine monophosphate (dB-cAMP) and 8-bromo cyclic AMP (8-Br-cAMP) on tumor growth and proliferating activity of human bile duct cancer serially transplanted in nude mice was evaluated. dB-cAMP or 8-Br-cAMP was subcutaneously injected daily for 14 or 28 days after inoculating cancer cells in nude mice. Tumor volume doubling time, mitotic index, labeling index by BrdU, nuclear DNA content and cell cycle by Flow Cytometry were investigated. Tumor growth was suppressed by these drugs. Mitotic index of the treatment groups for the 14 day study decreased compared to the control, but not for the 28 day study. Labeling index, DNA index, S fraction and proliferating index were not significantly changed by differentiation treatment.

KEY WORDS: cell differentiation, site-selective cyclic AMP, human bile duct cancer

INTRODUCTION

Bile duct cancer is frequently diagnosed as an advanced cancer and the majority of the patients with bile duct cancer cannot undergo surgical removal. The prognosis of bile duct cancer is extremely poor, even if the tumor is resected, because of infiltrative cancer spreading along intrahepatic bile ducts and microscopic cancer cells remaining on the dissection surface and multiple intrahepatic metastasis. Therefore, adjuvant therapeutic modalities such as irradiation and chemotherapy have been applied [1].

Of several kinds of cancer, cell differentiation induction therapy has been reported to be a useful therapy. The site-selective cyclic AMP analogue has been reported to induce the cell differentiation to benign property without cytotoxity [2].

The objective of this study is to evaluate the effect of the site-selective cAMP analogue on tumor growth and proliferating activities in human bile duct cancer xenografted in athymic nude mice.

MATERIALS AND METHODS

BALB/C nude mice, 6 weeks old at the beginning of the experiment, were used. Transplantable adenocarcinoma of human bile duct was inoculated into the subcutaneous tissue of the backs in nude mice. When a tumor measured 5 mm in their large dimension, subcutaneous injection of 0.1 ml of RPMI solution containing site-selective cAMP analogs at a final concentration of 1 mM or 2 mM was begun. Injection was performed daily for14 or 28 days. As control, RPMI solution without cAMP analogs was injected subcutaneously. Tumor size was measured three times per week. Nude mice were sacrificed by exsanguination with cardiac puncture under general anaesthesia after completion of injections.

Tumor growth curves were drawn using an approximate volume calculated with serial measurements of tumor size. The volume doubling time was calculated at a logarithmic phase on the tumor growth curve. Morphological differentiation was investigated with Hematoxylin-Eosin staining. The mitotic index (MI) was measured microscopically with H-E staining. For bromo-deoxyuridine (BrdU) labeling index, immunohistochemical staining was adopted by the avidin-biotin-peroxidase-complex method. Flow cytometry was utilized to evaluate the changes in cell cycle and nuclear DNA content of cancer cells.

RESULTS and DISCUSSION

Cyclic AMP has been reported to regulate cell growth and differentiation, however its precise role in growth regulation has not been clearly defined. Cyclic AMP functions by binding to its receptor protein, cAMP-dependent protein kinase and there are two identified isozymes for cAMP-dependent protein kinase, type I and type II. These isozymes are composed of dimeric regulatory subunits that contain two types of binding sites for cAMP, namely site 1 and site 2. cAMP analogs selectively bind to either one of two sites and these two kinds of site-selective cAMP are divided into two groups, C-2 or C-8 analog (site 1 selective) and C-6 analog (site 2 selective).

Concerning growth inhibition in human cancer, controversial results have been reported on the effect of cAMP on cancer cell growth by using cAMP analogs such as dB-cAMP and 8-Cl-cAMP. Katsaros et al [3] has evaluated the effect of 24 site selective analogs on the growth of human cancer cell lines such as breast, colon, lung cancer and fibrosarcoma. 8-Cl, N^6-benzyl, and N^6-phenyl-8-p-chlorophenyl-thio-cAMP were the three most potent analogs, but dB-cAMP (C-6) showed no growth inhibition. The combination of C-8 and C-6 analogs had synergistic effects in growth inhibition without sign of toxic effects in *in vitro* study.

Table 1   Tumor Doubling Time and Mitotic Index

Group Dosage	Injection	Doubling Time	Mitotic Index
dB-cAMP			
1mM	14 (days)	7.4(days)	$4.7 \pm 0.1 (^0/_{00})$
1mM	28	6.7	6.2 ± 2.8
2mM	28	6.6	4.6 ± 1.6
8-Br-cAMP			
1mM	14	8.3	4.1 ± 1.9
1mM	28	7.4	6.3 ± 1.0
Control		6.6	7.3 ± 3.3

Table 2   BrdU Labeling Index and Flow Cytometry

Group Dosage	BrdU L.I.(%)	Flow Cytometry		
		S (%)	P.I.(%)*	DNA Index
dB-cAMP				
1mM	2.84±1.1	13.0±4.0	18.0	1.61±0.03
8-Br-cAMP				
1mM	3.12±0.7	9.7±1.6	18.2	1.64±0.03
Control	2.85±2.2	9.5±6.1	17.6	1.63±0.02

*P.I. = [S + G_2/M] / [G_0/G_1 + S + G_2/M] x 100 (%)

The present study evaluated the effect of dB-cAMP and 8-Br-cAMP on the growth of human bile duct cancer xenografted in nude mice. The tumor growth was inhibited as shown in Table 1 indicating the changes of tumor doubling times. The morphological changes with formation of a large gland structure and papillary growth into the glandular cavity were seen sporadically in the treated groups. The mitotic index decreased in the treated groups, especially in the groups treated for 14 days. Accordingly, the tumor growth was more suppressed during the first two weeks for injections. The cell cycle analysis performed after 28 day injections showed no significant differences between the treated and untreated groups in BrdU labeling index, the fraction of S phase, or proliferating index. Also nuclear DNA content and DNA ploidy pattern were not changed. The fraction of S phase in dB-cAMP treatment group showed a higher value possibly due to a block in one phase of the cell cycle, while the growth inhibition produced by 8-Br-cAMP was not due to the toxic effect of the adenosine or its metabolites.

In conclusion, the site-selective cAMP analogs produce growth inhibition by slowing down cell cycle progression and probably promoting cell differentiation. Thus, cAMP analog could be a useful tool for the control of cancer growth in bile duct cancer.

REFERENCES

1. Koyama K, Tanaka J, Kato S, Asanuma Y (1989) New strategy for treatment of carcinoma of the hilar bile duct. Surg Gynecol Obstet 168: 523-530
2. Cho-Chung YS, Clair T, Tagliaferri P, Katsaros D, Tortora G, Neckers L, Avery TL, Crabtree GW, Robins RK (1989) Site-selective cyclic AMP analogs as new biological tools in growth control, differentiation, and proto-oncogene regulation. Cancer Invest 7:161-177
3. Katsaros D, Tortora G, Tagliaferri P, Clair T, Ally S, Neckers L, Robins RK, Cho-Chung YS (1987) Site-selective cyclic AMP analogs provide a new approach in the control of cancer cell growth. FEBS Lett 223:97-103

Immunotherapy

Significance of Membrane Lymphotoxin (mLT) Expressed on Killer Cells for Adoptive Immunotherapy

Yasuhito Abe, Atsushi Horiuchi, Katsuhiko Kimura, and Shigeru Kimura

The Second Department of Surgery, Ehime University School of Medicine, Shigenobu-cho, Onsen-gun, Ehime, 791-02 Japan

ABSTRACT

Cytotoxic cytokine, human lymphotoxin (LT/TNF-ß), is expressed on the membrane of human lymphokine-activated killer (LAK) cells of both natural killer and T cell origin. Human LAK cells express mLT and produce soluble LT. The levels of mLT expression were correlated with IL-2 concentration in culture media. mLT is lytically active, which is shown by paraformaldehyde fixation of LAK cells. Moreover, LAK cells without fixation showed cytotoxicity against L929 cells, which was partly neutralized by anti-LT but not anti-TNF antibody. mLT negative LAK cells, manipulated by 24 hours culture of mLT positive LAK cells using media without IL-2, partly lost the killing activity against several human tumor cell lines such as MIA PaCa human pancreatic cancer cell. Killing activity of mLT positive LAK cells against these tumor cell lines was partly neutralized by anti-LT but not anti-TNF antibody. Collectively, our data indicate that mLT is an important tumoricidal effector molecule expressed on LAK cells for adoptive immunotherapy.

KEY WORDS: membrane lymphotoxin, LAK cells, adoptive immunotherapy

INTRODUCTION

Human lymphotoxin (LT/TNF-β), a potent cytotoxic cytokine, is produced mainly by T lymphocytes *in vivo* and *in vitro*. Lymphotoxin is originally found in the supernatant of PHA-stimulated lymphocyte culture. The amino acid sequence was analyzed and cloned using human B lymphoblastoid cell line, RPMI 1788 with PMA stimulation. Human lymphotoxin was revealed to possess 30 % amino acid sequence homology with human tumor necrosis factor (TNF/TNF-α). Actually it binds the same receptors as TNF, and shares many biological activities with TNF (1,2).

Human TNF is now revealed to possess both membrane and soluble forms. The 26 kDa precursor molecule of TNF stacks into the plasma membrane via its leader sequence. Therefore, TNF is the type II protein of which the N-terminal exists outside of the membrane. Soluble form of TNF of which the molecular weight is 18 kDa is secreted by the clipping on the cell membrane by a putative protease (1,2).

LAK cells have potent cytocidal activity against wide range of tumor cells. LAK cells release some cytotoxic molecules such as perforin and proteases. The mechanism of target cell killing is thought to be common in LAK cells and CTL clones. However, the precise action of such molecules and other putative cytotoxic substances remains unclear (4).

Membrane lymphotoxin (mLT) was found on LAK cells (1). We suppose that this molecule exerts important role in target cell killing. Thus, we carried out the analysis of mLT expressed on LAK cells as an tumoricidal effector. The data obtained in this study strongly suggest that mLT on LAK cells is an important tumoricidal effector not only in long term killing but also in short term cytotoxicity.

MATERIALS AND METHODS

Reagents

Human recombinant LT was kindly donated by Kanegafuchi Biochemical Co. (Hyogo, Japan). Antisera against LT was raised against New Jealand White Rabbit. Blood was collected by venipuncture, and IgG fraction was separated by using Protein A-Cellulofine (Seikagaku Kougyou, Tokyo, Japan). For the flow cytometric analysis of LAK cells, anti-LT IgG was digested into F(ab')$_2$ fragment by 2 % pepsin (Sigma, St Louise, MO) treatment, and further affinity purified by using LT coupled with Cellulofine (Seikagaku Kougyou).

LAK cells

Blood was collected from healthy donors with heparinization. Peripheral blood mononuclear cells (PBMC) were separated using Hitopaque 1077 (Sigma). After washing PBMC with phosphate buffered saline (PBS), cells were cultivated by RPMI 1640 supplemented with 10 % fetal bovine serum (FBS: GIBCO, Grand Island, NY), and 800 IU/ml interleukin 2 (LAK media). After the third day of culture, LAK cells were passaged with the LAK media. Established LAK cells were cultured without IL-2 for 24 hours to obtain mLT negative LAK cells (4).

Flow cytometric analysis
LAK cells (0.5-1.0 x 10[6]) were incubated with 100 ng of anti-LT rabbit F(ab')$_2$ followed by the incubation with anti-rabbit IgG goat F(ab')$_2$ fragment conjugated with FITC (Tago, Bulingame, CO). After washing, the stained LAK cells were subjected to the analysis using FACScan (Becton Dickinson, Mountaindew, CA) and FACScan program (Becton Dickinson). For the negative control of anti-LT antibody, F(ab')$_2$ fragment from normal rabbit serum was used. Data was analyzed by mean channel shift from negative control.

51Cr release assay
Target cells (1.0 x 10[7]) were incubated with 100 µCi of Na$_2$[51]CrO$_4$ (ICN, Costa Mesa, CA) for 90 min at 37°C. After washing with culture media, labeled cells were incubated with LAK cells at various effector/target (E/T) ratio during the indicated periods. Supernatant was collected and the radioactivity was counted using γ–counter (Aloka, Tokyo, Japan). Percentages of the specific target cell lysis was calculated as follows:
Specific lysis (%) = (Sample count-Spontaneous count)/(Total count-Spontaneous count) x 100.

ELISA
LT was estimated using ELISA developed in our laboratory.

RESULTS AND DISCUSSION

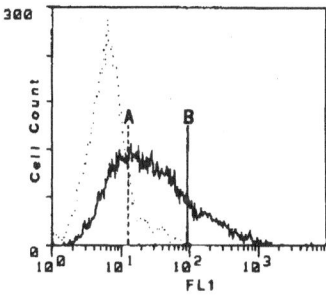

FIG. 1. Expression of mLT on LAK cells. LAK cells (day 8) express mLT as is typically shown in Fig. 1. mLT immunoreactivity was expressed by the mean channel shift (M.C.) calculated as (B-A), where A is the mean channel of negative control and B is that of mLT.

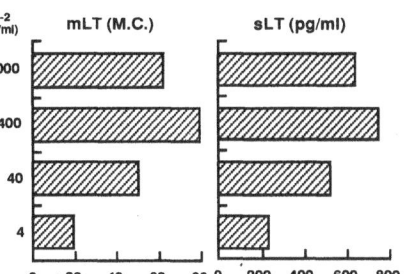

FIG. 2. The correlation of IL-2 levels, mLT expression, and sLT secretion by human LAK cells. Peripheral mononuclear cells were cultivated with various concentrations of IL-2 for 3 days. sLT levels and mLT expression was measured. mLT expression and sLT secretion was correlated with each other.

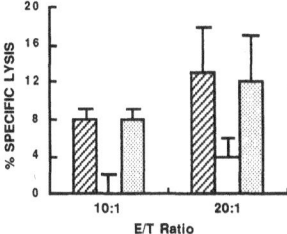

FIG. 3. Cell lytic activity of LAK cells against L929 cells was blocked by anti-LT but not anti-TNF antibody. LAK cells were incubated with ^{51}Cr-labeled L929 cells for 16 hrs at E/T ratio of 10:1 and 20:1. Percentages of specific lysis were expressed mean ± SD. In the assay, 10 µl of NRS (open bar), anti-LT (filled bar) or anti-TNF (dotted bar) antiserum was added.

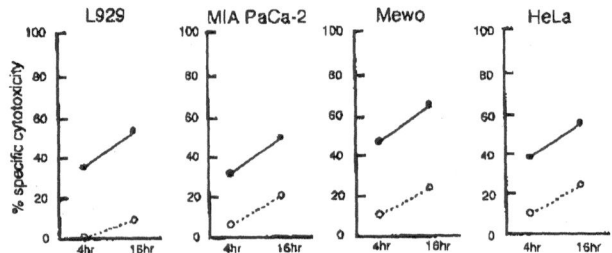

FIG. 4. Cytotoxicities of mLT positive (●—●) and mLT negative (○---○) LAK cells against various cancer cell lines. LAK cells were precultured for 24 hours with or without IL-2 to establish mLT positive and negative LAK cells *in vitro*. Target cells were labeled with ^{51}Cr and incubated with LAK cells during the indicated period at E/T ratio of 10:1. Percent specific lysis of target cells were calculated as in materials and methods. mLT negative LAK cells showed same cytotoxicity against K562 and Daudi cells (data not shown) as mLT positive cells. mLT negative LAK cells have lower cytotoxicity against these cell lines at 4 hr assay and 16 hr assay (above left).

TABLE 1

Cell	% specific lysis		% suppression
	NRS	anti-LT	
L929	32.4	16.1	50.3
MIA PaCa-2	53.3	42.5	22.3
Mewo	57.9	42.5	26.5
HeLa	39.7	31.9	19.6

Table 1. Anti-LT partly blocked LAK cell cytotoxicity against various cell lines. mLT positive LAK cells were incubated with ^{51}Cr labeled target cells and affinity prepared F(ab')$_2$ fragment of anti-LT or NRS F(ab')$_2$. Percent suppression was shown in the last column. Anti-LT evidently blocked LAK cell cytotoxicity.

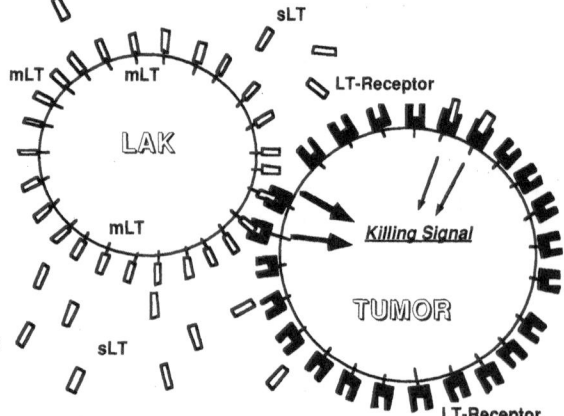

LAK cells express mLT but not mTNF (1). mLT is biologically active, which is established by paraformaldehyde fixation of LAK cell (2) and antibody blocking study of unfixed LAK cytotoxicity. This study revealed that mLT may be working as a tumoricidal effector in short term killing as well as long term killing. mLT negative LAK cells, which are basically the same as mLT positive LAK cells except mLT expression (data not shown), exert lower cytotoxicity (in 4 hr and 16 hr assay) against tumor cells than mLT positive LAK cells. Anti-LT (but not anti-TNF) partially blocked mLT positive LAK cell cytotoxicity even in the short term cytotoxic assay. Therefore, mLT is indicated to kill the target tumor cells directly (or via other unknown cytotoxic molecules) as is shown in the last figure.

REFERENCES

1. Abe Y, Miyake M, Horiuchi A, Kimura S, Hitsumoto Y (1991) Expression of membrane associated lymphotoxin/tumor necrosis factor-β on human lymphokine-activated killer cells. Jpn J Cancer 82: 23-26
2. Abe Y, Horiuchi A, Osuka Y, Kimura S, Granger GA, Gatanaga T (1992) Studies of membrane-associated lymphotoxin in human lymphokine-activated T-killer cells *in vitro*. Lymphokine Cytokine Res 11: 115-121
3. Abe, Y, Miyake M, Osuka Y, Kimura S, Granger GA, Gatanaga T (1992) Transforming growth factor-β$_1$ down-regulates expression of membrane-associated lymphotoxin and secretion of soluble lymphotoxin by human lymphokine-activated killer T cells *in vitro*. Lymphokine Cytokine Res 11: 245-251
4. Miyake M, Horiuchi A, Kimura K, Abe Y, Kimura S, Hitsumoto Y (1992) Correlation between killing activity towards the murine L929 cell line and expression of membrane-associated lymphotoxin-related molecule of human lymphokine-activated killer cells. Eur J Immunol 22: 2147-2152

The Generation of CD4 Cytotoxic T Lymphocyte Augmented by Immobilized Anti-CD3 Antibody and Interleukin-2

Masaji Tani, Hiroshi Tanimura, Hiroki Yamaue, Makoto Iwahashi, Shizuma Mizobata, Kohei Noguchi, Takuya Tsunoda, and Tsukasa Hotta

Department of Gastroenterological Surgery, Wakayama Medical College, Wakayama, 640 Japan

ABSTRACT

The DNA synthesis and the proliferative response of autologous tumor specific cytotoxic T lymphocytes (CTLs) induced by autologous mixed lymphocyte tumor cell culture, remarkably increased by activation with immobilized anti-CD3 Ab and IL-2 compared with IL-2 alone. The cytotoxicity of the activated CTLs was kept against autologous tumor cells, moreover was induced against KATO-III and Daudi. The cytotoxicity was inhibited by anti-HLA class I and anti-HLA-DR MoAb in 4-h CRA and anti-HLA-DR MoAb in 16-h CRA against autologous tumor cells. In addition, the cytotoxicity was inhibited by the elimination of $CD8^+$ cells for 4 h and that of $CD4^+$ cells in 16-h CRA using negative selection against autologous tumor cells. Major cell surface antigens of these CTLs was $CD3^+$, $CD4^+$, $CD25^+$, $CD45RA^-$, helper T cell, and the activated CTLs which produced IL-2. It is concluded that the CTLs activated with immobilized anti-CD3 Ab and IL-2 were $CD4^+$ CTLs having not only killer function but helper function and were one of the effective strategies in adoptive immunotherapy by the direct cytotoxicity and the induction of killer cells in vivo.

KEY WORDS: cytotoxic T lymphocyte, AMLTC, immobilized anti-CD3 antibody, helper/killer, adoptive immunotherapy

INTRODUCTION

Since Rosenberg and colleagues performed adoptive immunotherapy (AIT) to advanced cancer patients with lymphokine-activated killer (LAK) cells activated interleukin-2 (IL-2) in vitro [1], AIT has been one of useful strategies of cancer therapy. The generation of strong specific cytotoxicity against autologous tumor is important for available adoptive immunotherapy. We have reported AIT using tumor-infiltrating lymphocytes (TILs) activated IL-2 and IL-4, which have the strong cytotoxicity against autologous tumor cells compared with LAk cells, and clinical efficacy was 59%. However, all cases can not be induced TILs, so we investigated cytotoxic T lymphocytes (CTLs) induced by autologous mixed lymphocyte tumor culture (AMLTC) to overcome the problems of TILs. We investigated the propagation of CTLs induced by AMLTC with immobilized anti-CD3 monoclonal antibody combined with IL-2 and the characteristic analyses of this activated CTLs, and presented that these CTLs are available in AIT.

MATERIAL AND METHODS

Induction of CTL by AMLTC

Peripheral blood mononuclear cells (PBMC) of 30 patients with malignant tumors (1 breast cancer, 1 lung cancer, 13 gastric cancer, 1 leiomyosarcoma of the stomach, 8 colonic cancer, 1 gallbladder cancer, 1 bile duct cancer, 1 ovarian cancer, 1 malignant mesothelioma of the peritoneum, 1 origin unknown carcinomatous ascites) were separated from cancer patients by Ficoll-Hypaque gradient centrifugation, and were suspended at 2×10^6/ml in RPMI-1640 medium supplemented with 2 mM L-glutamine, 100 U/ml of penicillin, 100 μg/ml of streptomycin, 50 μM 2-mercaptoethanol and 5% heat-inactivated human AB serum. The PBMC (responder) were cultured with autologous tumor cells treated with 50 μg/ml of mitomycin C (MMC) at 37°C for 40 min (stimulator) for 5 days at various R/S ratios.

The DNA synthesis of CTL induced by AMLTC

The DNA synthesis of CTL was measured by the incorporarion of ^{3}H-thymidine (^{3}H-TdR). 2x10^5/well of responder with stimulator were cultured for 5 days in 96 well round-bottomed microtiter plate, 37.5 KBq/well of ^{3}H-TdR was added to each well during the last 18 hours of culture, harvested, and the radioactivity was determined.

Activation of the CTLs with immobilized anti-CD3 MoAb and IL-2

Culture wells were coated 1-2 hours at room temperature with 10 μg/ml of anti-CD3 MoAb (muromonab-CD3, IgG$_{2a}$, Orthoclone, USA) in 0.05M Tris/phosphate buffer saline (PBS) (pH 9.2). 5x10^5/ml of CTLs were activated with 10 μ g/ml immobilized anti-CD3 MoAb combined with IL-2 (S6820, Shionogi, Osaka, Japan) or none. The DNA synthesis was measured by the ^{3}H-TdR incorporation of 5x10^4/well of CTL pulsed ^{3}H-TdR during the last 18 hours of the 3 day's culture in 96 well flat-bottomed microtiter plate as described above.

Target cells

The target cells were autoogous tumor cells, KATO-III signet ring cell carcinoma cells of the stomach cell line, Daudi Burkitt lymphoma cell line and K562 chronic myelogenous leukemia cell line. The cell lines were maitained in RPMI-1640 medium supplemented with 10% fetal bovine serum (FBS). The autologous tumor cells were purified by enzymatic digestion as previously described [2].

Cytotoxic assay

A 4-h and 16- h ^{51}Cr-release assay was performed to assess killer cell cytotoxicity as described [2]. Briefly, the target cells were labeled with 3.7MBq of Na$_2$^{51}CrO$_4$. Then, 100 μl of ^{51}Cr-labeled tumor cells (1 × 10^5/ml) were added to 100 μl of effector cells (effector-to-target ratio 15:1) for 4 h and 16 h. After incubation, the radioactivity of supernatants was determined with a gamma counter.

Characterization of the activated CTL with immobilized anti-CD3 Ab and IL-2

The surface antigens of the CTLs were examined by flow cytometry, using a FITC- or PE- labelled anti-human CD3, CD4, CD8, CD16, CD25, CD45RA, TCR γ / δ and Mik-β1 monoclonal antibodies for a flow cytometric examination (FACStar, Becton Dickinson). The major histocompatibility complex (MHC) restrictions of the activated CTL were clarified by monoclonal antibodies. At time of 4-h and 16-h ^{51}Cr release assay, anti-HLA class I MoAb, anti-HLA-DR MoAb or mouse IgG as control was added to the microtiter plate at a final concentration of 1 μg/ml. Negative selection method was performed by immunomagnetic separation using sheep IgG as control, anti-CD4 or anti-CD8 monoclonal antibodies (IgG) with magnetic beads (M-450, Dynal, Oslo, Norway). After incubation at 4°C for 30 min with occasional shaking, CTLs were performed magnetic separation and assessed for cytotoxic activity in a 4-h and 16-h ^{51}Cr-release assay.

Determination of IL-2 activity of CTL

1x10^6/ml of activated CTLs were cultured for 24 hours, stimulated with 20 ng/ml of PMA and/or 500 ng/ml of A23187. 100 μl of the culture supernatant or standard IL-2 were added to 1x10^5/ml of CTLL-2 (IL-2 dependent T cell leukemia cell line) in microtiter plate. After 24 h culture, the IL-2 activity of CTLs was determined with the DNA synthesis of CTLL-2 by ^{3}H-TdR incorporration during the last 8 h culture of 24 h.

Results

The DNA synthesis was augmented by AMLTC at 100 of R/S ratio. The cytotoxicity against autologous tumor cells, KATO-III and K562 was 28.7%, 1.2% and 6.7% in a 4-h ^{51}Cr release assay, suggesting that autologous tumor specific

CTLs were induced by AMLTC, and these CTLs were T cells of CD3-positive but not NK cells. Although the ^{3}H-TdR incorporation of CTL induced by AMLTC was not significantly augmented by IL-2 alone, that was markedly augmented by the stimulation by immobilized anti-CD3 MoAb and IL-2. And the proliferative response with immobilized anti-CD3 Ab and IL-2 was remarkably stimulated. The optimal concentration of IL-2 was 250 IU/ml. The cytotoxicity against autologous tumor cells induced by AMLTC against autologous tumor cells was kept in 4-h and 16-h CRA by the activation of immobilized anti-CD3 MoAb and IL-2 (Fig. 1). However, the activated CTLs were generated not only autologous tumor specific cytotoxicity but also non-specific cytotoxicity. Next, we investigated the characteristic of the activated CTLs. The expression of activated CTLs' surface antigens was CD3-, CD4-, CD25- positive and CD45RA-negative, helper T cells. Moreover, the activated CTLs were not only HLA class I restricted but also HLA-DR restricted, and CD4-positive T cells exhibited the highly cytotoxicity against autologous tumor cells .

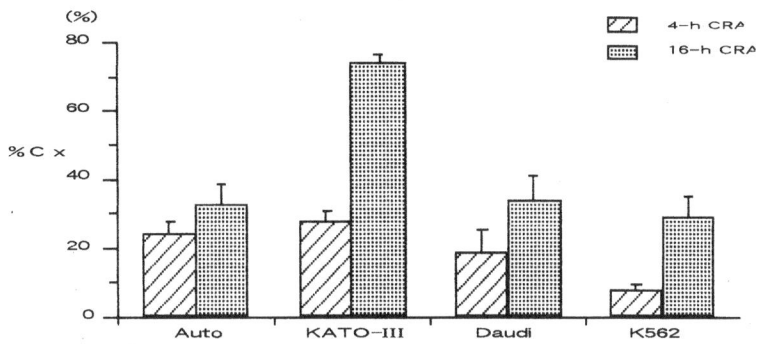

Fig. 1 The cytotoxicity of CTL induced by AMLTC

The activated CTLs generated from 2 patients with gastric cancer and 2 patients with colonic cancer produced 12, 15, 100 and 125 IU/ml of IL-2 by stimulation with PMA and A23187.

DISCUSSION

Autologous tumor specific CTLs were generated by AMLTC, and the activated CTLs with immobilized anti-CD3 Ab and IL-2 proliferated significantly. The cytotoxicity of activated CTLs kept against autologous tumor cells, moreover that was induced against KATO-III and Daudi. The activated CTLs were CD8 CTLs reported previously and CD4 CTLs having not only killer function but helper function. The CD4 CTLs were one of the effective strategies in adoptive immunotherapy by the direct cytotoxicity and the bystander killing by the induction of killer cells in vivo.

REFERENCES

1. S. A. Rosenberg, M. T. Lotze, L. M. Muul, S. Leitman, A. E. Chang, S. E. Ettinghausen, Y. M. Matory, J. M. Skibber, E. Shiloni, J. Veto, C. M. Seipp, C. Simpson and C. M. Reichert (1985) Observation on the systemic administration of autologous lymphokine-activated killer cells and recombinant interleukin-2 to patients with metastatic cancer. New Engl. J. Med. 313: 1485-1492
2. T. Tsunoda, H. Tanimura, H. Yamaue, M. Iwahashi, M. Tani, M. Tamai, K. Arii and K. Noguchi (1992) The promotive effect of interleukin 4 with interleukin 2 in the proliferation of tumor-infiltrating lymphocytes from patients with malignant tumor. Biotherapy 4: 9-15
3. M. Tani, H. Tanimura, H. Yamaue, M. Iwahashi, T. Tsunoda, M. Tamai, K. Noguchi and K. Arii (1992) In vitro generation of activated natural killer cells and cytotoxic macrophages with lentinan. Eur. J. Clin. Pharmacol. 42: 623-628

HLA-DR Expression on Cancer Cells and T Cell Reaction in Colorectal Carcinoma

Kanji Tanaka, Mika Morita, Shigeo Okamura, Tokio Okusa, Yasushi Nakane, Hideho Takada, and Koshirou Hioki

Second Department of Surgery, Kansai Medical University, Moriguchi, Osaka, 570 Japan

ABSTRACT

60 cases of colorectal adenocarcinoma were immunohistochemically examined to clarify the relationship between HLA−DR expression on tumor cells and T cell infiltration. The more HLA-DR$^+$ cancer cells in the carcinoma tissue increased, the more T cells tended to aggregate in both the infiltrating front of cancer tissue and the intracarcinomatuos stroma. We speculate that HLA−DR antigen on cancer cells might be immunoreactive and seems to be closely related with the cellular immunity in colorectal carcinoma.

KEY WORDS : HLA-DR, T cell, colorectal carcinoma

INTRODUCTION

HLA-DR is known as a class II antigen of the major histocompatibility complex (MHC) and has been reported to be expressed on many types of immunocompetent cells and an immunoreactive antigen, especially which is necessary for antigen presentation in T cell reaction. On the other hand, many studies showed HLA-DR was also observed on various kinds of cancer cells[1][2][3].
T cell reaction itself is commonly detected in tumor tissues, not only in the carcinomatous stroma but also on tumor cells. Some postulated that it played an important role for the host resistance to cancer cells and caused favorable effect on tumor bearing host.
In this study, we examined the relationship between HLA−DR expression and T cell reaction in human colorectal carcinoma.

MATERIALS AND METHODS

60 cases of colorectal adenocarcinoma were examined. All specimens were taken at the time of surgery, fixed in 10% formalin, embedded in paraffin, cut into serial sections 4 μm in thickness and were stained with the use of the indirect immunoperoxidase method. Mouse monoclonal antibody to HLA−DR (LN-3) was obtained from Histoclone (Seikagaku Kogyo Co., Tokyo, Japan) and to human T cell (UCHL−1) was purchased from Dakopatts (Kyowa Medics Japan, Tokyo, Japan). Fragments of horseradish peroxidase (HRP) − labeled goat F (ab')$_2$ to mouse IgG used as the second antibody were obtained from Tago Inc.(Cosmo Bio Co., Tokyo, Japan).
The grade of HLA−DR reactivity in tumor tissues (HLA−DR positivity) was divided into four classes, according to the proportion of positively stained tumor cells with HLA−DR as follows; 4 + : more than 80% of cancer cells were positively stained, 3 + : 50−80% stained, 2 + : 10−50% stained and 1 + : less than 10% stained. The number of infiltrating UCHL-1$^+$ cells were expressed as the mean number of cells per 0.16mm^2 of tissues at the following three sites : 1) the infiltrating front of carcinoma (IF), 2) the intracarcinomatous stroma (IS) and 3) normal tissue (NR).

820

The data were analyzed by the Student's T test.
All patients received no chemotherapy or radiation prior to operation and their preoperative clinical data revealed no abnormalities on laboratory testing of liver function parameters, serum immunoglobulin concentrations and cellular immunity.

RESULTS

1. All of colorectal tumor tissues showed positive staining of HLA – DR antigen with a variety of its positivity and intensity. The infiltration of T cells was observed around HLA – DR⁺ cancer cells (Figure 1, Table 1).
2. The number of infiltrating T cells increased gradually according to the increase of HLA – DR⁺ cancer cells in the tumor tissues with statistical significance, which was detected in not only the infiltrating front of carcinoma (IF) but also the intracarcinomatous stroma (IS) (Table 1).

Table 1. The correlation between HLA – DR staining grade and the number of infiltrating T cells

Sites of tissue	Number of T cells			
	[a]1 +	2 +	3 +	4 +
[b]IF	[c]146.4 ± 48.2	158.9 ± 39.3	159.2 ± 26.8*	183.9 ± 71.4***
IS	55.4 ± 21.4	78.6 ± 26.8*	112.5 ± 33.9	171.4 ± 67.9**
NR	10.7 ± 3.6	10.8 ± 3.9	14.3 ± 4.3	16.1 ± 3.2
total	n = 16	n = 16	n = 10	n = 18

a) Proportion of positively stained tumor cells ; 4 +, > 80 % of tumor cells positively stained ; 3 +, 50 – 80 % stained ; 2 +, 10 – 50 % stained ; 1 +, 10 % > stained.
b) IF ; the infiltrating front of carcinoma, IS ; the intracarcinomatous stroma, NR ; normal tissue.
c) Mean ± SD.
* There was a significant difference *** at $p < 0.001$, ** at $p < 0.01$ and * at $p < 0.05$: For IF : * between 2 + and 3 + ; *** between 3 + and 4 +. For IS : * between 1 + and 2 + ; ** between 2 + and 4 +.

DISCUSSION

HLA – DR was positive in all cases of colorectal carcinoma tissues in this study. HLA – DR has been reported to be present in other cancer tissues in gastrointestinal tract[1]. It has been also detected in other types of human malignant tissues such as meningioma, melanoma, lung cancer and so on[2]. We already showed that HLA – DR expression closely correlated with CEA distribution in colorectal cancer cells, i.e., the positivity of HLA – DR increased according to the change of the distribution of CEA, from its intracytoplasmic to intrastromal localization[3]. We also revealed that HLA – DR and secretory component (SC) related each other in gastric tumor cells, i.e., both HLA – DR and SC existed in almost same cancer cells[1]. As CEA and SC are well -known to be tumor-associated antigens, so HLA – DR also may be a tumor – related antigen. On the other hand, numerous studies have shown that HLA – DR was involved in a variety of immune reactions especially in antigen presentation. T lymphocytes were observed to aggregate around HLA – DR⁺ tumor cells. This seemed to indicate that the immnoreaction between HLA – DR⁺ tumor cells and T cells were under way in carcinoma tissue. The number of T cells increased according to the increase of HLA – DR⁺ cancer cells in the present study. The reason for this result remained unclear, but there might be a possible explanation as follows. That is, HLA – DR induced lymphoid infiltration because of its function relating to antigen presentation. T lymphocytes including IFN – γ⁺ cells caused the induction and augmentation of HLA – DR expression on tumor cells. These two HLA − DR⁺ cancer cells and T cells affected positively each other to work for the increase of mutual reaction.

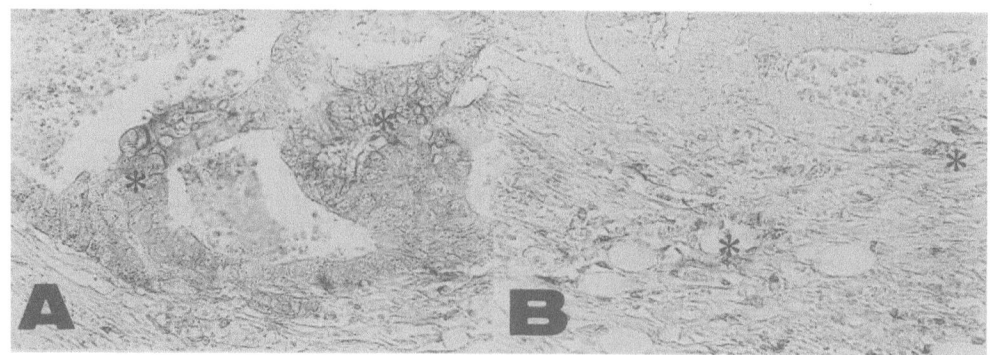

Figure 1. HLA − DR and T cells in colorectal carcinoma.
　　　　HLA − DR (A) is present on cancer cells (*) and T cells infiltrates
　　　　(B) around HLA − DR⁺ tumor cells (*).

REFERENCES

1. Hirozane N, Tanaka K, Nakane Y, Yamamura M, Hioki K, Nagura H, Yamamoto M (1991) Expression of HLA − DR and secretory component antigens and lymphocyte infiltration in human gastric nonmalignant and malignant tissues: an immunohistochemical study. J Surg Oncol 46 : 77 − 86
2. Rossi ML, Sanchez FC, Hughes JT, Esiri MM, Coakham HB (1988) Immunocytochemical study of the cellular immune response in meningiomas. J Clin Pathol 41 : 314 − 319
3. Tanaka K, Nagura H, Hamada H, Yamamura M, Hioki K, Yamamoto M (1988) Immunohistochemical evaluation of human colorectal neoplasms for CEA, HLA class II antigen and DNA polymerase α. Dig Organ Immunol. 21 : 209 − 213

Therapeutic Efficacy of a Tumor-Infiltrating Lymphocyte Clone in Combination with Soluble Tumor-Specific Transplantation Antigen and Cyclophosphamide

H. Komichi[1], H. Yamagishi[1], Y. Ueda[1], K. Ohmori[1], K. Kan[1], T. Hayashi[1], Y. Tanaka[1], T. Ueki[1], K. Naito[1], T. Oka[1], and B.D. Kahan[2]

[1]Second Department of Surgery, Kyoto Prefectural University of Medicine, Kyoto, 602 Japan
[2]Division of Immunology and Organ Transplantation, Department of Surgery, The University of Texas, Medical School at Houston, TX 77030, USA

ABSTRACT

Tumor-specific cytotoxic T lymphocyte (CTL) clones were selected for therapeutic use from bulk cultures (BC) of tumor-infiltrating lymphocytes (TILs) derived from the methylcholanthrene(MCA)-induced fibrosarcoma in C3H/He mice. The adoptive transfer of a tumor-specific TIL clone named CTL-8 (1×10^7 cells, intravenously on days 7 and 14) was combined in an immunotherapy model in which hosts bearing 4-day established MCA-F tumors were treated with weekly subcutaneous injections of isoelectrophoretically purified 1-butanol-extracted tumor-specific transplantation antigen (TSTA, 1μg) and intraperitoneal injections of low-dose cyclophosphamide (CY, 20mg/kg, days 4 and 11). This regimen (TSTA/CY+CTL-8) inhibited outgrowth of tumors more significantly than TSTA/CY treatment and greatly prolonged host survival. The effectors of TSTA/CY+CTL-8 bore Lyt2+ as well as L3T4+ in spleens of tumor bearing hosts, although the TSTA/CY regimen induced activated L3T4+ cells alone.

KEY WORDS: Tumor-specific transplantation antigen (TSTA), Tumor-infiltrating lymphocyte clone, Tumor-specific immunotherapy

INTRODUCTION

Tumor-specific transplantation antigen (TSTA)[1] may be extracted from methylcholanthrene(MCA)-induced fibrosarcomas with either potassium chloride (3MKCl) or butyl alcohol (1-butanol)[2,3,4]. Pretreatment of the murine host with tumor extracts protects against syngeneic tumor challenges[5]. Extracted materials evoke delayed-type hypersensitivity reactions in mice preimmunized with irradiated homotypic tumor cells[6]. TSTA, that is administered alone, does not retard but sometimes enhances neoplastic outgrowth[7,8]. However, TSTA combined with cyclophosphamide (CY), an agent that putatively diminishes suppressor T-cell generation[9,10], reduces the outgrowth of tumor challenges[11], as well as postsurgical experimental metastases[12,13]. We have established a specific CTL clone from tumor-infiltrating lymphocytes, and report herein that this clone potentiates the efficacy of TSTA/CY to reduce tumor growth, prolong the survival of susceptible syngeneic hosts, and amplify splenic T-effector cells.

MATERIALS AND METHODS

Female 10- to 15-week old C3H/HeJ mice were used. Three noncrossreactive MCA-induced sarcomas (MCA-F, MCA-D, MCA-SP) were maintained by cryopreservation and serial subcutaneous propagation for only seven transplant generations[2]. Two other tumor cell lines, namely EL-4 and YAC-1, were maintained in vivo.
The immunogenic fraction 16 of MCA-F tumor extracts that had been prepared with 2.5% butyl alcohol were purified by isoelectrical focusing (pI6.4), as previously described[3,4,14,15]. The TSTA activity of purified fractions was confirmed by in vivo immunoprotection tests[5]. The protein content of the extracts was determined with the Bio-Rad protein assay using an ovalbumin standard[16].
Tumor cells were harvested from subcutaneous neoplasms by triple enzymatic digestion[17]. The resultant single-cell suspension was used as a source of target cells or TILs.
In vitro cytotoxic activity was assessed in a 4-hour ^{51}Cr-release assay.
In vivo neutralization was determined in local adoptive transfer assays (LATA)

using subcutaneous inoculation of mixtures of 1×10^4 target tumor cells with various numbers of effector cells into normal syngeneic C3H/HeJ mice[18].

In the systemic adoptive transfer assays (SATA), the specific in vivo activities of T cells were assessed in mice bearing 3-day established subcutaneous tumors[19]. Varying numbers of effector cells were adoptively transferred via the tail vein. Tumor diameters were serially measured with vernier calipers.

To obtain a TIL-enriched population, single cells dispersed from 21-day-old MCA-F tumors as described above were depleted by adherence using plastic dishes and nylon wool. Nylon- and plastic-nonadherent cells were then cultured in the presence of 5 BRMP U/mL of recombinant human IL-2 (Genzyme) in RPMI 1640 with 10% fetal calf serum for 2 weeks. BC TILs were cloned immediately after being established using the limiting dilution at 0.3 cells/well. BC TILs or cloned TILs named CTL-8 were used as effectors for in vitro and in vivo experiments after a 5- to 7-day period of in vitro cultivation with irradiated tumor cells and normal splenic feeder cells for restimulation[20].

For the immunotherapy model, tumors were produced by inoculation of 1×10^5 MCA-F cells subcutaneously into the right flanks of syngeneic C3H/HeJ mice. Four days later the hosts were treated with weekly SC injections of TSTA ($1 \mu g$) and IP injections of low-dose cyclophosphamide (CY, 20mg/kg, days 4 and 11) and adoptive transfers of CTL-8 (1×10^7 cells iv on days 7 and 14).

For statistics, differences in mean tumor diameters were determined using Student's t test. Host survival times were analyzed using the Gehan modification[21] of the generalized Wilcoxon test.

RESULTS

Among 48 established TIL clones, three were tumor-specific, one of which denoted CTL-8 showed its more selective cytotoxicity toward MCA-F than other tumor cell lines in both an in vitro cytotoxicity assay and in vivo LATA, as well as its rapid in vitro proliferative ability. In SATA, CTL-8 effectively reduced MCA-F tumor growth at the 2.5×10^6-cell dose, but it did not alter outgrowth of MCA-D or MCA-SP neoplasms, even at the 2×10^7-cell dose. Both BC TILs and CTL-8 displayed the Thy1.2+, Lyt2+, L3T4- phenotype on flow cytometric analysis. CTL-8 was selected as the agent for specific immunotherapy because CTL-8, but not BC TILs, had specific activity as effectors of MCA-F tumor resistance.

Table: Therapeutic Effect of TSTA/CY+CTL-8 against 4-day-established Subcutaneous MCA-F Tumors*

Treatment	Mean (±SEM) Tumor Diameter# mm	P		Mean (±SEM) Survival Time$ days	P	
None	11.6 ± 1.3	--		39.6 ± 1.6	--	
TSTA	14.1 ± 0.6	NS		40.6 ± 1.6	NS	
CY	11.6 ± 1.3	NS		41.9 ± 1.6	NS	
CTL-8	12.1 ± 0.8	NS		37.0 ± 1.7	NS	
TSTA/CY	7.1 ± 1.3	<0.025	--	44.2 ± 1.9	<0.05	--
TSTA/CY+CTL-8	1.8 ± 0.5	<0.01	<0.01	57.2 ± 4.7	<0.01	<0.025

*Tumors were produced by inoculation of 1×10^5 MCA-F cells subcutaneously into the right flank of syngeneic C3H/HeJ mice. Four days later the hosts were randomized into six groups of 10 mice each. Group 1 included untreated control animals; group 2, those receiving weekly subcutaneous injections of $1 \mu g$ of tumor-specific transplantation antigen (TSTA) beginning on day 4; group 3, those treated with 20mg/kg of intraperitoneal cyclophosphamide (CY) on days 4 and 11; group 4, those receiving intravenous adoptive transfer of CTL-8 (1×10^7) on days 7 and 14; group 5, those receiving TSTA and CY; and group 6, those receiving TSTA and CY along with CTL-8. NS indicates not significant.

#Tumor sizes were measured 18 days after inoculation and differences in mean tumor diameters were determined using Student's t test.

$Host survival times within 80 days of observation were analyzed using the Gehan modification of the generalized Wilcoxon test.

In the immunotherapy model, each modality was ineffective when used alone. The combination of TSTA and CY moderately reduced outgrowth. Using transfers of CTL-8 cells combined with TSTA/CY, tumor diameter was further reduced. While

none of the single treatment modalities alone prolonged host survival, the combination of TSTA and CY moderately prolonged mean host survival and the triple regimen of TSTA/CY and CTL-8 further extended survival (Table).
To determine which lymphocyte population mediates the regression of MCA-F tumors in this setting, LATAs were performed using the splenocytes from hosts. The splenocytes were first fractionated with plastic-dish nonadherence. The adherent fraction was inactive; the nonadherent fraction mediated tumor resistance. The nonadherent fraction was subjected to negative depletion with anti-T cell monoclonal antibodies and complement. On the one hand, tumor-neutralizing activities of splenocytes from both the group that received no treatment and the group treated with TSTA/CY were reduced by treatment with either anti-Thy1.2 or anti-L3T4, but not anti-Lyt2 antibody, and complement. On the other hand, the effectors in splenocytes of hosts treated with TSTA/CY along with CTL-8 contained both Lyt2+ effector subpopulation and L3T4+ elements, because tumor-neutralizing activity was markedly reduced only by treatment with a combination of anti-L3T4 and anti-Lyt2 monoclonal antibodies and complement and not by treatment with each antibody alone.
In vitro cytotoxic assays using splenocytes after mixed lymphocyte-tumor culture with MCA-F cells showed that the adoptive transfer of CTL-8 cells was effective in inducing cytotoxic effectors in spleens irrespective of whether hosts were normal or tumor-bearing, or whether they were treated with TSTA/CY.

DISCUSSION

Multimodality cancer immunotherapy can harness active and adoptive approaches. Combination of extracted TSTA and low-dose CY retards tumor growth owing to the capacity of the former agent to amplify specific (L3T4+) helper-cell generation[13,22], and to that of the latter to inhibit suppressor T-cell generation[23,24] in the MCA model, an effect that was potentiated by adoptive transfer of a cloned T-cell line derived from BC TILs[20]. On the other hand, the activity of adoptive transferred Lyt2+ effectors may be reinforced by the chemoimmunotherapy with TSTA/CY because of the induction of IL-2-producing L3T4+ helper elements[25,26] in tumor-bearing mice.
The experiments presented herein showing establishment of CTL clones from TILs document a potential clinically relevant method to use surgically removed tumors to produce therapeutic reagents.

REFERENCES

1. Baldwin RW (1973) Adv Cancer Res 18: 1-76
2. Pellis NR, Tom BH, Kahan BD (1974) J Immunol 113: 708-711
3. LeGrue SJ, Kahan BD, Pellis NR (1980) J Natl Cancer Inst 65: 191-196
4. LeGrue SJ, Pellis NR, Riley LB, Kahan BD (1985) Cancer Res 45: 3164-3172
5. Pellis NR, Kahan BD (1975) J Immunol 115: 1717-1722
6. Macek CM, Kahan BD, Pellis NR (1980) J Immunol 125: 1639-1643
7. Fujimoto S, Greene MI, Sehon AH (1976) J Immunol 116: 791-799
8. Rao VS, Bonavida B (1976) Cancer Res 36: 1384-1391
9. North RJ (1982) J Exp Med 155: 1063-1074
10. Awwad M, North RJ (1988) Immunology 65: 87-92
11. Kahan BD, Pellis NR, LeGrue SJ, Tanaka T (1982) Cancer 49: 1168-1173
12. Nomi S, Pellis NR, Kahan BD (1984) J Natl Cancer Inst 73: 943-950
13. Nomi S, Pellis NR, Kahan BD (1985) Cancer 55: 1296-1302
14. Nomi S, Naito K, Kahan BD, Pellis NR (1986) Cancer Res 46: 5606-5610
15. LeGrue SJ, Allison JP, Macek CM, Pellis NR, Kahan BD (1981) Cancer Res 41: 3956-3960
16. Bradford MM (1976) Anal Biochem 72: 248-254
17. Rong GH, Grimm EA, Sindelar WF (1985) J Surg Oncol 28: 131-133
18. Pellis NR, Kahan BD (1978) Methods Cancer Res 14: 29-54
19. Naito K, Pellis NR, Kahan BD (1987) Cell Immunol 108: 483-494
20. Komichi H, Smith S, Kahan BD (1992) Arch Surg 127: 1417-1423
21. Gehan EA (1965) Biometrika 52: 203-223
22. Naito K, Pellis NR, Kahan BD (1988) Cell Immunol 111: 216-224
23. Ray PK, Raychaudhuri S (1981) J Natl Cancer Inst 67: 1341-1345
24. Mokyr MB, Dray S (1983) Cancer Res 43: 3112-3119
25. Wong RA, Alexander RB, Puri RJ, Rosenberg SA (1991) J Immunother 10: 120-130
26. Chou T, Shu S (1987) J Immunol 139: 2103-2109

Enhancement of Tumor Cell Susceptibility to Tumor-Infiltrating Lymphocyte by Treatment with Cisplatin

Kohei Noguchi, Hiroshi Tanimura, Hiroki Yamaue, Makoto Iwahashi, Masaji Tani, Tsukasa Hotta, Shizuma Mizobata, and Mikiko Tamai

Department of Gastroenterological Surgery, Wakayama Medical College, Wakayama, 640 Japan

ABSTRACT

The tumor cell susceptibility to tumor-infiltrating lymphocytes (TILs) was investigated to be augmented by pretreatment with CDDP in vitro. The susceptibility of autologous tumor cells and KATO-III cells was enhanced by treated with 2 µg/ml of CDDP for 12 h measured by 4-h and/or 16-h ^{51}Cr-release assay. And, on that time, the binding ratio to TILs was increased, although expression of surface antigens of CDDP-treated tumor cells were not altered. Thus, it was suggested that the effect of CDDP on tumor cells susceptibility to TILs caused by the enhancement of binding to effector cells.

KEY WORDS: CDDP, tumor-infiltrating lymphocytes, adoptive immunotherapy, tumor cells susceptibility, immunochemical modulation

INTRODUCTION

Cisplatin (CDDP; cis-diamminedichloroplatinum II) is an active agent available for the treatment of malignant tumors as a cytocidal drug. Recently, adoptive immunotherapy using tumor-infiltrating lymphocytes (TILs) has shown some efficacy in patients with advanced cancer; however, the clinical results are not yet adequate. Therefore, some techniques of enhancing the susceptibility of tumor cells to the TILs is required. In some patients received previous chemotherapy with CDDP, clinical responses to adoptive immunotherapy were observed. The present study was designed to examine whether tumor cell lysis by TILs was enhanced by pretreatment with CDDP in vitro, and also to clarify the mechanism underlying the effect of CDDP on tumor cells.

MATERIALS AND METHODS

Separation of TILs and Autologous Tumor Cells

Surgical specimens were obtained from 5 patients with gastrointestinal cancer, and malignant ascites were from 6 patients. Separation of TILs and autologous tumor cells were performed as previously described [1]. The purity of TILs reached 60-85%, and that of autologous tumor cells was usually more than 90%. The TILs were suspended in RPMI-1640 medium (GIBCO, Island, New York, USA) supplemented with 10% heat-inactivated human AB serum obtained from healthy donors, 2 mmol/L-glutamine, 100 U/ml of penicillin, 100 µg/ml of streptomycin, and 50 µM 2-mercaptoethanol (complete medium), and incubated with IL-2 (recombinant human IL-2, S-6820, Shionogi Pharmaceutical Co., Japan) in 24 well microtiter plates (Corning No.25820) for 3-4 weeks.

CDDP Treatment

CDDP (Nippon Kayaku Co., Tokyo, Japan) was suspended in complete medium at a concentration of 0.5 µg/ml. Tumor cells grown in culture flasks for 48 h before exposure to CDDP, so as to achieve a logarithmic growth phase. They were then incubated at 1×10^5 cells/ml in 6-well microtiter plates (Falcon No.3046) with 2 µg/ml of CDDP for 12 h at 37°C in a humidified 5% CO_2 atmosphere. Control wells were incubated simultaneously without CDDP. After incubation, the cells were harvested, washed and suspended in complete medium.

Assay for Cytotoxicity

A 4-h and 16-h ^{51}Cr release assay was performed as described elsewhere [1,2]. Effector to target ratios were fixed at 15:1, and the spontaneous release did not exceed 15% for KATO-III cells, or 25% for autologous tumor cells, of the maximum release that was obtained with 1 M HCl. The pretreatment of CDDP did not affect the spontaneous release of ^{51}Cr in this study. Percent cytotoxicity was calculated as described [1,2].

The Expression of Tumor Cell Surface Antigens with CDDP

The expression of tumor cell surface antigens were assessed by flow cytometric analysis as previously reported [3]. The antibodies used were anti-HLA Class I (Cosmobiol., No.0107), anti-HLA DR (Becton Dickinson, No.MA-7363), anti-β_2-microglobulin (Cosmobio., No.0114), anti-CD54 (intercellular adhesion molecule-1, ICAM-1) antibody (Cosmobio., No.0544), and VCAM-1 (biodesign, P4244M, Kennebunkport, USA), and as a secondary antibody, fluorescein-isothiocyanate-conjugated anti-mouse IgG (specific for heavy and light chains; no cross-reaction with human IgG, Cappel, USA).

Single-cell Assay for Tumor Cell Binding

A single-cell assay was used to determine the percentage of effector cells bound to target cells. Briefly, 4×10^5 target and effector cells were mixed at 1:1 ratio in the total volume of 1 ml of complete medium and incubated at 37°C for 5 min. The tube was then centrifuged at 100 g for 5 min, after which the pellet was resuspended gently with a pipette in 1% molten agarose at 37°C. After 5 min at room temperature, the percentage of tumor binding cells (%TBC) was determined by counting 200 effector cells. The %TBC was calculated as follows:

$$\frac{\text{No. of effector cells binding to tumor cells}}{\text{total number of effector cells (bound + unbound)}} \times 100$$

RESULTS

Table 1. Enhancement of susceptibility of CDDP-treated tumor cells to TILs (E/T=15)

assay	target	% cytotoxicity	
		untreated	CDDP-treated
4-h ^{51}Cr release assay	autologous tumor cells	5.3 ± 2.1	14.5 ± 4.7*
	KATO-III cells	41.7 ± 6.5	46.9 ± 6.8**
16-h ^{51}Cr release assay	autologous tumor cells	36.9 ± 12.1	45.4 ± 12.3*
	KATO-III cells	54.1 ± 6.1	63.1 ± 6.0**

The susceptibility of CDDP-treated autologous tumor cells and KATO-III cells was enhanced (*P<0.01, **P<0.05, compared to untreated tumor cells).

Table 1 shows the enhancement of the susceptibility of CDDP-treated autologous tumor cells and KATO-III cells to TILs by 4-h and 16-h ^{51}Cr release assay (P<0.05).

Table 2. Expression of tumor cell surface antigens after treatment with CDDP

(KATO-III cells)

	relative fluorescence intensity	
	untreated	CDDP-treated
HLA Class I	1664 ± 112	1670 ± 129
HLA-DR	1260 ± 159	1255 ± 147
β_2-microglobulin	1430 ± 120	1449 ± 118
ICAM-1	463 ± 147	470 ± 146
VCAM-1	0	0

The expression of tumor cell surface antigens was not changed by treatment with CDDP.

The expression of tumor cell surface antigens was not changed by treatment with CDDP (Table 2).

As shown in Table 3, tumor binding cells against CDDP-treated KATO-III cells was enhanced more than that against untreated KATO-III cells (P<0.05).

Table 3. Single cell binding assay

(n=4)

effector cells	% tumor binding cells	
	untreated KATO-III cells	CDDP-treated KATO-III cells
TILs (cultured with 1,500 IU/ml of IL-2 for 3-4 weeks)	18 ± 5.4	33 ± 9.6*

KATO-III cells were treated with 2 µg/ml of CDDP for 12 h. The percentage of tumor binding effector cells was enhanced by CDDP treatment (*P<0.01, compared to untreated tumor cells).

DISCUSSION

This paper shows the enhancement of tumor cell susceptibility to TILs by treatment with CDDP in vitro, and clarified that the mechanism underlying the high susceptibility of CDDP-treated tumor cells to TILs was exist regard to the enhancement of binding ratio to TILs without the alternation of expression of tumor cell surface antigens by CDDP-treatment. This result suggested that CDDP-treatment could affect the affinity of TILs and tumor cells without up-regulation of tumor cell surface antigens. Thus, the combination immunochemo-therapy with CDDP and TILs offers hope for improving the clinical response and the long-term survival in cancer patients.

REFERENCES

1. Tsunoda T, Tanimura H, Yamaue H, Iwahashi M, Tani M, Tamai M, Arii K, Noguchi K (1992) The promotive effect of interleukin 4 with interleukin 2 in the proliferation of tumor-infiltrating lymphocytes from patients with malignant tumor. Biotherapy 4:9-15
2. Yamaue H, Tanimura H, Noguchi K, Iwahashi M, Tsunoda T, Tani M, Tamai M, Hotta T, Mizobata S, Arii K (1991) Cisplatin treatment renders tumor cells more susceptibility to attack by lymphokine-activated killer cells. J Clin Lab Immunol 35:165-170
3. Iwahashi M, Tanimura H, Yamaue H, Tsunoda T, Tani M, Tamai M, Noguchi K, Hotta T (1992) Defective autologous mixed lymphocyte reaction (AMLR) and killer activity generated in the AMLR in cancer patients. Int J Cancer 51:67-71

Changes of Lymphocyte Subsets Following Various Surgical Stress

Shoichi Hazama[1], Masaaki Oka[1], Shigefumi Yoshino[1], Kohji Shimoda[1], Michinari Suzuki[1], Norio Iizuka[1], Kenji Wadamori[1], Wang Fang Xin[1], Takashi Suzuki[1], Yumiko Akitomi[2], Sachie Murata[2], Yukio Hattori[2], and Yuhzou Ooba[2]

[1]Department of Surgery II, [2]Department of Clinical Laboratory Science, Yamaguchi University School of Medicine, Ube, Yamaguchi, 755 Japan

ABSTRACT

This study evaluated some changes in the lymphocyte subsets after surgery in 42 patients with various malignant and benign diseases. The subsets were analyzed using monoclonal antibodies and flow cytometry and compared prior to surgery, and on days 3 and 7 following surgery.
After surgery, the percentages of $CD4^+$ cells increased, while two color analysis showed that those of suppressor inducer T-cells increased. The percentages of $CD8^+$ cells decreased, while those of cytotoxic T-cells decreased. The percentages of CD56 cells decreased after surgery. However, the proportion of interleukin-2 (IL-2) receptor positive cells increased. These results suggest that IL-2 administration may be one strategy to prevent postoperative immunosuppression.

KEY WORDS: surgical stress, lymphocyte subset, flow cytometric analysis

INTRODUCTION

In immune surveillance, lymphocytes play an important role in mediating the overall host defense response to microbial organisms and cancer. As a consequence of technologic developments, various monoclonal antibodies to lymphocyte subsets and flow cytometry systems are available. Furthermore, specific T-cell subsets such as helper, cytotoxic, suppressor inducer, and suppressor T-cell can be detected by two color analysis. Therefore, analysis of lymphocyte subsets may yield more precise information on postoperative immune status. For example, if cytotoxic T-cells decrease after surgery, postoperative trials to increase their numbers might improve the immune suppression. However, there are a few reports on the analysis of lymphocyte subsets in the postoperative patients (1-5).
The aim of this study was to identify the lymphocyte subsets which are impaired after surgery using various monoclonal antibodies to lymphocytes.

MATERIALS AND METHODS

Patients

Forty-two patients who underwent elective abdominal surgery under general anesthesia in our clinic were investigated in this study. The patients consisted of 27 males and 15 females, ranging in age from 24 to 86 years. The diagnoses of the patients are listed in table 1. Thirty-six patients had malignant disease for which hepatectomy, colectomy, rectal amputation, gastrectomy and so forth were performed, and 6 had benign disease such as chronic pancreatitis and intrahepatic gall stones. None of the patients with malignant disease received any chemotherapeutic agents prior to or after the operation. Surgical blood loss ranged from 70 mL to 32,000 mL (mean: 1905 mL), and the duration of the surgical procedure ranged from 120 minutes to 685 minutes (mean: 386 minutes).

Table 1. List of diseases

Diseases	No of patients	
Malignant disease		36
Hepatocellular carcinoma	10	
Colorectal cancer	9	
Gastric cancer	8	
Esophageal cancer	4	
Pancreatic cancer	3	
Carcinoma of the biliary tract	2	
Benign disease		6
Chronic pancreatitis	2	
Intrahepatic gall stones	2	
Esophageal varices	1	
Intestinal fistel	1	
Total		42

Peripheral blood preparation and flow cytometric analysis

Peripheral blood samples were collected aseptically from patients on day 0 (prior to surgery), and on days 3 and 7 after surgery. EDTA anticoagulants were used. For lysed whole blood preparations, 100 uL of whole blood was mixed with 5 uL of antibody reagent (see below) and incubated on ice for 30 minutes. After staining, the erythrocytes were lysed by Ortho-mune (Ortho Diagnostic System Inc., Raritan, NJ). After the lysis was complete, the leukocytes were washed three times at 4 C^O with phosphate-buffer saline (PBS). Two hundred uL of PBS was added and the samples were analyzed on EPICS flow cytometers (Coulter Electronics, Inc., Hialeah, FL), using a fluorescence excitation of 200 to 500 mW at 488 nm. For each sample, 5.000 lymphocytes were analyzed.

Antibody reagents

All antibodies were purchased from Coulter Immunology (Hialeah, FL). Fluorescein isothiocyanate (FITC)-conjugated anti-CD3 (T3), anti-CD4 (T4), anti-CD20 (B1), anti-CD25 (IL-2R1), anti-CD56 (NKH-1), anti-HLA-DR (I2) and anti-CD11b (MO1) were used. Phycoerythrin (PE)-conjugated anti-CD8 (T8) and TQ1 (cluster unknown) were also used. Two color analysis was performed by a combination of TQ1&CD4 and CD8&CD11b.

Statistical analysis

Statistical analysis was performed using Student's T test for paired means. Values of $p < 0.05$ were considered significant.

RESULTS (Table 2)

The percentages of CD4$^+$ cells (helper/inducer T-cells), CD25$^+$ cells (interleukin-2 (IL-2) receptor positive cells) and CD4$^+$/CD8$^+$ ratio increased significantly both on days 3 and 7 after surgery ($p < 0.002$). The percentages of CD20$^+$ cells (B-cells) and HLA-DR$^+$ cells (activated T-cells, monocytes, or B-cells) increased on day 3 and on day 7, respectively.
The percentages of CD8$^+$ cells (suppressor/cytotoxic T-cells) and CD56$^+$ cells (natural killer (NK) cells) decreased significantly both on days 3 and 7 ($p < 0.002$). The percentages of CD3$^+$ cells (pan T-cells) did not change following surgery.
Two color analysis revealed that there was a increase in the TQ1$^+$T4$^+$ cells(suppressor inducer T-cells) both on day 3 and day7, and a decrease in the T8$^+$MO1$^-$ cells (cytotoxic T-cells) both on day 3 and day 7. Thus, the increase in the CD4$^+$ cells implies an increase in the suppressor inducer T cells, while a decrease in the CD8$^+$ cells means a decrease in the cytotoxic T-cells.

Table 2. Changes in the lymphocyte subsets after surgical stress

Lymphocyte subset	day 0	day 3	day 7
CD3	63.4 $\pm$ 1.8	63.5 $\pm$ 1.8	66.4 $\pm$ 1.6
CD4	43.9 $\pm$ 1.6	49.6 $\pm$ 1.5*	50.9 $\pm$ 1.4*
CD8	27.6 $\pm$ 1.1	22.5 $\pm$ 1.2*	23.0 $\pm$ 1.2*
CD4/CD8	1.75 $\pm$ 0.12	2.57 $\pm$ 0.19*	2.48 $\pm$ 0.15*
CD20	8.8 $\pm$ 0.5	11.7 $\pm$ 0.9*	9.6 $\pm$ 0.6
CD25	5.2 $\pm$ 0.4	7.5 $\pm$ 0.5*	8.2 $\pm$ 0.5*
CD56	25.3 $\pm$ 1.6	17.6 $\pm$ 1.3*	18.2 $\pm$ 1.1*
HLA-DR	21.8 $\pm$ 1.5	24.9 $\pm$ 1.5	29.6 $\pm$ 1.6*
TQ1$^+$T4$^+$	29.5 $\pm$ 1.6	33.8 $\pm$ 1.7*	34.7 $\pm$ 1.5*
TQ1$^-$T4$^+$	10.1 $\pm$ 0.5	10.0 $\pm$ 0.6	10.5 $\pm$ 0.6
T8$^+$MO1$^+$	2.8 $\pm$ 0.3	2.7 $\pm$ 0.3	2.9 $\pm$ 0.3
T8$^+$MO1$^-$	28.1 $\pm$ 1.3	22.1 $\pm$ 1.4*	23.0 $\pm$ 1.2*

Values are mean $\pm$ S.E. (standard error). *:Preoperative values (day 0) vs. postoperative values (day 3 or day 7); $p < 0.002$.

DISCUSSION

Many investigators support the belief that surgical stress suppresses immunity. However, the mechanism of this immunosuppression following surgery remains controversial. Several previous reports have found changes in the lymphocyte subsets following surgery, ie, a decrease of helper T-cells to suppressor T-cells ratio(1) and NK cells (4).
Our data indicated that: 1)the overall percentage of helper/inducer T-cells increases. Since two color analysis revealed that the percentage of helper T-cells did not change and that the percentage of suppressor inducer T-cells increased, the increase in the helper/inducer T-cells is due to an increase in the suppressor inducer T-cells. These data are consistent with postoperative immunosuppression. 2)the percentage of suppressor/cytotoxic T-cells decreases. Since two color analysis showed that the percentage of suppressor T-cells did not change and that the percentage of cytotoxic T-cells decreased, the decrease in the suppressor/cytotoxic T-cells is due to a decrease in the cytotoxic T-cells. These data also are consistent with the postoperative immunosuppression. 3)the percentage of CD56 (NK cells) decreased after operation. Taken together, our data suggest that the prevention of postoperative immunosuppression may require both augmentation of the cytotoxic T-cells and NK cells and inhibition of the suppressor inducer T-cells. However, our data also showed that the proportion of IL-2 receptor positive cells increased. Therefore, the peri-operative administration of IL-2 may be effective in preventing postoperative immunosuppression.

REFERENCES

1. Hansbrough JF, Bender EM, Zapato-Sirvent R, Anderson J (1984) Altered helper and suppressor lymphocyte populations in surgical patients. Am J Surg 148:303-307
2. Grzelak I, Olszewski WL, Engeset A (1984) Influence of operative trauma on circulating blood mononuclear cells: Analysis using monoclonal antibodies. Eur Surg Res 16: 105-112
3. Hamid JM, Bancewicz J, Brown R, Ward C, Irving MH, Ford WL(1984) The significance of changes in blood lymphocyte population following surgical operations. Clin Exp Immunol 56: 49-57
4. Lennard TW, Shenton BK, Borzotta A (1982) The influence of surgical operations on components of the human immune system. Br J Surg 72: 771-776
5. Platt MPW, Lovat P, Watoson JG, Aynsely-Green A (1989) The effects of anesthesia and surgery on lymphocyte population and function in infants and children. J Pediatr Surg 24: 884-887

Others

Chemotherapy Induced Toxicity and Its Relation with Tissue DNA Synthesis: A Circadian Stage Dependent Study

Abdus Shakil, Naoki Hirabayashi, Masahiko Nishiyama, Kenjiro Aogi, and Tetsuya Toge

Department of Surgery, Research Institute for Nuclear Medicine and Biology, Hiroshima University, Hiroshima, Japan

ABSTRACT

Lethal and haematological toxicities of 5-fluorouracil and *cis* platinum investigated in female C3H mice were found to be related to their dosing time. Overall toxicity was greater in the early resting phase (3 HALO) (Hours After Light On) treated group among the four HALO points (3, 9, 15 and 21) investigated. Hematological toxicities were less pronounced with early activity span (15 HALO) treatment compared to others. Spleen and bone marrow DNA synthesis showed higher synthesis activity in the resting span and lower in the activity span in control animals. In the treated group synthesis activity was less affected when treated during the low synthesis period. This was well correlated with the toxic effects.

KEY WORDS : Chemotherapy, Circadian Rhythm, Dosing Time, Toxicity, DNA Synthesis

INTRODUCTION

Time dependent drug delivery systems have been a modern trend in cancer chemotherapy. The internal biological environment changes rhythmically during the 24 hours cycle which causes the host tissues to be affected by an anticancer agent in a time dependent pattern [1]. A number of factors or mechanisms are supposed to cause such variations, of which changes in the enzyme levels [2], tissue blood flow [3], cellular DNA synthesis [4] and functions of the different organ systems have been suggested. In the present study we have investigated the lethal and hematological toxicities of 5-fluorouracil (5-FU) and *cis* platinum (CDDP) in mice. We observed significant dosing time effect on lethality and hematological toxicities and found that the hematological toxicities are related to the DNA synthesis activity of the haematopoitic organs. The purpose of this study is to understand the underlying causes of the circadian variation of toxicity and to find out a safe dosing time.

MATERIALS AND METHODS

Six to 8 weeks old female C3H mice (Nihon Kurea, Japan) were housed in the animal facility room having 12 hours light alternating with 12 hours dark cycle (light on at 6:00 a.m. and off at 6:00 p.m.). They were synchronized to this cycle for at least 4 weeks prior to use in the experiment while food and water were supplied *ad libitum*. The experiment is shown in Table 1. 5-FU (Kyowa Hakko Kogyo Co. Ltd., Japan) or CDDP (Bristol-Meyer Squibb K.K., Japan), diluted in RPMI, were administered in intraperitoneal (i.p.) route at one of the four time points (3, 9, 15 and 21 HALO) (Fig 1) and sampled on the corresponding HALO time after indicated interval. Control groups received RPMI only. To investigate the DNA synthesis, the mice were injected 100 μCi of 3H-Thymidine (TdR) (NEN Biomedical Products, USA) i.p. one hour prior to a designated HALO time at which they were sacrificed. Femurs, spleens and other tissues were taken. Femurs were cut at both ends and their cavities flushed with RPMI, cell population was counted and filtered through glass fiber filter (Toyo Roshi, Japan) by negative suction. Filters were dried and vialed. Spleens were made 2 mm^3 pieces, weighed and acid soluble isotopes were removed by preserving the samples overnight in 5% trichloroacetic acid. Tissues were then washed, vialed and dissolved in NCS tissue soulblizer (Amersham, UK) for 6 hours. Scintillation cocktail was added to the vials and ^{3}H-TdR incorporation was measured in a liquid scintillation counter (Aloka, Japan). Statistical analysis of the data have been done by χ^2 and student's t test.

RESULTS

Lethal Toxicity : Mice were observed twice daily for a period of one month following treatment. Mortality following a single injection of an LD$_{50}$ dose of either drug showed a significant dosing time related effect (P < 0.05, 5-FU; < 0.01, CDDP) (Table 2). In both drug groups, early resting span (3 HALO) treatment showed higher mortality. A lower mortality was encountered with the late resting span (9 HALO) treatment. Mortality following the activity span treatment remained in the intermediate range and did not show any difference between early and late activity span dosing.

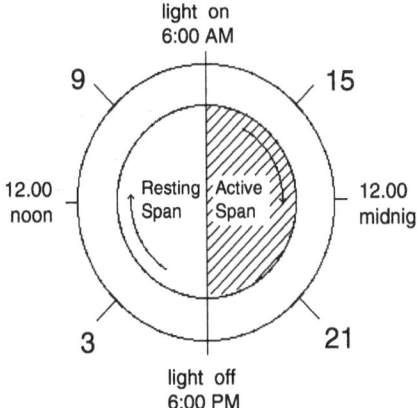

Fig. 1. Clock hours and HALO (Hours After Light On) Time. 3, 9, 15 and 21 HALO correspond with 9:00, 15:00, 21:00 and 3:00 hours, respectively.

Table 1 : Experimental Design.

Study[1]	Mice[2] per Study	Drug	Doses (mg/kg)	Toxicity Parameters
1†	140	5-FU[3]	300	Survival Rate
2†	120	CDDP[4]	16	Survival Rate
3†	40	5-FU	300	WBC count, Spleen size
4†	40	CDDP	16	WBC count, Spleen size
5†	48	5-FU	75	BMC[5] population
6†	48	CDDP	4	BMC population
7†	48	5-FU	75	DNA synthesis (Days 1, 4)
8†	48	CDDP	4	DNA synthesis (Days 2, 4)

[1] Each study was carried out for four HALO points. [2] Total number of mice in each study. [3] 5-fluorouracil. [4] cisplatinum. [5] Bone marrow cell. † Single dose treatment.

Haematological Toxicity : Figure 2 shows the 4th post treatment day peripheral WBC count carried out with the blood collected sectioning the tail. For CDDP, 15 HALO (early activity span) treatment showed an obvious leukocytosis, while leukopenia was induced by the drug with other HALO point treatments. In the case of 5-FU, drug induced leukopenia was less severe by 30% with 15 HALO treatment compared to other HALO points (P < 0.01).

DNA Synthesis : As measured by ^{3}H-TdR incorporation, both bone marrow and spleen cells showed higher synthesis activity during the resting span (Fig 3). Following treatment, drug induced suppression of synthesis activity was less and recovery from the suppression was higher in the 15 HALO treated group (P < 0.01).

Table 2 : Mortality following single LD$_{50}$ dose time dependent treatment with 5-FU or CDDP.

Drugs	Mice per HALO Gp.	Treatment Time (HALO)			
		3	9	15	21
		No. of Deaths (%)			
5-FU	35	16(45)	5(15)	11(31)	11(31)
CDDP	30	24(80)	3(10)	15(50)	15(50)

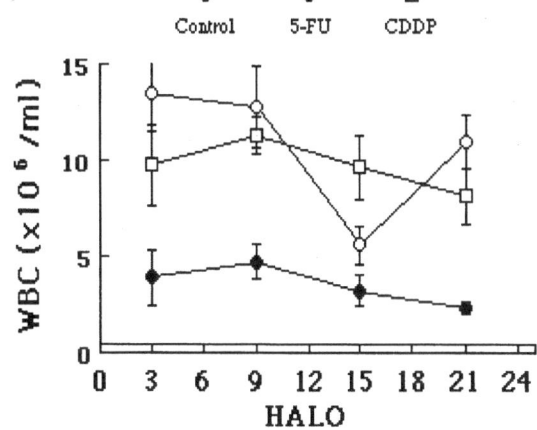

Fig. 2 : Post treatment day 4 peripheral WBC count. 15 HALO treated group show leukocytosis with CDDP and a less severe leukopenia with 5-FU.

DISCUSSION

Overall toxic pattern showed a greater drug induced toxicity following treatment at the early resting span (3 HALO) of mice. For 5-FU, the striking circadian variation of the activity of dihydropyrimidine dehydrogenase (DPD), the enzyme which catabolizes more than 80% of the dose administered [5], may be one of the causes. Peak and trough DPD activity has been shown during the late resting (9 HALO) and early resting (3 HALO) span, respectively, in rodents [2]. Therefore, the dose administered at the late resting span (9 HALO) gets rapidly catabolized leaving a little active drug to affect the target organs. The converse is true when the same dose is administered at the early resting span (3 HALO). Nevertheless, higher DNA synthesis activity during the early resting span may contribute to this fact which we have found in this experiment. As in the case of CDDP, if the death has been caused due to bone marrow suppression, a lower mortality with 9 HALO

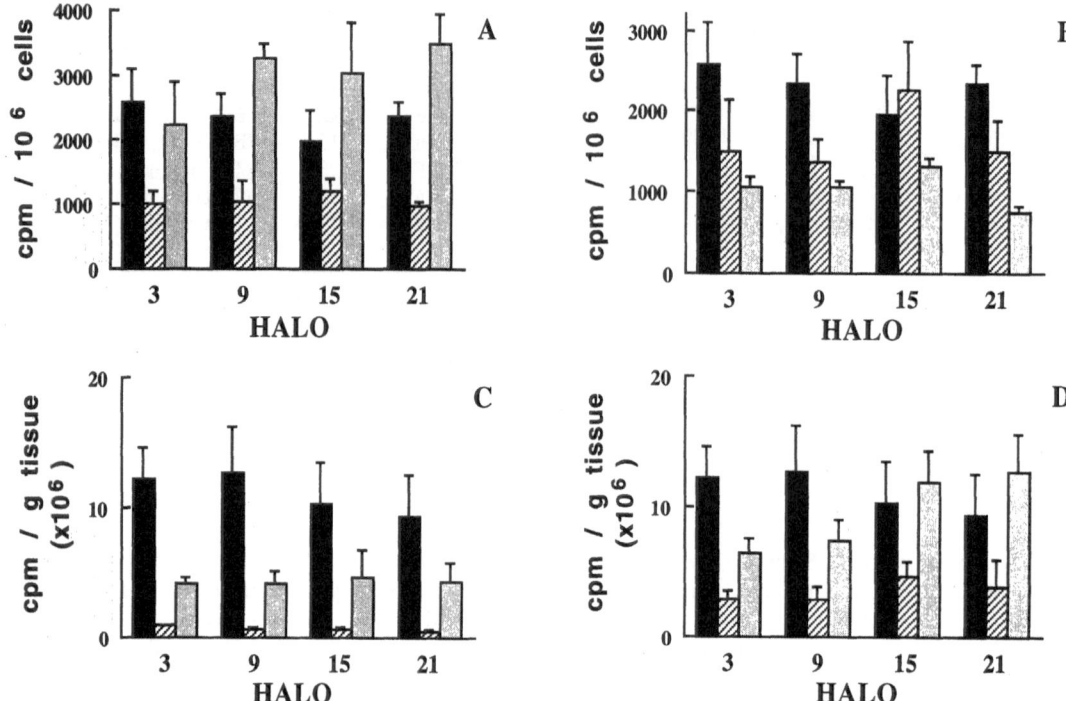

Fig. 3 : DNA synthesis activity measured by 3H-TdR incorporation in bone marrow cells (A, 5-FU; B, CDDP) and spleen cells (C, 5-FU; D, CDDP). The DNA synthesis in control animals is lower in the 15 HALO group and the drug induced suppression is less and recovery is higher with this HALO point treatment. The dark bar represents control, the striped bar represents 24 hours (5-FU) 48 hours (CDDP) after treatment and the light shaded bars represents 96 hours after treatment for both drugs.

treatment may be due to less suppression of the bone marrow DNA synthesis activity during this time. However, urinary functions have also been reported to play role for such variations [6]. Haematological toxicity which is likely to play a fatal role in chemotherapy found to be related to the degree of DNA synthesis. With both drugs, 15 HALO treatment showed less toxic effect during which the DNA synthesis activity is also less. Thus we conclude that variation of the DNA synthesis activity during the 24 hours cycle may play a significant role in causation of the circadian variation of toxicity.

REFERENCES

1. Levi FA, Mechkouri M, Roulon A, Bailleul A, Lemaigre G, Reinberg A and Mathe G. (1985) Europ. J. Clin. Oncol. 2: 1245-1251
2. Harris BE, Song R, Sen-jaw Soong and Diasio RB. (1990) Cancer Res. 50: 197-201
3. Hori K, Suzuki M, Tanda S, Saito S, Shinozaki M and Qiu-Hang Zhang. (1992) Cancer Res. 52: 912-916
4. Burns ER and Beland SS. (1984) Pharmacol. 28: 296-300
5. Chabner BA. (1982) In: Chabner BA (ed) Pharmacologic principles of cancer treatment, W.B. Saunders Philadelphia, pp 183-212
6. Hrushesky WJM, Borch R and Levi FA. (1983) Clin. Pharmacol. Ther. 32: 330-339

Leukopenia Due to 5-Fluorouracil (5-FU) Administration Is Improved by Glutamine Supplemented Elemental Diet (Gln-ED)

MOTAHAR H. AHMED, K. AOKI, and S. BABA

Second Department of Surgery, Hamamatsu University School of Medicine, Hamamatsu, Shizuoka, 431-31 Japan

ABSTRACT

We compared the effects of glutamine supplemented elemental diet (Gln-ED) on circulating white blood cells after administration of toxic doses of 5-FU (50 mg/kg daily for 3 consecutive days). Male wistar rats were maintained with isonitrogenous, isocaloric ED containing 3% Gln or 3% Glycine (control) through chronic indwelling intragastric feeding tubes (after gastrostomy). Three days after the administration of 5-FU through the feeding tube, circulating WBC count decreased by 41.6% in Glycine-ED group (2760+561) where as in rats infused with Gln-ED, total WBC count improved significantly (6400+291) which mimics the Sham control group (6633+378). In differential count of WBC, lymphocyte count was significantly increased in Gly-ED group than control group (Gln-ED gr. 70.0+3.6; Gly-ED gr. 54.4+5.2).

Key words: Glutamine, Elemental diet, 5-FU, Leukopenia

INTRODUCTION

5-FU, a chemotherapeutic drug have toxic side effects on rapidly proliferating white blood cells leading to leukopenia. Glutamine, the most abundant amino acid in mammalian blood is the major oxidative fuel for stimulated lymphocytes [1] and small intestine [2]. It may facilitate intestinal recovery after injury [3] and reduce endotoxemia [4]. By using lower concentration of glutamine parenteraly along with a lethal dose of 5-FU, it was reported that the toxicity on small intestinal mucosa but not leukopenia was improved [5]. We assumed that the doses used in the previous study [5] were too lethal to get any significant beneficial effect of glutamine on white cell count. Therefore we designed our study to use less lethal doses of 5-FU with higher concentration of glutamine in a modified model.

MATERIALS AND METHODS

Male wister rats weighing about 220 - 280 gm were divided into three groups:

```
    Gr. 1 : 5-FU + conventional ED + 3% glutamine (n=5)
    Gr. 2 : 5-FU + conventional ED + 3% glycine (n=5)
    Gr. 3 : normal sham control (n=3)
```

Indwelling intragastric feeding tube were placed aseptically by gastrostomy and were fitted with a swivel assembly to allow long term infusion in unrestraied rats. All were housed in individual metabolic cages and allowed water ad libitum and received a seven day continuous intragastric infusion (3 ml/hour) of an isonitrogenous, isocaloric ED containing 3% Glutamine (Gr. 1) and 3% Glycine (Gr. 2). From the 4th day of intragastric feeding, 50 mg/kg of 5-FU was administered daily for 3 consecutive days in Gr. 1 and Gr. 2. On 8th day, blood were sampled from all rats and analysed for total count of WBC and differential count of WBC, blood level of 5-FU and different aminoacids. We also measured the same parameters in Gr. 3 (5-FU untreated Sham control group). All the values were compared among the groups and analysed by student's t test.

RESULTS

Table 1 shows the total count (TC) and differential count of WBC in Gr. 1, 2 and 3. After the administration of 5-FU, circulating WBC count decreased by 41% in Gr. 2 (TC=2760+563, p<0.01) in compare to Gr. 3 (TC=6633+378). However, in Gr. 1 total WBC count were improved significantly (TC=6400+291, p<0.01). Lymphocyte count was found to be increased significantly in Gr. 1 compare to Gr. 2 and 3.

Table 1. Total count and differential count of WBC in three groups

Groups	Total count	PMN(%)	Lymphocyte(%)
Gr. 1	6400 + 291	25.8 + 3.5	70.0 + 3.6
Gr. 2	2760 + 563	40.4 + 3.9	54.4 + 5.2
Gr. 3	6633 + 378	43.3 + 3.0	51.3 + 3.0

Table 2 shows the blood levels of 5-FU in Gr. 1 and 2 after 3 days of starting 5-FU treatment. Table 3 represents the different aminoacids levels in Group 1 and 2.

Table 2. Blood levels of 5-FU

Gr. 1	5504 + 329 ng/ml
Gr. 2	4741 + 407 ng/ml

Table 3. Blood levels of different amino acids

Amino acids	Normal values (nmol/ml)	Gr. 1 (nmol/ml)	Gr. 2 (nmol/ml)
Glutamine	491-750	897.2 + 120	788.5 + 115
Glycine	202-307	127 + 20	1192.5 + 141
Ananine	255-591	461.4 + 168	501 + 152
Valine	207-591	243.2 + 33	250 + 28
Methionine	31- 39	50 + 6	54 + 11
Arginine	83-130	127.6 + 35	133 + 27
Phenylalanine	55- 71	59.6 + 21	84 + 23
Proline	146-267	135 + 11	153.5 + 16

DISCUSSION

5-Fluorouracil, a chemotherapeutic drug have toxic side effects on rapidly proliferating white blood cells leading to leukopenia. Glutamine had been shown to be an important oxidative fuel for stimulated lymphocytes and it may facilitate intestinal recovery after injury. It was reported that the toxicity on intestinal mucosa but not leukopenia was improved by glutamine supplemented total parenteralnutrition. Intragastrically supplied 5-FU maintained a good blood concentration (Table 2). Higher blood levels of glutamine and glycine were found after intragastrically supplied elemental diets. However glycine could not improve leukopenia as was improved by glutamine (Table 3). In differential count, Lymphocyte count was found to be increased significantly in Gln-ED group. Therefore we presume that Gln-ED improves leukopenia by increasing lymphocyte count revealing a possible involvement in immunological response.

REFERENCES

1. Salleh M, Ardawi M, Newsholme EA(1983) Glutamine metabolism in lymphocytes of the rat. Biochem.J. 212: 835-842

2. Windmueller HG, Spaeth AE (1974) Uptake and metabolism of plasma glutamine by the small intestine. J Biol Chem 249: 5070-5079

3. Fox AD, Kripke SA, De Paula JA, Berman JM, Settle RG, Rombeau JL (1988) The effect of a glutamine-supplemented enteral diet on methotrexate-induced enterocolitis. JPEN 12: 325-331

4. Fox AD, De Paula JA, Kripke SA (1988) Glutamine-supplemented elemental diets reduce endotoxemia in a lethal model of enterocolitis. Surg Forum 39: 46-48

5. O'Dwyer ST, Scott T, Smith RJ, Wilmore DW (1987) 5-Fluorouracil toxicity on small intestinal mucosa but not white blood cells is decreased by glutamine. Clin Res 35: 367a

Gianturco-Rosch Expandable Metallic Biliary Stent Applied for Treatment of Biliary Strictures

Hiroki Kanno, Eizo Okamoto, Naoki Yamanaka, Wataru Tanaka, and Chiaki Yasui

The First Department of Surgery, Hyogo College of Medicine, Nishinomiya Hyogo, 663 Japan

ABSTRACT

Thirty-five with obstructive jaundice were treated by Gianturco-Rosch type metallic stents nonsurgically during the period of 18 months from March 1991 to September 1992. The sububjects included 19 cases of primary biliary tract cancers, 10 cases of recurrences following hepatobiliary surgery, and 6 cases of benign biliary strictures. Mean jaundice-free period, jaundice free rate and survival rate at 6 months in the former two groups were 132 days, 72%, 72%, and 171 days,75%, 80% respectively. Patients with benign strictures are all alive without jaundice. Our experience shows the usefulness of metallic stent, which provides better quality of life as palliation in patients with inoperable malignant as well as benign biliary strictures.

KEY WORDS : biliary stricture, interventional procedure, prosthesis, obstructive jaundice

INTRODUCTION

We report clinical usefulness of self-expandable stainless steel stent in the treatment of patients with biliary stricture.

MATERIALS AND METHODS

Endoprosthesis

The self-expandable metallic stent (Giantuco-Rosch biliary"Z"stent, COOK,Bloomington) was constructed of stainless steel wire in a zigzag pattern. One hundred seventy four stents were inserted in 35 patients during the period of 18 months from March 1991 to September 1992.

Patient Population

Thirty-five patients with comfirmed biliary stricture had prostheses inserted. Nineteen patients (Gr-1),12 men and 7 women, ranging in age from 54 to 85 years, had inoperable malignant strictures. Seventeen patients had hilar bile duct cancer, 2 had gallbladder cancer. Ten patients (Gr-2), 8 men and 2 women, aged 41 to 75 years had cancer recurrences after surgery. Three patients had anastomotic recurrences at hepaticojejunostomy for hilar bile duct cancer. Three patients with gallbladder cancer, 3 with colon cancer, and 1 with gastric cancer had lymph node recurrences following hepatectomy. Twenty-one patients of Gr-1 and Gr-2 received external irradiation before stent placement. Six patients (Gr-3) , 5 men and 1 woman , aged 19 to 78 years , had benign stricture. One patient had chronic pancreatitis, and one had cholangitis. Four patients developed strictures after biliary surgery : One patient after pancreatoduodenectomy for gastric cancer , 2 after resection of extra hepatic bile duct for intrahepatic calculi and congenital biliary dilatation, and 1 after right hepatic lobectomy for hepatocellular carcinoma.

Technique

All patients were initially treated with echo guided percutaneous transhepatic biliary
drainage (PTBD). The stricture was passed with a guide wire and original 5fr.catheter
(Hyogo, COOK, Bloomington), and subsequently a dilator. After serum bilirubin level
decreased to less than 2 mg/dl, the stent was plased across the stricture and a 7 fr.
polyurethane catheter was advanced through the stent. One week later, after obtaining
a cholangiogram to chcek the position and patency of the stent,the 7 fr. catheter was
removed (Fig.1).

```
                  Malignant case  4~ 5 W
           ↗          Irradiation            ↘
PTBD                  Biliary dilation              Metallic stent    →    Removal of external
                                                    placement        1W    drainage tube
           ↘      Benign case     3 W       ↗
                  Biliary dilation
```

Fig.1 Treatment schedule for obstructive jaundiced patients using stents

RESULTS

Stents were placed successfully in 35 patients. The mean number of stents used per
patient was 5 (2-12) stents in Gr-1, 6 (2-12) in Gr-2, and 4 (2-6) in Gr-3.
The duration of survival and jaundice free after stent placement is shown in Table 1,
Table 2 and Fig. 2. The median jaundice free period was 200 (0-450) days for Gr-1 and
209 (30-360) days for Gr-2. Fifty-two percent of patiets in Gr-1 and Gr-2 died of
disease progression. Patients in Gr-3 were all alive without recurrence of jaundice.
In all patients , there were no major complications such as bleeding or biliary
infection ascribable to the stenting. Late complications occurred in 8 patients(23%)
were improved after immediate treatments(Table 3). However, occlusion of the stents
developed by ingrowth of the tumor in 6 (32%) of Gr-1 and in 6 (60%) of Gr-2.

Table 1 Patency and survival in 35 patients

Group	Average jaundice free period (day)	Jaundice free rate (%) at 6 months	at 12 months	Median survival period (month)
1	132.1 (0-450)	72 (72%)*	45 (16%)*	8
2	170.8 (30-360)	75 (80%)*	0 (23%)*	10
3	280.0 (60-480)	100 (100%)*	100 (100%)*	alive

( )* : Survival rate

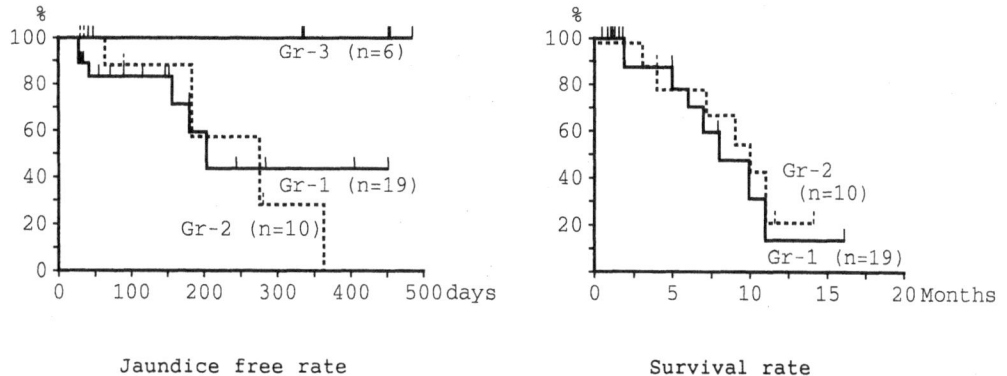

Jaundice free rate   Survival rate

Fig.2 Prognosis of patients after stent placement

Table 2 Results of stents in 20 patients with highlar bile duct cancer

	Jaundice free rate		Survival rate	
	at 6 months	at 12 months	at 6 months	at 12 months
With irradiation (n=17)	83 %	22 %	75 %	23 %
without irradiation (n=3)	67 %	0 %	67 %	0 %

Table 3 Complications

Problem	Incidence	Treatment
Migration of stent	2.9% (1/35)*	Additional stent placed
Occulusion within 30 days	11.4% (4/35)*	Additional stent placed (3), Drained alone (1)
Liver abscess	11.4% (4/35)*	Percutaneously drained
Cholangitis	2.9% (1/35)	Antibiotics

* : The cases overlapped each other.

DISCUSSION

Various prosthesis have been developed for malignant biliary strictures [1-3]. Reports on the average jaundice free period ranged from 4 to 9 months and the median survival time was 3 to 6 months [1-5]. The present procedure , using Giantuco-Rosch self-expandable metallc " Z " stents , provided more beneficial effect than did the other studies. Percutaneously inserted self-expandable metallic stent in combination with external radiation therapy was an useful non-surgical modality in managing malignant obstructive jaundice for palliation. Long-term follow-up is required to determine the role of stenting in the management of benign biliary strictures.

REFERENCES

1. Coons HG, Carey PH (1983) Large-bore,long biliary endoprostheses (biliary stents) for improved drainage. Radiology 148:89-94
2. Irving JD, Adam A, Dick R, Dondelinger RF, Lunderquist A, Roche A (1989) Gianturco expandable metallic biliary stents: results of a European clinical trial. Radiology 172:321-326
3. Yoshioka T, Sakaguchi H, Yoshimura H, Tamada T, Ohishi H, Uchida H, Wallace S (1990) Expandable metallic biliary endoprostheses: preliminary clinical evaluation. Radiology 177:253-257
4. Adam A, Chetty N, Roddie M, Yeung E, Benjamin IS (1991) Self-expandable stainless steel endoprosthesis for treatment of malignant bile duct obstruction. AJR 156:321-325
5. Yamamoto H, Nimura Y, Hayakawa N, Kamiya J, Kondo S, Nagino M (1993) Endoprosthesis under percutaneous transhepatic cholangioscopy (PTCS) for malignant biliary obstruction. J Jpn Biliary Assoc 7:43-50

Statistical Reappraisal of Cancer Staging System

Yoshihiro Yamazoe[1], Shunzou Maetani[2], Hisashi Onodera[1], Kazutomo Inoue[1], and Masayuki Imamura[1]

[1]The First Department of Surgery, Faculty of Medicine, [2]Research Center for Biomedical Engineering, Kyoto University, Kyoto, 606 Japan

ABSTRACT

Using data from 1116 gastric cancer and 905 colorectal cancer patients, respectively, a computer-assisted search was made for a better staging system for both types of cancer. All possible classifications in terms of T and N factors were evaluated by the Akaike Information Criterion (AIC). The results showed that for both types of cancer, substantial proportions of the generated classification systems were actually better than the conventional systems (21.4% and 93.8%, respectively). This was confirmed by a linear trend test, whose chi square value correlated well with the AIC. We conclude that computer-assisted statistical studies are essential for the critical reappraisal and evaluation of the conventional staging systems, and for the identification of better classification systems.

KEY WORDS: Akaike information criterion, linear trend test, stage classification, gastric cancer, colorectal cancer

INTRODUCTION

Many cancer stage classifications have been proposed for various types of cancer, and there can be a number of logically possible classifications even if the factors used are restricted. It is very difficult to exhaustively check which classification is the best for the prediction of survival without the aid of a computer. Thus, we created all logically possible classifications by a computer simulation, and selected the best classification by calculating and comparing the value of the Akaike Information Criteria (AIC) [1-3] using five year survival data from gastric cancer (GC) and cancer of the colon and rectum (CCR) patients. We also compared these classification systems to Japanese staging systems by linear trend chi square test [4].

ATIENTS AND METHODS

Patients

Data sets were obtained from 1116 patients with GC and 905 patients with CCR who were operated on in our department, and who were followed up. Each data set contained six items: survival time, depth of tumor penetration (T), lymph node metastasis (N), liver metastasis, distant metastasis, and peritoneal dissemination. The last five findings are predictor variables of survival time. All these findings were originally recorded according to the general rules proposed by the Japanese Research Society for Gastric Cancer (JRSGC) [5] or the Japanese Research Society for Cancer of the Colon and Rectum (JRSCCR) [6]. To represent the stage classification simply, T and N categories were grouped together and they were re-classified into three (T1-T3) and three (N0-N2) grades for GC, and four (T1-T4) and three (N0-N2) grades for CCR (**Table 1**). When we calculated the AIC value for each classification, we excluded patients whose stage was the worst possible (stage IV patients for GC and stage V patients for CCR). We also excluded patients who were not followed-up for at least five years, leaving 376 GC patients and 447 CCR patients. **Table 2** shows the T-N categories and the outcomes of these patients.

Table 1. Definitions of T and N categories for gastric and colorectal cancers

gastric cancer	colorectal cancer
T1: no prognostic serosal invasion (ps(-)).	T1: Tumor confined to the muscularis propria or more superficial layers.
T2: cancerous invasion extends to subserosa with infiltrative growth (ss γ).	T2: Slight extramuscular spread without serosal penetration
T3: cancer cells present on the serosal surface and exposed to the peritoneal cavity (se).	T3: Serosal penetration or extensive extramuscular spread without invasion of adjacent organs.
N0: No lymph node metastasis.	T4: Direct invasion of adjacent organs.
N1: Lymph node metastasis limited to the lymph nodes of Group 1*.	N0: No lymph node metastasis.
N2: Lymph node metastasis limited to the lymph nodes of Group 2*.	N1: Lymph node metastasis limited to the epicolic or paracolic nodes.
	N2: Lymph node metastasis beyond the paracolic level.

*: See The General Rules for the Gastric Cancer Study in Surgery and Pathology.

Generation of stage classifications

The stage classification systems according to the general rules proposed by the JRSGC is shown diagrammatically in **Fig. 1** by entering one of the numbers I, II, or III into a 3 x 3 T-N table while excluding the worst stage IV. Likewise, the stage classification proposed by the JRSCCR can also be shown by entering I, II, III, or IV into a 4 x 3 T-N table while excluding the worst prognostic stage V (**Fig. 2**). Therefore, any classification scheme can be created by allotting a number to each cell as a stage identifier [3]. By changing these numbers, all possible classifications were generated. In order to select only logical classifications, the following restrictions were made: (1) each number is chosen from the 9 (3 x 3, GC) or 12 (4 x 3, CCR) integers beginning from I; (2) the same number can be used repeatedly, but no skipping is allowed between I and the maximum number, which ranges from II to the total number of stages in that classification; (3) the cell in the left upper corner (T1N0) always represents stage I; and (4) the stage of a cell must be equal to or higher than the stage of all cells which lie to the left of and above it (i.e. the stage of $T_i N_j$ must be equal to or higher than the stage of $T_{i'} N_{j'}$ if $i >= i'$ and $j >= j'$).

Assessment of the prognostic value of classifications

Table 2. T-N categories and patient outcomes for gastric and colorectal cancer

gastric cancer		
	Death within 5 years	Survival over 5 years
T1N0	13	182
T1N1	22	39
T1N2	15	12
T2N0	7	4
T2N1	9	6
T2N2	9	4
T3N0	6	8
T3N1	17	7
T3N2	11	5

colorectal cancer		
	Death within 5 years	Survival over 5 years
T1N0	10	103
T1N1	0	14
T1N2	1	3
T2N0	20	93
T2N1	15	22
T2N2	16	17
T3N0	15	32
T3N1	13	18
T3N2	20	9
T4N0	5	5
T4N1	2	0
T4N2	13	1

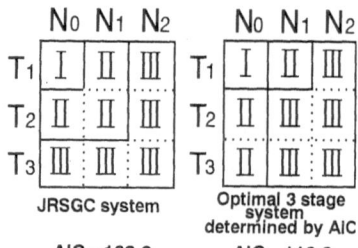

Fig 1. The JRSGC stage classification (left) and the optimal 3 stage classification determined by AIC (right) for gasrtric cancer, represented in a 3X3 table.

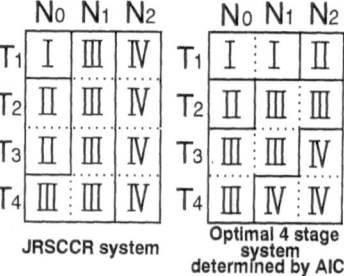

Fig 2. The JRSCCR stage classification (left) and the optimal 4 stage classification determined by AIC (right) for colorectal cancer, represented in a 4X4table.

The prognostic value of each classification was assessed by the AIC. The AIC was calculated as follows:

$$ AIC = -2 \sum_{i=0}^{1} \sum_{j=1}^{c} n(i,j) \cdot \log[n \cdot n(i,j) / \{n(i,*) \cdot n(*,j)\}] + 2(c-1) $$

where death within 5 years is indicated by $i = 0$, and 5-year survival by $i = 1$. c is the number of stages, n is the total number of patients, $n(i, j)$ is the number of patients with the i th outcome in the j th stage, $n(i, *)$ is the total number of patients with the i th outcome, and $n(*, j)$ is the total number of patients in the j th stage. The smaller (the more negative) the AIC value of a classification, the more information that classification provides, and hence the better it is. The AIC permits a straightforward comparison between classification schemes with different numbers of stages, e.g. between 4-stage and 5-stage models. All possible classification models were successively generated using a Hewlett-Packard computer (HP9000 series 300 model 382), evaluated by the AIC, and compared with each other as well as with the JRSGC and JRSCCR staging systems. We defined a classification mode as unsuitable if each stage did not have an observed rate of survival lower than the preceding (lower-ranked) group.

Comparison of the JRSGC and JRSCCR systems with our optimal model using life-table analysis

To assess the validity of our methods, our optimal 3-stage model (4-stage model when the worst stage IV was included) was compared to the JRSGC system using data from 1116 GC patients by calculating the chi square value of the linear trend test. Similarly, our optimal 4-stage model (5-stage model when stage V was included) was compared to the JRSCCR system using data from 905 CCR patients.

RESULTS

A total of 3,151 and 146,975 logical classification models were generated from the 3 x 3 and 4 x 3 tables, respectively. The number of stages ranged from 2 to 9 and from 2 to 12 (**Table 3**). Of these models, 2,595 and 128,268 were inconsistent with the survival data for GC and CCR (**Table 2**), respectively, in that a more advanced stage group showed a higher 5-year survival. Among the 556 and 18,707 suitable classifications, a total of 119 (21.4 %) and 17,552 (93.8 %) were better than the JRSGC and JRSCCR stage classifications, respectively. In the case of GC, if the number of stages was restricted to three, then 118 models were possible. Twelve of these classifications were inconsistent with our data, and 10 (9.4 %) had superior prognostic information (smaller AIC value) than the JRSGC system (AIC=-108.9). Out of all the logical classification systems, a total of 21.4 % were better than the JRSGC system. In the case of CCR, if the number of stages was restricted to four, then 2,362 models were possible, of which 1,849 were inconsistent with our data and 1,461 (76.9 %) were better than the JRSCCR system (AIC=-67.3). 93.8 % of all logical classifications were better than the JRSCCR system. **Figs. 1** and **2** diagrammatically represent these optimal models, which were selected to have the same number of stages as the JRSGC and JRSCCR stage systems.

Fig. 3 shows the survival curves of GC patients classified by the JRSGC and system by our optimal classification using the same number of stages. The chi square values for the two systems were 406.3 and 411.4, respectively. **Fig. 4** shows the survival curves of CCR patients classified by the JRSCCR system and by our optimal classification using the same number of stages. The chi square values for the two systems were 329.1 and 434.0, respectively. Compared to the survival curves generated by the JRSGC or JRSCCR system, those derived from our classification model are wider apart, thus indicating a greater differentiation between the stages.

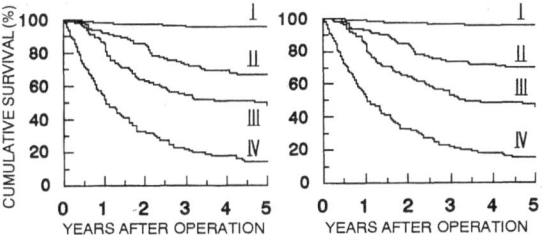

Fig.3 Survival curves for the JRSCCR stage system (left) and for our optimal model of the same number of stages (right).

DISCUSSION

It is noteworthy that 21.4 % of the logically possible classifications for GC were better than the JRSGC system and, surprisingly, 93.8 % of classifications for CCR were better than the JRSCCR system. It is true that the optimal models were a little more compli-cated, but one must consider the role of stage clas-sification as a prognostic tool in determining the survival of a patient with the greatest possible accuracy. If we think much of the simplicity, It would be practical to select the simplest model from many alternatives whose value of the AIC was nearly the same.

In this study, we checked the AIC values of all logical classification systems in order to determine which classifications are better than the JRSGC or JRSCCR systems. Since it is too time-consuming to check all the possible classifications [2], it seems more practical to use the algorithm previously reported [3] for the purpose of identifying the best model for a given number of stages. By using this algorithm, we generated the best model in a very short time. Since the best model determined by AIC showed good chi square value on the linear trend test, we confirmed the usefulness of this procedure. If the objective variable were changed to 1-year survival instead of 5-year, for example, a new staging system can easily be generated which represents the short-term prognosis more accurately.

Table 3. Number of classifcations for gastric (left) and colorectal (right) cancers.

gastric cancer			
Number of stages	Logical	Suitable	Better than JRSGC (%)
2	11	18	0 (0.0%)
3	118	106	10 (9.4%)
4	396	215	48(22.3%)
5	771	167	51(30.5%)
6	910	47	10(21.3%)
7	644	3	0 (0.0%)
8	252	0	
9	42	0	
TOTAL	3151	556	119(21.4%)

colorectal cancer			
Number of stages	Logical	Suitable	Better than JRSCCR(%)
2	33	33	3 (9.1%)
3	388	375	172(45.9%)
4	2362	1899	1461(76.9%)
5	8671	4739	4405(93.0%)
6	20707	6092	5963(97.9%)
7	33390	4031	4011(99.5%)
8	36778	1325	1324(99.9%)
9	27342	201	201 (100%)
10	13146	12	12 (100%)
11	3696	0	
12	462	0	
TOTAL	146975	18707	17552(93.8%)

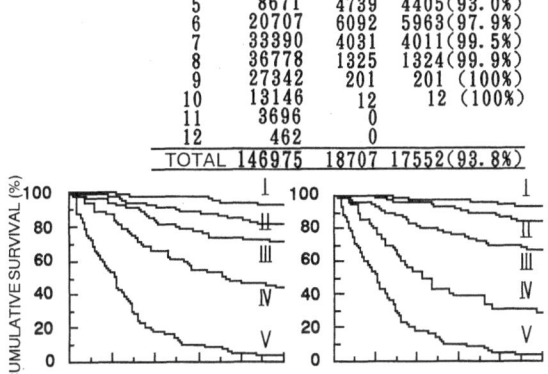

Fig 4. Survival curves for the JRSCCR stage system (left) and for our optimal model of the same number of stages (right).

REFERENCES

1. Akaike H (1973) A new look at the statistical model identification. IEEE Trans Autom Contr AC-19: 716-723
2. Maetani S, Onodera H, Nishikawa T, Tobe T (1991) Systematic computer-aided search of optimal staging system for colorectal cancer. J Clin Epidemiol 44: 285-291
3. Yamazoe Y, Maetani S, Onodera H, Nishikawa T, Tobe T (1992) Histopathological prediction of liver metastasis after curative resection of colorectal cancer. Surg Oncology 1: 237-244
4. Peto R, Pike MC, Armitage NE, Breslow NE, Cox DR, Howard SV, Mantel N, McPherson K, Peto J, Smith PG (1977) Design and analysis of randomized clinical trials requiring prolonged observation of each patient. II. Analysis and examples. Br J Cancer 35: 1-39
5. Japanese Research Society for Gastric Cancer (1981) The general rules for the gastric cancer study in surgery and pathology. Jpn J Surg 11: 127-145
6. Japanese Research Society for Cancer of the Colon and Rectum (1983) The general rules for clinical and pathological studies on cancer of the colon, rectum and anus. Jpn J Surg 13: 557-573

Study on the Central Mechanism of Indomethacin for Relieving GI Cancer Pain

Qi-Song Li, Xiao-Hong Hu, and Xuin-Fen Huan

Department of Neurobiology, Shanghai Medical University, Shanghai 200032, China

ABSTRACT

Based on the acceptable result of Indomethacin (Indo) suppository in controlling advanced GI cancer related pain,the aim of this study is to explain the central mechanism of Indo. Experiments found that: Indo 2mg.kg-1 iv. as well as Indo 50mg/rab. intracerebral ventricular(icv) significantly increased the visceral pain threshold (VPT) during 10-40min after injection. PGE2-Ab(1:600/2μl) icv significantly increase the VPT. However, VPT decreased obviously(p<0.05) when phentolamine 50μg/rat. was given icv 10min before Indo iv. Nalox-one 20 ug/2μl icv 10 min after Indo iv the VPT had no apparent change during 60 min. The concentration of central PGE2 was decreased after Indo iv injection, by contrast central NA was increased,and β-endorphine of the perfusate was no significantly change.

KEY WORD: Indomethacin, cancer related pain, rabbit visceral pain model, Phentolamine, Naloxone

INTRODUCTION

Since seventies Ferreira et al[1,2].found the existence of both central and periphral antialgesic action of aspirin-like drugs. Our previous work convinced that Indo suppsitory (50mg bid or 100mg qd),alone or combined with otheranalgesics, 80% of them reported being free of pain or only mild, tolerable discomfort. In the present paper we review the effect of Indo and try to explain its central mechanism using rabbit visceral pain model for study

MATERIALS AND METHODS

Preparation of Experimental Animal

Adult healthy rabbits either sex, weighing 1.6 to 2.5 kg from University Animal Center were used for developing visceral pain model.The number of animal is indicated in each experiment,(1) Visceral pain model:The rabbits were anesthesized by iv injection of 30mg.kg-1 Pentobarbital,and placed on the right position to expose the left major splanchnic nerve for setting a pair of two ends of an electric stimulator on it.(2) Implantation ofintracranial cannula: The anesthesized rabbits were placed onthe prone position with their head fixed on the steotaxic apparatus (coordinate: P-13, L/R-0.5, H-1). A stainless steel push-pull cannula with outer diameter of 0.65 mm and inner diameter of 0.40 mm was implantedin the 4th ventrical.

Measurement of Visceral Pain Threshold and Substance of Perfusate

An autoelectric stimulator was used with a train of 400-500 ms, consisted of 0.5 ms width,40 HZ of biphasic square waves each 0.1 ms in duration, through a constant current output. The intensity start from 0.1 mA every 5s then o.1 mA added by monitor screen for supervising and cut off while the escape response of the rabbit appeared, score the absolute value of mA as the Visceral Pain Threshold (VPT). The concentration of PGE2 measured by RIA and that of NA, b-endorphine of perfusate weredetermined by HPLC-chemical detector.

Preparation of Artificial CSF for Intraventricular Perfusion:

The artificial CSF was made of NaCl - 7.605g, KCl - 0.223g, NaH2PO4 .12 H2O- 0.014g, NaHCO3 - 2.10g, MgCl2 .6H2O - 0.162g, CaCl2 - 0.144g,titrated to pH 7.2-7.3,with phosphate in 4°C. Intraventricular perfusion was performed by a constant flow rate perfusator(B.Brawn,Germany),the CSF pass through into the push-pull cannula with a speed of 0.075/min The sample collection should 30 min after perfution for ballance.

Drugs for Intraventricular or Peripheral Injection:

Indomethacin (Sigma,U.S.A.) was dissolved in sodium bicarbonate (2g/100ml) and then titrated to PH 7.2 with sodium phosphate. Phentolaming and Naloxone (Institute of Pharmaceutical chemistry , Shanghai Medical University), were dissolved in normal saline (1/10).PGE2-Ab(Research Institute of Animal,Beijing) was dissolved in PBS solution. The volumedid not exceed 0.5 ml and doses are indicated in each experiment.

Experiment Protocol:

To test the analgesic effect of Indo, rabbits were divided at random into two groups, A and B. A was injected with the drug and B with the same volume of the solvent as control. The experiment began at one week after operation, when the rabbits got stable response to the electric stimulation and the push-pull cannula in the 4th ventricle was in good condition. Each session was tested every 10min for 40-90mim to determine the alteration of VPT.

Data Analyses:

The data obtained from each session before and after injection of drug or placebo according to the alteration of VPT (mA).All values were expressed as X̄±SD. The data were statistically analyzed by student 't' test, and statistical significance was accepted at p< 0.05.

RESULTS:

1. The Effect of iv or icv Injection of Indo on VPT of Rabbits

As shown in Fig. 1 the VPT of group A after Indo injection(2 mg.kg-1)produced a progressively increasing, with the maximal point at 20 min, then stepwise decreasing. After the same volume of solvent injection in group B,it appeared to decrease slightly over the course. The difference between the two groups were significant at 10, 20, 30, and 40 min.In Fig.2 shows the group A after Indo icv(50μg/10μl per rabbit),the VPT appeared to increase with two peaks at 10, and 40min, 40 min later it subsided progressively,however,there was no obvious alteration in the group B.

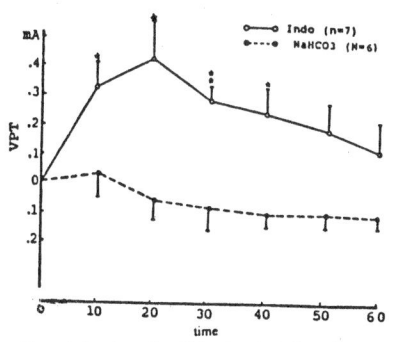

Fig. 1 Analgesic Effect of Indo (iv) on VPT.X̄±SD mA *P< 0.05, **P< 0.01 VS Control.

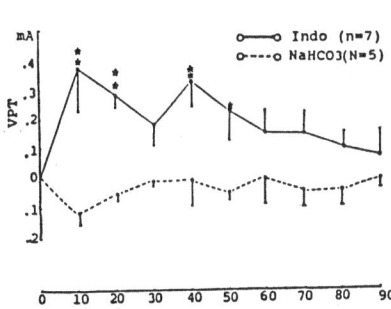

Fig. 2 Analgesic Effect of Indo (i.c.v) on VPS X̄±SD mA *P< 0.05, **P< 0,01 VS Control.

2. The Effect of PGE2-Ab icv Injecion on VPT and Influence of Phentolamine or Naloxone on the Aantialgesic Eeffect of Indo

Fig. 3 shows after icv injection (PGE2-Ab 1:600/20μl) the VPT of group A significantly increased and with two peaks at 30 ans 50 min, but there was no apparent change in the B group. It revealed that the central PGE2 play a role of exerting hyperalgesia.
Fig. 4 shows the interaction between phentolamine and Indo, as the phentolamine (a NA receptor antagonist) 50μg/10μl was icv injected before iv of Indo (2mg.kg-1) the VPT of group A significantly decreased at 30 and 40 min when compared with Indo iv alone (upper line). andcomparedwith icv Phentolamine alone(lowerline).Itmeans thatthe antialgesic effect of Indo was inhibited by a-NA antagonist. The interaction between Indo and naloxone, appeared no difference between them, so the analgesic effect of Indo unaffected. Suggesting that Indo exerts its analgesic effect probably by the existence of a NA receptor, and dos not exert its action by either endogenous opioid or acting directly through the opioid receptors.

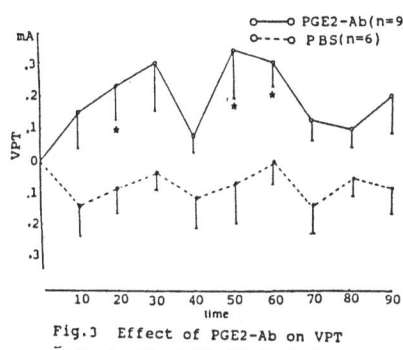

Fig.3 Effect of PGE2-Ab on VPT X̄±SD mA, *P< 0.05, VS Control

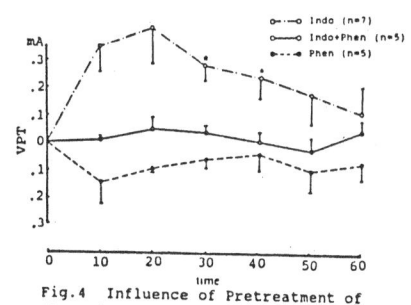

Fig.4 Influence of Pretreatment of Phentolamine on The Analgesic Effect of i.v. administration of Indo X̄±SD *P< 0.05 VS Indo+Phen

3. The Concentration of PGE2 , NA, and b- Endorphine of Perfusate

Table showes that Indo iv injection leading to the increase of VPT was associate with decreased level of endogenous PGE2,by contrast, with increased level of NA and no difference in β-endorphine. This results indicated that Indo exerts its antialgesic effect positively related to NAlevel and negatively related to central PGE2 level.

Table 1 VPT And Concentration of NA, B-Ep, PGE2 in CSF before And 25-35 min after iv administration of Indo

		VPT (mA)	NA (ng/40 μl)	VPT (mA)	β-Ep(pg/ml)	VPT (mA)	PGE2(pg/100μl)
Indomethacin	B	1.08±0.09	18.10±3.6	1.07±0.07	12.5±3.8	1.14±0.08	103.03±56.08
	A	1.48±0.16*	31.16±2.75*	1.37±0.16	16.0±4.3	1.52±0.15	81.69±57.89*
Control	B	0.96±0.12	24.96±2.86	1.03±0.12	14.1±3.3	1.02±0.08	83.39±34.55
	A	1.00±0.13	24.41±5.19	1.05±0.05	17.9±3.0	1.06±0.15	101.26±27.29

DISCUSSION

Indo is a potent antialgesic drug [3,4] which was the first of the newer NSAIDs and is used extensively in Europe[5] and in China[6] for the treatment of pain secondary to bone metastasis and primary liver cancer metastasis. However, the antialgesic action of NSAIDs have long been regarded to be an indirect consequence of the antiedema or antiinflamatory activity of these compounds[7,8]. Ferreira raised the central effect of Indo thereafter many reports controversly[9,10,11] so the mechanism of Indo for control visceral pain is not clear, further, study of mechanism in controlling visceral pain is a difficult and complicated task.Methods for producing visceral pain model included mechanical, chemical, ischemic and electrical nerve/organ stimulation,however,there are merits and demerits in each method[12].Deleo(1989) found that systemic Indo had a marked analgesic effect in the duodenal distension model but not be found in other traditional NSAIDs. He suggested that a duodenal distension stimulus does not have a pheripheral prostaglandine E2-mediated nociceptive mechanisn, the effect of Indo support an alternate, possibly central nonprostanoid visceral antinociceptive action[13]. Our results indicated that both Indo iv and icv injection had marked analgesic effect in the left major splanchnic nerve stimulation which activated afferents from the esophagus, stomach, small intestine, colon ,liver, gallbladder,pancreas, spleen and some pelvic organs. David[1982] first found the third postganglionic component in the left major splanchnic nerve in cat by a wide field electronmicroscopic anaysis[14].Thus believing that selecting the left major splanchnic nerve stimulation as GI noxious model is proper acceptable.Our data revealed that the central analgesic effect of Indo exerts its activity by the existence of a NA receptor coodinated with the increase of NA level in the 4th ventricle c.s.f. the central effect of Indo was affected by the central PGE2 [table].   The present results suggested that use proper dose of Indo in suppsitoty modality combined with other analgesics by clock offord successful efficacy for relieving CI cancer related pain.the central mechanism of Indo may be related to the existence of a NA receptor and central PGE2 can inhibit the analgesic effect of Indo. However, the comprehensive interaction among The PGE2, NA ,opioid substance and central effect of Indo remain to be further study.

REFERENCE

1. Ferreira SH, Lorenzetti BB and Correa (1978) Central and peripheral antialgesicaction of aspirin-like drugs. Eur J Pharmacol 53:39-48
2. Ferreira SH (1983) Prostaglandins: peripheral and central analgesia. In: JJ Bonica ed al(eds): Advences in Pain Research and Therapy,Vol.5, Raven Press, New York pp.627-634
3. Li D, Wang JP, Yang XY and Wang YM (1985) Determination of indomethacin concentration inserum by High Performance Liquid Chromatography. Acta Aca-demiae Medicinae Primae Shanghai 12:270-274
4. Capetola RJ, Rosenthale ME, Dubinsky B and McGuire JL (1983) Peripheral antialgesics: A review. Clin Pharmacol 23:545-546
5. Beaver WT (1990) Nnsteroidal antiinflammation druges in cancer pain. In: Foley KM et al(eds) Advances in pain research and therapy,Vol. 16. Raven Press, USA, pp. 109-128
6. Li QS, Hang XF. Ma HJ and Cheng MH (1992) Palliative treatment of ad-vanced cancer related pain. J Pract Oncol 7:70-71
7. Gilfoil T, Klavins J (1965) 5-Hydroxytryptamine, bradykinin and histamine as mediators of inflammatory hyperesthesia. Am J Physiol, 208:867
8. Guzman F,Braun C,LIm RKS,Potter GD and Rodgers DW (1964) Narcotic and non-narcotic analgesicwhich block visceral pain evoked by intra-arterial injection ofbreadykinin and other algesic agents.Arch Int Pharmacodyn 149:571-585
9. Winter CA, Kling PJ (1980) Analesic action of indomethacin in rats with trypsin-induced hyperalgesia. J Pharm Pharmacol 32:875-876
10. Hendler NH, Long DM, Wise TN (1982) Diagnosis and treatment of chronic pain. John Wright. PSG Inc, U.S.A pp 183-198
11. Taiwo YO and Levine JD (1986) Indomethacin blocks central nociceptive effects of PGF2a. Brain Research 373:81-84
12. Gebhart CF; Ness TT (1991) Mechanisms of visceral pain. In: MR Bone, JE Charton and CJ Woolf (Eds.) Proceedings of The VIth World Congress on Pain. Elsevier Science Publishoers B.V, Netherlands. pp351-363
13. Deleo JA, Colburn RW, Coombs DW, Ellis MA (1989) The differentiation of NSAIDs and prostaglandin action using a mechanical visceral pain model in the rat. Pharmacol Behav 33:253-255
14. Kuo DC,Yong GCH, Yamasaki DS and Kranrhamer GM (1982) A wide field electron microscopic analysis of the fiber constituents of the major splanchnic nerve incat.J Comparative Neurology 210:49-58

Effects of TPN or Enteral Nutrition on Gallbladder Motor Function in Postoperative Gastric Cancer Patients

Yozo Aoki, Hirohisa Nakatsuka, Masafumi Nakamura, Sumikazu Oka, Naohisa Yamade, and Masayuki Tsukiyama

Department of Surgery, Hashimoto Municipal Hospital, Hashimoto, Wakayama, 648 Japan

ABSTRACT

In totally gastrectomized patients on enteral nutrition (EN) or total parenteral nutrition (TPN), we studied the gallbladder (GB) image ultrasonographically on the 14th postoperative day, and compared its contractibility with each other by nutritional supports. In EN group, the GB began to contract 20 min after the beginning of EN ($P<0.01$, vs before EN), and reached its peak 40 min later ($P<0.001$). In TPN group, significant contraction could not be observed compared with the initial GB size and intravesical sludge continued to exist throughout the experiment. Thus, EN seems to be a more physiological nutritional method from a viewpoint of GB motor function.

KEY WORDS: gastric cancer, total gastrectomy, enteral nutrition, total parenteral nutrition, gallbladder motor function

INTRODUCTION

EN via jejunostomy and TPN are effective and often life-saving means of providing adequate nutrition for various conditions. These two nutritional supports are sometimes indicated for postgastrectomy patients to tide over critical situations in postoperative acute stage. In surgery for gastric malignancy, hepatic branch of the vagal nerve, which innervate the GB, is necessarily transected in regional lymph node dissection, and transection of the branch may result sometimes in GB dysfunction that leads to biliary dilation, sludge and gallstone formation [1]. Similar diseases have also been reported in association with TPN [2]. In this study, we surveyed the GB image ultrasonographically in order to investigate the GB motor function in totally gastrectomized patients on EN or TPN.

MATERIALS AND METHODS

Twelve patients with pre- and intraoperative normal biliary tract comfirmed by ultrasound (US), liver function tests, inspection and palpation enrolled in this study. All patients underwent total gastrectomy with regional lymph node dissection for gastric cancer and reconstructed with Roux-en-Y fashion. They consisted of 2 groups ; one involved 5 patients (4 men, 1 woman, aged 59 ~ 64 yr [mean 63.2 yr]) who were placed on cyclic constant rate EN via jejunostomy (which had been made in gastric surgery). The second group consisting of 7 patients (4 men, 3 women, aged 57 ~ 71 yr [mean 62.9 yr]) were fed with TPN immediately postoperatively. Two kinds of commercial nutrients (SNN-6010, Snow Brand, or T-330, Terumo, Japan) were selected as enteral tube-feeding solutions. An enteral feeding pump was used to provide an accurate and consistent formula infusion (100 ml/hr, 1 kcal/ml). TPN consisted of a commercial solution (Hicaliq-2, Terumo, Japan). The daily caloric input provided by the EN or TPN was 1,400 ~ 2,100 kcal.

Between the 10th and 14th postoperative days, when the delivery of nutrients had reached their full strength, the study was undertaken. A US machine (Aloka ECHO CAMERA, SSD-650, Japan) was used with a 3.5-MHz transducer to study GB size. Timing of GB contraction measurements was set at 0, 1, 3, 5, 10, 20, 30, 40, 50, 60, 90, and 120 min and the GB area on the image was analogized from the product of its maximal length and its maximal intersecting width. The contraction rate was calculated from the following formula ;

Contraction rate (%) = $(1 - GB_n/GB_0) \times 100$, where GB_0 and GB_n mean the basal GB area and a given GB area for a given time, respectively.

Difference between means were evaluated by unpaired t test (2 sided). Informed consent was obtained from all subjects studied.

RESULTS

EN Group

Fig. 1 shows time-dependent contractile activity of the GB in 5 subjects. US image before EN showed enlarged GB and intravesical sludge. Intravesical sludge and bile stasis were observed till 10 min after EN. Thereafter, these findings disappeared within 20 min after EN and movement of intravesical bile began to be observed at about the same time. These changes on US image were observed as the GB contracted. The GB began to contract 20 min after EN (P<0.01, vs before EN). Contraction rate reached its peak at 40 min (45.5%, P<0.001, vs before EN) and was 30.7% (P<0.01, vs before EN) even after 120 min.

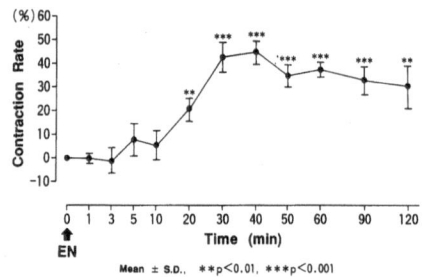

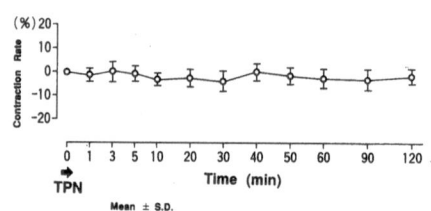

Fig.1 Changes of the contraction rate of the gallbladder in EN group

Fig.2 Changes of the contraction rate of the gallbladder in TPN group

TPN Group

Changes of the contraction rate of the GB in 7 cases is shown in Fig. 2. At the beginning of observation, the GB distended and intravesical sludge was clearly demonstrated, and these findings were constantly seen for 120 min. Significant contraction compared with the initial size could not be observed throughout the experiment.

DISCUSSION

EN and TPN have become important in the management of surgical patients who are unable to maintain nutritional needs by the oral route. EN can be used if the intestinal tract is functioning because : 1. patients have no sepsis owing to intravenous catheter infection, 2. lower grade of atrophy in intestinal villi, and 3. portal pathway of nutrient absorption. When a gastric cancer patient undergoes total gastrectomy, truncal vagotomy is inevitable with critical dissection of regional lymph nodes. Truncal vagotomy accompanied with total gastrectomy has been intraoperatively confirmed in all our subjects.

Total gastrectomy with regional lymph node dissection and postoperative TPN predispose the patients to functional lack of the GB [3]. Messing et al [4] used real-time US to study the development of gallstone during TPN. They found that GB sludge developed in 50% in TPN patients between the 4th and 6th week and was evident in all 23 patients receiving TPN for a period longer than the 6th week. Gallstones were demonstrated in 6 of the 14 patients with biliary sludge, and 3 underwent cholecystectomy.

Using serial US studies, Gafá et al [5] evaluated the incidence and development of sludge and lithiasis formation of the biliary tract in 12 patients who underwent total gastrectomy and postoperative TPN. Sludge of the GB was demonstrated in 5 of the 12 patients after a minimum period of 9 days after the operation, and in 4 of them, microlithiasis of the GB was subsequently revealed. In all instances, sludge and microlithiasis were completely "silent", however, Gafá et al [5] indicated the necessity for preventive measures against the possible and serious complications of these diseases. Baker et al [6] recommended cyclic TPN, administration of glucagon and cholecystokinin (CCK), and oral feeding when the patient's clinical state permits as one of the counterplan.

Contrary to the fact that no significant contraction was noted in cases on TPN, the maximum contraction rate of GB in patients who were placed on EN was 45.5%. These results explain a possibility that nutrients administered via jejunostomy tube irritate the intestinal mucosa, which leads to the GB contraction.

What are the causative factors of GB contraction ? There is no possibility of regeneration or recommunication of the hepatic branch of the vagal nerve which has already been transected in surgery. It should be taken into consideration that nutrients administered stimulate the intestinal mucosa, which promote secretion of some gut hormones, and provoke the GB contraction by its humoral effect. CCK is a potential contributing factor to the GB contractibility. This is secreted by CCK-secreting cell, I cell which distributes 62.5% in the duodenum, 26.0% in the upper small intestine and, in part, 3.0% in the lower small intestine [7].

Thus, EN can be said to be a more physiological nutritional method from a viewpoint of GB motor function in postgastrectomy patients.

REFERENCES

1. Rehnberg O, Haglund U (1985) Gallstones disease following antrectomy and gastroduodenostomy with or without vagotomy. Ann Surg 201:315-318
2. Quigley EMM, Marsh MN, Shaffer JL, Markin RS (1993) Hepatobiliary complications of total parenteral nutrition. Gastroenterology 104:286-301
3. Pitt HA, King III W, Mann LL, Roslyn JJ, Berquist WE, Ament ME, DenBesten L (1983) Increased risk of cholelithiasis with prolonged total parenteral nutrition. Am J Surg 145:106-112
4. Messing B, Bories C, Kunstlinger F, Bernier JJ (1983) Does total parenteral nutrition induce gallbladder sludge formation and lithiasis ? Gastroenterology 84:1012-1019
5. Gafá M, Sarli L, Meselli A, Pietra N, Carreras F, Peracchia A (1978) Sludge and microlithiasis of the biliary tract after total gastrectomy and postoperative total parenteral nutrition. Surg Gynecol Obstet 165:413-418
6. Baker AL, Rosenberg IH (1987) Hepatic complication of total parenteral nutrition. Am J Med 82:489-497
7. Bloom SR, Polak JM (1978) In: Bloom SR (ed) Gut hormones. Churchill Livingstone, London, pp 3-18

Surgical Management of Digestive Cancers in Chronic Hemodialysis Patients

YOSHITAKA WAKIZAKA[1,2], YOSHIMI NAKANISHI[2], and JUNICHI UCHINO[1]

[1]First Department of Surgery, Hokkaido University School of Medicine, Sapporo, 060 Japan
[2]Department of Surgery, Sapporo City General Hospital, Sapporo, 060 Japan

ABSTRACT

We studied the causative factor of increased incidence of digestive cancer and the appropriate methods of surgical management in our 12 hemodialysis patients with digestive cancers. The fact that they usually ate meals, which contained low fibrous and high fatty components is probably one of the main causes of the high incidence rate of colorectal cancer. Because the common subjective symptoms complained by these patients were often found in the unbalanced syndrome of chronic hemodialysis, it was difficult to distinguish these malignancies from a severe renal failure state. Thus, all cases were already in the advanced stages at the initial discovery point. Various risk factors (anemia, low serum protein, bleeding tendency, immuno-compromised state, etc.) caused postoperative complications, and preoperative appropriate adjustment of these abnormalities reduced the incidence of postoperative complications. Several modified therapeutic methods (hemodialysis without heparin, complete parenteral nutrition to recent advances in postoperative management of digestive cancers in chronic hemodialysis patients.

KEY WORDS: chronic hemodialysis patients, digestive cancer, perioperative management, postoperative complications

INTRODUCTION

The incidence of malignant tumors, especially digestive cancers in chronic hemodialysis patients is usually higher than in normal control persons [1-3]. The highest incidence rate of malignancies was found in the digestive tract of chronic hemodialysis patients at the Kidney Center of Sapporo City General Hospital. Over the last 7 years, we have operated on 12 patients receiving chronic hemodialysis therapy for gastrointestinal cancers. The pathogenetic factor of this increased incidence of digestive cancer and the appropriate methods of surgical management are not well known. Therefore, we have undertaken analysis of the records of these 12 patients to solve these problems.

MATERIAL AND METHODS

Analysis was performed on 12 patients who received surgery for gastrointestinal cancer. All of these patients were hemodialyzed at the Kidney Center of Sapporo City General Hospital during the last 7 years. Surgical disorders in these patients were gastric cancer (1 case),

Table 1
Summary of clinical features in 12 hemodialysis patients who developed gastrointestinal cancer

No.	Sex	Age on discovery of gastrointestinal cancer	Original renal disease	Months on hemodialysis to discovery of gastrointestinal cancer (Months)	Type of digestive cancer	year
1	M	75	Chronic glomerulonephritis	75	Rectum	1985
2	F	72	Nephrosclerosis	1	Ascending colon	1985
3	M	64	Diabetic nephropathy	50	Ascending colon	1986
4	M	43	Diabetic nephropathy	2	Rectum	1986
5	M	54	Chronic glomerulonephritis	42	Rectum	1987
6	M	51	Polycystic kidney	3	Stomach	1988
7	M	65	Diabetic nephropathy	100	Ascending colon	1988
8	F	67	Chronic glomerulonephritis	73	Rectum	1989
9	M	52	Chronic glomerulonephritis	7	Ascending colon	1989
10	M	58	Chronic glomerulonephritis	31	Sigmoid colon	1990
11	M	40	Focal glomerulorsclerosis	50	Transverse colon	1991
12	F	53	Chronic glomerulonephritis	114	Cecum	1992

Figure 1

The standard regimens of surgery and perioperative hemodialysis in chronic hemodialysis patients with digestive cancers

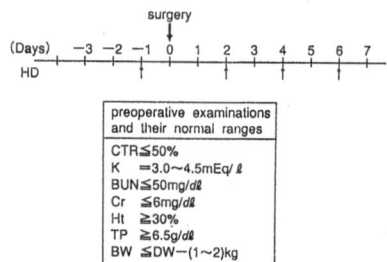

preoperative examinations and their normal ranges
CTR≦50%
K =3.0~4.5mEq/ℓ
BUN≦50mg/dℓ
Cr ≦6mg/dℓ
Ht ≧30%
TP ≧6.5g/dℓ
BW ≦DW−(1~2)kg

colon cancer (7 cases) and rectal cancer (4 cases). The clinical features in these 12 hemodialysis patients are shown in Table 1.During the postoperative periods, hemodialysis was performed 3 times per week after the second day of operation. We performed hemodialysis using gabexate mesilate (Millacrit) or nafamostat mesilate (FUTHAN) as a anticoagulant, without heparin, associated with transfusion of packed red blood cells and fresh frozen plasma in order to elevate the patients' hematocrit value to higher than 30 percent. The standard regimen of surgery and perioperative hemodialysis in these patients is shown in Figure 1.

RESULTS

The results below from our study showed that:
(1) The incidence of digestive cancers, especially colorectal cancer in these hemodialysis patients was higher than that in normal persons. At the time of initial discovery, the clinical stages of digestive cancer in these patients were highly advanced and the prognosis was usually poor [1].
(2) The mean dialysis period of these patients before their operations was three years and 9 months. Malignancies were found within one year from the beginning of maintenance dialysis in 4 patients (33.3%), and were found within 5 years in 8 patients (66.7%). There was a significant negative correlation between the relative risk of digestive cancer appearance and the length of time in the dialysis program [3].
(3) The initial subjective symptoms in these patients were appetite loss, anemia, nausea and vomiting, weight loss, etc.. They were often found in an unbalanced syndrome of chronic hemodialysis or chronic renal failure state. All of these 12 patients ate meals which contained low fibrous and high fatty components and tended not to eat enough vegetables and fruits. Eleven of these 12 patients complained of being constipated during the preoperative periods. This fact reflects the westernization of dietary regimens and a decrease in dietary fiber intake in Japanese hemodialysis patients.
(4) The highest incidence rate of postoperative complication was seen in various types of infection, i.e., sepsis, pneumonia, wound infection, etc.. Disturbance of wound healing, i.e., wound dehiscence, breakdown of the anastomosis or anastomotic dehiscence, anastomotic leakage, occurred in 4 patients. Only one patient needed additional surgery due to postoperative hemorrhage and hematoma. In 8 out of 12 patients that underwent surgical treatment, satisfactory results were obtained (Table 2).

Table 2
Postoperative complications and their frequencies in chronic hemodialysis patients with digestive cancers

Postoperative complication	Frequency(%)
sepsis or pneumonia	5/12 (42)
hyperkalemia	3/12 (25)
wound dehiscence or anastomotic leak	4/12 (33)
gastrointestinal bleeding	1/12 (8)
overhydration	2/12 (17)
Arrhythmia or cardiac complications	1/12 (8)

Table 3
Preoperative problems and their management in choronic hemodialysis patients with digestive cancers

Preoperative risk factors	Frequency(%)	Managements
anemia	9/12 (75)	blood transfusion
low serum protein	11/12 (92)	transfusion of fresh frozen plasma, administration of serum protein products
bleeding tendency	12/12 (100)	hemodialysis using gabexate mesilate (FOY) or nafamostat mesilate, without heparin
disturbance of wound healing	6/12 (50)	complete parenteral nutrition using the 50-70% glucose solution, amino acid solution such as AIMU, etc.
immunocompromised state	12/12 (100)	prophylactic administration of aitibiotics (cephlosporins or penicillins to avoid nephrotoxicity)
susceptibility to infection	6/12 (50)	
metabolic acidosis	6/12 (50)	administration of Meylon, etc.
hyperkalemia	6/12 (50)	administration of Kayexalate, etc.

DISCUSSION

It has been reported that hemodialysis patients had a higher incidence rate of malignancies and especially digestive cancer showed the highest incidence rate among these malignancies [1-3]. In our analysis the same result was obtained, thus the incidence rate or colorectal cancer was highest among all kinds of malignancies associated with hemodialysis. Only one case was Dukes A and B cases were Dukes C among these 11 colorectal cancer patients. As many as 7 of the 12 patients died from cancer. In this way, almost all cases were already in advanced stages at the initial discovery point, and their prognosis was usually very poor [1].
In general, various risk factors in these hemodialysis patients caused postoperative complications. In our results, anemia (75%), low serum protein (92%), bleeding tendency (100%) and immunological suppression (100%) [4,5] had higher incidences in all preoperative disturbances. However, appropriate adjustment of these abnormalities (transfusion of blood

and fresh frozen plasma, administration of serum protein products, etc.) reduced these preoperative problems.

Also, the incidence of postoperative complication had usually been said to be higher than in normal persons. In our study, sepsis or pneumonia (42%) and wound dehiscence or anastomotic leakage (33%) had the highest incidence rate of all postoperative complications. Especially hemodialysis without heparin using gabexate mesilate (FOY) or nafamostat mesilate and complete parenteral nutrition contributed to the advances in postoperative management of digestive cancers in chronic hemodialysis patients. After surgery, complete parenteral nutrition using 50-70% glucose solution, an amino acid solution such as AMIU, etc., was performed with careful attention to overhydration. However, disturbance of wound healing, i.e., wound dihiscence, breakdown of the anastomosis, anastomotic dehiscence or anastomotic leakage, occurred in 4 patients. We also used various other hemopurification methods such as, peritoneal dialysis, etc. We usually used cephalosporins or penicillins as the antibiotics and avoided the use of aminoglycosides or tetracyclines which have high nephrotoxicity side effects (Table 3).

Because the number of patients or all ages receiving hemodialysis has been significantly rising recently, the number of reports of such patients with digestive cancers will increase. Therefore, efforts to rule out the likelihood of digestive cancers at an early stage should be made using ultrasonography, GI series and determination of serum tumor markers and so on. Because digestive cancers of the colon and rectum, which are often detected by hemorrhage, occur frequently in hemodialysis patients, examination of the lower digestive tract as well as careful history-taking and digital examination of the rectum are important in these patients.

Chronic renal failure in itself has a poor prognosis; thus when we surgically treat hemodialysis patients with cancers, careful attention should be paid to the indications for surgery and perioperative management.

REFERENCES

1. Miach PJ, Dawborn JK, Xipell J (1976) Neoplasia in patients with chronic renal failure on long-term dialysis. Clinical Nephrology 5:101-104
2. Lindner A, Farewell VT, Sherrard DJ (1981) High incidence of neoplasia in uremic patients receiving long-term dialysis (Cancer and long-term dialysis). Nephron 27:292-296
3. Riambau E, Roma J, Aubia J, Lloveras J, Masramon J (1987) Malignant disorders and long-term survival in haemodialysis patients. The Lancet 28:754-755
4. Matas AJ, Simmons RL, Kjellstrand CM, Buselmeier TJ (1975) Increased incidence of maliganancy during chronic renal failure. The Lancet 19:883-885
5. Penn I, Starzl TE (1972) Malignant tumors arising de novo in immunosuppressed organ transplant recipients. Transplantation 14:401-417

List of Contributors

Abe, R. 726
Abe, Yasuhito 517, 814
Abe, Yoshishige 428
Adachi, K. 487
Adachi, Y. 660
Ahmed, M.H. 837
Aikou, T. 277
Aizawa, K. 619
Akagi, Y. 493
Akamo, Y. 360, 693
Akay, H. 436
Akgül, H. 339
Akimoto K. 663
Akimoto, S. 663
Akitomi, Y. 829
Akiyama, S. 218, 508
Amakawa, Y. 499
Amano, S. 579
Amioka, K. 529
Amuro, Y. 657
Anazawa, S. 444
Ando, K. 579
Anzai, R. 406
Aogi, K. 834
Aoki, H. 499
Aoki, K. 24
Aoki, Kunio 837
Aoki, Tatsuya 699
Aoki, Teruaki 369
Aoki, Toshiaki 699
Aoki, Y. 849
Arai, K. 275, 342
Arakawa, A. 333
Arakawa, Y. 604, 622
Araki, Y. 493
Arii, K. 619
Arima, K. 357
Arima, N. 484
Arima, S. 570
Arimoto, Y. 239
Asaki, S. 461
Asano, G. 403
Asano, Y. 657
Asanuma, T. 406
Asanuma, Y. 759, 807
Ashizawa, N. 487
Awane, M. 610
Azuma, M. 490

Baba, H. 160

Baba, M. 277
Baba, S. 547, 690, 705, 837
Barreto, R.Z. 442
Beral, V. 38
Bernal, F.S. 442
Beyler, A.R. 436
Bhuiya, M.M.R. 795
Bose, S.M. 544
Burger, M.M. 7

Carr, B. 121
Chai, J.-C. 210
Chen, Z.-P. 210, 292
Chida, T. 333
Chung, Y.-S. 239, 242, 260, 743,
    762, 768, 788

Deguchi, H. 717
Deguchi, Y. 366, 425, 532
Demirci, S. 339
Doki, Y. 171, 254, 439, 452
Dökmeci, A. 601
Dönderici, Ö. 601
Douglass, Jr., H.O. 148
Dumlu, S. 601

Eckhardt, S. 2
Endo, M. 64, 174, 185, 449
Endou, Y. 372
Esaki, Y. 468
Etchegaray, A. 185
Eto, T. 792

Fujii, H. 585, 684
Fujii, T. 177
Fujikawa, T. 740
Fujimaki, M. 179, 221, 471
Fujimori, T. 369
Fujimoto, Jiro 380
Fujimoto, Jiro 640
Fujimoto, T. 366, 425, 532
Fujimura, M. 419
Fujimura, T. 236, 372, 412
Fujio, N. 654, 678
Fujioka, N. 425, 532
Fujioka, T. 324, 388

Fujita, H. 177
Fujita, I. 215, 403
Fujita, Masahide 576
Fujita, Masato 628, 663
Fujita, T. 306
Fujita, Y. 564
Fukazawa, S. 634
Fukuda, I. 482
Fukuda, R. 487
Fukuhara, K. 637
Fukumoto, S. 487
Fukunaga, M. 386
Fukuoka, T. 684
Fukushima, S. 610
Fukushima, T. 634
Fukushima, W. 613
Fukuzawa, K. 514
Funabiki, H. 354
Funatsuka, M. 737
Furukawa, H. 422, 455, 496
Furukawa, K. 625, 640
Futami, K. 570

Gao, Z.-M. 292
Garduño, I. 442
Goi, T. 484, 511
Gotoda, A. 348
Gotoh, I. 604, 622
Gotoh, M. 666, 669
Gouchi, A. 774
Gungor, A. 436
Gunji, Y. 377
Güngör, A. 203
Gupta, B.D. 544

Hada, R. 336
Hada, T. 657
Hagiwara, A. 324, 388, 431
Hakama, M. 38
Hamada, Y. 257
Hanyu, F. 643, 751, 777
Hara, H. 801
Hara, T. 616
Harada, N. 751, 777
Harada, T. 409
Hasegawa, H. 785
Hasegawa, M. 535
Hashimoto, T. 487

855

Kato, Yujiro 807, 810
Katoh, R. 315
Katsumori, T. 628, 663
Katsumoto, Y. 386
Katsuragawa, H. 643
Kawabata, S. 245
Kawachi, Y. 538, 672
Kawaguchi, S. 616
Kawai, J. 619
Kawai, S. 538
Kawamura, E. 625, 640
Kawano, T. 64, 174, 185, 449
Kawarada, Y. 779
Khanna, S.K. 544
Kido, K. 714
Kikuti, K. 594
Kim, C.B. 303, 552
Kim, I.C. 345
Kim, J.-P. 19, 154
Kim, K.-S. 260, 762
Kim, S.H. 782
Kim, S.M. 782
Kim, Y.S. 762, 768, 788
Kimura, H. 372
Kimura, Katsuhiko 517, 814
Kimura, Kozaburo 394, 699
Kimura, S. 517, 814
Kinoshita, F. 564
Kinoshita, H. 168, 654, 678
Kinoshita, K. 372
Kinoshita, T. 109, 227, 272, 300
Kiriyama, K. 508
Kishimoto, H. 591
Kitamura, K. 115, 567, 582, 771
Kitamura, M. 275, 342
Kitamura, Yoshio 283
Kitamura, Youichi 269
Kitao, Y. 474
Kito, T. 294
Kiyama, T. 403
Ko, S. 714
Kobari, M. 87
Kobashi, K. 471
Kobayashi, H. 643
Kobayashi, I. 576
Kobayashi, Kenji 439, 452
Kobayashi, Kenji 693
Kobayashi, M. 720
Kobayashi, N. 648
Kobayashi, O. 383
Kobayashi, S. 643
Kobayashi, Seibi 51
Kobayashi, Shigeru 56
Kobori, O. 194
Kodaira, S. 499
Kodama, I. 245
Kodama, Masashi 248
Kodama, Masashi 333
Koh, T. 657
Kohno, H. 607
Kohno, K. 397
Koitabashi, H. 315
Koito, K. 348

Koizumi, Y. 266
Kojima, O. 591
Komichi, H. 720, 823
Kondo, K. 218, 508
Kondo, S. 795
Kondo, Yasuyuki 242, 260, 743, 762, 768
Kondo, Yukifumi 348
Kondoh, Y. 230, 400
Konishi, T. 464, 702
Konn, M. 336, 708
Konno, H. 690, 705
Kontani, T. 523
Koo, B.-H. 782
Koseki, H. 406
Kotani, T. 567, 582, 771
Koufuji, K. 245
Kouzmitchev, V.A. 377
Kouzu, T. 377
Koyama, Hiroki 422
Koyama, Hiroshi 631, 723
Koyama, K. 333, 759, 807, 810
Koyama, Y. 726
Koyanagi, Y. 394, 699
Kuang, Y.-L. 210
Kubo, N. 263
Kubo, S. 654, 678
Kubota, Y. 555
Kuge, Y. 732
Kumagai, K. 363
Kumegawa, H. 245
Kurihara, M. 132, 594
Kurita, A. 321
Kuroda, C. 666
Kuroda, D. 573
Kuromizu, J. 520
Kurosu, Y. 579
Kusama, M. 394
Kusama, S. 681
Kusanagi, H. 206
Kusunoki, M. 588
Kuwano, H. 160
Kuwata, K. 474
Kuzu, I. 339, 436
Kwon, S.-J. 300

Lavery, I.C. 104
Lee, J.S. 345
Lee, K. 529
Levin, B. 29
Li, L. 409
Li, Q.-S. 846
Lin, Z.-Y. 81
Liu, S.-H. 354
Lu, J.-Z. 81
Lu, W.-Q. 289

Ma, X.C. 248
Ma, Z.-C. 81
Machimura, T. 94
Madariaga, J.R. 121

Maeda, K. 239, 242, 743
Maeda, T. 567, 628, 663
Maehara, M. 484, 511
Maetani, S. 535, 843
Mafune, K. 464
Mai, M. 366, 425, 532, 681
Makuuchi, H. 94
Maniwa, Y. 523
Maruiwa, M. 245
Marukawa, O. 529
Marukawa, T. 666
Maruo, Y. 705
Maruta, M. 520
Maruyama, C. 643
Maruyama, K. 109, 227, 272, 300
Masaki, K. 479, 502
Masuda, Y. 280, 549
Masuo, K. 363
Matai, K. 306
Matin, A.F.M. 547
Matsubara, S. 637
Matsui, S. 171, 254, 452
Matsukawa, M. 132, 594
Matsukawa, S. 735
Matsuki, N. 372
Matsukura, N. 215, 403
Matsumoto, A. 514
Matsumoto, H. 412
Matsumoto, Masayuki 477
Matsumoto, Muneyuki 684
Matsumoto, S. 375
Matsumoto, Y. 397, 607
Matsuno, S. 87, 406, 558, 637, 687
Matsuno, T. 604
Matsushige, H. 297
Matsuura, A. 51
Matsuura, S. 479
Matumoto, H. 236
Matuno, T. 774
Mettlin, C. 46
Mieno, H. 98
Migita, T. 558
Mikami, Yasunori 336
Mikami, Youshi 477
Min, J.S. 303, 552
Minamoto, T. 532
Minato, H. 324, 388
Minu, A.R. 174
Misawa, K. 675
Mishima, Y. 538, 672
Misumi, A. 357
Mitomi, T. 94, 230, 400
Mitsuoka, T. 468
Miura, K. 406, 558
Miura, S. 499
Miura, Y. 482
Miwa, K. 236, 412
Miwa, M. 482
Miya, K. 711
Miyagaki, T. 115, 567
Miyaishi, S. 753
Miyaji, M. 230, 400
Miyajima, N. 520

Key Word Index